A Systematic Approach To Shoulder Rehabilitation

Bryce W. Gaunt, PT, SCS
George M. McCluskey III, MD
Illustrations by Carol Capers, MSMI

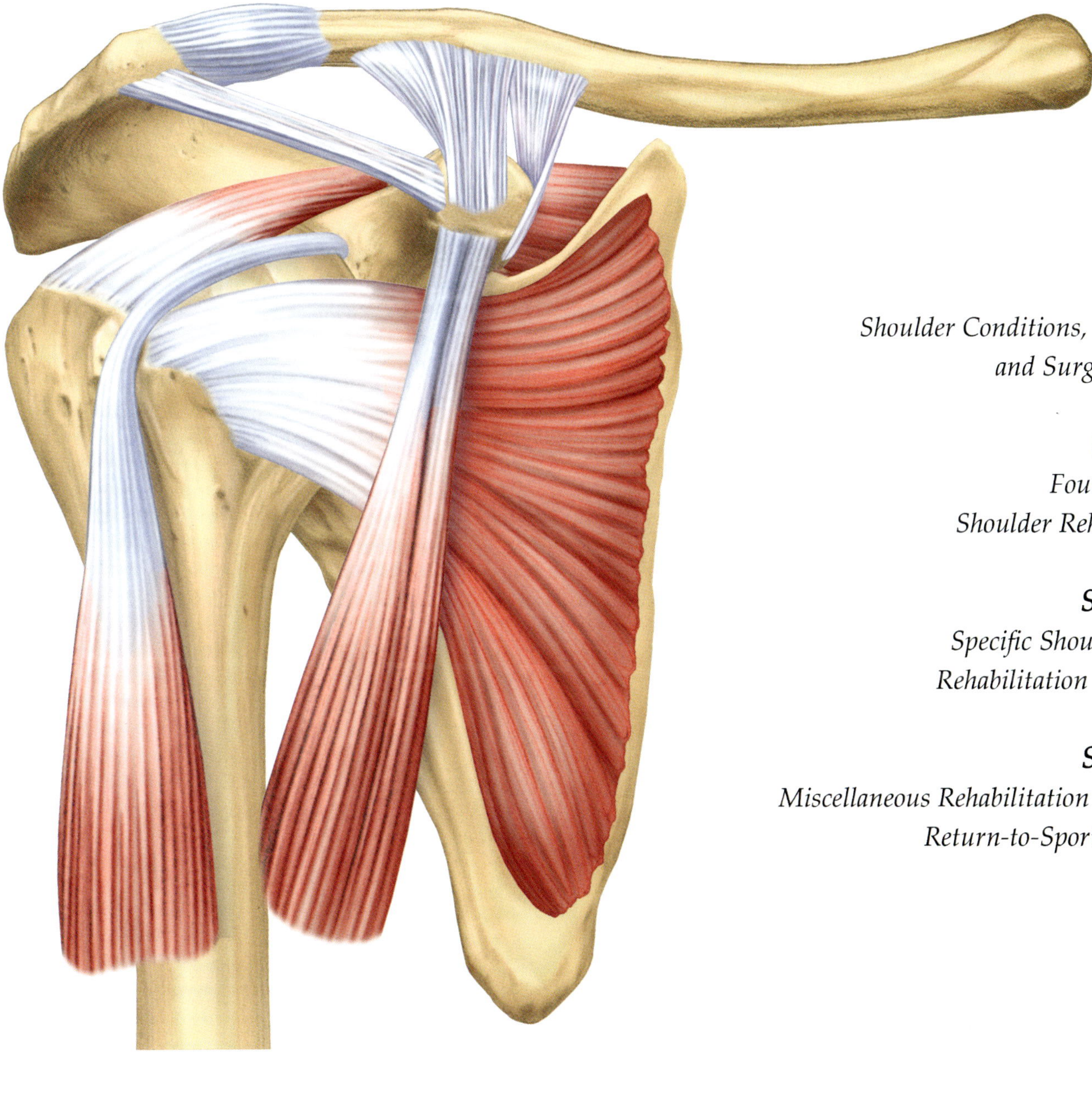

Section I
Shoulder Conditions, Treatment, and Surgical Repair

Section II
Foundations of Shoulder Rehabilitation

Section III
Specific Shoulder Girdle Rehabilitation Guidelines

Section IV
Miscellaneous Rehabilitation Topics and Return-to-Sport Programs

HPRC
Your progress. Our excellence.
Together we will.

Corporate Office
6298 Veterans Parkway, Suite 5A
Post Office Box 8068
Columbus, GA 31908-8068

A Systematic Approach To Shoulder Rehabilitation

ISBN 978-0-9855961-0-1

NOTICES

Knowledge and best practice in this field are constantly changing. As new research and experience broaden our understanding, changes in research methods, professional practices, or medical treatment may become necessary.

Practitioners and researchers must always rely on their own experience and knowledge in evaluating and using any information, methods, compounds, or experiments described herein. In using such information or methods, they should be mindful of their own safety and the safety of others, including parties for whom they have a professional responsibility.

With respect to any drug or pharmaceutical products identified, readers are advised to check the most current information provided on procedures featured or by the manufacturer of each product to be administered to verify the recommended dose or formula, the method and duration of administration, and contraindications. It is the responsibility of practitioners, relying on their own experience and knowledge of their patients, to make diagnoses, to determine dosages and the best treatment for each individual patient, and to take all appropriate safety precautions.

To the fullest extent of the law, neither the publisher nor the authors, contributors, or editors assume any liability for any injury and/or damage to persons or property as a matter of product liability, negligence, or otherwise or from any use or operation of any methods, products, instructions, or ideas contained in the material herein.

ISBN 978-0-9855961-0-1

$150.00
ISBN 978-0-9855961-0-1
59999>
9 780985 596101

HPRC
Your progress. Our excellence.
Together we will.

Printed in the United States.

Foreward

I was honored to be asked by Bryce Gaunt and George McCluskey III to write this foreword. This book represents more than 20 years of working together and learning from each other regarding the management of patients with shoulder injuries. I personally was blessed to be present at the beginning of this collaboration; however, I take my hat off to both of these gentleman and their collaborators, as they have done a tremendous service for all rehabilitation specialists. They have addressed what often is missing in our literature recently; they have focused on the details of how they do their rehabilitation. The authors provide the reader with several clinical pearls. They discuss their philosophy based on both the clinical experience of working together and the available literature that supports their approach. Clinical experience is part of the original definition of evidence-based medicine by Sackett et al[1]; however, it is often not shared with the level of detail that is presented in this book.

A Systematic Approach to Shoulder Rehabilitation focuses on rehabilitation for shoulder injuries and covers a wide variety of pathologic conditions and surgical interventions. The purpose of the book is to provide a detailed understanding for general physical therapists about the current best practice of shoulder rehabilitation. It provides excellent insight for all therapists, in particular for our young colleagues who are trying to capture the nuances of exercise progression. Chapters focus on nonoperative and postoperative rehabilitation programs with very specific detail and criteria to progress. The illustrations are clear and colorful, which will be beneficial when educating patients about their shoulder conditions.

I have read many articles over the last 25 years in the orthopaedic and sports medicine journals in which the authors have described the shoulder pathologic condition, mechanism of injury, and clinical assessment; have detailed the surgical intervention; and then have skimmed over the rehabilitation section with a few sentences. We now have a shoulder book that provides clear rehabilitation principles to explain the logic behind the intervention. I believe readers will truly enjoy reading this book and learning the details of shoulder rehabilitation from these outstanding clinical experts.

Tim L. Uhl, PhD, PT, ATC, FNATA
Associate Professor
Co-Director of Musculoskeletal Laboratory
Department of Rehabilitation Sciences
College of Health Sciences
University of Kentucky, Lexington, KY

1. Sackett DL, Rosenberg WMC, Gray JAM, Haynes RB, Richardson WS. Evidence based medicine: what it is and what it isn't. *BMJ*. 1996;312(7023):71–72.

Dedications

To George M. McCluskey, Jr, PT

My father, my mentor, and my hero.
Your unconditional love for your family, your work ethic, and your character are unparalleled.
I am proud to be your son.

George M. McCluskey III, MD

To my wife, Becky, and son, Davis, for supporting me and sacrificing our time together during the years it took to complete this project. I love you both all the much in the world! I also want to give a special thank you to 3 people who have had a profound influence on my professional development. To Tim Uhl, PhD, PT, ATC, FNATA, for mentoring me and inspiring me toward clinical excellence, nonstop professional growth, and sharing the knowledge I have with others. You were the best first boss a young therapist could ever have. To George M. McCluskey III, MD, for believing in me, teaching me, challenging me to grow and excel, and for being the visionary for this wonderful project. Finally, to Mr. McCluskey, I wish I could have learned from you working side by side, but I thank you for setting the standard and expectation of excellence!

Bryce W. Gaunt, PT, SCS

Preface

Our reason for writing *A Systematic Approach to Shoulder Rehabilitation* is to provide a detailed understanding about the current best practice of shoulder rehabilitation to the student or clinician who does not specialize in shoulder girdle rehabilitation. We believe this book is timely because it has taken us 20 years of working together as a shoulder surgeon and physical therapist in a high-volume specialty shoulder practice to define, refine, and mature a systematic approach to shoulder rehabilitation that works efficiently with athletes and the elderly alike. We remember the labors, frustrations, and disappointments of searching and creating rehabilitation strategies and guidelines that are consistently effective, scientifically based, logical, easy to teach other clinicians, and well tolerated by patients. The goal of this book is to shorten the learning curve of rehabilitation specialists by educating them about many common and challenging conditions and surgical procedures of the shoulder and providing an easy-to-understand systematic progression of therapeutic exercise that can be applied successfully to treat patients with a broad spectrum of shoulder disorders.

Our focus is placed on a criteria-based advancement and the "why" behind our clinical decision making. Detailed rehabilitation guidelines with specific exercise choices also are included to help augment your clinical decision making. Special situations are addressed for patients from youth athletes to the elderly. Clinical pearls of wisdom are highlighted so the reader can easily identify concepts and hints that are essential to understand or that improve the speed of the patient's recovery.

This book differs from other books on shoulder rehabilitation that have multiple contributors in several respects. Whereas each author presents his or her individual tricks of the trade and rehabilitation preferences, a large degree of synergy exists in the central tenets of rehabilitation. Authors were carefully selected, and a large number of chapters were written in-house so consistency in our systematic approach would be present among chapters.

Rehabilitation is an afterthought or the rehabilitation of athletes alone is emphasized in many collaborate reference books involving surgeons and rehabilitation specialists. We recognize the value of and include the shoulder surgeon's perspective of anatomy, pathophysiology, clinical evaluation, and nonoperative and operative decision making, including an overview of common surgical procedures, in this book. However, our emphasis is on the rehabilitation of all types of shoulder injuries, and we recognize that most patients who are seen by rehabilitation providers for shoulder conditions are not athletes. We include an entire section on the foundations of our system of shoulder rehabilitation to give the reader a detailed understanding of the core principles and progressions of our system, and in later sections of the book, the reader can learn how these principles are applied to specific problems.

Many reference books include general rehabilitation guidelines that provide the framework for rehabilitation and allow the rehabilitation provider to use the specific interventions they prefer. We purposely have taken a different approach and have chosen to include specific rehabilitation protocols that give great detail on exercise selection and progression and give suggestions on exercise frequency and volume. We do recognize that individualizing the exercise prescription for each patient is important, and we recognize that many interventions can be used to accomplish the same goal. However, over our 20 years of examining evidence, learning from others, refining and maturing our systematic progression, and sharing our patients with their hometown therapists, we have found a specific selection and progression of exercises that works the most efficiently and most effectively in our hands and have chosen to share that. For the student or clinician who is in the process of establishing his or her rehabilitation preferences, we believe these specific protocols will be an invaluable asset. Seasoned shoulder therapists should enjoy comparing their approach to rehabilitation with our method, critically examining both to sharpen and refine their clinical decision-making skills.

Finally, we believe this book differs from other shoulder reference books in the quality and number of illustrations thanks to the skills of Carol Capers, MSMI, CMI. Carol is a certified member of the Association of Medical Illustrators and has won numerous awards for her illustration and design work, which is evident as you examine her more than 1000 different images contained in this book. Her illustrations make difficult concepts easy to understand and bring action to static images. These images alone make this book a must have reference.

A very special word of thanks and gratitude cannot fully express our appreciation to Elizabeth Harbison, our medical writer. Her dedication to this project and uncompromising standards are an essential ingredient to this project and provide an invaluable benefit to the reader.

A special thank you also is due to the contributors to this book who believed in this project and graciously gave of their time to share their expertise.

Bryce W. Gaunt, PT, SCS
Clinical Director of Physical Therapy
HPRC at St. Francis Rehabilitation Center
Columbus, Georgia

George M. McCluskey III, MD
Director, St. Francis Shoulder Center
Director, St. Francis Shoulder Fellowship Program
St. Francis Hospital
Columbus, Georgia

Contributors

Bryce W. Gaunt, PT, SCS
Clinical Director of Physical Therapy
HPRC at St. Francis Rehabilitation Center
Columbus, Georgia

George M. McCluskey III, MD
Director, St. Francis Shoulder Center
Director, St. Francis Shoulder Fellowship Program
St. Francis Hospital
Columbus, Georgia

Lane Bailey PT, DPT, CSCS
Doctoral Candidate
Department of Physical Therapy
Arnold School of Public Health
University of South Carolina
Columbia, South Carolina

Jo A. Barker, PT
HPRC at St. Francis Rehabilitation Center
Columbus, Georgia

John J. Basti, PT
Lecturer, College of Physicians & Surgeons
Columbia University
New York, New York

Consultant
Department of Orthopaedics
Center for Shoulder, Elbow and Sports Medicine
Columbia University Medical Center
New York, New York

Andrew Beach, PT, ECS
HPRC
Columbus, Georgia

Turner A. "Tab" Blackburn, Jr, MEd, PT, ATC
Vice President of Corporate Development
Clemson Sports Medicine and Rehabilitation
Clemson, South Carolina

Clinical Director
Sports Plus Physical Therapy
Manchester, Georgia

Adjunct Assistant Professor
University of St. Augustine
School of Physical Therapy
St. Augustine, Florida

Thomas Boers, PT, MT
Human Performance and Rehabilitation Center
Columbus, Georgia

Cari Lee Cordell, MD
Shoulder and Elbow Specialist
Hand and Microvascular Specialist
St. Joseph's Mercy Hospital
Hot Springs, Arkansas

Jeff R. Fraser, PT, MS, ECS, CNIM
Director, Clinical Electrophysiology
HPRC
Columbus, Georgia

Sachiko T. Garner, PT, MS
HPRC at St. Francis Rehabilitation Center
Columbus, Georgia

Michael J. Griesser, MD
Orthopaedic Surgery Sports Medicine Fellow
The Cleveland Clinic
Cleveland, Ohio

Joshua D. Harris, MD
Orthopaedic Surgery Resident
The Ohio State University
Columbus, Ohio

Jacqueline B. Henson
Bachelor of Science Candidate
Davidson College
Davidson, North Carolina

John A. Hinson, MD
Assistant Professor, Department of Orthopaedic Surgery
Georgia Health Sciences University
Augusta, Georgia

Kristine Jankowski, PT, DPT, CPI
Clinical Director and Owner
Full Circle Health, LLC
Palm Beach Gardens, Florida

Grant L. Jones, MD
Associate Professor
Department of Orthopaedic Surgery
Team Physician
Department of Athletics
The Ohio State University
Columbus, Ohio

Martin J. Kelley, PT, DPT, OCS
Penn Presbyterian Medical Center
University of Pennsylvania Health System
Philadelphia, Pennsylvania

Joseph H. Kostuch, PT, SCS
HPRC at St. Francis Rehabilitation Center
Columbus, Georgia

Kevin G. Laudner, PhD, ATC, FACSM
Professor of Athletic Training Education at Illinois State University
Normal, Illinois

Director of Research
Texas Metroplex Institute for Sports Medicine and Orthopedics
Arlington, Texas

Michael T. Lebec, PT, PhD
Associate Professor
Department of Physical Therapy and Athletic Training
Northern Arizona University
Flagstaff, Arizona

Brian G. Leggin, PT, DPT, OCS
Good Shepherd Penn Partners
Penn Therapy and Fitness
Penn Presbyterian Medical Center
Philadelphia, Pennsylvania

Steven D. Levin, MD
Assistant Professor
Department of Orthopaedic Surgery
University of Chicago Pritzker School of Medicine
NorthShore University HealthSystem
Evanston, Illinois

Robert G. Lewis, MD
Director, St. Francis Sports Medicine Center
St. Francis Shoulder Center
St. Francis Hospital
Columbus, Georgia

Shannon B. Lucas, PTA
HPRC at St. Francis Rehabilitation Center
Columbus, Georgia

Brian J. Phillips, PT, DPT
HPRC at St. Francis Rehabilitation Center
Columbus, Georgia

Michael S. Potter, MD
PCRMC Medical Group
Rolla, Missouri

Howard D. Routman, DO, FAOAO
Director, Palm Beach Shoulder Service
Attending Physician, Atlantis Orthopaedics
President, Palm Beach Shoulder and Sports Medicine Foundation
Associate Clinical Professor, Nova-Southeastern University
North Palm Beach, Florida

Matthew A. Schwartz, MD
Carolina Orthopaedic Associates
Rock Hill, South Carolina

Amee L. Seitz, PT, PhD, DPT, OCS
Assistant Professor, Department of Physical Therapy
Bouvé College of Health Sciences
Northeastern University
Boston, Massachusetts

Stephanie M. Squitieri, PT, DPT, CSCS
Senior Physical Therapist
PRO Sports Physical Therapy of Westchester
Scarsdale, New York

Joel B. Stenslie, PT
HPRC at St. Francis Rehabilitation Center
Columbus, Georgia

Chuck Thigpen, PhD, PT, ATC
Clinical Research Scientist
Proaxis Therapy
Greenville, South Carolina

Assistant Consulting Professor
Doctor of Physical Therapy Division
Department of Community and Family Medicine
Duke University School of Medicine
Durham, North Carolina

Adjunct Assistant Professor
Clemson Bioengineering Department
Clemson University
Clemson, South Carolina

Adjunct Assistant Professor
Department of Physical Therapy
Arnold School of Public Health
University of South Carolina
Columbia, South Carolina

Todd J. Twiss, MD
Freeman Orthopaedic Surgery and Sports Medicine
Freeman Hospital
Joplin, Missouri

Timothy F. Tyler, MS, PT, ATC
Clinical Research Associate
Nicholas Institute of Sports Medicine and Athletic Trauma
New York, New York

Contents

Shoulder Conditions, Treatment, and Surgical Repair

Section I

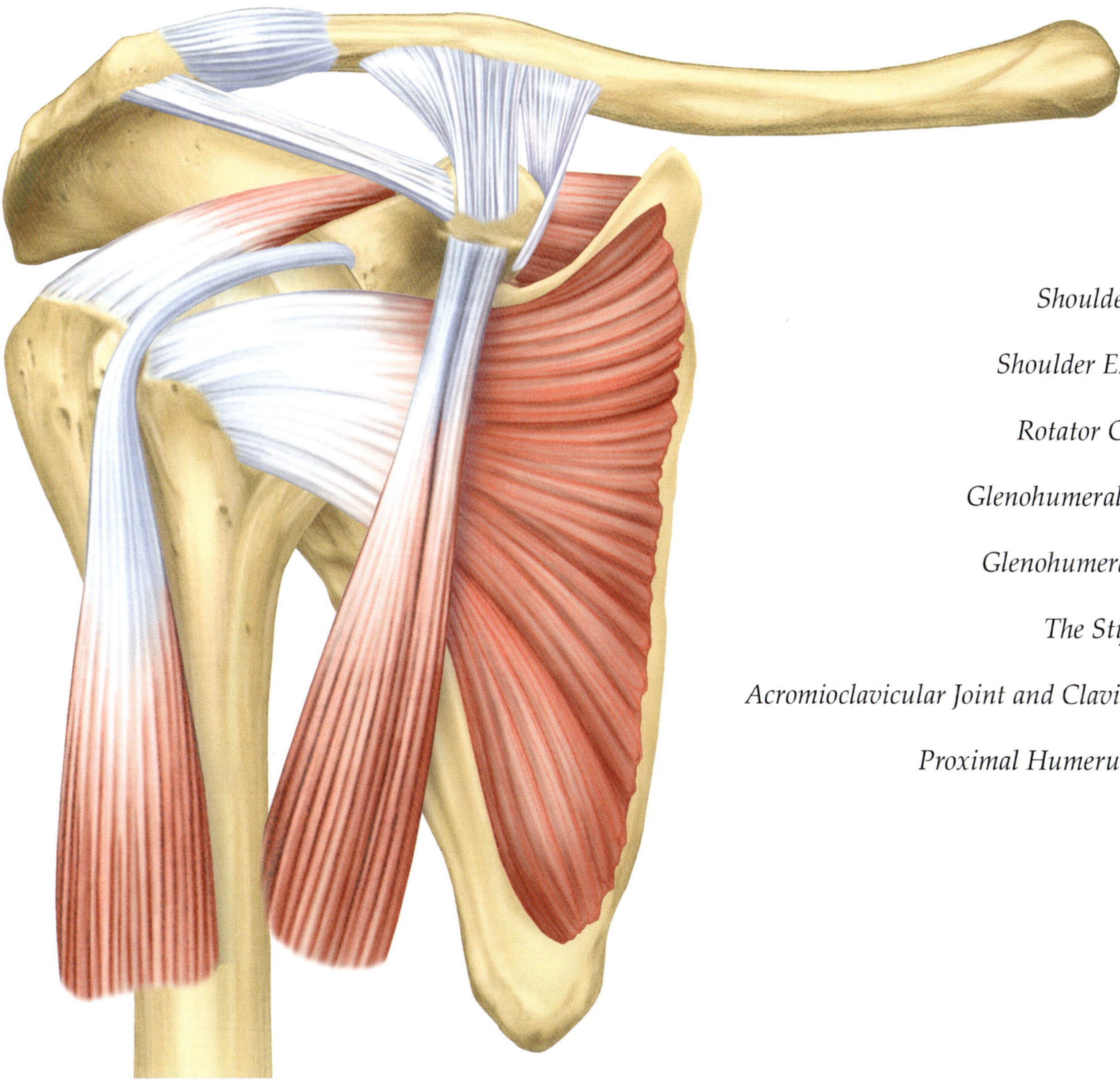

Shoulder Anatomy

Michael S. Potter, MD; Jacqueline B. Henson; Matthew A. Schwartz, MD; and George M. McCluskey III, MD

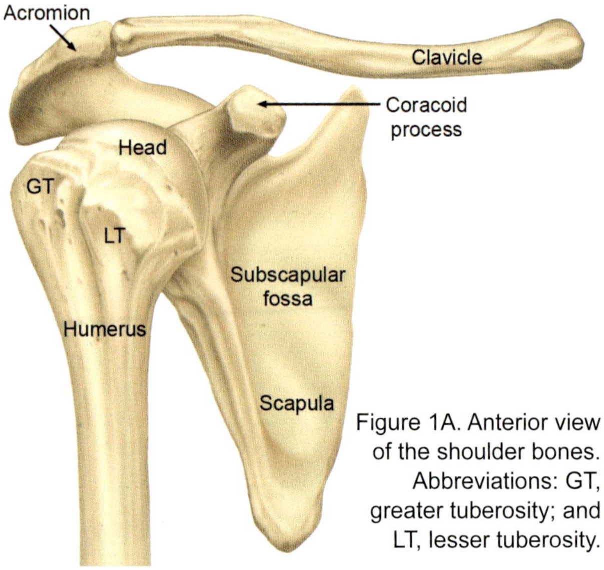

Figure 1A. Anterior view of the shoulder bones. Abbreviations: GT, greater tuberosity; and LT, lesser tuberosity.

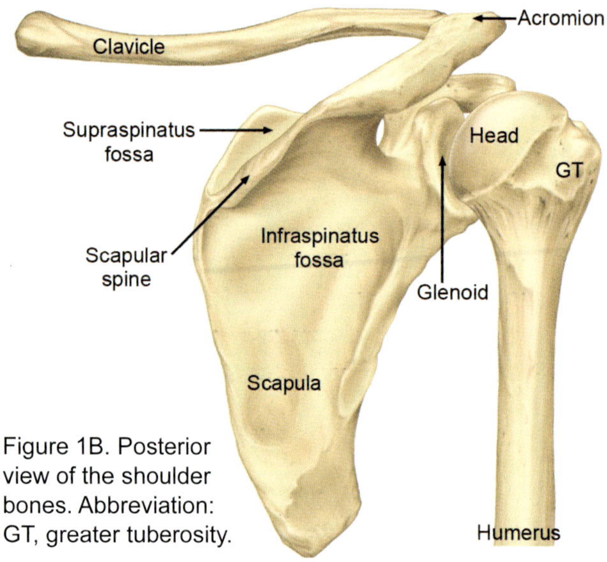

Figure 1B. Posterior view of the shoulder bones. Abbreviation: GT, greater tuberosity.

BONY ANATOMY

The shoulder is a complex joint that involves 3 main bony structures: the scapula, clavicle, and proximal humerus (Figures 1A and 1B). It has the greatest range of motion of any joint in the body and is the least congruous with little inherent bony stability, making it the most frequently dislocated joint in the human body. The shoulder relies on a complex arrangement of soft tissues, including its capsule and ligamentous and muscular restraints to achieve stability. These complexities lead to interesting challenges for rehabilitation providers and surgeons as they address the many disease processes that occur in this joint. A fundamental understanding of the anatomic structures involved is indispensable in appreciating and rehabilitating patients' shoulders.

Scapula

The scapula forms the posterior portion of the shoulder girdle. It is roughly triangular in shape, and its ventral surface is concave to accommodate the dorsum of the thorax. It is situated between the second and seventh ribs posteriorly. Surrounded by a muscular envelope and free of any bony attachments, it has a wide excursion across the posterior aspect of the rib cage. The 3 fossae and 4 processes composing the scapula are integral in anchoring the key shoulder girdle muscles that accomplish the shoulder's complex and unique motion.

Anteriorly, the large subscapularis fossa houses the subscapularis muscle, whereas posteriorly, the spine of the scapula separates the supraspinatus and infraspinatus fossae, which contain the origins of these

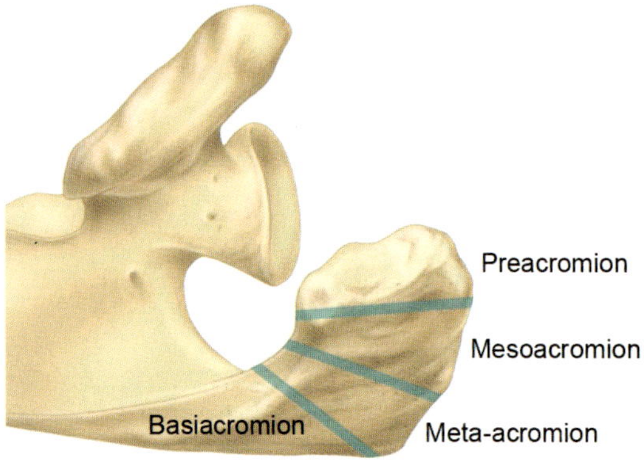

Figure 2. Acromion ossification centers.

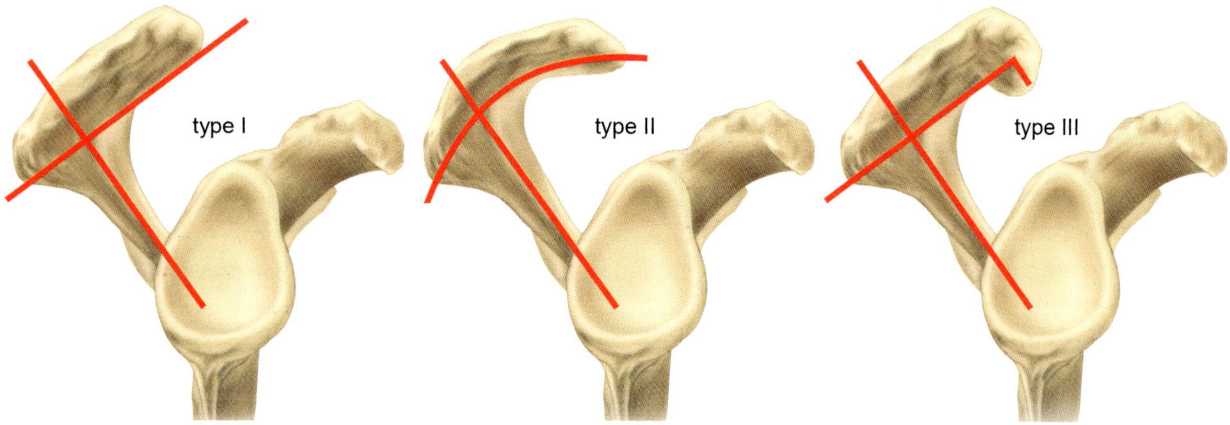

Figure 3. Three types of acromions.

muscles, respectively. In addition, the posterior deltoid and trapezius muscles insert on the scapular spine. The acromion process is the termination of the spine of the scapula and forms the summit of the shoulder. It protects the humeral head from direct trauma superiorly and serves as an insertion point for the deltoid anteriorly and laterally. During puberty, 3 ossification centers arise to form the bony acromion.[1] These centers generally fuse by age 22 years, but an unfused apophysis can lead to an os acromiale and can be a source of impingement on the supraspinatus tendon as a preacromion, mesoacromion, meta-acromion, or basiacromion (Figure 2).[2]

The acromion process, particularly the appearance of its undersurface, is perhaps the most widely studied portion of the scapula. Bigliani et al[3] classified acromions into 3 types and found correlations between these and the incidence of impingement and rotator cuff lesions (Figure 3). Type I acromion has a relatively smooth undersurface and presents the least encroachment into the supraspinatus outlet. Type II acromion has a more prominently curved undersurface. Type III acromion has a hooked undersurface and has been found to have the highest correlation with rotator cuff lesions from an external impingement process.[4]

The acromion is also the attachment of many major ligaments within the shoulder complex. Between the apex of the acromion and the coracoid, the coracoacromial ligament is a critical structure that forms the roof of the coracoacromial arch (Figure 4). Loss of

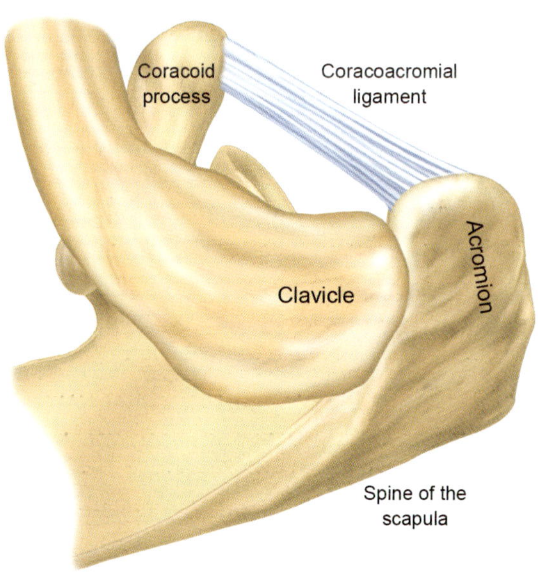

Figure 4. Aerial view of the coracoacromial ligament.

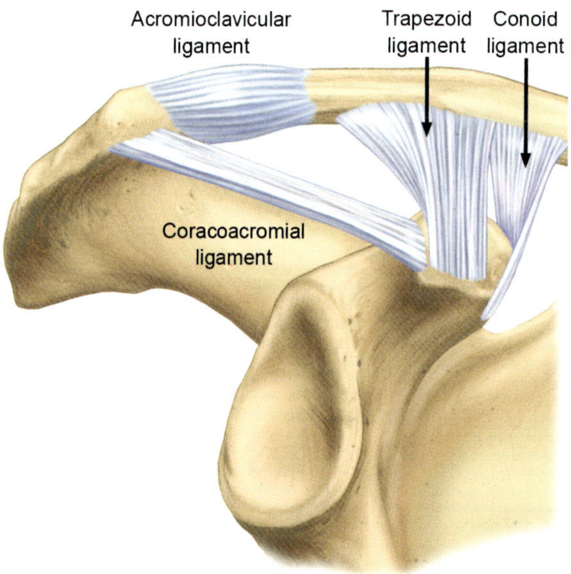

Figure 5. Ligamentous attachments to the coracoid.

this arch with large to massive rotator cuff tears leads to superior migration of the humeral head and further dysfunction of glenohumeral joint kinematics.

The coracoid process arises from the neck of the scapula just medial to the glenoid. This curved appendage to the scapula has been termed the *lighthouse to the shoulder* and serves as the attachment site for both ligaments and muscles in and around the shoulder girdle. It has strong connections to the clavicle through the conoid and trapezoid ligaments and is linked to the humerus by the coracohumeral ligament (CHL) (Figure 5). It is the origin of the short head of the biceps brachii and the coracobrachialis muscles and is the insertion of the pectoralis minor muscle.

At the base of the coracoid is the suprascapular notch. The suprascapular ligament forms its roof. Here, the suprascapular nerve travels beneath the ligament while the vessels accompanying the nerve travel above it (Figure 6). The nerve gives off 2 branches to the supraspinatus muscle then winds around the lateral border of the scapular spine to the spinoglenoid notch, passing under the spinoglenoid ligament. At this point, the nerve enters the infrapsinatus fossa and provides branches to the muscle. Damage to the nerve at one of

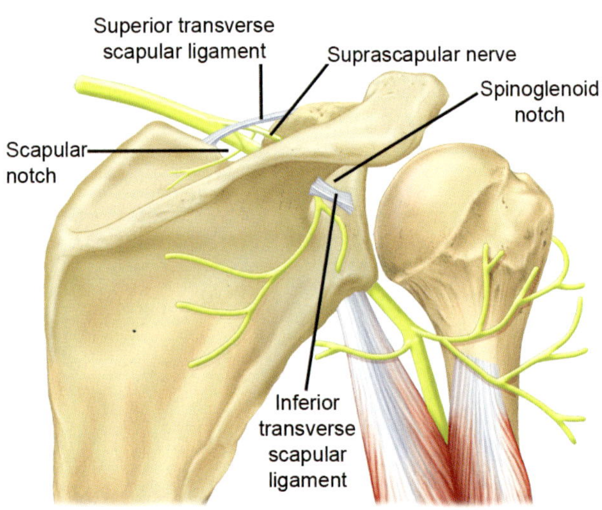

Figure 6. Anatomy in the area of the suprascapular nerve.

these locations by compression or traction can result in differing patterns of injury to the infraspinatus alone or to the supraspinatus and infraspinatus together.

The glenoid cavity is a shallow fossa shaped like an inverted comma. It is narrow superiorly and wide at its base. Hyaline cartilage, which is thickest at the periphery, lines it, whereas the center has the least amount of

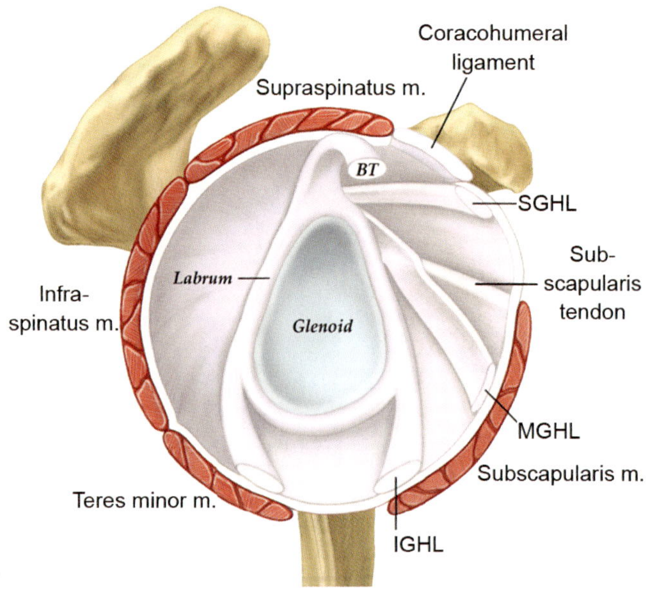

Figure 7. Lateral view of the glenohumeral ligaments. Abbreviations: BT, biceps tendon; SGHL, superior glenohumeral ligament; MGHL, middle glenohumeral ligament; and IGHL, inferior glenohumeral ligament.

articular cartilage, often developing a bare area with age.[5] It articulates with the humeral head to form the glenohumeral joint. The outer margins of the glenoid are lined by the labrum, which is a thick fibrous ring (Figure 7). Varying in thickness, it serves as an attachment site for several static ligamentous restraints within the shoulder joint complex, such as the superior glenohumeral ligament (SGHL), middle glenohumeral ligament (MGHL), and inferior glenohumeral ligament (IGHL). In addition, the labrum deepens the glenoid's articular surface to accommodate the much larger humeral head. Two tubercles on the bony glenoid serve as attachment sites for muscles that act indirectly on the glenohumeral joint. Inferiorly, the long head of the triceps originates from the inferior glenoid tubercle, whereas the long head of the biceps arises from the apex of the glenoid at the superior glenoid tubercle. The glenoid can be anteverted or more commonly retroverted with respect to the orientation of the scapula; average retroversion is approximately 1.23°.[6] However, with respect to the coronal plane of the body, the glenoid is anteverted between 30° and 40° because the scapula sits anterior to this plane.[7] It generally is tilted superomedially to inferolaterally when viewed in the anteroposterior (AP) plane. This relative upward-facing orientation is thought to contribute to the shoulder joint's overall stability.

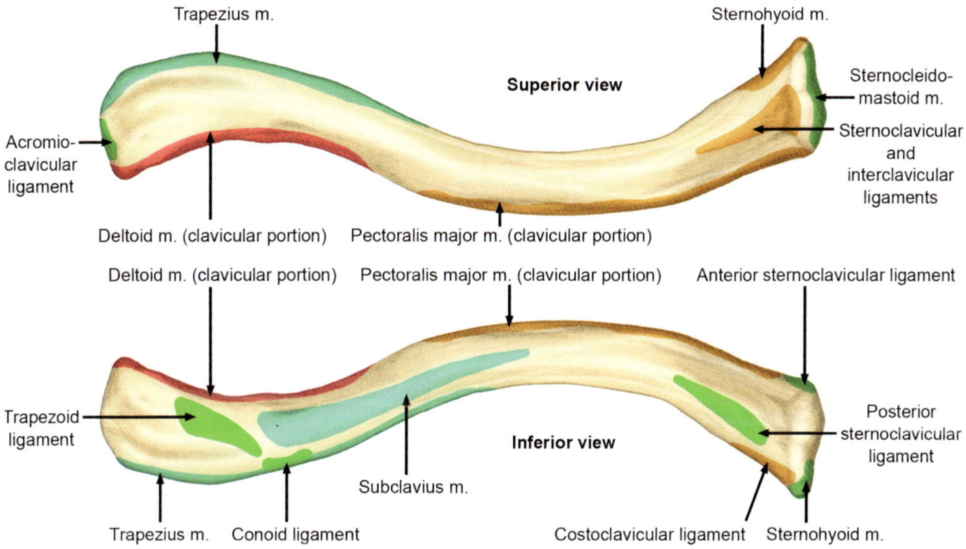

Figure 8.
Superior and inferior views of the clavicle with ligamentous and muscular attachment sites.

Clavicle

The clavicle, or collar bone, is the first bone in the skeleton to ossify, and this occurs around the fifth week of gestation. It also possesses the last ossification center in the human body to fuse. This occurs medially with the shaft of the clavicle between the ages of 22 and 25 years. Formed primarily by intramembranous ossification, it has a double curve: convex medially at its sternal border and concave toward the acromion (Figure 8). This unique geometry allows the clavicle to rotate on its long axis like a crankshaft to place the upper extremity in many functional positions. Through the clavicle, the upper extremity is suspended from the thorax, acting as a strut, and primarily serves as a site of attachment for muscles, including the deltoid, trapezius, pectoralis major, and sternocleidomastoid. It articulates laterally with the scapula at the acromioclavicular (AC) joint and medially with the axial skeleton at the sternoclavicular joint. It protects the subclavian artery and vein traveling on its undersurface and the brachial plexus that is situated posteriorly. The position of the clavicle relative to the scapula is maintained at the AC joint with its superior and inferior ligaments and joint capsule and through the coracoclavicular ligaments, conoid, and trapezoid.

Proximal Humerus

The humerus is a long bone that connects the elbow and the shoulder. It articulates proximally with the glenoid cavity of the scapula and distally with the radius and ulna. The proximal humerus consists of the humeral head, the greater and lesser tuberosities, and the bicipital groove (Figure 9).

The proximal humerus is roughly spherical in shape and is covered by hyaline cartilage over approximately one-third of its surface that articulates with the glenoid. The greater and lesser tuberosities are lateral to the humeral head and function as attachment sites for the rotator cuff muscles. The greater tuberosity has 3 facets (superior, middle, and inferior) upon which the supraspinatus, infraspinatus, and teres minor insert. It is larger and situated more posteriorly than the lesser tuberosity, which receives the subscapularis insertion. The bicipital groove runs between the greater and lesser tuberosities and holds the long head of the biceps tendon.

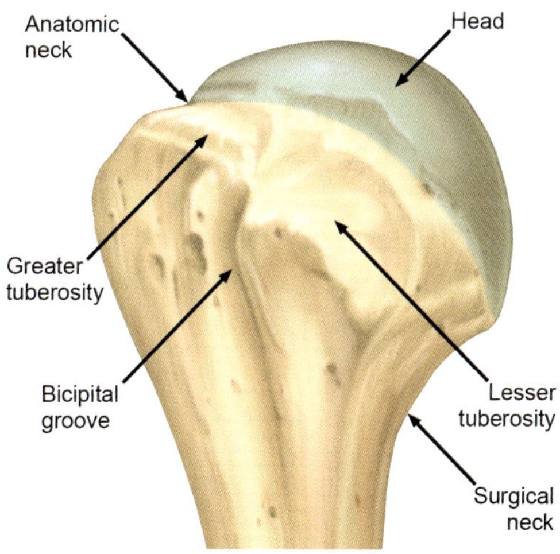

Figure 9. Anatomic landmarks for the proximal humerus.

The proximal humerus arises from 3 ossification centers: 1 for the head, 1 for the greater tuberosity, and 1 for the lesser tuberosity. The angle formed by the upward-pointing articular surface and the shaft of the humerus varies from 130° to 160°.[8] Relative to the transepicondylar axis of the elbow, the proximal humerus is retroverted on average 33° on the dominant side and 29° on the nondominant side.[9] The 2 tuberosities are separated by the intertubercular or bicipital groove where it lodges the tendon of the long head of the biceps as it travels away from the superior glenoid. Between the superior edge of the tuberosities and the articular margin of the humeral head is a deep sulcus that delineates the anatomic neck of the humerus and is obscured by the footprint of the rotator cuff. The surgical neck lies just inferior to the tuberosities and is the most common site of fractures of the proximal humerus.

JOINTS AND LIGAMENTS

Joints are the junctions at which 2 bones come together, allowing certain motions and prohibiting others. The motions that are permitted are determined by the bony structures, ligaments, and surrounding musculature. Because of the complex arrangement of its 4 joints, the shoulder has the greatest range of motion of any joint in the human body.

Glenohumeral Joint

The glenohumeral joint is formed by the shallow glenoid and the much larger humeral head. It is more akin to a golf ball on a tee rather than a true ball-and-socket joint (Figure 10). It has the greatest range of motion of any joint in the body and is the least congruous with little inherent bony stability. A complex arrangement of soft tissues, including its capsule and ligamentous and muscular restraints, provide stability. Therefore, this joint is the most frequently dislocated in the human body. The glenohumeral joint works in concert with the sternoclavicular, AC, and scapulothoracic articulations to rotate the upper extremity within and relative to the sagittal and coronal planes of the body. The relative contributions of glenohumeral and scapulothoracic motion in the movement of the shoulder joint complex have been studied widely. The ratio has been determined to be generally 2:1, with the larger contribution initially coming from the glenohumeral joint.[10,11] During the first 30° of shoulder elevation, motion at the scapulothoracic joint is variable and often absent.[12] With greater elevation, the relationship between the 2 articulations becomes more linear with more equal contributions from each.

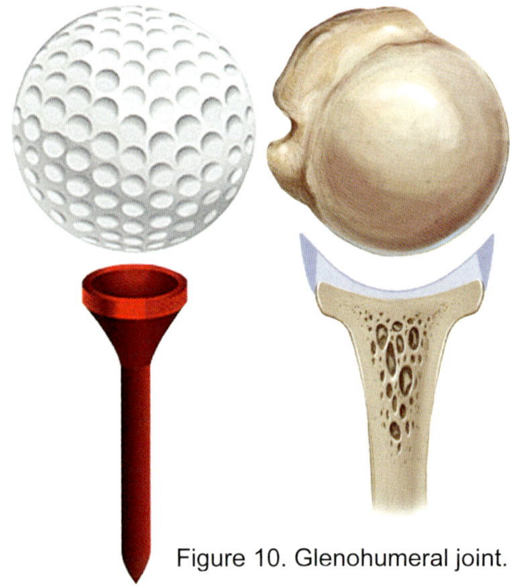

Figure 10. Glenohumeral joint.

As the curved scapula moves along the curved surface of the posterior aspect of the rib cage, multiple muscles retract, protract, or tilt it to provide a stable base for the upper extremity to generate force and power. Motion of the scapula, in turn, elevates the acromion to allow free tendon excursion of the rotator cuff muscles. A complex and coordinated effort by the periscapular muscles is required to accomplish this positioning of the scapula. This delicate balance has profound implications on glenohumeral mechanics because of their intimate relationship. Any aberration in muscle function or in the bony anatomy of the posterior thorax, as in scoliosis, can create nonrhythmic or disorganized motion at this joint and can lead to what Kibler and McMullen[13] termed *scapular dyskinesia*.

Capsule and Static Stabilizers

The shoulder capsule is large relative to the humeral head and can cover an area roughly twice that of the articular surface of the proximal humerus (Figure 11). It is reflected from the margin of the glenoid cavity over the labrum and as far as the anatomic neck of the humerus, blending with the articular surface at its margin. Anteriorly and inferiorly, the capsule is loose

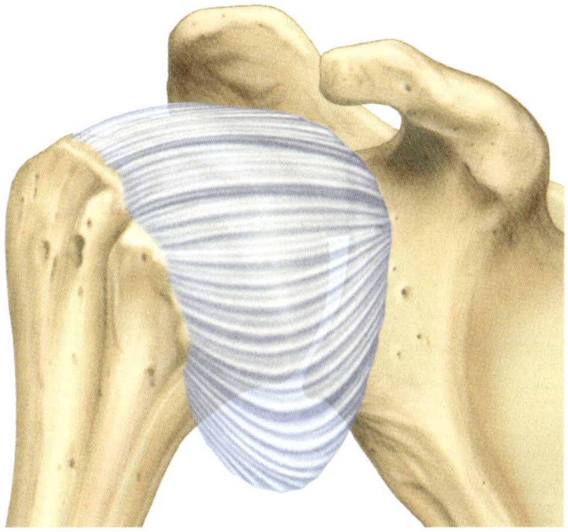

Figure 11. Anterior view of the shoulder capsule.

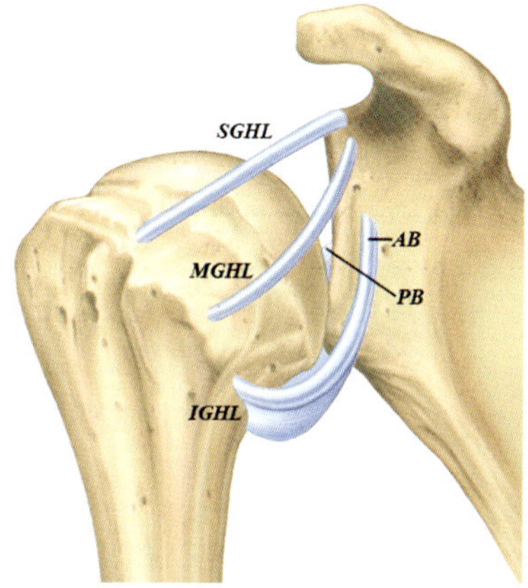

Figure 13. Superior (SGHL), middle (MGHL), and inferior (IGHL) glenohumeral ligaments with the shoulder at 0° of abduction. Abbreviations: AB, anterior band; and PB, posterior band.

and redundant. This redundancy or slack in the capsule is taken up as the upper extremity is abducted. One of the unique characteristics of the capsule is its negative intra-articular pressure created by osmotic differences in the surrounding soft tissues. This process pulls water away from the articular surfaces and draws the capsule inward. In doing so, it contributes to the stability of the glenohumeral joint. In the resting state, the shoulder joint capsule has approximately 1 mL of synovial fluid; however, it can accommodate up to 30 mL and even more in cases of excessive shoulder laxity. In pathologic states, such as adhesive capsulitis, it might only be able to contain 5 mL of fluid.

Discrete thickenings or condensations within the capsule anteriorly and inferiorly provide most of the static restraint to dislocation of the glenohumeral joint. They are the SGHL, MGHL, and IGHL (Figure 12).

The SGHL has 2 sites of origin: the superior glenoid tubercle just anterior to the long head of the biceps and the base of the coracoid. It inserts onto the lesser tuberosity and is present in more than 90% of individuals.[14,15] Working in concert with the middle glenohumeral and CHL ligaments, it provides a restraint to inferior and posterior translation of the humerus within the glenoid at 0° of shoulder abduction (Figure 13).

The MGHL is the most variable of the capsular ligaments. It is absent in approximately 27% of shoulders and can demonstrate morphologic differences between individuals.[16] One of these variants is the Buford complex. This consists of a cord-like MGHL that originates high off the glenoid rim and is associated with a sublabral foramen at the anterosuperior glenoid that is devoid of any labral tissue.[17] The MGHL originates from either the bony glenoid or labrum just inferior to the SGHL and inserts medial to the lesser tuberosity (Figure 14). It is a secondary restraint to inferior trans-

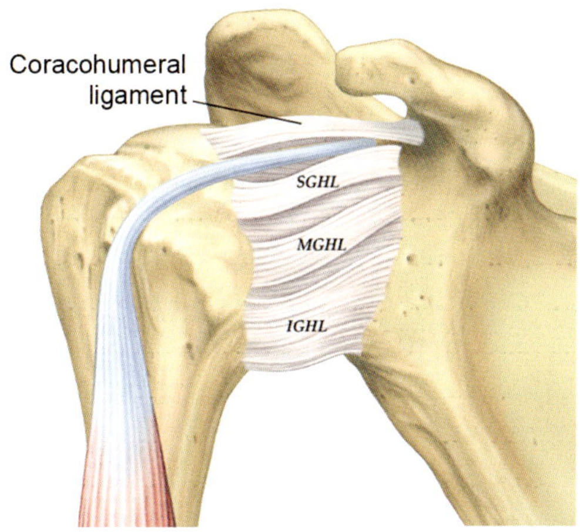

Figure 12. Anterior view of the superior (SGHL), middle (MGHL), and inferior (IGHL) glenohumeral ligaments.

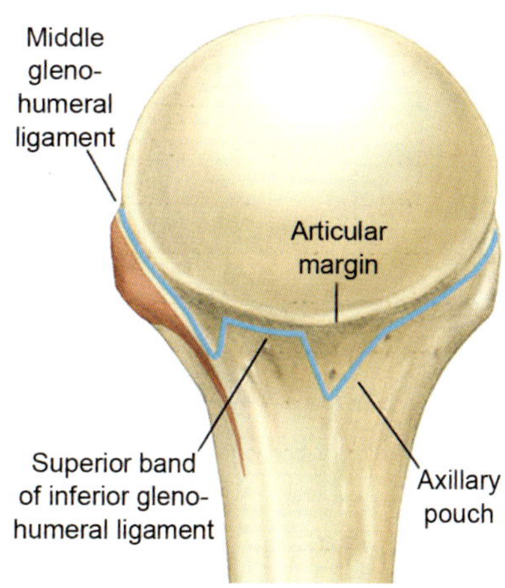

Figure 14. Humeral insertion sites of the middle and inferior glenohumeral ligaments.

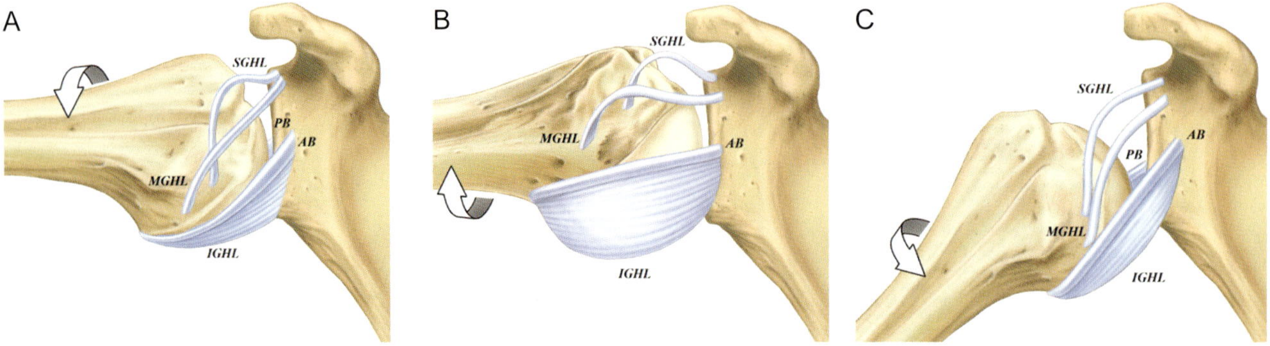

Figure 15. Inferior glenohumeral ligament (IGHL). A, 90° of abduction and internal rotation. B, 90° of abduction and external rotation. C, 45° of abduction and internal rotation. Abbreviations: SGHL, superior glenohumeral ligament; PB, posterior band; AB, anterior band; and MGHL, middle glenohumeral ligament.

lation of the glenohumeral joint in the adducted and externally rotated extremity and also limits anterior translation with the extremity between 45° and 90° of abduction.[18]

The IGHL is the most important static restraint within the shoulder joint complex. More than just a solitary ligament, this complex structure consists of anterior and posterior bands and an intervening axillary pouch. It originates from the glenoid rim and neck from the 3 o'clock position anteriorly to the 9 o'clock position posteriorly. The IGHL complex is the primary restraint to dislocation of the humeral head, having a reciprocating relationship between the 2 bands as the upper extremity is taken from internal to external rotation in the abducted position (Figure 15). With the extremity in 90° of abduction and in maximum external rotation, the anterior band fans out and tightens to resist anterior translation of the humerus, and the posterior band becomes lax. In an acute anterior shoulder dislocation, the anterior band often is avulsed from the anterior glenoid as a soft tissue tear or Bankart lesion or with a portion of the glenoid rim in the form of a bony Bankart lesion. As the extremity is rotated internally in the abducted position, the posterior band tightens and fans out to support the humeral head and resist posterior translation. As this occurs, conversely the anterior band relaxes. The IGHL complex also provides stability to an inferiorly directed force with the upper extremity in an abducted position and is the major restraint at 90° of abduction.[14,19]

The CHL is an extra-articular structure that arises at the base of the coracoid at its lateral margin. It passes obliquely downward and outward to insert on the lesser and greater tuberosities, spanning the bicipital groove. Its fibers are associated intimately with those of the capsule and ultimately blends with the tendon of the supraspinatus.[18] The role of the CHL in stabilizing the glenohumeral joint is still largely unknown, but it and the MGHL are believed to provide a restraint to inferior translation with the upper extremity in adduction. Some investigators believe that it suspends the humeral head in the glenoid with the extremity at the side.[5] As the upper extremity is brought into abduction, the ligament relaxes and loses its ability to support the humerus.[5]

The rotator interval (RI) is a triangular portion of the shoulder capsule that is situated between the upper border of the subscapularis and the anterior border of the supraspinatus tendons (Figure 16). It comprises fibers of the subscapularis and supraspinatus tendons, CHL, SGHL, and glenohumeral joint capsule. The RI closes down with internal rotation of the humerus

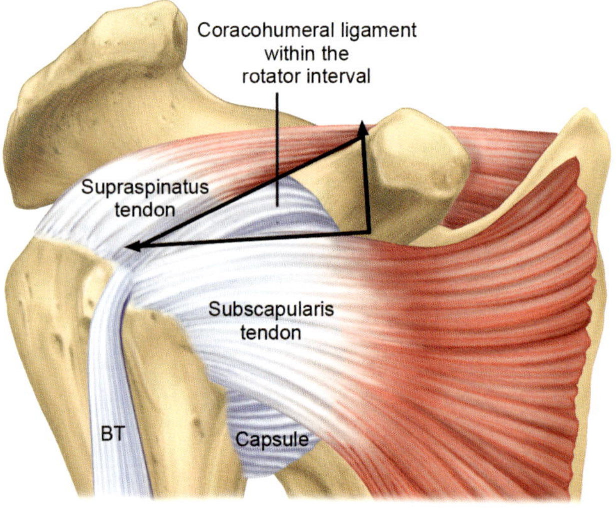

Figure 16. Rotator interval. Abbreviation: BT, biceps tendon.

and opens with external rotation. Therefore, it plays a prominent role in the treatment of shoulder laxity. By closing this interval through open surgery or arthroscopically, the effective volume of the glenohumeral joint is decreased, and subsequently stability is increased. Harryman et al [20] found that by sectioning the RI, posterior translation of the glenohumeral joint increased by 50% and inferior translation increased by 100%.

Sternoclavicular Joint

The sternoclavicular joint is the only articulation between the axial skeleton and the upper extremity, and as with other joints around the shoulder, very little of the inherent stability is borne by the shape of its bony ends. The joint is stabilized by a surrounding capsule, anterior and posterior sternoclavicular ligaments, interclavicular and costoclavicular (CC) ligaments, and an intra-articular fibrocartilage disc (Figure 17).[21] It acts as a ball and socket by affording movement in all planes. The fibrocartilage disc plays a key role in freedom of movement, whereas the AC joint has an intra-articular disc that is often rudimentary and, when present, often is perforated in the center. The disc divides the joint into 2 cavities, each of which has its own synovial membrane and provides a shock absorber to medially directed blows to the sternum. The anterior and posterior sternoclavicular ligaments attach at the periphery of the disc. The posterior ligament is the strongest stabilizer of the joint to inferior depression of the lateral clavicle, and the anterior and posterior ligaments work together to resist rotation of the clavicle as it is depressed during shoulder elevation. The interclavicular ligament runs between the medial ends of the clavicles. Its fibers mesh with those of the joint capsule superiorly, and it also contributes to the stability of the joint as the lateral clavicle is depressed. The CC ligaments provide a firm attachment from the medial clavicle to the first rib. The anterior CC ligament acts as a checkrein to lateral displacement of the clavicle on the ribcage, whereas the posterior ligament works to resist medial displacement.[5] The sternoclavicular joint is somewhat protected by its medial location, and because it possesses greater stability compared with the AC joint, it is often the less injured of the 2. Injury can include anterior or, less commonly, posterior dislocation or physeal fracture due to the late closure of the medial clavicle epiphysis, as mentioned.

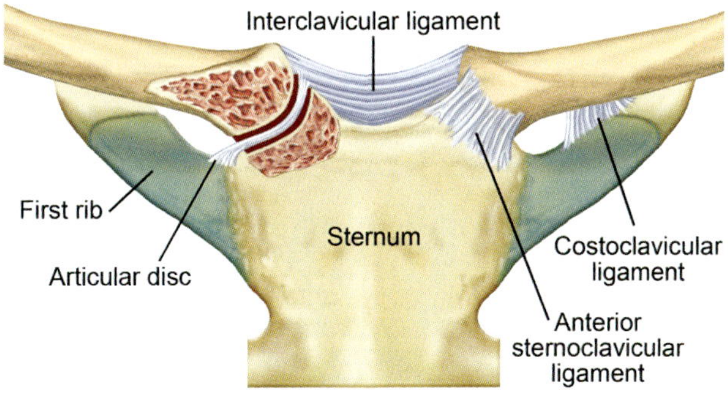

Figure 17. Sternoclavicular joint.

Acromioclavicular Joint

This diarthrodial joint is situated between the lateral or distal clavicle and the acromion. It allows the acromion to glide in the AP plane as the scapula is retracted and protracted, the clavicle to rotate up to 20°, and the acromion to tilt as the extremity is abducted and adducted.[5] When present, an intra-articular disc separates the articular surfaces of the clavicle and acromion. Stability of the joint is provided primarily by the strong coracoclavicular ligaments. They provide a restraint to vertical translation of the clavicle relative to the acromion. These ligaments are not part of the true articulation of the joint, but because they lead to dysfunction of the joint when disrupted, they always are included in its discussion. The trapezoid ligament sits lateral relative to the conoid ligament and slightly anterior (Figure 18).[21] Its fibers are confluent with those of its counterpart and pass obliquely from

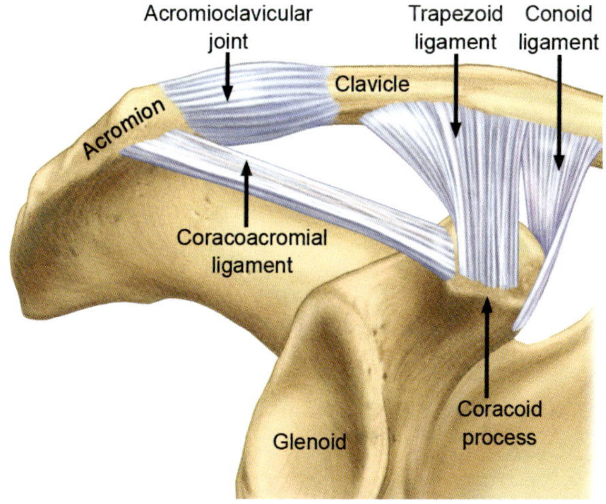

Figure 18. Acromioclavicular joint.

the coracoid to the undersurface of the clavicle. The conoid ligament, which is more medial and posterior, is the more important and stronger of the 2 ligaments. It comprises dense fascicular bands and originates from a shallow depression at the base of the coracoid process. In addition to being a checkrein on superior migration of the clavicle, these ligaments limit rotation of the scapula; the trapezoid limits forward rotation, and the conoid limits posterior rotation.[22] The superior and inferior AC ligaments provide horizontal stability in the AP plane. They are continuous with one another anteriorly and posteriorly to form a complete capsule around the joint. The superior ligament is the main stabilizer because it is considerably thicker than the inferior ligament and has fibers that interlace with those of the trapezius and deltoid muscles. Injury to this joint is among the most common that can occur around the shoulder.

Scapulothoracic Articulation

During many motions of the shoulder, the scapula can be protracted or retracted, moving laterally or medially against the chest wall. This articulation between the anterior concave surface of the scapula with the posterior convex surface of the chest wall constitutes the scapulothoracic articulation, which is the fourth joint of the shoulder. Because the only osseous connection between the scapula and the axial skeleton is with the clavicle, the stability of the scapula primarily is provided by its muscular attachments.

Intrinsic Scapular Ligaments

Coracoacromial Ligament. The coracoacromial ligament spans the space between the coracoid process and the acromion, forming the coracoacromial arch. This arch serves as an important structure in preventing superior migration of the humeral head. The subacromial bursa is situated below the coracoacromial arch, separating it from the supraspinatus muscle of the rotator cuff.

Superior Transverse Scapular Ligament. The superior transverse scapular ligament travels from the base of the coracoid process to the upper border of the scapula, forming a foramen over the suprascapular notch. The suprascapular nerve runs beneath it (Figure 19).

Inferior Transverse Scapular Ligament. The inferior transverse scapular ligament stretches from the lateral border of the scapular spine to the posterior edge of the glenoid. It forms a foramen over the spinoglenoid notch, through which the suprascapular nerve travels.

MUSCLES

Muscles are tissues of contractile fibers that provide force to organs, resulting in motion. When a muscle is stimulated, it contracts, shortening its length and exerting a force. Where the force is applied depends on the origin and insertion points of the muscle. Through different combinations of forces, skeletal muscles give motion to the skeletal system and stability to its joints. The muscles of the shoulder interact with its bones, scapula, clavicle, and humerus to provide it with a wide range of motion and dynamic stability.

Muscles of the Shoulder Joint Complex

The coordination of 20 muscles is needed to achieve motion that is smooth and rhythmic at the glenohumeral joint. Many of these muscles, such as the deltoid, infraspinatus, and pectoralis, have multiple segments that accomplish different tasks in both stabilizing and moving the shoulder. The glenohumeral joint is essentially an unconstrained joint working with the scapula. As it "floats" along the rib cage posteriorly, it is capable of placing the upper extremity in many functional positions in space, and with each position, the relationship among these various muscles changes. They can be grouped into muscles that act directly on the glenohumeral joint, such as the deltoid and rotator

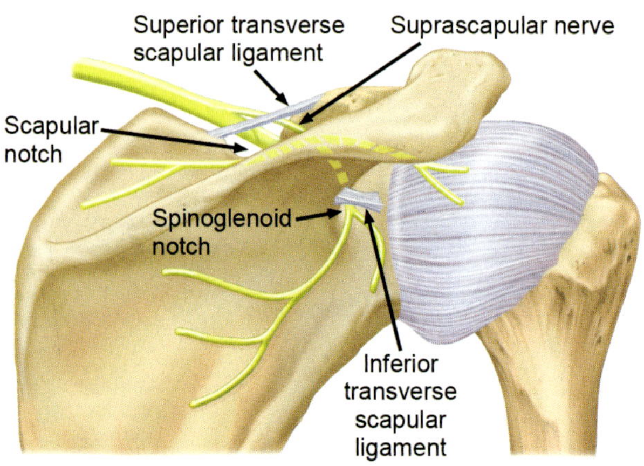

Figure 19. Intrinsic scapular ligaments.

cuff; muscles that act indirectly, such as the pectoralis and biceps brachii; and muscles of the scapulothoracic articulation that move and stabilize the scapula on the posterior thorax.

Deltoid

Every discussion of the muscles that act on the shoulder joint must begin with the most important one: the deltoid. This triangular-shaped muscle takes its name from its resemblance to the Greek letter Δ. It

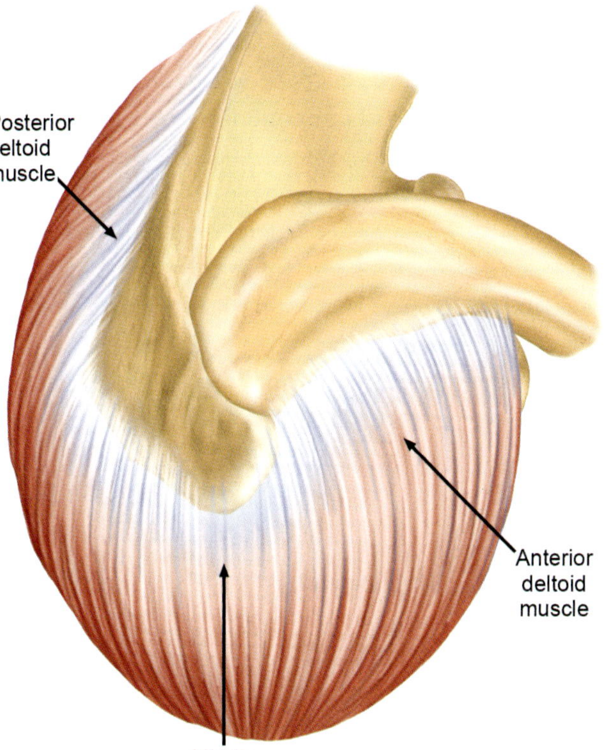

Figure 20. Three divisions of the deltoid muscle.

forms the rounded contour of the shoulder and principally functions to abduct the upper extremity. The deltoid comprises 3 divisions (anterior, middle, and posterior) that are separated by a raphe and work synergistically with each other and the muscles of the rotator cuff to raise the extremity overhead (Figure 20). The neurovascular bundle supplying the deltoid runs on its undersurface and consists of the axillary nerve and posterior humeral circumflex artery. The nerve and artery travel posterior to anterior, entering the posterior aspect of the shoulder through the quadrilateral space. Here, the axillary nerve gives off fibers to the teres minor as it continues to wind around anteriorly. Knowledge of the distance that the axillary nerve lies in relation to the acromion is of great interest to surgeons who work around the shoulder joint. It has been found to be variable throughout its course, running approximately 5 cm from the posterior acromion and approximately 6 cm from the anterior acromion.[23,24]

The anterior division of the deltoid originates from the lateral-third of the clavicle, whereas the middle division arises from the acromion. Together, their primary role is in abduction of the upper extremity and elevation in the scapular plane.[5] The posterior division works in concert with the anterior and middle divisions but contributes less to these functions. The posterior division originates from the scapular spine, works to extend the extremity, and aids in externally rotating the humerus. Likewise, the anterior division has a role in internally rotating the humerus. All 3 divisions fuse to form a common tendon that inserts on the deltoid tuberosity at the lateral humeral shaft.

For normal elevation of the upper extremity to be accomplished, both the deltoid and supraspinatus muscles must be functioning synchronously. This has been confirmed in studies in which simultaneous axillary and suprascapular nerve blocks made active shoulder abduction impossible.[25] Investigators believe that with the upper extremity at the side, the supraspinatus initiates abduction of the shoulder, whereas the deltoid muscle with its dominant force directed vertically provides most of the remaining force required to bring the extremity to and above shoulder level. This pull of the deltoid creates a vertical shear force at the glenohumeral joint that is offset by an inferiorly directed force generated by the infraspinatus and teres minor muscles. The moment arm of the deltoid progressively improves as the extremity is brought into more abduction.[26]

Rotator Cuff

The rotator cuff is an intimate arrangement of muscle tendons that play a central role in motion at the shoulder joint. Although often considered by its individual parts, it functions as a cohesive unit. Each of the tendons of 4 muscles (supraspinatus, infraspinatus, teres minor, and subscapularis) that compose it fans out from its muscle belly to form 1 continuous insertion onto the proximal humerus (Figure 21). In the layered configuration of the shoulder, the rotator cuff lies just superficial to the capsule of the glenohumeral joint. The muscles that compose the tendinous portion of the cuff originate from the scapula and insert onto the lesser and greater tuberosities surrounding the humeral head.

The rotator cuff muscles work in concert with the surrounding and supporting musculature of the shoulder joint complex to allow its great range of motion. They act as dynamic stabilizers by maintaining the humeral head centered in the glenoid throughout shoulder motion. They accomplish this by joint compression and humeral head depression because of their orientation and vector of pull relative to the glenoid. When intact, these vector relationships develop force couples between opposing muscles. In turn, this creates a stable fulcrum for balanced and fluid motion at the glenohumeral joint.[5]

Supraspinatus. The supraspinatus originates from the superior scapula, occupying nearly the entire supraspinatus fossa. It passes over the humeral head through the supraspinatus outlet to insert onto the greater tuberosity. At its insertion, the tendon of the supraspinatus becomes confluent with that of the infraspinatus. During all phases of shoulder elevation, the muscle is active and mainly functions to assist the deltoid first by initiating abduction and second by compressing the humeral head within the glenoid to balance the upward force of the deltoid.[27]

The supraspinatus muscle is innervated by the suprascapular nerve, which branches from the upper trunk of the brachial plexus with contributions from the C5 and C6 nerve roots. It enters the supraspinatus fossa, passes beneath the muscle, curves around the spine of the scapula, and enters the infraspinatus fossa. Within the supraspinatus fossa, it supplies 2 branches to the muscle while providing 3 or 4 branches to the infraspinatus within its fossa.[28] The suprascapular nerve also provides small branches to innervate the capsule and glenohumeral joint.

Infraspinatus and Teres Minor. The infraspinatus and teres minor are the primary external rotators of the humerus, with the infraspinatus playing a dominant role. In addition to the teres minor assisting in this task, the posterior aspect of the deltoid contributes.[25] The infrapsinatus and teres minor muscles are innervated by the suprascapular and posterior divisions of the axillary nerves, respectively, both of which receive contributions from the C5 and C6 nerve roots. The 2 muscles originate from the scapula: the infraspinatus from its fossa and the teres minor from the midportion of the lateral border of the scapula (Figure 22). The infraspinatus is a bipennate muscle with a distinct raphe separating the 2 segments. This can present confusion because it often is mistaken for the intermuscular interval between the 2 external rotators.

Subscapularis. The subscapularis is a triangular-shaped muscle that originates from the whole subscapularis fossa at the anterior aspect of the scapula. This largest and most powerful of the rotator cuff muscles has a multipennate architecture that terminates into a tendon inserting onto the lesser tuberosity. It is the only rotator cuff muscle that inserts here and also has portions of the tendon that insert onto the medial humeral neck.[29] The fibers of the subscapularis tendon become intermingled with those of the capsule before its insertion. The muscle is an active internal rotator of the humerus and acts as a passive restraint to anterior translation of the humeral head by its mass and location.[30] As the upper extremity is raised, it also draws

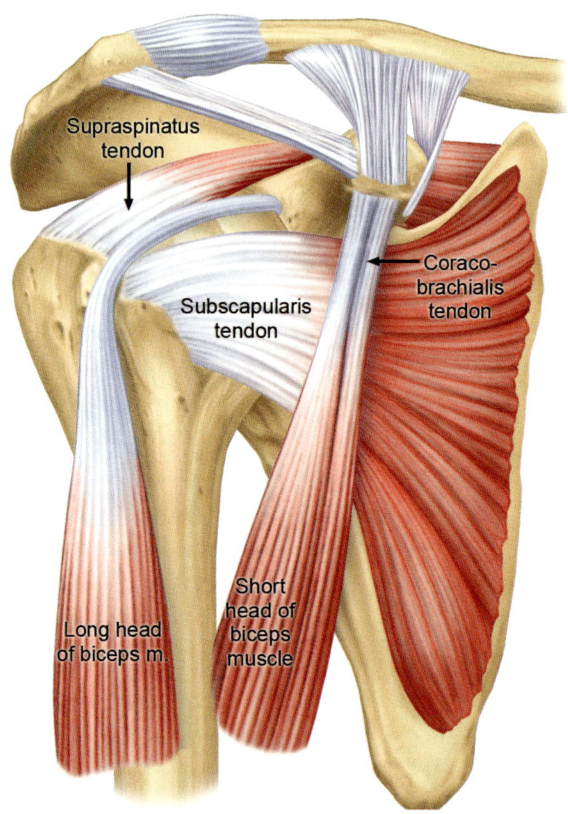

Figure 21. Anterior view of the rotator cuff muscles.

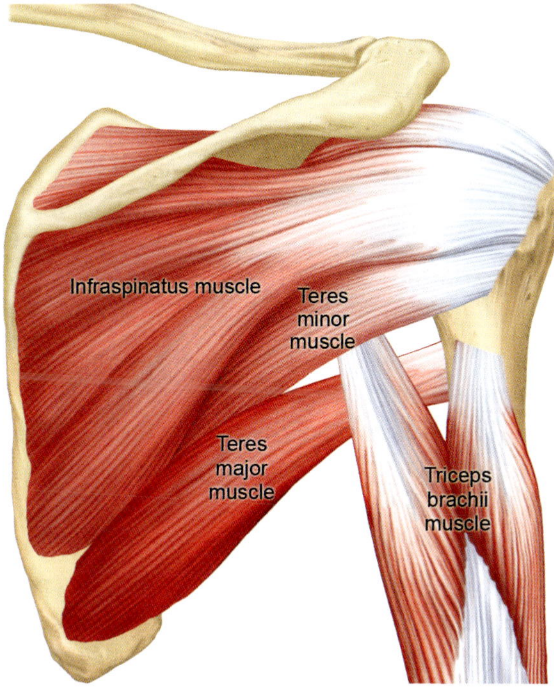

Figure 22. Posterior view of the rotator cuff muscles.

the humerus downward because of the orientation of its fibers and vector of pull. The subscapularis has a dual innervation from the upper and lower subscapular nerves, which arise from the posterior cord of the brachial plexus, and as the other muscles of the cuff, it is supplied by the C5 and C6 nerve roots.

Biceps Brachii

The biceps is a long fusiform muscle composed of 2 heads (long and short), each of which have a separate origin around the shoulder girdle. The short head arises from the coracoid at its apex along with the coracobrachialis. The long head of the biceps originates from the superior glenoid tubercle and labrum and occupies the bicipital groove, traveling between the greater and lesser tuberosities as it exits the glenohumeral joint. The 2 heads join to form a common tendon with 2 distal insertions. Laterally, the tendon inserts into the radial tuberosity, and medially, it becomes continuous with the deep fascia of the volar forearm musculature.

The biceps is innervated by the musculocutaneous nerve with contributions primarily from the C5 and C6 nerve roots. Primarily a muscle of the elbow functioning mainly as a supinator of the forearm and elbow flexor, its role at the shoulder joint has generated considerable debate. Electromyographic analysis of the biceps during shoulder motion with the forearm and elbow fixed has shown that the muscle is quiet during these activities.[31]

Triceps Brachii

The triceps occupies the entire posterior aspect of the humerus. It comprises 3 heads (lateral, medial or deep, and long heads). The lateral and medial heads originate from the posterior humerus; the lateral, from the proximal one-half; and the medial, from the inferior two-thirds. The long head arises from the infraglenoid tubercle, but it is not intra-articular as the long head of the biceps tendon is. The 3 heads have a common insertion onto the proximal aspect of the ulna at the olecranon process.

The triceps is innervated by the radial nerve, with contributions from C6, C7, C8, and T1 nerve roots. It extends the elbow joint and is the direct antagonist to the biceps and brachialis muscles. Although it has a very peripheral role in shoulder motion, researchers have found in electromyography studies that it is active during the phases of pitching.[32] In addition, the triceps is believed to function in shoulder adduction by offsetting shear forces that the main shoulder adductors generate.[5]

Lastissimus Dorsi

The latissimus dorsi is a broad flat muscle with an origin that posteriorly covers a large surface area. It arises from the inferior 6 thoracic vertebrae, all 5 lumbar vertebrae, portions of the sacrum and iliac crest, and a small portion of the inferior angle of the scapula. Its muscle fibers pass in different directions from these varied origins and form the posterior contour of the axillary fold. These fibers converge into a common tendon that twists upon itself to ultimately insert onto the floor of the intertubercular groove just anterior to the tendon of the pectoralis major muscle.

The latissimus dorsi is innervated by the thoracodorsal nerve from the posterior cord of the brachial plexus, with nerve roots C6, C7, and C8 supplying contributions. It extends, adducts, and internally rotates the humerus at the shoulder joint and draws the inferior angle of the scapula inferiorly, effectively moving the shoulder downward and backward.

Teres Major

The teres major originates from the dorsal aspect of the inferior angle of the scapula. Its fibers extend outward and upward to insert onto the humerus at the intertubercular groove medial to the insertion of the latissimus dorsi. The 2 tendons are intimately associated with one another and are separated by a synovial bursa. The teres major works synergistically with the latissimus to extend, adduct, and internally rotate the humerus at the shoulder joint. It is innervated by the lower subscapular nerve from the posterior cord of the brachial plexus with fibers from the fifth, sixth, and seventh nerve roots.

Pectoralis Major

The pectoralis major is a broad, triangular muscle that originates in 2 divisions from the anterior thoracic region. The superior half, or clavicular head, arises from the medial clavicle and upper part of the sternum (Figure 23). The sternal head is the inferior half and arises from the distal end of the sternum, the external oblique aponeurosis, and the costal cartilage of the first 6 ribs. From each origin, the muscle fibers are directed laterally, converge, and rotate 90° onto one another. The confluence of these fibers inserts onto the humeral shaft at the crest of the intertubercular groove in a broad, flat, and bilaminar tendon.[33] The anterior lamina comprises fibers primarily from the clavicular head, and the posterior lamina comprises fibers from the sternal head and portions of the external oblique aponeurosis. At its insertion, the most inferior fibers insert more proximally, and the superior fibers insert more distally. Whereas the latissimus makes up the contour of the posterior axillary fold, the pectoralis provides its shape anteriorly.

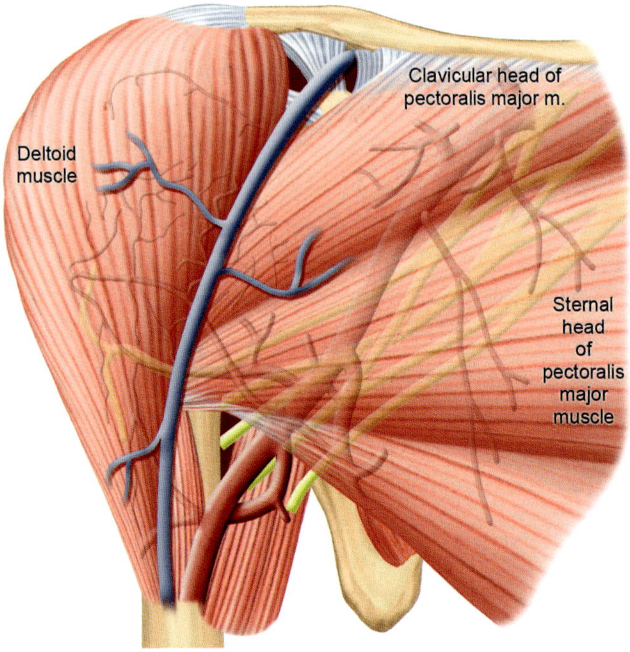

Figure 23. Pectoralis major muscle.

The pectoralis major has a dual innervation from the lateral and medial pectoral nerves, which arise from the lateral and medial cords of the brachial plexus, respectively. The lateral pectoral nerve innervates the clavicular head and the medial portion of the sternal head and has contributions from the C5, C6, and C7 nerve roots. The medial pectoral nerve, which comprises fibers from the C8 and T1 nerve roots, supplies the lateral portion of the sternal head and supplies branches to the pectoralis minor where the nerve first enters on its undersurface.[34] This muscle is a powerful adductor, flexor, and internal rotator of the upper extremity and is active during extension of the extremity from a flexed position as it is brought to neutral.[5]

Scapulothoracic Muscles

Eighteen muscles link the scapula to the humerus and the cervical and thoracic regions that allow for coordinated and fluid glenohumeral motion. Of these, the levator scapulae, rhomboids major and minor, serratus anterior, omohyoid, pectoralis minor, and trapezius are the scapulothoracic muscles (Figure 24). They work in concert to provide a stable scapular platform from which movement of the upper extremity is accomplished. Dysfunction within these muscles either individually or collectively leads to winging of the scapula and scapular dyskinesia.[13]

The trapezius is the largest and most superficial of the scapulothoracic muscles. It has 3 divisions, each having a different effect on the scapula. The upper division inserts into the spine of the scapula laterally, as well as the acromion and distal clavicle. It works synergistically with the levator scapulae to elevate the scapula cranially and to elevate its lateral angle. This action results in the shoulder shrug. The middle portion of the trapezius inserts medially on the scapular spine and helps to stabilize it and to initiate upward rotation of the scapula to face the glenoid cavity supe-

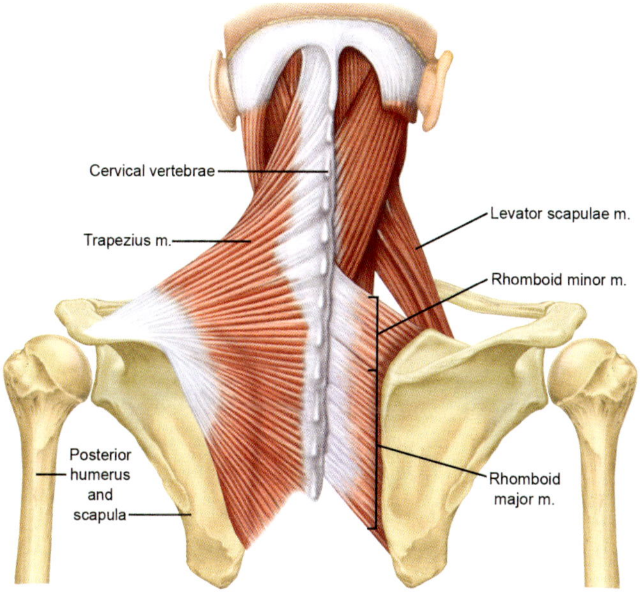

Figure 24. Scapulothoracic muscles that can be viewed from the posterior aspect.

riorly. In addition, the middle trapezius and rhomboids major and minor work to retract the scapula. The inferior division of the trapezius inserts more medially than the middle division and provides inferior stability to the scapula. It also plays a role in rotating the scapula superiorly and in maintaining the spine in extension and drawing the acromion posteriorly. It is innervated by the accessory spinal nerve (cranial nerve XI), which runs in the medial 50% of the muscle.[35]

The rhomboids major and minor along with the levator scapulae rotate the scapula inferiorly, which effectively elevates its medial border. This action places the glenoid cavity in a downward-facing position. Protraction of the scapula is accomplished by the serratus anterior and pectoralis minor with some contribution from the pectoralis major.

Levator Scapulae

The levator scapulae muscle originates on the transverse processes of the C1 to C3 vertebrae and inserts on the superior angle of the scapula just above the insertion of the rhomboid minor. When it contracts, it elevates the superior angle and, in conjunction with the serratus anterior, upwardly rotates the scapula. As the rhomboids, the levator scapulae is innervated by the dorsal scapular nerve and receives its blood supply from the dorsal scapular artery.

Serratus Anterior

The serratus anterior originates from the anterior surface of the ribs and inserts on the anterior surface of the medial border of the scapula (Figure 25). It functions to protract the scapula and, along with the levator scapulae, produces upward rotation. The long thoracic nerve supplies innervation.

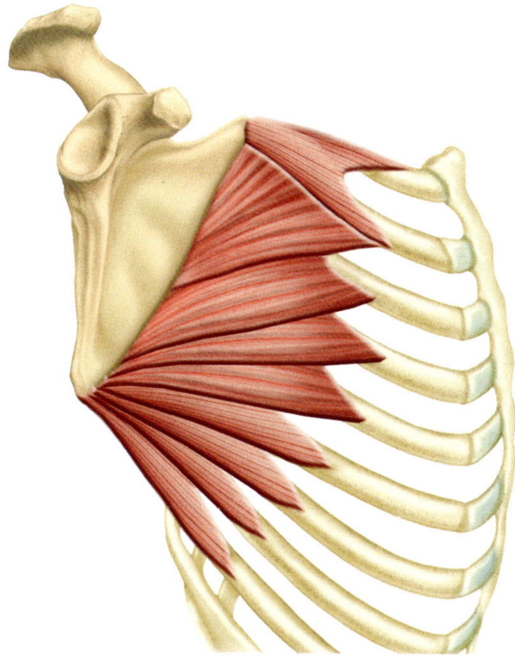

Figure 25. Serratus anterior muscle.

BURSAE

Bursae are small, synovial, fluid-filled sacs that often are found in joints. They lie between bones, ligaments, muscles, and tendons at points of friction, providing a smooth surface over which they can glide. Bursae can become infected, which is a condition called bursitis.

Synovial bursal membranes are found interposed between anatomic layers that move upon one another throughout the human body. Within the complex arrangement of the muscles of the shoulder girdle, these bursae create an efficient gliding mechanism. The superficial sleeve of musculature around the shoulder comprising the deltoid and teres major can move freely over the deeper rotators of the glenohumeral joint because of these biologic cushions.

The subacromial bursa adheres at its base to the greater tuberosity and rotator cuff, whereas the roof of the bursa is attached to the acromion on its under-

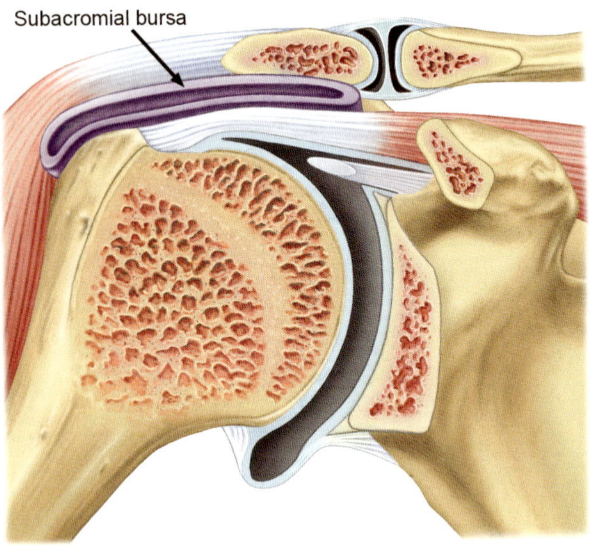

Figure 26. Subacromial bursa.

surface (Figure 26).[36] Under normal circumstances, it does not communicate with the glenohumeral joint unless a defect exists in the musculotendinous cuff. Often considered an extension of the subacromial bursa, the subcoracoid bursa and subscapularis bursa work together to offset friction that the superior fibers of the subscapularis generate against the scapular neck, humeral head, and coracoid process.

NERVES

Nerves are bundles of axons of neurons that conduct electrochemical signals between the central nervous system and the organs of the body. Injury to nerves can cause a loss of motion if muscle denervation results. The branches of the brachial plexus innervate the shoulder.

Neural Structures Around the Shoulder

According to Hilton's Law, a nerve that supplies a joint, including the skin overlying that joint, tends to supply the muscles that move the joint. This seems to hold true for the shoulder girdle. The primary movers of the glenohumeral joint are the axillary, musculocutaneous, suprascapular, and subscapular nerves. All provide contributions to the ligaments, capsule, and synovium of the shoulder joint. In addition, the supraclavicular nerves from the C3 and C4 nerve roots supply the skin above the clavicle and over the acromion and portions of the deltoid. The posterior shoulder girdle has cutaneous innervation supplied by the dorsal rami of the spinal nerves in that region following a dermatome distribution.

Brachial Plexus

Innervation of the shoulder primarily is provided by the brachial plexus, which is a network of nerve fibers running from the spinal cord through the neck and axilla to the upper extremity. It is organized into roots, trunks, divisions, cords, and branches (Figure 27).

The 5 roots of spinal nerves C5 to T1 merge to form 3 trunks. The upper trunk is formed by the C5 and C6 roots; the middle trunk, by the C7 root; and the lower trunk, by the C8 and T1 roots. Each of these trunks is split into anterior and posterior divisions. As the brachial plexus passes below the clavicle into the axilla, these divisions merge to form cords, which are named relative to their positions to the axillary artery. The posterior cord consists of the posterior divisions of all 3 trunks. The medial cord contains only the anterior division of the lower trunk. The remaining anterior divisions form the lateral cord. The branches of the brachial plexus split off of these cords.

Axillary Nerve. The axillary nerve branches off of the posterior cord of the brachial plexus, traveling into the quadrilateral space (Figure 28), which is formed medially by the long head of the triceps, laterally by the shaft of the humerus, superiorly by the teres minor, and inferiorly by the teres major. From the quadrilater-

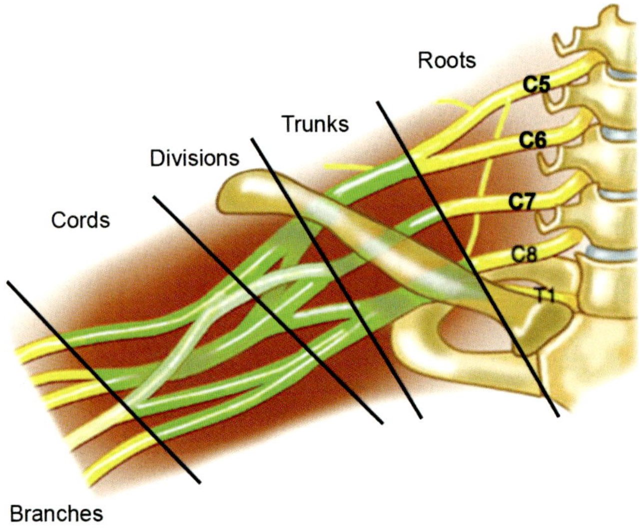

Figure 27. Brachial plexus organization.

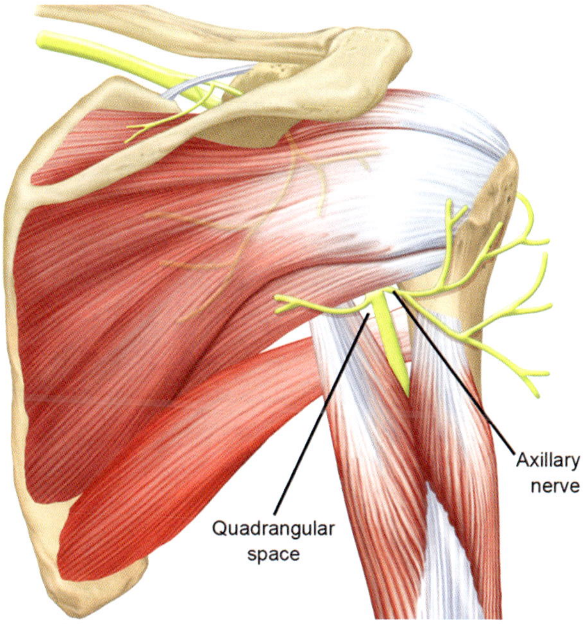

Figure 28. Axillary nerve in the quadrangular space.

al space, its anterior branch innervates the deltoid, and its posterior branch terminates at the teres minor.

Musculocutaneous Nerve. The musculocutaneous nerve branches high off of the lateral cord of the brachial plexus, traveling through the upper extremity. It passes through the coracobrachialis muscle and between the biceps brachii and brachialis, innervating them. The musculocutaneous nerve terminates distally in the forearm as the lateral antebrachial cutaneous nerve.

Suprascapular Nerve. The suprascapular nerve branches off of the upper trunk of the brachial plexus. It transverses the suprascapular notch, traveling under the superior transverse scapular ligament, and innervates the supraspinatus. It then courses through the spinoglenoid notch to the infraspinous fossa where it innervates the infraspinatus. Compression of the suprascapular nerve at the suprascapular notch causes denervation of both muscles, whereas compression at the spinoglenoid notch causes denervation of only the infraspinatus.

Long Thoracic Nerve. The long thoracic nerve branches off of the brachial plexus before it reaches the clavicle. It courses downward and innervates the serratus anterior muscle. Injury to this nerve causes medial scapular winging.

Spinal Accessory Nerve. The spinal accessory nerve is the 11th cranial nerve, originating in the brain. It travels posteriorly to innervate the sternocleidomastoid and trapezius. Injury to the nerve leads to lateral scapular winging.

VASCULAR ANATOMY

Arteries course through the body to bring oxygenated blood and nutrients to tissues, allowing them to perform necessary metabolic processes. Cells require oxygen to perform cellular respiration, converting sugar into energy. This is especially important in muscles, which require large amounts of energy for muscle contraction. The axillary artery and its branches supply the tissues of the shoulder, most importantly its muscles (Figure 29).

Perfusion of the upper extremity begins with the subclavian artery. It arises from the innominate, or brachiocephalic, artery on the right side of the body and from the arch of the aorta on the left side. From here, the rich vascular tree around the shoulder girdle branches from this artery. It emerges above the first rib and is divided into 3 parts based on its relationship to the anterior scalene muscle, where it passes between it and the middle scalene. The vertebral and internal mammary arteries come off the subclavian and the thyrocervical and costocervical trunks. The dorsal scapular artery to the rhomboids can branch directly from the subclavian or, at times, arises from the thyrocervical trunk. From this axis also arises the

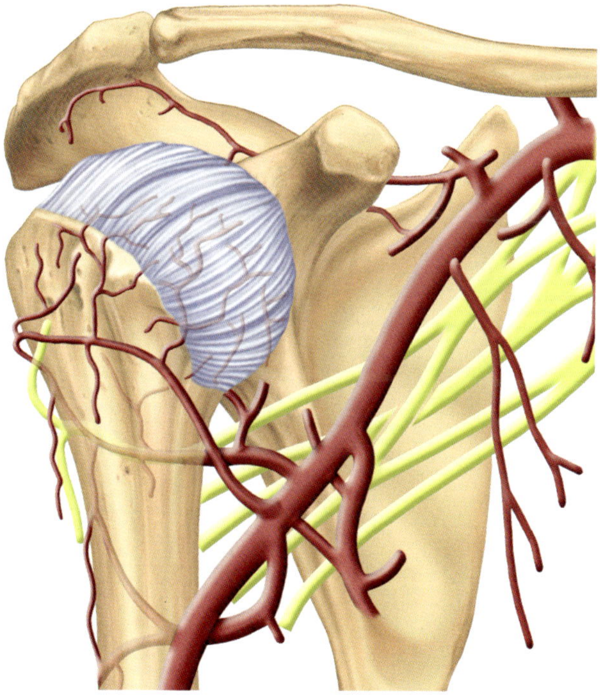
Figure 29. Neurovascular structures.

suprascapular artery as it passes obliquely in front of the anterior scalene toward the scapula. The artery travels above the transverse scapular ligament superior to the suprascapular notch, and the suprascapular nerve lies below it. As the artery passes into the supraspinatus and infraspinatus fossae, it becomes the principle blood supply to those muscles.

Between the first rib and the inferior border of the teres major muscle, the subclavian becomes the axillary artery. Three portions traditionally are designated to the axillary artery based on its relationship with the pectoralis minor muscle (Figure 30). The first portion is above the pectoralis minor, the second is behind it, and the third is below the muscle. Here, the axillary artery travels alongside the brachial plexus with its cords intimately involved with the second and third portions of the artery.

The first portion of the axillary artery gives off only 1 branch: the superior thoracic artery. It passes between the pectoralis minor and major muscles, providing small contributions to each and ultimately anastomosing with the internal mammary and intercostal arteries. The thoracoacromial artery branches from the start of the second portion, providing several branches to structures around the shoulder girdle. From this arterial axis, the acromial, deltoid, pectoral, and clavicular arteries arise. The second branch from this portion of the axillary artery is the lateral thoracic artery. This branch shows considerable variability in its origin, at times arising from thoracoacromial artery. It passes along the inferior border of the pectoralis minor and primarily supplies this muscle and the pectoralis major and serratus anterior muscles.

The third portion of the axillary gives off the subscapular artery, its largest branch, and the humeral circumflex arteries

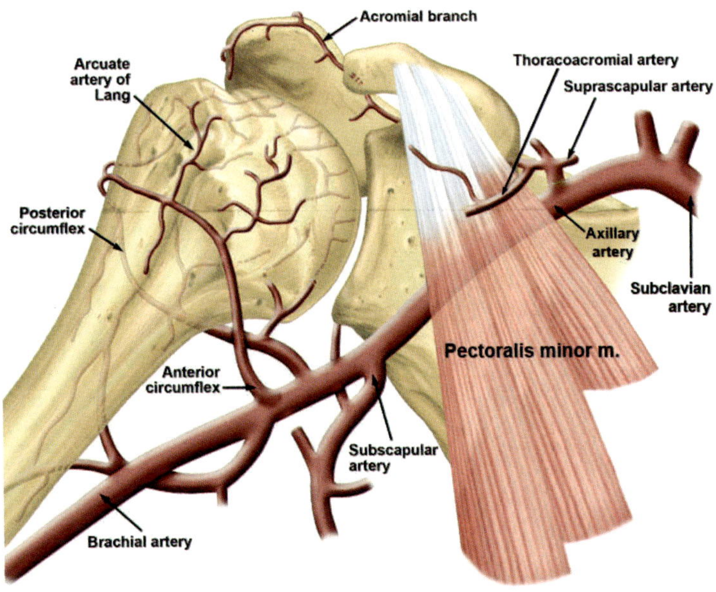

Figure 30. Branches of the axillary artery and its relationship to the pectoralis minor muscle insertion.

anteriorly and posteriorly. From its origin the subscapular artery passes posteriorly and almost immediately gives off the circumflex scapular artery, winding around the lateral border of the scapula to enter the infraspinatus fossa. The final 2 branches of the axillary artery are the anterior and posterior humeral circumflex arteries. The posterior humeral circumflex wraps around the humeral neck posteriorly and enters the quadrangular space traveling with the axillary nerve. The anterior humeral circumflex is the smaller of the 2 branches and provides the principle blood supply to the humeral head. The ascending branch of the artery enters the bone in the area of the intertubercular groove as the arcuate artery. Before penetrating the humeral head, it supplies portions of the greater and lesser tuberosities. In addition, the arterial branches of the axillary provide blood supply to the capsule of the glenohumeral joint and top of the labrum and supporting ligaments.[5] The axillary then becomes the brachial artery as it travels beyond the lower border of the teres major muscle and into the upper extremity.

REFERENCES

1. Liberson F. Os acromiale: a contested anomaly. *J Bone Joint Surg*. 1937;19(3):683–689.
2. Bigliani LU, Norris TR, Fischer J, Neer CS. The relationship between the unfused acromial epiphysis and subacromial impingement lesions. *Orthop Trans*. 1983;7:138.
3. Bigliani LU, Morrison DS, April EW. The morphology of the acromion and its relationship to rotator cuff tears. *Orthop Trans.* 1986;10:288.
4. Morrison DS, Bigliani LU. The clinical significance of variations in acromial morphology. *Orthop Trans*. 1987;11:234.
5. Rockwood CA Jr, Matsen FA III, Wirth MA, Lippitt SB, eds. *The Shoulder*. 4th ed. Philadelphia, PA: Saunders Elsevier; 2009.
6. Churchhill RS, Brems JJ, Kotschi H. Glenoid size, inclination, and version: an anatomic study. *J Shoulder Elbow Surg*. 2001;10(4):327–332.
7. De Wilde LF, Berghs BM, VandeVyver F, Schepens A, Verdonk RC. Glenohumeral relationship in the transverse plane of the body. *J Shoulder Elbow Surg*. 2003;12(3):260–267.

8. Iannotti JP, Gabriel JP, Schneck SL, Evans BG, Misra S. The normal glenohumeral relationships: an anatomical study of one hundred and forty shoulders. *J Bone Joint Surg Am.* 1992;74(4):491–500.
9. Kronberg M, Broström LA, Söderlund V. Retroversion of the humeral head in the normal shoulder and its relationship to the normal range of motion. *Clin Orthop Relat Res.* 1990;253:113–117.
10. Inman VT, Saunders JBDM, Abbott LC. Observations on the function of the shoulder joint. *J Bone Joint Surg.* 1944;26(1):1–20.
11. Harryman DT II, Walker ED, Harris SL, Sidles JA, Jackins SE, Matsen FA III. Residual motion and function after glenohumeral or scapulothoracic arthrodesis. *J Shoulder Elbow Surg.* 1993;2(6):275–285.
12. Freedman L, Munro RR. Abduction of the arm in the arm in the scapular plane: scapular and glenohumeral movements. A roentgenographic study. *J Bone Joint Surg Am.* 1966;48(8):1503–1510.
13. Kibler WB, McMullen J. Scapular dyskinesis and its relation to shoulder pain. *J Am Acad Orthop Surg.* 2003;11(2):142–151.
14. Steinbeck J, Liljenqvist U, Jerosch J. The anatomy of the glenohumeral ligamentous complex and its contribution to anterior shoulder stability. *J Shoulder Elbow Surg.* 1998;7(2):122–126.
15. DePalma AF, Callery G, Bennett GA. Shoulder joint: variational anatomy and degenerative lesions of the shoulder joint. *Instr Course Lect.* 1949;6:255–281.
16. O'Brien SJ, Warren RF, Schwartz E. Anterior shoulder instability. *Orthop Clin North Am.* 1987;18(3):395–408.
17. Williams MM, Snyder SJ, Buford D Jr. The Buford complex: the "cord-like" middle glenohumeral ligament and absent anterosuperior labrum complex. A normal anatomic capsulolabral variant. *Arthroscopy.* 1994;10(3):241–247.
18. Burkart AC, Debski RE. Anatomy and function of the glenohumeral ligaments in anterior shoulder instability. *Clin Orthop Relat Res.* 2002;400:32–39.
19. Urayama M, Itoi E, Hatakeyama Y, Pradhan RL, Sato K. Function of the 3 portions of the inferior glenohumeral ligament: a cadaveric study. *J Shoulder Elbow Surg.* 2001;10(6):589–594.
20. Harryman DT II, Sidles JA, Harris SL, Matsen FA III. The role of the rotator interval capsule in passive motion and stability of the shoulder. *J Bone Joint Surg Am.* 1992;74(1):53–66.
21. DePalma AF. Surgical anatomy of the acromioclavicular and sternoclavicluar joints. *Surg Clin North Am.* 1963;43:1541–1550.
22. Fukuda K, Craig EV, An KN, Cofield RH, Chao EY. Biomechanical study of the ligamentous system of the acromioclavicular joint. *J Bone Joint Surg Am.* 1986;68(3):434–440.
23. Cetik O, Uslu M, Acar HI, Comert A, Tekdemir I, Cift H. Is there a safe area for the axillary nerve in the deltoid muscle? A cadaveric study. *J Bone Joint Surg Am.* 2006;88(11):2395–2399.
24. Beals TC, Harryman DT II, Lazarus MD. Useful boundaries of the subacromial bursa. *Arthroscopy.* 1998;14(5):465–470.
25. Colachis SC Jr, Strohm BR. Effect of suprascapular and axillary nerve blocks on muscle force in upper extremity. *Arch Phys Med Rehabil.* 1971;52(1):22–29.
26. Perry J. Biomechanics of the shoulder. In: Rowe CR, ed. *The Shoulder.* New York, NY: Churchill Livingstone; 1988:1–15.
27. Howell SM, Imobersteg AM, Seger DH, Marone PJ. Clarification of the role of the supraspinatus muscle in shoulder function. *J Bone Joint Surg Am.* 1986;68(3):398–404.
28. Rengachary SS, Burr D, Lucas S, Hassanein KM, Mohn MP, Matzke H. Suprascapular entrapment neuropathy: a clinical, anatomical, and comparative study: part 2. Anatomical study. *Neurosurgery.* 1979;5(4):447–451.
29. Hinton MA, Parker AW, Drez D Jr, Altchek D. An anatomic study of the subscapularis tendon and myotendinous junction. *J Shoulder Elbow Surg.* 1994;3(4):224–229.
30. Symeonides PPL. The significance of the subscapularis muscle in the pathogenesis of recurrent anterior dislocation of the shoulder. *J Bone Joint Surg Br.* 1972;54(3):476–483.
31. Levy AS, Kelly BT, Lintner SA, Osbahr DC, Speer KP. Function of the long head of the biceps at the shoulder: electromyographic analysis. *J Shoulder Elbow Surg.* 2001;10(3):250–255.
32. Jobe FW, Moynes DR, Tibone JE, Perry J. An EMG analysis of the shoulder in pitching: a second report. *Am J Sports Med.* 1984;12(3):218–220.
33. Marmor L, Bechtol CO, Hall CB. Pectoralis major muscle function of sternal portion and mechanism of rupture of normal muscle: case reports. *J Bone Joint Surg Am.* 1961;43(1):81–87.
34. Klepps SJ, Goldfarb C, Flatow E, Galatz LM, Yamaguchi K. Anatomic evaluation of the subcoracoid pectoralis major transfer in human cadavers. *J Shoulder Elbow Surg.* 2001;10(5):453–459.
35. Jobe CM, Kropp WE, Wood VE. Spinal accessory nerve in a trapezius-splitting surgical approach. *J Shoulder Elbow Surg.* 1996;5(3):206–208.
36. Strizak AM, Danzig L, Jackson DW, Resnick D, Staple T. Subacromial bursography: an anatomical and clinical study. *J Bone Joint Surg Am.* 1982;64(2):196–201.

RECOMMENDED READING

Bramhall JP. Functional anatomy of the shoulder. In: Andrews JR, Zarins B, Wilk KE, eds. *Injuries in Baseball.* Philadelphia, PA: Lippincott-Raven; 1998:39–45.

Galatz LM, ed. *Orthopaedic Knowledge Update: Shoulder and Elbow 3.* Rosemont, IL: American Academy of Orthopaedic Surgeons; 2008.

Gray H. *Anatomy of the Human Body.* 29th American ed. Goss CM, ed. Philadelphia, PA: Lea & Febiger; 1973.

Hatch GF III, Costouros JC, Millet PJ, Warner JJP. Shoulder labral tears and instability. In: Johnson DH, Pedowitz RA, eds. *Practical Orthopaedic Sports Medicine & Arthroscopy.* Philadelphia, PA: Lippincott Williams & Wilkins; 2007:171–199.

Iannotti JP, Williams G Jr, eds. *Disorders of the Shoulder: Diagnosis & Management.* 2nd ed. Philadelphia, PA: Lippincott Williams & Wilkins; 2007.

Lieberman JR, ed. *AAOS Comprehensive Orthopaedic Review*. Rosemont, IL: American Academy of Orthopaedic Surgeons; 2009.

Mudge MK, Wood VE, Frykman GK. Rotator cuff tears associated with os acromiale. *J Bone Joint Surg Am*. 1984;66(3):427–429.

I-2

Clinical Examination of the Shoulder

Todd J. Twiss, MD; John A. Hinson, MD; and George M. McCluskey III, MD

A complete clinical examination of the shoulder includes a thorough history, physical examination, and appropriate imaging studies. The examination begins with a proper clinical history, which will guide all further investigation. Gathering a complete, directed, and proper history is an art that requires experience and patience. In a short period, the clinician must ask appropriate questions and actively listen to the patient's responses to guide further investigation. Each patient will tell you exactly what is wrong if correctly prompted and you are listening. Historical data, such as age, chief concern, sex, specifics of pain, instability, neurovascular symptoms, and associated medical conditions, will provide an initial differential diagnosis, then a directed physical examination can confirm clinical suspicion.

Too often in a busy clinical environment, relying on technology to establish a diagnosis seems easier, but as clinicians, we must not forget that we are evaluating the patient and not the imaging studies or other diagnostic tests. Each detail provided in the clinical examination must be placed in the proper context to arrive at the correct diagnosis. The patient's history along with a thorough examination and appropriate imaging studies must support a specific pathologic process. That is, the examiner is gathering details for the patient's clinical story. When each element of that story supports a specific diagnosis, the probability that we are prescribing the right intervention increases exponentially.

As with examination of other parts of the body, a complete shoulder examination has several basic tenets that, when followed, will increase the clinician's diagnostic acumen. Shoulder conditions can be caused by problems intrinsic and extrinsic to the shoulder. For problems intrinsic to the shoulder, 5 basic principles for musculoskeletal evaluations apply, including inspection, palpation, range of motion, strength, and special tests. Along with a dedicated shoulder examination, a complete general evaluation of the patient and cervical spine, neurologic, and vascular examinations can eliminate extrinsic causes of shoulder conditions.

GENERAL EXAMINATION

A directed shoulder examination usually does not include thorough examination of all body systems, but a focused global examination can highlight systemic disease, which can cause shoulder problems. Details gathered from a patient's history focus the global examination. Visceral concerns, trauma, systemic disease, effects of medication, and neurologic disease can cause shoulder pain or weakness.

Cardiac, pulmonary, liver, kidney, and visceral problems can result in referred shoulder pain. Pleurisy, a pneumothorax, or a Pancoast tumor can cause referred pain in the ipsilateral shoulder and upper trapezius. Myocardial ischemia is notorious for leading to left pectoral, shoulder, and upper extremity pain. Liver abscess, peptic ulcer, kidney, and splenic ruptures have been known to refer pain to the shoulder. Any details in the history of atypical shoulder pain and visceral concerns can guide the examiner to look at the cardiac, respiratory, or abdominal systems.

Any patient with shoulder concerns after a major trauma requires a complete evaluation in line with the advanced trauma life support protocol. They should have a complete airway, breathing, circulatory, and neurovascular examination. In addition, the clinician should palpate all musculoskeletal prominences in the upper and lower extremities and should thoroughly examine the skin for ecchymosis to guide further treatment.

Reports of pain and weakness in the shoulder can be caused by problems intrinsic to the shoulder, spine conditions, systemic disease, congenital abnormalities, or side effects of medication. Cervical spine conditions cause referred pain to the shoulder and upper extremity and will be described in detail in another section. Systemic demylenating disorders, such as amyotrophic lateral sclerosis, can result in shoulder weakness. Patients with shoulder pain and weakness along with multiple systemic concerns must be evaluated for polymyositis, fibromyalgia, collagen vascular disease, Lyme disease, rheumatoid arthritis, and other rheumatologic disorders. History of oral steroid use for conditions, such as ulcerative colitis, Crohn disease, psoriasis, and rheumatoid disorders, can result in avascular necrosis in the shoulder and other locations. Finally, the examiner should expose the patient to evaluate the skin and generalized musculoskeletal symmetry. Skin lesions consistent with psoriasis can be related to shoulder pain due to psoriatic arthritis. Medication, such as warfarin, clopidogrel, aspirin, and other blood-thinning agents, can cause multiple superficial ecchymosis and affect further surgical or invasive medical treatment. Finally, congenital abnormalities, such as absence of the pectoralis, Sprengel deformity, and Turner syndrome, can be identified easily with appropriate exposure.

Because of the close relationship between the shoulder and neck, every complete shoulder examination should include a complete neck examination. Shoulder problems can cause neck pain and neck problems, which cause shoulder and upper extremity pain. The neck should be inspected from both anterior and posterior aspects. Evidence of neck and shoulder girdle asymmetry, muscle mass, scars, and deformity provide clues about substantial cervical spine conditions. Range of motion, including flexion, extension, rotation, and bending, is assessed. Exact measurements of motion are difficult to assess, but difficulty with active motion and lack of motion in particular planes highlight neck conditions.

The Spurling test is used to assess the patient for discogenic disorders. Standing behind the patient, the examiner places the cervical spine in extension and rotation toward the affected side (Figure 1). Reproduction of shoulder and upper extremity concerns with an axial load on the spine is considered a positive response.

NEUROLOGIC AND VASCULAR EXAMINATION

A complete neurologic examination is not required with every shoulder examination, but a focused upper extremity neurologic and vascular examination should be performed for each patient. A focused examination of upper extremity strength, sensation, and reflexes is required with a complete shoulder examination. By assessing deltoid, biceps, triceps, wrist extension, and intrinsic hand function, the examiner tests all cervical nerve roots to the upper extremity. Reflex testing should be performed bilaterally to compare for hyperflexia or hyporeflexia, which signify an upper or lower motor neuron lesion. The biceps reflex is used to test the C5 nerve root; brachioradialis, C6; and triceps, C7. In addition, sensory testing can highlight focal nerve deficits, systemic problems, or regional nerve deficits. Light touch sensation with differentiation between sharp and dull sensations can be used to test typical dermatomal patterns.

Vascular problems of the upper extremity can be manifested as changes in sensation, skin, temperature, or hair loss. Palpating pulses or listening for bruits can reveal major vascular compromise. Thoracic outlet syndrome involves compression of the neurovascular bundle as it exits from the superior thoracic outlet between the anterior and middle scalene muscles. Compression of the subclavian vessels or the brachial plexus can cause referred shoulder pain and peripheral symptoms that are positional. Maneuvers to elicit thoracic outlet syndrome include the Adson maneuver and Wright test along with several others. Each maneuver must be interpreted with caution because the patient

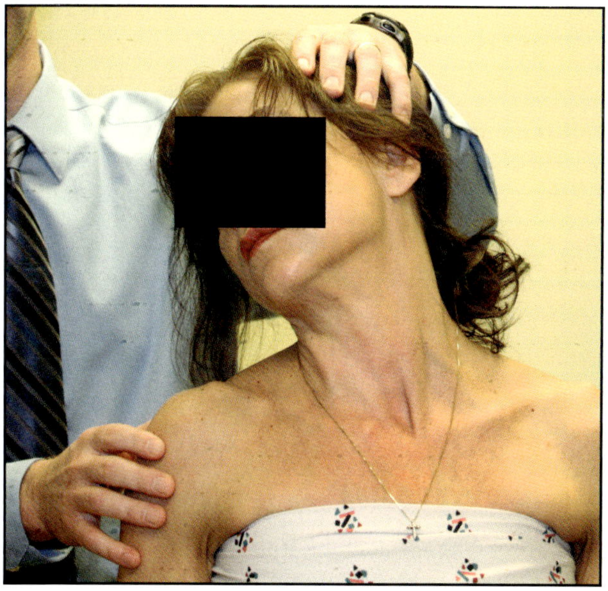

Figure 1. Spurling test.

must state without prompting that the test reproduces the symptoms. The Adson maneuver is performed with the examiner behind the patient. The shoulder is extended, and the neck is turned to the affected side. (Figure 2) A positive test reproduces symptoms and obliterates the radial pulse. To perform the Wright test, the examiner brings the upper extremity into abduction and external rotation and instructs the patient to hold his or her breath (Figure 3). A positive test reproduces symptoms and reduces the radial pulse. With each provocative examination, the clinician attempts to replicate the neurovascular compression at the superior thoracic outlet.

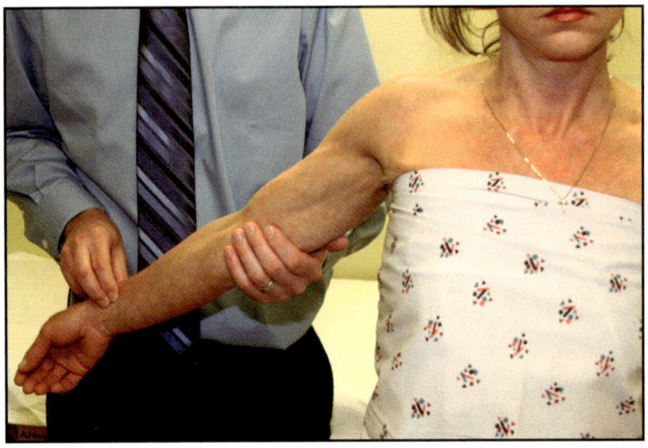

Figure 2. Adson maneuver.

SHOULDER EXAMINATION

Inspection

As in other areas of the body, the physical examination of the shoulder begins with a thorough and systematic inspection. Although often difficult to do in a busy practice, the patient should be observed while walking into the examining room. Posture, body habitus, and attitude of the shoulder should be assessed. Any obvious asymmetry should be noted. The inability to reach out normally to shake hands at the initial greeting can indicate the severity of the shoulder concern.

After taking a thorough history, the examiner instructs female patients to change into a gown and male patients to disrobe from the waist up (Figure 4). All aspects of the shoulder girdle and upper extremity to be examined should be visible and unclothed. The skin is

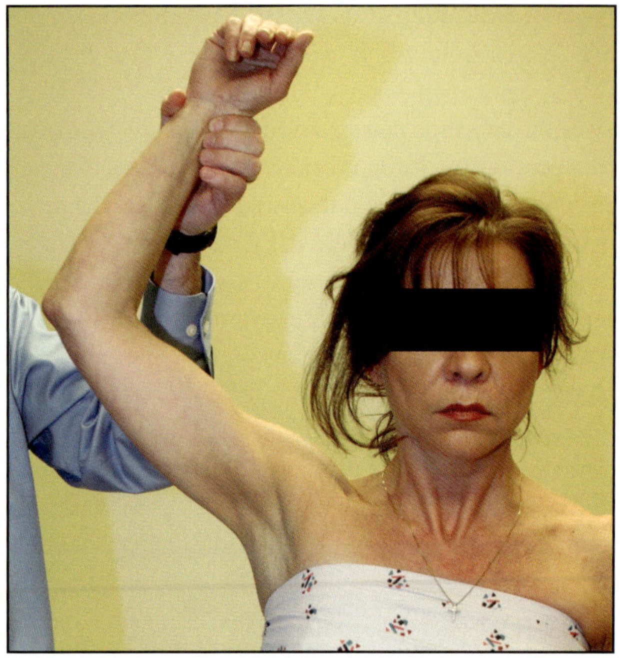

Figure 3. Wright test.

inspected first. The examiner should look for swelling, redness, or other signs of infection. Both traumatic and surgical scars should be documented. The examiner also should note bruising from previous trauma and should note masses or other skin conditions that might

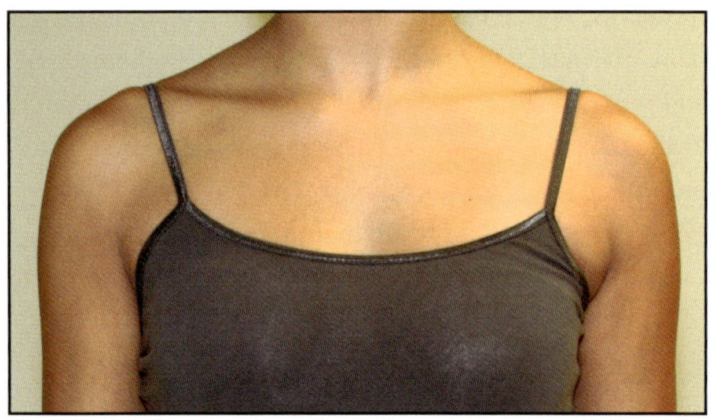

Figure 4A. The female patient should be adequately exposed while maintaining her modesty.

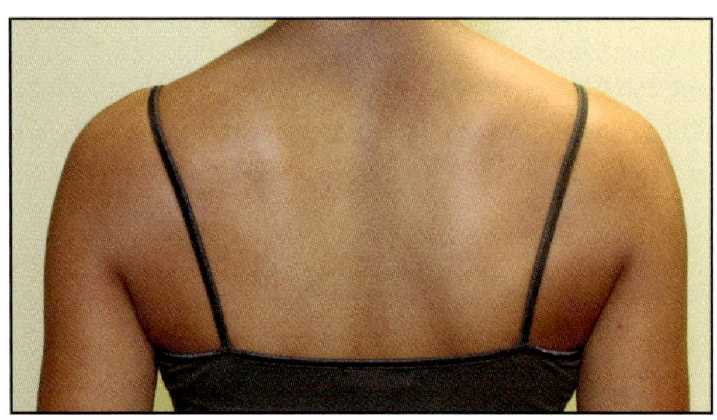

Figure 4B. Both shoulders are exposed to allow comparison for any asymmetry.

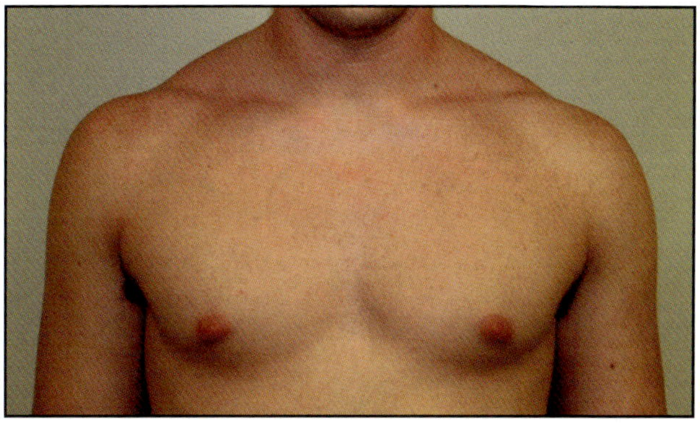

Figure 4C. Inspecting the anterior aspect of the shoulder.

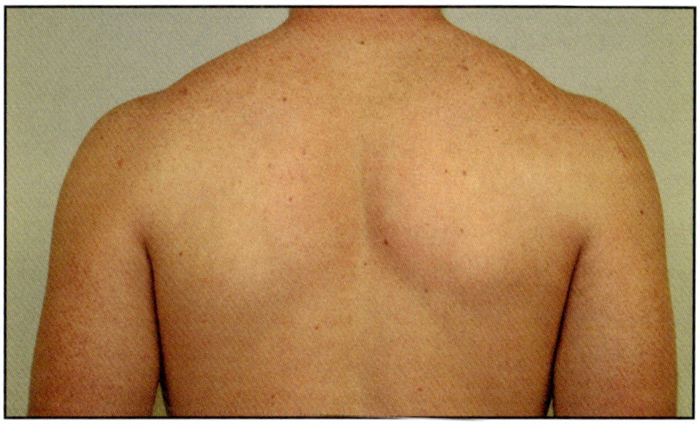

Figure 4D. Inspecting the posterior aspect of the shoulder.

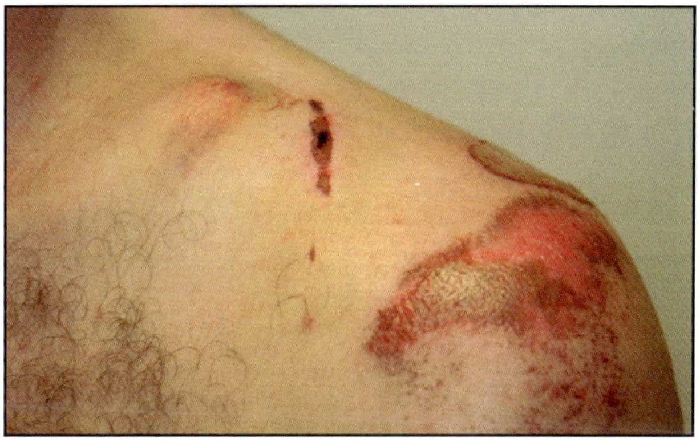

Figure 5. The patient has multiple abrasions and lacerations and a clavicle fracture sustained in a motorcycle accident. Treatment of the fracture was delayed until the skin healed.

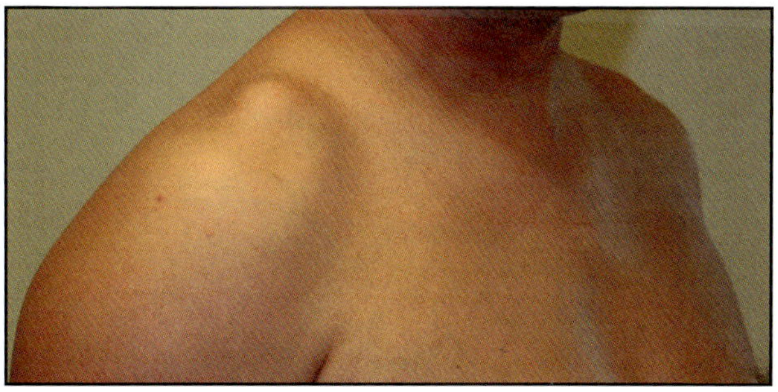

Figure 6. This patient with a grade V acromioclavicular joint separation shows an obvious deformity with elevation of the distal clavicle relative to the acromion.

affect treatment options or the underlying shoulder concern (Figure 5). Deformity at either the acromioclavicular (AC) or sternoclavicular (SC) joint also should be identified (Figure 6).

Close scrutiny should be given to the overall contour of the upper extremity to be examined. The deltoid, pectoralis, and trapezius muscles compose the visible framework of the anterior shoulder girdle, whereas the latissimus dorsi, periscapular, and rotator cuff muscles compose the posterior shoulder girdle. Muscle atrophy around the shoulder girdle that is visible to the examiner is an important finding because it can indicate a chronic condition or could represent a more serious neurologic deficit (Figure 7). While examining the patient from behind, the clinician should note any scapular winging because it can indicate a neurologic lesion or could be a compensatory mechanism for dysfunction elsewhere within the shoulder girdle musculature. The upper arm contour should be inspected for evidence of biceps rupture (Figure 8). The presence of a spinal deformity, such as scoliosis or kyphosis, affects shoulder function because it can change the position of the scapula relative to the humerus, and it should be documented.

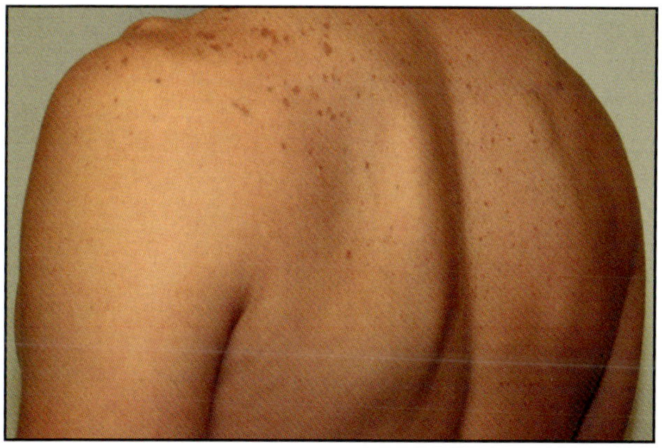

Figure 7. Infraspinatus atrophy.

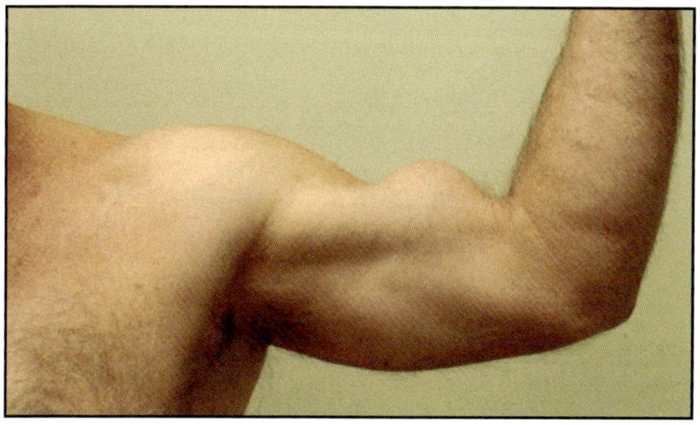

Figure 8. Popeye deformity.

Palpation

The examination of the shoulder should proceed in a stepwise fashion. After a thorough inspection of the patient and the extremity of interest, the examiner should palpate the relevant bony prominences and soft tissue zones to gather additional information that will lead to a clinical diagnosis. To efficiently accomplish this, the examiner stands behind the patient. The most medial structures are assessed first. The suprasternal notch and SC joint are palpated (Figure 9). Moving laterally along the shaft of the clavicle, the examiner encounters the AC articulation. Tenderness or a prominence here could represent either an AC separation or perhaps joint arthrosis (Figure 10). Just distal and medial to this area, the coracoid process can be felt as it projects from the anterior scapula deep to the pectoralis musculature (Figure 11). Moving laterally from this point leads the examiner to the bicipital groove, which is bounded medially by the lesser tuberosity and laterally by the greater tuberosity (Figure 12). Tenderness here could indicate disorders in the long head of the biceps as it travels away from its intra-articular origin at the supraglenoid tubercle. In this same area, palpation along the anterolateral aspect of the proximal humerus occasionally can enable the examiner to detect a defect in the supraspinatus tendon that is indicative of a massive rotator cuff tear.[1] Just superior to this point is the summit of the shoulder: the acromion (Figure 13). Its contour should be assessed beginning anteriorly, continuing to the posterior aspect of the acromion and along the spine of the scapula, and concluding with palpation of the medial and lateral borders of the scapula (Figure 14). The supraspinatus and infraspinatus

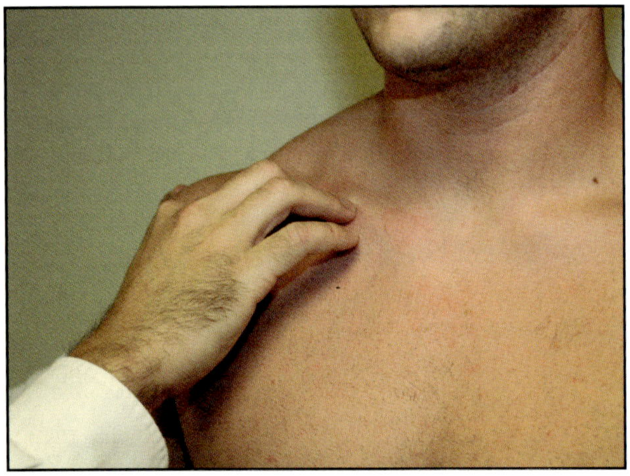

Figure 9. Palpation of the sternoclavicular joint.

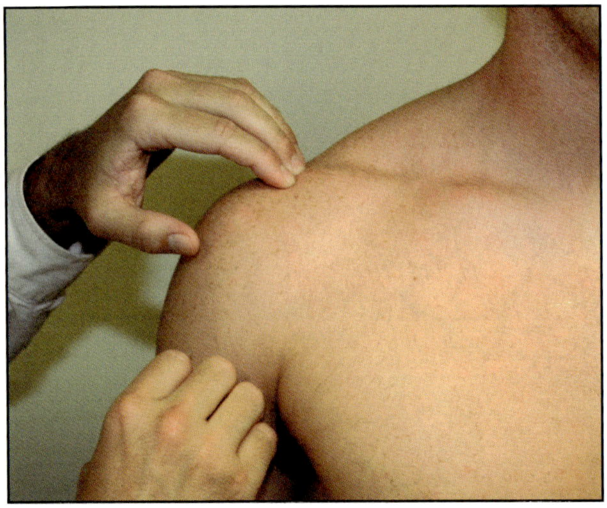

Figure 10. Palpation of the acromioclavicular joint.

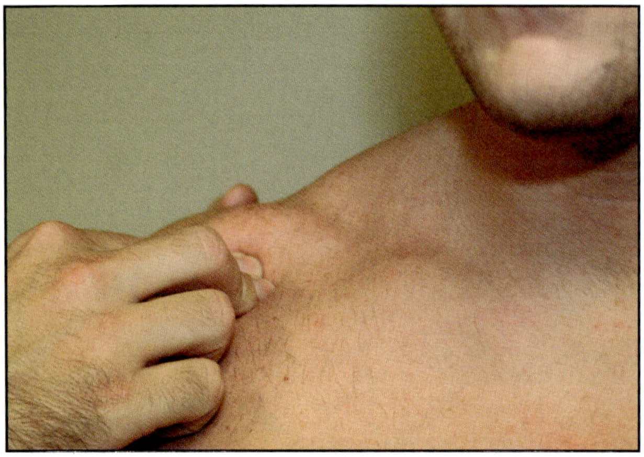

Figure 11. Palpation of the coracoid process.

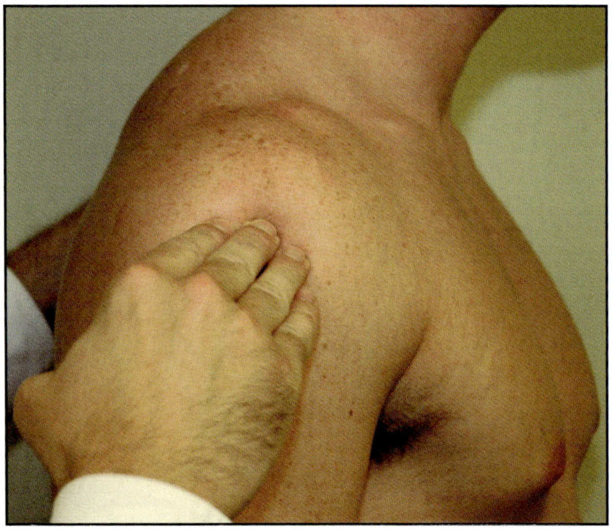

Figure 12. Palpation along the anterolateral aspect of proximal humerus at the bicipital groove.

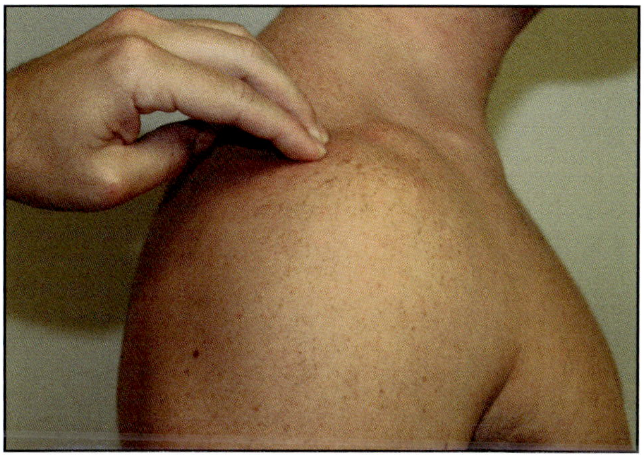

Figure 13. Palpation of the acromion.

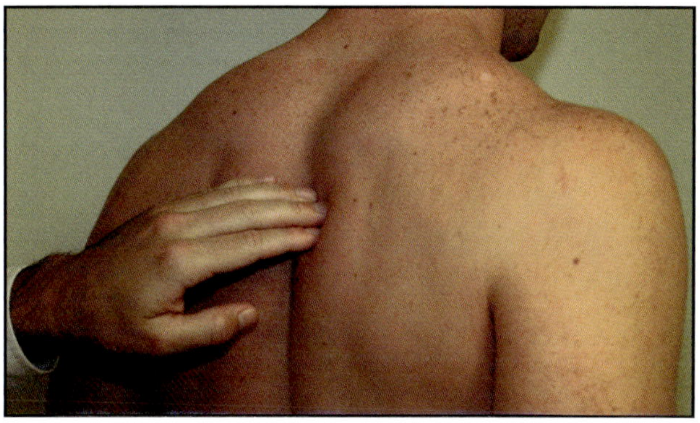

Figure 14. Palpation of the medial border of the scapula.

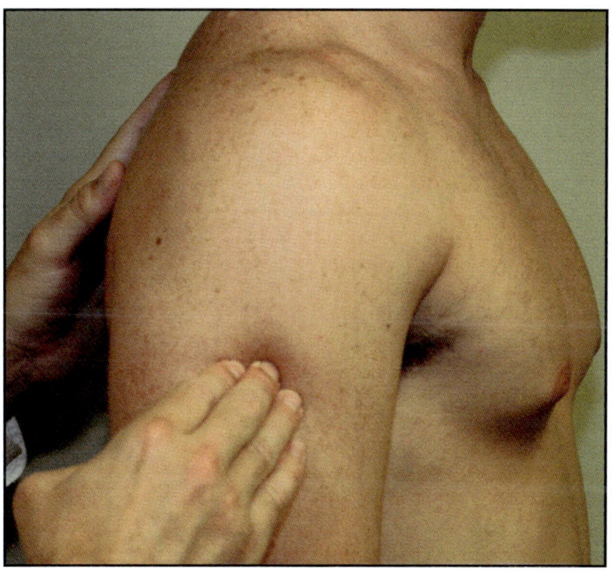

Figure 15. Palpation of the deltoid insertion.

muscle bellies lie within their respective fossae, which are superior and inferior to the spine of the scapula. A hollow depression indicates that these muscles have atrophied from disuse, chronic rotator cuff conditions, or neurologic injury. A thorough examination also should include the deltoid insertion at the lateral aspect of the upper extremity (Figure 15) and a thorough assessment of the trapezius and paracervical musculature.

While palpating the shoulder girdle, the clinician can elicit diagnostic clues by passively moving the patient's upper extremity and instructing him or her to place the affected extremity in certain positions. In this way, crepitus can be felt in the subacromial space or glenohumeral joint and in the AC and SC joints. Abducting the patient's upper extremity facilitates examination of the axilla. The palpable lymph nodes can point to possible infection in or around the shoulder joint. Manipulating the patient's cervical spine causes the sternocleidomastoid muscle to become more prominent; this is another important location where swollen lymph nodes can be detected. Having the patient actively flex them against resistance enhances inspection and palpation of the large muscles around the shoulder girdle. This measure can aid in detecting rupture of the long head of the biceps or singling out disorders in 1 of the 3 segments of the deltoid. The scapular stabilizers, such as the rhomboids major and minor, also can be examined more easily by having the patient, with the shoulder in internal rotation, push posteriorly against resistance.

Range of Motion

Passive and active methods for testing shoulder range of motion should be used in the clinical setting. Limitation to motion in any plane is an important finding and requires accurate documentation. The techniques used to obtain these measurements involve the use of handheld devices, such as a goniometer or inclinometer, or visual estimation. The latter method is probably the most widely used because it is easy, quick, and cost effective. Factors that influence shoulder range of motion, such as sex, age, upper extremity dominance, and pathologic process, should be considered when assessing a patient. Shoulder motion decreases with age, and McFarland[2] reported that women have an overall greater range of motion (approximately 8%) in abduction than men. In addition, measurements can be taken with the patient standing, sitting, or lying supine. Motion also can be affected by the position of the extremity relative to the torso. For example, external and internal rotation can be assessed with the upper extremity at the side or abducted from the body 90°. The most useful tool to eliminate all of these variables is to compare the affected extremity with the contralateral side. Asymmetry noted by inspection, by palpation, or when testing for shoulder range of motion should raise a red flag to the examiner.

The basic measurements that should be documented when evaluating shoulder range of motion are elevation within the plane of the scapula, internal rotation and external rotation, and less commonly shoulder extension.

Elevation. Elevation of the upper extremity is accomplished as a coordinated function of the glenohumeral and scapulothoracic articulations. This motion occurs in a 2:1 ratio with 1° of motion at the scapula for every 2° at the glenohumeral joint. The scapula rests on the thoracic cavity along the rib cage and is posteriorly angled approximately 30° anterior relative to the coronal plane. Elevation within this direction of the scapula is called *scaption*. Traditionally, researchers have reported that the shoulder elevates through an arc of 180°; however, researchers using computed tomography scans have estimated that true elevation of the humerus on average is between 150° and 170°.[3,4]

The clinician instructs the patient to initiate elevation of the shoulder with the thumb facing upward and assesses the maximum height that can be reached (Figure 16). By placing the hand in this position, the humerus externally rotates, allowing the greater tuberosity to clear the acromion. With the thumb in the down position, shoulder elevation is underestimated falsely. The clinician continues to advance the shoulder passively after the patient actively has reached maximum height (Figure 17). The ability to force the upper extremity into additional flexion without causing pain could indicate weakness. If no further motion can be achieved, then extrinsic or intrinsic joint stiffness should be considered. Both measurements should be documented.

External Rotation. The clinician begins by assessing external rotation with the patient standing and the upper extremity at the side in 0° of abduction (Figure 18). To isolate the glenohumeral joint, the clinician holds the patient's elbow with one hand and gently externally rotates the extremity with the other, guiding the patient at the wrist. It will be evident that an end point has been reached when the patient's upper

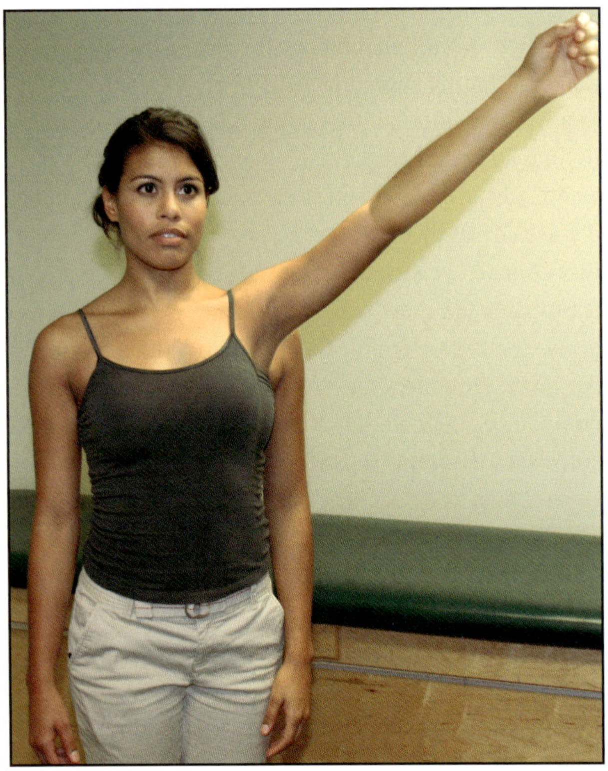

Figure 16. Active forward elevation.

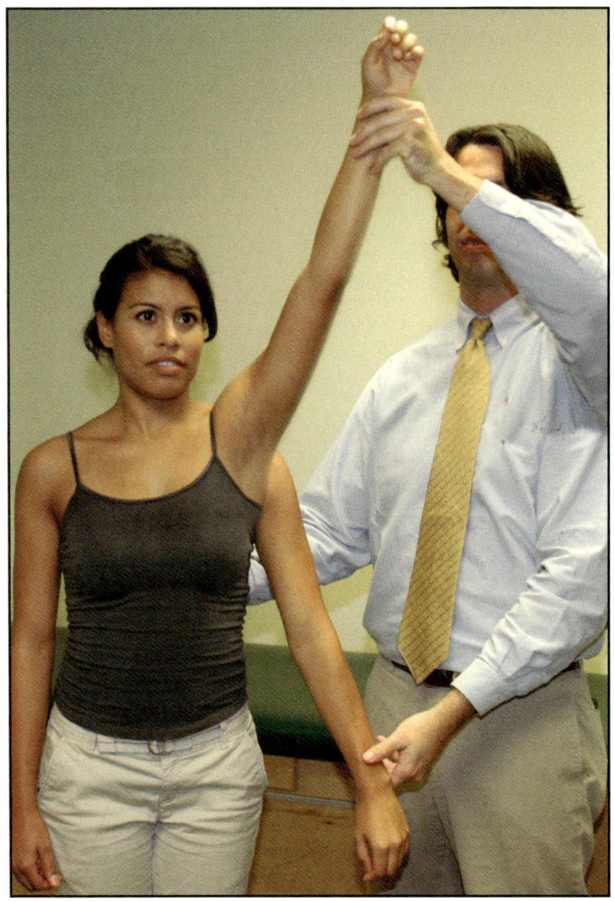

Figure 17. Passive forward elevation.

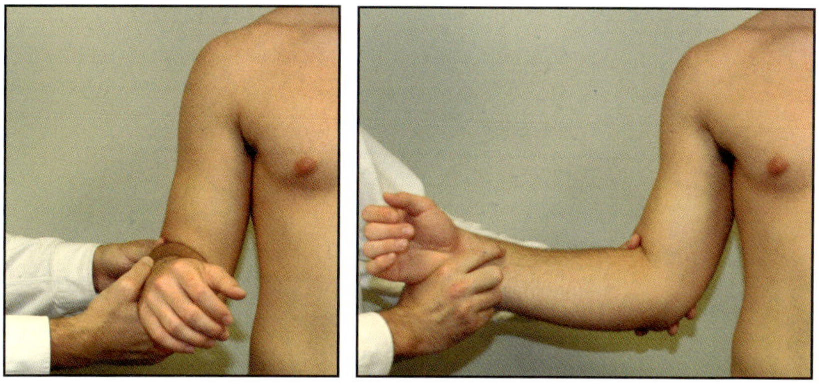

Figure 18. Assessing external rotation at the glenohumeral joint.

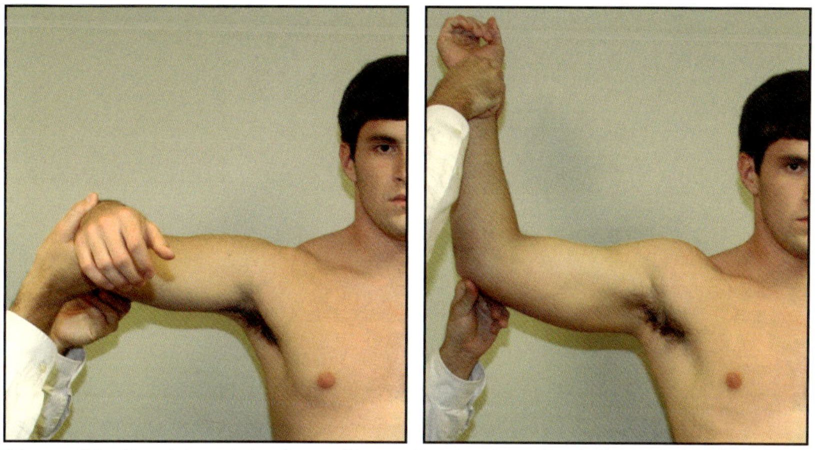

Figure 19. Shoulder abduction with maximal external rotation might elicit pathologic conditions of the glenohumeral joint or labrum.

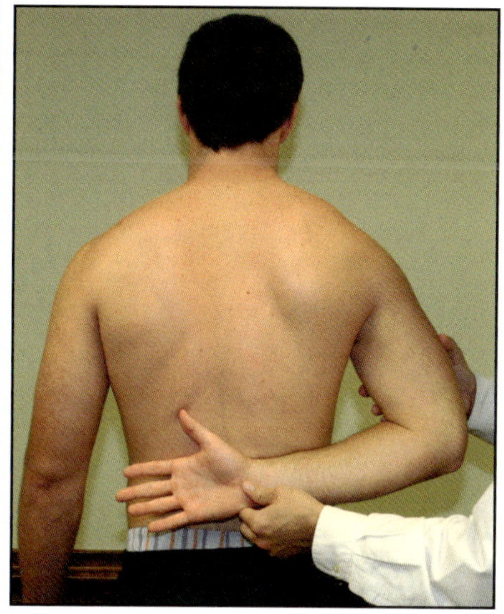

Figure 20. "Thumb up back" test.

body begins to turn in the direction of rotation. From this position, the shoulder should move through an arc of approximately 50°. Next, the clinician abducts the shoulder to 90° and beginning with the forearm parallel to the ground, he or she brings the shoulder to maximum external rotation (Figure 19). One hand is used to support the patient's elbow; the other, to guide the wrist and hand through the motion. In patients who are not overhead athletes, approximately 90° of motion should be obtained. The clinician notes any tenderness elicited with this maneuver because it might indicate instability within the glenohumeral joint or labral conditions. Accomplished overhead athletes, such as tennis players and pitchers, often can achieve much greater than 90° of external rotation in this position.

Internal Rotation. In 1994, the American Shoulder and Elbow Society recommended that shoulder internal rotation should be determined by the "thumb up back" test.[2] During this maneuver, the patient places his or her hand as far up the back as possible with the palm facing outward and the thumb pointing superiorly (Figure 20). The highest spinal level that the thumb can reach is recorded as a measure of maximum internal rotation. However, it has been shown that this test does not isolate glenohumeral internal rotation and actually violates the normal 2:1 ratio of glenohumeral to scapular motion. A fair amount of elbow motion also is required to accomplish this maneuver.

As with external rotation, internal rotation can be evaluated with the shoulder in 90° of abduction. The patient's forearm again is positioned parallel to the floor. While supporting the elbow with one hand, the examiner internally rotates the shoulder, gently pushing the hand toward the ground. On average, the shoulder will move through an arc of only 20° to 25° from this position. This motion also can be assessed with the patient in the lateral decubitus position. In this way, steadying the scapula against the examination table isolates the glenohumeral joint. This technique has been advocated by some to more accurately evaluate the overhead athlete for the presence of glenohumeral internal rotation deficit (or GIRD) (Figure 21). When compared with the opposite nondominant shoulders, the affected shoulders of many athletes who engage in

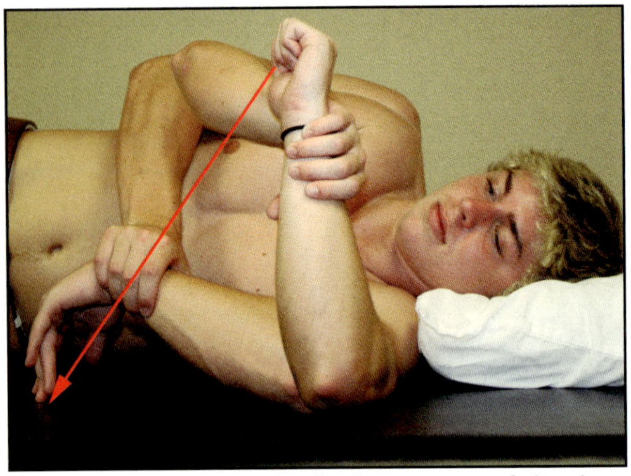

Figure 21. Maneuver testing for the presence of glenohumeral internal rotation deficit.

aggressive and repetitive overhead throwing will demonstrate a loss of internal rotation and an increase in external rotation. This has been theorized to create abnormal motion within the glenohumeral joint, leading to internal impingement, partial-thickness rotator cuff tears, and superior labrum anterior-posterior lesions.

Strength. Strength testing of the shoulder girdle musculature is central to a comprehensive physical examination of the shoulder. Evaluating the shoulder and ruling out the countless other disease processes that can mimic shoulder disorders, including degenerative and acute disorders of the cervical spine, neurologic diseases (eg, Parkinson and multiple sclerosis), and tumors within the central and peripheral nervous system, is critical. When pain is not an accompanying concern, looking for other sources of weakness is particularly important.

Muscle grading systems are additional tools used within the examination that allow clinicians to communicate examination findings in a consistent and accepted format. The most commonly used scale is depicted in the Table. It uses a 5-point scale to grade muscle strength relative to resistance applied to the extremity with gravity and with gravity eliminated. A plus can be added at the discretion of the examiner to convey additional information.

Variables, such as the patient's age, hand dominance, and sex, need to be considered when manual testing of the shoulder musculature is performed. The examiner also needs to be cognizant of his or her own strength relative to that of the patient so false conclusions about weakness are not drawn.

Given the complex and coordinated effort required to produce motion at the glenohumeral joint, isolating individual muscles around the shoulder girdle is particularly difficult. Tests designed to single out certain muscles and even segments within larger muscles, such as the deltoid, have been designed and studied throughout the literature. Testing groups of muscles that produce a certain motion about the shoulder joint, such as internal and external rotation and shoulder flexion and extension, often is more useful. We describe some of the most used and studied tests within the shoulder examination and focus on the basic motions of the shoulder and the muscles that produce that motion.

Shoulder Elevation (Flexion) and Extension

Supraspinatus. The supraspinatus can be torn completely, but the patient can exhibit full range of motion in the shoulder. Often, with a large rotator cuff tear involving the supraspinatus, pain is the limiting factor preventing full shoulder elevation. One of the most commonly used tests for supraspinatus strength is the Jobe empty-can test. It is performed with the patient standing and the upper extremity at 90° of abduction and 30° anterior to the coronal plane. This position places the upper extremity within the plane of the scapula. The thumbs are pointed toward the ground in the empty-can position (Figure 22). The examiner provides downward pressure at the wrists while the patient exerts upward resistance. Both extremities should be tested using the contralateral side for comparison. In addition, this test can be performed with the thumbs

Table. Muscle Grading System[5]

Muscle Grade	Description
5-Normal	Complete range of motion against gravity with full resistance
4-Good	Complete range of motion against gravity with some resistance
3-Fair	Complete range of motion against gravity
2-Poor	Complete range of motion with gravity eliminated
1-Trace	Evidence of slight contractility and no joint motion
0-Zero	No evidence of contractility

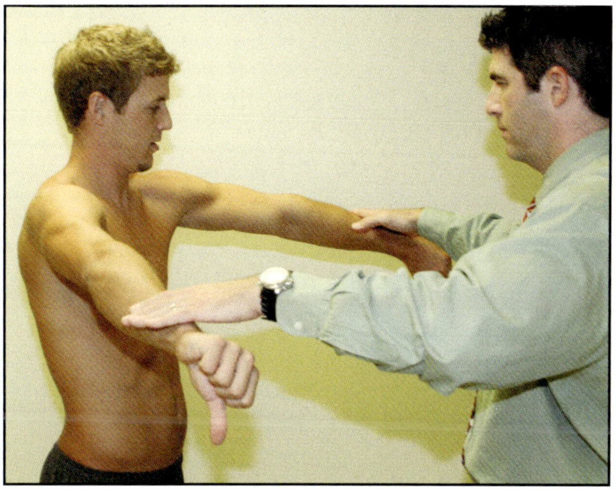

Figure 22. Jobe empty-can test.

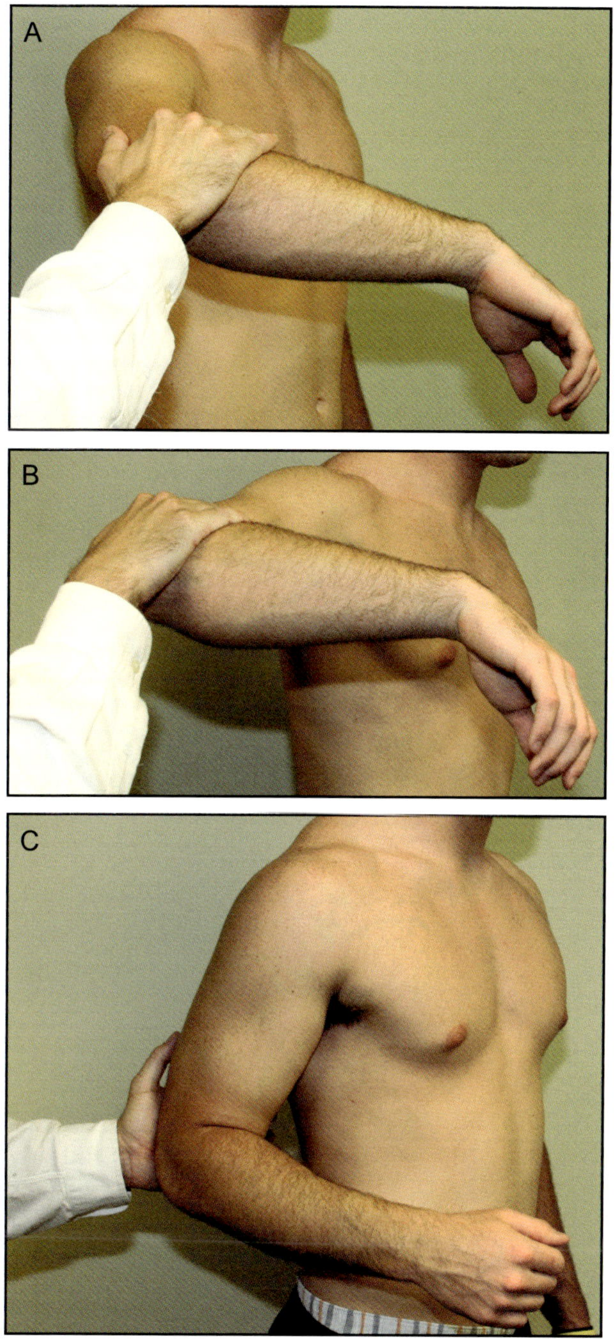

Figure 23. Maneuvers to test the anterior deltoid, A, middle deltoid, B, and posterior deltoid, C.

up in the full-can position and with patient lying prone. Some clinicians advise keeping the hands in a neutral position to alleviate some of the discomfort that can be caused by internally and externally rotating the upper extremity in this position.[2]

Deltoid. The primary function of the deltoid is to elevate the humerus. It comprises 3 segments, each of which can be isolated and tested effectively. To test the anterior deltoid, the patient can sit or stand. The clinician holds the upper extremity slightly anterior to the frontal plane of the body and in approximately 70° of abduction with the elbow bent or in full extension. The examiner exerts a downward force at the forearm while the patient attempts to flex the upper extremity forward (Figure 23A). From this same starting position, the examiner can apply a force directed toward the patient's torso at the elbow while the patient attempts to abduct the upper extremity. This effectively will isolate and test the middle deltoid (Figure 23B). The posterior deltoid extends the humerus. It can be tested in the same position and with the patient upright in a standing position. The examiner is positioned beside the patient and applies pressure to the elbow from a posterior to anterior direction as the patient attempts to force the shoulder into extension (Figure 23C).

Latissimus Dorsi. The latissimus works to adduct the humerus and contribute to shoulder extension along with the posterior deltoid and teres major. In clinical practice, it is tested less commonly and is not often the source of shoulder concerns; however, in the larger clinical picture, it could present clues to a neurologic deficit around the shoulder girdle. It can be tested with the patient in the prone position. With the arm resting on the examination table, the patient elevates the upper extremity into extension. The upper extremity naturally will move into slight internal rotation. The examiner grasps the forearm near the wrist and, as the patient attempts to adduct the extremity, applies resistance (Figure 24).

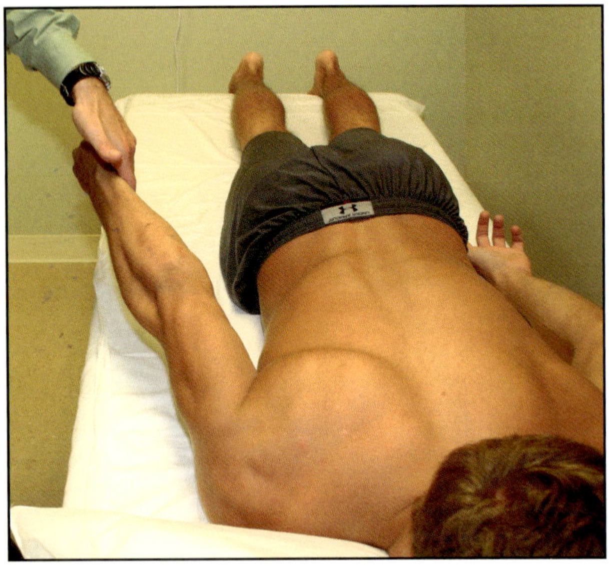

Figure 24. Examination for latissimus dorsi strength.

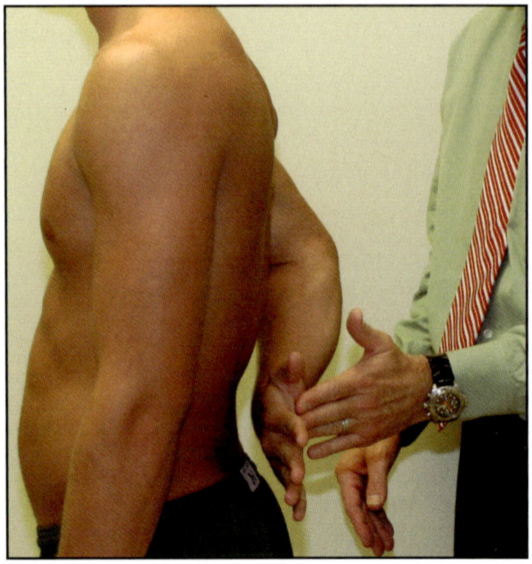

Figure 25. Examination for subscapularis strength.

Internal and External Rotation

Subscapularis. The subscapularis is the largest and most powerful rotator cuff muscle.[6] It occupies the entire subscapularis fossae at the anterior aspect of the scapula and primarily serves to internally rotate the shoulder. It and tests that have been designed to evaluate the strength and integrity of this muscle have been studied widely. The lift-off test is the best examination tool to assess the strength of the subscapularis muscle.[7] To perform this maneuver, the patient places the hand behind himself or herself with the shoulder in maximum internal rotation. With the palm facing posteriorly, the patient lifts the hand from the lumbar region of the back and holds it away from the body. The test is positive if the patient cannot carry this out or cannot lift the hand against resistance provided by the examiner (Figure 25). Accuracy of this test depends on the ability of the patient to initially place the hand in this position. Limitations to range of motion for mechanical reasons or because of pain would preclude the patient from performing this examination.

The belly-press test, or Napoleon sign, can be used for patients who cannot internally rotate the shoulder. This test can be done with the patient sitting or standing. The patient is instructed to place the hand on the abdomen and press inward (Figure 26). If his or her wrist volar flexes during this maneuver, the test is determined to be positive because the wrist is compensating for a weak subscapularis that cannot internally rotate the shoulder. The belly-press test has been shown in electromyography studies to activate the upper subscapularis to a greater extent than the lower portion of the muscle.[8] In contrast, Tokish et al[8] also demonstrated that the lift-off test activated the lower subscapularis to a greater extent than the belly-press test. Both were found to be valid measures of subscapularis function.

With a positive belly-press test, an additional clue to the severity of subscapularis weakness is a positive belly-off sign.[9] With the patient's hand resting on the abdomen and palm facing inward, the examiner brings the upper extremity into maximum internal rotation with the elbow flexed to 90° and the wrist supported. The patient is instructed to maintain the shoulder in internal rotation as the wrist is released. This test is positive for substantial subscapularis weakness if he or

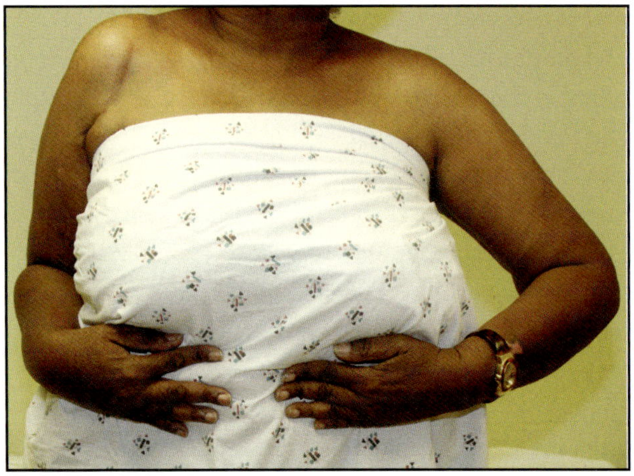

Figure 26. Napolean sign.

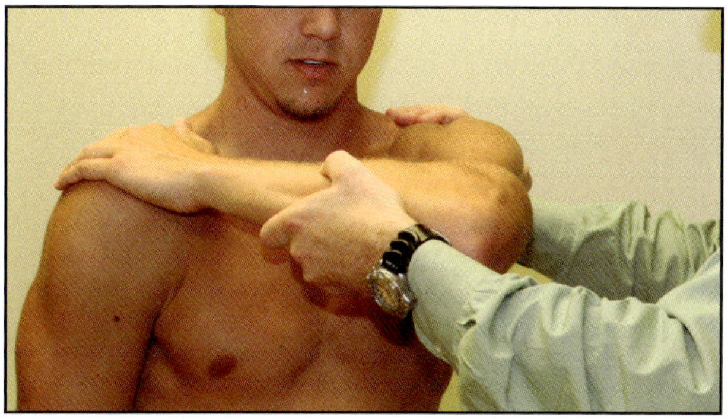

Figure 27. Bear-hug test.

she cannot hold this position and the hand moves away from the abdomen.

Recently, the bear-hug test has been described to assess subscapularis strength.[10] To perform this test, instruct the patient to place the hand of the affected extremity on the opposite shoulder in maximum internal rotation. The fingers should be in extension, and the elbow should be translated as far anterior as possible. The examiner is positioned in front of the patient and attempts to remove the hand from the shoulder by moving the shoulder into external rotation (Figure 27). The test is positive if the patient is either unable to maintain this position or unable to resist the examiner.

Pectoralis Major. The pectoralis major primarily functions as a shoulder adductor. However, it also contributes to internal rotation. Rupture of the pectoralis either within the substance of the muscle or at its insertion on the medial humerus commonly is seen in weight trainers.[11] When encountered acutely, substantial swelling and ecchymosis often accompany it. However, if the injury is remote, it is often less obvious. To accentuate the deformity produced when rupture of the pectoralis is suspected, instruct the patient to stand with the hands clasped in front of himself or herself and to push the hands together (Figure 28). A visible sulcus will be evident in the area of the anterior axillary fold where the tendon inserts (Figure 29).

Strength testing of the pectoralis is not performed as commonly as strength testing of other muscles of the shoulder girdle, such as the rotator cuff. The upper and lower portions of the muscle can be tested with the patient standing and the upper extremity elevated to 90° in front of the patient. With the upper extremity held in slight internal rotation, the examiner applies force to the medial forearm as the patient attempts to adduct the extremity. By lowering the upper extremity slightly

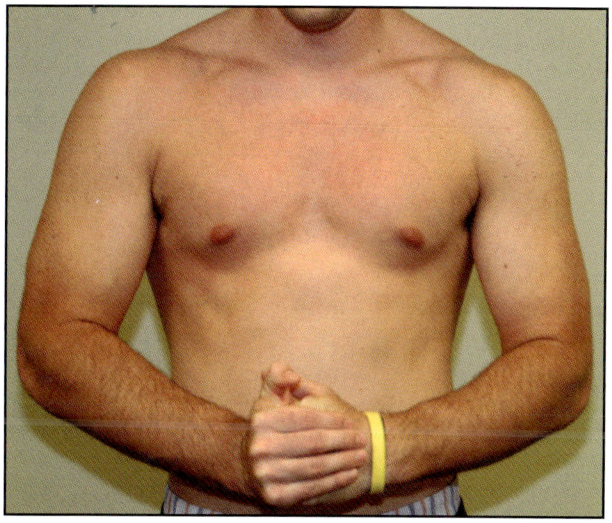

Figure 28. Pectoralis major rupture test.

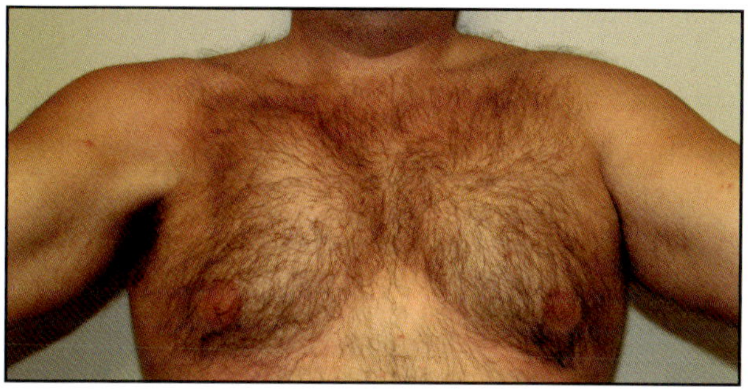

Figure 29. Pectoralis major rupture with visible sulcus in the anterior axillary fold.

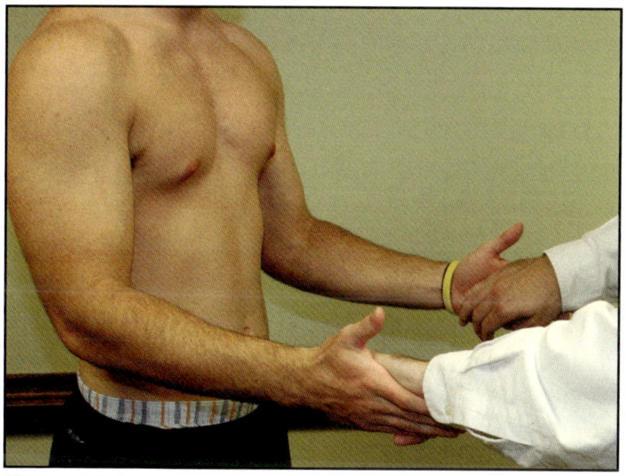

Figure 30. Strength testing of the pectoralis muscle.

in less forward flexion, the examiner also can assess the lower portion of the pectoralis (Figure 30).

Infraspinatus and Teres Minor. The primary external rotators of the shoulder are the teres minor and infraspinatus muscles. A small contribution comes from the posterior deltoid.[12] The teres minor is the smallest of the rotator cuff muscles and rarely causes shoulder pain or dysfunction in isolation. Tests have

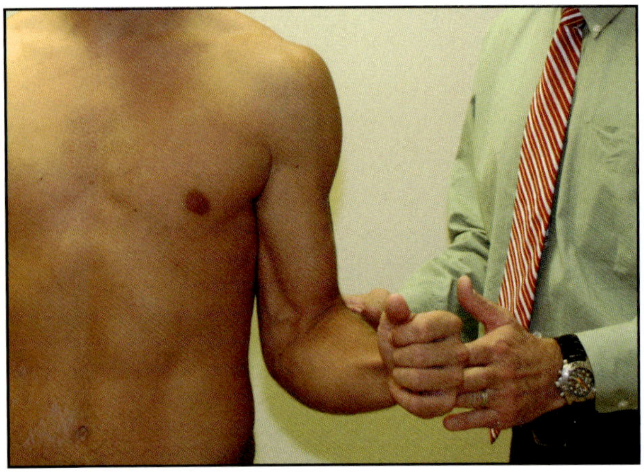

Figure 31. Infraspinatus strength test.

been designed specifically to evaluate this muscle, but they rarely are performed in a clinical setting. The infraspinatus is involved more commonly when shoulder pain and dysfunction are the chief concern. To test its integrity, the patient holds the upper extremities at the sides in 0° of abduction or a neutral position. With elbows flexed to 90°, the patient pushes out against the examiner's hands as he or she tries to resist external rotation (Figure 31). This test can be done with the patient sitting or standing. The patient must maintain the elbows at the sides so he or she does not abduct the shoulders to gain a mechanical advantage.[2]

Scapular Stabilizers

Trapezius and Serratus Anterior. Roughly triangular in shape, the trapezius is the largest of the scapulothoracic muscles. It cloaks the deeper scapular stabilizers and forms the contour of the posterior shoulder girdle. The trapezius comprises upper, middle, and lower portions, and when dysfunction becomes clinically important, the upper trapezius generally is involved. The primary function of the trapezius, along with the levator scapulae, is to elevate the scapula. Having the patient perform a shoulder shrug against resistance can enable the examiner to easily assess both muscles. The examiner stands behind the patient, firmly rests both hands on the shoulders over each acromion, and instructs the patient to shrug the shoulders while providing downward resistance (Figure 32). As with other aspects of the shoulder examination, any asymmetry should be noted.

The spinal accessory nerve innervates the trapezius. A complete or partial lesion within the nerve can cause the scapula to tilt laterally due to paralysis of the upper trapezius (Figure 33). This lateral scapular winging is distinct from medial scapular winging caused by paralysis of the serratus anterior from injury to the long thoracic nerve.

When the serratus anterior muscle contracts, it moves the scapula anterior on the thoracic cage. This movement is called *protraction*, and to test for it and for the competency of the muscle, the examiner instructs the patient to perform a push-up or to push against a wall while standing upright and leaning slightly forward. The examiner observes the patient from behind. If the serratus anterior cannot hold the scapula against the thoracic cavity, medial rotation and protrusion of the inferior angle of the scapula will be evident, and this is medial scapular winging (Figure 34). Alternatively, scapular protraction can be tested in isolation by resisting the patient's attempt to "reach" forward. To perform this maneuver, the examiner stands behind the patient with one hand resting on the thoracic spine to stabilize the patient and the other hand supporting the patient's elbow. The patient holds the upper extremity in 90° of flexion and with his or

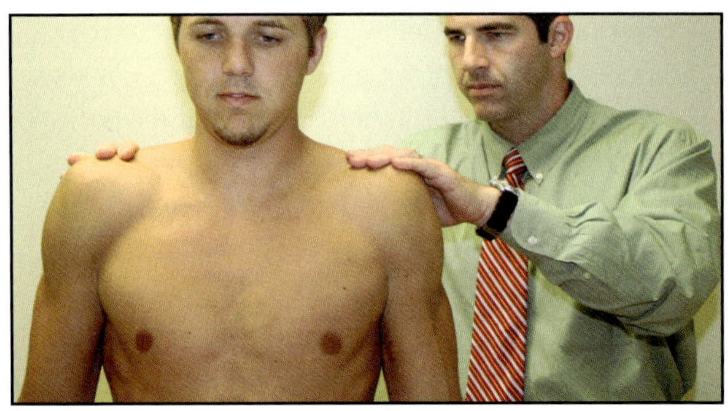

Figure 32. Shoulder shrug test for trapezius strength.

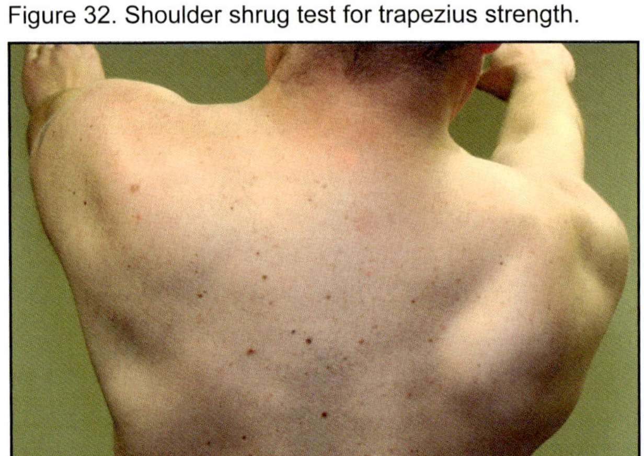

Figure 33. Lateral translation of the scapula in a patient with a spinal accessory nerve palsy.

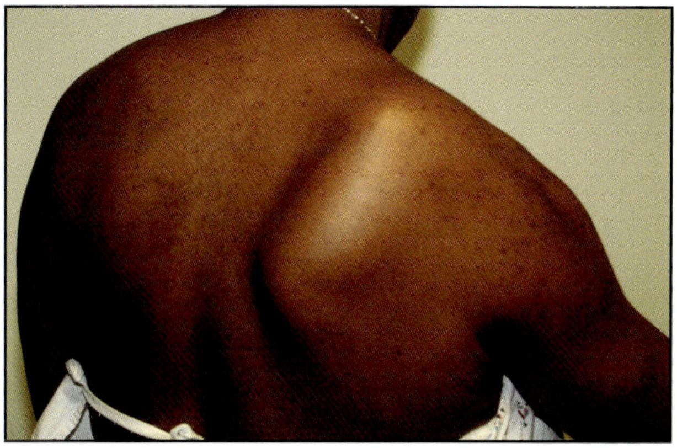

Figure 34. Medial scapular winging.

her hand on the opposite shoulder. Next, the patient forces the bent upper extremity forward in an attempt to touch the wall with his or her elbow. If the serratus anterior is not competent, the scapula will protrude and rotate medially.

Rhomboids Major and Minor. In contrast to the action of the serratus anterior that moves the scapula anteriorly or protracts the scapula relative to the thoracic cage, the rhomboids retract the scapula. The rhomboids major and minor and a small contribution from the trapezius allow the shoulders to be pulled back into the position of attention. To test for this, the examiner stands in front of the patient with his or her hands resting securely on the patient's shoulders. The patient is instructed to pull the shoulders back into the position of attention while the examiner provides gentle resistance, attempting to bend the shoulders forward (Figure 35).

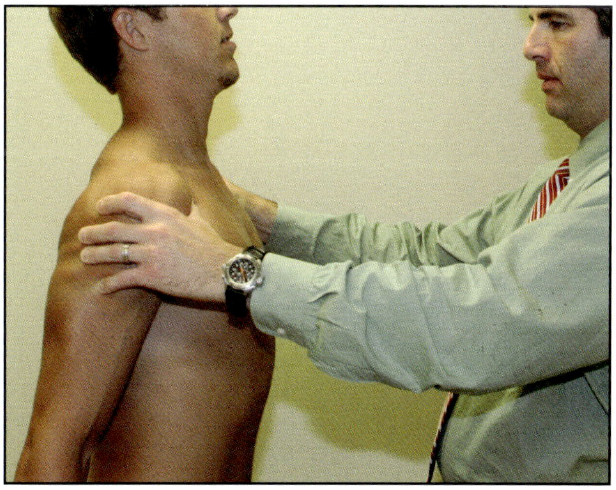

Figure 35. Strength testing of the rhomboids.

SPECIAL TESTS

Rotator Cuff and Impingement

Neer[13] described that impingement from the anterior aspect of the acromion contributed to rotator cuff lesions. He suggested that osteophyte formation and lesions within the coracoacromial ligament and AC joint would encroach upon the subacromial space and lead to degenerative wear of the rotator cuff and, in particular, the supraspinatus tendon. Later, Bigliani et al[14] described the role of acromial morphology on this process. This phenomenon of external impingement is more prevalent in an aging population; however, other forms of impingement have been described.

Walch et al[15] and Jobe[16] described internal impingement in the overhead athlete. They theorized that contact between the posterosuperior glenoid and the undersurface of the rotator cuff leads to tendon damage as the upper extremity repeatedly is placed in abduction and external rotation, such as in the late cocking phase of pitching. An increase in glenohumeral joint laxity that often is found in elite athletes is believed to be the inciting event to allow this abnormal motion within the shoulder. Early in this process, the athlete experiences stiffness and is slow to warm up. This progresses to pain at the posterior aspect of the shoulder due to tightness in the posterior capsule.[17] Often, provocative tests for labral lesions and instability, such as the anterior apprehension and relocation tests (described later in this chapter), are positive. Rehabilitation is often difficult if this posterior capsular tightness is left uncorrected.[17] The internal rotation resistance stress test is used to differentiate between internal and external impingement. The examiner stands behind the patient. The extremity is positioned in 90° of abduction and 80° of external rotation. The patient is instructed to perform isometric resistance to external rotation followed by isometric resistance to internal rotation (Figure 36). The examiner compares the resistance. A patient with good strength in external rotation and weakness in internal rotation is considered to have a positive test for internal impingement. Good strength in internal rotation but relative weakness in external rotation is considered a positive finding for external impingement.

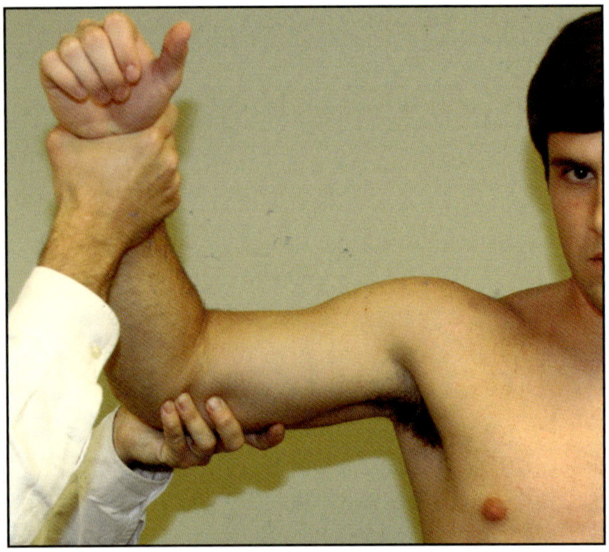

Figure 36. Internal rotation resistance stress test.

Coracoid or subcoracoid impingement has been described. This encroachment of the coracoid process on the anterior humeral structures is believed to cause pain that can mimic rotator cuff lesions and radiate into the upper extremity, mimicking cervical radiculopathy.[18] The exact mechanism has not been elucidated, and making the diagnosis clinically is often difficult. The Kennedy-Hawkins position with the upper extremity positioned at 90° of forward flexion and internal rotation has been found to evoke pain when this entity is present.[2] The Gerber subcoracoid impingement test is used to diagnose coracoid impingement syndrome. The shoulder is forward flexed to 90° and internally rotated (Figure 37). Adduction of the upper extremity brings the lesser tuberosity further into contact with the tip of the coracoid and is added to the flexion and internal rotation maneuver. A positive test elicits pain at the anterior aspect of the shoulder in the area of the coracoid. Patients might have a palpable click on testing. These patients will be tender to palpation over the coracoid.

Signs of Impingement. Neer[13,19] described the impingement sign as pain elicited with passive forward elevation of the upper extremity. The examiner stands behind the patient with one hand stabilizing the scapula and the other hand guiding the upper extremity into maximum forward elevation. Evocation of pain indicates a positive finding (Figure 38). However, it is somewhat nonspecific and can be positive with other shoulder conditions. In addition, he described the painful arc of motion as indicative of this impingement process and rotator cuff disease. Again, the examiner passively moves the patient's extremity through a range of motion from maximum forward elevation to to a resting position, and the pain that is produced between 70° and 120° of elevation indicates lesions within the subacromial space.

The impingement test was described as an adjunct to the Neer sign to aid in confirming pain originating from the subacromial space. The examiner injects a local anesthetic, often lidocaine, into this area and documents whether pain is relieved after the maneuver is performed again. Quantifying the percentage of relief gained can help determine the extent of disease that is present.

The Kennedy-Hawkins sign is performed with the examiner positioned to the side of the patient who is

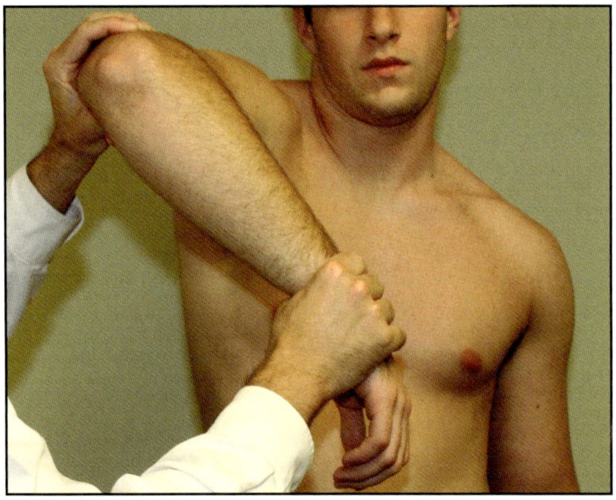

Figure 37. Gerber subcoracoid impingement test.

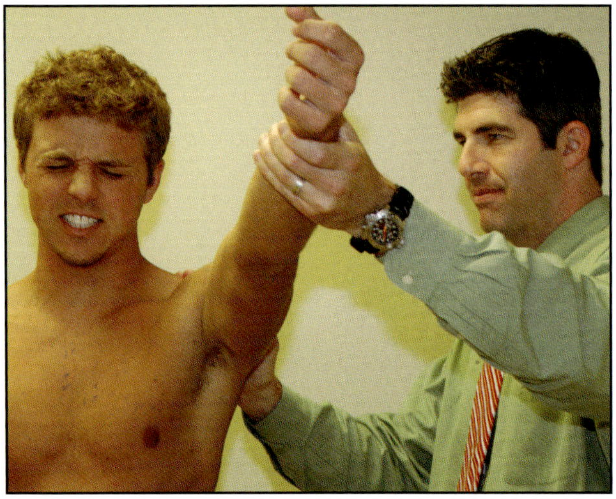

Figure 38. Neer impingement sign.

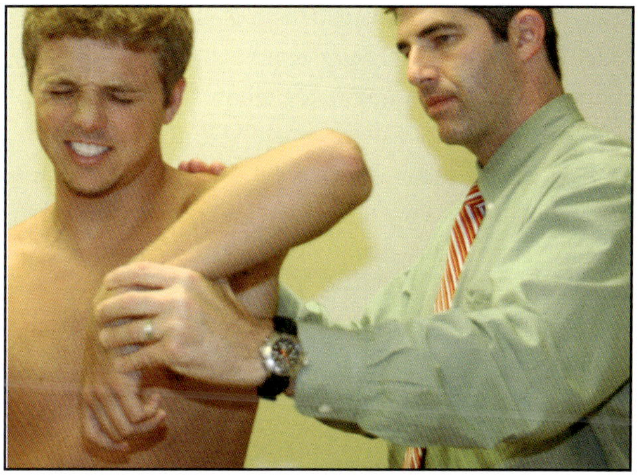

Figure 39. Kennedy-Hawkins impingement test.

either sitting or standing. The patient flexes the upper extremity to 90°, and the examiner moves the upper extremity into maximum internal rotation (Figure 39). Again, one hand stabilizes the scapula as the other hand guides the patient's extremity. Pain elicited here is believed to come from the greater tuberosity as it is brought into close contact with the undersurface of the acromion and the coracoacromial ligament. This sign is believed to more accurately indicate the impingement process and rotator cuff disease if it is performed with the upper extremity in forward flexion rather than abduction.[2]

Signs of a Torn Rotator Cuff. Clues to lesions within the rotator cuff usually are evident during the strength testing portion of the physical examination. In addition, local tenderness around the shoulder girdle and a palpable rent can be appreciated at the anterosuperior aspect of the humeral head during the examination. The defect in the supraspinatus tendon can be felt by palpating the insertion of the supraspinatus just distal to the edge of the acromion (Figure 40). This often will elicit pain from the patient, as well. Another nonspecific sign commonly present with a torn rotator cuff is subacromial crepitus. This crepitus can be painful to the patient and can be evoked by taking the patient's extremity through passive internal and external rotation with the upper extremity at the side. However, the location of pain as described by the patient has not been found to accurately point to the location of the tear within the rotator cuff.[19]

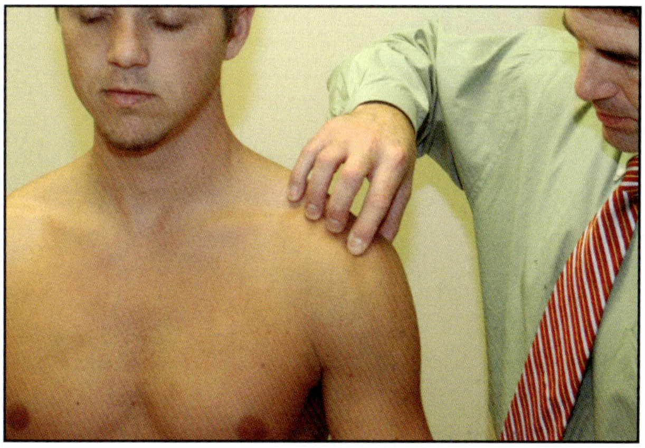

Figure 40. Test for supraspinatus rent sign.

Dramatic signs can be present with a massive rotator cuff tear. A prominence at the anterosuperior aspect of the shoulder on inspection could indicate a superiorly migrated humeral head or anterosuperior escape, which also occurs when the coracoacromial arch has been compromised. Egress of synovial fluid through a large defect in the rotator cuff also can be seen as swelling at the superior aspect of the shoulder. Signs of atrophy within the infraspinatus and supraspinatus are discernible as depressions at the posterior aspect of the shoulder within the infraspinatus and supraspinatus fossa, respectively (Figure 41). In contrast, signs of acute traumatic injury to the shoulder resulting in massive rotator cuff tears are swelling, ecchymosis, and preservation of the substance of the involved muscles.[1] Specific signs within the physical examination have been described and are used to develop a clinical picture when evaluating patients with large to massive rotator cuff tears.[19]

The external rotation lag sign was described by Hertel et al[20] as a measure of competence of the infra-

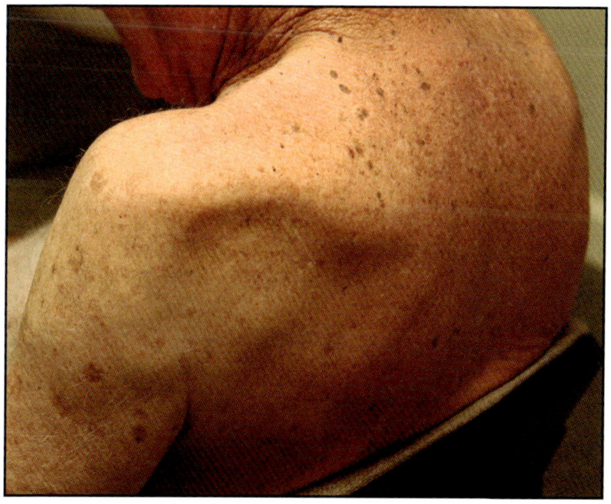

Figure 41. Patient demonstrates signs of atrophy of the supraspinatus. Note the depressions.

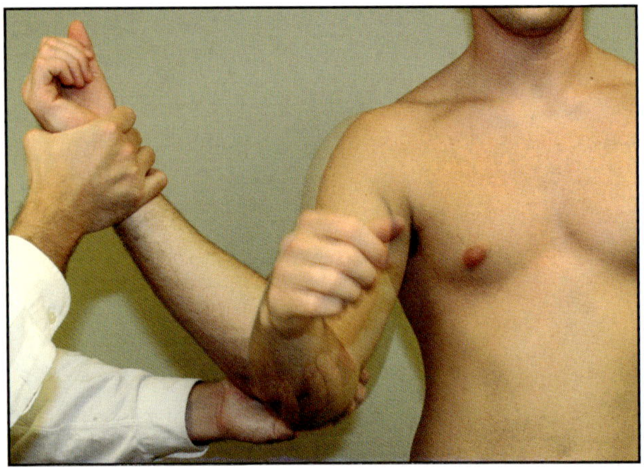

Figure 42. External rotation lag test.

spinatus and supraspinatus. The test can be performed with the patient seated or standing and the examiner positioned at the patient's side. The examiner holds the patient's extremity in slight flexion to approximately 20° with the elbow flexed to 90° and moves the upper extremity into maximum external rotation. The patient is instructed to hold this position (Figure 42). The upper extremity falling back into internal rotation is a positive sign. The magnitude of lag or drop from maximum external rotation is recorded to within the nearest 5°. The ability of the patient to hold the extremity in external rotation at 20° of flexion has been shown to depend more on a fully functioning supraspinatus than deltoid.[21]

The internal rotation lag sign, which Hertel et al[20] also described, tests the integrity of the subscapularis. This test, in conjunction with tests for subscapularis function described earlier, provides additional clues to create an overall clinical picture when assessing the patient for large to massive rotator cuff tears. To perform this test, the examiner is situated at the patient's side. He or she holds the affected extremity in maximum internal rotation with the elbow flexed to 90° and the extremity in approximately 20° of elevation and 20° of extension. The hand of the patient, which is resting on the abdomen, is lifted away from the body. The patient is instructed to maintain this position as the examiner releases the wrist (Figure 43). The magnitude of the drop is recorded to the nearest 5°.

The drop sign[22] also is used to evaluate the infraspinatus. The examiner, who is positioned behind the seated patient, holds the affected extremity in an abducted and externally rotated position as close to 90° as tolerable. The extremity is elevated within the plane of the scapula, and the patient is instructed to hold this position as the examiner relinquishes support of the extremity (Figure 44). If a lag occurs and the upper extremity falls into internal rotation, the infraspinatus is determined to be incompetent. Again, the lag is measured and recorded to within the nearest 5°.

The drop-arm sign is manifested by the patient's inability to hold up the upper extremity against gravity. It can be performed 2 different ways. The first way is for the examiner to passively elevate the upper extremity to 90° and instruct the patient to hold this position. The inability to hold up the upper extremity against gravity indicates a positive test. The second way to perform the test is for the examiner to instruct the patient to actively elevate the shoulder. When the shoulder is maximally elevated, the examiner instructs the patient to lower the upper extremity in a controlled manner. The inability to lower the upper extremity in a slow, controlled fashion is a positive test. In addition,

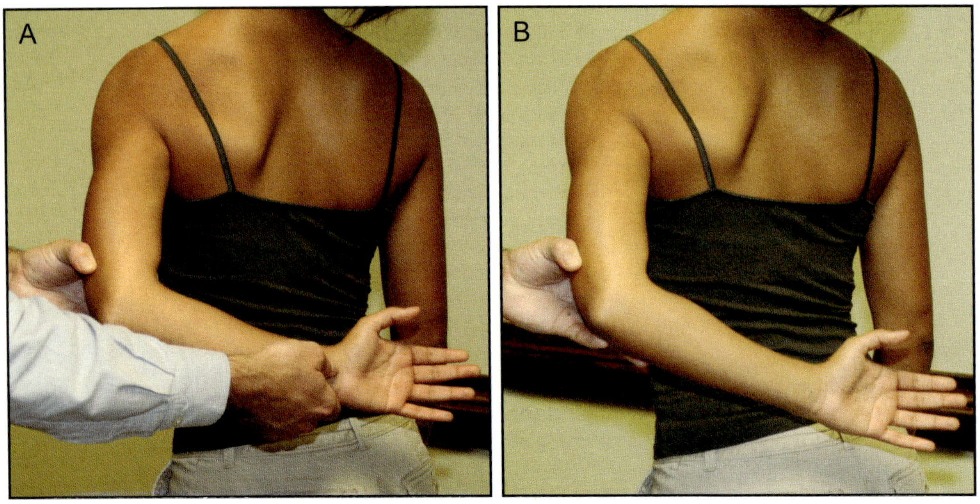

Figure 43. A, Internal rotation lag test. B, Negative sign.

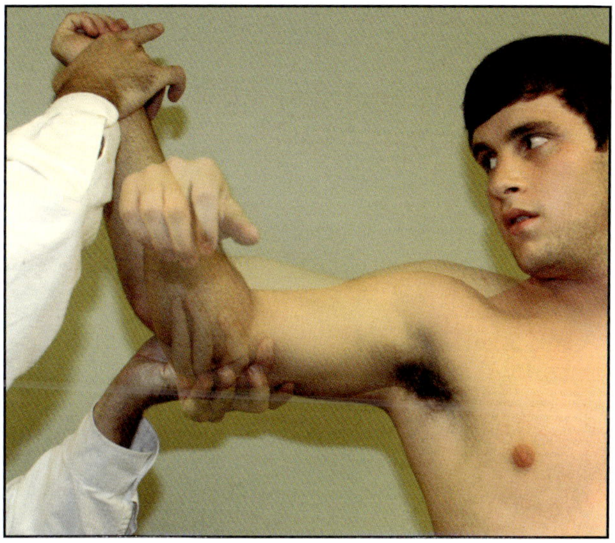

Figure 44. Positive drop sign, or lag sign, for an incompetent infraspinatus muscle.

patients with massive rotator cuff tears can lose the ability to actively raise the upper extremity to shoulder level. This loss of forward elevation is called pseudoparalysis (Figure 45).

The hornblower's sign is positive in patients with large to massive rotator cuff tears involving the supraspinatus and infraspinatus. It was first described by Walch et al[22] and is based on the observed phenomenon that when instructed to bring the hand to the mouth, a patient with substantial rotator cuff lesions will elevate the elbow because he or she cannot actively externally rotate the upper extremity to achieve the task. Because the patient cannot do this, he or she must elevate the upper extremity to 90° then allow the upper extremity to fall into internal rotation, thus bringing the hand to the mouth (Figure 46). Again, this test is used as an adjunct to the remainder of the examination and helps to solidify the clinical picture when determining to what extent the rotator cuff is diseased.

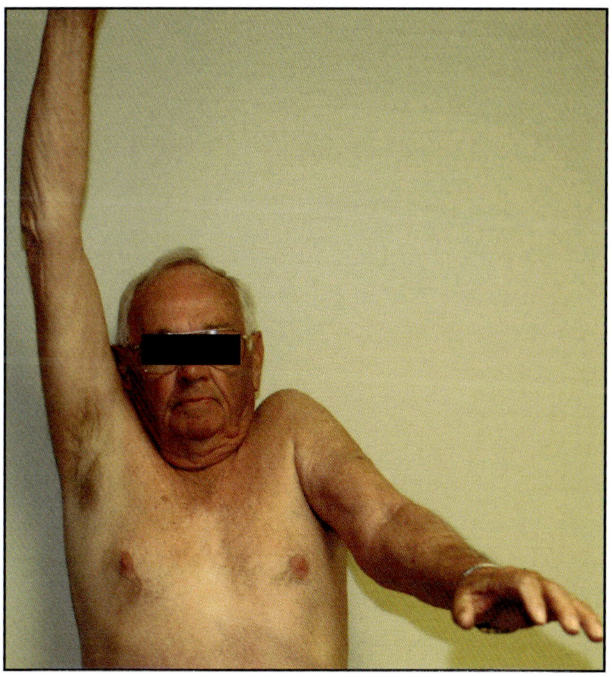

Figure 45. This patient with a massive rotator cuff tear and pseudoparalysis cannot raise his left extremity to shoulder level.

Biceps and Labrum

The biceps anchor is the origin of the long head of the biceps brachii and is fixed firmly atop the superior glenoid. It has attachments to both the bony glenoid at the supraglenoid tubercle and the superior labrum spreading out both anteriorly and posteriorly.[23] It is a common site of injury within the shoulder, particularly in the overhead athlete, and seldom is found in isolation. The superior labrum anterior-posterior (SLAP) lesion originally was described by Andrews et al[24] and later classified by Snyder et al.[25] Much interest since its identification has been focused on physical examination tests that might single out this condition and differentiate it from other sources of shoulder pain. To date, this endeavor has been elusive. However, certain provocative tests can be useful, particularly when taken in combination, to create an overall clinical picture and aid in diagnosis.

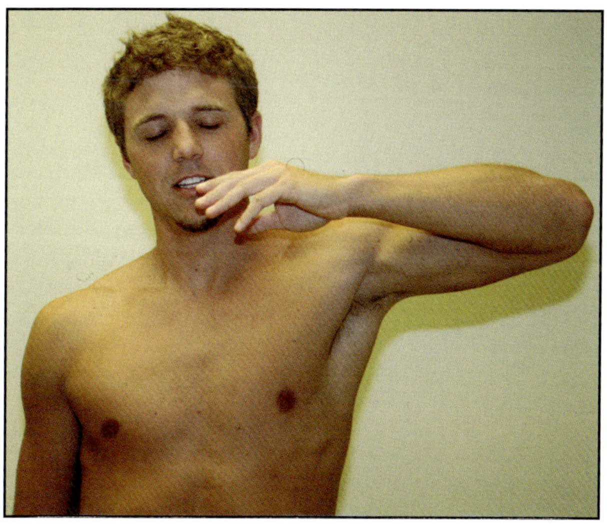

Figure 46. Negative hornblower's sign.

The O'Brien, or active compression, test was described earlier for diagnosing conditions within the AC joint[26]; however, when deep pain is elicited or the patient feels a painful "click," a SLAP lesion can be suspected. The test is performed with the patient standing and the upper extremity in 90° of flexion and 10° to 30° of adduction. The examiner instructs the patient to point his or her thumb toward the floor and resist a downward force that the examiner applies. Next, the examiner instructs the patient to externally rotate the upper extremity so the forearm is supinated (Figure 47). The maneuver is repeated, and in the presence of a SLAP lesion, the patient should experience pain relief.[27]

Parentis et al[28] showed the Yergason supination test has a specificity of 92.7% in diagnosing SLAP lesions. The test is performed with the examiner positioned at the patient's side and supporting the extremity. The elbow is flexed to 90°, and the forearm is in full pronation. The patient is instructed to supinate the forearm while the examiner provides resistance by holding the wrist (Figure 48). Reproduction of the patient's pain is a positive result.

The Speed test is often positive in the presence of a biceps tendon lesion and can be useful in identifying SLAP lesions. It is performed with the patient sitting upright, the upper extremity positioned in 90° of flexion, and the forearm positioned in full supination. The examiner provides a downward force directed at the midforearm as he or she instructs the patient to elevate the upper extremity against resistance (Figure 49). Again, pain elicited with this maneuver indicates a positive finding.

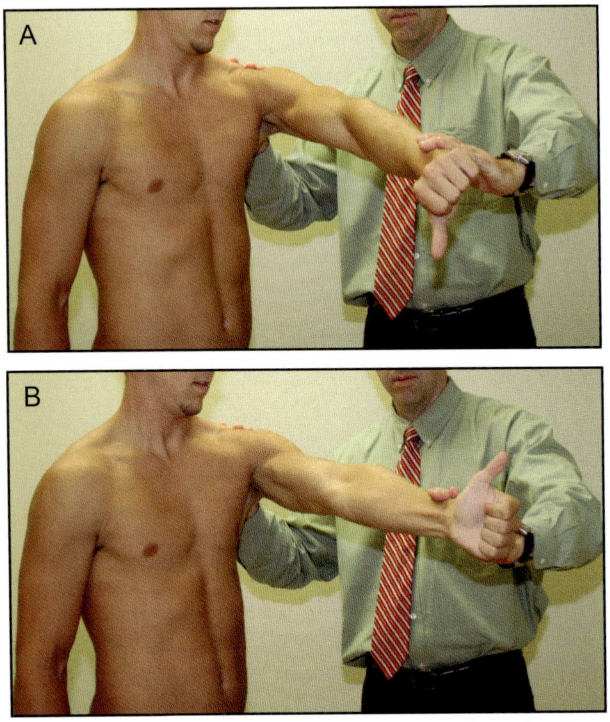

Figure 47. O'Brien test with internal rotation, A, and external rotation, B.

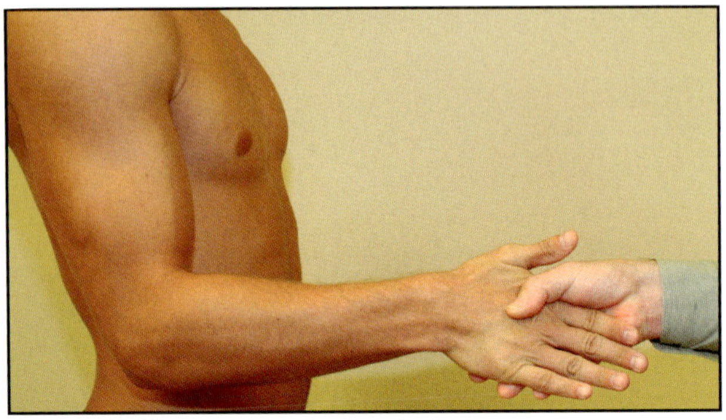

Figure 48. Yergason supination test.

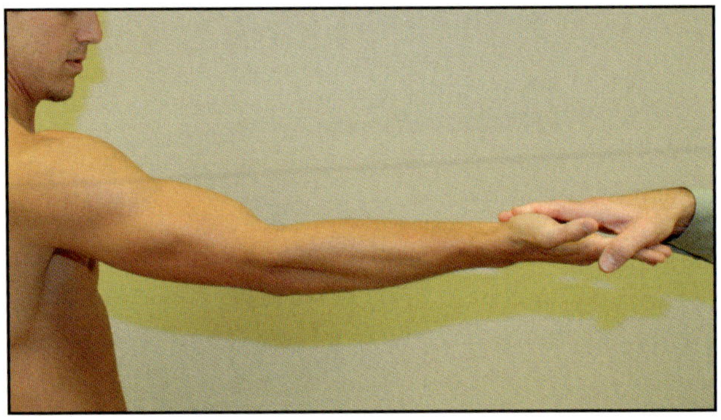

Figure 49. Speed test.

The Kibler test or anterior glide test[29] is performed with the patient standing. He or she is instructed to place the hand upon the hip with the thumb facing posteriorly. The examiner, who is positioned at the side of the patient, stabilizes the scapula with one hand while using the other hand to provide an axial load directed toward the glenohumeral joint. Next, he or she directs this force in an anteroposterior direction, applying shearing forces across the superior glenoid (Figure 50). In the presence of a tear at the superior labrum, pain or a click should be elicited.

Myers et al[30] described the resisted supination external rotation test for diagnosing SLAP lesions. This test was designed in an attempt to re-create the "peel back" mechanism seen at the superior labrum arthroscopi-

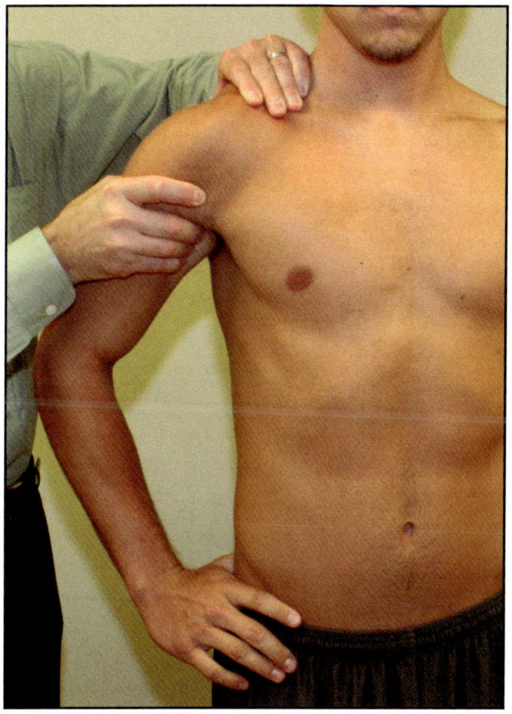

Figure 50. Kibler test.

cally in the presence of a SLAP lesion. It is performed with the patient lying supine and the scapula resting firmly on the examination table. The examiner stands to the side of the patient, supporting the extremity in 90° of abduction. The elbow is flexed to between 65° and 70°, and the forearm is held in slight pronation or neutral rotation. The patient is instructed to supinate the forearm while the examiner provides resistance. As the patient performs this action, the examiner gently moves the shoulder into maximum external rotation (Figure 51). The test is positive if the patient feels anterior or deep shoulder pain or if a clicking or catching sensation is appreciated.

Instability

Laxity Versus Instability. The glenohumeral joint is the most freely mobile of all joints of the human body. The soft tissue architecture around the shoulder contributes more to its stability than the bony relationship of the humerus contributes to the glenoid cavity.[31] When evaluating a patient for lesions related to the glenohumeral joint, the examiner needs to differenti-

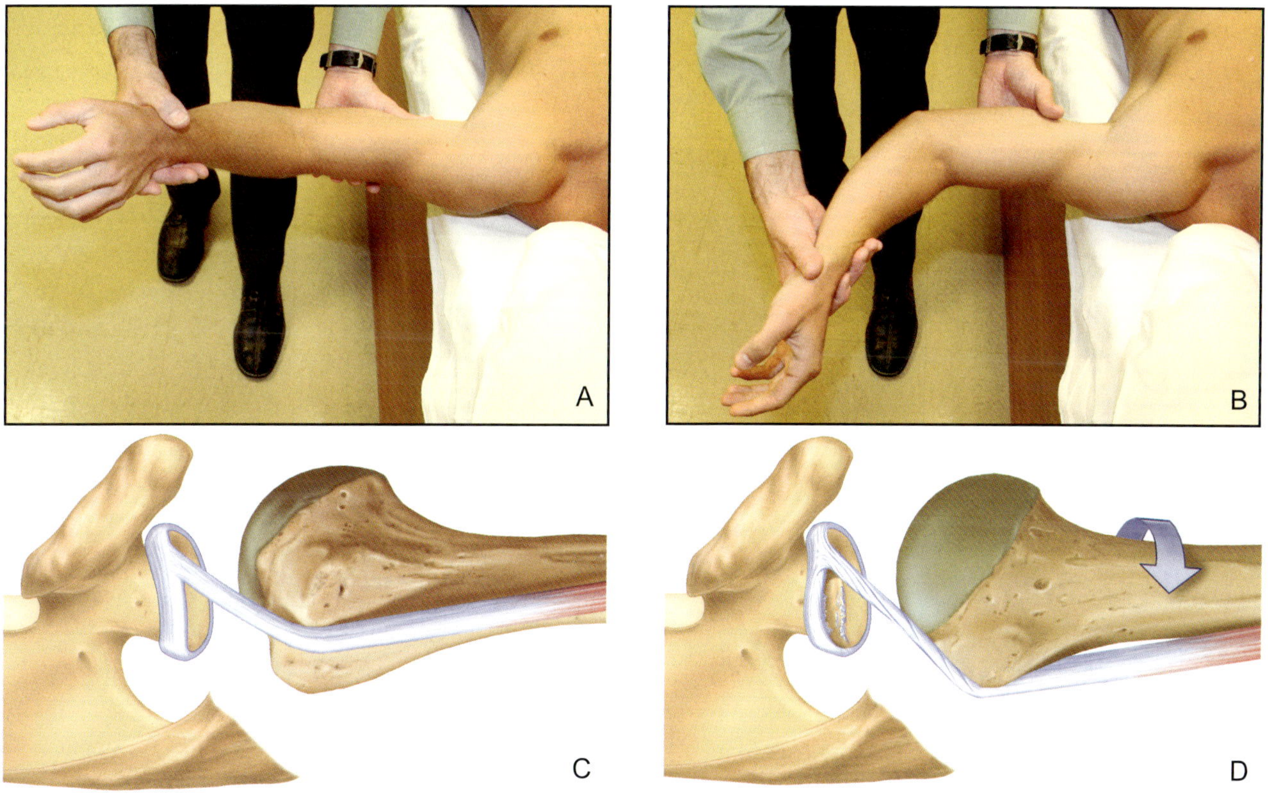

Figure 51. Resisted supination external rotation test. A, Neutral rotation. B, Maximum external rotation. C, Superior labrum in neutral rotation. D, Superior laburm in maximum external rotation demonstrating the “peel back” sign.

ate between laxity, which can be inherent to the patient and often functional, and instability, which can be debilitating. In general, laxity can be considered a trait inherent to the individual, whereas instability is its pathologic variant.

Motion that occurs between 2 bones is a byproduct of their bony architecture and the position and condition of the ligaments between them. This interaction makes up a joint, and the movement that takes place there is the laxity of the joint.[2] Often, a patient will exhibit a generalized ligamentous laxity. Clinical signs of hyperlaxity include the ability to touch the thumb to the forearm, recurvatum of the elbow, and recurvatum of the knee (Figure 52). Evidence of hyperlaxity often is seen in patients with multidirectional instability of the shoulder. Determining this before performing provocative maneuvers for shoulder laxity will help create an overall clinical picture.

The process of evaluating the shoulder joint for laxity or instability should begin with the method reported by Richards et al.[32] This method has been adopted by the American Shoulder and Elbow Society and

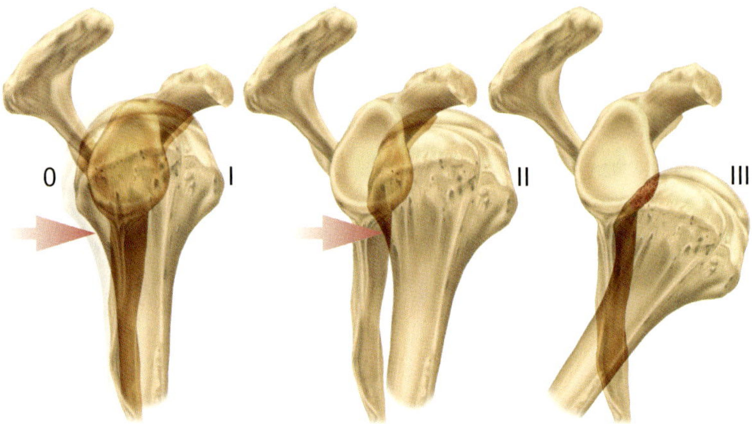

Figure 53. Grades I, II, and III shoulder instability.

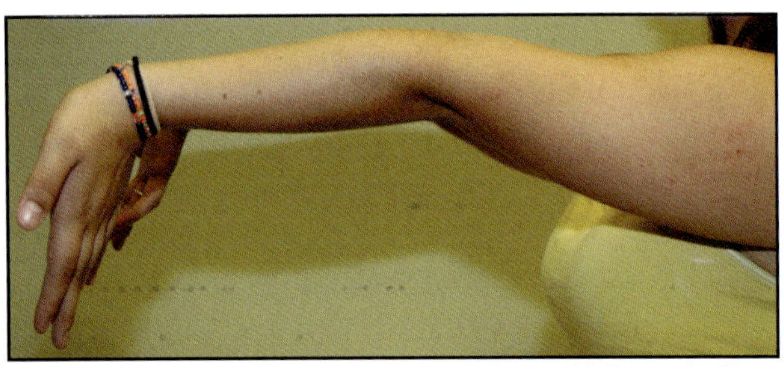

Figure 52A. Elbow recurvatum in patient with hyperlaxity.

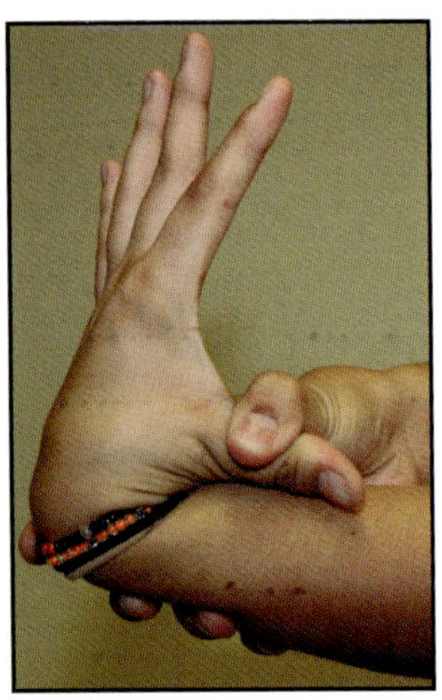

Figure 52B. The same patient demonstrates the ability to touch her thumb to her forearm due to hyperlaxity.

grades laxity within the joint from 0 to III based on what the examiner feels when attempting to manually sublux the humeral head over the anterior glenoid rim. Grade 0 constitutes normal translation; grade I, translation of the humeral head to the anterior glenoid rim; grade II, translation of the humeral head just over the rim; and grade III, the ability to move the humeral head over the rim so that the humeral head remains out of the joint when force applied by the examiner is released (Figure 53).[2]

The anterior and posterior drawer tests[33] can be performed in the supine position with the patient's scapula firmly resting on the examination table and the upper extremity positioned free over the side. To begin the anterior drawer test, the examiner stands at the patient's side and holds the extremity between 80° and 120° of abduction, between 0° and 20° of forward flexion, and between 0° and 30° of external rotation. One of the examiner's hands stabilizes the scapula and applies pressure over the anterior aspect of the acromion and humeral head, and the other hand manipulates the proximal humerus in a joystick fashion, translating the humeral head anteriorly and posteriorly. The examiner stabilizes the patient's extremity during this maneuver by holding the hand in his or her axilla (Figure 54).

The posterior drawer test is performed similarly; however, the examiner flexes the elbow of the extremity to 120° and slightly internally rotates the upper extremity. The examiner uses the hand to stabilize the scapula to force the humeral head posteriorly by employing gentle pressure with the thumb just lateral

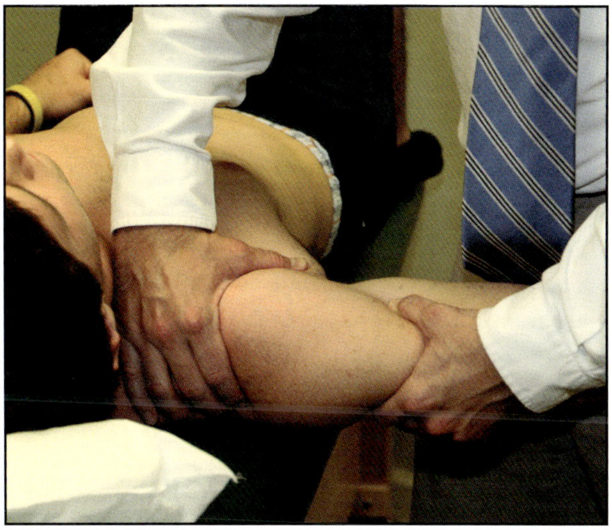

Figure 54. Anterior drawer test.

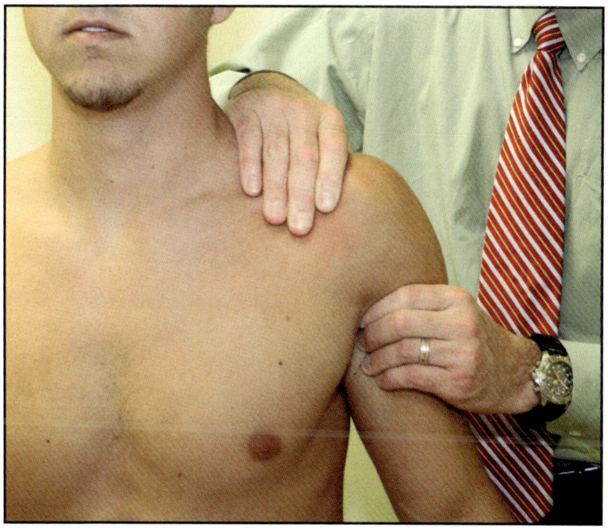

Figure 56. Load-and-shift test.

to the coracoid (Figure 55). This maneuver is designed to translate the head over the posterior glenoid rim. In cases of extreme laxity or instability, the head can remain out of the joint after pressure is relieved.

The load-and-shift test as described by Silliman and Hawkins[34] can be performed with the patient either seated or positioned supine. The examiner is positioned behind the extremity and holds it in approximately 20° of flexion and 20° of abduction. He or she stabilizes the patient's scapula with one hand and grasps the proximal humerus with the other hand. The examiner then provides an axial load to the proximal portion of the upper extremity to seat the humerus

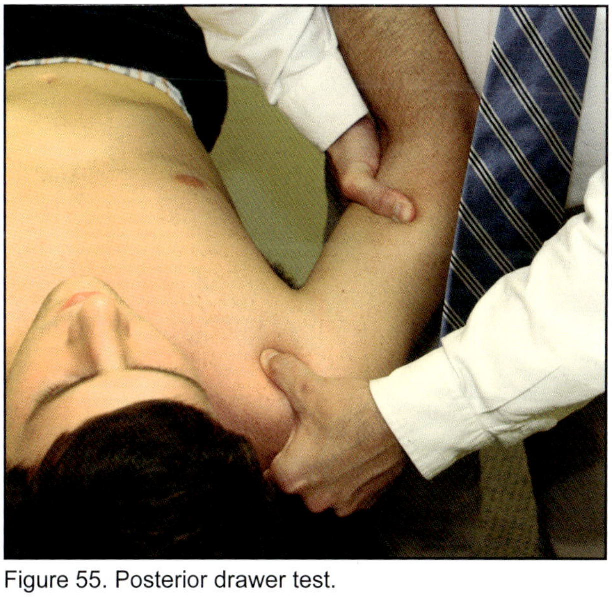

Figure 55. Posterior drawer test.

within the glenoid. Next, he or she applies both anterior and posterior forces to assess for translation of the humeral head across the anterior and posterior glenoid faces, respectively (Figure 56). As with the anterior and posterior drawer tests, this test is used to develop an overall clinical picture and is not graded to determine any specific degree of shoulder laxity or instability.

The sulcus sign[35] is designed to test for inferior laxity. The maneuver is performed with the patient seated, supine, or standing. While positioned in front of the patient, the examiner grasps both extremities just proximal to the elbows and applies a downward force. If inferior shoulder laxity is present, a sulcus will be evident at the anterior portion of the shoulder as the humerus is distracted inferiorly away from the glenoid. The sulcus sign indicates inferior laxity; if it elicits pain, it indicates instability.[2] The distance between the lateral edge of the acromion and the humeral head is observed. With the patient in a sitting position, the upper extremity is first tested with the shoulder internally rotated and the hand resting in the lap. Both upper extremities can be tested simultaneously. Second, the upper extremity is tested in external rotation, and the examiner looks for a change in the magnitude of the sulcus sign (Figure 57). If the patient demonstrates continued increased translation in external rotation, a rotator interval lesion is suspected. Laxity can be graded by measuring the degree of laxity in centime-

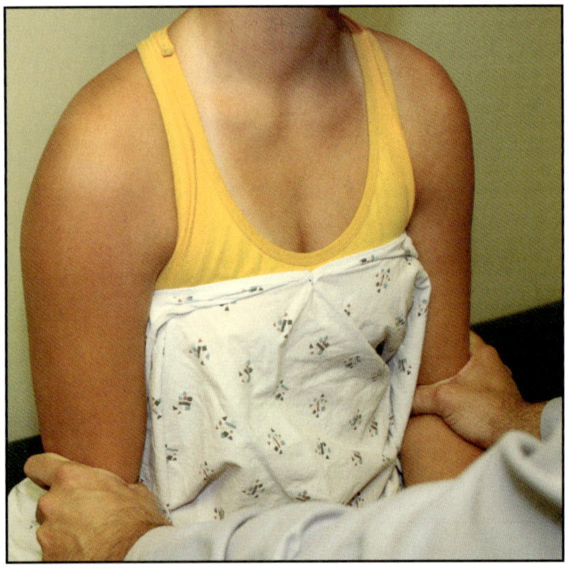

Figure 57A. The sulcus sign tests for inferior laxity.

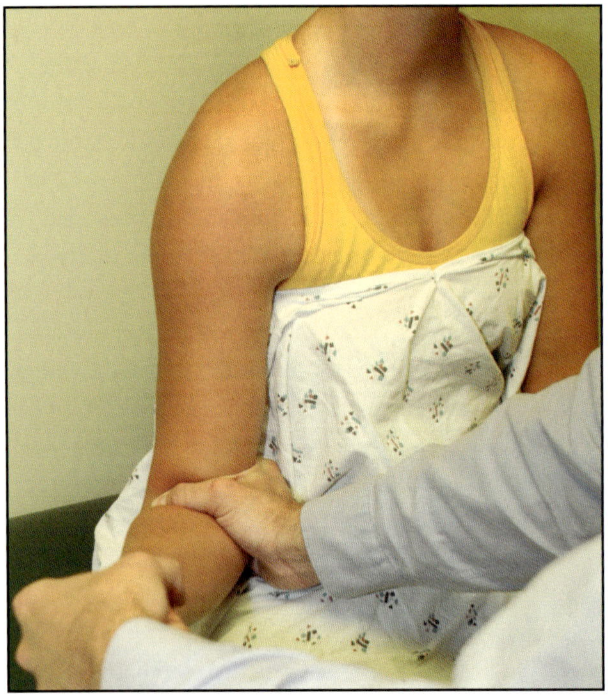

Figure 57B. In external rotation, the sulcus test indicates a rotator interval lesion.

ters. This commonly is classified as grade I (<1.5 cm), grade II (1.5–2.0 cm), and grade III (>2.0 cm). Grading is sometimes simplified to low (<1.5 cm) and high (>1.5 cm). The sulcus sign generally is considered to be a test for evidence of laxity and is not a clinical test for instability.

Instability and Labral Injury. Pathologic shoulder instability is due to a traumatic event or is the cumulative effect of repetitive microtrauma within the glenohumeral joint. Depending on the pattern of instability and direction of stress to which the joint is subjected, the labral tear can be anterior or posterior or can involve the biceps anchor at the superior labrum. When the patient's chief concern centers on painful chronic or traumatic instability, it can be prudent to forego laxity testing for provocative tests that help identify the presence of structural injury to the joint.

In a maneuver similar to the McMurray test for meniscal tears within the knee, the humerus can be manipulated within the glenohumeral joint to elicit pain and an audible and palpable click or "clunk." This maneuver is called the *compression rotation test*[36] and is performed with the patient lying supine. The examiner, who is positioned behind the patient, supports the affected extremity at the elbow and wrist. Gentle compressive force is applied to seat the humerus within the joint as the shoulder is passively circumducted (Figure 58). When a torn labrum is present, the humeral head often captures a flap of tissue as it comes in contact with the glenoid rim, producing this labral click.[37]

The examiner should test for anterior instability with the patient lying supine to allow for a full complement of maneuvers to be accomplished at once while keeping the patient as relaxed as possible. The apprehension test[38] is performed with the examiner standing to the side of the patient and supporting the extremity in abduction and external rotation (Figure 59). As the upper extremity is brought into this "cocking" position, the patient often feels anxiety or apprehension because of the stresses placed on the anterior restraints of the shoulder, making it vulnerable to subluxation or dislocation. When subtle instability is present, the shoulder can be moved into more extreme abduction and external rotation, and an anterior force can be applied to the humerus to elicit discomfort.

Popularized by Jobe et al,[17] the relocation test is used as an adjunct to this maneuver. It is performed with the patient lying supine and the scapula resting firmly on the examination table. The examiner is positioned at the patient's side and supports the affected extremity in abduction and external rotation (Figure 60). The examiner exerts a posteriorly directed force on the proximal humerus, providing a stabilizing force within the glenohumeral joint. Resolution of the feeling of

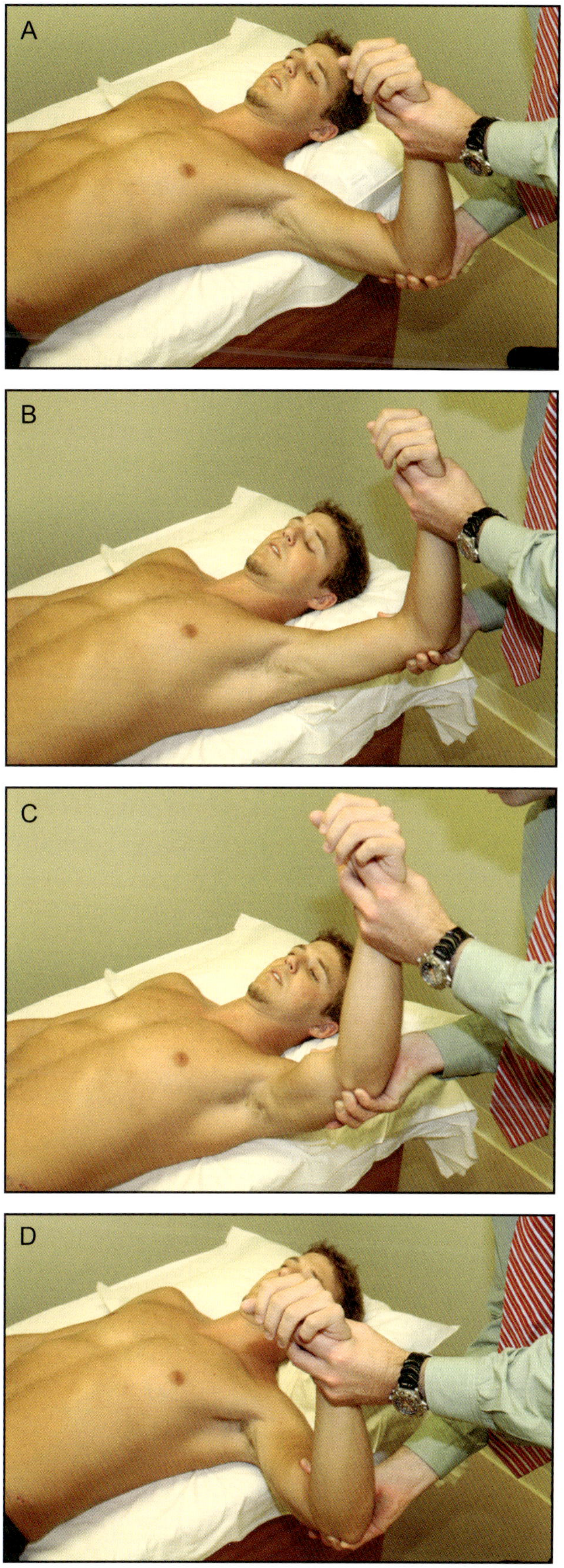

Figure 58 A-D. Compression rotation test.

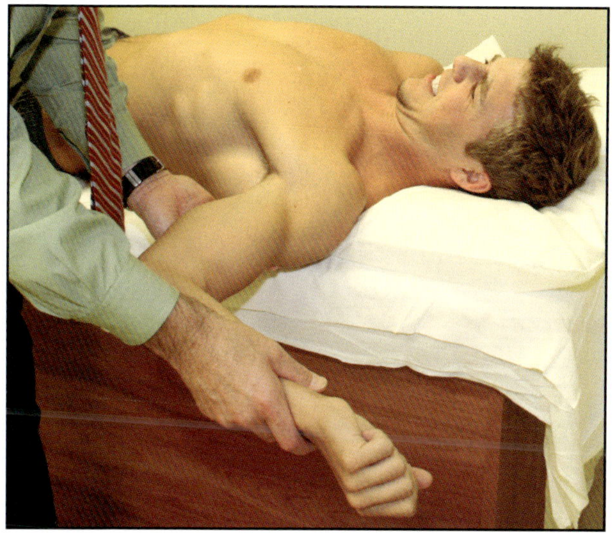

Figure 59. Apprehension test.

apprehension and relief of pain with this maneuver is believed to support the presence of anterior instability. With the posteriorly directed force applied, the examiner should be able to take the extremity into more extreme external rotation if instability rather than other shoulder lesions is the cause of pain.

The surprise,[34] or release, test is performed to help build a case for anterior instability. While positioned at the patient's side, the examiner releases the posteriorly directed force on the proximal humerus (Figure 61). The sudden return of apprehension or pain is a positive finding and supports the diagnosis of anterior shoulder dysfunction.

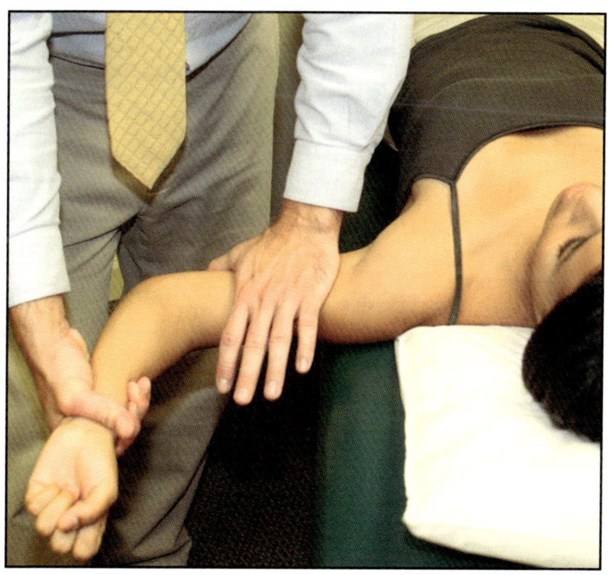

Figure 60. Relocation test.

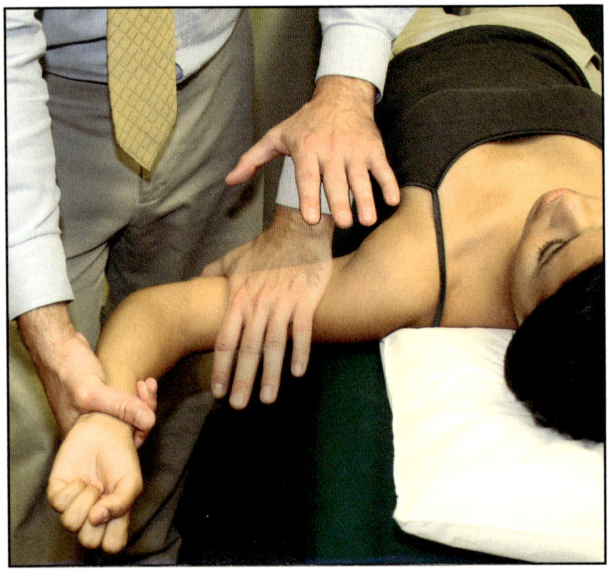

Figure 61. Surprise, or release, test.

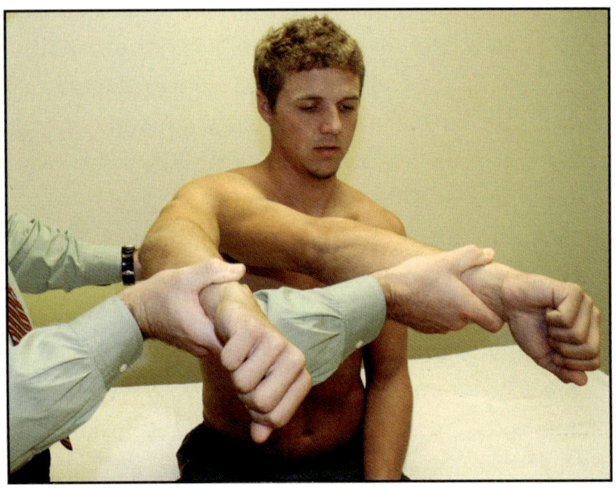

Figure 62. Posterior apprehension test.

Lo et al[39] studied the apprehension, relocation, and surprise tests and found that of the 3, the surprise test most accurately predicted instability and the relocation test was the least reliable in differentiating instability from other forms of shoulder conditions, such as rotator cuff tears. The tests were not performed in isolation but rather in succession, and positive findings on all 3 examinations were highly specific for anterior shoulder instability.[39] This finding supports the notion that this portion of the examination can be considered as 1 test with 3 maneuvers rather than individual tests. The apprehension test should be conducted first to determine the position that elicits the most discomfort. In this way, the relocation and surprise tests provide more useful and accurate information.

Isolated posterior instability and labral lesion is much less commonly encountered in clinical practice. With the posterior apprehension sign described by Kessel, the examiner attempts to elicit pain by placing the extremity in a position to stress the posterior restraints of the shoulder and recreate an episode of instability.[2] The examiner stands to the side of the patient and holds the extremity in 90° of flexion and slight adduction and internal rotation. Next, he or she exerts a posteriorly directed force in an attempt to force the humeral head over the posterior glenoid rim (Figure 62). As in the apprehension test for anterior instability, the patient experiences pain or the feeling of impending shoulder dislocation or subluxation. From this same position, the examiner can perform the jerk test.[19,40] As the humeral head is forced over the posterior glenoid rim, the patient experiences a painful "jerk." The examiner then extends the upper extremity away from the body back to a neutral position. As the humerus reduces back into the glenohumeral joint, a second painful jerk might be elicited from the patient.

Kim et al[41] described the Kim lesion as a superficial tearing of the posterior labrum and glenoid articular cartilage without complete detachment of the labrum. They reported that this "marginal crack" within the labrum was limited to the posteroinferior quadrant of the glenoid in patients with posterior shoulder instability. Kim et al[42] reported on a novel examination to test for this lesion within the posterior labrum. The Kim test is performed with the patient sitting and the examiner positioned beside the patient. The examiner holds the elbow and proximal aspect of the upper extremity sup-

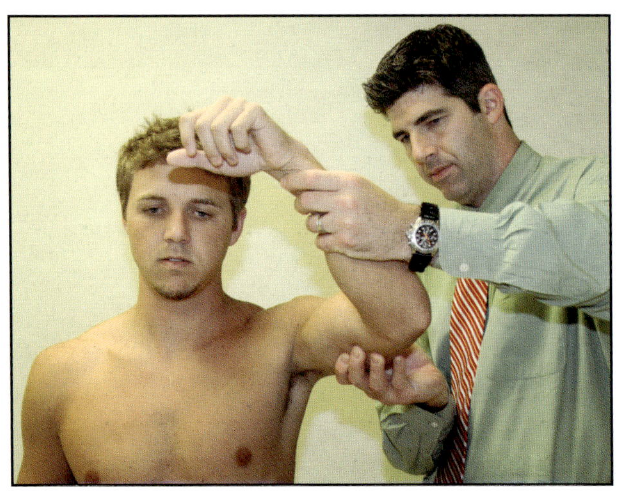

Figure 63. Kim test.

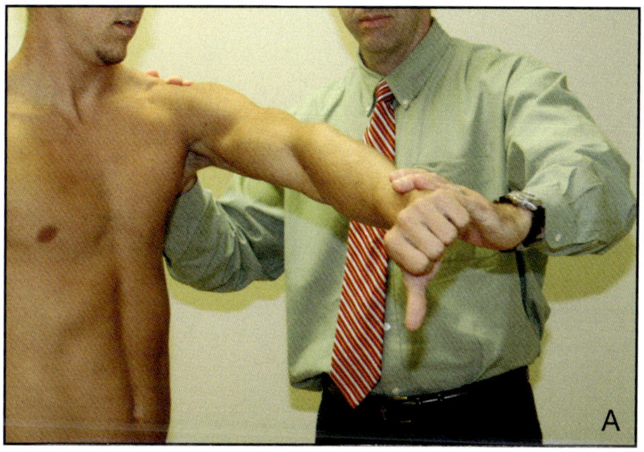

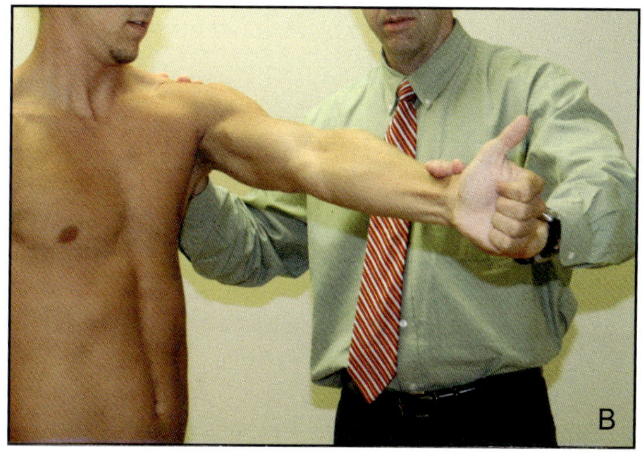

Figure 64. O'Brien test. A, Internal rotation. B, External rotation.

ported in 90° of abduction and angled approximately 45° upward in the frontal plane of the body. He or she then applies a posteroinferiorly directed force to the proximal aspect of the extremity (Figure 63). Even in the absence of an audible or palpable clunk, pain elicited with this maneuver is believed to indicate the presence of this posterior labral injury. Compared with the jerk test for detecting posterior labral lesions, the Kim test was found to be a slightly more sensitive but less specific measure. In addition, they found that when combined, the sensitivity of the 2 tests was 97% for detecting injury to the posteroinferior labrum.[42]

Acromioclavicular Joint

One of the most useful tools to employ when evaluating a patient for AC joint lesions is observation. Swelling or a prominence at the AC joint could indicate recent trauma, infection, and tumor or advanced joint arthrosis. Unlike pain associated with rotator cuff lesions, the patient often feels AC joint pain directly over the joint. When patients who have isolated AC joint disease are asked from where their pain is originating, they commonly point directly to that area of the shoulder.[2] Pain relief provided by an injection of local anesthetic into the AC joint can be a useful diagnostic tool and therapeutic measure.

O'Brien et al[26] described the active compression test (O'Brien test) as a maneuver to detect both AC joint lesions and SLAP lesions. The test is performed in 2 stages both with the patient standing and the examiner positioned either behind or beside the patient. He or she instructs the patient to hold the affected extremity at 90° of forward flexion and slight adduction. With the patient's thumb pointing toward the floor (Figure 64A), the examiner exerts a downward force as the patient resists. Pain generated by this maneuver and felt at the superior aspect of the shoulder is thought to originate from the AC joint; if felt deep within the shoulder, a superior labrum lesion is suspected. Next, the test is repeated with the palm facing upward or in the "thumb up" position (Figure 64B), and a decrease in the level of discomfort should be observed.

The cross-body adduction test is another tool that can help develop a clinical picture when an AC joint lesion is suspected. The examiner stands beside the patient and holds the affected extremity at 90° of forward flexion. The upper extremity then is taken into maximum adduction across the patient's body (Figure 65). This action compresses the AC joint and should reproduce the patient's pain if disease is present there. In addition, the overhead adduction, or cuff integrity, test can be used to assess for contribution of the AC joint to shoulder pain. To perform the overhead adduc-

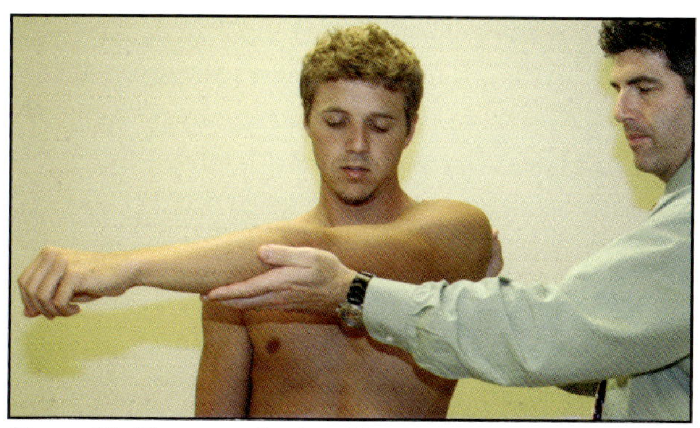

Figure 65. The cross-body adduction test.

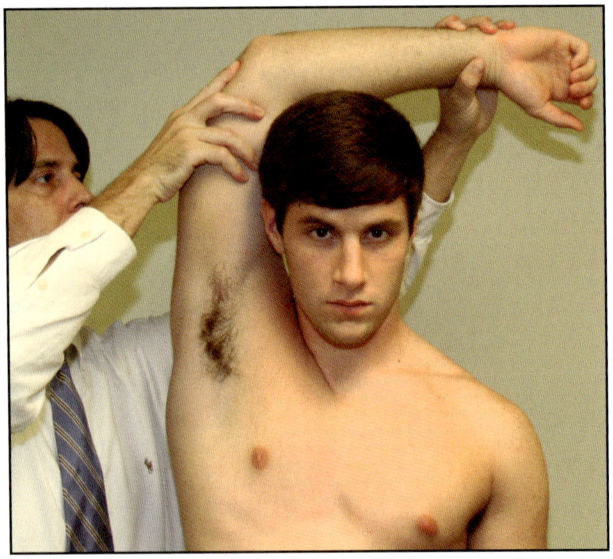

Figure 66. The overhead adduction, or cuff integrity, test.

tion test, the upper extremity is forward flexed to near maximum elevation. Next, it is adducted over the head (Figure 66). A positive test again is marked by pain. Localization of lesions to the AC joint can be accomplished by injection of the joint with local anesthetic. If this relieves the pain found on examination, it identifies the AC joint as the source of pain.

Walton et al[43] described the Paxinos sign to evaluate the AC joint. To perform this test, the examiner stands behind the patient who is either sitting or standing with the upper extremity resting comfortably at the side. The examiner places his or her hand atop the affected shoulder with the thumb positioned on the posterolateral aspect of the acromion and the index finger positioned on the distal clavicle. He or she then applies a gentle force in an anterosuperior direction to the acromion and inferior pressure with the index finger (Figure 67). A positive finding with this test was believed to aid in differentiating pain originating from the AC joint from other forms of shoulder dysfunction.[43] Interestingly, these researchers also showed that, in the presence of a positive Paxinos sign and a positive bone scan indicating AC joint disease, the examiner could have 99% confidence that the AC joint was the source of the shoulder pain.[43]

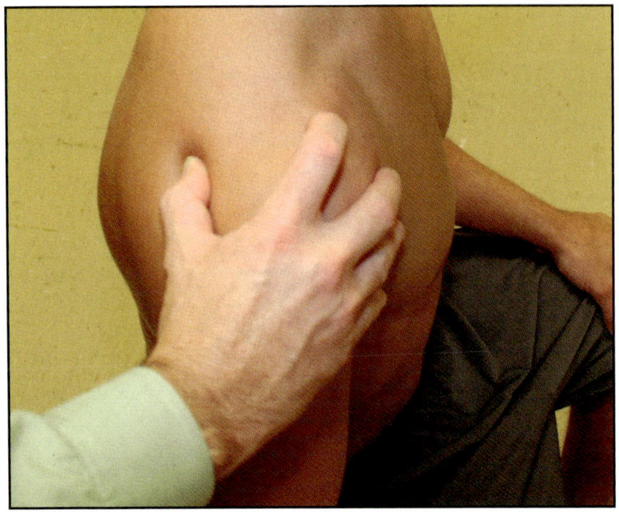

Figure 67. Paxinos sign.

Sternoclavicular Joint

Injuries to the SC joint are infrequent, and the evaluation is fairly routine compared with that of other areas of the shoulder. A history of trauma, including fracture, dislocation, and subluxation, is usually paramount for typical SC joint issues. Inspecting the SC joint and comparing it with the contralateral side provides evidence of swelling and asymmetry with subluxation or anterior dislocation (Figure 68). With posterior dislocation, compression of the great vessels and neck structures can distend neck veins; cause unilateral upper extremity swelling; or affect speaking, breathing, or swallowing. Erythema, tenderness, and warmth around the distal clavicle signify an inflammatory process, such as infection, Freiberg avascular necrosis, tumors, or osteitis condensans. In patients who have had surgery or have generalized ligamentous laxity, voluntary subluxation or crepitus can be demonstrated with simple shoulder movements.

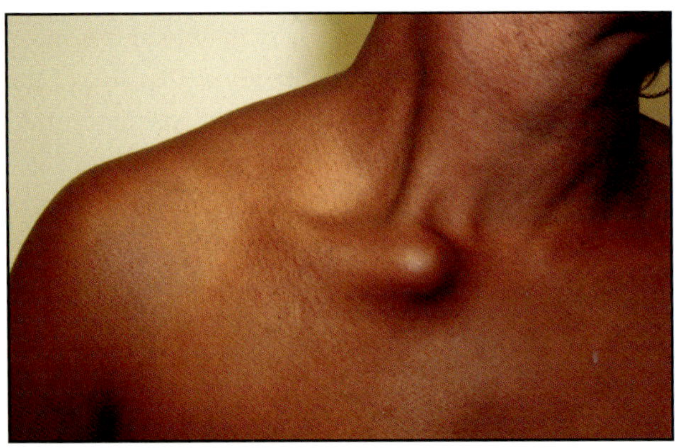

Figure 68. Sternoclavicular joint dislocation.

Scapulothoracic Dysfunction

Although often overlooked, pathologic conditions of the scapula substantially contribute to shoulder dysfunction. Synchronous movement of the glenoid and humerus, contributions of the glenohumeral ligaments and labrum to static stability, and the dynamic stabilizing effect of the rotator cuff on the shoulder have long been the focus of primary shoulder conditions. Asynchronous movements and inhibition or disorganization of activation patterns of scapulothoracic musculature can result from numerous injuries to the shoulder. In addition, primary conditions of the scapulothoracic articulation can manifest in secondary functional shoulder problems.

Examination of scapular movement can be accomplished mostly by simple observation from the posterior aspect. Several specific tests have been derived to make this observation more scientific, but the most accurate measure of scapulothoracic dysfunction combines overall observation for distant contributions to scapular lesions, dynamic evaluation of motion, activation, and corrective maneuvers. Excessive cervical lordosis, increased thoracic kyphosis, increased pelvic tilt, and hip rotational abnormalities can lead to difficulty with scapular protraction and retraction. Long-standing scapular winging can be observed easily in the resting position on the posterior aspect of the thorax. Pure serratus anterior muscle weakness from a long thoracic nerve palsy will create a prominent superomedial border and a depressed acromion (Figure 69). Isolated trapezius weakness from a spinal accessory nerve palsy causes a protracted inferior border and elevated acromion (Figure 70). Motion of the scapula should be assessed by both raising and lowering of the extremity. More subtle scapular dyskinesis can manifest itself as a "hitch," clunk, or jump while lowering the upper extremity. Several cycles should be observed to view true scapular movement and rhythm. Scapular dyskinesis can be classified as type I (prominent inferomedial border), type II (prominent medial scapular border), or type III (prominent superomedial border).[44]

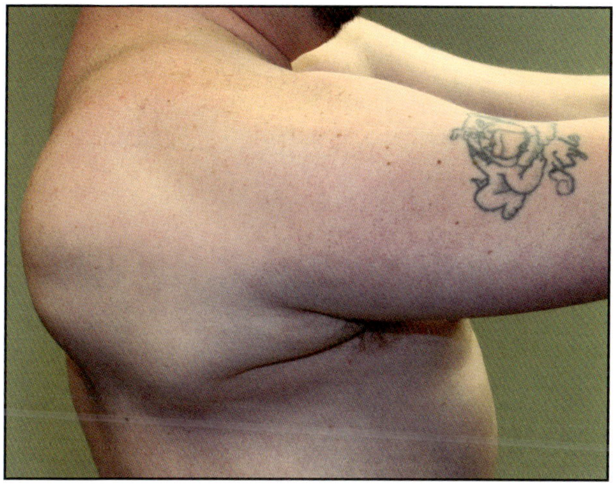

Figure 70. Lateral scapular winging.

Several trigger points can exist where abnormal scapular posture has caused tightness and scarring of certain muscles. Pain with palpation over the coracoid tip signifies a tight pectoralis minor and short head of the biceps associated with scapular dyskinesis. In addition, pain or crepitus over the superomedial border of the scapula can signify an inflamed levator scapulae or trapezius insertion with scarring of the scapulothoracic bursa. Tenderness throughout the course of the trapezius and along the medial border of the scapula also is common with scapular dysfunction. Scapular strength

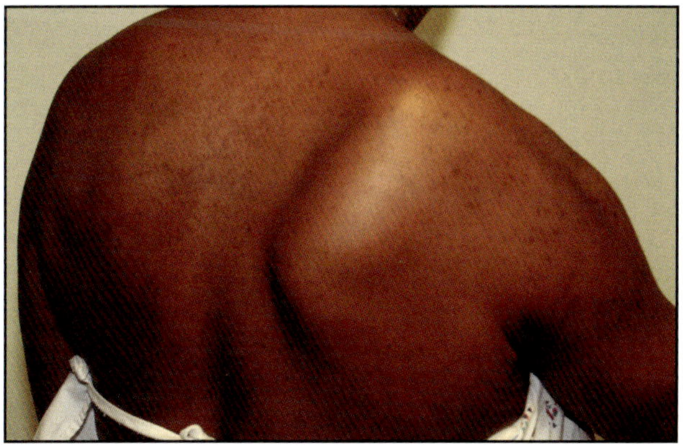

Figure 69. Medial scapular winging.

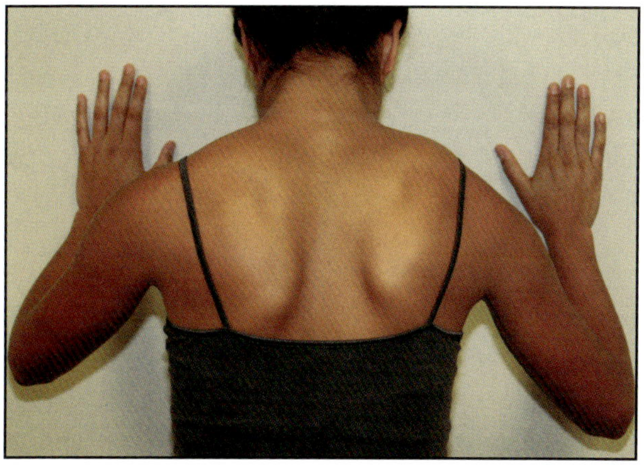

Figure 71. Wall push-ups.

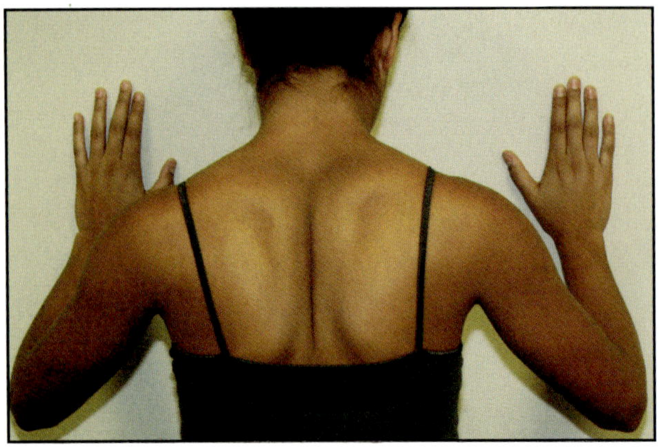

Figure 72. Forced scapular retraction.

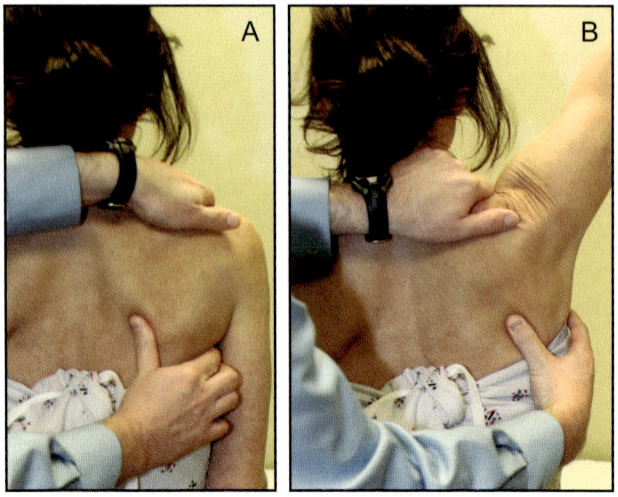

Figure 73 A and B. Scapular assistance test.

is difficult to assess, but wall push-ups and scapular retraction can indicate periscapular muscular strength (Figure 71). Forced scapular retraction, in which both medial borders are pinched together, should be maintained easily (Figure 72). If burning pain occurs after 15 seconds of this maneuver, scapular weakness should be suspected. In addition, scapular winging can become more prominent after 10 wall push-ups in a patient with scapular weakness.

Special tests to assess for scapular contribution to shoulder lesions include the scapular assistance test, scapular flip sign, and scapular retraction test. With the scapular assistance test, contributions of scapular motion abnormalities to impingement are assessed. The examiner manually stabilizes the scapula while rotating the inferior border of the scapula laterally as he or she brings the upper extremity into forward elevation (Figure 73). This motion simulates the force couple of the serratus anterior and trapezius, and elimination of impingement symptoms indicates that these muscles should be the focus of a directed rehabilitation program. The scapular flip sign can be assessed from behind the patient. The examiner resists external rotation of the upper extremity with the extremity in adduction and elbow bent to 90°. Abnormal rotation of the scapula can be observed in various causes of shoulder lesions and indicates poor scapular stabilization (Figure 74). Finally, the scapular retraction test is assessed as the examiner stabilizes the medial border of the retracted scapula and the patient brings the upper extremity into forward elevation (Figure 75). Relief of impingement symptoms indicates a positive test and poor scapular stabilization.

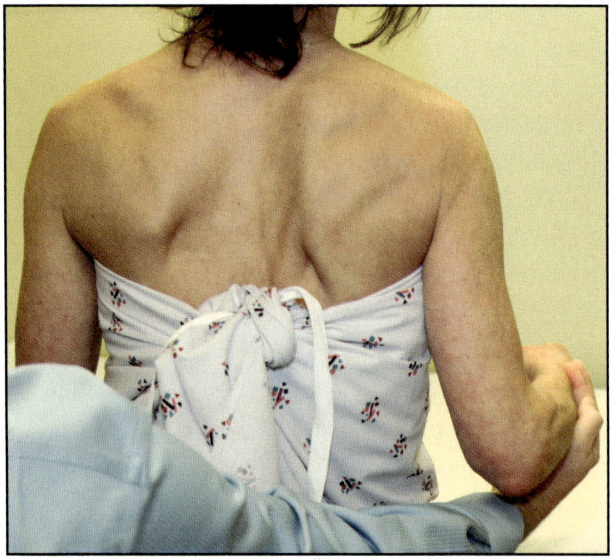

Figure 74. Scapular flip sign.

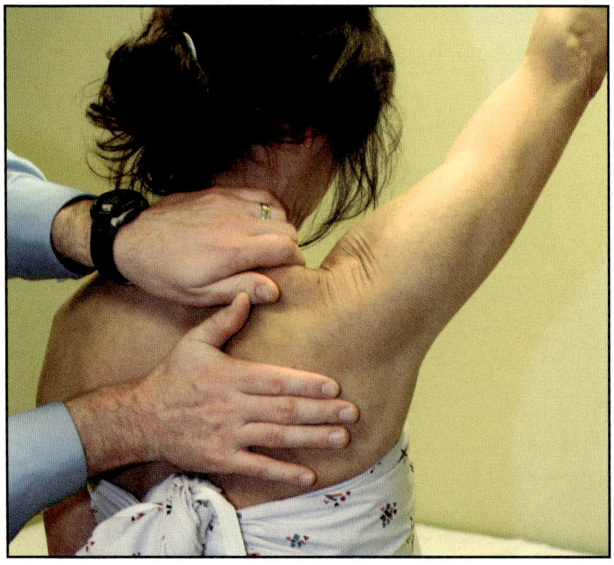

Figure 75. Scapular retraction test.

CONCLUSIONS

The shoulder is a complex joint in which pathologic conditions can be caused by disease processes intrinsic and extrinsic to the shoulder. After an appropriate and efficient clinical history, a complete physical examination can confirm clinical suspicion. By combining the clinical history with a focused general examination and combining the shoulder examination with appropriate inspection, palpation, range of motion, strength, and special tests, the probability increases that the examiner will provide the correct diagnosis and treatment. Whereas each physical examination test holds its own individual merit, the examiner must place all information into the appropriate clinical context to arrive at the correct diagnosis. Imaging studies and ancillary tests can help confirm a diagnosis, but a complete history and physical examination remain the cornerstone in the evaluation of shoulder lesions.

REFERENCES

1. Green A. Chronic massive rotator cuff tears: evaluation and management. *J Am Acad Orthop Surg*. 2003;11(5):321–331.
2. McFarland EG. *Examination of the Shoulder: The Complete Guide*. New York, NY: Thieme Medical Publishers; 2006.
3. Fung M, Kato S, Barrance PJ, et al. Scapular and clavicular kinematics during humeral elevation: a study with cadavers. *J Shoulder Elbow Surg*. 2001;10(3):278–285.
4. McClure PW, Michener LA, Sennett BJ, Karduna AR. Direct 3-dimensional measurements of scapular kinematics during dynamic movements in vivo. *J Shoulder Elbow Surg*. 2001;10(3):269–277.
5. Rockwood CA Jr, Matsen FA III, Wirth MA, Lippitt SB. *The Shoulder*. 3rd ed. Philadelphia, PA: Saunders; 2004.
6. Lyons RP, Green A. Subscapularis tendon tears. *J Am Acad Orthop Surg*. 2005;13(5):353–363.
7. Gerber C, Krushell RJ. Isolated rupture of the tendon of the subscapularis muscle: clinical features in 16 cases. *J Bone Joint Surg Br*. 1991;73(3):389–394.
8. Tokish JM, Decker MJ, Ellis HB, Torry MR, Hawkins RJ. The belly-press test for the physical examination of the subscapularis muscle: electromyographic validation and comparison to the lift-off test. *J Shoulder Elbow Surg*. 2003;12(5):427–430.
9. Scheibel M, Magosch P, Pritsch M, Lichtenberg S, Habermeyer P. The belly-off sign: a new clinical diagnostic sign for subscapularis lesions. *Arthroscopy*. 2005;21(10):1229–1235.
10. Barth JR, Burkhart SS, De Beer JF. The bear-hug test: a new and sensitive test for diagnosing a subscapularis tear. *Arthroscopy*. 2006;22(10):1076–1084.
11. Petilon J, Carr DR, Sekiya JK, Unger DV. Pectoralis major muscle injuries: evaluation and management. *J Am Acad Orthop Surg*. 2005;13(1):59–68.
12. Hoppenfeld S. *Physical Examination of the Spine and Extremities*. East Norwalk, CT: Appleton-Century-Crofts; 1976.
13. Neer CS II. Anterior acromioplasty for the chronic impingement syndrome in the shoulder: a preliminary report. *J Bone Joint Surg Am*. 1972;54(1):41–50.
14. Bigliani LU, Morrison DS, April EW. The morphology of the acromion and rotator cuff impingement. *Orthop Trans*. 1986;10:288.
15. Walch GA, Boileau P, Noel E, Donell ST. Impingement of the deep surface of the supraspinatus tendon on the posterosuperior glenoid rim: an arthroscopic study. *J Shoulder Elbow Surg*. 1992;1(5):238–245.
16. Jobe CM. Posterior superior glenoid impingement: expanded spectrum. *Arthroscopy*. 1995;11(5):530–536.
17. Jobe CM, Coen MJ, Screnar P. Evaluation of impingement syndromes in the overhead-throwing athlete. *J Athl Train*. 2000;35(3):293–299.
18. Gerber C, Terrier F, Ganz R. The role of the coracoid process in the chronic impingement syndrome. *J Bone Joint Surg Br*. 1985;67(5):703–708.
19. Itoi E, Minagawa H, Yamamoto N, Seki N, Abe H. Are pain location and physical examinations useful in locating a tear site of the rotator cuff? *Am J Sports Med*. 2006;34(2):256–264.
20. Hertel R, Ballmer FT, Lombert SM, Gerber C. Lag signs in the diagnosis of rotator cuff rupture. *J Shoulder Elbow Surg*. 1996;5(4):307–313.
21. Otis JC, Jiang CC, Wickiewicz TL, Peterson MG, Warren RF, Santner TJ. Changes in the moment arms of the rotator cuff and deltoid muscles with abduction and rotation. *J Bone Joint Surg Am*. 1994;76(5):667–676.
22. Walch GA, Boulahia A, Calderone S, Robinson AH. The "dropping" and "hornblower's" signs in evaluation of rotator-cuff tears. *J Bone Joint Surg Br*. 1998;80(4):624–628.
23. Nam EK, Snyder SJ. The diagnosis and treatment of superior labrum, anterior and posterior (SLAP) lesions. *Am J Sports Med*. 2003;31(5):798–810.
24. Andrews JR, Carson WG Jr, McLeod WD. Glenoid labrum tears related to the long head of the biceps. *Am J Sports Med*. 1985;13(5):337–341.
25. Snyder SJ, Karzel RP, Del Pizzo W, Ferkel RD, Friedman MJ. SLAP lesions of the shoulder. *Arthroscopy*. 1990;6(4):274–279.
26. O'Brien SJ, Pagnani MJ, Fealy S, McGlynn SR, Wilson JB. The active compression test: a new and effective test for diagnosing labral tears and acromioclavicular joint abnormality. *Am J Sports Med*. 1998;26(5):610–613.
27. D'Alessandro DF, Fleischli JE, Connor PM. Superior labral lesions: diagnosis and management. *J Athl Train*. 2000;35(3):286–292.
28. Parentis MA, Glousman RE, Mohr KS, Yocum LA. An evaluation of the provocative tests for superior labral anterior posterior lesions. *Am J Sports Med*. 2006;34(2):265–268.
29. Kibler WB. Specificity and sensitivity of the anterior slide test in throwing athletes with superior glenoid labral tears. *Arthroscopy*. 1995;11(3):296–300.
30. Myers TH, Zemanovic JR, Andrews JR. The resisted supination external rotation test: a new test for the diagnosis of superior labral anterior posterior lesions. *Am J Sports Med*. 2005;33(9):1315–1320.
31. Steinbeck J, Liljenqvist U, Jerosch J. The anatomy of the glenohumeral ligamentous complex and its contribution to anterior shoulder stability. *J Shoulder Elbow Surg*. 1998;7(2):122–126.

32. Richards RR, An KN, Bigliani LU, et al. A standardized method for the assessment of shoulder function. *J Shoulder Elbow Surg*. 1994;3(6):347–352.
33. Gerber C, Ganz R. Clinical assessment of instability of the shoulder: with special reference to the anterior and posterior drawer tests. *J Bone Joint Surg Br*. 1984;66(4):551–556.
34. Silliman JF, Hawkins RJ. Classification and physical diagnosis of instability of the shoulder. *Clin Orthop Relat Res*. 1993;291:7–19.
35. Neer CS II, Foster CR. Inferior capsular shift for involuntary inferior and multidirectional instability of the shoulder: a preliminary report. *J Bone Joint Surg Am*. 1980;62(6):897–908.
36. Snyder SJ, Karzel RP, Del Pizzo W, Ferkel RD, Friedman MJ. SLAP lesions of the shoulder. *Arthroscopy*. 1990;6(4):274–279.
37. Satterwhite YE. Evaluation and management of recurrent anterior shoulder instability. *J Athl Train*. 2000;35(3):273–277.
38. Magee DJ. *Orthopaedic Physical Examination*. 2nd ed. Philadelphia, PA: WB Saunders; 1992.
39. Lo IK, Nonweiler B, Woolfrey M, Litchfield R, Kirkley A. An evaluation of the apprehension, relocation, and surprise tests for anterior shoulder instability. *Am J Sports Med*. 2004;32(2):301–307.
40. Kim SH, Park JC, Park JS, Oh I. Painful jerk test: a predictor of success in nonoperative treatment of posteroinferior instability of the shoulder. *Am J Sports Med*. 2004;32(8):1849–1855.
41. Kim SH, Ha KI, Yoo JC, Noh KC. Kim's lesion: an incomplete and concealed avulsion of the posteroinferior labrum in posterior and multidirectional posteroinferior instability of the shoulder. *Arthroscopy*. 2004;20(7):712–720.
42. Kim SH, Park JS, Jeong WK, Shin SK. The Kim test: a novel test for posteroinferior labral lesion of the shoulder. A comparison to the jerk test. *Am J Sports Med*. 2005;33(8):1188–1192.
43. Walton J, Mahajan S, Paxinos A, et al. Diagnostic values of tests for acromioclavicular joint pain. *J Bone Joint Surg Am*. 2004;86(4):807–812.
44. Kibler WB, Uhl TL, Maddux JW, Brooks PV, Zeller B, McMullen J. Qualitative clinical evaluation of scapular dysfunction: a reliability study. *J Shoulder Elbow Surg*. 2002;11(6):550–556.

I-3

Rotator Cuff Lesions

Cari L. Cordell, MD, and George M. McCluskey III, MD

PERTINENT ANATOMY

The rotator cuff comprises a group of 4 muscles: the supraspinatus, infraspinatus, teres minor, and subscapularis (Figure 1). The tendon of each muscle is attached to a specific location on the humerus to assist in range of motion of the shoulder. The rotator cuff also collectively compresses the humeral head into the glenoid fossa and stabilizes the glenohumeral joint (Figure 2). The supraspinatus arises from the superior aspect of the scapula above the scapular spine, extends laterally, and inserts onto the anterosuperior aspect of the greater tuberosity (Figure 2). Its main action is forward elevation with maximum effort at 30° of elevation. The infraspinatus originates from the scapula below the scapular spine and inserts onto the greater tuberosity posterior to the supraspinatus (Figure 3). This muscle is 1 of the 2 main external rotators of the humerus. The teres minor, which is the other main

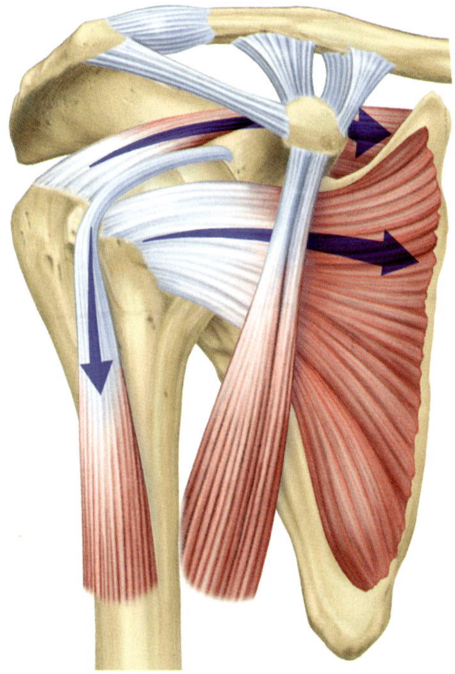

Figure 2. Anterior view of glenohumeral joint rotator cuff muscle force couples causing humeral head compression.

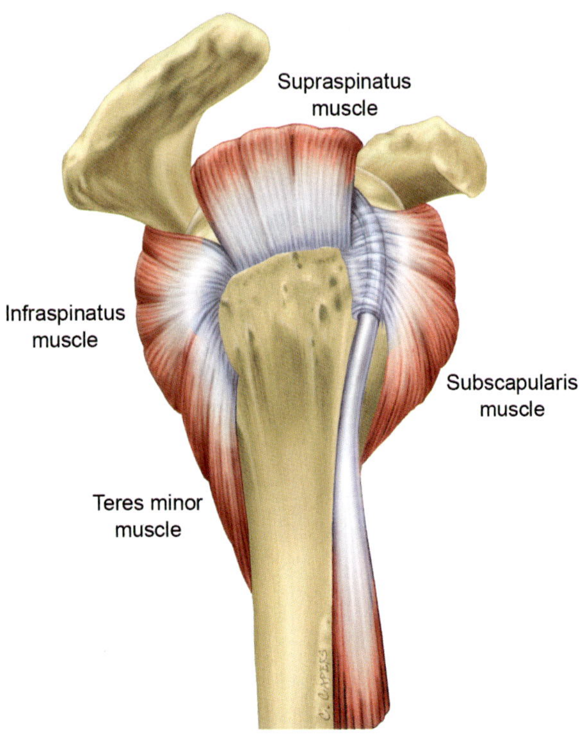

Figure 1. Lateral view of rotator cuff muscle insertions.

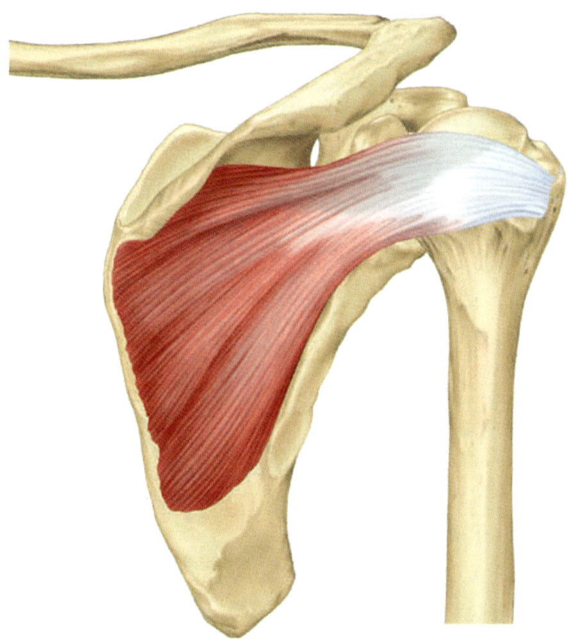

Figure 3. Posterior view of infraspinatus muscle origin and insertion.

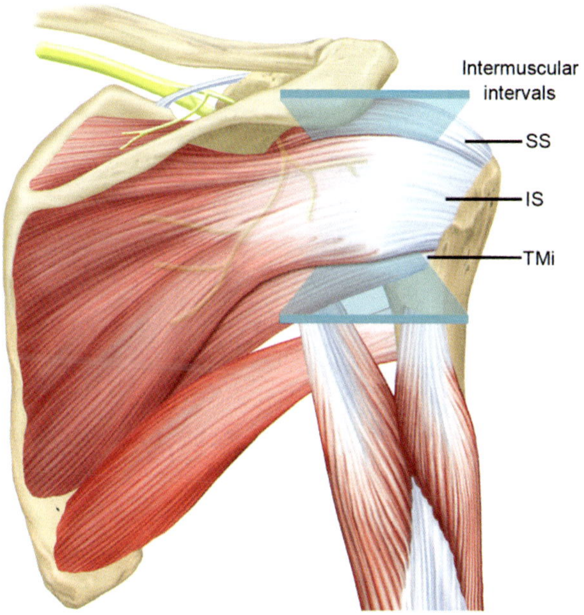

Figure 4. Teres minor muscle (TMi) origin and insertion and its relationship to the supraspinatus (SS) and infraspinatus (IS) tendon insertions.

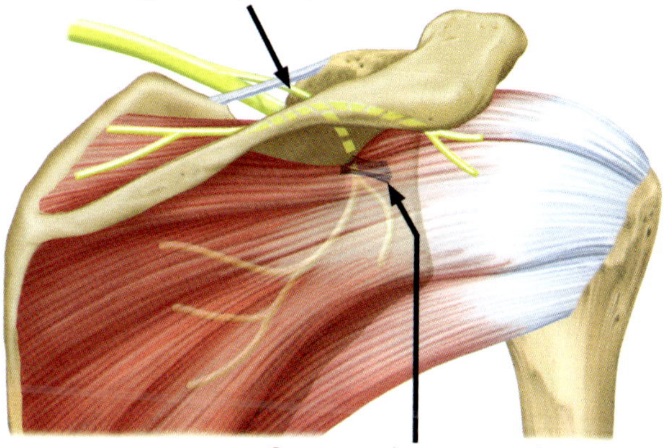

Figure 6. Suprascapular innervation of the supraspinatus and infraspinatus muscles.

external rotator, arises from the lateral border of the scapula and inserts on the lower portion of the posterior aspect of the greater tuberosity (Figure 4). The subscapularis originates from the anterior surface of the scapula. Most of the tendon inserts on the lesser tuberosity, and a smaller portion inserts below the lesser tuberosity on the humerus (Figure 5). It functions as an internal rotator of the humerus.

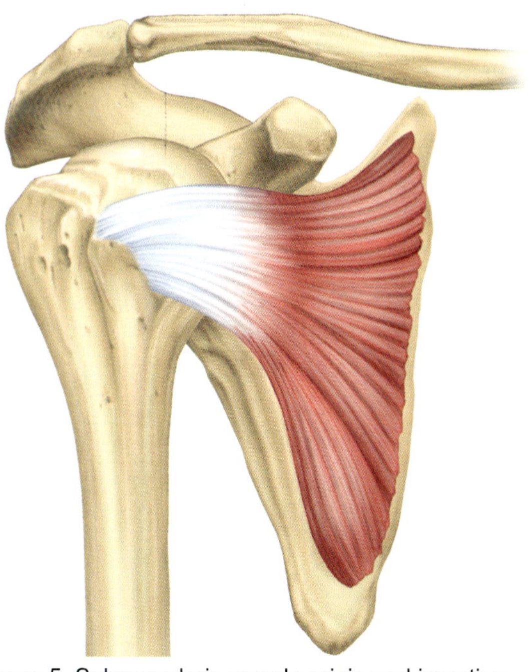

Figure 5. Subscapularis muscle origin and insertion.

The suprascapular nerve supplies both the supraspinatus and infraspinatus muscles. The supraspinatus is supplied by the nerve after it passes through the suprascapular notch, and the infraspinatus is supplied after the nerve passes through the spinoglenoid notch. A branch of the axillary nerve supplies the teres minor. The upper and lower subscapular nerves supply the subscapularis muscle (Figure 6).

Five distinct histologic layers of the rotator cuff have been described.[1] The second and third layers comprise tendinous fibers. The fibers are oriented parallel to the axes of the supraspinatus and infraspinatus in the second layer and are oriented obliquely in the third layer. The first, fourth, and fifth layers comprise loose connective tissue and have an abundance of arterioles. This possibly could predispose the inner and outer layers to partial tearing. Investigators have shown that the tensile strength is lower in the articular side than the bursal side of the supraspinatus, further predisposing it to tearing.[2]

The clinician must know the measurements of the rotator cuff footprint to determine the size and percentage of the partial-thickness rotator cuff tear. This information helps direct treatment. Dugas et al[3] determined the medial insertion of the supraspinatus tendon averages 12.7 mm and the lateral insertion averages 12.1 mm. Therefore, they concluded a tear of greater than 7 mm represents a partial-thickness tear of greater than 50% of the tendon's thickness. Mochizuki et al[4] suggested the supraspinatus footprint is smaller, with a medial-to-lateral insertion width equal to 6.9 mm and an anterior-to-posterior width equal to 12.6 mm. The authors stated the infraspinatus covered most of the tuberosity.[4] Most investigators agree that a tear equal to or greater than 6 mm represents a tear of 50% of the tendon's thickness. These findings suggest a normal variation in the thickness of the tendon and the insertional footprint.

The vascularity of the cuff has been studied in great detail (Figure 7). When investigating the blood supply of the rotator cuff, Rothman and Parke[5] revealed contributions from the suprascapular artery and the anterior and posterior circumflex arteries. Moseley[6] described a rich anastomosis between osseous and tendonous vessel. However, a hypovascular area of the supraspinatus tendon near its insertion site also has been described.[7] Researchers have found this hypovascular area is on the articular side of the cuff.[8,9] In their cadaveric study, Rathbun and Macnab[10] revealed that perfusion of the rotator cuff depended on the position of the upper extremity and proposed that in earlier studies in which researchers suggested hypovascularity of the rotator cuff, the upper extremity was positioned in adduction. In contrast, more recent investigators performing laser Doppler studies have shown substantial blood flow at the critical zone of insertion and an increase in blood flow at the margin of cuff tears.[11] Authors of histologic studies also have shown no areas of avascularity of the supraspinatus tendon.[1,12,13] However, when using ultrasound to evaluate 31 shoulders, Rudzki et al[14] found decreased blood flow to the supraspinatus tendon in patients more than 40 years of age. They also noted increased blood flow in all patients with exercise.[14]

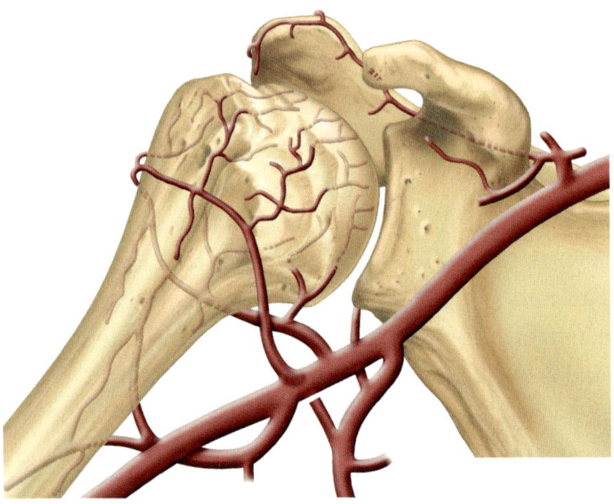

Figure 7. Vascularity of the humeral head.

PATHOPHYSIOLOGY

The pathogenesis of rotator cuff tears is multifactorial. Factors associated with tears largely can be divided into 2 main groups. Extrinsic factors are associated with tears that are not related to the rotator cuff tendon. Intrinsic factors are associated with changes within the tendon.

Genetic factors might play a role in the development of a rotator cuff tear. Researchers have suggested a possible predisposition to tendon degeneration due to apoptosis and regenerative capacity.[15,16] When comparing siblings with unrelated individuals, full-thickness tears were more likely present in asymptomatic siblings with documented tears than in unrelated participants.[16] The size of full-thickness tears also was more likely to progress in siblings.

Demographics also play an important role in developing a rotator cuff tear. Most importantly, increasing age greatly increases the risk. Using ultrasound to evaluate both shoulders in 588 patients with unilateral shoulder pain, Yamaguchi et al[17] found a high correlation between the onset of rotator cuff disease and increasing age. Onset occurred at an average age of 48.7 years for patients with no rotator cuff tears, 58.7 years for patients with unilateral tears, and 67.8 years for patients with bilateral tears. Patients who had a symptomatic tear after 60 years of age had a 50% chance of having a rotator cuff tear in the other shoulder. In patients who had symptomatic rotator cuff tears in one shoulder and asymptomatic tears in the other shoulder, the symptomatic tears were 30% larger than the asymptomatic tears. Overall, patients who presented with full-thickness, symptomatic tears had a 35.5% prevalence of full-thickness tears on the contralateral side.[17]

Wendelboe et al[18] reported that body mass index (BMI) is associated with the development of a rotator cuff tear. An elevated BMI is associated with an increased risk for rotator cuff tendinitis and the need for surgery to treat rotator cuff lesions. People with BMIs greater than 35 had the highest odds ratio, and the risk increased with the degree of obesity.

Coexisting medical conditions also play a role in the development of a rotator cuff tear. Northover et al[19] found that a history of diabetes increased the risk. Chen et al[20] compared the results of patients who had type 1 diabetes and rotator cuff tears and of patients who did not have diabetes.[20] Ninety percent of the group with diabetes and 93% of the control group had good-to-excellent results. The authors found that although the results were similar, the group with diabetes had more postoperative complications.[20]

Hypercholesterolemia recently has been associated with the development of rotator cuff disease. Abboud and Kim[21] obtained the cholesterol levels of 160 patients evaluated for shoulder pain and found rotator cuff tears in 74 patients. Sixty-three percent of the patients with rotator cuff tears and 28% of patients without tears had elevated cholesterol. In the rotator cuff tear group, triglycerides and low-density lipoprotein concentrations were higher, and high-density lipoprotein were lower. The mechanism that investigators have proposed suggests normal connective tissue is susceptible to focal deposition of cholesterol in the elderly population. This creates cholesterol deposits in the tendon that effectively alter the mechanical properties, contributing to the intrinsic mechanism of tendon failure. The increased cholesterol also alters the extracellular matrix, which might lead to increased tendon injury and impaired healing.

Cigarette smoking increases the risk for developing a rotator cuff tear.[22,23] In their ultrasound examination of 586 consecutive patients with shoulder pain, Baumgarten et al[22] found that 375 patients had rotator cuff tears. The association between smoking and the presence of a rotator cuff tear was strong and was dependent on dose and time. A history of smoking and smoking within the 10 years before the study was correlated with an increased risk for a rotator cuff tear.

Kane et al[23] evaluated the shoulders of and performed lung biopsies for 72 cadavers to determine the incidence of rotator cuff disease in smokers and nonsmokers. They found rotator cuff lesions in 36 shoulders; 23 shoulders were from smokers, and 13 were from nonsmokers. The authors concluded the incidence of rotator cuff tears is almost double in smokers than nonsmokers.

A cycle exists between intrinsic and extrinsic factors. Intrinsic factors include age-related tendon changes. A loss of cellularity occurs, and the vascularity is altered with time. The fibrocartilage mass at the insertion is altered and might become calcified. With age, the collagen fibers become thin and disoriented. Myxoid and hyaline degeneration and fatty infiltration occur. Chondroid metaplasia is seen at the rotator cuff insertion site. Age-related changes in the bone, including a disruption of Sharpey fibers and the development of osteoporotic bone at the insertion site, occur.

The collagen is altered in a diseased cuff. In a healthy cuff, the central zone is mostly type 1 collagen with smaller amounts of type 3.[24] The fibrocartilagenous zone of insertion is type 2 collagen, which can withstand compressive loads. In the diseased cuff, an increase in type 3 collagen and decrease in type 2 are found at the fibrocartilagenous zone of insertion. Degenerative changes primarily occur in the middle and articular layers of the torn rotator cuff. Shear forces with loading have been found to be the greatest at the articular layer near the insertion site.[24] Granulation tissue at the site further weakens the cuff tissue.

Another intrinsic mechanism is microtrauma. Mechanical stress causes small injuries to the rotator cuff tendon in the form of microtears. Before healing occurs, a second insult leads to more damage. If the microtears occur in the leading edge of the supraspinatus tendon, more load is placed across the adjacent tendon fibers, and less insult is necessary to exceed the load to failure. This is known as the *zipper phenomenon*.

In the rat model, overuse from eccentric muscle loading causes changes in the supraspinatus tendon. An added insult to overuse leads to changes in the histologic and mechanical properties of the rotator cuff. Other researchers have shown an accumulation of reactive oxygen species ultimately leads to increased apoptosis or cell death.[25] Yuan et al[26] reported a 34% increase in the proportion of apoptotic cells at the edge of a rotator cuff tear compared with the proportion in the control group. Researchers have shown an imbalance of muscle-fiber diameter and distribution in the supraspinatus muscles of patients with symptomatic rotator cuff tears.[27] Fast-twitch muscle fibers are affected more than slow-twitch fibers. Therefore, the form and function of the rotator cuff is altered. This leads to dynamic instability of the rotator cuff.

Nho et al[25] described the neural theory of tendinopathy as a potential mechanism for rotator cuff tears. According to their theory, overuse leads to neural overstimulation with increased glutamate-signaling proteins, increased apoptosis, and increased substance P. Recruitment of inflammatory cells and reorganization of rotator cuff architecture result. Structural weakness within the rotator cuff followed by damage occurs.

Extrinsic changes involve processes outside of the tendon. Subacromial impingement was first postulated by Neer and Poppen[28] based on their intraoperative observations (Figure 8). They described swelling of the tendon and thickening of the subacromial bursa. They also noted spurring on the acromion and insertion of the coracoacromial ligament. Bigliani et al[29] described the 3 types of acromions based on cadaveric dissections. They noted type I, or a flat acromion, represented 17% of the specimens; type II, or curved, represented 43%; and type III represented 39% (Figure 9). Researchers have debated about whether the type of acromion is congenital or developmental. Yazici et al[30] suggested that types II and III are acquired with age and result from traction spurs that lie within the coracoacromial ligament. Neer introduced this concept, but more recently, specimens from surgery of the coracoacromial ligament have shown chondroid metaplasia near the acromial insertion, suggesting this ligament becomes the hook by enchondral ossification.

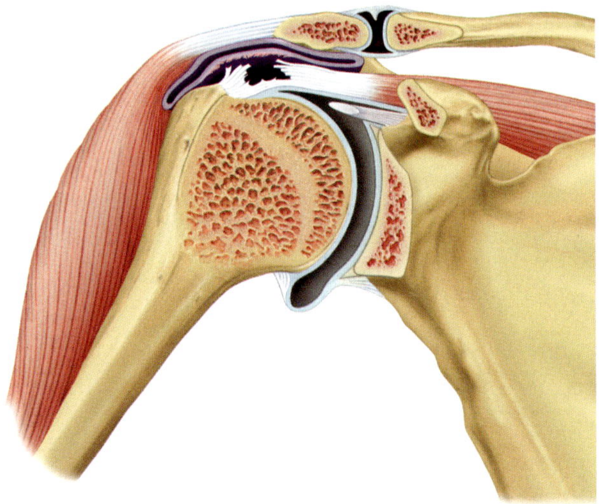

Figure 8. Extrinsic changes include subacromial impingement, subacromial bursa thickening, and acromial spurs.

Internal, or posterosuperior, impingement involves the posterosuperior glenoid rim, capsule, and rotator cuff (Figure 10). The possible causes include a tight posterior capsule, anterior instability, microinstability, reduced humeral retroversion, and scapular dyskinesis.

Gerber and Sebesta[31] described anterosuperior internal impingement due to combined lesions of the biceps pulley and the superior articular surface of the subscapularis tendon (Figure 11). The biceps pulley includes the superior glenohumeral ligament and the coracohumeral ligament. The authors showed that impingement of the undersurface of the pulley and of the subscapularis tendon occurs against the anterosuperior glenoid rim in a position of flexion and internal rotation of the extremity.[31] When lesions of the pulley or the subscapularis tendon were present, they could be shown to contact corresponding lesions of the anterosuperior glenoid labrum in the flexion and internal position of the extremity.

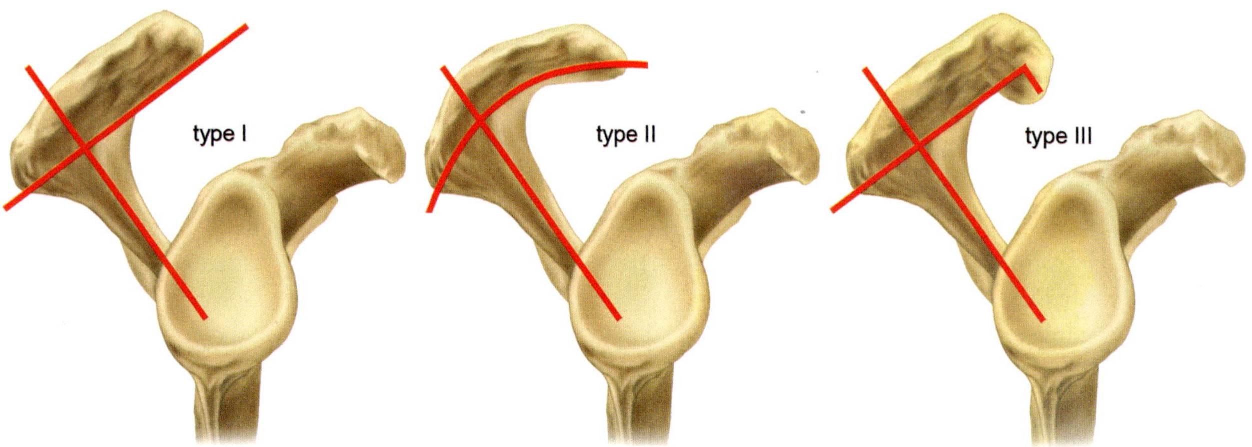

Figure 9. Three types of acromions.

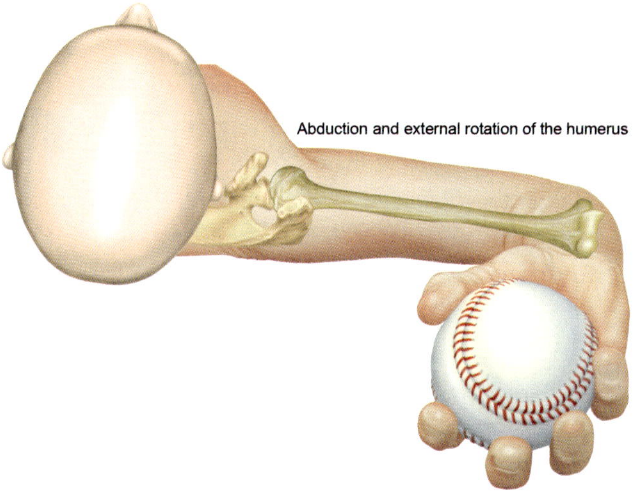

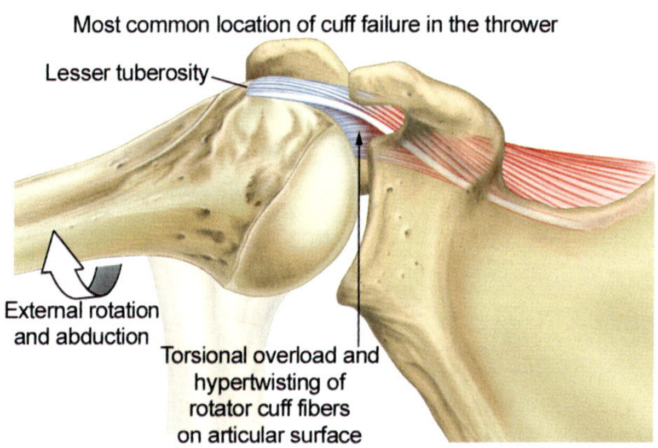

Figure 10. Posterosuperior external impingement.

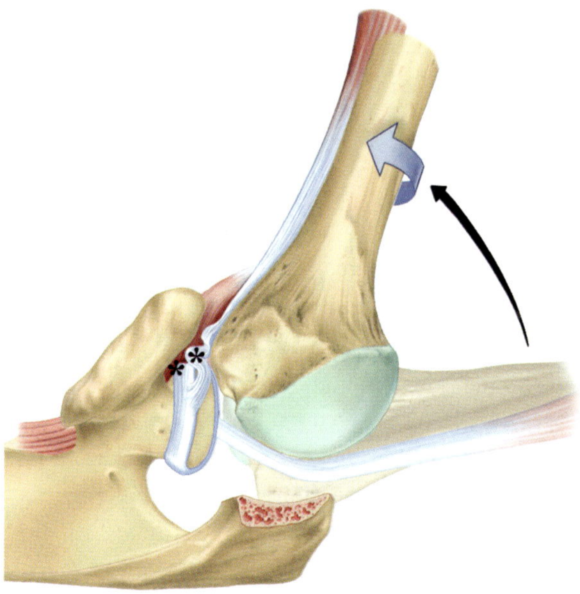

Figure 11. Anterosuperior internal impingement. * Point of impingement at the undersurface of the biceps pulley and subscapularis tendon against the anterosuperior glenoid rim during flexion and internal rotation of the extremity.

Direct trauma is a well-known cause of rotator cuff injury (Figure 12). A fall or a dislocation can cause a rotator cuff tear. The incidence of a rotator cuff tear with a dislocation is correlated directly with increasing age. Individuals have a 30% chance of sustaining a rotator cuff tear with a dislocation in the fourth decade of life, and the risk increases to 60% in the sixth decade of life. In other words, as patients age, they are more likely to develop a cuff tear with an anterior shoulder dislocation.

NATURAL HISTORY

The natural history of rotator cuff tears has been studied in great detail. Little evidence for spontaneous healing of a full-thickness tear exists in humans. A small partial-thickness tear has the greatest potential to heal. Based on scientific data, a tear most likely will progress with time, but the rate of progression is highly variable.

In their review of patients with asymptomatic tears, Yamaguchi et al[32] found the rate of progression was 50% at 5 years if the tear became symptomatic. In other words, 51% (23 of 45 patients) of the previously asymptomatic patients developed symptoms at a mean of 2.8 years. The rate of progression was 22% at 5 years if the tear remained asymptomatic. No patient in their study had a decrease in the size of the tear. The authors concluded the risk of tear size progression increases with time.

In contrast, Yamanaka and Matsumoto[33] studied patients with partial-thickness rotator cuff tears at 1 year after treatment and found the tears had enlarged in 50% of the patients and had progressed to full-thickness

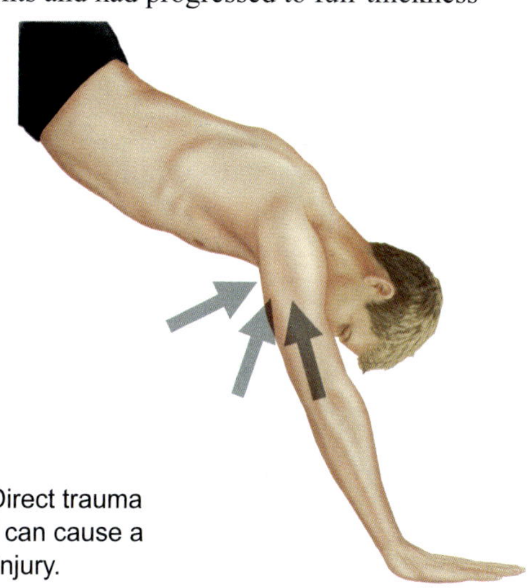

Figure 12. Direct trauma due to a fall can cause a rotator cuff injury.

tears in 25%. The tear was smaller in 10% of patients, and the partial-thickness tear had healed in 10%. Clinical and functional scores improved for all groups at 1-year follow-up.

Structural changes occur within the torn rotator cuff tendon and muscle. Retraction of the tendon from the bone occurs with time and is related more to the configuration than the size of the tear (Figure 13). The muscle becomes denervated, and muscle atrophy develops. Fatty infiltration within the muscle becomes evident (Figure 14); therefore, the rotator cuff becomes stiff and loses its elasticity. After an unknown period, some patients develop rotator cuff arthropathy.

Meyer et al[34] used magnetic resonance imaging (MRI) to evaluate the asymmetric atrophy of the supraspinatus tendon after a rotator cuff tear. With MRI, they examined the distribution of muscle atrophy and fatty infiltration in 64 shoulders and found that the muscular changes were asymmetric. The muscle portion originating from the fascia primarily atrophied, whereas the muscle portion originating from the scapula primarily underwent fatty infiltration. In contrast, atrophy with disuse or denervation is symmetric.

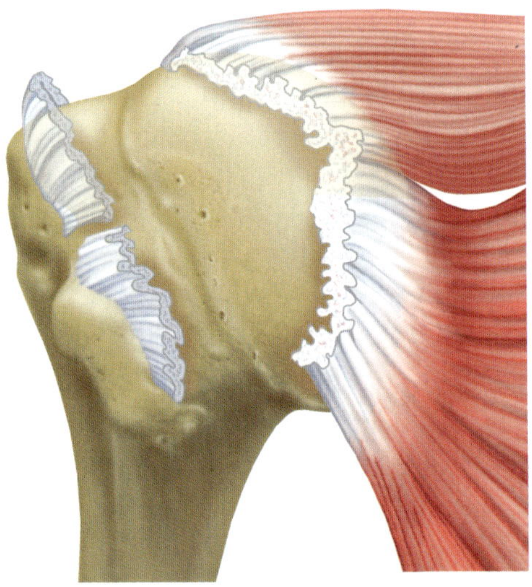

Figure 13. Retraction of tendon from bone.

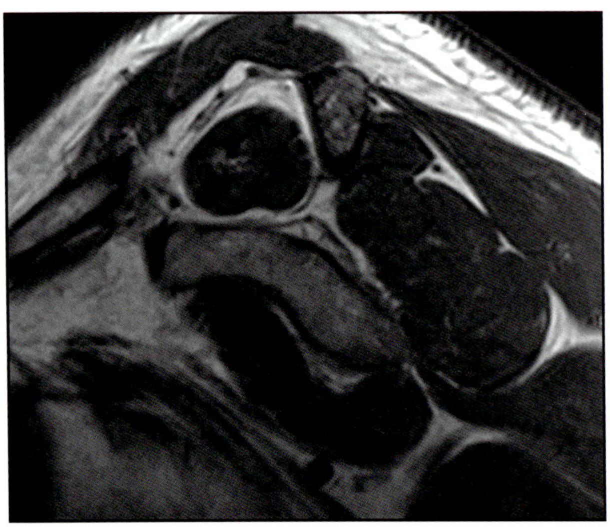

Figure 14. Fatty infiltration within the torn muscle.

Fatty infiltration and muscle atrophy are believed to be irreversible.[35,36] Authors of animal studies have shown changes at 6 to 12 weeks after detachment.[35,36] In the canine model, Safran et al[35] surgically detached the infraspinatus tendon to determine the effect on the muscle. After 12 weeks, the stiffness of the tendon had increased. In the first 6 weeks, muscle volume had decreased, but intramuscular fat had increased. When compared with reattachment at 12 weeks, reattachment at 6 weeks prevented an increase in fat accumulation. However, Uhthoff et al[36] showed the delay before reattaching the tendon did not lead to greater muscle atrophy.

In a retrospective review of 1688 human patients with rotator cuff tears, Melis et al[37] found moderate fatty infiltration at 4 years and severe fatty infiltration by 6 years with all types of rotator cuff tears. When isolating patients with traumatic rotator cuff tears, they found moderate fatty infiltration at 3 years and severe fatty infiltration at 5 years. Progression of fatty infiltration was faster when more than 1 tendon was torn.

Rotator cuff tear arthropathy is rare (Figure 15). When the supraspinatus and infraspinatus are torn, the spacer effect of the rotator cuff is lost. Superior displacement of the humeral head results, and the load on the biceps tendon increases. The subscapularis eventually tears, and this leads to destabilization of the biceps tendon. The upward pull of the deltoid becomes unresisted, and the upper glenoid and labrum become degenerated. The humeral head migrates more superiorly as the rotator cuff tendon becomes a head elevator. Humeral articular cartilage is lost secondary to contact with the corocoacromial arch. On a molecular level, a proposed biomechanism involves an increase in the amount of cartilage-degrading enzymes, which Kim et al[38] found increased in the synovial fluid of patients with rotator cuff tears. They also found an increase in the cartilage catabolic markers in the synovial fluid, which was proportionate to tear size.

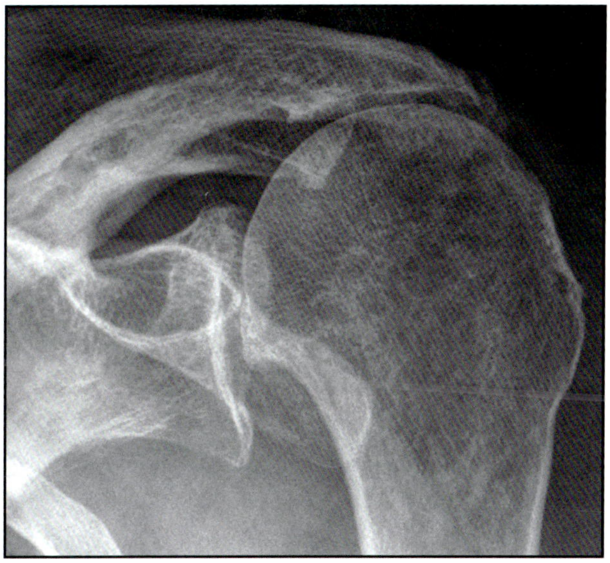

Figure 15. Rotator cuff arthropathy.

DIAGNOSIS AND CLINICAL EVALUATION

The diagnosis of a rotator cuff tear is based on history and physical examination and usually is confirmed by MRI. The patient most often reports pain. The location of the pain varies but commonly occurs on the anterolateral aspect of the shoulder with radiation laterally over the deltoid and at the deltoid insertion. The pain typically does not radiate below the elbow. Pain at night and with activity are very common. Patients describe pain with overhead activities or activities in which the affected upper extremity is outstretched behind them, especially with the addition of weight in the upper extremity. Patients, especially those with large to massive, full-thickness rotator cuff tears, also might report weakness in the upper extremity.

On physical examination, the patient could have evidence of atrophy of the supraspinatus or infraspinatus, which suggests the tear is chronic and potentially massive (involving more than 1 tendon) and includes a large amount of retraction (Figure 16). Inspection should include evaluation for a torn biceps tendon, which suggests a large to massive cuff tear with subscapularis involvement. The patient has tenderness in various areas but often over the greater tuberosity. Palpation in the area of the greater tuberosity could reveal a palpable rotator cuff defect through the overlying skin and deltoid. Some patients have tenderness to palpation over the deltoid insertion. When the subscapularis tendon is involved, pain in the anterior aspect of the shoulder can occur. Both active and passive range of motion should be examined. Range of motion is variable, but most patients with rotator cuff tears have no loss of motion. For patients who have rotator cuff tears and also have developed synovitis, range of motion is limited. Pain also can limit range of motion. A patient with a full-thickness tear might not have a smooth arc of motion and might find lowering the upper extremity from an elevated position more difficult than actively elevating the upper extremity.

The strength of the rotator cuff muscles can help determine which tendons are involved and to what extent they are involved. The strength of the supraspinatus is tested with the upper extremity in 90° of forward elevation in the plane of the scapula and the upper extremity in slight internal rotation (Figure 17). The external rotation strength of the infraspinatus

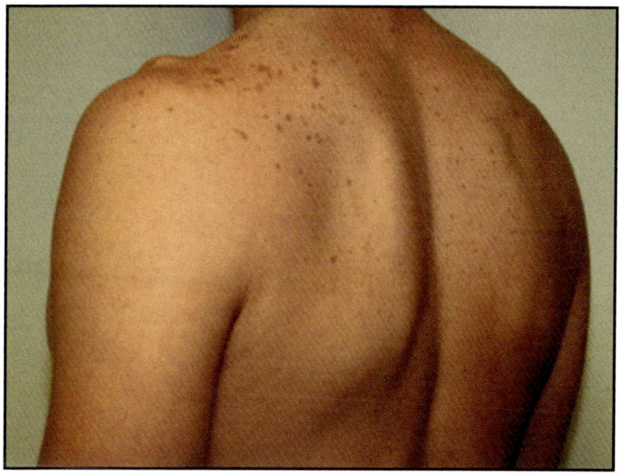

Figure 16. Visual inspection of infraspinatus atrophy.

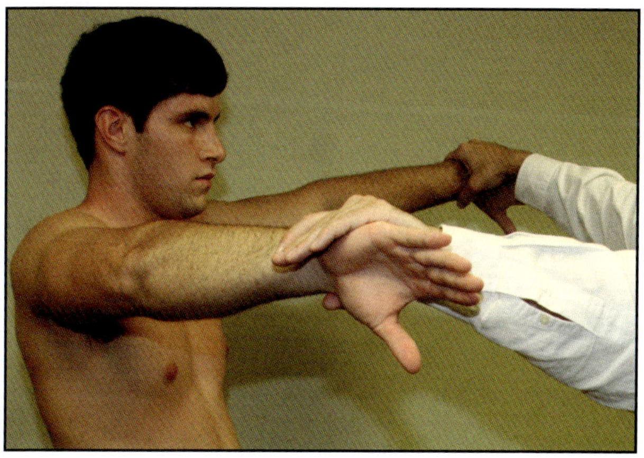

Figure 17. Supraspinatus strength test.

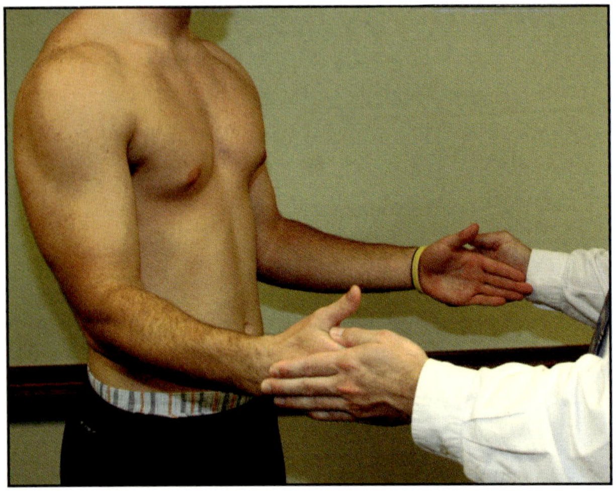

Figure 18. External rotation strength test.

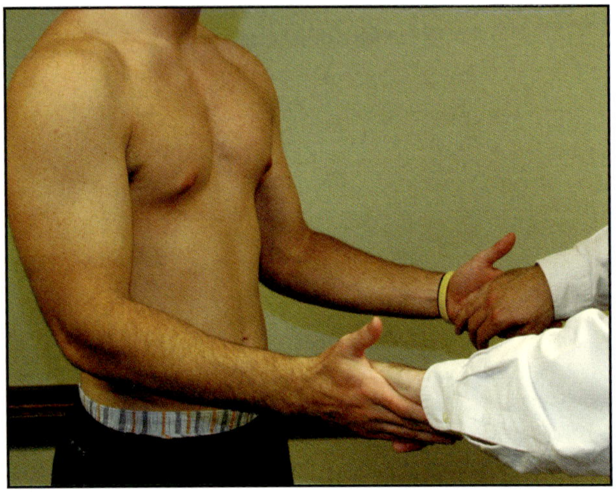

Figure 19. Internal rotation strength test.

is tested with the upper extremity adducted and the elbow flexed to 90° (Figure 18). A positive external rotation lag sign, in which the patient cannot hold the upper extremity in external rotation, suggests weakness or a tear involving the infraspinatus or teres minor, or both. Internal rotation strength is tested with the upper extremity adducted and the elbow flexed to 90° (Figure 19). Specific testing for the subscapularis includes the lift-off and belly-compression tests. In the lift-off test, the patient pushes the hand away from the lumbar spine against resistance. Patients who have difficulty have a weak, partially torn, or completely torn subscapularis. A positive belly-compression test occurs when the patient presses the hand into the abdomen, and the elbow drops backward due to internal rotation weakness (Figure 20). A positive internal rotation

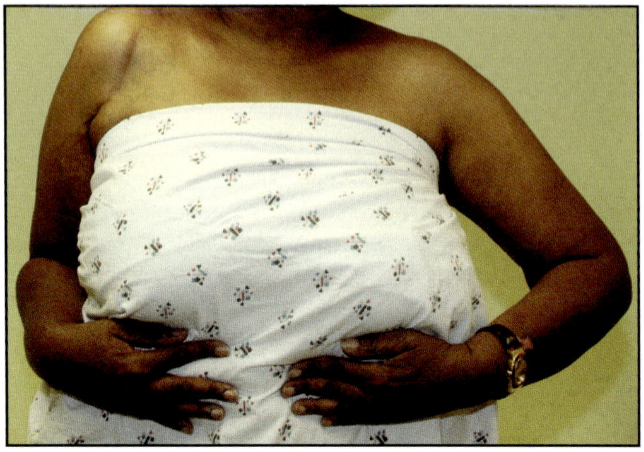

Figure 20. Lift-off and belly-compression test.

lag sign, in which the patient cannot hold the upper extremity in internal rotation, suggests weakness or a tear of the subscapularis. Recurrent anterior instability can result from an acute, complete subscapularis tear. Patients with massive rotator cuff tears can have pseudoparalysis of the upper extremity that prevents them from actively raising it. A positive drop-arm test suggests a rotator cuff tear. A positive hornblower's sign signifies a massive rotator cuff tear and severe loss of infraspinatus and external rotation strength of the teres minor. The patient cannot hold the upper extremity in abduction and external rotation.

Imaging Evaluations

Each patient should have plain radiographs performed at the time of initial presentation. For example, a true anteroposterior view, an axillary lateral view, and an anterolateral view of the impingement site are obtained at the initial clinic visit (Figures 21–23). These are necessary to evaluate the bony anatomy. Plain radiographs allow the clinician to evaluate the type of acromion and the possibility of osteophyte formation on the undersurface of the acromion, suggesting impingement in addition to rotator cuff disease. The acromioclavicular joint is examined for degenerative changes that need to be addressed at the time of surgery if they cause symptoms. Patients who have had a rotator cuff tear for a prolonged period have sclerosis and osteophyte formation involving the greater tuberosity. Often, if a massive rotator cuff tear is present, the space between the acromion and superior aspect of the humeral head, or the acromiohumeral distance, is

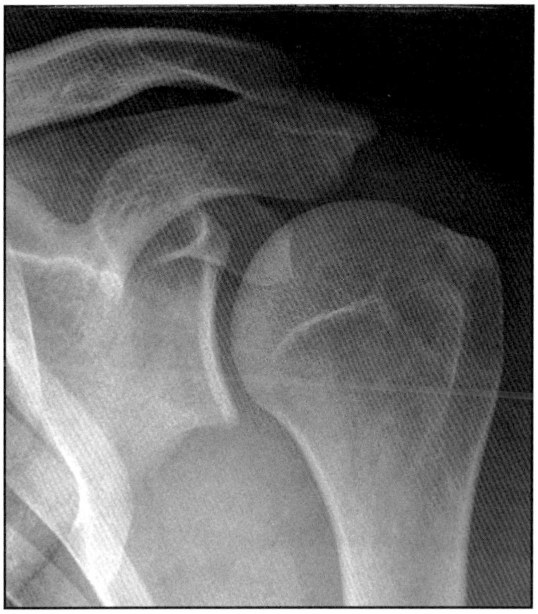

Figure 21. True anteroposterior radiographic view.

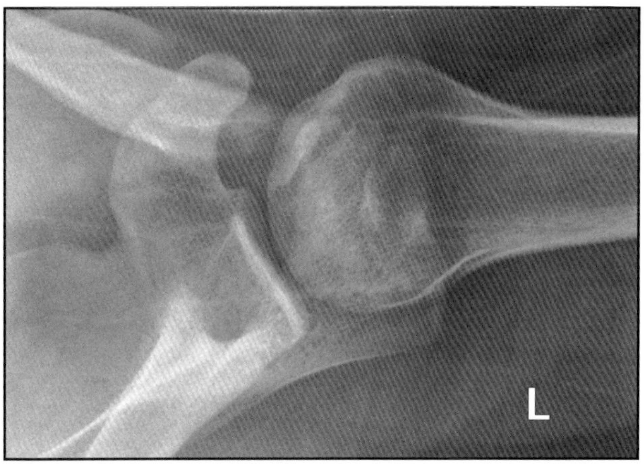

Figure 22. Axillary lateral radiographic view.

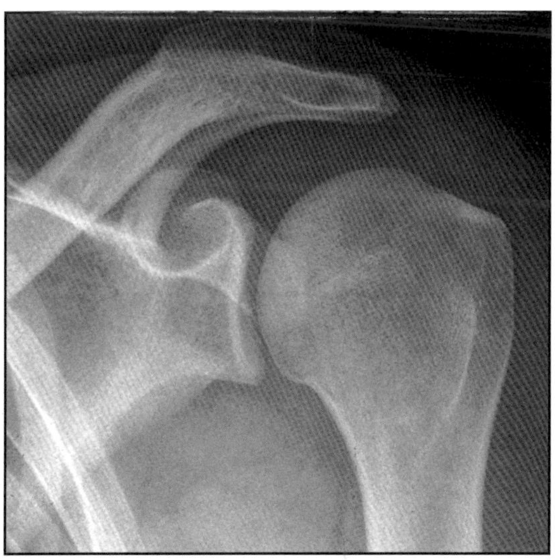

Figure 23. Anterolateral view of the impingement site.

decreased (Figure 24). The clinician must ensure primary or secondary osteoarthritis is not causing the pain in addition to a rotator cuff tear or an obvious bone or soft tissue tumor.

Arthrography, which once was the criterion standard, largely has been replaced by MRI. It most often is performed when a patient cannot have an MRI. The findings on MRI can help direct treatment recommendations. After plain films are obtained and interpreted and any potential additional pathologic conditions are ruled out, the clinician often obtains an MRI of the shoulder to evaluate the extent of the soft tissue injury. Important factors discovered with MRI include the size of the tear; which tendons were

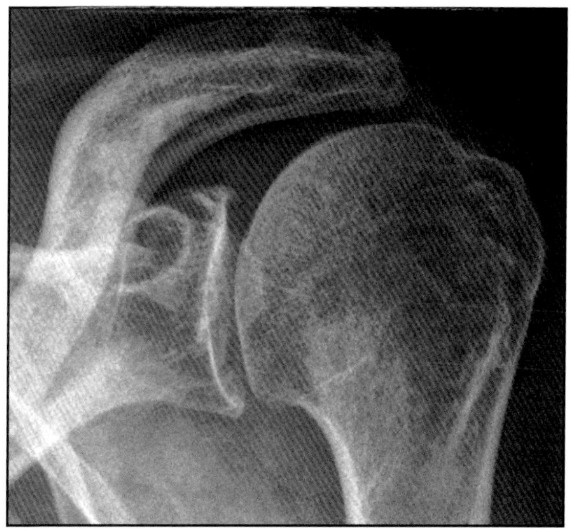

Figure 24. Radiograph shows decreased acromiohumeral space, indicating a massive rotator cuff tear.

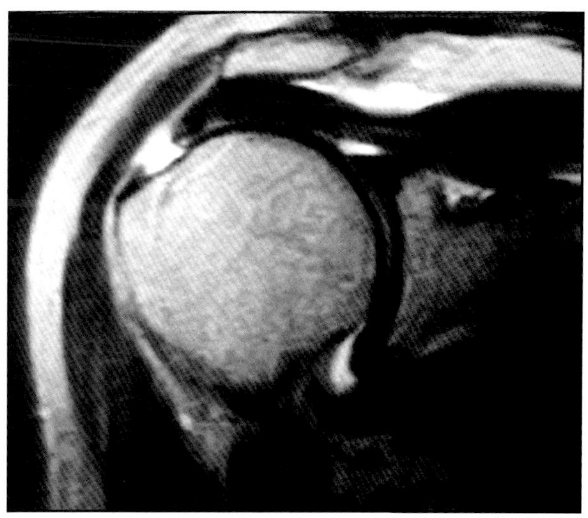

Figure 25. Magnetic resonance imaging is used to determine the extent of soft tissue injury.

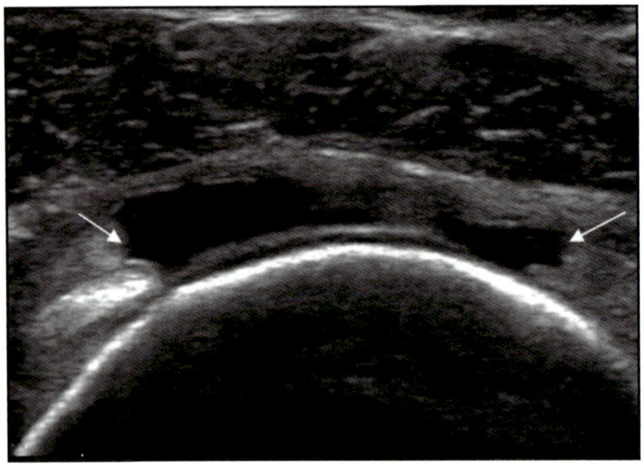

Figure 26. Ultrasound of the rotator cuff.

involved; the presence or absence of retraction of the tear; and the amount of atrophy, if present (Figure 25). The percentage of involvement of the rotator cuff tendon in patients with partial-thickness rotator cuff tears is important to help direct treatment. Additional pathologic lesions, such as degenerative labral tears, the presence of substantial acromioclavicular arthrosis, or the extent of glenohumeral osteoarthritis if present, often can be identified.

Ultrasound examination of the rotator cuff has become increasingly popular (Figure 26). The convenience of performing an ultrasound in the clinic, performing bilateral ultrasounds, and performing an interactive examination of the rotator cuff has made this an appealing option for evaluating rotator cuff tears. It also is estimated to be one-eighth of the cost of an MRI. It is very safe and noninvasive, but because it is difficult, the ultrasoundographer must be experienced with evaluating the rotator cuff. When comparing ultrasound and MRI with arthroscopic findings as the criterion standard, Teefey et al[39] found the accuracy for both modalities was 87%. The authors found no difference in distinguishing full-thickness from partial-thickness tears.[39] They also found no difference in predicting tear size and tendon retraction between MRI and ultrasound.[39] However, the criterion standard for diagnosis is direct visualization with diagnostic arthroscopy.

Patient Selection

Patients who have evidence of a full-thickness rotator cuff tear have a surgical problem in the shoulder. For elderly patients who have multiple medical problems or patients who are not adequate candidates for surgery because of multiple medical problems, a trial of nonoperative treatment is appropriate. Surgery is recommended for patients who are candidates for operative treatment and have full-thickness rotator cuff tears causing levels of pain and loss of function that are unacceptable to them. If the tear is acute (eg, the result of a shoulder dislocation), surgery should be performed within 3 to 4 weeks. For a patient who has a chronic tear, surgery can be performed as an elective procedure in a reasonable amount of time and when it is convenient for the patient. For a patient with a large partial-thickness tear, recommendations are based on the patient and his or her activity level. For an active patient whose pain is interfering with activities, surgery is recommended. For elderly, less-active patients, a trial of therapy is acceptable. Patients with small partial-thickness tears often improve with therapy. Patients who do not improve should consider surgery.

OPERATIVE TREATMENT OPTIONS

For a full-thickness rotator cuff tear, operative treatment options include open, mini-open, and arthroscopic rotator cuff repair. When repair cannot be performed because of the amount of retraction or poor-quality tissue, a debridement or partial repair of the rotator cuff tear is performed.

An open repair typically is performed through a superior approach in which the skin incision is made just off the lateral border of the acromion (Figure 27). Traditionally, the deltoid is detached from the acromion to improve visualization of the rotator

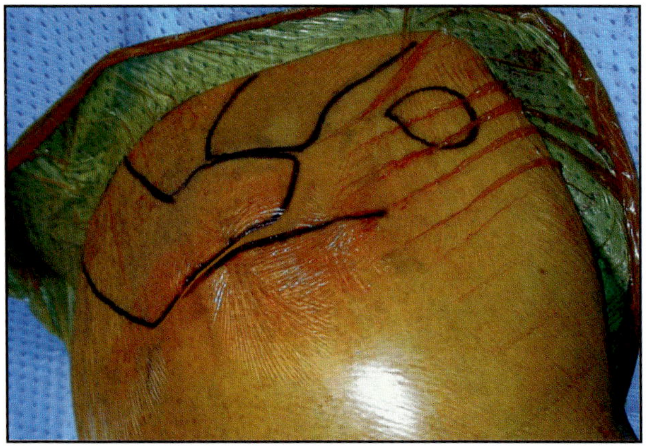

Figure 27. Anatomic landmarks and skin incision for the superior approach for an open repair.

cuff tear. The rotator cuff can be repaired through bone tunnels but most often is repaired using suture anchors. Open repair restores function, reduces pain, and provides long-term relief of symptoms. Adequate repair of the deltoid is important to avoid deltoid detachment, which would compromise patient outcome. Because arthroscopy is not used with this technique, a disadvantage is not being able to adequately visualize and address associated glenohumeral lesions. A more extensive surgical dissection must be performed, which potentially will increase postoperative pain and the risk of infection.

Mini-open repair involves repairing the rotator cuff tear through a smaller incision than the open technique (Figure 28). Arthroscopy is used to visualize the tear and treat additional lesions within the glenohumeral joint or subacromial space, such as evaluating and treating degenerative labral tears or biceps tendon tears or performing a subacromial decompression. This technique avoids the need to detach the deltoid. Results of the mini-open repair have been equal to those of an open repair at 1 and 2 years after surgery.[40]

With the development of new technology and improved surgical skill, an all-arthroscopic rotator cuff repair now is commonly performed. The theoretical advantages of the repair, which is performed through small portal incisions, include decreased immediate postoperative pain, decreased surgical insult to the deltoid, and decreased postoperative stiffness. This could result in increased patient satisfaction. Single-row and double-row repair constructs are used, and the technique chosen depends on the surgeon (Figure 29). Some researchers have shown that a double-row repair

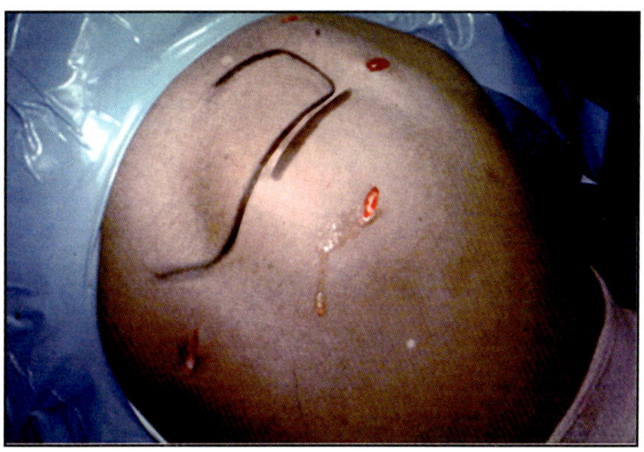

Figure 28. Anatomic landmarks and skin incision for a mini-open rotator cuff repair via a much smaller incision.

with medial and lateral sutures improves biomechanical strength.[41] The improved biomechanical properties of a double-row repair over a single-row repair include decreased strain over the footprint area, increased stiffness, and increased ultimate load to failure.[41] Mazzocca et al[42] did not show a difference in load to failure, cyclic displacement, and gap formation but found that a double-row repair consistently restored a larger footprint than the single-row repair did. A single row of anchors restores only 67% of the original footprint, whereas adding the second row increases the contact area by 60%, which restores more normal footprint anatomy.[43] Brady et al[44] found that after isolated lateral row repair, 52.7% of the rotator cuff footprint was left uncovered. On average, the double-row repair offered more than twice the footprint coverage yielded by a single-row repair. The double-row repair is more technically demanding than the single-row repair and might not necessarily improve patient satisfaction or functional outcome.[45]

For patients with partial-thickness rotator cuff tears that have not improved with nonoperative treatment, surgery is recommended. Operative treatment includes both debriding and repairing the partial-thickness tear. Park et al[46] used debridement to treat a tear comprising less than 50% of the thickness of the tendon and subacromial decompression in 37 patients; 24 patients had an articular-sided tear, and 13 had a bursal-sided tear. At 6 months after surgery, pain and function had improved in patients with bursal-sided tears, but they found no difference in pain and function at 1- and 2-year follow-up.[46] Cordasco et al[47] used debridement and subacromial decompression to treat 105 patients who had partial-thickness tears comprising less than 50% of the thickness of the tendon. They reported patients with articular-sided tears had a 3% failure rate, whereas patients with bursal-sided tears had a 29% failure rate.[47] Weber[48] used debridement or repair to treat 65 patients who had grade 3A or 3B tears and found repair resulted in significantly improved outcomes. The difference was greater with the bursal-sided tear subgroup. He concluded that bursal-sided tears were not treated adequately with debridement alone.[48]

Mazzocca et al[49] created articular-sided, partial-thickness tears comprising 25%, 50%, and 75% of the thickness of the supraspinatus tendon of cadav-

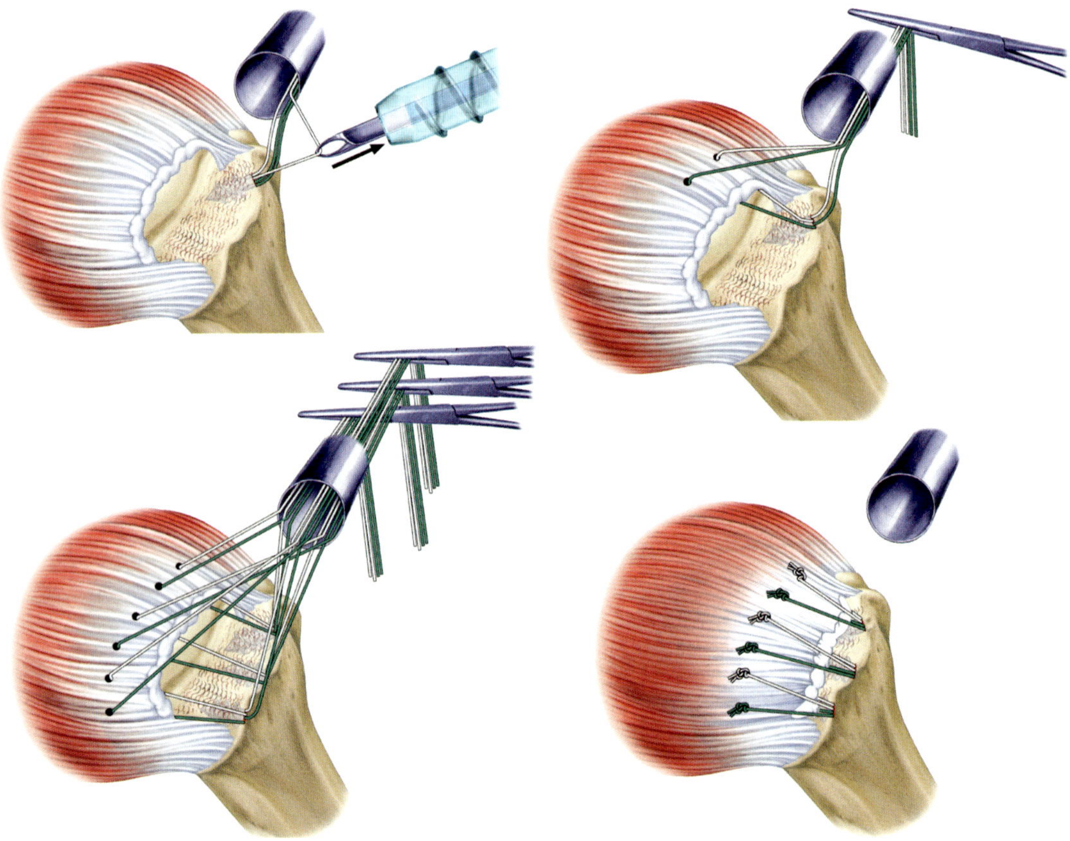

Figure 29A. Arthroscopic rotator cuff repair using a single-row construct.

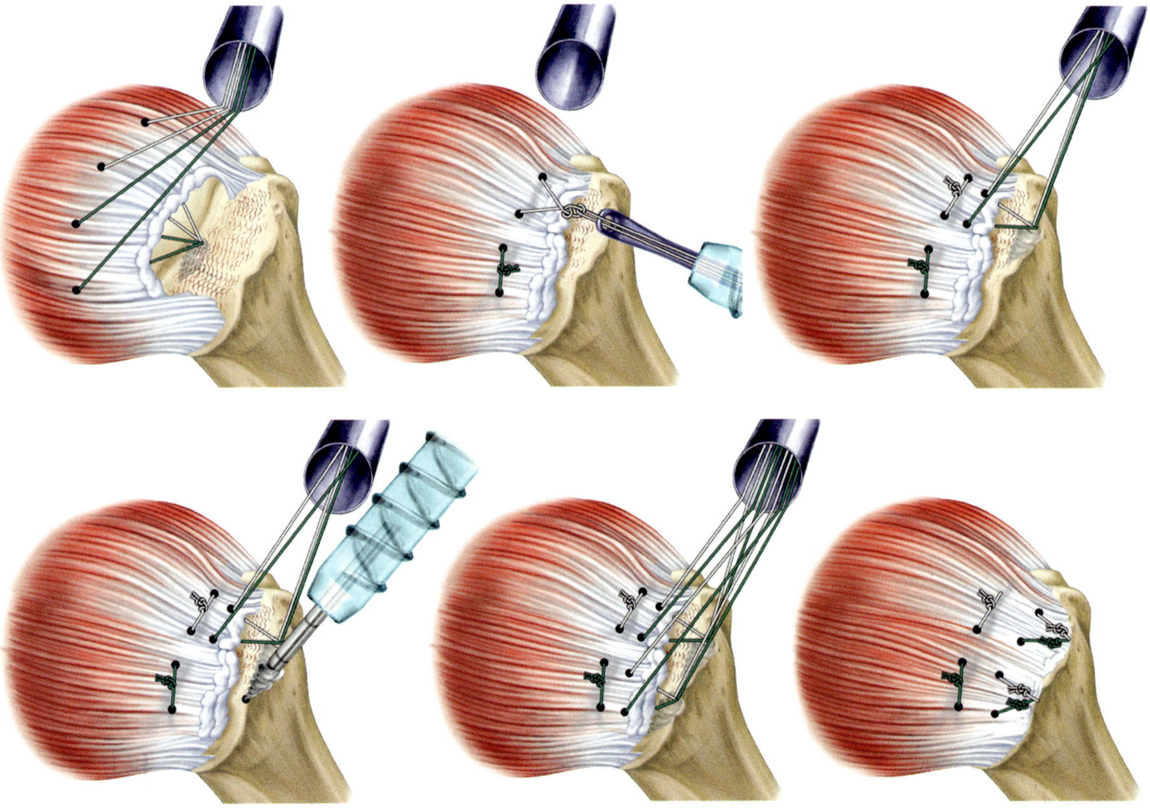

Figure 29B. Arthroscopic rotator cuff repair using a double-row construct.

ers; measured strain at glenohumeral angles of 45°, 60°, and 90°; repaired the tears; and measured strain again. They found an increase in rotator cuff strain between the intact rotator cuff tendon and partial-thickness tears comprising 50% and 75% of the thickness of the tendon. After repair, the strain returned to that with the intact state. The effect of the tear on strain increased as the abduction angle increased. The authors suggested that a biomechanical basis exists for repairing a partial-thickness tear greater than 50% of the footprint.[49]

Multiple techniques for repairing partial-thickness rotator cuff tears have been described. Lo and Burkhart[50] described a transtendon technique using suture anchors to repair partial-thickness, articular-sided rotator cuff tears, which also are known as partial articular supraspinatus tendon avulsion lesions (Figure 30). Conway[51] described a transcutaneous mattress suture repair. Wolff et al[52] illustrated a technique for repairing bursal-sided tears in which the articular side is left intact. They explained that 3 goals are achieved with this repair: the intact articular fibers act as an internal splint to protect the bursal-sided repair; a wide, anatomic footprint is recreated; and the length-tension mismatch is minimized because the tissue is not lateralized excessively. At 24-month follow-up, the 15 patients treated with this technique had excellent results.[52] The other treatment option involves converting a partial-thickness tear to a full-thickness tear and performing a standard repair of the rotator cuff.

For partial-thickness tears involving the subscapularis, treatment involves not only repairing the partial-thickness tear with suture anchors and recreating an anatomic footprint, but also addressing the potential cause of the defect within the tendon. A coracoplasty is performed in patients whose plain films and MRIs

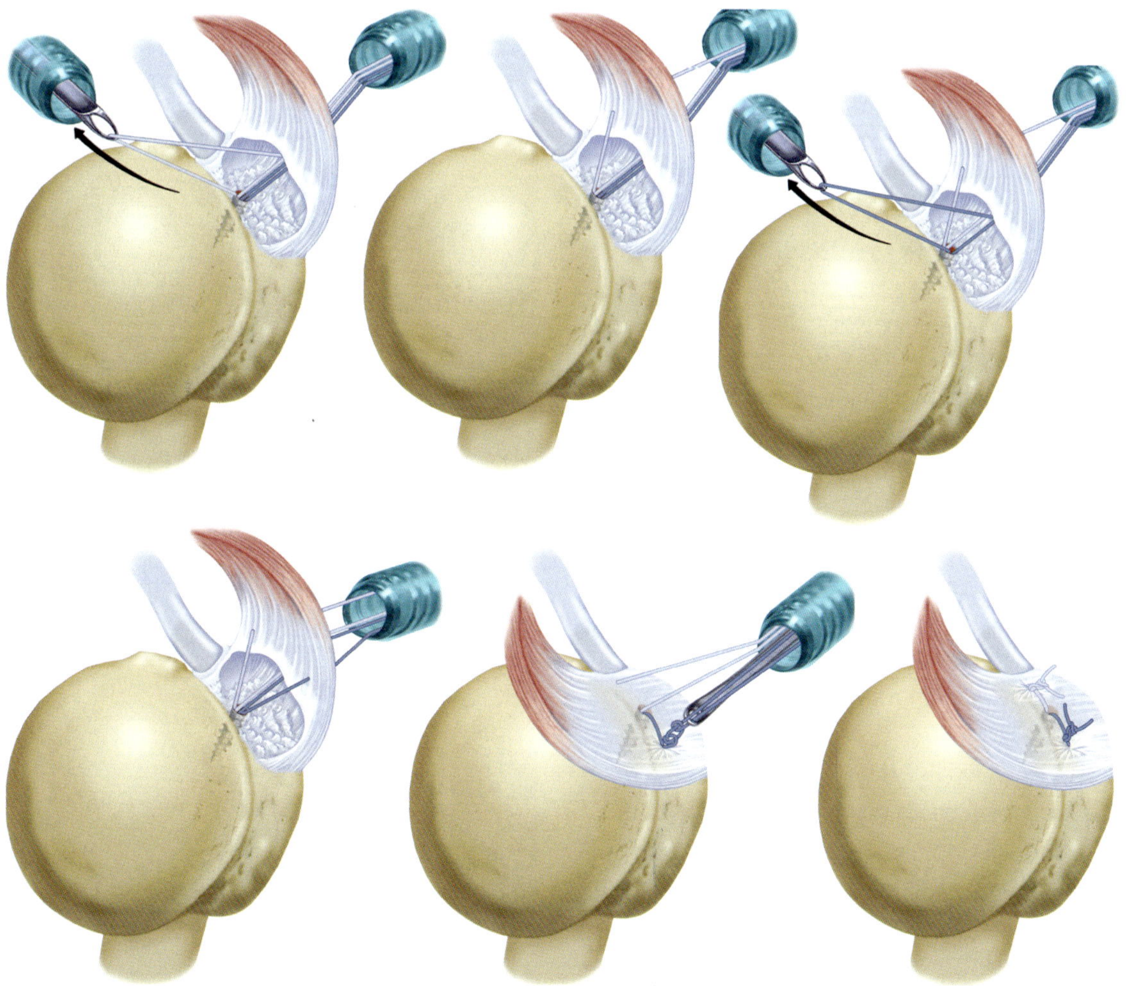

Figure 30. Transtendon technique for repairing partial-thickness rotator cuff tears.

show decreased distance between the tendon defect and the coracoid (Figure 31).

A partial-thickness tear in the overhead athlete is unique, and the appropriate treatment has been debated. The overhead athlete usually develops a partial articular tear with intratendinous extension lesion due to posterosuperior impingement. Failure occurs on the undersurface of the posterior portion of the supraspinatus and anterior portion of the infraspinatus with intratendinous delamination.[53] This is best visualized on the abduction-external rotation view. In their study of 67 professional pitchers treated with debridement alone, Reynolds et al[54] found 76% returned to competitive pitching, but only 55% returned to the same level or higher of competition. Lo and Burkhart[50] described a new technique for arthroscopic intratendinous repair for a delaminated, articular-sided rotator cuff tear. The normal anatomy of the articular side of the rotator cuff is restored, and the delamination component also is repaired, preventing overconstraint of the shoulder. Results are promising, but only 5 months of follow-up have been reported.

Many investigators have compared the different repair techniques available for partial-thickness rotator cuff tears. In their biomechanical study, Gonzalez-Lomas et al[55] compared a transtendon repair and a tear completion followed by repair. The transtendon repair showed less gapping and also had a higher mean ultimate failure strength. Park et al[56] compared the transtendon repair with 2 isolated mattress configurations. Gap formation in the anterior tendon was lower in the isolated mattress configuration but did not exceed 0.5 mm. The authors found no difference in linear stiffness, yield, ultimate load, or energy absorbed to failure. They concluded that the interimplant mattress cuff repair for articular-sided, partial-thickness tears involving 50% of the footprint has biomechanical characteristics similar to those of a repair using 2 isolated mattress sutures.[56]

Using an ovine model, Peters et al[57] compared no repair; transtendon repair; completion of the tear with tension-band, single-row repair; and completion of the tear with double-row repair for articular-sided, partial-thickness tears. They measured the footprint contact pressure and the ultimate load to failure and found footprint contact pressures were 3 times greater for the transtendon and double-row repairs than the single-

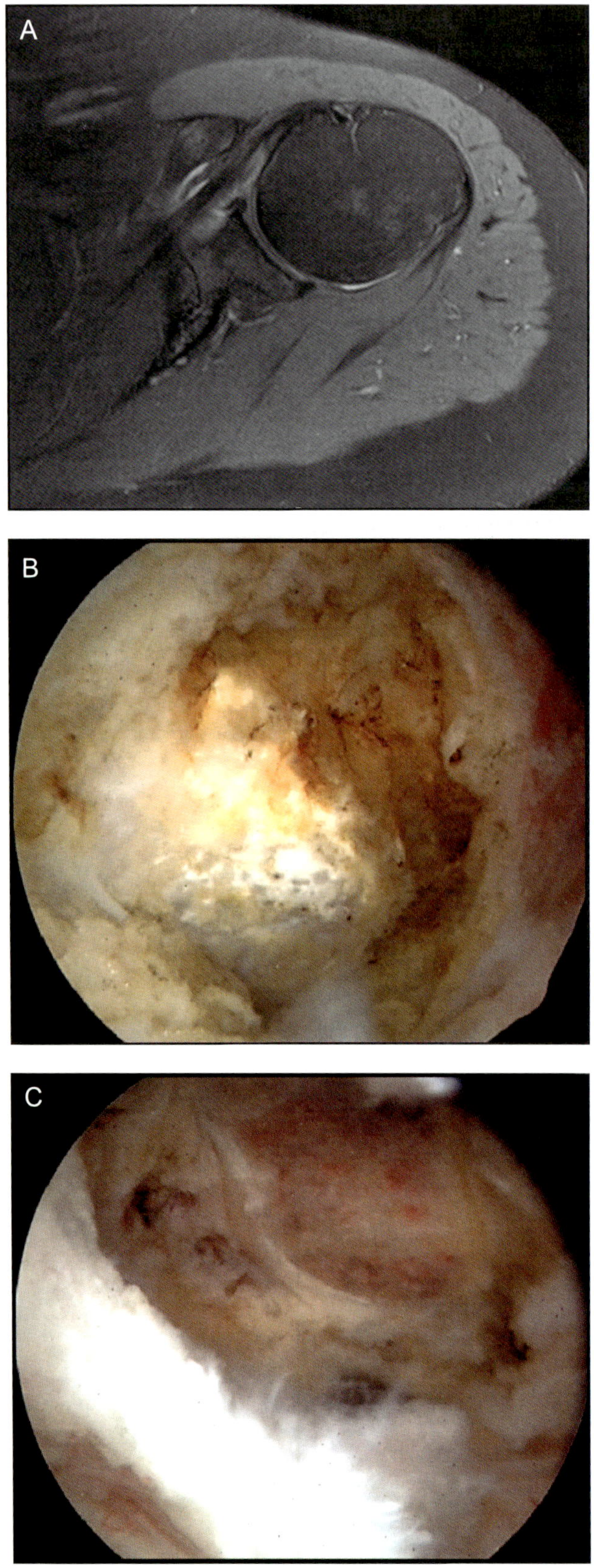

Figure 31. A, Magnetic resonance imaging scan shows decreased space between the subscapularis tendon defect and the coracoid. B and C, Arthroscopic view of coracoidplasty.

row and no repairs. Ultimate load to failure was more than 3 times greater for the transtendon repair than for the double-row and single-row repairs. The authors concluded that the transtendon repair biomechanically outperformed tear completion and repair in the ovine model. This type of repair showed the best combination of high footprint contact pressure and high ultimate failure load. Technical failure of the transtendon repair was seen in 3 of the 15 shoulders. These were excluded, and 3 more were performed for comparison. The authors believed this was related to the anchor they used and further evaluation should be performed in this area.[57]

NONOPERATIVE TREATMENT

Nonoperative treatment options for full-thickness rotator cuff tears are appropriate for patients who want to relieve pain and avoid surgery or for patients in whom surgery is not an option because of medical problems. Treatment includes taking nonsteroidal anti-inflammatory drugs; participating in a specific exercise program to maintain the range of motion; and strengthening the remaining intact rotator cuff, deltoid, and scapular muscles. If the patient has developed stiffness, exercises focus on regaining passive range of motion. Patients should avoid aggravating activities that cause discomfort. Avoiding sleeping on the affected shoulder often helps, and sleeping in a recliner can be more comfortable. Some patients report a decrease in symptoms after a corticosteroid injection, but little evidence is available to support this method of treatment for full-thickness rotator cuff tears. Patients who have had symptoms for more than 6 to 12 months and patients who have tears greater than 3 cm often have poor outcomes with nonoperative treatment. Strength rarely improves clinically with nonoperative treatment, but patients who mainly report pain and not weakness often are satisfied with the results of nonoperative treatment. Surgery is an option for patients who do not improve after a trial of nonoperative treatment and are candidates for this treatment.

For a partial-thickness rotator cuff tear, initial treatment should include a period of nonoperative management, especially if the partial-thickness tear involves less than 50% of the thickness of the tendon. Treatment includes modification of activities and potentially starting a nonsteroidal anti-inflammatory medication if the patient has no medical contraindications. Physical therapy includes a strict exercise program for capsular stretching, balancing shoulder dynamics, and strengthening the rotator cuff and periscapular musculature. A cortisteroid injection into the subacromial bursa might decrease inflammation in this area and pain; however, Koester et al[58] did not find evidence to support the use of a subacromial corticosteroid injection. If nonoperative treatment is unsuccessful after 6 to 12 months, the surgeon should consider operative intervention. Relative indications for repairing a partial rotator cuff tear include acute traumatic tears, bursal-sided tears, and a physically active patient.

POTENTIAL COMPLICATIONS

Based on a large review of 40 published studies on rotator cuff tears, the complication rate after rotator cuff repair is estimated at 10%.[59] The most common complication is a retear of the rotator cuff after repair. Several researchers have documented tearing of the rotator cuff after all types of repairs, with an estimated overall rate of 6%. However, tendon retear does not necessarily mean the patient will have a return of pain or poor functional outcome.[60,61] The rate of retear with arthroscopic repair is higher when the tear is greater than 3 cm. Smaller tears have a similar rate of retearing when comparing open and arthroscopic repairs. Nerve injury is rare; it is estimated to occur in 1% to 2% of patients and usually involves the axillary nerve. With open procedures, careful dissection is necessary to avoid this injury. Traction on the upper extremity and forceful manipulation also is associated with nerve injury and must be limited. Infection occurs in 1% of patients after rotator cuff repair. Using antibiotics before the procedure and enforcing sterile surgical technique reduce the risk of infection. After open repair, deltoid detachment is a postoperative complication in less than 1% of patients (Figure 32). Careful repair and protection during rehabilitation help avoid detachment. Stiffness might occur after repair. An early rehabilitation protocol and patient compliance help prevent postoperative loss of range of motion.

Figure 32. Deltoid detachment postoperative complication.

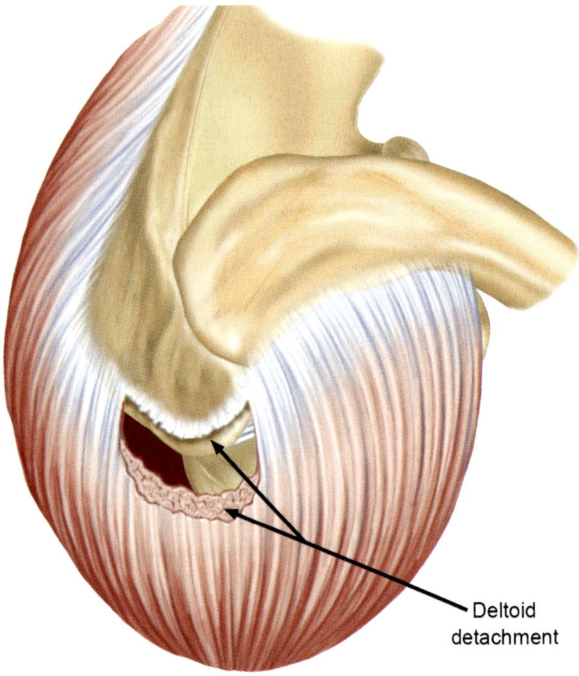

EXPECTED OUTCOMES

Patients who have a rotator cuff repair generally can expect improved function and decreased pain. Gore et al[62] found subjective improvement in 95% of shoulders with repaired cuffs at an average follow-up of 5.5 years. Most patients had marked relief of pain and minimal or no problems with activities of daily living. Results were better in patients with tears that were less than 2.5 cm than in patients with larger tears. Jost et al[63] showed that pain, function, strength, and patient satisfaction even after structural failure remained better after surgery than before surgery. Smith et al[64] found that involvement of the infraspinatus in the rotator cuff tear, female sex, and worker's compensation claims were correlated with decreased shoulder function.

In their systematic review, Lindley and Jones[65] revealed no difference in postoperative American Shoulder and Elbow Surgeons standardized shoulder assessment scores, University of California-Los Angeles shoulder rating scores, or pain scores or the incidence of recurrent rotator cuff tears between rotator cuffs repaired all arthroscopically and those repaired using the mini-open technique. Patients who have an arthroscopic repair might have decreased short-term pain.

Papadopoulos et al[66] studied the functional outcome and structural integrity after mini-open repair of large and massive rotator cuff tears. The 27 patients who underwent a repair of their rotator cuff tears returned at a minimum of 3 years for a follow-up functional evaluation and ultrasound investigation of rotator cuff integrity. The rotator cuff was healed in 48.1% (n = 13) of patients, whereas recurrent defects were detected in the remaining 51.9% (n = 14). In 92.5% (n = 12) of patients with a retear, the tear was smaller than the previous tear. Only 7.5% (n = 2) had a tear larger than the original tear. Despite the high rate of retear, the functional scores improved. Only large retears were correlated with poorer functional outcome. The preoperative tear size was negatively associated with tendon healing. On average, patients with intact rotator cuff tears were 15 years younger than patients who sustained recurrence of a tear.[66]

The outcome of a rotator cuff repair in patients with large to massive tears and pseudoparalysis is promising. Oh et al[67] found that 75% of patients with pseudoparalysis had postoperative improvements in range of motion, with only 24.1% demonstrating pseudoparalysis postoperatively. All outcome scores improved by final follow-up. Among 37 patients who underwent computed tomography arthrography, rotator cuff healing was achieved in 33.3% in the pseudoparalytic group and 47.4% in the nonpseudoparalytic group. Recovery from pseudoparalysis after surgery in patients with large to massive cuff tears was evident in a large portion of the study group, and postoperative function and rotator cuff healing were not different according to the presence of pseudoparalysis.[67] Warrender et al[68] showed that obesity negatively affects the operative time of arthroscopic rotator cuff repairs, length of hospitalization, and functional outcomes. However, although the obese group had greater limitations and lower rates of satisfaction at final follow-up than their nonobese counterparts, they still reported improvements after the surgery.

The outcome after treatment for a partial-thickness rotator cuff has been evaluated. Norlin and Adolfsson[69] conducted a 10- to 13-year follow-up involving 162 of 181 patients who had arthroscopy and subacromial decompression to treat impingement. They reported that patients with isolated full-thickness tears of the supraspinatus had the best results followed by patients with partial-thickness tears. These authors concluded that decompression might prevent further rotator cuff deterioration and the repair might be unnecessary. However, the patients only were evaluated clinically, and no imaging was performed. Although the patients improved clinically, this did not show the rotator cuff spontaneously healed.

In a retrospective review of 33 patients who underwent debridement of a partial-thickness rotator cuff tear with acromioplasty, Kartus et al[70] revealed that 35% had a full-thickness tear on ultrasound examination at 101 months after surgery. Their findings suggest that acromioplasty and debridement of a partial-thickness tear do not protect the rotator cuff from further degeneration.

Researchers have reported successful results after the partial-thickness rotator cuff tear is completed and repaired. In 41 patients whose partial-thickness tears were greater than 50% (80% articular-sided tears), Deutsch[71] converted the tears to full-thickness tears then repaired them. All patients had improved range of motion and strength. Strength measurements were not different between the shoulders treated operatively and nonoperatively. Improvements were seen in the American Shoulder and Elbow Surgeons standardized shoulder assessment scores and pain relief. Forty of 41 patients were satisfied with their outcomes. Porat et al[72] reported improvement in forward elevation and abduction for 51 patients in their study treated with completion of the tear and repair. All patients had improved University of California-Los Angeles shoulder rating scores, and no patient had a poor result. In a study of 41 patients with partial-thickness tears treated with completion of the tear and repair, Kamath et al[73] showed by ultrasound examination that at 11 months, 88% of patients had an intact rotator cuff. Five of 41 patients had full-thickness defects within the tendon. The American Shoulder and Elbow Surgeons standardized shoulder assessment scores improved, with an overall patient satisfaction rate of 93%. The average age of patients with intact cuffs was 51.8 years, whereas the average age for patients with persistent defects was 62.6 years. The authors concluded arthroscopic repair of a high-grade partial-thickness tear results in a high rate of tendon healing, and patient age is an important factor.

Ide et al[74] followed 17 patients for 39 months after a transtendon repair. Postoperative scores improved in all patients after the repair, and no patient had a poor result. Of the 6 overhead athletes in the study, 2 returned to the same level of competition, 3 returned to a lower level, and 1 baseball pitcher was unable to return. Huberty et al[75] described postoperative stiffness after a transtendon repair of a partial-thickness tear. With the transtendon repair, sutures are tied on the tip of the bursal surface, potentially overtightening the bursal portion of the rotator cuff and causing postoperative stiffness. In response, Spencer[76] described an all-inside repair technique for articular-sided, partial-thickness tears. All 20 patients treated with this technique had improved Penn Shoulder Scale scores. Only 1 patient returned to the same level or higher of play. No one had postoperative stiffness.

CONCLUSIONS

Patients can expect improvements in function and decreased pain after repair of full-thickness and partial-thickness rotator cuff tears. Patients who undergo an arthroscopic repair usually have less pain in the immediate postoperative period. The complication of deltoid pull-off with an open procedure is not a risk factor for patients who undergo an arthroscopic repair of the rotator cuff. Despite this potentially devastating complication, most patients who have an open repair of the rotator cuff in which the deltoid is repaired appropriately are satisfied with the surgical outcome.

REFERENCES

1. Clark JM, Harryman DT II. Tendons, ligaments, and capsule of the rotator cuff: gross and microscopic anatomy. *J Bone Joint Surg Am.* 1992;74(5):713–725.
2. Nakajima T, Rokuuma N, Hamada K, Tomatsu T, Fukuda H. Histologic and biomechanical characteristics of the supraspinatus tendon: reference to rotator cuff tearing. *J Shoulder Elbow Surg.* 1994;3(2):79–87.
3. Dugas JR, Campbell DA, Warren RF, Robie BH, Millett RJ. Anatomy and dimensions of rotator cuff insertions. *J Shoulder Elbow Surg.* 2002;11(5):498–503.
4. Mochizuki T, Sugaya H, Uomizu M, et al. Humeral insertion of the supraspinatus and infraspinatus: new anatomical findings regarding the footprint of the rotator cuff. *J Bone Joint Surg Am.* 2008;90(5):962–969.
5. Rothman RH, Parke WW. The vascular anatomy of the rotator cuff. *Clin Orthop Relat Res.* 1965;41:176–186.
6. Moseley HF. The vascular supply of the rotator cuff. *Surg Clin North Am.* 1963;43:1521–1522.

7. Lindblom K. On pathogenesis of ruptures of the tendon aponeurosis of the shoulder joint. *Acta Radiol*. 1939;20(6):563–577.
8. Uhthoff HK, Loehr J, Sarkar J. The pathogenesis of rotator cuff tears. In: *Proceedings of the Third International Conference on Surgery of the Shoulder, Fukuora, Japan, October 27, 1986*. Reading, UK: International Congress of Shoulder and Elbow Surgery; 1986:211–212.
9. Lohr JF, Uhthoff HK. The microvascular pattern of the supraspinatus tendon. *Clin Orthop Relat Res*. 1990;254:35–38.
10. Rathbun JB, Macnab I. The microvascular pattern of the rotator cuff. *J Bone Joint Surg Br*. 1970;52(3):540–553.
11. Swiontkowski MF, Iannotti JP, Boulas HJ, Esterhai JL. Intraoperative assessment of rotator cuff vascularity using laser Doppler flowmetry. In: Post M, Morrey BF, Hawkins RJ, eds. *Surgery of the Shoulder*. St Louis, MO: Mosby-Year Book; 1990:208–212.
12. Clark JC. Fibrous anatomy of the rotator cuff. Presented at: Annual Meeting of the American Academy of Orthopaedic Surgeons; March 1998; New Orleans, LA.
13. Clark J, Sidles JA, Matsen FA. The relationship of the glenohumeral joint capsule to the rotator cuff. *Clin Orthop Relat Res*. 1990;254:29–34.
14. Rudzki JR, Adler RS, Warren RF, et al. Contrast-enhanced ultrasound characterization of the vascularity of the rotator cuff tendon: age- and activity-related changes in the intact asymptomatic rotator cuff. *J Shoulder Elbow Surg*. 2008;17(1 suppl):96S–100S.
15. Harvie P, Ostlere SJ, Teh J, et al. Genetic influences in the aetiology of tears of the rotator cuff: sibling risk of a full-thickness tear. *J Bone Joint Surg Br*. 2004;86(5):696–700.
16. Gwilym SE, Watkins B, Cooper CD. Genetic influences in the progression of tears of the rotator cuff. *J Bone Joint Surg Br*. 2009;91(7):915–917.
17. Yamaguchi K, Ditsios K, Middleton WD, Hildebolt CF, Galatz LM, Teefey SA. The demographic and morphological features of rotator cuff disease: a comparison of asymptomatic and symptomatic shoulders. *J Bone Joint Surg Am*. 2006;88(8):1699–1704.
18. Wendelboe AM, Hegmann KT, Gren LH, Alder SC, White GL Jr, Lyon JL. Associations between body-mass index and surgery for rotator cuff tendinitis. *J Bone Joint Surg Am*. 2004;86(4):743–747.
19. Northover JR, Lunn P, Clark DI, Phillipson M. Risk factors for the development of rotator cuff disease. *Int J Shoulder Surg*. 2007;1(3):82–86.
20. Chen AL, Shapiro JA, Ahn AK, Zuckerman JD, Cuomo F. Rotator cuff repair in patients with type I diabetes mellitus. *J Shoulder Elbow Surg*. 2003;12(5):416–421.
21. Abboud JA, Kim JS. The effect of hypercholesterolemia on rotator cuff disease. *Clin Orthop Relat Res*. 2010;468:1493–1497.
22. Baumgarten KM, Gerlach D, Galatz LM, et al. Cigarette smoking increases the risk for rotator cuff tears. *Clin Orthop Relat Res*. 2010;468:1534–1541.
23. Kane SM, Dave A, Haque A, Langston K. The incidence of rotator cuff disease in smoking and nonsmoking patients: a cadaveric study. *Orthopedics*. 2006;29(4):363–366.
24. Kumagai J, Sarkar K, Uhthoff HK. The collagen types in the attachment zone of rotator cuff tendons in the elderly: an immunohistochemical study. *J Rheumatol*. 1994;21(11):2096–2100.
25. Nho SJ, Yadav H, Shindle HK, Macgillivray JD. Rotator cuff degeneration etiology and pathogenesis. *Am J Sports Med*. 2008;36(5):987–993.
26. Yuan J, Wang MX, Murrell GA. Cell death and tendinopathy. *Clin Sports Med*. 2003;22(4):693–701.
27. Irlenbusch U, Gansen HK. Muscle biopsy investigations on neuromuscular insufficiency of the rotator cuff: a contribution to the functional impingement of the shoulder joint. *J Shoulder Elbow Surg*. 2003;12(5):422–426.
28. Neer CS, Poppen NK. Supraspinatus outlet. *Orthop Trans*. 1987;11:234.
29. Bigliani LU, Morrison D, April EW. The morphology of the acromion and its relationship to rotator cuff tears. *Orthop Trans*. 1986;10:228.
30. Yazici M, Kopuz C, Gülman B. Morphologic variants of acromion in neonatal cadavers. *J Pediatr Orthop*. 1995;15(5):644–647.
31. Gerber C, Sebesta A. Impingement of the deep surface of the subscapularis tendon and the reflection pulley on the anterosuperior glenoid rim: a preliminary report. *J Shoulder Elbow Surg*. 2000;9(6):483–490.
32. Yamaguchi K, Tetro AM, Blam O, Evanoff BA, Teefey SA, Middleton WD. Natural history of asymptomatic rotator cuff tears: a longitudinal analysis of asymptomatic tears detected sonographically. *J Shoulder Elbow Surg*. 2001;10(3):199–203.
33. Yamanaka K, Matsumoto T. The joint side tear of the rotator cuff: a follow up study by arthrography. *Clin Orthop Relat Res*. 1994;304:68–73.
34. Meyer DC, Pirkl C, Pfirrmann CW, Zanetti M, Gerber C. Asymmetric atrophy of the supraspinatus muscle following tendon tear. *J Orthop Res*. 2005;23(2):254–258.
35. Safran O, Derwin KA, Powell K, Iannotti JP. Changes in rotator cuff muscle volume, fat content, and passive mechanics after chronic detachment in a canine model. *J Bone Joint Surg Am*. 2005;87(12):2662–2670.
36. Uhthoff HK, Matsumoto F, Trudel G, Himori K. Early reattachment does not reverse atrophy and fat accumulation of the supraspinatus: an experimental study in rabbits. *J Orthop Res*. 2003;21(3):386–392.
37. Melis B, Wall B, Walch G. Natural history of infraspinatus fatty infiltration in rotator cuff tears. *J Shoulder Elbow Surg*. 2010;19(5):757–763.
38. Kim YS, Bigliani LU, Fujisawa M. Stromal cell-derived factor-1 (SDF-1, CXCL 12) is increased in the subacromial bursitis and downregulated by steroid and nonsteroidal anti-inflammatory agents. *J Orthop Res*. 2006;24(8):1756–1764.
39. Teefey SA, Rubin DA, Middleton WD, Hildebolt CF, Leibold RA, Yamaguchi K. Detection and quantification of rotator cuff tears: comparison of ultrasonographic, magnetic resonance imaging, and arthroscopic findings in seventy-one consecutive cases. *J Bone Joint Surg Am*. 2004;86(4):708–716.
40. Mohtadi NG, Hollinshead RM, Sasyniuk TM, Fletcher JA, Chan DS, Li FX. A randomized clinical trial comparing open to arthroscopic acromioplasty with mini-open rotator cuff repair for full-thickness rotator cuff tears: disease-specific quality of life outcome at an average 2-year follow-up. *Am J Sports Med*. 2008;36(6):1043–1051.
41. Kim DH, Elattrache NS, Tibone JE, et al. Biomechanical comparison of a single-row versus double-row suture anchor technique for rotator cuff repair. *Am J Sports Med*. 2006;34(3):407–414.

42. Mazzocca AD, Millett PJ, Guanche CA, Santagelo SA, Arciero RA. Arthroscopic single-row vs double-row suture anchor rotator cuff repair. *Am J Sports Med.* 2005;33(12):1861–1868.
43. Apreleva M, Ozbaydar M, Fitzgibbons PG, Warner JJ. Rotator cuff tears: the effect of reconstruction method on three dimensional repair site area. *Arthroscopy*. 2001;18(5):519–526.
44. Brady PC, Arrigoni P, Burkhart SS. Evaluation of residual rotator cuff defects after in vivo single- versus double-row rotator cuff repairs. *Arthroscopy*. 2006;22(10):1070–1075.
45. Wall LB, Keener JD, Brophy RH. Clinical outcomes of double-row versus single-row rotator cuff repairs. *Arthroscopy*. 2009;25(11):1312–1318.
46. Park JY, Yoo MJ, Kim MH. Comparison of surgical outcome between bursal and articular partial thickness rotator cuff tears. *Orthopedics*. 2003;26(4):387–390.
47. Cordasco FA, Backer M, Craig EV, Klein D, Warren RF. The partial-thickness rotator cuff tear: is acromioplasty without repair sufficient? *Am J Sports Med.* 2002;30(2):257–260.
48. Weber SC. Arthroscopic debridement and acromioplasty versus mini-open repair in the treatment of significant partial-thickness rotator cuff tears. *Arthroscopy*. 1999;15(2):126–131.
49. Mazzocca AD, Rincon LM, O'Connor RW, et al. Intra-articular partial-thickness rotator cuff tears: analysis of injured and repaired strain behavior. *Am J Sports Med.* 2008;36(1):110–116.
50. Lo IK, Burkhart SS. Transtendon arthroscopic repair of partial-thickness, articular surface tears of the rotator cuff. *Arthroscopy*. 2004;20(2):214–220.
51. Conway JE. Arthroscopic repair of partial-thickness rotator cuff tears and SLAP lesions in professional baseball players. *Orthop Clin North Am*. 2001;32(3):443–456.
52. Wolff AB, Magit DP, Miller SR, Wyman J, Sethi PM. Arthroscopic fixation of bursal-sided rotator cuff tears. *Arthroscopy*. 2006;22(11):1247.e1–1247.e4.
53. Brockmeier SF, Dodson CC, Gamradt SC, Coleman SH, Altchek DW. Arthroscopic intratendinous repair of the delaminated partial-thickness rotator cuff tear in overhead athletes. *Arthroscopy*. 2008;24(8):961–965.
54. Reynolds SB, Dugas JR, Cain EL, McMichael CS, Andrews JR. Débridement of small partial-thickness rotator cuff tears in elite overhead throwers. *Clin Orthop Relat Res*. 2008;466:614–621.
55. Gonzalez-Lomas G, Kippe MA, Brown GD, et al. In situ transtendon repair outperforms tear completion and repair for partial articular-sided supraspinatus tendon tears. *J Shoulder Elbow Surg*. 2008;17(5):722–728.
56. Park MC, Jun BJ, Park CJ, Oh JH, Lee TQ. Biomechanical analysis of a knotless transtendon interimplant mattress repair for partial-thickness articular-sided rotator cuff tears. *Am J Sports Med.* 2009;37(1):2427–2434.
57. Peters KS, Lam PH, Murrell GA. Repair of partial-thickness rotator cuff tears: a biomechanical analysis of footprint contact pressure and strength in an ovine model. *Arthroscopy*. 2010;26(7):877–884.
58. Koester MC, Dunn WR, Kuhn JE, Spindler KP. The efficacy of subacromial corticosteroid injection in the treatment of rotator cuff disease: a systematic review. *J Am Acad Orthop Surg*. 2007;15(1):3–11.
59. Mansat P, Cofield RH, Kersten TE, Rowland CM. Complications of rotator cuff repair. *Orthop Clin North Am*. 1997;28(2):205–213.
60. Liu SH, Baker CL. Arthroscopically assisted rotator cuff repair: correlation of functional results with the integrity of the cuff. *Arthroscopy*. 1994;10(1):54–60.
61. Harryman DT II, Mack LA, Wang KY, Jackins SE, Richardson ML, Matsen FA III. Repairs of the rotator cuff: correlation of functional results with integrity of the cuff. *J Bone Joint Surg Am*. 1991;73(7):982–989.
62. Gore DR, Murray MP, Sepic SB, Garner GM. Shoulder-muscle strength and range of motion following surgical repair of full-thickness rotator cuff tears. *J Bone Joint Surg Am*. 1986;68(2):266–272.
63. Jost B, Zumstein M, Pfirrmann CW, Gerber C. Long-term outcome after structural failure of rotator cuff repairs. *J Bone Joint Surg Am*. 2006;88(3):472–479.
64. Smith KL, Harryman DT II, Antoniou J, Campbell B, Sidles JA, Matsen FA III. A prospective, multipractice study of shoulder function and health status in patients with documented rotator cuff tears. *J Shoulder Elbow Surg*. 2000;9(5):395–402.
65. Lindley K, Jones GL. Outcomes of arthroscopic versus open rotator cuff repair: a systematic review of the literature. *Am J Orthop (Belle Mead NJ)*. 2010;39(12):592–600.
66. Papadopoulos P, Karataglis D, Boutsiadis A, Fotiadou A, Christoforidis J, Christodoulou A. Functional outcome and structural integrity following mini-open repair of large and massive rotator cuff tears: a 3–5 year follow-up study. *J Shoulder Elbow Surg*. 2011;20(1):131–137.
67. Oh JH, Kim SH, Shin SH, et al. Outcome of rotator cuff repair in large-to-massive tear with pseudoparalysis: a comparative study with propensity score matching. *Am J Sports Med.* 2011;39(7):1413–1420.
68. Warrender WJ, Brown OL, Abboud JA. Outcomes of arthroscopic rotator cuff repairs in obese patients. *J Shoulder Elbow Surg*. 2011;20(6):961–967.
69. Norlin R, Adolfsson L. Small full-thickness tears do well ten to thirteen years after arthroscopic subacromial decompression. *J Shoulder Elbow Surg*. 2008;17(1 suppl):12S–16S.
70. Kartus J, Kartus C, Rostgård-Christensen L, Sernert N, Read J, Perko M. Long-term clinical and ultrasound evaluation after arthroscopic acromioplasty in patients with partial rotator cuff tears. *Arthroscopy*. 2006;22(1):44–49.
71. Deutsch A. Arthroscopic repair of partial-thickness tears of the rotator cuff. *J Shoulder Elbow Surg*. 2007;16(2):193–201.
72. Porat S, Nottage WM, Fouse MN. Repair of partial thickness rotator cuff tears: a retrospective review with minimum two-year follow-up. *J Shoulder Elbow Surg*. 2008;17(5):729–731.
73. Kamath G, Galatz LM, Keener JD, Teefey S, Middleton W, Yamaguchi K. Tendon integrity and functional outcome after arthroscopic repair of high-grade partial-thickness supraspinatus tears. *J Bone Joint Surg Am*. 2009;91(5):1055–1062.
74. Ide J, Maeda S, Takagi K. Arthroscopic transtendon repair of partial-thickness articular-side tears of the rotator cuff: anatomical and clinical study. *Am J Sports Med.* 2005;33(1):1672–1679.
75. Huberty DP, Schoolfield JD, Brady PC, Vadala AP, Arrigoni P, Burkhart SS. Incidence and treatment of postoperative stiffness following arthroscopic rotator cuff repair. *Arthroscopy*. 2009;25(8):880–890.
76. Spencer EE Jr. Partial-thickness articular surface rotator cuff tears: an all-inside repair technique. *Clin Orthop Relat Res*. 2010;468:1514–1520.

I-4

Glenohumeral Instability

Todd J. Twiss, MD, and George M. McCluskey III, MD

The inherently unstable shoulder joint sacrifices stability at the cost of mobility. It has the greatest range of motion and highest dislocation rate of any major joint. Recent advances in the understanding of anatomy, pathophysiology, biomechanics, clinical evaluation, and imaging studies have resulted in great advances in the understanding and treatment of the unstable shoulder. Current goals of restoration of normal anatomy and shoulder function are an improvement over outdated treatment methods, which blocked physiologic motion to prevent recurrent instability.

PERTINENT ANATOMY

A combination of both dynamic and static restraints provides shoulder stability. Static restraints include articular congruence, articular version, the glenoid labrum, and capsuloligamentous restraints. The rotator cuff, biceps tendon, deltoid, and scapular stabilizer muscles provide a dynamic restraint to instability.

The shoulder joint is an articulation of the proximal humerus and glenoid fossa. The glenoid is pear-shaped and relatively flat, with a radius of curvature greater than that of the humeral head. It is retroverted 1.23° relative to the scapular plane.[1] The humeral head has an average retroversion of 19° to the humeral shaft and a 130° to 140° neck-shaft angle. The humeral head is substantially larger than the glenoid, and the relationship has been compared with that of a golf ball on a tee (Figure 1). This difference results in an unconstrained articulation with little inherent bony stability.

The labrum is a triangular fibrocartilaginous ring around the circumference of the glenoid (Figure 2). It provides a site of attachment for the capsule and glenohumeral ligaments, deepens the glenoid fossa, increases the surface area of the glenoid, and acts as a chock block to prevent translation of the humeral head. Several anatomic variations, particularly of the superior labrum, exist, and the long head of the biceps tendon shares its origin with labral tissue at the supraglenoid tubercle.

Along with the bony structures and labrum, the joint capsule and glenohumeral ligaments are static restraints (Figure 3). The glenohumeral ligaments are merely thickenings of the capsule, and both primarily are composed of type 1 collagen. Major ligamentous structures include the coracohumeral ligament, superior, middle, and inferior glenohumeral ligament complex (IGHLC). Both the coracohumeral and superior glenohumeral ligaments restrain external rotation and inferior translation in an adducted extremity.[2] The middle glenohumeral ligament prevents translation and external rotation with abduction of 45° to 60°, and the inferior glenohumeral ligament stabilizes the shoulder in 90° of abduction and external rotation.[2] Overall, the IGHLC is the most important restraint to external rotation of the shoulder.[2,3] Recent cadaveric data have shown that the capsule and ligamentous structures do

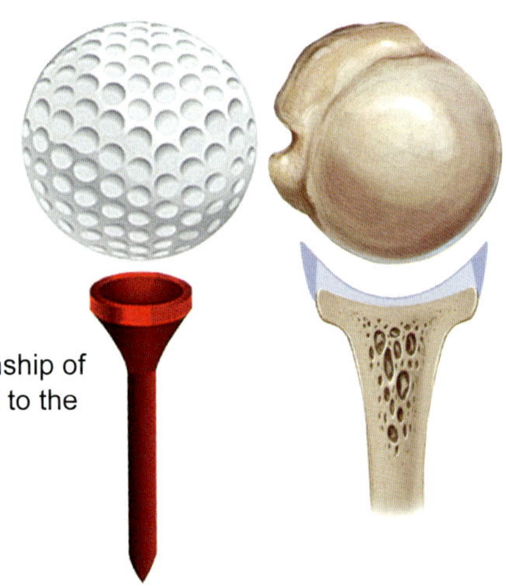

Figure 1. Relationship of the humeral head to the glenoid.

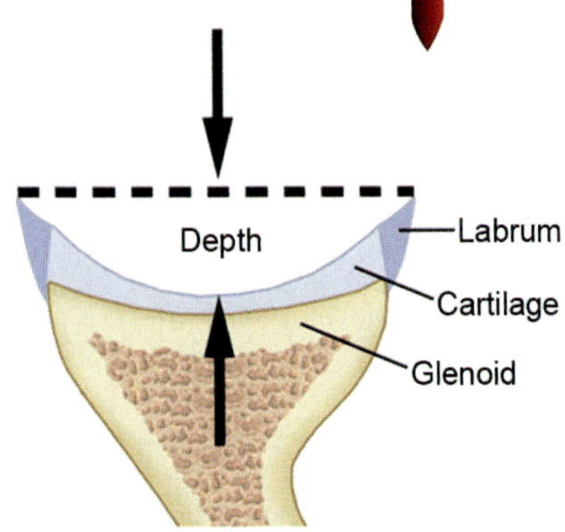

Figure 2. Glenoid labrum.

Glenohumeral Instability

Figure 3. Glenohumeral ligament complex. Abbreviations: BT, biceps tendon; SGHL, superior glenohumeral ligament; MGHL, middle glenohumeral ligament; and IGHL, inferior glenohumeral ligament.

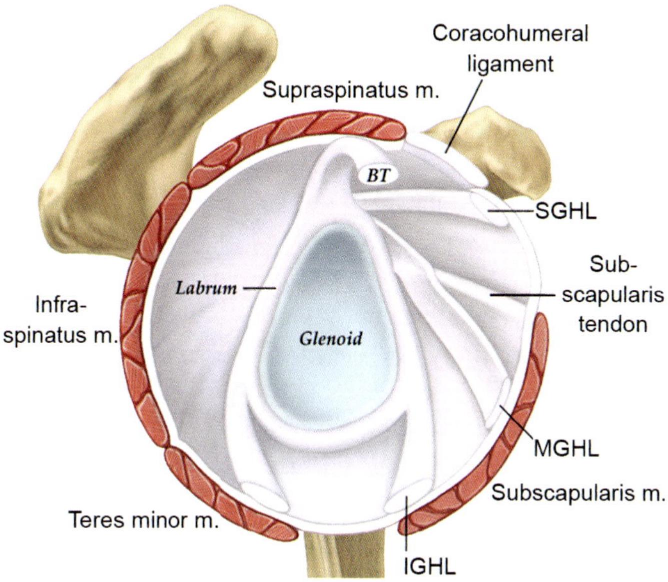

not act in isolation but behave like a cylinder, undergoing strain in multiple areas during rotation and translation.[3] An intact capsule maintains a negative intra-articular pressure to further stabilize the shoulder.

Finally, the rotator interval is a region of the glenohumeral joint capsule between the superior border of the subscapularis and anterior border of the supraspinatus, which also is a static stabilizer (Figure 4). This region contains the superior glenohumeral ligament, coracohumeral ligament, and long head of the biceps tendon and provides stability to inferior translation and external rotation with the upper extremity at the side.[1]

As a general rule, the static stabilizers of the shoulder function to restrict translation and rotation at extreme positions of motion, and dynamic factors provide stability throughout the midranges of motion when static structures are relaxed. Muscle forces around the shoulder compress the humeral head against the concave glenoid surface, allowing concentric rotation of the humeral head.[4]

The rotator cuff consists of the subscapularis, supraspinatus, infraspinatus, and teres minor muscles, which originate from the scapula and insert onto the proximal humerus. The function of each tendon depends on its line of pull. Together, they internally rotate, externally rotate, and stabilize the humerus to initiate forward elevation and abduction. This dynamic action creates a balanced concavity-compression effect on the shoulder

Figure 4. Rotator interval.

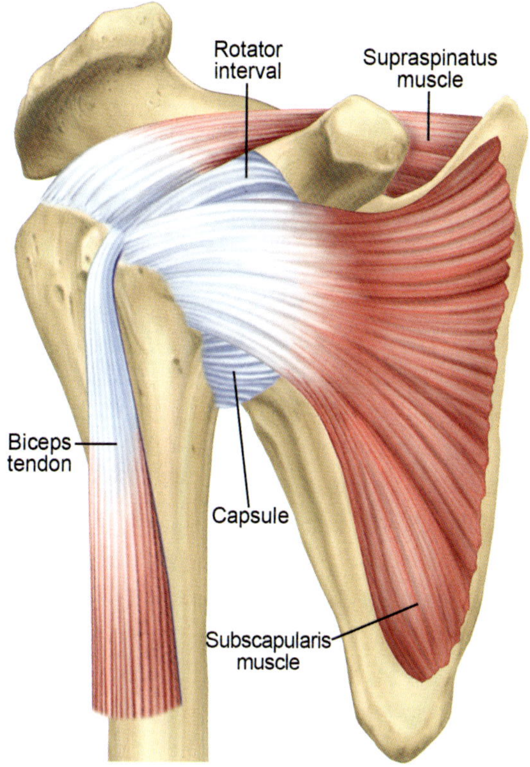

joint throughout the range of motion (Figure 5), and it directs a net joint-reaction force within the glenoid arc.[4]

Other muscular stabilizing forces include the deltoid, scapular rotators, and biceps tendon. The deltoid resists inferior translation and creates a compression

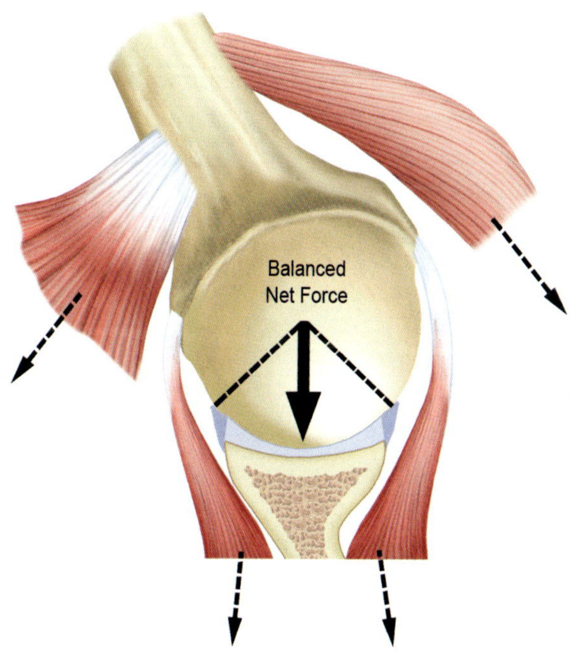

Figure 5. Rotator cuff concavity-compression effect and net joint-reaction force.

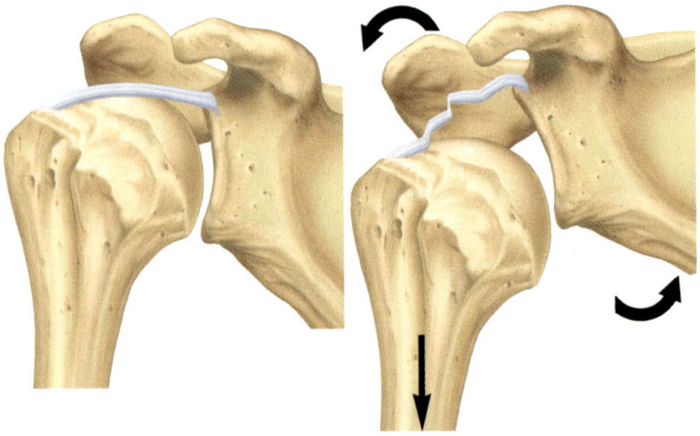

Figure 6. Scapular dumping.

force on the glenoid at 60° of abduction in the scapular plane.[4] The scapular rotators position the scapula on the chest wall, creating a stable glenoid platform for coordinated glenohumeral and scapulothoracic motion. Muscular forces of the trapezius, rhomboids, serratus anterior, and levator scapulae control the posture of the scapula. Alteration of this posture can reduce normal tension of the capsule and ligaments, resulting in scapular dumping (Figure 6).[5] The long head of the biceps tendon travels through the bicipital groove, travels into the rotator interval, and inserts onto the supraglenoid tubercle. Researchers believe it is a secondary depressor of the humeral head and centers the humeral head on the glenoid during the end ranges of rotational motion.[1]

Finally, mechanoreceptors located throughout the shoulder joint act as dynamic stabilizers. Structures, including the inferior glenohumeral ligament, middle glenohumeral ligament, subscapularis tendon, biceps tendon, supraspinatus, and labrum contain mechanoreceptors that carry proprioceptive information to the brain via the dorsal columns of the spinal cord.[6]

PATHOPHYSIOLOGY

To examine the pathoanatomy of glenohumeral instability, a clear definition of instability and the degree, mechanism, and chronicity of instability must be established. Confusion exists between the terms *laxity* and *instability*. Glenohumeral laxity is an asymptomatic translation of the humeral head outside the glenoid arc, which is not a pathologic condition. Instability is a pathologic condition in which translation of the humeral head on the glenoid results in symptoms of pain and apprehension. Instability can result from various degrees of translation. A subluxation refers to symptomatic incomplete or partial dislocation usually with spontaneous reduction, whereas a dislocation occurs when the joint becomes displaced or malaligned, often requiring a reduction. Mechanisms of glenohumeral instability can be simplified into traumatic and atraumatic causes. Outdated descriptive acronyms include TUBS (traumatic event that is unidirectional associated with Bankart lesion requiring surgery) and AMBRI (atraumatic, multidirectional, bilateral, responds to rehabilitation and inferior capsular shift). These acronyms can be misleading because a traumatic event can result in a multidirectional problem, and a patient with joint hyperlaxity can sustain trauma, causing unidirectional instability. Chronicity determines the type of lesions associated with instability. Acute instability usually results from a macrotrauma and specific anatomic insult, but chronic instability causes repetitive microtrauma and specific tissue changes.

Disruption of the static or dynamic restraints produces the pathoanatomy responsible for shoulder instability. The old concept of an "essential lesion" is outdated, and multiple factors related to both mechanism of injury and patient factors lead to instability. Authors of clinical and experimental studies have shown that no single factor is responsible for stability and no single lesion can cause instability.[7–10] Instability results after an insult to multiple structures in the shoulder, and both bony and soft tissue structures are affected.[7–10]

Bony lesions associated with glenohumeral instability can result from acute trauma or repetitive wear. Traumatic insults can result in fractures to either the proximal humerus or glenoid. Acute anterior dislocation can cause a Hill-Sachs defect, which is a compression fracture of the posterolateral humeral head (Figure 7), or a bony Bankart lesion, which is a fracture of the anteroinferior glenoid rim (Figure 8). Greater tuberosity fractures also are seen in patients who have sustained anterior dislocations (Figure 9). Chronic or recurrent anterior dislocation can result in erosion of the anteroinferior glenoid rim, causing an "inverted-pear" glenoid and larger engaging Hill-Sachs lesions (Figures 10 and 11).[11] Acute posterior dislocation can cause posterior glenoid-rim defects, reverse Hill-Sachs lesions, and concomitant surgical neck or complex proximal humerus fracture (Figure 12). Recurrent posterior dislocation results in posterior glenoid erosion.[12] Chronic or locked dislocations result in substantial

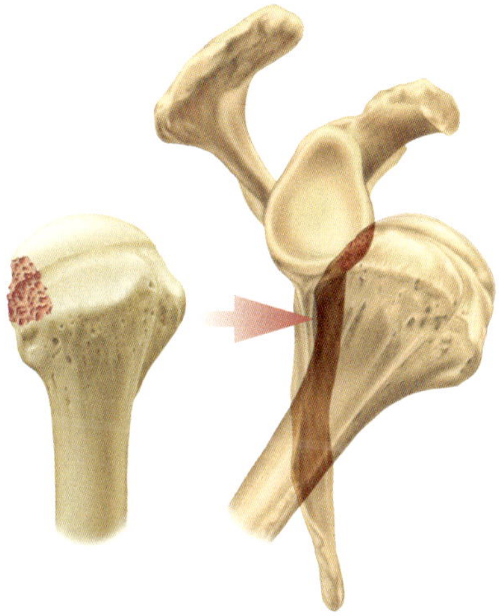

Figure 7. Hill-Sachs lesion.

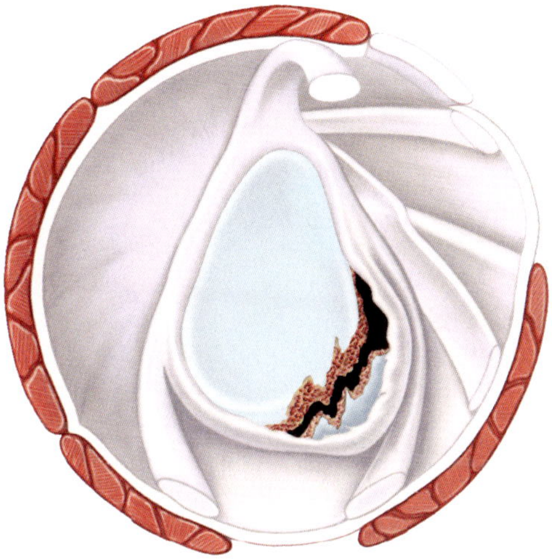

Figure 8. Bony Bankart lesion.

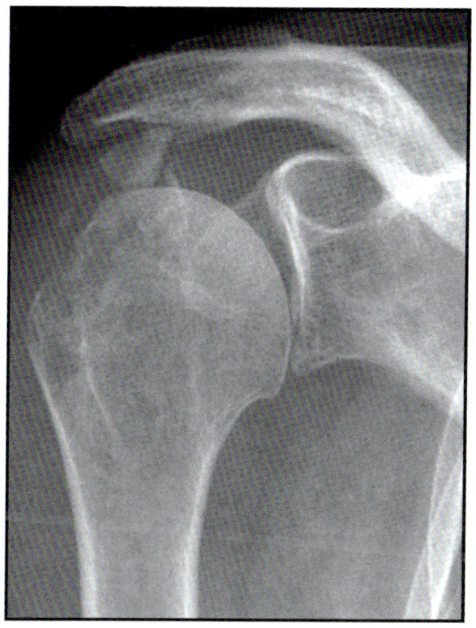

Figure 9. Greater tuberosity fracture with dislocation.

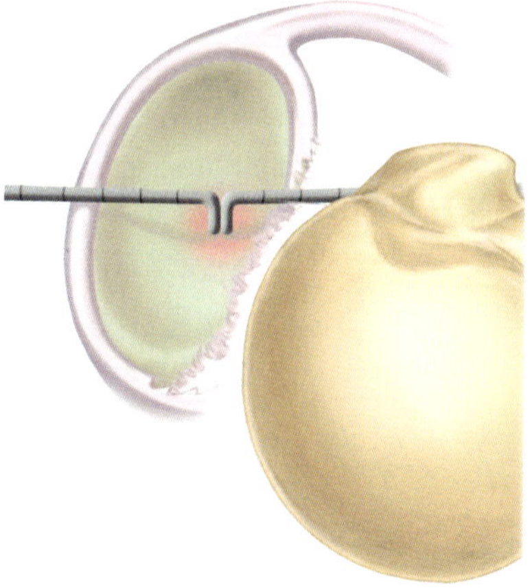

Figure 10. Inverted-pear glenoid.

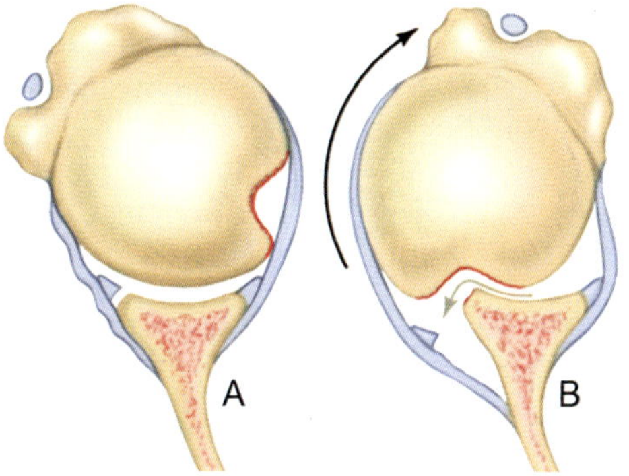

Figure 11 A and B. Hill-Sachs lesion engaging.

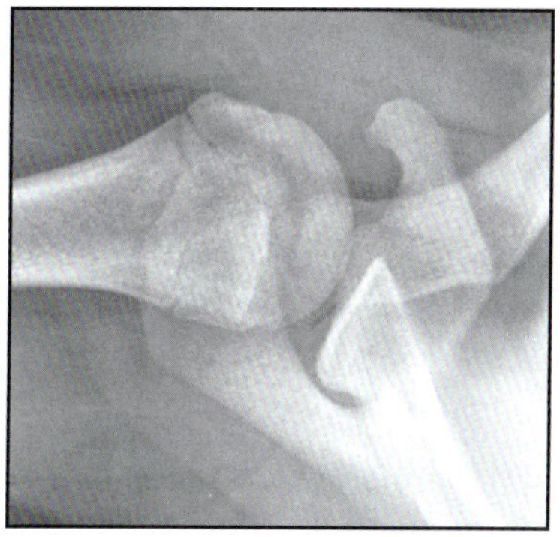

Figure 12. Increased glenoid retroversion and posterior glenoid erosion with posterior instability.

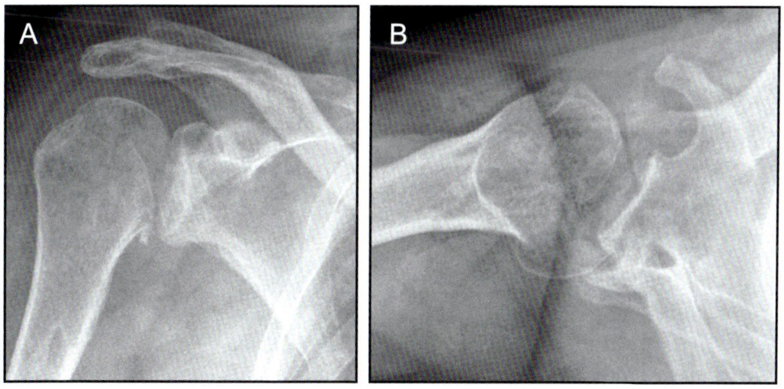

Figure 13. Chronic dislocation. A, Anteroposterior view. B, Axillary view.

bony defects, and locations of the defects depend on the direction of dislocation (Figure 13).

Soft tissue lesions can include pathologic changes of the labrum, capsule, glenohumeral ligaments, rotator cuff, and dynamic muscular stabilizers. Classically, the Bankart lesion, which is an avulsion of the anteroinferior labrum and IGHLC from the glenoid rim, was viewed as the essential lesion for anterior dislocation (Figure 14).[2,7,8] This results in decreased glenoid depth and reduction in force required for dislocation. Cadaveric and clinical data have shown that although it is seen in most anterior dislocations, a Bankart lesion alone is not sufficient to cause dislocation.[8] An anterior labroligamentous periosteal sleeve avulsion lesion results after the labrum, IGHLC, and periosteum displace and heal medially along the scapular neck (Figure 15). This more chronic lesion results in a substantially higher risk of recurrent instability.[13] Lesions of both the supe-

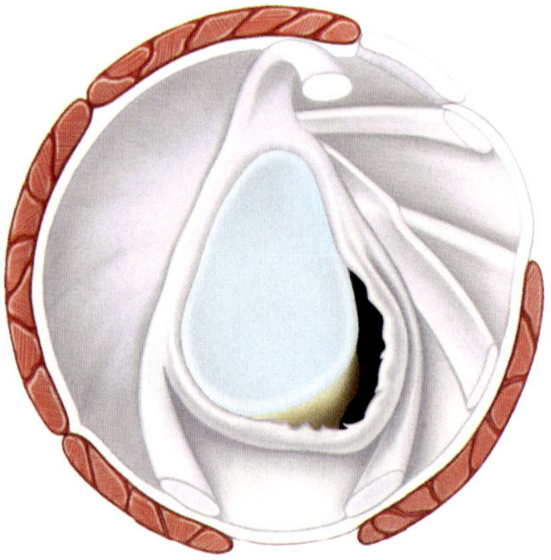

Figure 14. Bankart lesion.

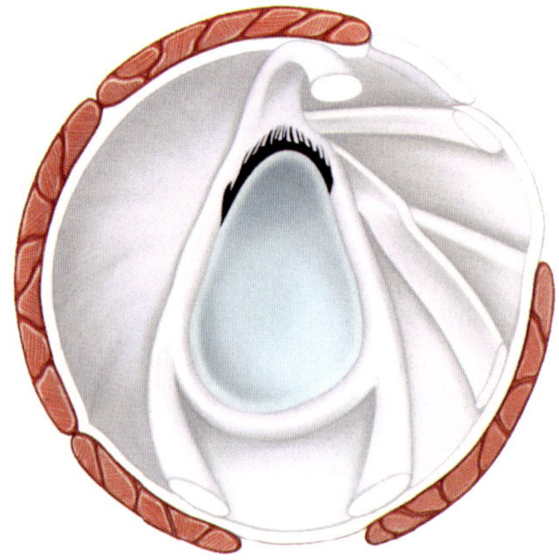

Figure 16. Superior labrum anterior-posterior lesion.

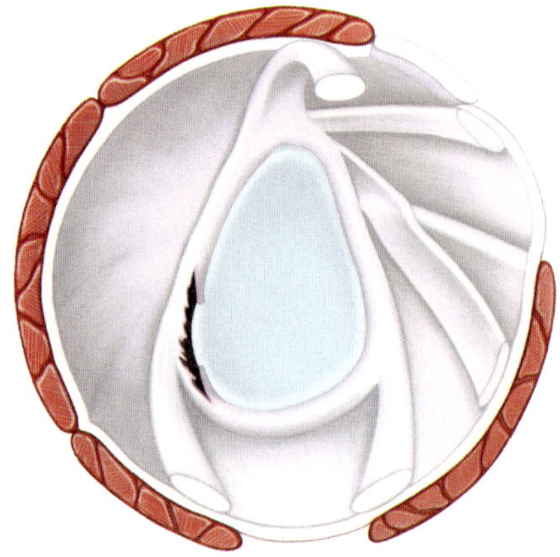

Figure 17. Posterior labral tear and Kim lesions.

Figure 15. Anterior labroligamentous periosteal sleeve avulsion lesion.

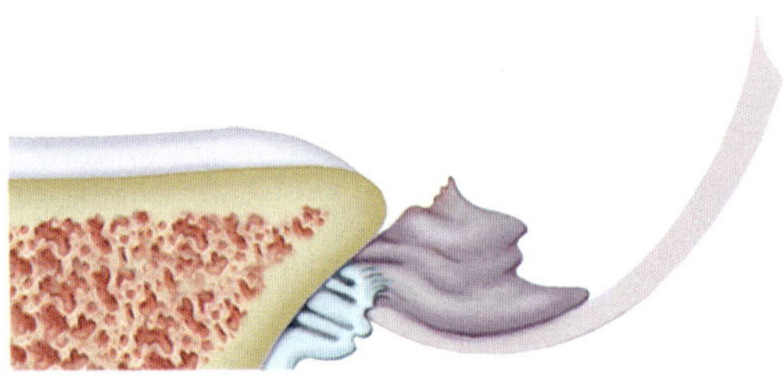

rior and posterior labrum also result in glenohumeral instability. Superior labrum anterior-posterior (SLAP) lesions can cause increased glenohumeral translation and result in instability (Figure 16).[14] Correlations can be seen in patients who are less than 40 years of age and have concomitant SLAP tears and Bankart lesions.[15] Posteroinferior labral tears can be seen with posterior dislocations, and concealed avulsions of the posteroinferior labrum or Kim lesions occasionally can result in posterior and multidirectional instability (Figure 17).[16]

A capsular lesion can result after either acute traumatic or repetitive microtrauma. In cadaveric studies, researchers have shown that failure of the IGHLC can occur in multiple locations with instability. It occurs at the glenoid or humeral insertions or in the intrasubstance 40%, 25%, and 35% of the time, respectively.[7] Humeral avulsion of the glenohumeral ligament lesions can occur after substantial trauma with or without concomitant lesions of the labrum (Figure 18).[17] Capsular tears also can be seen in patients with acute dislocations. Repetitive microtrauma and capsular stretch occur in overhead athletes secondary to overuse.[10] Fatigued dynamic stabilizers allow increased strain to the capsuloligamentous restraints. This results in plastic deformation of the capsule over time (Figure 19). In addition, atraumatic instability in patients with hyperlaxity is secondary to excessive capsular laxity and either macrotraumatic or microtraumatic insult.

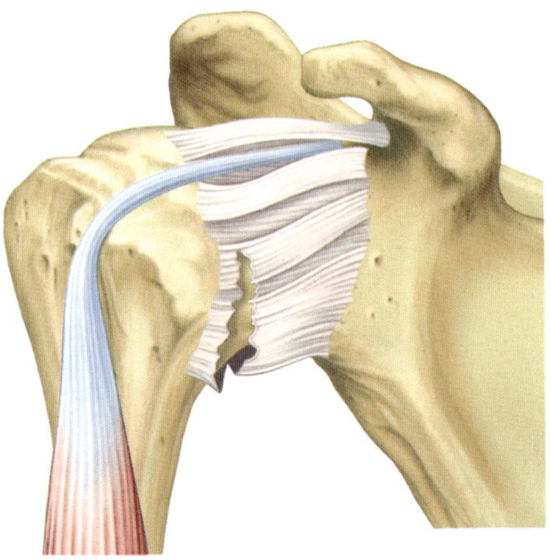

Figure 18. Humeral avulson of the glenohumeral ligament lesion.

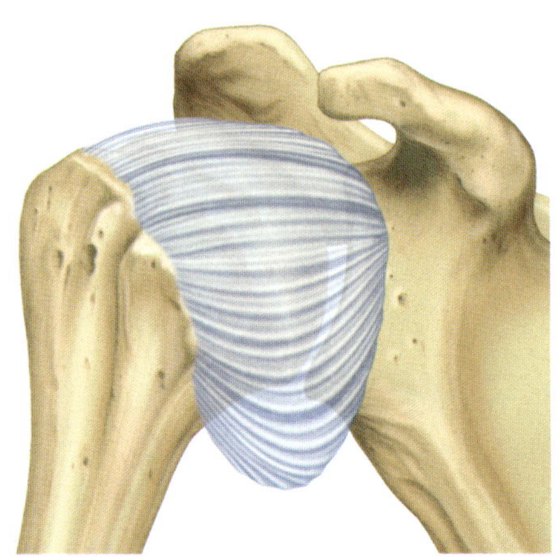

Figure 19. Patulous inferior capsule.

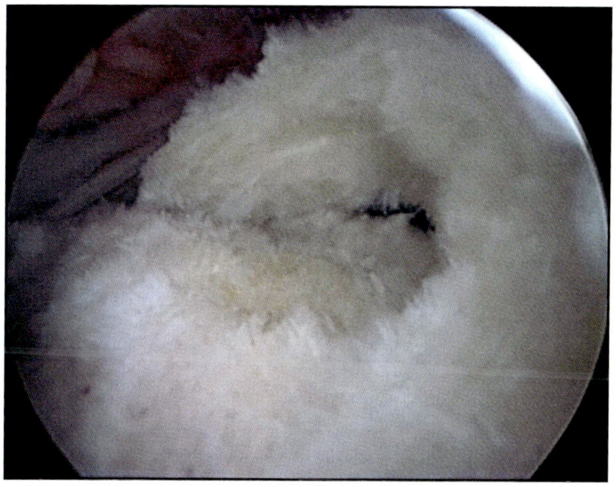

Figure 20. Rotator cuff tear.

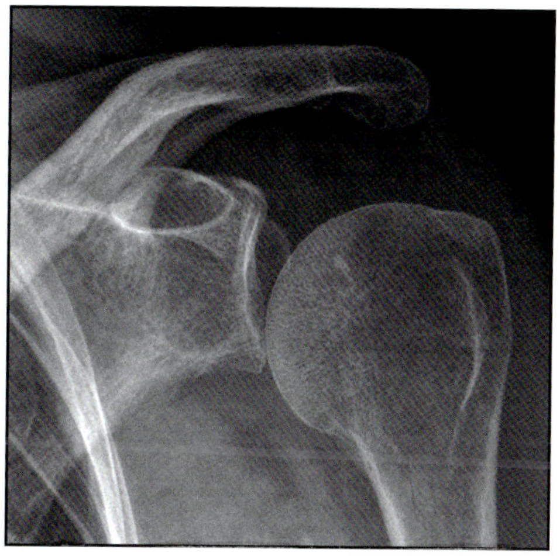

Figure 21. Axillary nerve palsy with inferior humeral subluxation.

With glenohumeral instability, the rotator cuff and other muscular stabilizers can be abnormal. Patients who are more than 40 years of age typically present with complete rotator cuff tears after dislocations (Figure 20).[18] Anterior dislocations can cause tearing of the subscapularis and supraspinatus, and chronic superior subluxation of the glenohumeral joint is seen with massive rotator cuff tears. Abnormal muscular coordination and activity can be seen in patients with multidirectional instability. Electromyography can display abnormal firing of the deltoid and shoulder girdle musculature associated with multidirectional instability.[19]

Neurologic imbalance also occurs with glenohumeral instability. Electric shock and seizure can cause posterior dislocation. With sustained firing of all muscles of the shoulder girdle, the relatively stronger internal rotators overpower the external rotators, resulting in posterior dislocation. Nerve injury results in approximately 48% of the population after an acute episode of instability (Figure 21).[20] The axillary and suprascapular nerves are the most commonly affected, with an average recovery time of 12 to 45 weeks. Nearly complete nerve recovery can be expected in most patients, but a substantial loss of motion results too.[20]

DIAGNOSIS

Accurate diagnosis of glenohumeral instability requires a complete knowledge of pertinent anatomy, pathophysiology, patient history, physical examination, and appropriate imaging. As mentioned, glenohumeral instability is a pathologic condition in which translation of the humerus outside the glenoid arc causes symptoms of pain and apprehension. Many different classification systems have been proposed. Factors examined include cause, direction, chronicity, and combinations thereof. Gerber and Nyffeler[21] proposed an elegant classification system, which distinguishes among static, dynamic, and voluntary dislocation. Static instability is diagnosed with radiographs and describes a degenerative condition that has resulted in fixed anterior, superior, or posterior subluxation of the humeral head.[21] Dynamic lesions are either unidirectional or multidirectional and either are or are not associated with hyperlaxity.[21] Individuals who voluntarily dislocate the shoulder fall into 3 groups: muscular, positional, and psychiatric dislocators.[21] Accurate diagnosis allows communication among orthopaedic surgeons and implementation of appropriate treatment.

Clinical and Imaging Evaluation

A thorough history and physical examination are paramount to the diagnosis of glenohumeral instability. Multiple imaging techniques, examination under anesthesia, and arthroscopy are tools that help establish a diagnosis when the cause of instability is unclear, but nothing is a substitute for a clinical diagnosis. Determining the exact details surrounding the onset and initial incident of instability is important. Factors, such as age, mechanism, position, and direction of instability provide important guides to treatment. In addition, types of previous treatment, including rehabilitation, immobilization, or operations, help delineate the problem. Finally, ongoing symptoms, including apprehension, shoulder pain, positional issues, neck pain, and voluntary or habitual dislocation guide treatment.

Physical examination has an important role in the diagnosis of shoulder instability. A complete musculoskeletal evaluation, including inspection, palpation, range of motion, strength testing, neurologic evaluation, cervical spine evaluation, shoulder stability testing, and other special tests, is essential. Visual inspection will uncover any signs of collagen disorders, such as widened scars, atrophy that indicates nerve injury, scapular dyskinesis, or a sulcus sign pointing toward multidirectional instability (Figure 22). Any difference between active and passive range of motion, as well as in strength, should be assessed. Patients with anterior instability usually have tenderness over the posterior capsule, and patients with multidirectional instability generally display tenderness over the medial border of the scapula. Concomitant rotator cuff lesions present as weakness, tenderness over the greater tuberosity, or crepitation throughout the range of motion. Signs, such as thumb hyperabduction and finger, elbow, and knee hyperextension, point toward global ligamentous laxity (Figure 23). Special tests to elucidate the cause of instability include the sulcus sign, load and shift, apprehension, and relocation.

The sulcus sign is performed with the patient's extremity at the side in neutral rotation and adduction (Figure 24). The examiner places inferiorly directed force on the humerus and measures the distance between the humeral head and acromion. A distance of greater than 2 cm is considered a positive test and indicates inferior instability. A positive sulcus sign is a requirement for a diagnosis of multidirectional instability. In addition, the test can be performed with the extremity at the side in maximum external rotation. This maneuver will tension the anterior capsule and rotator interval, and the persistence or resolution of a sulcus sign in external rotation highlights pathologic lesions in these structures.

Figure 23 A and B. Generalized ligamentous laxity.

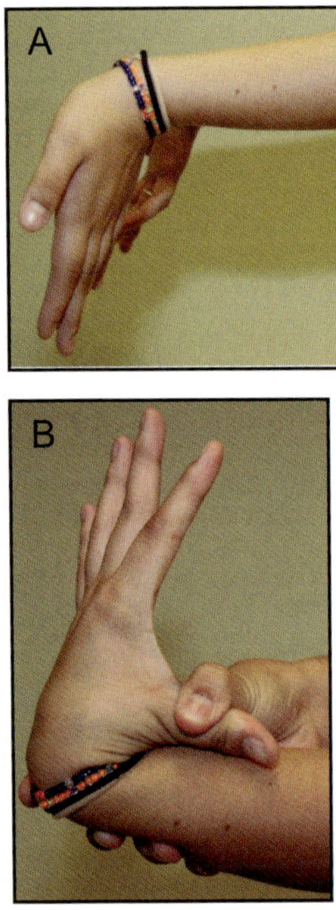

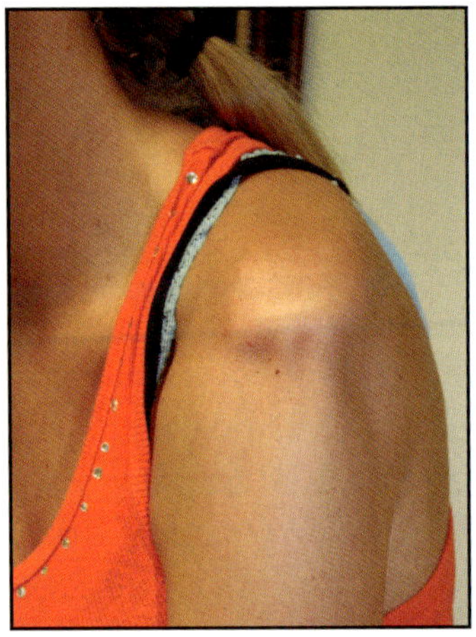

Figure 24. Sulcus sign.

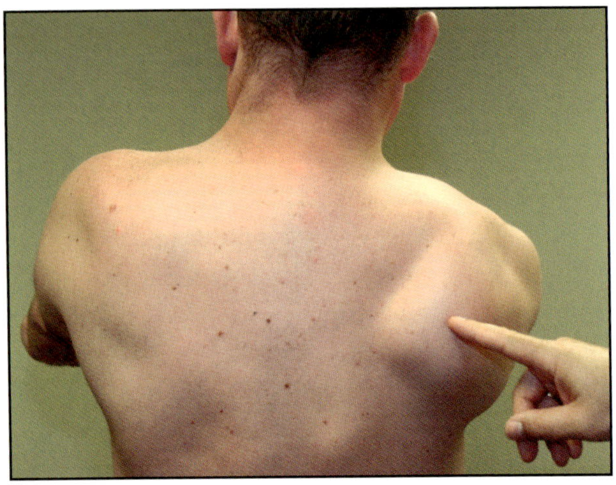

Figure 22. Scapular winging.

Load-and-shift testing establishes clinically important translation of the humeral head on the glenoid. The test is performed either in the seated or supine position. The supine position with the scapula stabilized will effectively eliminate scapulothoracic motion (Figure 25). The upper extremity is placed in the scapular plane in 20° of abduction and forward flexion, and the humeral head is loaded. An anterior, posterior, and inferior stress is placed, and clinically important translation is graded. Grade 0 indicates minimal movement; grade I+, the humeral head rides onto the labrum; grade II+, the humeral head subluxes but spontaneously reduces; and grade III+, the humeral head dislocates and remains dislocated (Figure 26).

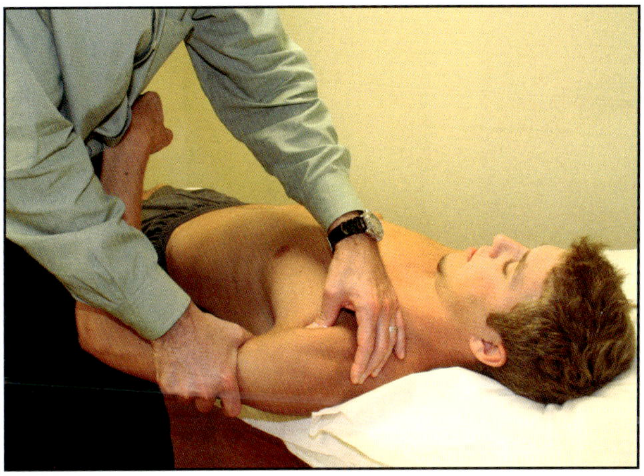

Figure 25. Load-and-shift test.

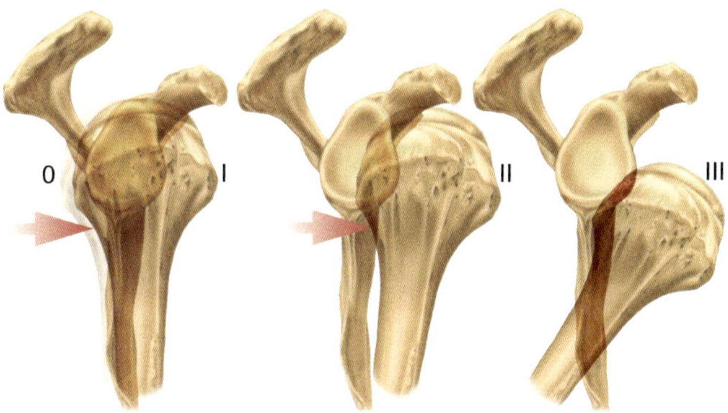

Figure 26. Grades of glenohumeral joint translation.

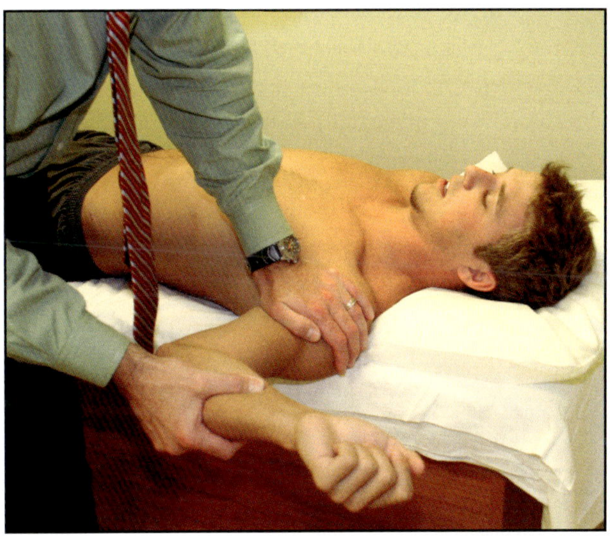

Figure 27. Apprehension and relocation test.

Apprehension and relocation are best tested in the supine position (Figure 27). The upper extremity is placed in 90° of abduction and maximum external rotation. The patient will express a feeling of apprehension or impending instability either through oral cues, facial expressions, or protectively contracting their muscles. Relocation can be assessed in conjunction with apprehension by placing a posteriorly directed force on the proximal humerus. Both apprehension and pain should disappear. The presence and relief of pain only with apprehension and relocation are associated with conditions other than instability, but the relief of apprehension with relocation substantially increases the accuracy of the test for instability.[22,23] For posterior apprehension, the shoulder is adducted, internally rotated, and flexed to 90°, and a posterior force is applied. In addition, a posterior jerk test and novel Kim test can be used to assess the shoulder for posterior instability with a symptomatic posterior labral tear.[24,25] The jerk test is performed with the patient seated. The examiner applies an axial force to the extremity in 90° of abduction and internal rotation. The extremity is horizontally adducted with axial force maintained. Pain and a "clunk" are indicative of a positive test (Figure 28).[24] The Kim test is performed

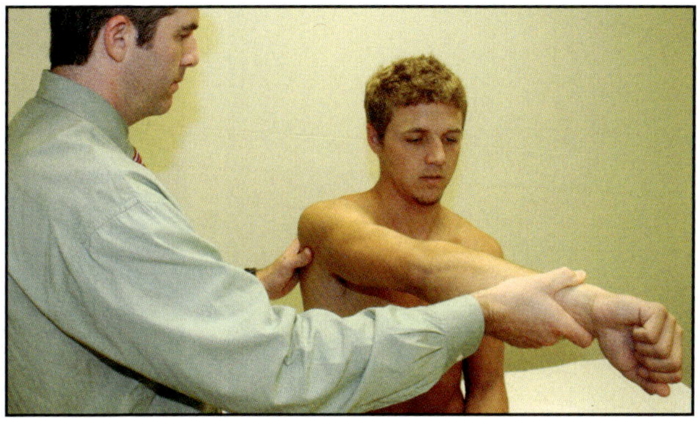

Figure 28. Jerk test.

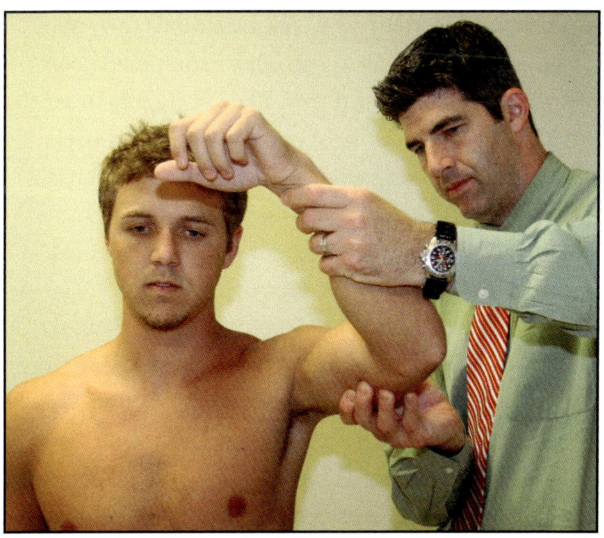

Figure 29. Kim test.

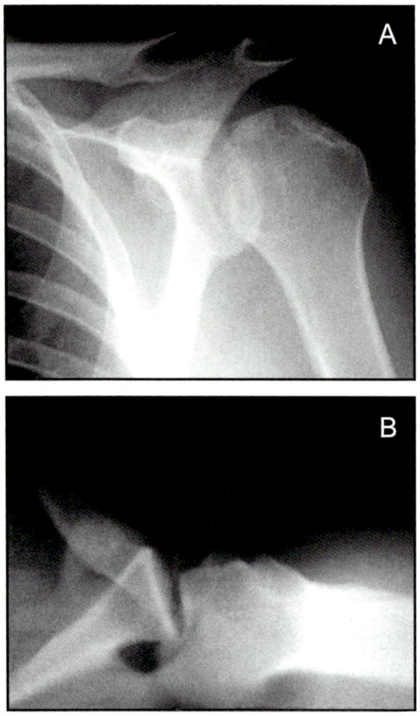

Figure 30. Posterior dislocation. A, Anteroposterior view. B, Axillary-lateral view provides the best view.

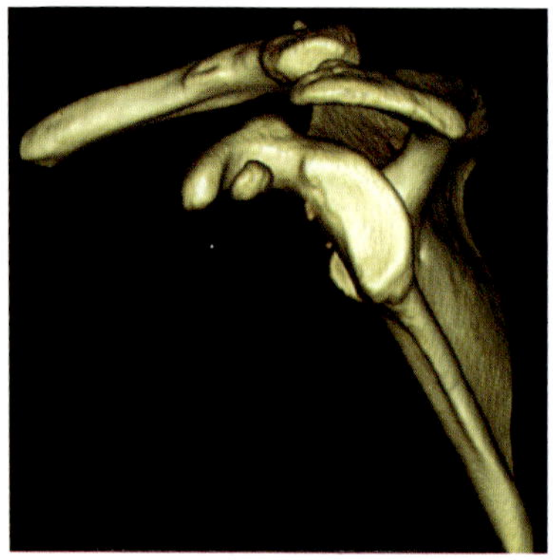

Figure 31. Three-dimensional computed tomography scan shows glenoid bone loss.

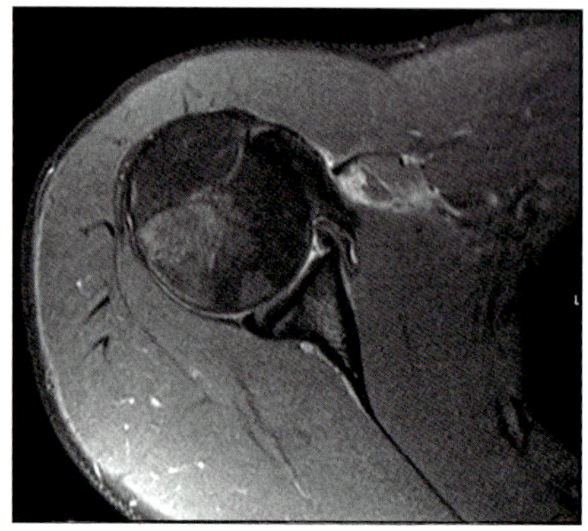

Figure 32. Magnetic resonance imaging scan demonstrates a labral tear.

with the patient seated and the upper extremity in 90° of abduction. The examiner holds the elbow and places a strong posterior and inferior force on the extremity while placing an axial load and diagonally elevating the extremity to 45°. Sudden onset of shoulder pain indicates a positive test (Figure 29).[25] When painful, the posterior jerk test can indicate future failure of nonoperative management.[24] The jerk test combined with the novel Kim test has a sensitivity of 97% at detecting a substantial posteroinferior labral lesion.[25]

Imaging can provide more information to the complete evaluation of instability. Plain radiographs are the initial imaging modality of choice to assess concentricity of the glenohumeral joint and bony pathologic lesions, such as bone loss or fracture. For an acute instability episode, radiographic views must include true anteroposterior (AP) and axillary-lateral views of the shoulder (Figure 30). Without an axillary-lateral view, an acute dislocation can be missed, especially if it occurs in the posterior direction. Special views, such as the West Point, Stryker notch, or AP in internal rotation views, highlight bony defects, such as bony Bankart or Hill-Sachs lesions.[26] Ultimately, computed tomography scan with 3-dimensional reconstruction views provide the most accurate detail of bony anatomy and should be obtained if clinically important bone loss is suspected (Figure 31).

Magnetic resonance imaging remains the criterion standard for imaging of the shoulder in patients with instability (Figure 32). Advantages of magnetic resonance imaging include superior soft tissue resolution, multiplanar images, no ionizing radiation, and the ability to view the rotator cuff and intra-articular structures. Injection of intra-articular contrast, or magnetic resonance arthrography, increases the sensitivity and accuracy in the diagnosis of subtle labral and ligamentous lesions, anterior labral tears, SLAP lesions, partial-thickness rotator cuff tears, and both acute and chronic labroligamentous lesions.[27]

Patient Selection

Decisions for treatment of instability are based on several factors, including mechanisms, chronicity, age, direction, classification, and patient factors. Nonoperative management is appropriate for many instability patterns. Patients with atraumatic episodes, voluntary instability, posterior instability, multidirectional instability, and certain cases of chronic dislocations and patients who are children or athletes in season can be treated successfully with nonoperative measures. Principles of nonoperative management include treatment with reduction, a period of immobilization, and directed physical therapy. Operative treatment is recommended for irreducible or open dislocations, recurrent dislocations, substantial bony defects with recurrence, and failure of nonoperative management for patients with anterior, posterior, or multidirectional instability. Because of high rates of redislocation and poor functional outcomes, patients who are less than 25 years of age and have acute initial dislocations are candidates for acute arthroscopic stabilization.[28,29]

OPERATIVE TREATMENT

Anterior Instability

The goal of operative treatment for anterior instability is to address any clinically important bone lesions, to repair the Bankart lesion, to restore tension on the anteroinferior glenohumeral ligament, and to retension the capsule with appropriate capsulorrhaphy. Various treatments have been employed throughout the years, but recent advances in both the understanding of basic science principles and shoulder biomechanics and operative technique have improved patient outcomes.

Open procedures can be grouped into anatomic and nonanatomic repairs. Nonanatomic repairs retension structures, such as the subscapularis and capsule, to limit external rotation. Although these procedures effectively eliminate redislocation, they have high rates of patient dissatisfaction and osteoarthritis.[30] On the other hand, open anatomic procedures, such as open Bankart-type repairs, provide the criterion standard by which all other techniques are compared (Figure 33).[30] Open capsulolabral repair has low rates of dislocation, good preservation of range of motion, reasonable return to function, and high ratings of patient satisfaction.[30] Despite these outcomes, concerns over the need to detach and reattach the subscapularis have prompted interest in arthroscopic methods.[31] For recurrent anterior instability, anterior capsular shift with and without Bankart repair allows anatomic reconstruction of the damaged capsule and labrum while avoiding detaching the subscapularis, which reduces operative time, decreases blood loss, and improves cosmesis.[30] The procedure is performed through standard posterior, anterosuperior, and anteroinferior arthroscopic portals. The labral-ligamentous complex is mobilized from a scarred and nonanatomic position, anchors are placed on the glenoid rim from inferior to superior, sutures are passed to shift the capsule and labrum from an inferior to superior position, and secure arthroscopic knots are tied. Modern arthroscopic techniques have rates of recurrence equal to those of traditional open repair, with increases in patient satisfaction.[30,32] Currently, primary indications for open repair include capsular or subscapularis deficiency, humeral avulsions of the glenohumeral ligament, and substantial bone loss.

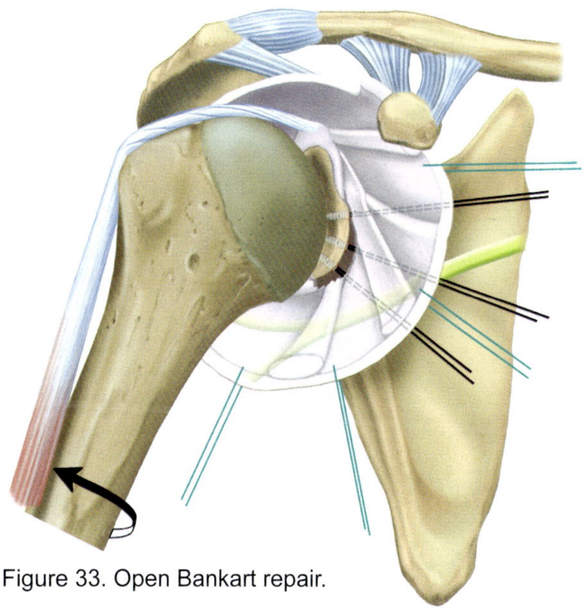

Figure 33. Open Bankart repair.

Accepted criteria for substantial bone loss are defects of the anteroinferior glenoid rim of greater than 20% to 30% and an engaging Hill-Sachs lesion.[11] Various treatments for an engaging Hill-Sachs lesion include allograft reconstruction, impaction grafting, rotational osteotomy, prosthetic replacement, and arthroscopic remplissage. Purchase and associates[33] described the novel technique of arthroscopic remplissage, which insets the infraspinatus into the humeral head defect. This procedure can be used for large- to moderate-sized Hill-Sachs lesions without glenoid bone loss and for moderate-sized Hill-Sachs lesions with less than 25% glenoid bone loss.[34] The technique involves placing suture anchors in the humeral head defect and performing a "capsulotenodesis" of the posterior capsule and infraspinatus tendon.[35] The procedure makes the Hill-Sachs lesion extra-articular and eliminates engagement of the defect with the anterior glenoid rim.[36] There is some concern over loss of range of motion and posterosuperior pain after this technique. However, recurrence rates, patient satisfaction scores, and range of motion do not seem to differ substantially between patients who received this technique and patients who received Bankart repair alone for recurrent anterior instability with an engag-

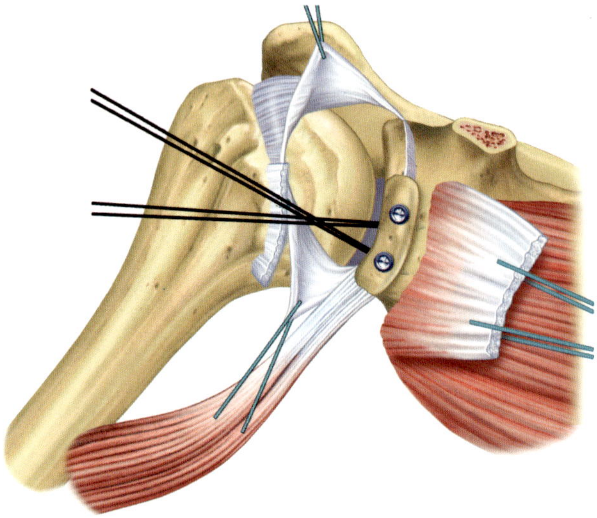

Figure 34. Latarjet procedure.

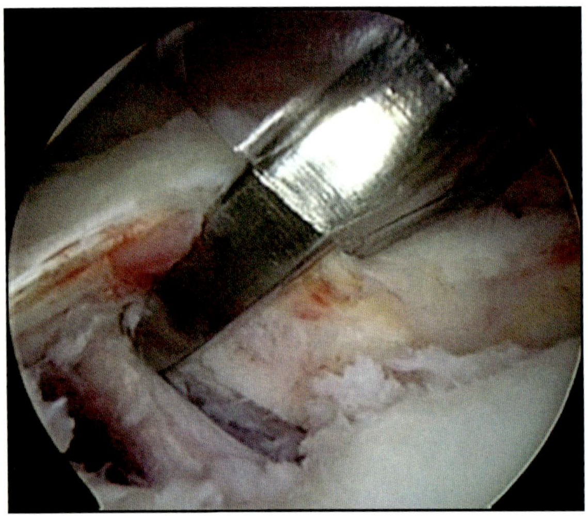

Figure 35. Arthroscopic view of Bankart lesion.

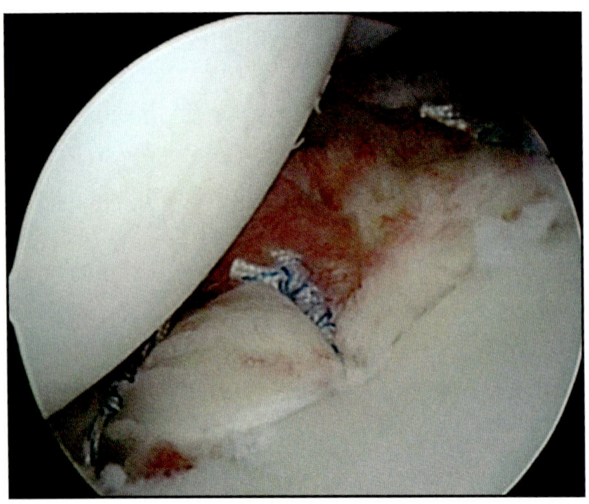

Figure 36. Arthroscopic Bankart repair.

ing Hill-Sachs lesion.[37] Despite their high prevalence, defects in the humeral head are usually smaller and do not require operative treatment.[38] Defects of the antero-inferior glenoid rim create the inverted-pear glenoid, which leads to failure of soft tissue repair alone and high rates of recurrence.[11] Again, multiple options exist for treatment of glenoid deficiency, including allograft reconstruction, iliac crest autograft augmentation, and various methods of coracoid process transfers.

The preferred method for treating anteroinferior glenoid deficiency is the Latarjet procedure. With this procedure, the coracoid process is transferred with the conjoined tendon and reattached to the anterior glenoid neck through a split in the subscapularis tendon, and the remaining capsule is repaired to the conjoined tendon (Figure 34). The procedure provides a triple-blocking effect, with the bone block providing support, the conjoined tendon acting as a sling in abduction and external rotation, and the repair of the capsule to the conjoined tendon providing stability.[39,40] Overall, the procedure has a low rate of recurrence of anteroposterior glenoid deficiency, high rate of patient satisfaction, high rate of return to sport, and low rate of arthritis if the graft is placed without too much lateral overhang.[39–41]

Arthroscopic treatment of anterior shoulder instability has emerged as the preferred method of treatment because of its advantages over the open approach, such as improved visualization, reduced operative trauma, decreased postoperative pain, and ability to address additional pathologic lesions (Figures 35 and 36). Initial attempts at arthroscopic repair of instability had high rates of failure, but with advances in technology, operative technique, and surgeon expertise, rates of recurrence and patient satisfaction with properly indicated arthroscopic treatment exceed those with an open approach.[30,32] Principles of arthroscopic repair mirror those of an open approach, with specific focus on anatomic reduction of the labrum and restoration of appropriate capsular tension. In addition, arthroscopic techniques can address other pathologic lesions, including SLAP lesions, rotator cuff tears, and bone loss. Techniques, such as arthroscopic bony Bankart repair and arthroscopic remplissage for Hill-Sachs lesions, can be used for bony defects in combination with soft tissue repair.

Posterior Instability

Patients with involuntary recurrent posterior instability are acceptable candidates for operative intervention. As with anterior instability, operative intervention for this condition is focused on treating both the bony and soft tissue lesions. Interventions can be either arthroscopic or open. Indications for arthroscopic repair include traumatic posterior Bankart lesions (Figure 37).[42] Relative contraindications to arthroscopic intervention include failed arthroscopic stabilization, glenoid erosion, and excessive glenoid retroversion.[12] The typical arthroscopic soft tissue procedure includes a labral repair with posterior capsulorrhaphy.

Open procedures typically are used in revision surgery, excessive glenoid retroversion or bone loss, and failure of nonoperative management with persistent posterior displacement of the humeral head relative to the glenoid.[12] A posteroinferior capsular shift is analogous to an anteroinferior shift in which the posterior capsule is detached from the humerus and flaps are created for suturing in a pants-over-vest fashion (Figure 38). This effectively reduces a patulous posterior capsular volume and restores normal glenohumeral articulation. If bone loss or excessive retroversion is present, this capsular shift is combined with a bone-block–type procedure. Glenoid osteotomy with opening-wedge bone graft or augmentation of the posterior glenoid with allograft or autograft effectively restores normal glenoid version. Unfortunately, high recurrence rates can be seen with these posterior bone-block–type procedures.[12] Finally, in patients who are having revision procedures and have profound posterior soft tissue deficiency, augmentation with Achilles tendon allograft can provide a checkrein to posterior subluxation.

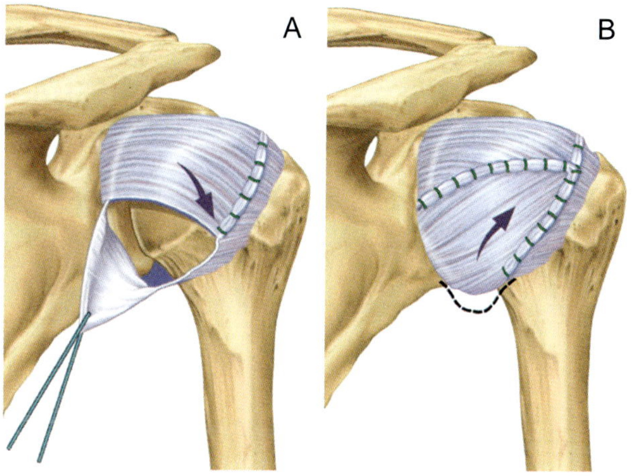

Figure 38 A and B. Open posterior capsular shift.

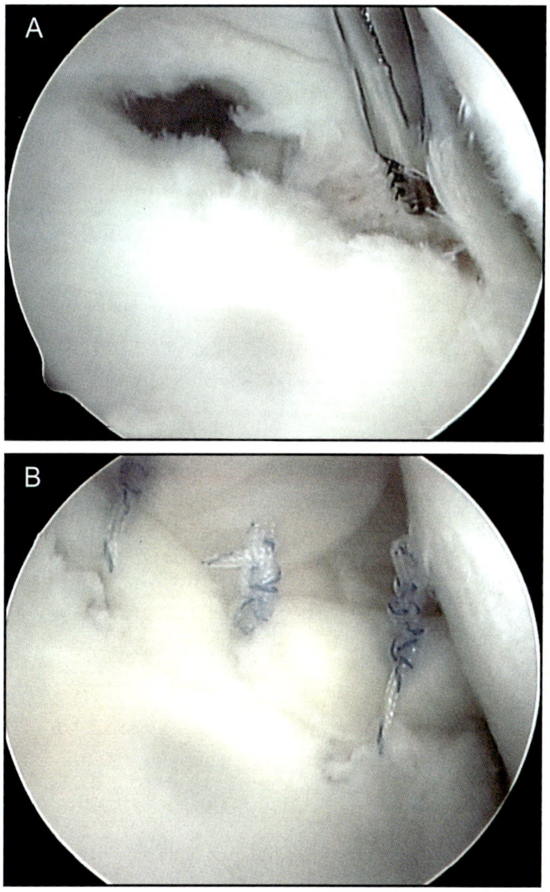

Figure 37 A and B. Arthroscopic view of posterior labral tear and repair.

Multidirectional Instability

Pathologic lesions of multidirectional instability are inferior capsular redundancy with rotator interval lesions. Inferior instability is the universal finding, with instability in at least one other direction: anterior or posterior.[43] These patients also can be treated with an open or arthroscopic approach. Both approaches aim to reduce capsular volume and treat the rotator interval lesion, if indicated. In patients with extreme multidirectional instability, anterior and posterior capsulorrhaphy are performed in addition to rotator interval closure. Despite advances in arthroscopic techniques,

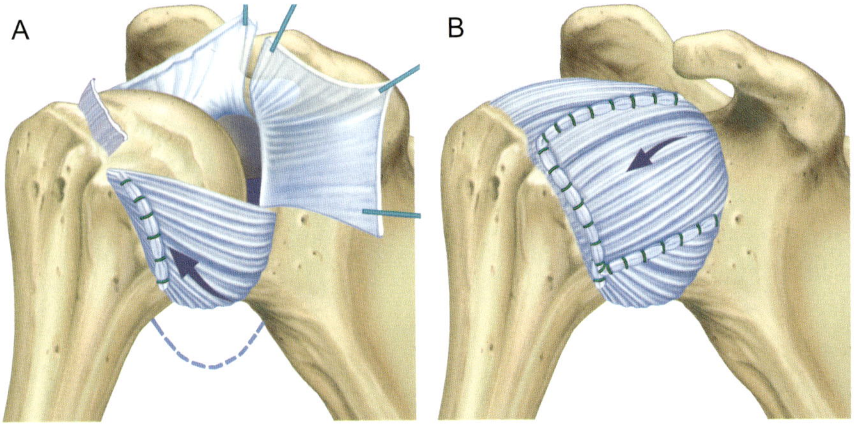

Figure 39 A and B. Open anteroinferior capsular shift.

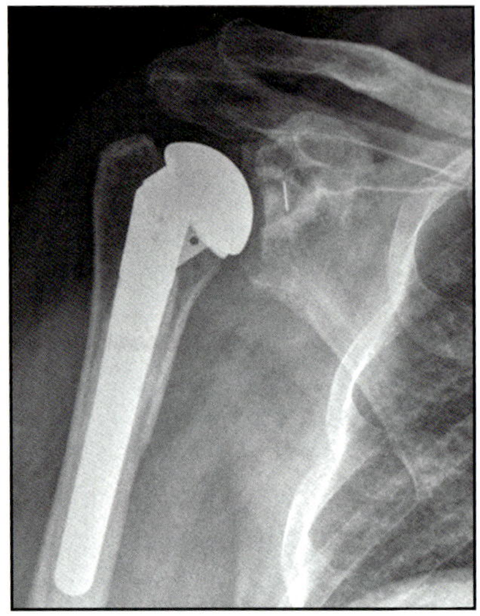

Figure 40. Chronic dislocation treated with prosthesis.

open inferior capsular shift remains the criterion standard for reduction of capsular volume and treatment of multidirectional instability (Figure 39).[44]

Chronic or Neglected Dislocations

With chronic dislocations, the operative treatment depends on multiple patient- and injury-specific factors. If the patient is suitable for operative treatment, various options exist to treat both chronic anterior and posterior dislocations. For both types, closed reduction is recommended only if the injury is less than 3 weeks old, and the humeral head has no substantial structural damage.[45] All other cases require open treatment.

For posterior dislocations, both the time from injury and the size of the humeral head defect and articular surface guide treatment. For patients who have acute injuries with defects less than 20% to 40% of the humeral head, open reduction with disimpaction grafting is recommended.[46] A reconstructive operation is required to treat more chronic injuries. Allograft reconstruction or subscapularis and lesser tuberosity transfers can provide stability. Finally, a prosthetic replacement is required to treat patients who have chronic injuries with more than 50% involvement of the head or severe articular cartilage destruction (Figure 40).[46] Similarly, chronic anterior dislocations require open reduction with treatment of the bony and soft tissue lesions. If the reduction is stable, only a capsulolabral repair is required, but if the reduction is unstable, the bony lesion must be addressed. Hill-Sachs defects and anterior glenoid bone loss can be treated with either local autograft transfers or structural allograft.[45] If involvement of the humerus or glenoid is more than 50% and is associated with substantial degenerative joint disease, a prosthetic reconstruction is required.[46]

NONOPERATIVE TREATMENT OPTIONS

Principles of nonoperative management involve concentric reduction of the glenohumeral joint, a period of immobilization, and directed physical therapy with guided return to activities. Acute dislocations require emergent reduction. Several techniques have been described to treat both anterior and posterior dislocations. For any reduction, attempts should be as atraumatic as possible with adequate analgesia provided to allow muscle relaxation and a rapid and relatively painless restoration of a concentric glenohumeral joint. Although many methods exist, the traction-countertraction method commonly is used (Figure 41). With the patient positioned supine, a sheet is placed around the chest to supply countertraction while the surgeon provides traction in the direction of the deformity. Gentle rotation disengages the humeral head from the glenoid. Researchers have reported success with alternative techniques, such as the external rotation and Milch methods (Figure 42).[47,48] With a posterior dislocation, the upper extremity must be forward flexed, internally rotated, and adducted to disengage the humeral head from the glenoid followed by longitudinal traction, pressure on the humeral head, and external rotation to reduce the joint. Posterior dislocations are associated with anterior compression fractures of the humeral head, and larger bony deficits place the patient at greater risk for redislocation.

For years, the shoulder has been placed in a standard sling for various periods after reduction of an anterior dislocation of the shoulder (Figure 43A). Both duration of immobilization and position seem to affect the rate of recurrence. When comparing short (1-week) and prolonged (3-week) immobilization in a young patient population, Hovelius et al[49] reported immobilization did not change the ultimate prognosis at long-term follow-up. In addition, recent evidence has supported immobilizing the shoulder in external rotation after an anterior dislocation (Figure 43B).[50,51] Cadaveric data have shown better reduction of the labrum with external rotation, and authors of prospective randomized studies have shown a reduced rate of recurrent instability with immobilization in external rotation.[50,51] After posterior dislocation, longer periods of immobilization and an extremity position of extension and external rotation relaxes the posterior capsule and allows healing in a shortened position.

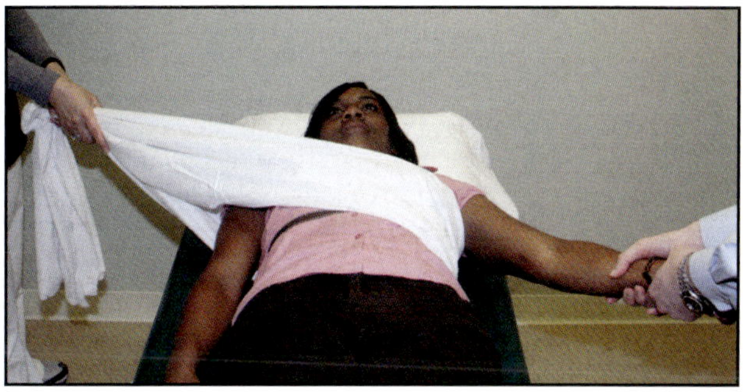

Figure 41. Traction and countertraction reduction method.

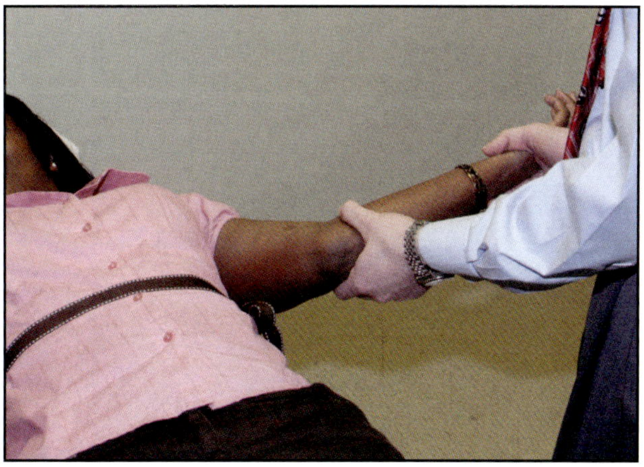

Figure 42. External rotation reduction method.

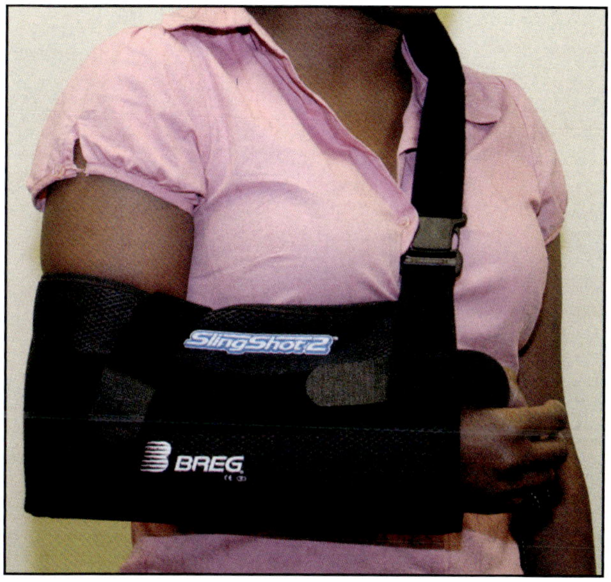

Figure 43A. Standard sling.

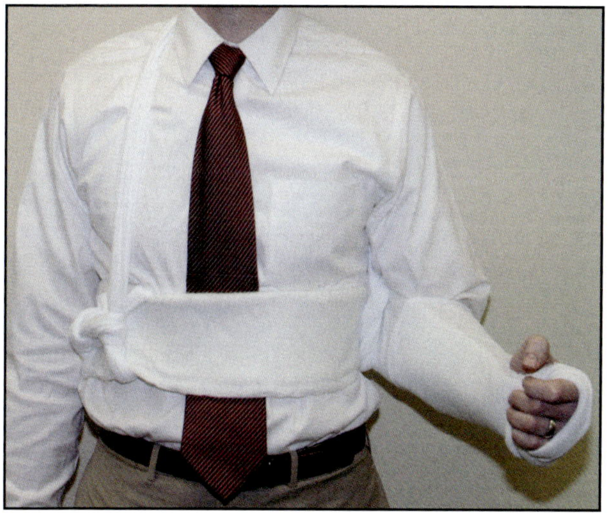

Figure 43B. External rotation bracing.

After reduction and proper immobilization, directed physical therapy allows restoration of glenohumeral joint function. Rehabilitation protocols should focus on avoiding provocative positions, restoring normal range of motion, strengthening the dynamic and periscapular stabilizers, and re-establishing proprioception and neuromuscular control. For anterior instability, a strict rehabilitation protocol and appropriate bracing allows athletes to return to sport and complete their seasons.[52] Anterior instability protocols focus on avoiding abduction and external rotation, restoring functional and pain-free range of motion, and strengthening the rotator cuff and periscapular stabilizers so they can substitute for damaged static restraints.

All patients with multidirectional instability are given a prolonged course of nonoperative management as a first line of treatment. Again, the specific focus of each protocol is to avoid positions that stress the shoulder in an inferior direction and strengthen the rotator cuff and periscapular musculature to restore concavity compression. The ultimate focus is to restore normal muscle-firing patterns and proprioception. In addition, scapulothoracic and glenohumeral motions must be symmetric and coordinated. Proper patient education is paramount to ensure understanding of the disease process and compliance with the rigorous physical therapy program. Compliance with this rigorous nonoperative routine has yielded high rates of success.[53]

Nonoperative management also has a high rate of success with posterior instability.[54] Positions of posterior instability, forward flexion, adduction, and internal rotation are avoided. Dynamic stabilizers, such as the posterior deltoid, periscapular muscles, and infraspinatus, are strengthened to substitute for the damaged static stabilizers.

POTENTIAL COMPLICATIONS

Although treatment for glenohumeral instability results in high rates of success, complications can be challenging for the surgeon and debilitating for the patient. Recurrence of instability is the primary outcome measure to judge instability treatment, but secondary complications, such as loss of motion, capsulorrhaphy arthropathy, hardware complications, neurovascular injury, and infection, also can occur. As treatment is specific for each form of instability, complications are specific to each intervention for instability. Generally, failed repair of instability results from incorrect diagnosis, incorrect procedure, or technical error.

Depending on the procedure, recurrent instability ranges from 3% to 50% after operations to treat anterior instability.[55] If patients with posterior or multidirectional instability are misdiagnosed, arthroscopic or open procedures to treat anterior instability will asymmetrically tighten nonpathologic structures and exacerbate the true direction of instability (Figure 44). In a series of failed repairs of instability, Boone and Arciero[55] found that not recognizing the direction of instability was a major cause of failure. In addition, inappropriate procedures did not address structures with pathologic changes and resulted in recurrence of instability. Both pathologic capsulolabral changes and bony deficits must be addressed with anterior procedures. Failure to recognize and treat both bony and soft tissue lesions results in high rates of failure.[56] Complications specific to open operations for anterior

Figure 44. Asymmetric capsular tightening.

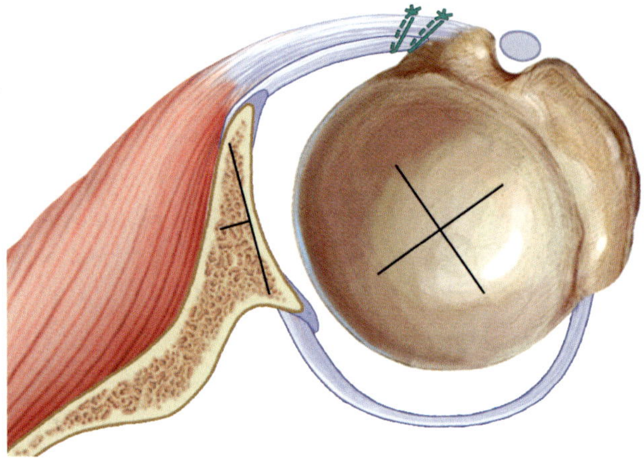

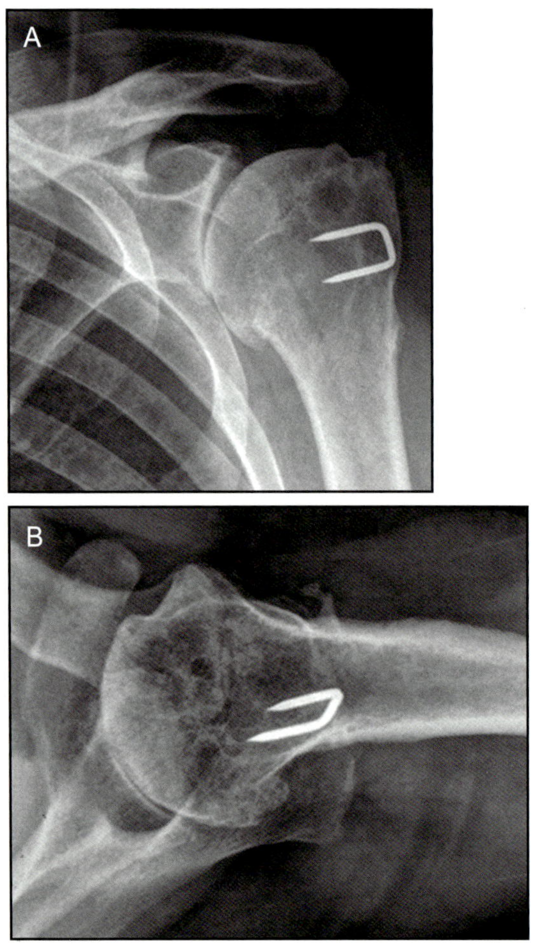

Figure 45 A and B. Capsulorrhaphy arthropathy.

instability revolve around subscapularis management. The subscapularis tendon is taken down from the lesser tuberosity for open capsulolabral reconstruction, and subscapularis insufficiency has been reported as a cause of operative failure and postoperative instability.[31] Asymmetric tightening can result in limits of external rotation and abnormal glenohumeral mechanics and might lead to capsulorrhaphy arthropathy (Figure 45).[57] Any hardware placed around the glenoid, whether for fixation of bone blocks or suture anchors for soft tissue reconstruction, can loosen or become prominent and can irreversibly damage the articular surface (Figure 46). The axillary nerve, which courses under the inferior capsule, also is at particular risk during repair for anterior instability. Success rates with modern arthroscopic techniques equal those with open intervention. The primary mode of failure results from unrecognized substantial bone loss, which can result in recurrence of up to 67%.[11]

Major complications after posterior repair include recurrence, degenerative arthritis, and coracoid impingement syndrome. The rate of recurrence is higher after procedures to treat posterior instability than after procedures to treat anterior or multidirection instability.[12,54] Factors affecting recurrence rates include misdiagnosis, failure to address all components of instability, and failure of rehabilitation. Patients with posterior instability typically have components of multidirectional instability that, if untreated, cause failure.[16,58] All structures with lesions, including the labrum, capsule, glenoid retroversion, and the rotator interval, must be addressed to avoid recurrence. In addition, for at least 6 weeks after the operation, the patient must avoid placing the shoulder in positions of flexion, adduction, and internal rotation to prevent recurrence. Glenoid osteotomy to correct glenoid retroversion can result in premature degenerative joint disease if the articular surface is violated (Figure 47).[12] In addition, if glenoid version is overcorrected, the humeral head can take an anteromedial orientation and impinge on the coracoid process.[12]

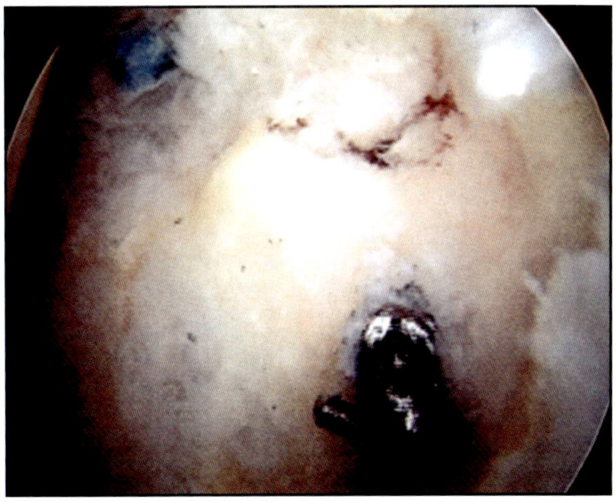

Figure 46. Prominent hardware after instability repair.

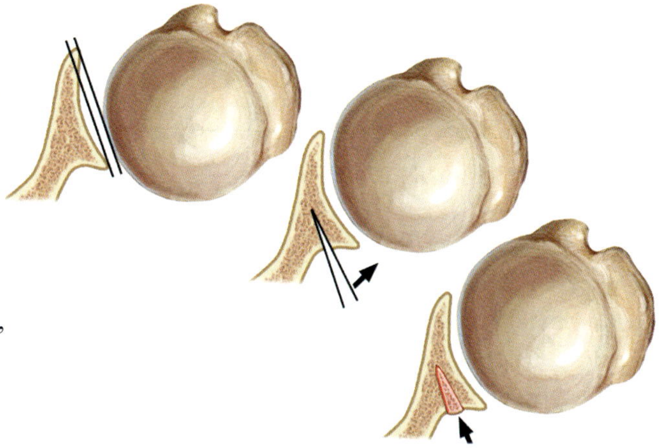

Figure 47. Posterior glenoid osteotomy.

Treatment of multidirectional instability has high rates of success, but recurrence can result in persistent and end-stage instability. Thermal capsulorrhaphy has high rates of failure and the need for revision surgery when used to treat multidirectional instability.[59] Capsular necrosis, residual capsular laxity, and chondrolysis result from the use of thermal capsulorraphy.[60]

EXPECTED OUTCOMES

In general, patients with glenohumeral instability can expect return of nearly normal function with appropriately selected nonoperative or operative intervention. Nonoperative management is successful for patients with atraumatic instability, posterior instability, or multidirectional instability. Success rates for these individuals with appropriately tailored nonoperative treatment regimes are between 63% and 88%.[53,54] The age of the patient at first dislocation and the risk for recurrence are directly correlated, with younger patients having a higher risk of recurrence than older patients. For primary traumatic anterior dislocation, high rates of redislocation and decreased functional outcomes in young patients have caused some authors to recommend immediate arthroscopic stabilization.[28,29] Hovelius et al[49] reported that after 25-year follow-up, half of the primary anterior shoulder dislocations that had been treated nonoperatively in patients aged 12 to 25 years had not recurred or had become stable over time. From this data, authors determined that immediate surgery for the treatment of all first-time dislocations in patients less than 25 years of age would result in a 30% to 50% rate of unnecessary operations.[49] Patients with a traumatic anterior shoulder dislocation can expect a slight decrease in function, increased risk of arthropathy, and 17% risk of dislocation of the contralateral shoulder.[50,61]

Operative treatment of recurrent anterior instability can reliably return patients to pretraumatic levels of function, reduce rates of redislocation, and provide satisfactory results. Long-term follow-up of open Bankart repair has shown a 10% rate of recurrence, complete return to preinjury sporting level, and high rates of patient satisfaction.[62] The operation does not prevent the development of arthritis and does decrease range of motion and function compared with the contralateral extremity.[32,62] The results of modern arthroscopic techniques are equal to those of open Bankart repairs in terms of recurrence rates (around 10%), patient satisfaction, and return to activities.[32,63,64] Advantages of arthroscopic repair include better subscapularis function, range of motion, and functional scores than open Bankart repair.[31,32,63,64] If a bone-block procedure is required, excellent results can be obtained with the Latarjet procedure (Figure 48). Hovelius et al[40] reported a 98% rate of satisfaction with a 4% rate of redislocation and a 9% risk of persistent apprehension at long-term follow-up. The risk of developing arthritis depends on appropriate graft placement. The risk of developing moderate to severe arthritis with appropriate graft placement is 8%, and the risk with nonoptimum positioning is 17%.[41]

Success also can be achieved with open and arthroscopic repair of both multidirectional and posterior instability. Neer and Foster[43] reported satisfaction rates of 98% with open inferior capsular shift and only 1 recurrent subluxation at 7 months after surgery. Hamada et al[65] found an 88% rate of satisfactory outcomes with open inferior capsular shift at long-term follow-up. Arthroscopic treatment of multidirectional instability has yielded 94% good-to-excellent results at 2- to 5-year follow-up.[66] At long-term follow-up, Wolf et al[67] found open posterior capsular shift yielded an 84% rate of satisfaction and 19% rate of recurrence. Bradley et al[68] showed arthroscopic techniques in athletes with symptomatic unidirectional posterior instability allowed 89% to return to sport and substantial improvements in stability, pain, and function. Results for chronic dislocations do not equal those of acute dislocations, but researchers have shown that operative intervention provides improved functional results in appropriately selected patients.[45,46]

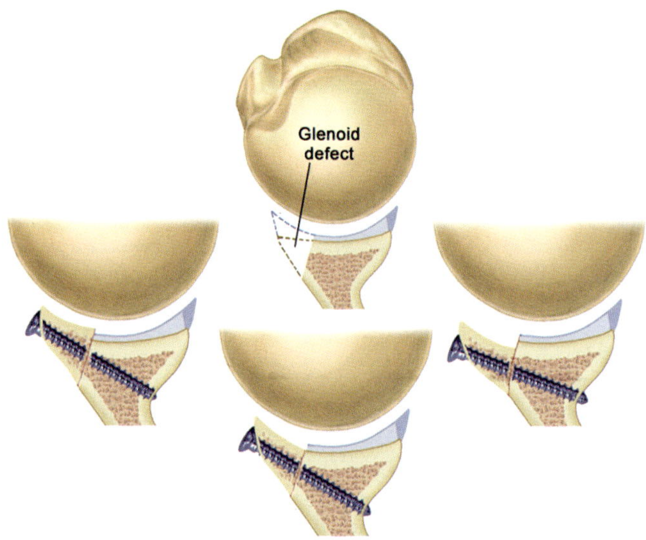

Figure 48. Latarjet graft placement.

REFERENCES

1. Park MC. Anatomy and function of the shoulder structures. In: Galatz LM, ed. *Orthopaedic Knowledge Update: Shoulder and Elbow 3*. Rosemont, IL: American Academy of Orthopaedic Surgeons; 2008:3–14.

2. Burkart AC, Debski RE. Anatomy and function of the glenohumeral ligaments in anterior shoulder instability. *Clin Orthop Relat Res*. 2002;400:32–39.

3. Kuhn JE, Huston LJ, Soslowsky LJ, Shyr Y, Blasier RB. External rotation of the glenohumeral joint: ligament restraints and muscle effects in the neutral and abducted positions. *J Shoulder Elbow Surg*. 2005;14(1 suppl S):39S–48S.

4. Labriola JE, Lee TQ, Debski RE, McMahon PJ. Stability and instability of the glenohumeral joint: the role of shoulder muscles. *J Shoulder Elbow Surg*. 2005;14(1 suppl S):32S–38S.

5. McCluskey GM III. Classification and diagnosis of glenohumeral instability in athletes. *Sports Med Arthrosc Rev*. 2000;8(2):158–169.

6. Lephart SM, Warner JJP, Borsa PA, Fu FH. Proprioception of the shoulder joint in healthy, unstable, and surgically repaired shoulders. *J Shoulder Elbow Surg*. 1994;3(6):371–380.

7. Bigliani LU, Pollock RG, Soslowsky LJ, Flatow EL, Pawluk RJ, Mow VC. Tensile properties of the inferior glenohumeral ligament. *J Orthop Res*. 1992;10(2):187–197.
8. Pouliart N, Marmor S, Gagey O. Simulated capsulolabral lesion in cadavers: dislocation does not result from Bankart lesion only. *Arthroscopy*. 2006;22(7):748–754.
9. Taylor DC, Arciero RA. Pathologic changes associated with shoulder dislocations: arthroscopic and physical examination findings in first-time, traumatic anterior dislocations. *Am J Sports Med*. 1997;25(3):306–311.
10. Werner AW, Lichtenberg MD, Schmitz H, Nikolic A, Habermeyer P. Arthroscopic findings in atraumatic shoulder instability. *Arthroscopy*. 2004;20(3):268–272.
11. Burkhart SS, De Beer JF. Traumatic glenohumeral bone defects and their relationship to failure of arthroscopic Bankart repairs: significance of the inverted-pear glenoid and the humeral engaging Hill-Sachs lesion. *Arthroscopy*. 2000;16(7):677–694.
12. Millett PJ, Clavert P, Hatch GF III, Warner JJ. Recurrent posterior shoulder instability. *J Am Acad Orthop Surg*. 2006;14(8):464–476.
13. Ozbaydar M, Elhassan B, Diller D, Massimini D, Higgins LD, Warner JJ. Results of arthroscopic capsulolabral repair: Bankart lesion versus anterior labroligamentous periosteal sleeve avulsion lesion. *Arthroscopy*. 2008;24(11):1277–1283.
14. Panossian VR, Mihata T, Tibone JE, Fitzpatrick MJ, McGarry MH, Lee TQ. Biomechanical analysis of isolated type II SLAP lesions and repair. *J Shoulder Elbow Surg*. 2005;14(5):529–534.
15. Kim TK, Queale WS, Cosgarea AJ, McFarland EG. Clinical features of the different types of SLAP lesions: an analysis of one hundred and thirty-nine cases. *J Bone Joint Surg Am*. 2003;85(1):66–71.
16. Kim SH, Ha KI, Yoo JC, Noh KC. Kim's lesion: an incomplete and concealed avulsion of the posteroinferior labrum in posterior or multidirectional posteroinferior instability of the shoulder. *Arthroscopy*. 2004;20(7):712–720.
17. Richards DP, Burkhart SS. Arthroscopic humeral avulsion of the glenohumeral ligaments (HAGL) repair. *Arthroscopy*. 2004;20(2 suppl):134–141.
18. Porcellini G, Paladini P, Campi F, Paganelli M. Shoulder instability and related rotator cuff tears: arthroscopic findings and treatment in patients aged 40 to 60 years. *Arthroscopy*. 2006;22(3):270–276.
19. Morris AD, Kemp GJ, Frostick SP. Shoulder electromyography in multidirectional instability. *J Shoulder Elbow Surg*. 2004;13(1):24–29.
20. Visser CP, Coene LN, Brand R, Tavy DL. The incidence of nerve injury in anterior dislocation of the shoulder and its influence on functional recovery: a prospective clinical and EMG study. *J Bone Joint Surg Br*. 1999;81(4):679–685.
21. Gerber C, Nyffeler RW. Classification of glenohumeral joint instability. *Clin Orthop Relat Res*. 2002;400:65–76.
22. Tzannes A, Paxinos A, Callanan M, Murrell GA. An assessment of the interexaminer reliability of tests for shoulder instability. *J Shoulder Elbow Surg*. 2004;13(1):18–23.
23. Farber AJ, Castillo R, Clough M, Bahk M, McFarland EG. Clinical assessment of three common tests for traumatic anterior shoulder instability. *J Bone Joint Surg Am*. 2006;88(7):1467–1474.
24. Kim SH, Park JC, Park JS, Oh I. Painful jerk test: a predictor of success in nonoperative treatment of posteroinferior instability of the shoulder. *Am J Sports Med*. 2004;32(8):1849–1855.
25. Kim SH, Park JS, Jeong WK, Shin SK. The Kim test: a novel test for posteroinferior labral lesions of the shoulder. A comparison to the jerk test. *Am J Sports Med*. 2005;33(8):1188–1192.
26. Itoi E, Lee SB, Amrami KK, Wenger DE, An KN. Quantitative assessment of classic anteroinferior bony Bankart lesions by radiography and computed tomography. *Am J Sports Med*. 2003;31(1):112–118.
27. Waldt S, Burkart A, Imhoff AB, Bruegel M, Rummeny EJ, Woertler K. Anterior shoulder instability: accuracy of MR arthrography in the classification of anteroinferior labroligamentous injuries. *Radiology*. 2005;237(2):578–583.
28. Kirkley A, Griffin S, Richards C, Miniaci A, Mohtadi N. Prospective randomized clinical trial comparing the effectiveness of immediate arthroscopic stabilization versus immobilization and rehabilitation in first traumatic anterior dislocations of the shoulder. *Arthroscopy*. 1999;15(5):507–514.
29. Handoll HH, Almaiyah MA, Rangan A. Surgical versus non-surgical treatment for acute anterior shoulder dislocation. *Cochrane Database Syst Rev*. 2004;(1):CD004325.
30. Millett PJ, Clavert P, Warner JJ. Open operative treatment for anterior shoulder instability: when and why? *J Bone Joint Surg Am*. 2005;87(2):419–432.
31. Sachs RA, Williams B, Stone ML, Paxton L, Kuney M. Open Bankart repair: correlation of results with postoperative subscapularis function. *Am J Sports Med*. 2005;33(10):1458–1462.
32. Fabbriciani C, Milano G, Demontis A, Fadda S, Ziranu F, Mulas PD. Arthroscopic versus open treatment of Bankart lesion of the shoulder: a prospective randomized study. *Arthroscopy*. 2004;20(5):456–462.
33. Purchase RJ, Wolf EM, Hobgood ER, Pollock ME, Smalley CC. Hill-Sachs "remplissage": an arthroscopic solution for the engaging Hill-Sachs lesion. *Arthroscopy*. 2008;24(6):723–726.
34. Ochoa E Jr, Burkhart SS. Glenohumeral bone defects in the treatment of anterior shoulder instability. *Instr Course Lect*. 2009;58:323–336.
35. Koo SS, Burkhart SS, Ochoa E. Arthroscopic double-pulley remplissage technique for engaging Hill-Sachs lesions in anterior shoulder instability repairs. *Arthroscopy*. 2009;25(11):1343–1348.
36. Deutsch AA, Kroll DG. Decreased range of motion following arthroscopic remplissage. *Orthopedics*. 2008;31(5):492.
37. Nourissat G, Kilinc AS, Werther JR, Doursounian L. A prospective, comparative, radiological, and clinical study of the influence of the "remplissage" procedure on shoulder range of motion after stabilization by arthroscopic Bankart repair. *Am J Sports Med*. 2011;39(1):2147–2152.
38. Kazel MD, Sekiya JK, Greene JA, Bruker CT. Percutaneous correction (humeroplasty) of humeral head defects (Hill-Sachs) associated with anterior shoulder instability: a cadaveric study. *Arthroscopy*. 2005;21(12):1473–1478.
39. Allain J, Goutallier D, Glorion C. Long-term results of the Latarjet procedure for the treatment of anterior instability of the shoulder. *J Bone Joint Surg Am*. 1998;80(6):841–852.

40. Hovelius L, Sandström B, Sundgren K, Saebö M. One hundred eighteen Bristow-Latarjet repairs for recurrent anterior dislocation of the shoulder prospectively followed for fifteen years: study I. Clinical results. *J Shoulder Elbow Surg.* 2004;13(5):509–516.
41. Hovelius L, Sandström B, Saebö M. One hundred eighteen Bristow-Latarjet repairs for recurrent anterior dislocation of the shoulder prospectively followed for fifteen years: study II. The evolution of dislocation arthropathy. *J Shoulder Elbow Surg.* 2006;15(3):279–289.
42. Williams RJ III, Strickland S, Cohen M, Altchek DW, Warren RF. Arthroscopic repair for traumatic posterior shoulder instability. *Am J Sports Med.* 2003;31(2):203–209.
43. Neer CS II, Foster CR. Inferior capsular shift for involuntary inferior and multidirectional instability of the shoulder: a preliminary report. *J Bone Joint Surg Am.* 1980;62(6):897–908.
44. Cohen SB, Wiley W, Goradia VK, Pearson S, Miller MD. Anterior capsulorrhaphy: an in vitro comparison of volume reduction. Arthroscopic plication versus open capsular shift. *Arthroscopy.* 2005;21(6):659–644.
45. Goga IE. Chronic shoulder dislocations. *J Shoulder Elbow Surg.* 2003;12(5):446–450.
46. Griggs SM, Holloway GB, Williams GR Jr, Iannotti JP. Chronic dislocations. In: Iannotti JP, Williams GR Jr, eds. *Disorders of the Shoulder: Diagnosis & Management.* 2nd ed. Philadelphia, PA: Lippincott Williams & Wilkins; 2007:461–486.
47. Eachempati KK, Dua A, Malhotra R, Bhan S, Bera JR. The external rotation method for reduction of acute anterior dislocations and fracture-dislocations of the shoulder. *J Bone Joint Surg Am.* 2004;86(11):2431–2434.
48. O'Connor DR, Schwarze D, Fragomen AT, Perdomo M. Painless reduction of acute anterior shoulder dislocations without anesthesia. *Orthopedics.* 2006;29(6):528–532.
49. Hovelius L, Olofsson A, Sandström B, et al. Nonoperative treatment of primary anterior shoulder dislocation in patients forty years of age and younger: a prospective twenty-five-year follow-up. *J Bone Joint Surg Am.* 2008;90(5):945–952.
50. Miller BS, Sonnabend DH, Hatrick C, et al. Should acute anterior dislocations of the shoulder be immobilized in external rotation? A cadaveric study. *J Shoulder Elbow Surg.* 2004;13(6):589–592.
51. Itoi E, Hatakeyama Y, Sato T, et al. Immobilization in external rotation after shoulder dislocation reduces the risk of recurrence: a randomized control trial. *J Bone Joint Surg Am.* 2007;89(10):2124–2131.
52. Buss DD, Lynch GP, Meyer CP, Huber SM, Freehill MQ. Nonoperative management for in-season athletes with anterior shoulder instability. *Am J Sports Med.* 2004;32(6):1430–1433.
53. Burkhead WZ Jr, Rockwood CA Jr. Treatment of instability of the shoulder with an exercise program. *J Bone Joint Surg Am.* 1992;74(6):890–896.
54. Fronek J, Warren RF, Bowen M. Posterior subluxation of the glenohumeral joint. *J Bone Joint Surg Am.* 1989;71(2):205–216.
55. Boone JL, Arciero RA. Management of failed instability surgery: how to get it right the next time. *Orthop Clin North Am.* 2010;41(3):367–379.
56. Tauber M, Resch H, Forstner R, Raffl M, Schauer J. Reasons for failure after surgical repair of anterior shoulder instability. *J Shoulder Elbow Surg.* 2004;13(3):279–285.
57. Levine WN, Arroyo JS, Pollock RG, Flatow EL, Bigliani LL. Open revision stabilization surgery for recurrent anterior glenohumeral instability. *Am J Sports Med.* 2000;28(2):156–160.
58. Kim SH, Noh KC, Park JS, Ryu BD, Oh I. Loss of chondrolabral containment of the glenohumeral joint in atraumatic posteroinferior multidirectional instability. *J Bone Joint Surg Am.* 2005;87(1):92–98.
59. D'Alessandro DF, Bradley JP, Fleischli JE, Connor PM. Prospective evaluation of thermal capsulorrhaphy for shoulder instability: indications and results, two- to five-year follow-up. *Am J Sports Med.* 2004;32(1):21–33.
60. Park HB, Yokota A, Gill HS, El Rassi G, McFarland EG. Revision surgery for failed thermal capsulorrhaphy. *Am J Sports Med.* 2005;33(9):1321–1326.
61. Robinson CM, Howes J, Murdoch H, Will E, Graham C. Functional outcome and risk of recurrent instability after primary traumatic anterior shoulder dislocation in young patients. *J Bone Joint Surg Am.* 2006;88(11):2326–2336.
62. Pelet S, Jolles BM, Farron A. Bankart repair for recurrent anterior glenohumeral instability: results at twenty-nine years' follow-up. *J Shoulder Elbow Surg.* 2006;15(2):203–207.
63. Tjoumakaris FP, Abboud JA, Hasan SA, Ramsey ML, Williams GR. Arthroscopic and open Bankart repairs provide similar outcomes. *Clin Orthop Relat Res.* 2006;446:227–232.
64. Carreira DS, Mazzocca AD, Oryhon J, Brown FM, Hayden JK, Romeo AA. A prospective outcome evaluation of arthroscopic Bankart repairs: minimum 2-year follow-up. *Am J Sports Med.* 2006;34(5):771–777.
65. Hamada K, Fukuda H, Nakajima T, Yamada N. The inferior capsular shift operation for instability of the shoulder: long-term results in 34 shoulders. *J Bone Joint Surg Br.* 1999;81(2):218–225.
66. Gartsman GM, Roddey TS, Hammerman SM. Arthroscopic treatment of multidirectional glenohumeral instability: 2- to 5-year follow-up. *Arthroscopy.* 2001;17(3):236–243.
67. Wolf BR, Strickland S, Williams RJ, Allen AA, Altchek DW, Warren RF. Open posterior stabilization for recurrent posterior glenohumeral instability. *J Shoulder Elbow Surg.* 2005;14(2):157–164.
68. Bradley JP, Baker CL III, Kline AJ, Armsfield DR, Chhabra A. Arthroscopic capsulolabral reconstruction for posterior instability of the shoulder: a prospective study of 100 shoulders. *Am J Sports Med.* 2006;34(7):1061–1071.

I-5

Glenohumeral Arthritis

Howard D. Routman, DO, FAOAO

Arthritis is a term that refers to a group of conditions that affect the joints and cause pain, deformity, and loss of function. Osteoarthritis (OA) is the most common type of arthritis and is considered to be the most common joint disorder overall. Many people who are more than age 65 years display clinical or radiographic signs of OA. In this chapter, I present an overview of different types of shoulder arthritis.

OSTEOARTHRITIS

The understanding of the basic science of OA has been advancing for some time. Articular cartilage damage and loss long have been considered the primary causes of OA. In more recent work, researchers have supported the idea that degenerative arthrosis and arthrosis related to repeated injury have different mechanisms in terms of the protein-fluid shifts at the microscopic level but have similar end results. Increased vascularity to the subchondral bone, increased stiffness in the subchondral plate, and a change in the water-protein balance in the cartilage matrix are the hallmarks of the arthritic process. This leads to sclerosis, formation of osteophytes (bone spurs), subchondral cystic changes, loss of cartilage thickness, and subsequent joint-space narrowing. The amount of compressive stress that articular cartilage can handle is very particular. Experimental canine models have shown that a higher-than-normal, single, compressive load reliably can result in progressive arthritic changes. This might explain the predisposition for shoulder arthritis in certain patient populations, such as heavy weight trainers who tend to apply substantial force across the joint surface (particularly in heavy bench pressing).

Osteoarthritis of the shoulder is the most common arthritic condition of the shoulder and has a very typical clinical presentation. Most patients with OA maintain an intact rotator cuff despite the degenerative condition of the joint surface. Patients with OA of the shoulder report pain in the shoulder region that ranges from the deltoid insertion to the posterior joint line, upper trapezius, and bicipital groove. Most patients describe that their shoulders were functioning well and recently have had a decrease in motion, increase in pain, and loss of functional internal rotation. Less commonly, patients recognize that the shoulder was not moving well and recently has become more stiff and painful. Sometimes, the pain is not the primary issue. Stiffness and loss of motion, especially internal and external rotation, can be a functional problem and can result in the desire to seek treatment. Pain is typically worse at night, and difficulty getting to sleep and staying asleep is not uncommon. Common concerns of patients with OA of the shoulder are listed in Table 1.

Clinical Examination

Findings of the rehabilitation provider during clinical examination of a patient with shoulder OA are consistent with the pathophysiology of the osteoarthritic shoulder. Because the rotator cuff in most patients is intact, strength testing of the shoulder is usually good. Passive range of motion (ROM) and active ROM are usually similar as long as the scapula is stabilized during active ROM testing. Pure glenohumeral scaption with the scapula stabilized usually is decreased (Figure 1). External rotation in neutral abduction usually is limited. The end feel of these 2 losses of passive ROM are characteristic. Unlike the rubbery and frequently very painful end feel of external rotation ROM in the patient with adhesive capsulitis, the end feel of rotation in the shoulder with OA is typically bony, which is due to osteophyte contact inside the joint. The exam-

Table 1. Common Concerns in Patients With Osteoarthritis

Shoulder pain
Difficulty closing a brassier behind the back
Difficulty placing a wallet in the back pocket
Difficulty tucking in a shirt behind the back
Difficulty using the upper extremity to apply a seatbelt
Difficulty sleeping
Difficulty dressing
Difficulty toileting
Difficulty with feeding

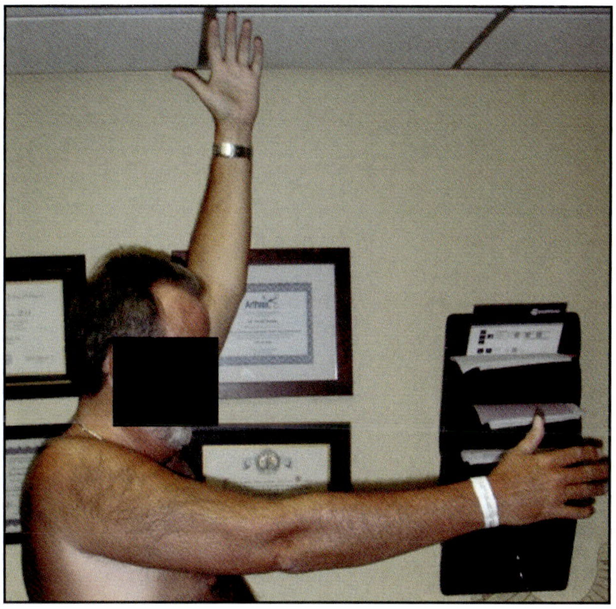

Figure 1. Loss of elevation from glenohumeral arthritis.

iner will have the sense that even if he or she applies further force to the joint, the only motion that will continue will be from the scapulothoracic articulation. Similar to adhesive capsulitis, the pain at end ROM can vary. Depending on the degree of inflammation, some patients will have no pain at end-range external rotation, and the examiner will experience only the solid osseous end point palpably. Other patients might have a degree of discomfort toward the end of the range and pain at the terminus of motion. However, it is very uncommon for the patient to express the same degree of apprehension or guarding that a patient with inflamed adhesive capsulitis typically can demonstrate. Palpable crepitus from the glenohumeral joint can range from the sensation of grinding fine sandpaper to large, loud, popping and clunking sounds that can be painful. Sometimes, the coracoid process can have the appearance of being more prominent, and this is a sign that the OA process has become more severe and that the humeral head has subluxed posteriorly and eroded the posterior glenoid. As characteristic as the examination for this problem can be, good-quality radiographs are required to avoid missing more unusual problems.

Radiographic Findings

To discuss the abnormal findings of OA of the shoulder, the examiner first must understand the normal radiographic appearance of a nonarthritic shoulder. The nonarthritic glenohumeral joint has adequate spacing both between the humeral head and the glenoid and between the humeral head and the acromion (Figure 2). The humeral head is round and smooth, and on radiographs, the transition from the proximal aspect of the medial metaphysis of the humerus to the articular surfaces of the humeral head is a smooth contour. The humeral head is centered on the glenoid on radiographs. The imaginary line drawn along the lateral border of the scapula and continuing under the glenoid neck and to the glenoid face easily should be able to continue along the medial border of the humerus down the shaft without any substantial breaks in the line. In

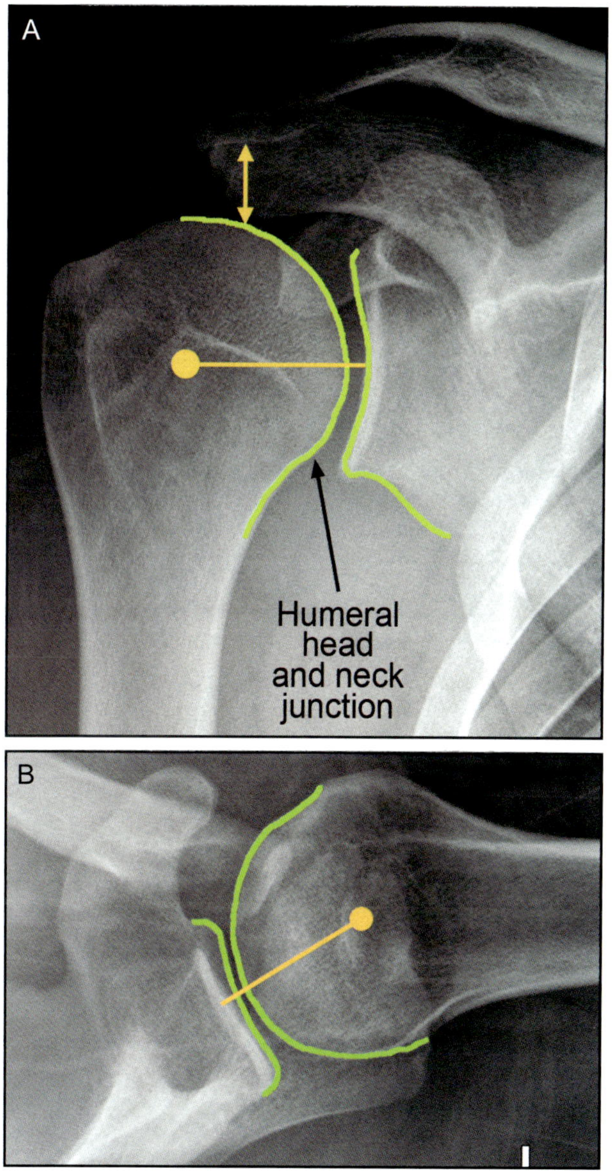

Figure 2. A, Anteroposterior, or Grashey, radiographic view demonstrates a glenohumeral joint without arthritis. B, Axillary view.

contrast, the osteoarthritic shoulder displays irregular joint surfaces with, at times, large bone spurs typically along the inferior one-half of the head (Figure 3). These are termed the *goat's beard osteophytes* and can cause the loss of rotation associated with OA. The humeral head has the tendency to sublux posteriorly in the osteoarthritic shoulder and can cause posterior glenoid bone erosion and loss. The space between the humeral head and the glenoid can be obliterated completely, but the space between the humeral head and the acromion typically is preserved; this is another indicator of the relatively protected status of the rotator cuff in the shoulder with OA. This acromiohumeral interval is the location where the supraspinatus muscle and tendon resides. Narrowing of this interval reduces the space for the supraspinatus and is seen in the shoulder with rotator cuff deficiency. The rotator cuff is not as likely to be intact in most of the other arthritic conditions of the shoulder except in avascular necrosis. Although most of the radiographically important diagnostic information can come from well-performed plain radiographs, more advanced imaging in select patients has a role.

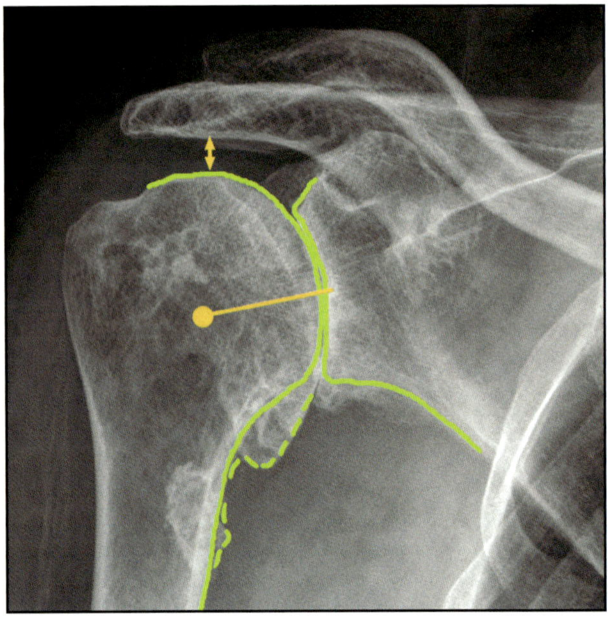

Figure 3. The radiograph shows that the subacromial space (yellow double-headed arrow) is maintained in a patient with osteoarthritis. The arch depicted in green also indicates cuff integrity. The typical goat's beard osteophyte is noted in the area outlined by the green dashed line.

As the humeral head flattens and the force across the joint changes in progressive OA of the glenohumeral joint (Figure 4A), the glenoid can experience substantial pressure and develop different patterns of wear. Plain radiographs can demonstrate these different patterns, but for some patients, a computed tomography scan is needed to understand this deformed anatomy. Having a good preoperative sense of this wear is critical because the surgical technique, which is described elsewhere in this text, needs to be catered to the preexisting glenoid and humeral deformity. The typical wear patterns for OA are mostly posterior (Figure 4B),

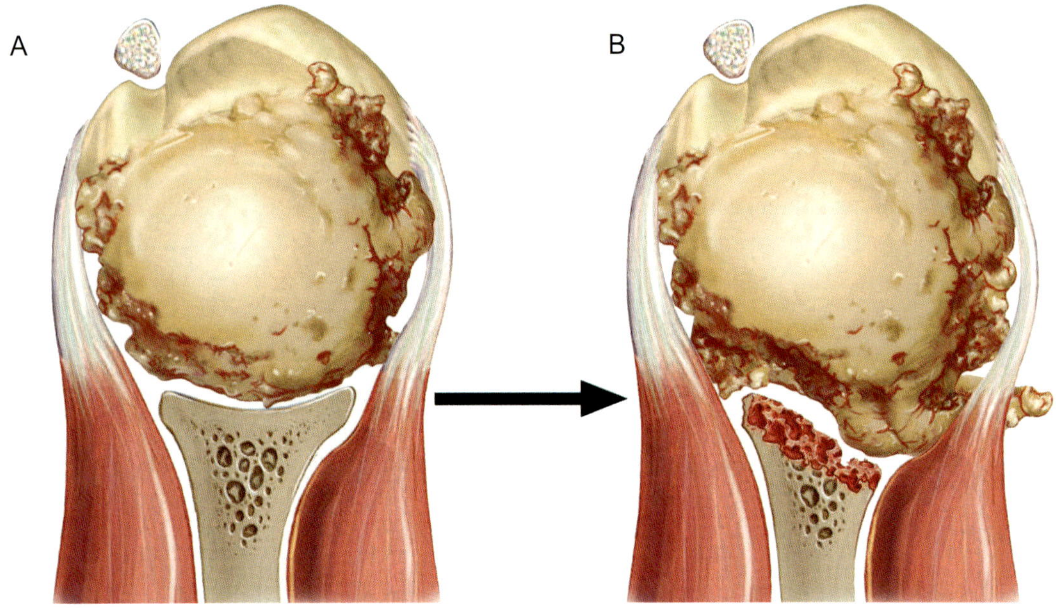

Figure 4. Arthritic conditions of the shoulder joint. Osteoarthritis leads to sclerosis, formation of osteophytes, subchondral cystic changes, loss of cartilage thickness, and joint-space narrowing, A, and demonstrates irregular joint surfaces, goat's beard osteophytes, and posterior glenoid bone erosion and loss, B.

and occasionally the surgeon encounters glenoid erosion that is so severe that re-creating the glenoid with bone graft is the only way to reconstruct the joint.

Treatment

Initial treatment with medications, including nonsteroidal anti-inflammatory drugs, is typical. After the disease progresses, patients might experience pain relief from injections of corticosteroids or from viscosupplements. Arthroscopic intervention has not been shown to be dramatically successful in patients with OA. Shoulder arthroplasty can result in substantial relief of pain and restoration of function in these patients. Total shoulder arthroplasty, in which both the humeral head and the glenoid are replaced, is preferred to treat OA because relief of pain is more reliable when both sides of the joint are addressed than when only the humeral head is replaced (hemiarthroplasty) (Figure 5).[1] A satisfactory rotator cuff is required to obtain the best result when total shoulder arthroplasty is used to treat OA.[2]

RHEUMATOID ARTHRITIS

Another arthritis-related source of shoulder discomfort is rheumatoid arthritis (RA). With this soft tissue disease, the formation of pannus in the joint causes erosive changes and pain. The pannus can erode into the surrounding soft tissues and bone around the shoulder joint, eventually wearing through the rotator cuff and causing enzymatic degradation of the articular surfaces. This clinical syndrome is characterized by morning stiffness, periarticular soft tissue swelling around 3 or more joints, and swelling of the fingers and wrists that is typically symmetric. When RA affects the shoulder, the pattern of arthritic change in that joint is substantially different from the pattern that typically is seen in OA. Contrary to OA, osteophyte formation is not very common, and the erosive pattern on the glenoid is typically more central than posterior (Figure 6A). The rotator cuff status (intact or not intact) of the patient with RA and shoulder pain is always a concern. As the disease progresses, the rotator cuff can be more involved, and it is not uncommon for patients with RA to present with a combination of substantial central bone loss of the glenoid and dramatic rotator cuff deficiency, making their management more challenging.

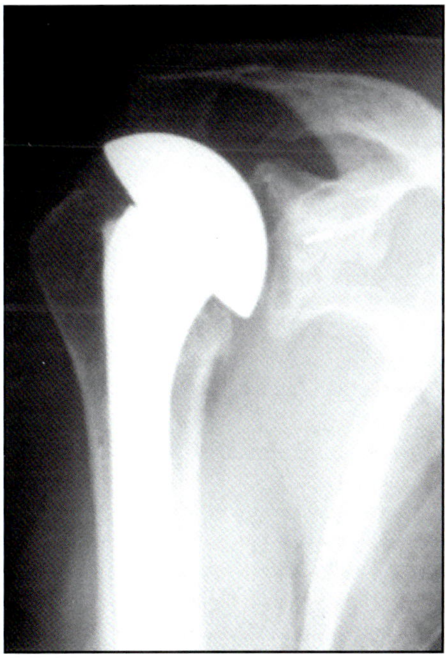

Figure 5. Anteroposterior radiographic view of a total shoulder replacement.

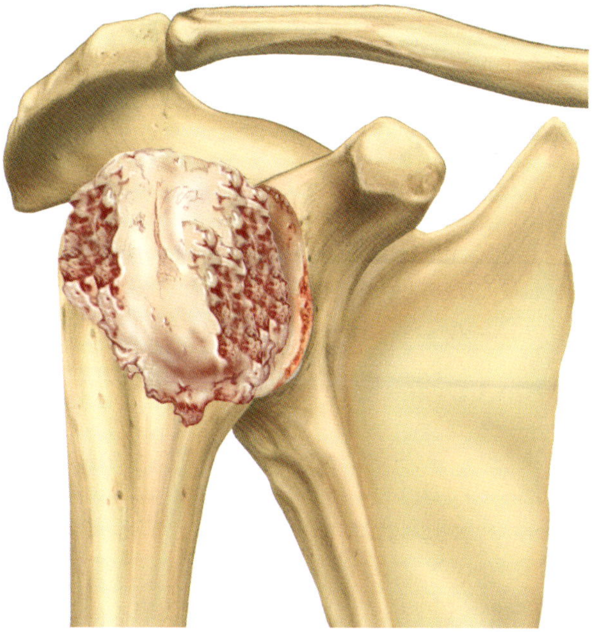

Figure 6A. Erosive changes associated with rheumatoid arthritis.

The bone quality in the patient with RA typically is poor. Large cysts can form within the humeral head and glenoid, resulting in a humeral head that is nothing more than a shell. This alteration of bony strength needs to be taken into account when operatively treating these patients. In addition, arthritic disease of the elbow is more common in the population with RA, and operative treatment for RA affecting the shoulder needs to be performed with the understanding that elbow replacement in that patient is possible in the future.

Frequently, a window of time exists when patients with RA have substantial synovitis without dramatic joint-space narrowing. In those patients, less invasive procedures, such as arthroscopic synovectomy, might be successful. However, after the joint space narrows and bony destruction begins, the role of joint-preserving procedures is limited.

Physical Examination

The findings on physical examination when severe RA has affected the glenohumeral joint can be similar to those that are identified in OA. In RA, the examination for rotator cuff deficiency must be performed. Whereas most patients with OA have a strong rotator cuff on examination, patients with RA might or might not have a strong rotator cuff, and this is important to document at the time of examination. In addition to the integrity of the rotator cuff, the stability of the shoulder and the size and strength of the surrounding rotator cuff musculature should be tested. Because RA is a systemic disease, the integrity of the surrounding joints in addition to the glenohumeral joint should be documented. The acromioclavicular, sternoclavicular, and elbow joints should be evaluated for loss of mobility and synovitis at the time of initial evaluation.

Radiographic Findings

The characteristic osteophytes of OA usually are not present, but smaller and less dramatic osteophytes can be present. The humeral head can appear to be less dense or osteopenic on radiographs, and segmental collapse of the articular surface can exist (Figure 6B). When present, cysts in the humeral head and glenoid can be visible on radiographs but are visualized more easily with more sophisticated imaging techniques, such as magnetic resonance imaging or computed tomography scan (Figure 6C). Glenoid erosion and bone loss can be present, making reconstructive glenoid surgery more challenging at times in these patients. The humeral head can appear to be subluxed superiorly in the joint when the rotator cuff is deficient, which is much more common in RA than in OA.

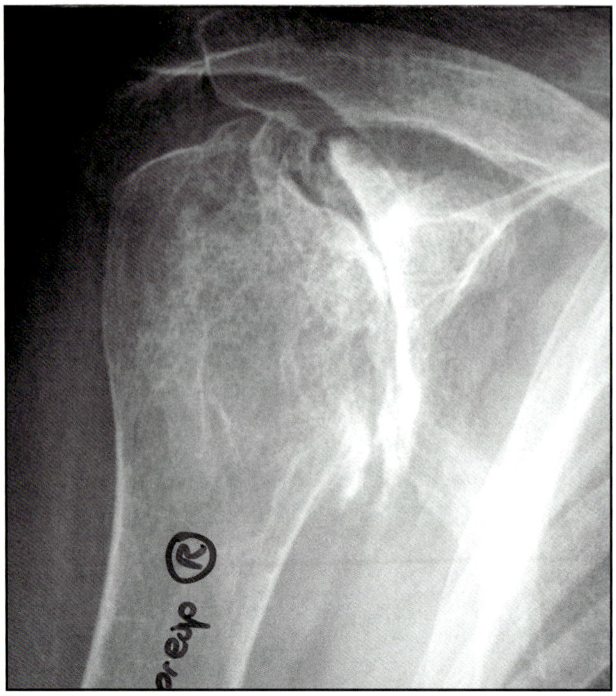

Figure 6B. Anteroposterior radiographic view of a shoulder with rheumatoid arthritis demonstrates a less-dense or osteopenic humeral head with segmental collapse of the medial articular surface.

Treatment

Management can range from medications through injections to arthroscopic debridement and to joint replacement procedures. Total shoulder arthroplasty can be considered in the older patient with satisfactory rotator cuff integrity. If the rotator cuff is not intact and the patient has progressed to the point where arthroplasty can be considered, hemiarthroplasty or reverse

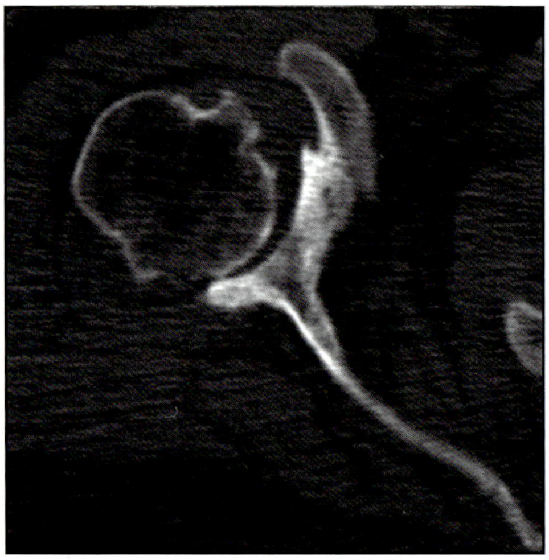

Figure 6C. The computed tomography scan shows severe medial erosion of the glenoid in rheumatoid arthritis.

shoulder arthroplasty can be performed. Hemiarthroplasty is preferred in the younger patient; reverse arthroplasty, in the older patient.

AVASCULAR NECROSIS

Avascular necrosis can be divided into posttraumatic and metabolic sources. It occurs when the bone that supports the cartilage of the humeral head is absorbed due to a loss of blood supply to this area. Loss of architectural and structural support of the cartilage result, and irregularity of the cartilage ensues. The cartilage can detach, and flaps of cartilage can act as loose or foreign bodies within the shoulder, resulting in mechanical catching and pinching that causes substantial pain (Table 2).

In the posttraumatic environment, the blood supply to the humeral head can be damaged, particularly with displaced fractures of the proximal humerus. The ascending branch of the circumcised vessel that penetrates into the humeral head can be violated during fracture-dislocations of the proximal humerus, resulting in an immediate vascular insult that might not manifest for months after the original injury.

Metabolic sources of avascular necrosis function to "choke off" the blood supply to the humeral head. The areas of humeral head necrosis might be global or segmental. A segmental or limited area of humeral head necrosis does not always produce symptoms. Patients might have small areas of avascular necrosis or osteonecrosis of the humeral head without symptoms.

Radiographic Findings

In early avascular necrosis, the glenoid can have a normal radiographic appearance as the humerus begins to collapse. As the disease progresses and the structural support below the cartilage goes away, the humeral head collapse can become more dramatic on radiographs (Figure 7). As the surfaces become roughened, the glenoid cartilage also can be injured, and disease can be appreciated on both sides of the joint.

Table 2. Causes of Avascular Necrosis

Alcoholism
Caisson disease
Steroid use
Vascular compression
Vasculitis
Embolism or thrombosis
Radiation damage
Sickle cell anemia
Trauma

Treatment

Not all avascular necrosis causes symptoms, and if the patient is comfortable, no treatment may be needed. After structural joint changes develop, arthroplasty can be considered. Because avascular necrosis can be very localized in the humeral head, sometimes a localized resurfacing can be used to address this specific loss of bone. Otherwise, the entire humeral head can be replaced (hemiarthroplasty), or both sides of the joint can be replaced (total shoulder arthroplasty), depending on the status of the glenoid and rotator cuff.

In patients who sustain fractures to the proximal humerus in which complete devascularization of the humeral head has occurred, operative replacement of the humeral head is considered. After the size of the avascular necrosis resulting in collapse of the humeral head is beyond the patient's threshold of pain, the management of this problem typically requires operative reconstruction. Partial resurfacing, complete resurfacing, or shoulder arthroplasty can be considered in these patients.

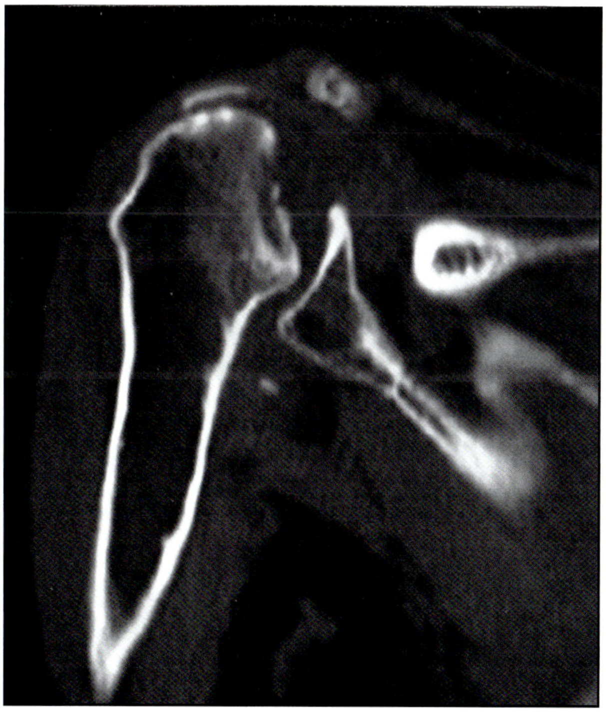

Figure 7. Anteroposterior radiographic view of a shoulder with avascular necrosis demonstrates humeral head collapse due to lack of structural support from cartilage.

POSTTRAUMATIC OR POSTOPERATIVE ARTHRITIC CONDITIONS

In the past, operative reconstruction for instability of the shoulder resulted in substantial tightening of the front portion of the shoulder to avoid extreme external rotation, which was thought to contribute to instability.[3] These procedures that alter the ability of the upper extremity to reach a certain position in space are considered nonanatomic reconstructions. In addition to the expected loss of motion, one of the problems with nonanatomic reconstruction is the anticipated muscle-force imbalance that occurs when the shoulder is over-tightened intentionally. Patients who have undergone these tightening procedures can develop increased compressive forces across the posterior aspect of their shoulders and develop substantial arthritic changes over time. These patients are different from patients with standard OA because in addition to the bony and cartilaginous changes that occur in the arthritic process, postoperative contracture associated with the arthritic changes can make the operative correction more challenging. In fact, the results for replacement of a shoulder with posttraumatic arthritis usually are not as good as the results for replacement of a shoulder with standard idiopathic OA.

Posttraumatic arthritis can comprise mixed clinical findings. Patients can have classic arthritic stiffness combined with rotator cuff deficiency and postoperative scarring. Some patients can have a degree of neurologic injury, and a detailed nerve evaluation can be helpful during the initial evaluation.

Radiographic Findings

Radiographic findings of the shoulder with posttraumatic or postoperative arthritic changes vary. Combinations of avascular necrosis, retained fracture hardware, rotator cuff deficiency, and capsular loss are not uncommon.

Treatment

Treatment is based on the age, glenoid status (arthritic or not arthritic), and rotator cuff status (intact or not intact) of the patient. In younger patients with good-quality glenoid and rotator cuff, hemiarthroplasty options can be considered, but in the older patient with substantial rotator cuff deficiency and glenoid loss, reverse arthroplasty can be successful. Posttraumatic or postoperative arthritis can be the most challenging surgical problem faced by surgeons who perform shoulder replacements and is very similar in difficulty to revision shoulder replacement surgery.

ROTATOR CUFF DEFICIENCY ASSOCIATED WITH ARTHRITIS

Neer et al[4] described rotator cuff tear arthropathy as a distinct diagnosis. It is a pathologic entity that has typical radiographic and clinical findings. Typically, patients gradually lose elevation, rotation, and abduction as the disease progresses, and on radiographs, the greater tuberosity can appear to be eroded, a paucity of osteophytes usually exist on the humeral neck, and the humeral head usually has migrated superiorly and can articulate with the acromion and acromioclavicular joint (Figure 8).

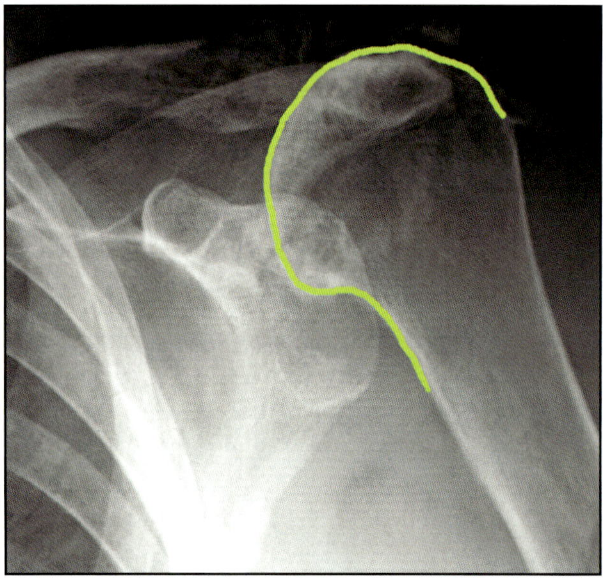

Figure 8. Rotator cuff tear arthropathy. Note the superior migration, indicating massive rotator cuff deficiency.

Rotator cuff deficiency associated with arthritis of any type is a separate category and deserves specific mention. Under normal circumstances, total shoulder arthroplasty requires satisfactory rotator cuff integrity and rotator cuff balance and function for the upper extremity to move well and function appropriately. When the rotator cuff has functional deficiencies, the ability to elevate the extremity in space is affected, and the balance of forces across the prosthetic glenoid causes sheer toggle on the prosthetic-bone interface and can cause loosening of the glenoid component. Therefore, total shoulder arthroplasty typically is avoided in patients with massive cuff deficiency.

Rotator cuff deficiency can occur with OA, resulting in the typical erosions of the glenoid and formation of humeral osteophytes. It also can occur with virtually any other type of shoulder arthropathy, including RA, posttraumatic arthritis, and postoperative arthritis. The physical examination reveals a combination of motor weakness from the cuff deficiency and stiffness related to articular incongruity.

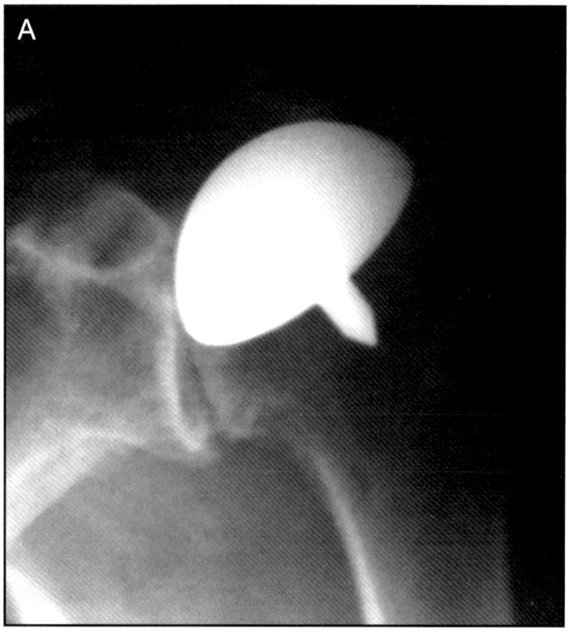

Figure 9. Surgical options for treating glenohumeral arthritis include resurfacing arthroplasty, A, stemmed hemiarthroplasty, B, total shoulder arthroplasty, C, and reverse total shoulder arthroplasty, D.

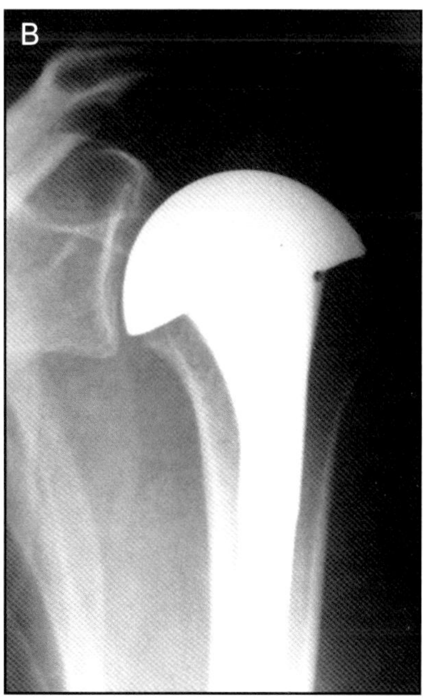

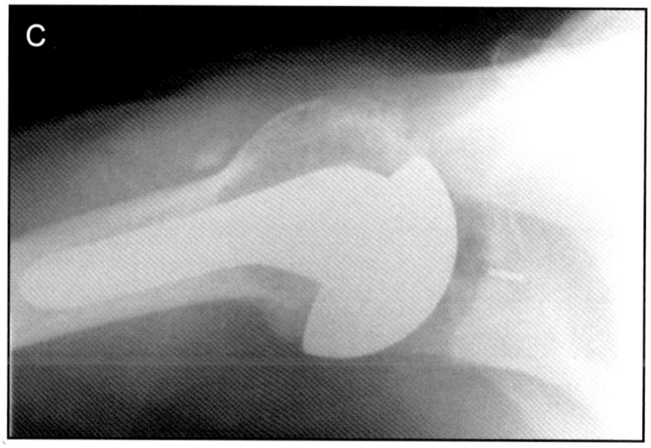

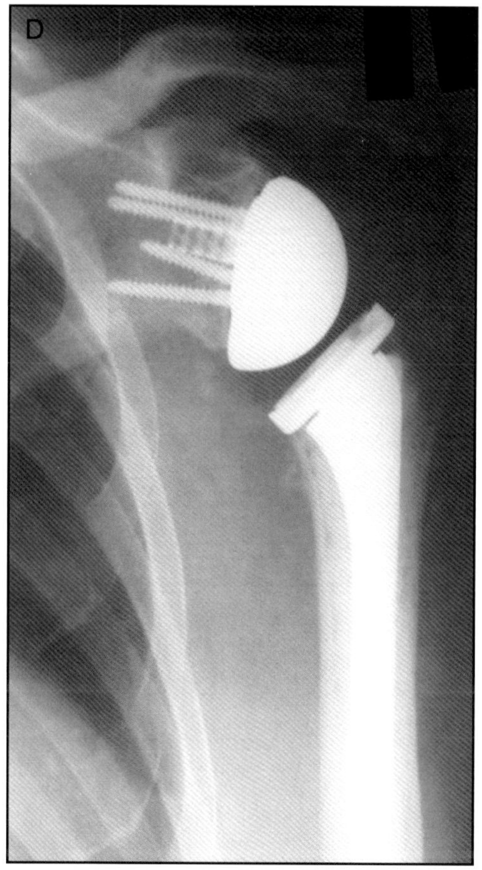

Hemiarthroplasty of the shoulder has been the standard treatment for some time. It is a reasonable consideration in patients who have rotator cuff deficiency, can elevate the extremity overhead, and have pain from arthropathy. The procedure can be performed with a stemmed or nonstemmed device. When a nonstemmed device is used, hemiarthroplasty frequently is called *resurfacing* of the shoulder (Figure 9).

Recently, reverse shoulder arthroplasty has become a more mainstream option that is applied for this indication. When true pseudoparalysis of the shoulder is present, hemiarthroplasty typically cannot restore overhead elevation, so reverse shoulder arthroplasty can be considered. An elderly patient with good-quality deltoid bulk, a functioning deltoid, satisfactory passive ROM with loss of active ROM secondary to massive cuff deficiency, and arthritis of the shoulder is the ideal candidate for reverse shoulder arthroplasty.

Reverse shoulder arthroplasty involves replacing the shoulder joint with a ball on the glenoid and a socket on the humeral side. Although the geometry of the shoulder is inverted, the function that can be restored is remarkable. This design allows the deltoid to contact a stable fulcrum and allows the humerus to rotate around the scapula, enabling overhead elevation and use of the extremity in space. The amount of external rotation that a patient can achieve after a reverse arthroplasty largely is based on the degree of the posterior rotator cuff that is present at the time of surgery. External rotation strength is not expected if a patient has massive cuff deficiency, including the infraspinatus and teres minor. Postoperatively, patients might regain elevation overhead but have persistent external rotation weakness (Figure 10).

MISCELLANEOUS ARTHRITIC CONDITIONS OF THE SHOULDER

Many other conditions can lead to progressive shoulder arthritis. Inflammatory conditions are not limited to RA. Gouty arthropathy develops when sodium monourate crystals deposit in the shoulder and inflammation results. Pseudogout results from calcium pyrophosphate deposition in the shoulder that leads to inflammation and progressive loss of the articular surfaces. Infection of the joint can cause rapid destruction of the articular surfaces as enzymatic degradation of the cartilage occurs due to the release of toxins from the immune system. White blood cells that migrate to the joint to clear an infection also damage the cartilage itself.

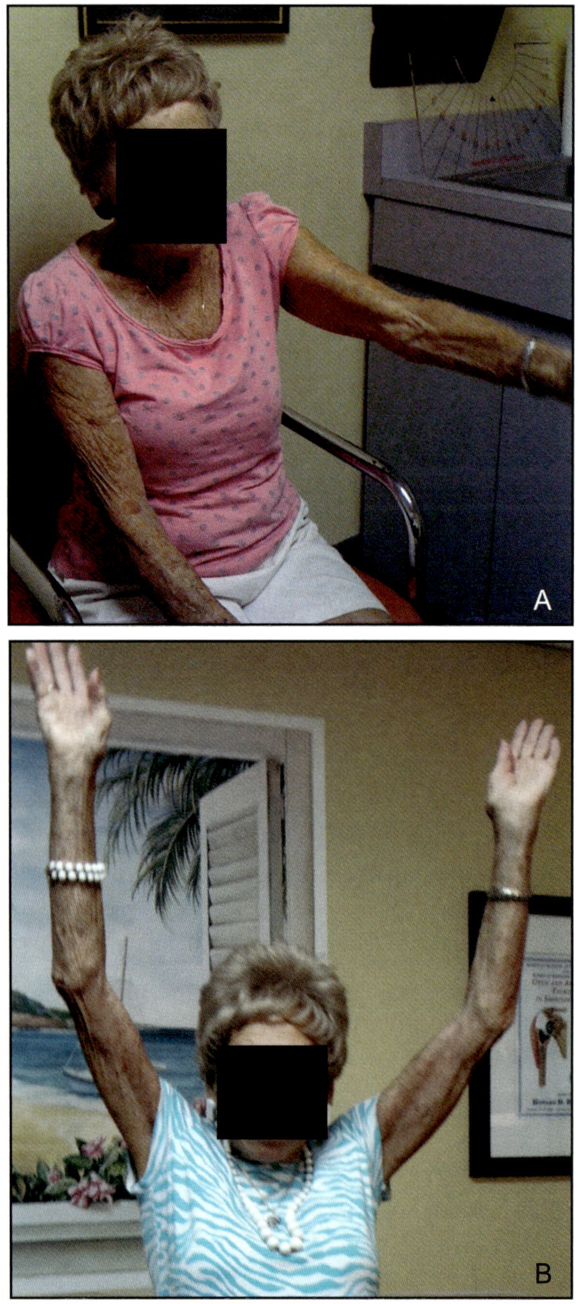

Figure 10. Preoperative, A, and postoperative, B, clinical photographs show improved range of motion after successful reverse shoulder replacement for rotator cuff tear arthropathy.

Treatment for these miscellaneous arthritic conditions is predicated primarily on treating the underlying disorder and secondarily on addressing the glenohumeral consequences. Infections of the shoulder need to be taken very seriously and treated with surgical debridement and lavage and with intravenous antibiotics. An arthroplasty can be performed safely only after the infection has been cleared from the joint. Even after an infection appears to be cleared, the risk of reinfection still exists.

REVISION ARTHROPLASTY

A shoulder arthroplasty can fail, and each case of failure must be addressed individually. Among the challenges that the surgeon might encounter are soft tissue deficiency, bone loss, neurologic injury, and infection. The treatment for revision arthroplasty can be prescribed only after the surgeon thoroughly understands these challenges and has developed a surgical treatment plan to address all factors that are present. Reverse shoulder arthroplasty has become a good salvage procedure for complex failed shoulder arthroplasty indications.

CONCLUSIONS

Arthritic conditions of the shoulder have many causes. From a rehabilitation standpoint, the ability to recognize the different types of arthritic conditions of the shoulder can be helpful because the treatment options vary. Total shoulder arthroplasty for OA, RA, and avascular necrosis is a reliable and effective operation; however, rehabilitation after these procedures is critical to the final outcome. Reverse shoulder arthroplasty for rotator cuff deficiency with arthritis and for revision arthroplasty can result in dramatic improvement in function and substantial relief of pain when executed appropriately.

REFERENCES

1. Gartsman GM, Roddey TS, Hammerman SM. Shoulder arthroplasty with or without resurfacing of the glenoid in patients who have osteoarthritis. *J Bone Joint Surg Am*. 2000;82(1):26–34.
2. Edwards TB, Boulahia A, Kempf JF, Boileau P, Nemoz C, Walch G. The influence of rotator cuff disease on the results of shoulder arthroplasty for primary osteoarthritis: results of a multicenter study. *J Bone Joint Surg Am*. 2002;84(12):2240–2248.
3. Hawkins RJ, Angelo RL. Glenohumeral osteoarthrosis: a late complication of the Putti-Platt repair. *J Bone Joint Surg Am*. 1990;72(8):1193–1197.
4. Neer CS II, Craig EV, Fukuda H. Cuff-tear arthropathy. *J Bone Joint Surg Am*. 1983;65(9):1232–1244.

I-6

The Stiff Shoulder

Steven D. Levin, MD

CLASSIFICATION AND DEFINITION

The stiff shoulder is a common yet poorly understood disorder of the glenohumeral joint or extra-articular shoulder. It often is called *frozen shoulder* or *adhesive capsulitis*. The descriptive terminology of the condition is confusing because of its close overlap with other shoulder conditions that cause similar dysfunction, including painful loss of active and passive range of motion of the shoulder joint. Frozen shoulder is a syndrome that encompasses different causes resulting in the same pathologic condition and dysfunction. Historically, *periarthritis of the shoulder* was the term used to describe painful shoulders for which the symptoms could not be explained by glenohumeral arthritis.[1] Codman[2] later posited that frozen shoulder is "a condition difficult to define, difficult to treat and difficult to explain from the point of view of pathology." He also believed that *frozen shoulder* was a term used to describe a condition of tendinitis with secondary involvement of the subacromial bursa. He noted, "the term applies to many other conditions which cause spasm of the short rotators or adhesions about the joint or bursae."[2] The current consensus definition of the American Shoulder and Elbow Society is, "A condition of uncertain etiology characterized by significant restriction of both active and passive shoulder motion that occurs in the absence of a known intrinsic shoulder disorder."[3]

Although many people have stiff shoulder, the diagnosis and understanding of the condition are difficult and limited. Neviaser and Neviaser[4] described the term *frozen shoulder* as a "waste can diagnosis" because it often was overused and misapplied to patients with a stiff and painful shoulder. Neviaser[5] also noted that other painful conditions of the shoulder, such as calcific tendinitis, bicipital tenosynovitis, glenohumeral and acromioclavicular (AC) joint arthritis, and tears of the rotator cuff, can lead to a stiff and painful shoulder. Other authors have defined *primary frozen shoulder* as an idiopathic condition and *secondary frozen shoulder* as one associated with a known intrinsic, extrinsic, or systemic pathologic condition.[6]

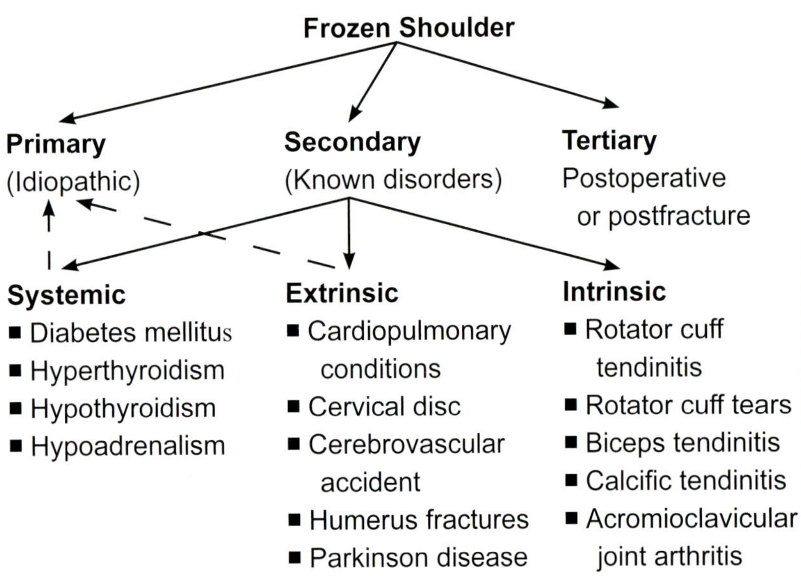

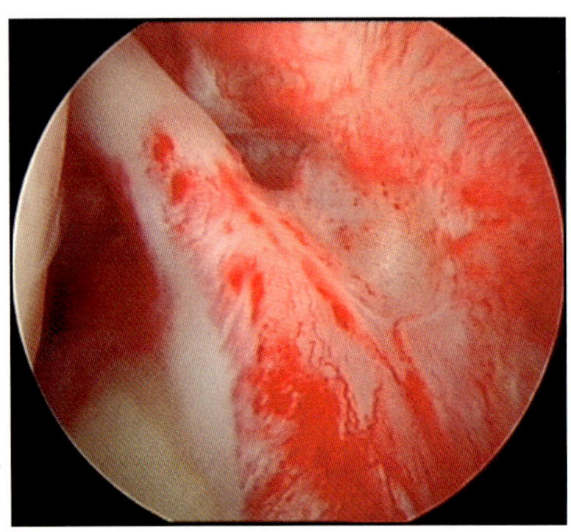

Figure 1. Proposed pathways for the development of frozen shoulder syndrome.

Zuckerman and Rokito[7] recently polled 190 members of the American Shoulder and Elbow Society to review their proposed definition of *frozen shoulder* and its classification into primary and secondary types, with secondary frozen shoulder further subdivided into 3 types (Figure 1). The proposed definition is that "frozen shoulder is a condition characterized by a functional restriction of both active and passive shoulder motion for which radiographs of the glenohumeral joint are essentially unremarkable except for the possible presence of osteopenia or calcific tendinitis."[7] Primary frozen shoulder is considered a diagnosis for all cases for which an underlying cause or associated condition cannot be identified. Secondary frozen shoulder includes all cases of frozen shoulder in which an underlying cause or associated condition can be identified. This secondary type is further subdivided into intrinsic, extrinsic, and systemic types. Intrinsic includes limitation of active and passive range of motion that occurs in association with rotator cuff disorders (tendinitis and partial-thickness or full-thickness tears), biceps tendinitis, or calcific tendinitis. Extrinsic includes cases for which an association with an identifiable abnormality remote to the shoulder itself exists. Examples include limitation of active and passive motion found in association with previous ipsilateral breast surgery; cervical radiculopathy; chest wall tumor; previous cerebrovascular accident; or more local extrinsic problems, including previous humeral shaft fracture, scapulothoracic abnormalities, AC joint arthritis, or clavicle fracture. Systemic cases occur in association with systemic disorders, including but not limited to diabetes mellitus, hyperthyroidism, hyperparathyroidism, hypoadrenalism, or any other condition that has been documented to have an association with development of frozen shoulder.

Most of those surveyed agreed with the proposed definition of *frozen shoulder* and the division into primary and secondary, as well as the subdivision of secondary into intrinsic, extrinsic, and systemic types. For the purposes of this chapter, this represents the accepted classification of frozen shoulder.

EPIDEMIOLOGY

The incidence of frozen shoulder is difficult to assess secondary to its overlying and confounding diagnoses with other shoulder conditions. Nonetheless, it is a common disorder that often is reported by many researchers to affect approximately 2% to 5% of the general population.[8–10] Many of these researchers included populations with specific comorbid conditions and a higher incidence of frozen shoulder than the general population.[8,10] Therefore, it is often an overinflated estimate of the incidence. The condition commonly affects people from 40 to 60 years of age[8,9] and more commonly affects women than men.[11] The nondominant extremity is involved more frequently,[9,12] but it often presents bilaterally and commonly affects the contralateral side years after onset of symptoms in the first shoulder.[8,9,13,14] No one has reported racial predilection. Twenty percent to 30% of patients report a history of minor or major trauma to the shoulder.[9,12] The ensuing stiffness is often largely due to immobility of the affected shoulder. The immobility, which usually is due to protection from motion-induced pain, allows for scarring and disuse contracture of the microtraumatized capsule and other soft tissue.

The question of whether a genetic predisposition for frozen shoulder exists has arisen. Researchers studying twins have shown that it occurs 2 to 3 times more commonly than by chance.[15] Whether an environmental component exists is unclear. Some researchers have shown a strong association between adhesive capsulitis and Dupuytren disease (fibrotic hand contracture),[16,17] which also is believed to have a heritable component. Smith et al[17] showed that Dupuytren disease is 8.27 times more common in patients with frozen shoulder than the general population. However, they did not fully explain the association.

NORMAL SURGICAL ANATOMY

The shoulder joint has more degrees of freedom and motion than any other joint. Therefore, the glenohumeral joint is a minimally constrained, loose articulation. Other than the loose bony constraint of the small glenoid and nearly perfect congruence of the large humeral head, the soft tissues, including the capsule, labrum, rotator cuff, and scapular muscles, provide secondary stabilization for the shoulder girdle. Matsen et al[18] proposed the theory of concavity compression: a stabilizing mechanism in which compression of the convex humeral head into the concave glenoid fossa

Figure 2. Soft tissue and bony restraints providing stabilization and concavity compression of the shoulder joint.

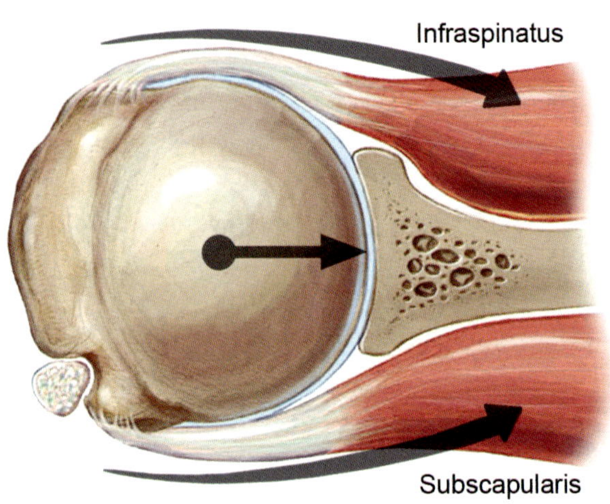

stabilizes it against translating forces. This offers further stability guided by the surrounding capsule and soft tissues, such as the rotator cuff (Figure 2). The glenohumeral ligaments and capsule, which normally are lax or under minimal tension during most shoulder rotations, function mainly at the extremes of rotation and translation to statically constrain the joint against excessive movement of the humeral head on the glenoid.[19]

During normal shoulder motion, tightening and loosening of the glenohumeral ligaments and capsule encircling the humeral head are accompanied by lengthening and shortening of the rotator cuff and deltoid.[20] Loss of shoulder motion can be the result of any condition (intrinsic, extrinsic, or systemic) that directly affects these structures or their ability to move relative to each other. Many traumatic maladies can alter shoulder anatomy in a way that prevents normal shoulder motion (ie, glenohumeral fractures; malunited fractures; Bankart lesions; or soft tissue conditions, such as rotator cuff tears or labral tears). Arthritis and neurologic lesions, as well as the myriad of other extrinsic and systemic pathologic conditions listed in Figure 1, can alter normal smooth glenohumeral motion.

PATHOPHYSIOLOGY

The pathophysiology of frozen shoulder is poorly understood. Several theories have been proposed, and basic science studies are limited. Nonetheless, the role of various biologic factors,[16,21,22] stresses, and neovascularity[16,23] have been supported.

Neviaser[24] used the term *adhesive capsulitis* to describe pathologic findings he discovered in open surgery. He commonly found capsular and synovial inflammation, adhesions, and adherence of the axillary fold to itself and lower down on the anatomic neck of the humerus. With the advent of arthroscopy, Wiley[25] shared that thickening of the capsule and contracture of the inferior capsule occurs rather than an adherence of the axillary fold. Contracture of the soft tissue capsule and ligaments that constrain the glenohumeral joint leads to decreased volume and, therefore, restriction of motion. Neer et al[26] proposed that when contracted, the coracoacromial ligament caused substantial restraint to external rotation (Figure 3). Ozaki et al[27] showed that external rotation was restored when released in patients who had adhesive capsulitis. Using MR arthrography Kim et al[28] found that patients with adhesive capsulitis had much less rotator interval volume than normal control patients (Figure 4).

On a microscopic level, frozen shoulder is thought to be due to synovial inflammation and capsular fibrosis. Biopsy of capsule and synovium specimens from patients with frozen shoulder have shown that cytokines, such as transforming growth factor B, interleukin 1B, platelet-derived growth factor, and tumor necrosis factor α, are involved in synovial hyperplasia and capsular fibrosis.[22] Increased neovascularization and vascu-

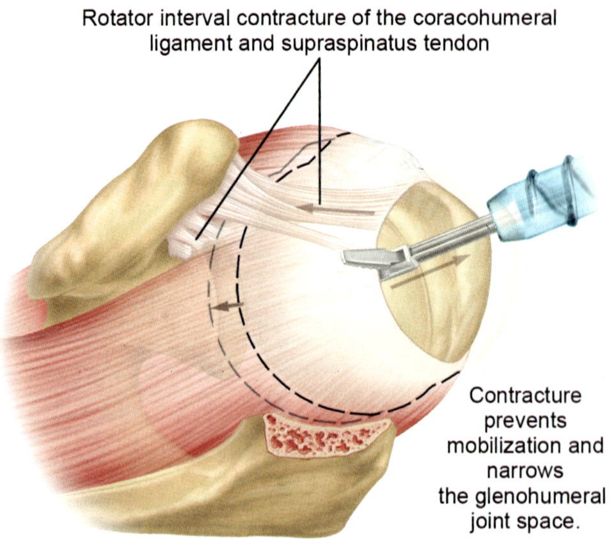

Figure 3. Contracted coracohumeral ligament and narrowed glenohumeral joint.

Figure 4. Diagram of rotator interval borders. Abbreviations: SS, supraspinatus; SSc, subscapularis.

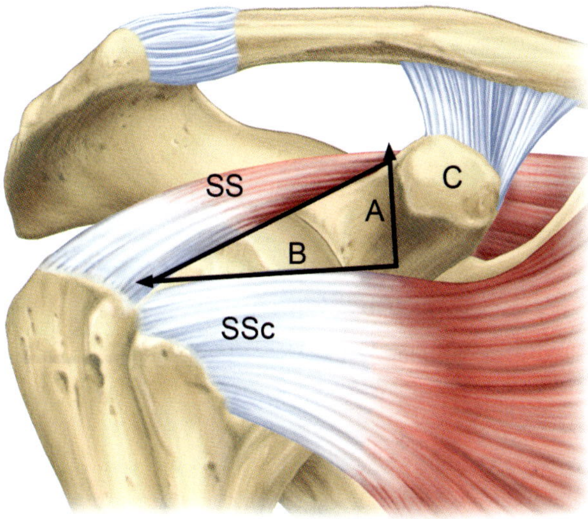

Figure 5. Stages of frozen shoulder.

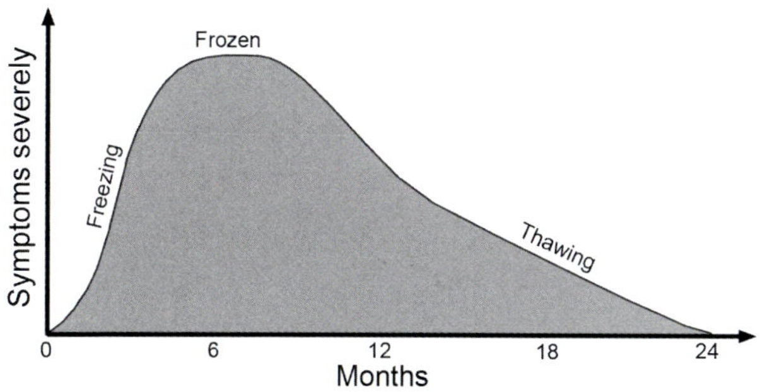

lar endothelial growth factor in the synovium of people who have diabetes and frozen shoulder have been demonstrated.[23] Histologic examination has shown increased synovial vascularization and has shown inflammation with collagen-containing high cellularity of mainly fibroblasts and myofibroblasts.[29]

Neviaser and Hannafin[30] and Neviaser and Neviaser[4] described 4 stages of increased frozen shoulder based on physical examination and arthroscopic examination. Frozen shoulder Stage 1 typically lasts less than 3 months and presents clinically with pain referred to the deltoid, which usually is most prominent at night. Clinical signs include capsular pain in deep palpation with an empty end feel at extremes of motion. These patients have full range of motion under anesthesia. Arthroscopic examination demonstrates inflamed synovium with fibrinous appearance and no capsular contracture or adhesions. This is obviously an early stage, so the anatomic contracture has not occurred yet. Hannafin et al[31] presented histopathologic progression of the disease in capsular biopsies from patients in the various stages. Patients in Stage 1 had rare inflammatory infiltrates with hypervascular and hypertrophic synovium yet normal capsular tissue.

Patients in Stage 2 have symptoms of pain at night and stiffness. This often is referred to as the *freezing stage* (Figure 5). Physical examination commonly reveals restricted forward flexion, abduction, and internal and external rotation. Some loss of motion under anesthesia begins to manifest itself. Arthroscopic appearance is that of marked erythematous synovium with the beginning of loss of the axillary fold (Figure 6). Biopsy specimens demonstrate synovitis similar to

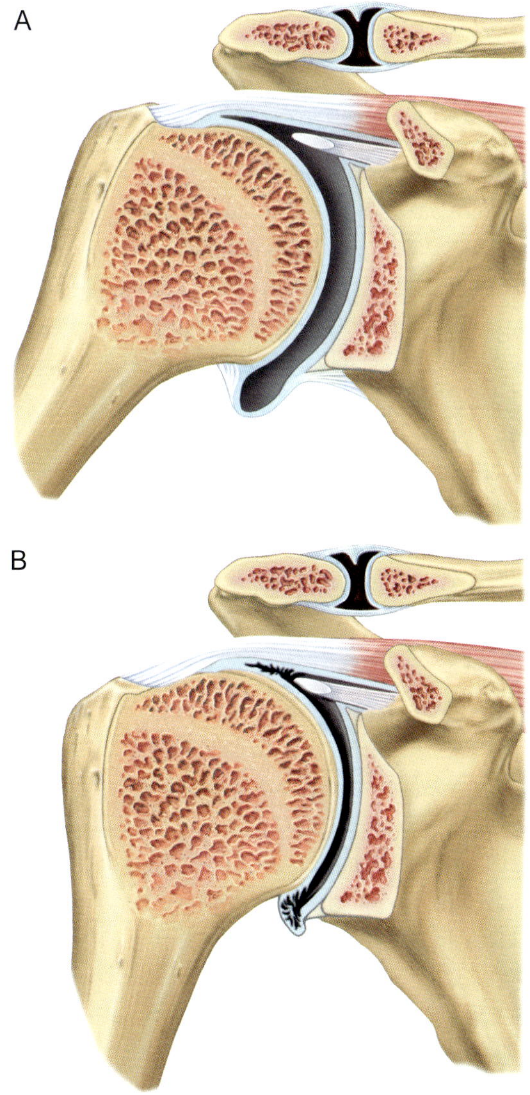

Figure 6. A, Normal axillary fold. B, Contracted axillary fold.

that in Stage 1 with the beginning of perivascularization and subsynovial capsular scar.

Stage 3, which is the maturation stage (Figure 5), presents with symptoms of extreme stiffness and pain at end ranges of motion. The physical signs are substantial loss of motion in all planes and no improvement under anesthesia. Patients come to a mechanical block on forced passive range of motion. Arthroscopic appearance is that of complete loss of axillary fold and a very tight glenohumeral joint, often making difficult the entrance into the joint with the arthroscope. Minimal synovitis with more capsular thickening is present. Biopsy specimens show hypercellular collagen with a thin synovial layer and increased fibrosis.

Stage 4, which is chronic frozen shoulder,[4] is referred to as the *thawing stage*.[13] Symptoms are profound stiffness with diminishing pain. Signs include substantial loss of motion but with gradual improvement. Arthroscopically, the surgeon sees mature scar tissue and adhesions, a tight glenohumeral joint, synovitis, and sometimes cartilage wear. Histopathology has not been reported because most patients who have been recalcitrant to nonoperative treatment have either refused operative intervention or have had their operation before the advent of this stage.

The freezing phase lasts from 10 to 36 weeks and is followed by the frozen phase that lasts from 4 to 12 months. The recovery, or thawing, phase generally can last from 5 to 26 months, with longer thawing associated with longer freezing phases. Reeves[13] described that the full duration of the disease process to last from 1 to 3.5 years, with a mean of about 30 months.

CAUSES

Whatever the underlying cause of frozen shoulder (idiopathic, intrinsic, extrinsic, or systemic), the disease process seems to follow the 4 stages described. Various endocrine disorders, such as thyroid, adrenal, and diabetes mellitus, follow these stages and are associated with frozen shoulder. The incidence of frozen shoulder is much higher in people with diabetes than in people without diabetes. Bridgman[8] reported the incidence of frozen shoulder in patients with diabetes was 10.8% and 2.3% in 600 control patients without diabetes. The exact association between cause and pathophysiology is unclear, but Lequesene et al[32] found abnormal glucose tolerance tests in 28% of patients with frozen shoulder and in 12% of age-matched and sex-matched controls with other rheumatologic conditions. This leads one to posit a correlation with hyperglycemia and the development of capsular contracture. Clearly, more randomized controlled studies are needed.

Trauma has been shown to be a common cause of frozen shoulder, especially when accompanied by prolonged periods of immobilization.[33] Often, patients are not conscious that they are protecting their injured shoulders, and because of the pain elicited by motion, patients substantially limit the amount of motion of their shoulders. This microtrauma causes fibrosis and eventual contracture of the capsule. If the shoulder is not moved appropriately, the scar can organize and thus limit the volume of the shoulder joint, resulting in loss of motion. However, most patients who sustain limited or minimal trauma to their shoulders, even when immobilized for a brief period, do not develop frozen shoulder. This has led some investigators to conclude that some patients possess a "constitutional" predisposition to develop frozen shoulder.[34] The theory is further supported by the substantial incidence of bilateral frozen shoulder.[6,35–37]

Psychological factors have been postulated to play a role in the development of frozen shoulder. Certain personality types and disorders, along with stressful life situations, can serve as a predisposing precipitating factor to its development.[38–41] Coventry[38] described a periarthritic personality that is prone to developing frozen shoulder. He observed a subset of patients who had "a peculiar emotional constitution in which they were unable to tolerate pain, expected others to get them well, and refused to take any personal initiative in their recovery." Other researchers have found no such correlation.[36,37] Nonetheless, it is at least a contributing factor in some patients who develop this disorder.

CLINICAL EVALUATION

Most patients with frozen shoulder do not seek medical attention until long after the onset of pain or stiffness. This is partly due to the insidious onset and the slow adaptation to the discomfort initially and loss of range of motion. As the symptoms progress and activities of daily living are compromised, patients ultimately seek treatment. Upon presentation, a thorough and careful history and physical examination must be taken. Questions to determine systemic causes, as well as trauma, must be asked. Intrinsic and extrinsic factors must be elicited in the history. The criteria for inclusion in most studies of frozen shoulder include insidious onset, pain elicited by isolated scapulohumeral passive motion, pain at night, painful restriction of passive scapulohumeral elevation to less than 90° to 100° and external rotation to less than one-half normal, and a radiograph excluding other pathologic processes (Figure 7).[29]

As with any physical examination, the clinician must observe the patient and in particular the shoulder girdle to elicit any signs of muscular atrophy. Examining both shoulders for comparison is imperative to get a sense of the range of motion in the unaffected shoulder. A careful examination of the cervical spine and a complete neurologic workup is essential to rule out any confounding neurologic cause for the shoulder pain and loss of motion. The clinician also must note any motor or sensory loss, which might be due to a neurologic lesion. Because the clinical hallmark of a stiff shoulder is loss of motion, an assessment of the active and passive range of motion of the shoulder must be done.

Active range of motion is assessed by simply instructing the patient to move his or her shoulder in the

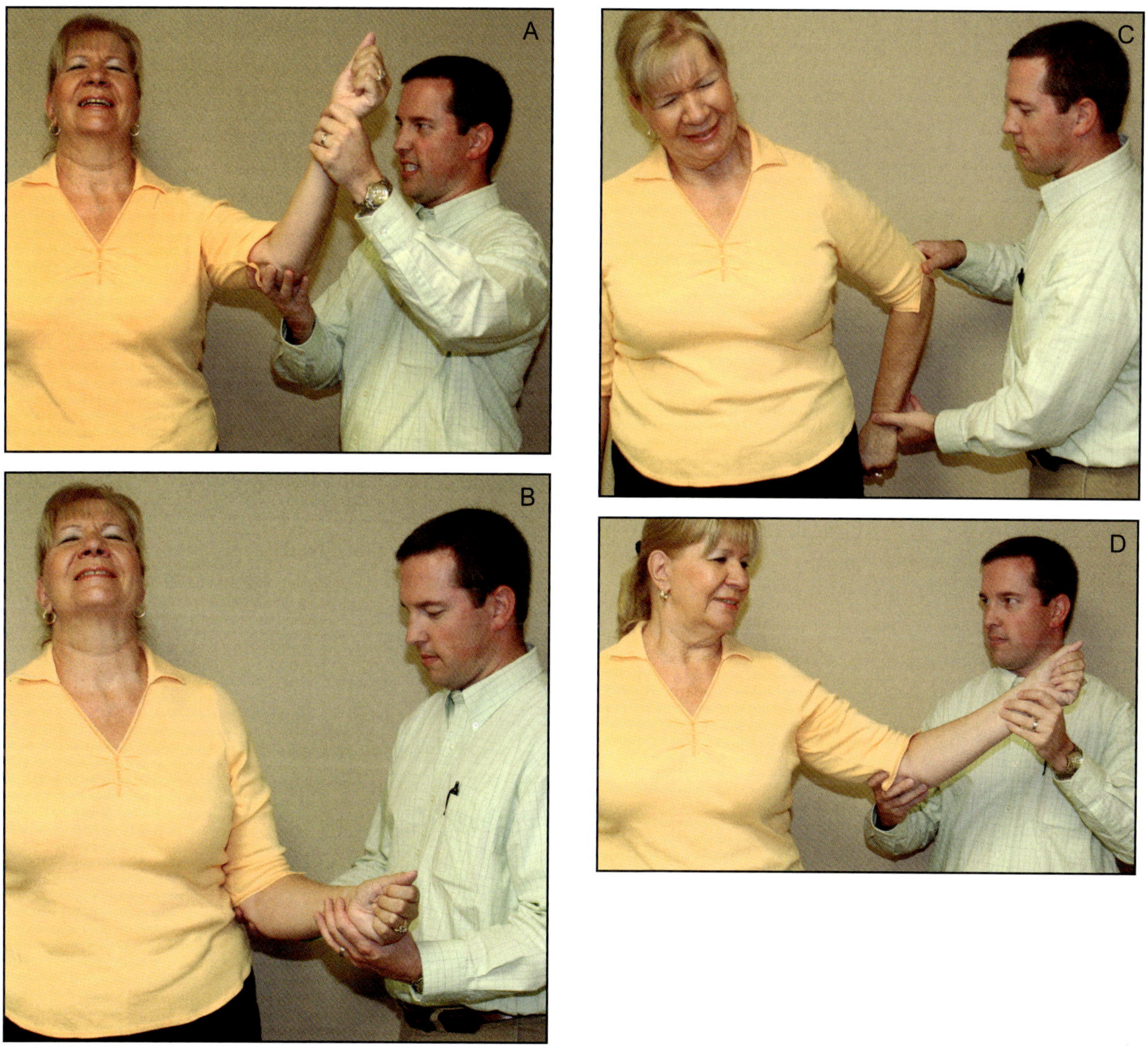

Figure 7. Decreased active range of motion with limited forward flexion, A, external rotation, B, internal rotation, C, and abduction, D.

Figure 8. Stabilization of the scapula while examining shoulder range of motion.

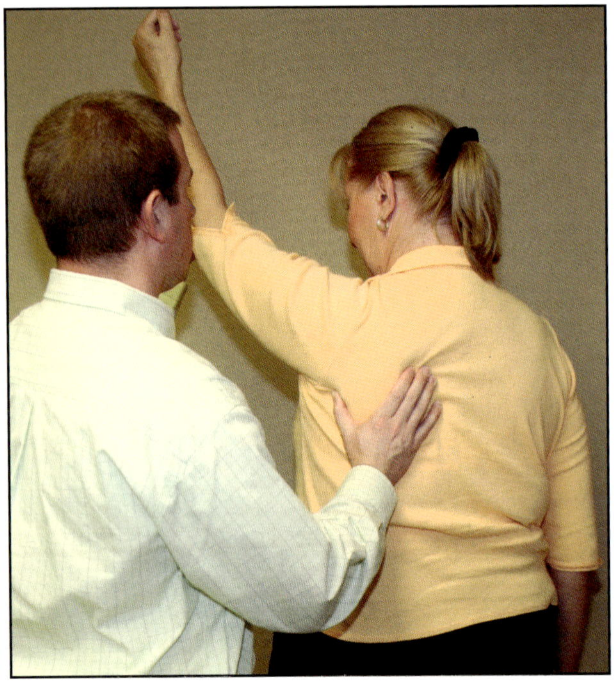

direction being assessed: forward flexion, abduction, and internal and external rotation. The values should be recorded and compared with those of the contralateral side. After active range of motion is recorded, passive range of motion should be evaluated. The clinician needs to record pure passive glenohumeral shoulder motion by eliminating any contributory or compensatory scapulothoracic motion. This is done by manually stabilizing the scapula while passively moving the glenohumeral joint in the desired direction (Figure 8). If a stiff scapulothoracic joint is present, it also must be evaluated and recorded. Active shoulder elevation typically is measured in the plane of the scapula with the patient seated. A firm end point or block to motion often is appreciated and seen with pain at extremes. The degree of loss of shoulder motion in making the diagnosis of frozen shoulder has little consensus.[42,43] Passive range of motion of the shoulder ideally is measured with the patient in the supine position, again guarding for scapulothoracic substitution by stabilizing the scapula. A firm end point must be distinguished from guarding secondary to pain to get a precise measurement. Documenting baseline active and passive range-of-motion readings at each office visit is important to monitor the patient's progress with regard to physical therapy.

Next, a generalized shoulder examination should ensue. Observation of the shoulder girdle, including noting previous surgical scars, bony deformities, and muscle atrophy, should be recorded. Palpation about the AC joint, rotator cuff, biceps tendon, and deltoid insertion should be performed, and elicitation of pain should be observed. This should be followed by all other commonly known provocative shoulder tests, such as Neer and Hawkins impingement tests, Speed, Yergason, active compression, apprehension and relocation, and scapular winging by observation with push-up against a wall. Measurement of active strength against resistance needs to be documented.

Specific patterns of motion loss frequently are commensurate with the cause of the stiffness. Primary adhesive capsulitis usually is accompanied by global loss of range of motion, whereas postoperative or posttraumatic adhesive capusulitis might be only in a plane affected by the operation or trauma. Rotator cuff lesions or subacromial impingement or adhesions might present with predominant loss in forward flexion or abduction with accompanying weakness or pain. This must be differentiated carefully from other patterns seen with different causes. Recognition of these various patterns of motion loss is important for helping determine the specific cause of stiffness and eventual treatment of it.

Loss of motion often is associated with the location of capsular contracture.[34] Limitation of external rotation with the upper extremity in the abducted position usually is associated with scarring in the anteroinferior region of the capsule, whereas limitation in the adducted shoulder is associated with contracture in the anterosuperior region of the capsule in the rotator interval.[26,27,44] Limitation of internal rotation in adduction and abduction is associated with scarring in the posterior portion of the capsule, which is reflected in loss of horizontal cross-chest adduction.[45] Subacromial bursitis can cause contractures consistent with an impingement process. Subdeltoid bursitis and subcoracoid impingement can cause scarring of tissue planes with resultant global contractures.

A lidocaine injection test can be helpful in determining the cause of shoulder stiffness. It can be given to not only the subacromial space, but also the AC joint, biceps tendon sheath, and glenohumeral joint to help determine the cause of pain or stiffness. For example, with subacromial impingement, the clinician can inject the subacromial space and record differences in range of motion, as well as responses to pain. If the pain is decreased but range of motion is still inhibited, it likely is due to subacromial adhesions, which contribute to frozen shoulder. Similarly, if the clinician injects the AC joint and normal adduction increases secondary to decreased pain, it likely is due to an intrinsic AC joint pathologic condition, such as AC joint arthritis. If the glenohumeral joint is injected and range of motion remains unchanged, it likely is due to intrinsic glenohumeral contracture. The use of lidocaine in the glenohumeral joint rarely is needed to make the diagnosis, but it can be used as an adjunct in cases that are difficult to diagnose. The clinician must proceed with caution in injecting the glenohumeral joint with any of the –caines.

Recently, researchers have revealed chondrolysis with the use of bupivacaine in the glenohumeral joint.[46,47] Deleterious affects of one-time lidocaine injection on the cartilage of the shoulder joint have not been reported, but recently, several investigators have documented chondrolysis with the use of continuous-flow –caines, such that the clinician should proceed with caution when injecting any of the –caines directly into the joint.

LABORATORY STUDIES

Routine laboratory testing of the blood for presumed systemic frozen shoulder is helpful but not always diagnostic. For example, people who have diabetes and frozen shoulder should have fasting blood glucose tests. Similarly, thyroid function tests should be assessed in patients who have frozen shoulder and suspected thyroid disease. Other helpful tests include complete blood count, chemistry profile, rheumatoid factor, and serology. Erythrocyte sedimentation rate is a nonspecific test that has been shown to be positive in 20% of patients.[42,43] Controversy exists about the relevance of increased levels of immune complexes in patients with adhesive capsulitis.[35,48,49] Serum triglycerides and cholesterol levels also have been shown to be elevated in patients with frozen shoulder compared with levels in age-matched and sex-matched controls.[50] Elevated levels of C-reactive protein occasionally have been seen in patients with frozen shoulder, but again this has not been shown to be diagnostic.[48]

IMAGING

Plain radiographs, including standard anteroposterior (AP), Y-view, axillary, and true AP views, in most cases are not helpful in diagnosing the cause of idiopathic frozen shoulder. However, they can help rule out other causes, such as disuse osteopenia, posttraumatic arthritis, degenerative arthritis and other arthritides, fracture malunion, and even nonarthritic glenohumeral joint narrowing. Radiographs also can be used to exclude other causes of shoulder stiffness and pain and thus can be complementary in making a diagnosis of calcific tendinitis, neoplastic processes, impingement, superior migration of the humeral head seen in rotator cuff tear arthropathy, glenohumeral osteoarthritis, and AC joint arthritis.

Arthrography is another diagnostic tool that has been shown not only to be helpful in diagnosing frozen shoulder, but also to be somewhat helpful in treating it. Neviaser[51] established, "… in true adhesive capsulitis arthrography shows a very definite decrease in joint capacity with obliteration of the axillary fold. In many cases the subscapular bursa is decreased in size or not visualized at all." He believed that the procedure could serve as a diagnostic aid to differentiate true adhesive capsulitis from stiffness and a painful shoulder due to other causes. Other authors have asserted that *decreased joint capacity*, defined as the inability of the joint to accept 5 to 10 mL of contrast or dye, is essential in making a diagnosis of adhesive capsulitis.[4,52] The normal glenohumeral joint capacity is around 15 mL. The severity of shoulder range-of-motion restriction also might be associated with reduction of joint volume.[6] Binder et al[11] noted that arthrographic findings do not indicate the type of onset (ie, primary or secondary or the rate or extent of recovery). Others have confirmed that such findings also have not had any predicted value in terms of the severity or prognosis of the disease.[53,54] Historically, others have used arthrography to document tearing of the capsule during manipulation under anesthesia.[6,55] However, with more modern accepted treatment techniques of arthroscopically guided manipulation and/or release, this recently has been used less commonly.

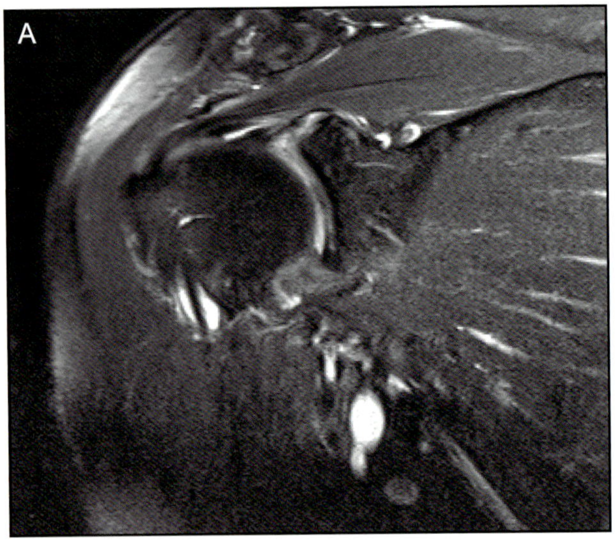

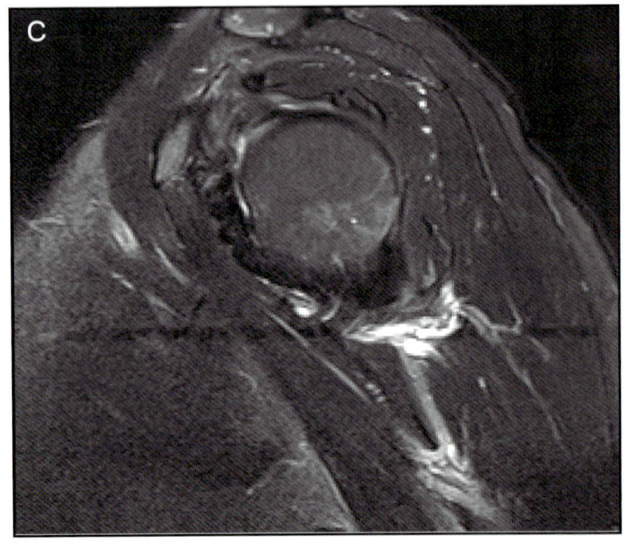

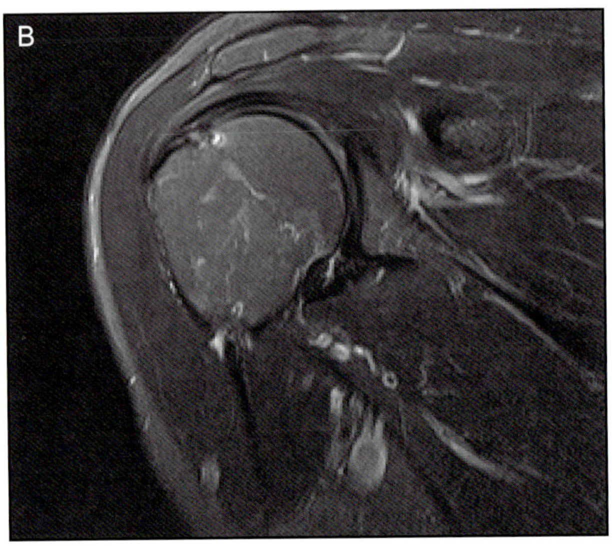

Figure 9. Magnetic resonance imaging or magnetic resonance arthrogram of classic findings of frozen shoulder: thickened coracohumeral ligament, decreased glenohumeral joint volume, and obliteration of subcoracoid fat. A and B, Coronal views show a thick inferior glenohumeral ligament. C, Sagittal view shows increased T2 signal in the rotator interval.

Ultrasound also has been shown to be helpful in the diagnosis of frozen shoulder. Thickness of the coracohumeral ligament can be measured in many shoulders, and thickening suggests adhesive capsulitis. This is very operator dependent and, therefore, difficult to rely on in many centers.

Although not commonly used, technetium scanning can be a useful adjunctive test in the diagnosis of frozen shoulder. Increased uptake in those patients usually is due to hypervascularity. Binder et al[42] noted that more than 90% of their patients had increased uptake on the diphosphonate scans, with 29% having more than 50% increased uptake compared with the opposite shoulder. The bone scan findings were of limited use in determining severity of the disease process, cause, or duration of symptoms and, therefore, seldomly are used.

No true criterion standard imaging study exists in diagnosing frozen shoulder, but magnetic resonance (MR) imaging and MR arthrography seem to produce the most reliable results and information. The findings have been shown to correlate well with operative findings.[56–58] In particular, thickening of the coracohumeral ligament and joint capsule in the rotator interval has been demonstrated with MR imaging and MR arthrography.[59,60] Obliteration of the subcoracoid fat between the coracohumeral ligament and coracoid can be present and is known as the *subcoracoid triangle sign* (Figure 9).[57] Generalized decrease of joint volume can be seen with MR imaging and, in particular, MR arthrography. Typically, MR imaging is ordered to rule out rotator cuff pathologic lesions in patients who present with signs and symptoms similar to those of patients with frozen shoulder. It is used more commonly, therefore, as an adjunct to rule out other intra-articular pathologic conditions.

MANAGEMENT OF FROZEN SHOULDER

Treatment for frozen shoulder begins with nonoperative therapy and is followed by more invasive treatments in recalcitrant cases. The level of evidence of most studies of treatment for frozen shoulder is limited due to many factors: varying causes, different presentation times of the phases of frozen shoulder, and difficulty in making a diagnosis. Therefore, most studies are case series or retrospective studies in which investigators have analyzed a specific treatment regimen.

Most patients present for treatment primarily because of pain followed by stiffness or loss of motion. Therefore, the first line of treatment is aimed at pain control so the patient can endure the second line of simultaneous treatment: aggressive physical therapy. Because the pathophysiology of frozen shoulder is poorly understood and the causes are many, a multimodal approach to treatment is often necessary. The treatment can be extensive and continue over a prolonged period. It must be adjusted constantly according to the patient's reaction and progress. Pain relief often is accomplished with analgesia and transcutaneous electrical nerve stimulation in the early stages of the disease process.[41,43] Use of narcotics generally is avoided because of dependence and because it could mask the effects of the patient's tolerance for the exercise therapy program. With any treatment regimen for frozen shoulder in patients with severe pain or pain out of proportion to objective findings, seeking advice from anesthesia pain consultants is often a good idea. Their aid in controlling the level of pain in patients is essential in helping patients comply with the necessary physical therapy program.

Nonsteroidal anti-inflammatory drugs (NSAIDs) often are used empirically for the treatment of frozen shoulder, but well-controlled studies are limited. Nevertheless, NSAIDs seem to help control inflammation in patients who present in the early phases of the disease process. Oral corticosteroids have been shown to help with pain[43] and, in some instances, early range of motion. However, little evidence is available to support their long-term use.[42,43] The stage of the disease process commonly is not delineated in these studies, so drawing valid conclusions about oral steroid use is difficult. The potential for systemic side effects with long-term use must be considered because many of these patients would use them for prolonged periods. Therefore, if they are used, they should be administered and monitored with extreme caution.

Codman[2] originally described a self-limited course of frozen shoulder, and many patients are treated with supervised neglect and analgesia, supervised physical therapy, and/or steroid injection. Injection therapy has been studied extensively and documented with Level I studies. Local intra-articular and subacromial corticosteroid injections have been used for relieving pain and less frequently for improving range of motion.[42,61,62] These injections are particularly helpful in the early freezing stages of the disease process[11,54] when pain prohibits the necessary participation in physical therapy.

Rizk and Pinals[41] compared a symptomatic group that received intra-articular methylprednisolone and lidocaine with an intra-articular lidocaine placebo and 2 control groups that received the same injections in the subacromial space. Patients had had symptoms for more than 6 months before injection. Follow-up lasted up to 6 months, with weekly checks for the first 11 weeks. The authors found no differences with blinded evaluation of pain and range of motion between the groups, but patients treated with intra-articular steroid showed more rapid improvement in pain. The difference was transient, lasting 2 to 3 weeks. Nonetheless, this could be seen as an important adjunct in patients with frozen shoulder in the early stages because it helps them better tolerate the rigors of physical therapy.

Shah and Lewis[63] performed a systematic review of randomized controlled studies. Nine randomized controlled trials were identified, and 4 were rated as high quality. Three showed benefit in association with the use of multiple corticosteroid injections as measured on the basis of pain reduction, improved function, and increased range of motion. The results suggested that multiple injections were beneficial until 16 weeks after the date of the first injection. No evidence was found to support giving more than 6 injections; as many as 3 injections were shown to be beneficial.

Bulgen et al[64] randomized 42 patients into 4 treatment groups: (1) intra-articular injection of methylprednisolone, (2) physical therapy with a supervised physical therapist, (3) ice and exercise, and (4) no treatment. All had persistent motion deficits at 6 months, but patients treated with injection had the most marked improvement in range of motion at 4 weeks. However, the difference was equalized at 6 months. These results have been duplicated by Bal et al.[65]

In a Level IV retrospective study, Hazleman[66] showed that intra-articular injection of hydrocortisone was correlated inversely with duration of symptoms. Thus, it is more helpful in the early stages of the disease process than in the later stages when frank capsular contracture has occurred. Many other researchers have pointed to the same conclusion[67–69] that (1) injections are beneficial in the early stages of the disease process; (2) the results taper off after 2 to 3 weeks; and (3) the injections allow for pain relief early, facilitating tolerance of physical therapy. Otherwise, remaining evidence of the benefit of injections remains equivocal. Steroid injections have not been shown to improve the rate of return of shoulder motion.[6,70] Injections should be used with caution because repeated injections have potentially deleterious and toxic side effects on the tendons, connective tissue, and cartilage.

Griesser et al[71] recently published a systemic review of the effectiveness of intra-articular corticosteroid injections for adhesive capsulitis. They only included Level I and II studies. Their hypothesis that the results for intra-articular steroid injection would engender substantial improvement in the short term but would show no difference compared with other treatments in the long term was confirmed.

The next and most commonly effective mode of treatment for frozen shoulder is physical therapy; as for most patients, a supervised physical therapy program will successfully treat primary adhesive capsulitis.[14,72,73] The therapy could last several months, consists of aggressive stretching and strengthening 2 to 3 times per week, and is supplemented with a strict home exercise program. The details of the actual therapy protocols are detailed elsewhere. However, in contrast to primary adhesive capsulitis, postoperative or posttraumatic shoulder stiffness is more recalcitrant to this regimen.[72,74–78] This might be due to other contributing factors, such as iatrogenic overtightening of the capsule in surgery to treat instability, physical block of range of motion secondary to malunion or nonunion of fracture, loose bodies, and development of scar tissue secondary to previous surgery or genetic predisposition. Therefore, determining the pathologic process responsible for the stiff shoulder is important to guide the specific physical therapy necessary to treat it.

An attempt at nonoperative physical therapy almost universally is accepted as first-line treatment in patients who have had stiff shoulders for less than 6 months and no previous treatment. The exceptions are those rare cases in patients with clear and obvious anatomic deformities that preclude physical therapy.

Most investigators have supported the use of physical therapy for treatment of the stiff shoulder.[79,80] Griggs et al[81] showed a 90% satisfactory rate with a stretching program for Stage 2 disease. In only approximately 10% of cases in most series, patients do not respond to these protocols.[9,12,81] Therefore, a carefully planned physical therapy program is employed almost universally. The program begins with an active-assistive range-of-motion exercise regimen with gentle passive stretching exercises. These exercises should be performed frequently and throughout the day rather than during prolonged single sessions. This allows for the adhesions to break up and stretch and not to reform. Patients need to go up to and beyond the point of pain to make and keep incremental increases in range of motion. This often necessitates controlling pain and seeking advice from pain anesthesia consultants. Further details on exact physical therapy exercises, techniques, and protocols are detailed in other chapters.

Suprascapular nerve blocks have been used as an adjunct to aggressive physical therapy. Anesthesiologists in pain clinic settings traditionally have provided them. Newer techniques recently have been used in office settings.[82] Advocates of their use have shown disruption of the normal pain pathways, allowing for greater tolerance of physical therapy and thus increased range of motion.[83] This has allowed tolerance of physical therapy and range-of-motion exercises, which has translated to increased early range of motion in symptomatic compared with control groups. It is an invasive procedure with potential side effects and complications and, therefore, usually is used in extreme recalcitrant cases. Better higher-level studies are needed to confirm its beneficial use.

Hydrodilitation or brisement also has been used as an alternative treatment for frozen shoulder. This is a method of capsular expansion with the injection of fluid or contrast material to distend the contracted capsule. Thus, the diagnostic test of arthrography or MR arthrography can be used as an aid in treating frozen shoulder. This rarely is used solely as a line of treatment and often is used in conjunction with physical therapy or manipulation. Therefore, its effectiveness alone has been difficult to quantify and is not recommended without adjunctive therapies. Using fluid-containing lidocaine, cortisone, and dye, Rizk and Pinals[41] showed that patients with frozen shoulder derived great benefit from the injection. The arthrographic results showed capsular tears in all cases, and in 13 of 16 patients, immediate pain relief and increased range of motion was experienced with improvement lasting over a 6-month period. The disruption of the contracted capsule was believed to be responsible for the relief of symptoms in these patients.

After 6 to 12 months of chronic stiffness and pain recalcitrant to all nonoperative measures described, more aggressive measures are considered. The next line of treatment that has been used historically is manipulation under anesthesia. The indication for the timing of its use generally includes demonstration of lack of forward flexion to 90° after at least 3 to 6 months of supervised physical therapy. Each case is individualized, so the timing can be altered depending on the various factors, such as cause, degree of pain, and severity of motion loss. Manipulation under anesthesia has been shown to improve range of motion and provide pain relief in patients who do not improve with a supervised rehabilitation program or who exhibit progression of stiffness while still undergoing a nonoperative treatment regimen.[4,84–86]

The procedure generally is done in the beach-chair position under general or regional anesthesia. Paralysis is necessary during the procedure to allow for complete release of contractures. Regional anesthesia, such as scalene nerve block, allows for pain relief immediately after manipulation. This is advantageous because the patient can move directly into a continuous passive motion (CPM) machine so he or she does not lose any of the motion gains made immediately at the time of surgery. Hospitalizing the patient for at least 1 to 2 days is imperative so an anesthesia pain consultant can maintain the block with an indwelling catheter and can monitor pain levels.[87,88] A long-acting agent, such as bupivacaine, usually is used. This has the added benefit of decreasing the amount of narcotics the patient might require.

Proper technique is critical to avoid potential complications. Complications, such as glenoid fracture and transient brachial plexus block, have been reported.[89] Subscapularis rupture, humeral head fracture, labral tears, rotator cuff tears, and biceps tendon injuries, also have been reported, so performing the procedure safely is critical.[90,91] Arthroscopically guided manipulation under anesthesia offers the advantage of enabling the surgeon to visualize the process as it occurs so he or she can avoid iatrogenic injury.

Neviaser and Neviaser[4] described their methods. The scapula is stabilized with one hand, while the arm is grasped above the elbow with the other. The extremity is moved gently through external rotation and internal rotation, while audible and palpable break-up of adhesions occurs. Warner[78] believed that after rotatory motion is regained, recovering flexion and abduction is easier if the greater tuberosity can be rotated out from under the acromion. If external rotation cannot be recovered, flexion is attempted followed by abduction and then external and internal rotation. To gain further range of motion by tearing the anterior capsule, the surgeon can abduct the upper extremity to 90° while applying an external rotation moment to it. This aids in breaking up the anterior and inferior scar and capsule.

After motion is attained through manipulation under anesthesia, maintaining it in the early postoperative period is critical. For this reason, patients typically are hospitalized and have nerve blocks or indwelling catheters, pain consults, and CPM machines. No authors of long-term Level I studies have documented their efficacy, but they do help with early motion in the functional range. The patient must not rely solely on the CPM machine but should use it as an adjunct to aggressive range of motion in physical therapy. After being discharged from the hospital, the patient must be enrolled in a supervised, aggressive physical therapy program 2 to 3 times per week until painless full range of motion is obtained. Details of the therapy protocol are described in other chapters.

In a long-term Level IV study, Ferrell et al[90] showed that treatment of idiopathic frozen shoulder by manipulation under anesthesia led to sustained improvement in shoulder motion and function at a mean of 15 years after surgery. Twenty-five patients had a mean of 6 months of physical therapy before manipulation under anesthesia. Significant improvements were seen in forward flexion (range, 104°–168°) and external rotation (range, 23°–67°). No complications were noted. Sixteen patients reported no or minimal pain, and 18 required no further surgery.

Dodenhoff et al[92] reported the results of manipulation under anesthesia in 37 patients (39 shoulders) in a prospective Level IV study. All patients with primary adhesive capsulitis had improvement in Constant scores from 24 before manipulation under anesthesia to 69 at 6 months after the procedure. Ninety-four percent of patients were satisfied secondary to increased ability to perform activities of daily living.

In a recent blinded, randomized controlled trial with 1-year follow-up, Kivimäki et al[93] evaluated 125 patients with frozen shoulder. Patients were divided into a group that received manipulation under anesthesia and home exercises or a group that received home exercises alone. At 3 months, the manipulation group had greater forward flexion, but no differences were observed for other outcomes. They concluded that in patients with frozen shoulder, manipulation under anesthesia did not confer additional benefit to that obtained with a home exercise program.

Researchers who performed arthroscopy after manipulation under anesthesia showed hemarthrosis in all shoulders, superior labrum anterior-posterior lesions, partial subscapularis tendon tears, anterior labral tears, and middle glenohumeral tears.[91] This lends further evidence to support arthroscopically controlled manipulation under anesthesia.

Haggart et al[94] studied 97 patients treated with manipulation under anesthesia and found 95% had excellent or good results with 4- to 9-year follow-up. Harmon[95] reviewed 400 manipulated shoulders and found full, painless range of motion in 64% to 94% of patients 2 to 3 years after manipulation. Therefore, it generally is accepted in patients who do not improve after a prolonged course of nonoperative treatment lasting more than 6 months. Manipulation under anesthesia is a safe procedure that substantially can shorten the course of the disease process. It allows patients to return to a more normal lifestyle with activities of daily living and work sooner than the reported natural history of this condition would indicate.[85]

Historically, manipulation under anesthesia has been the recommended treatment of choice after failure of the nonoperative modalities I have outlined. However, given the potential for iatrogenic complications, arthroscopically guided manipulation under anesthesia or manipulation with arthroscopically guided capsular release has been recommended more recently. The earliest description of arthroscopic release was by Conti[96] in 1979. Arthroscopic release offers many advantages over manipulation under anesthesia alone. The surgeon more easily can diagnose the stage of the disease process and can gain an idea of the cause by enabling visualization of the pattern of contracture. If necessary, therefore, a lesser procedure, such as synovectomy instead of manipulation and capsular release, can be performed if the pathologic condition encountered dictates it. Although many researchers have shown that a multimodal nonoperative treatment program is effective for most patients with adhesive capsulitis, arthroscopic release is intended for the minority who do not improve with this approach.[12,97]

Arthroscopy allows for a controlled release of structures that are directly responsible for the shoulder contracture and loss of motion. It is performed with careful, sequential manipulation so only the structures that need to be released are addressed. This is in contrast to simple manipulation under anesthesia, which can tear or injure other anatomic structures that might not necessarily need to be released. It also aids in avoiding iatrogenic injury and avoids the potential need for open release that clearly introduces other potential morbidities.

The procedure typically involves either scalene nerve block or indwelling catheter for postoperative pain relief so the patient can maintain the range of motion achieved from the release with pain control. The patient is admitted to the hospital for 1 to 3 days and uses a CPM machine with aggressive physical therapy 2 to 3 times per day while in the hospital. The procedure can be accomplished in the lateral decubitus or beach-chair position; I prefer the beach-chair position because in this position, the anatomy is oriented normally. After documenting the preoperative passive range of motion of the anesthetized patient before the procedure begins, the surgeon establishes a standard posterior viewing portal. Great caution must be taken when inserting the arthroscope in a patient with adhesive capsulitis because the glenohumeral joint always is contracted, and the surgeon must avoid potential iatrogenic injury to the articular cartilage of the humeral head and glenoid. Forceful manipulation now is not recommended before insertion of the arthroscope. The arthroscope should be inserted first to assess the exact pathologic lesion or affected structures, and after the exact pathologic condition is determined, it should be addressed with careful, controlled arthroscopic release of the affected structures with gentle, progressive manipulation. This technique decreases the incidence of wanton, unnecessary tearing of important soft tissue structures that heretofore were damaged before arthroscopy.

After the arthroscope is inserted, an anterosuperior outflow portal is developed so a probe can be inserted for palpation and inspection. The surgeon performs a systematic diagnostic arthroscopy to evaluate all aspects of the glenohumeral joint. It allows for assessment and evaluation of the shoulder for simply severe synovitis versus capsular contracture and other anatomic abnormalities. After the arthroscopic diagnosis is made and all structures are evaluated carefully, the surgeon decides how to proceed according to the pathologic conditions encountered. If capsular contracture is found, a surgical release is necessary. When all the synovitis and inflammatory tissue are debrided and ablated, the capsule and rotator interval are addressed. A thickened capsule, contracted coracohumeral ligament, and decreased rotator interval usually are encountered. Capsular division is started superiorly and proceeds inferiorly just a few millimeters off the labrum. This is done with radiofrequency ablation or electrocautery with a needle tip bovie. The release starts just anterior to the biceps tendon. As the division of the capsule proceeds, the surgeon gently externally rotates the upper extremity to aid with and monitor the range of motion gained (Figure 10). Release of the coracohumeral ligament at the coracoid base is especially important for gaining external rotation. Neer et al[26] and Ozaki et al[27] showed that such a release performed through an open approach is successful in restoring external rotation in patients with refractory frozen shoulder. The release proceeds from anterosuperior to anteroinferior. After the surgeon is past the equator of the glenoid, he or she must use extreme caution to avoid iatrogenic injury to the axillary nerve. If the release is performed within 1 to 3 mm of the glenoid labrum, it is usually safe. After the muscle fibers of the subscapularis are visualized, no further release medially is necessary. At this point, further release, if necessary, is done with an arthroscopic scissors to continue the dissection in a controlled manner to preclude the potential for thermal injury to the axillary nerve. At this point, the extremity is manipulated more and farther in degrees of forward flexion, in forward flexion and abduction, and in external rotation to gauge the adequacy of the release and need for further dissection. Restriction to cross-body adduction and internal rotation at this point indicates posterior capsular contracture, which warrants posterior capsular release.

In these cases, switching sticks are used to exchange viewing and working portals so the posterior capsule

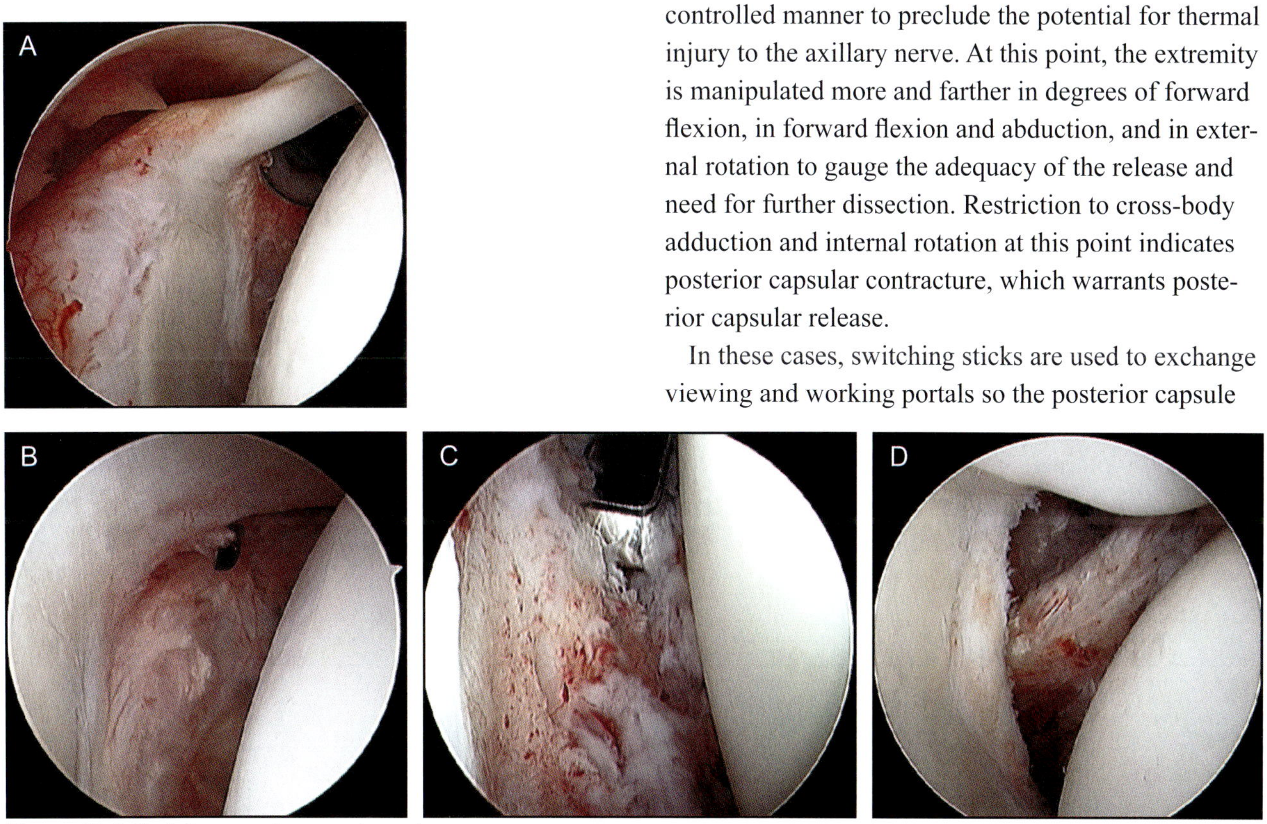

Figure 10 A-D. Arthroscopic capsular release.

can be addressed. The posterior release is performed in a similar manner as that described for the anterior release. The release posteriorly also must be done just off the labrum at the glenoid rim. The posterior capsule is thin, and the infraspinatus is superficial. Therefore, if the release is performed more laterally, iatrogenic injury to the infraspinatus tendon is more likely. After the posterior release is performed, a forced internal rotation moment is placed on the upper extremity with the arthroscope viewing from anterior to monitor the motion obtained.

After the desired internal rotation is reached, the dissection and manipulation is halted, and the surgeon inspects the subacromial space. The same posterior viewing portal used for glenohumeral release is used for initial inspection of the subacromial space. A midlateral portal is created as the working portal. The surgeon performs a meticulous bursectomy, taking care to avoid injuring the suprascapular nerve by venturing too far medially. A thorough bursectomy is performed, and all adhesions to the rotator cuff are taken down and debrided. If the surgeon determines preoperatively that the patient has impingement syndrome concomitantly, then he or she takes down the thickened coracoacromial ligament to the base of the coracoid and uses the cutting-block technique to accomplish an arthroscopic subacromial decompression. Any associated lesions, such as calcific deposits, AC joint arthritis, and rotator cuff tears that can contribute to shoulder stiffness, also can be addressed at this time.

Wiley[25] performed arthroscopic release in 37 patients with primary frozen shoulder. Pain relief was striking. Arthroscopic appearance was uniform; a patchy vascular reaction around the biceps and opening into the subscapularis bursa consistently was seen. Joint capacity always was reduced.

Uitvlugt et al[98] reviewed 20 cases of patients with frozen shoulder who underwent manipulation under anesthesia after 6 months of unsuccessful nonoperative treatment. The joint capsule was difficult to penetrate with the arthroscope because of the thickness of capsular tissue and contracted joint space. Vascular synovitis was found intra-articularly. The glenohumeral joint accepted less than the normal amount of fluid, but after manipulation, the joint accepted more fluid. Immediate postoperative second-look arthroscopy showed synovitis and capsular hemorrhage indicative of capsular tearing from manipulation.

Zanotti and Kuhn[99] defined anatomic consideration for capsular release in a cadaveric model. Anatomic dissection after circumferential release revealed an average distance from capsular release to axillary nerve of 7.04 mm, to posterior humeral circumflex artery of 8.2 mm, and to brachial artery of 15.97 mm. They believed that a safe margin between the capsule and neighboring neurovascular structures can be obtained by release within 1 cm of the glenoid rim (Figure 11).

In a multicenter retrospective study of arthroscopic release of the glenohumeral joint, Beaufils et al[100] evaluated the technical feasibility, results, and potential correlations between results and causes of stiffness. Motion gains were 86° for forward flexion, 72° for abduction, 34° for external rotation, and 6 spinous processes for internal rotation in 25 patients (26 shoulders). Gains in range of motion were independent from cause of shoulder stiffness, but global results were better in primary frozen shoulder in terms of pain and strength.

In an important study in which they further evaluated the results and differing causes, Elhassan et al[101] showed that patients with idiopathic and posttraumatic shoulder stiffness have better outcomes than patients with postoperative shoulder stiffness with arthroscopic capsular release. One hundred fifteen patients were

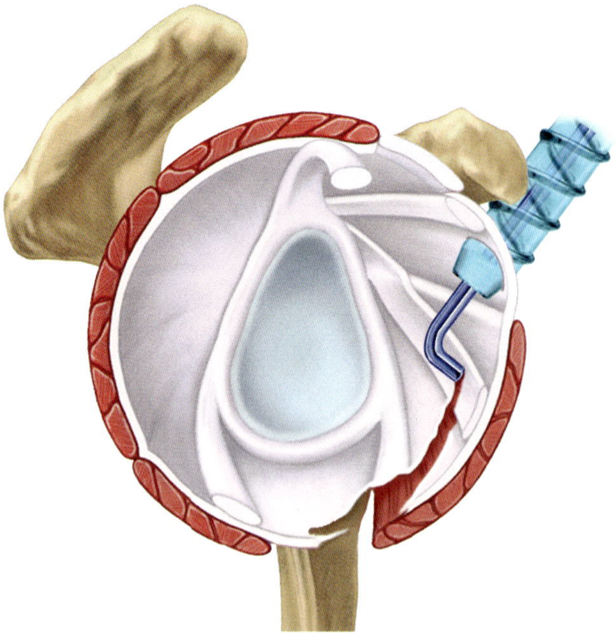

Figure 11. Capsular release with electrocautery device.

reviewed retrospectively. Arthroscopic capsular release was performed in all patients who underwent an average of 9 months of physical therapy. The Constant scores and subjective shoulder values were lower in the postoperative groups than the idiopathic and post-traumatic groups. This partly might be due to extrinsic contractures and scarring that cannot be addressed arthroscopically. Holloway et al[102] discovered similar findings in their study. Arthroscopic capsular release was as effective for improving range of motion in patients with postoperative shoulder contracture as it was for treating idiopathic contracture; however, the postoperative group had less improvement in subjective scores for pain, function, and patient satisfaction.

Arthroscopic release with manipulation under anesthesia is the treatment of choice for shoulder stiffness recalcitrant to all other nonoperative treatments. In rare cases, open release is entertained: stiffness on the basis of scarring among the subscapularis, strap muscles, and deltoid usually in patients who have undergone previous surgery. Patients with severe osteopenia based on risk of fracture of the proximal humerus also might be candidates for open release.[34] However, open release mostly is considered a historic treatment option, but it does merit analysis in this review. Great insight can be obtained from studying open releases to gain an appreciation of the anatomic considerations and the advantages of arthroscopic release in certain cases. In 1989, Ozaki et al[27] first reported the results of open release for recalcitrant cases of frozen shoulder with complete relief of pain and restoration of full range of motion in 16 of 17 patients. Omari and Bunker[103] reported on 25 patients with adhesive capsulitis and found open release was useful in severe cases.

Warner[78] elegantly described his technique in the rare cases of frozen shoulder that require open release. Most of these cases are usually postoperative. A deltopectoral approach is used, and adhesions between the humeral head and deltoid are released bluntly. The axillary nerve lies 3 to 5 cm below the lateral border of the acromion, so caution must be exercised. Dissection is easier if the upper extremity is abducted because this allows the deltoid to be more lax. The conjoined tendon is separated from scar to the subscapularis. This can be done with blunt or sharp dissection. The dissection should proceed lateral to the musculocutaneous nerve.

The rotator interval then is released from the humerus to the coracoid.[26] The shoulder should be manipulated as the dissection proceeds. If marked limitation of external rotation due to scar between the subscapularis and capsule still is present, the subscapularis is split in line with its fibers, and an elevator is used to release these adhesions. Ultimately, if restriction in external rotation still exists, a Z-plasty lengthening can be performed (Figure 12).

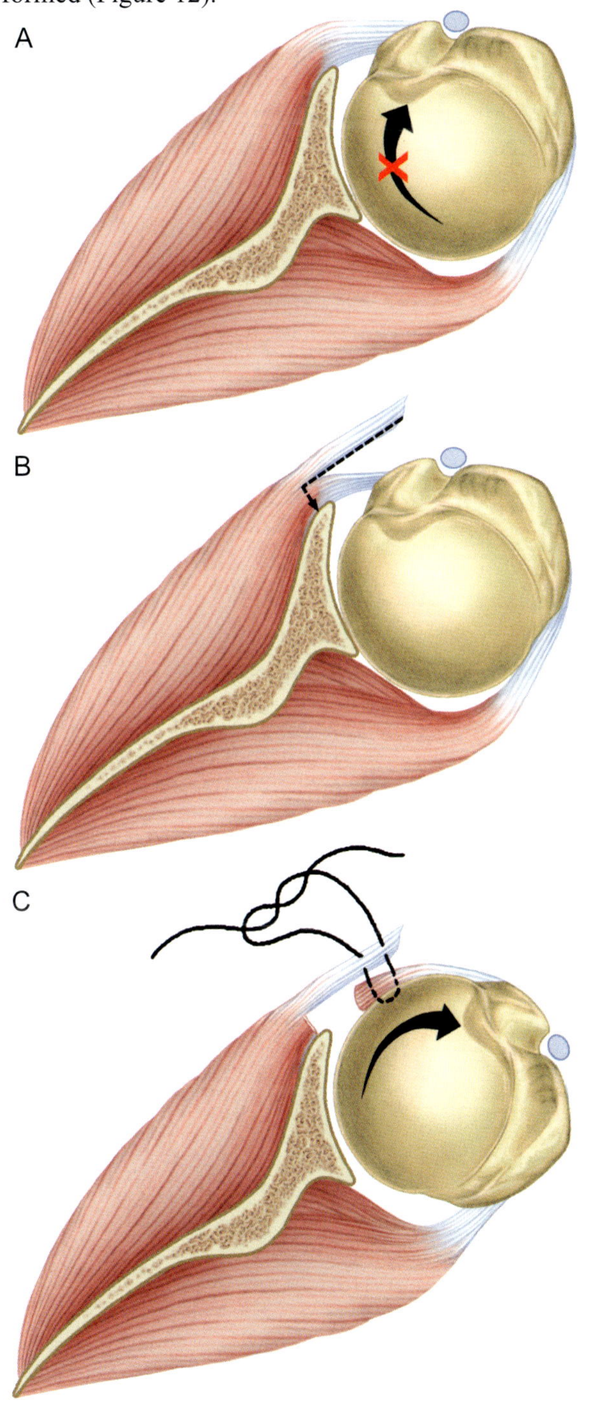

Figure 12 A–C. Z-plasty lengthening of the subscapularis.

If abduction and internal rotation remain limited, the inferior and posterior capsule can be released through the joint (Figure 13). A humeral head retractor and inferior glenoid retractor are placed to protect the axillary nerve. The capsule is released under direct visualization from inferior to posterior and superior. Retractors are removed, and motion is assessed. The extremity is postioned in maximum external rotation that will allow closure of the Z-plasty.

Postoperative physical therapy is administered during in-patient hospitalization twice a day (in the morning and afternoon) for the first 2 days. Pain is controlled with scalene nerve block or indwelling catheter monitored by anesthesia pain consultants. Patients undergo full, aggressive passive and active-assistive range-of-motion exercises under the supervision of a physical therapist and advance to active range of motion and strengthening. Detailed therapy protocols are discussed in more detail in other chapters. Use of CPM machines are recommended between sessions. Appropriate narcotic analgesia is dispensed on hospital discharge.

Open operative release needs to be protected especially if Z-plasty was performed. The position at which the Z-plasty was tightened in closure needs to be documented and conveyed to the physical therapist so he or she can guide the range of motion cautiously and appropriately. Passive range of motion usually is instituted for the first 4 weeks for this reason.

Patients are encouraged to use the upper extremity for activities of daily living. A home stretching program is instituted with outpatient physical therapy 2 to 3 times per week. Additional physical therapy after 4 to 6 weeks is individualized to the patient's specific needs. After pain-free full range of motion is attained for 1 to 3 months, the strengthening phase then ensues. Further details of this program are outlined in other chapters.

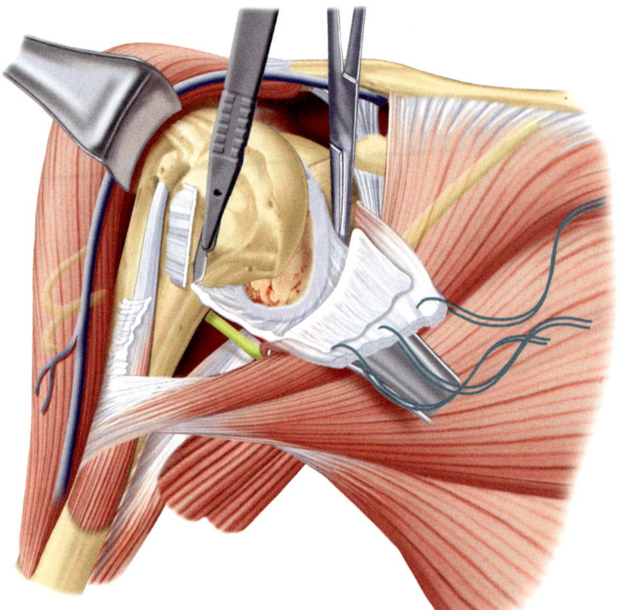

B

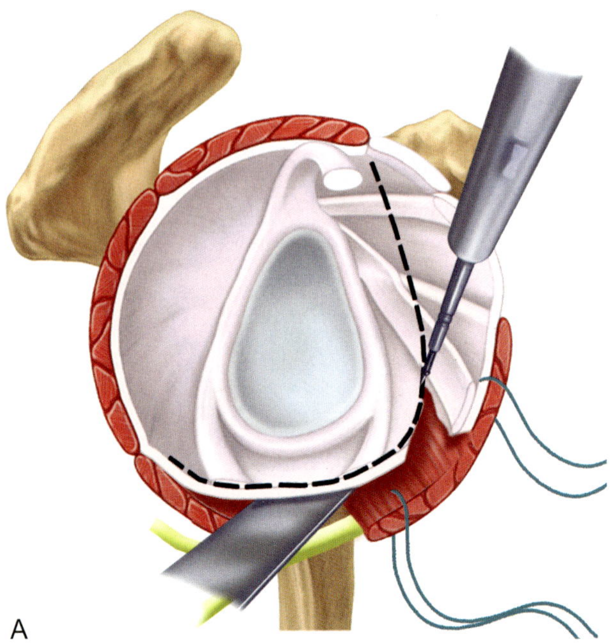

A

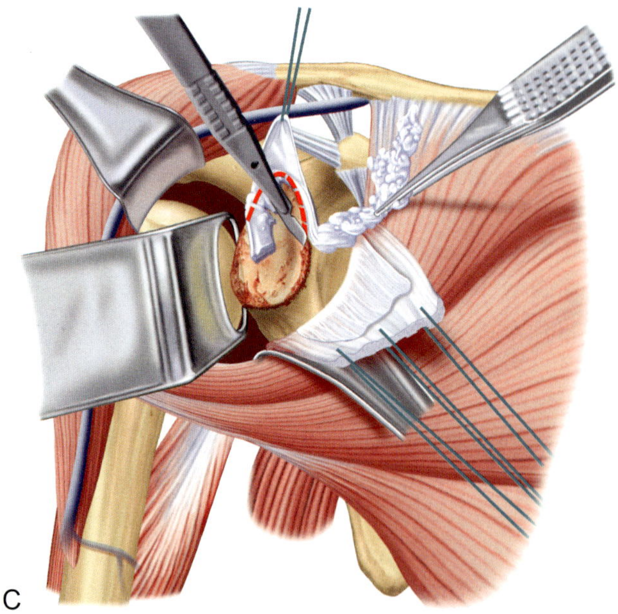

C

Figure 13 A-C. Circumferential open capsular release.

REFERENCES

1. Duplay ES. De la periarthrite scaulohumerale et.des raideurs de l'epaulequi en son la Consequence. *Arch Gen Med.* 1872;20:513–542.
2. Codman EA. *The Shoulder: Rupture of the Supraspinatus Tendon and Other Lesions in or About the Subacromial Bursa.* Boston, MA: Thomas Todd; 1934.
3. Zuckerman J, Cuomo F, Rokito S. Definition and classification of frozen shoulder: a consensus approach. *J Shoulder Elbow Surg.* 1994;3(suppl):S72.
4. Neviaser RJ, Neviaser TJ. The frozen shoulder: diagnosis and management. *Clin Orthop Relat Res.* 1987;223:59–64.
5. Neviaser RJ. Painful conditions affecting the shoulder. *Clin Orthop Relat Res.* 1983;173:63–69.
6. Lundberg BJ. The frozen shoulder: clinical and radiographical observations. The effect of manipulation under general anesthesia: structure and glycosaminoglycan content of the joint capsule. Local bone metabolism. *Acta Orthop Scand Suppl.* 1969;119:1–59.
7. Zuckerman JD, Rokito A. Frozen shoulder: a concensus definition. *J Shoulder Elbow Surg.* 2011;20(2):322–325.
8. Bridgman JF. Periarthritis of the shoulder and diabetes mellitus. *Ann Rheum Dis.* 1972;31(1):69–71.
9. Hand C, Clipsham K, Rees JL, Carr AJ. Long-term outcome of frozen shoulder. *J Shoulder Elbow Surg.* 2008;17(2):231–236.
10. Wolf JM, Green A. Influence of comorbidity on self-assessment instrument scores of patients with idiopathic adhesive capsulitis. *J Bone Joint Surg Am.* 2002;84(7):1167–1173.
11. Binder AI, Bulgen DY, Hazleman BL, Tudor J, Wraight P. Frozen shoulder: an arthrographic and radionuclear scan assessment. *Ann Rheum Dis.* 1984;43(3):365–369.
12. Levine WN, Kashyap CP, Bak SF, Ahmad CS, Blaine TA, Bigliani LU. Nonoperative management of idiopathic adhesive capsulitis. *J Shoulder Elbow Surg.* 2007;16(5):569–573.
13. Reeves B. The natural history of the frozen shoulder syndrome. *Scan J Rheumatol.* 1975;4(4):193–196.
14. Shaffer B, Tibone JE, Kerlan RK. Frozen shoulder: a long-term follow-up. *J Bone Joint Surg Am.* 1992;74(5):738–746.
15. Hakim AJ, Cherkas LF, Spector TD, MacGregor AJ. Genetic associations between frozen shoulder and tennis elbow: a female twin study. *Rheumatology (Oxford).* 2003;42(6):739–742.
16. Bunker TD, Anthony PP. The pathology of frozen shoulder: a Dupuytren-like disease. *J Bone Joint Surg Br.* 1995;77(5):677–683.
17. Smith SP, Devaraj VS, Bunker TD. The association between frozen shoulder and Dupuytren's disease. *J Shoulder Elbow Surg.* 2001;10(2):149–151.
18. Matsen FA III, Lippitt SB, Sidles JA, Harryman DT II. *Practical Evaluation and Management of the Shoulder.* Philadelphia, PA: WB Saunders; 1994:1–111.
19. Harryman DT II, Sidles JA, Clark HM, McQuade KJ, Gibb TD, Matsen FA III. Translation of the humeral head on the glenoid with passive glenohumeral motion. *J Bone Joint Surg Am.* 1990;72(9):1334–1343.
20. Warner JJP, Caborn DNM, Berger R, Fu FH, Seel M. Dynamic capsuloligamentous anatomy of the glenohumeral joint. *J Shoulder Elbow Surg.* 1993;2(3):115–133.
21. Bunker TD, Reilly J, Baird KS, Hamblen DL. Expression of growth factors, cytokines and matrix metalloproteinases in frozen shoulder. *J Bone Joint Surg Br.* 2000;82(5):768–773.
22. Rodeo SA, Hannafin JA, Tom J, Warren RF, Wickiewicz TL. Immunolocalization of cytokines and their receptors in adhesive capsulitis of the shoulder. *J Orthop Res.* 1997;15(3):427–436.
23. Ryu JD, Kirpalani PA, Kim JM, Nam KH, Han CW, Han SH. Expression of vascular endothelial growth factor and angiogenesis in the diabetic frozen shoulder. *J Shoulder Elbow Surg.* 2006;15(6):679–685.
24. Neviaser JS. Adhesive capsulitis of the shoulder (the frozen shoulder). *Med Times.* 1962;90:783–807.
25. Wiley AM. Arthroscopic appearance of frozen shoulder. *Arthroscopy.* 1991;7(2):138–143.
26. Neer CS II, Satterlee CC, Dalsey RM, Flatow EL. The anatomy and potential effects of contracture of the coracohumeral ligament. *Clin Orthop Relat Res.* 1992;280:182–185.
27. Ozaki J, Nakagawa Y, Sakurai G, Tamai S. Recalcitrant chronic adhesive capsulitis of the shoulder: role of contracture of the coracohumeral ligament and rotator interval in pathogenesis and treatment. *J Bone Joint Surg Am.* 1989;71(10):1511–1515.
28. Kim KC, Rhee KJ, Shin HD. Adhesive capsulitis of the shoulder: dimensions of the rotator interval measured with magnetic resonance arthrography. *J Shoulder Elbow Surg.* 2009;18(3):437–442.
29. Hsu JE, Anakwenze OA, Warrender WJ, Abboud JA. Current review of adhesive capsulitis. *J Shoulder Elbow Surg.* 2011;20(3):502–514.
30. Neviaser AS, Hannafin JA. Adhesive capsulitis: a review of current treatment. *Am J Sports Med.* 2010;38(11):2346–2356.
31. Hannafin JA, Chiaia TA, Wickiewicz TL, et al. Adhesive capsulitis: capsular fibroplasia of the glenohumeral joint. *J Shoulder Elbow Surg.* 1994;39(5 suppl):435.
32. Lequesene M, Dang N, Bensasson M, Mery C. Increased association of diabetes mellitus and capsulitis of the shoulder and shoulder-hand syndrome. *Scand J Rheumatol.* 1977;6(1):53–56.
33. DePalma AF. Loss of scapulohumeral motion (frozen shoulder). *Ann Surg.* 1952;135(2):193–204.
34. Cuomo F. Diagnosis, classification, and management of the stiff shoulder. In: Ianotti JP, Williams GR, eds. *Disorders of the Shoulder: Diagnosis and Management.* Lippincott Williams & Wilkins; 1999:397–417.
35. Bulgen DY, Hazleman BL, Voak D. HLA-B27 and frozen shoulder. *Lancet.* 1976;1(7968):1042–1044.
36. Oesterreicher W, Van Dam G. Social and psychological researches into brachialgia and periarthritis. *Arthritis Rheum.* 1964;7:670–683.
37. Wright V, Haq AM. Periarthritis of the shoulder: I. Aetiological considerations with particular reference to personality factors. *Ann Rheum Dis.* 1976;35(3):213–219.
38. Coventry MB. Problem of painful shoulder. *J Am Med Assoc.* 1953;151(3):177–185.
39. Fleming A, Dodman S, Beer TC, Crown S. Personality in frozen shoulder. *Ann Rheum Dis.* 1975;35(5):456–457.
40. Lorenz TH, Musser MJ. Life, stress, emotions and painful stiff shoulder. *Ann Intern Med.* 1952;37(6):1232–1244.
41. Rizk TE, Pinals RD. Frozen shoulder. *Semin Arthritis Rheum.* 1982;11(4):440–452.

42. Binder AI, Bulgen DY, Hazleman BL, Roberts S. Frozen shoulder: a long-term prospective study. *Ann Rheum Dis*. 1984;43(3):361–364.
43. Binder A, Hazleman BL, Parr G, Robert S. A controlled study of oral prednisolone in frozen shoulder. *Br J Rheumatol*. 1986;25(3):288–292.
44. Neviaser JS. Adhesive capsulitis of the shoulder: a study of pathological findings in periarthritis of the shoulder. *J Bone Joint Surg*. 1945;27(2):211–222.
45. Harryman DT II, Sidles JA, Harris SL, Matsen FA III. The role of the rotator interval capsule in passive motion and stability of the shoulder. *J Bone Joint Surg Am*. 1992;74(1):53–66.
46. Busfield BT, Romero DM. Pain pump use after shoulder arthroscopy as a cause of glenohumeral chondrolysis. *Arthroscopy*. 2009;25(6):647–652.
47. Rapley JH, Beavis RC, Barber FA. Glenohumeral chondrolysis after shoulder arthroscopy associated with continuous bupivacaine infusion. *Arthroscopy*. 2009;25(12):1367–1373.
48. Bulgen DY, Hazleman B, Ward M, McCallum M. Immunological studies in frozen shoulder. *Ann Rheum Dis*. 1978;37(2):135–138.
49. Kessel L, Bayley I, Young A. The upper limb: the frozen shoulder. *Br J Hosp Med*. 1981;25(4):334–339.
50. Bunker TD, Esler CN. Frozen shoulder and lipids. *J Bone Joint Surg Br*. 1995;77(5):684–686.
51. Neviaser JS. Arthrography of the shoulder joint: study of the findings in adhesive capsulitis of the shoulder. *J Bone Joint Surg Am*. 1962;44(7):1321–1359.
52. Janda DH, Hawkins RJ. Shoulder manipulation in patients with adhesive capsulitis and diabetes mellitus: a clinical note. *J Shoulder Elbow Surg*. 1993;2(1):36–38.
53. Itoi E, Tabata S. Range of motion and arthrography in the frozen shoulder. *J Shoulder Elbow Surg*. 1992;1(2):106–112.
54. Loyd JA, Loyd HM. Adhesive capsulitis of the shoulder: arthrographic diagnosis and treatment. *South Med J*. 1983;76(7):879–883.
55. Andren L, Lundberg BJ. Treatment of rigid shoulders by joint distension during arthrography. *Acta Orthop Scand*. 1965;36:45–53.
56. Connell D, Padmanabhan R, Buchbinder R. Adhesive capsulitis: role of MR imaging in differential diagnosis. *Eur Radiol*. 2002;12(8):2100–2106.
57. Mengiardi B, Pfirrmann CW, Gerber C, Hodler J, Zanetti M. Frozen shoulder: MR arthrographic findings. *Radiology*. 2004;233(2):486–492.
58. Sofka CM, Ciavarra GA, Hannafin JA, Cordasco FA, Potter HG. Magnetic resonance imaging of adhesive capsulitis: correlation with clinical staging. *HSS J*. 2008;4(2):164–169.
59. Carillon Y, Noel E, Fantino O, Perrin-Fayolle O, Tran-Minh VA. Magnetic resonance imaging findings in idiopathic adhesive capsulitis of the shoulder. *Rev Rhum Engl Ed*. 1999;66(4):201–206.
60. Tamai K, Yamato M. Abnormal synovium in the frozen shoulder: a preliminary report with dynamic magnetic resonance imaging. *J Shoulder Elbow Surg*. 1997;6(6):534–543.
61. Lee M, Haq AM, Wright V, Longton EB. Periarthritis of the shoulder: a controlled trial of physiotherapy. *Physiotherapy*. 1973;59(10):312–315.
62. Roy S, Oldham R. Management of painful shoulder. *Lancet*. 1976:19(1):1322–1324.
63. Shah N, Lewis M. Shoulder adhesive capsulitis: systematic review of randomized trials using multiple corticosteroid injections. *Br J Gen Pract*. 2007;57(541):662–667.
64. Bulgen DY, Binder AI, Hazleman BL, Dutton J, Roberts S. Frozen shoulder: prospective clinical study with an evaluation of three treatment regimens. *Ann Rheum Dis*. 1984;43(3):353–360.
65. Bal A, Eksioglu E, Gulec B, Aydog E, Gurcay E, Cakci A. Effectiveness of corticosteroid injection in adhesive capsulitis. *Clin Rehabil*. 2008;22(6):503–512.
66. Hazleman BL. The painful stiff shoulder. *Rheumatol Phys Med*. 1972;11(8):413–421.
67. Carette S, Moffet H, Tardif J, et al. Intraarticular corticosteroids, supervised physiotherapy, or a combination of the two in the treatment of adhesive capsulitis of the shoulder: a placebo-controlled trial. *Arthritis Rheum*. 2003;48(3):829–838.
68. Marx RG, Malizia RW, Kenter K, Wickiewicz TL, Hannafin JA. Intra-articular corticosteroid injection for the treatment of idiopathic adhesive capsulitis of the shoulder. *HSS J*. 2007;3(2):202–207.
69. van der Windt DA, Koes MW, Devillé W, Boeke AJ, de Jong BA, Bouter LM. Effectiveness of corticosteroid injections versus physiotherapy for treatment of painful stiff shoulder in primary care: randomised trial. *BMJ*. 1998;317(7168):1292–1296.
70. Quin CE. "Frozen shoulder": evaluation of treatment with hydrocortisone injections and exercises. *Ann Phys Med*. 1965;8:22–25.
71. Griesser MJ, Harris JD, Campbell JE, Jones GL. Adhesive capsulitis of the shoulder: a systematic review of the effectiveness of intra-articular corticosteroid injections. *J Bone Joint Surg Am*. 2011;93(18):1727–1733.
72. Harryman DT II. Shoulders: frozen and stiff. *Instr Course Lect*. 1993;42:247–257.
73. Murnhaghan JP. Frozen shoulder. In: Rockwood CA Jr, Matsen FA III, eds. *The Shoulder*. Philadelphia, PA: WB Saunders; 1990:837–862.
74. Hawkins RJ, Angelo RL. Glenohumeral osteoarthritis: a late complication of the Putti-Platt repair. *J Bone Joint Surg Am*. 1990;72(8):1193–1197.
75. Kieras DM, Matsen FA III. Open release in the management of refractory frozen shoulder. *Orthop Trans*. 1991;15:801.
76. Lusardi DA, Wirth MA,Wurtz D, Rockwood CA Jr. Loss of external rotation following anterior casulorrhaphy of the shoulder. *J Bone Joint Surg Am*. 1993;75(8):1185–1192.
77. Macdonald PB, Hawkins RJ, Fowler PJ, Miniaci A. Release of the subscapularis for internal rotation contracture and pain after anterior repair for recurrent anterior dislocation of the shoulder. *J Bone Joint Surg Am*. 1992;74(5):734–737.
78. Warner JJ. Frozen shoulder: diagnosis and management. *J Am Acad Orthop Surg*. 1997;5(3):130–140.
79. Green S, Buchbinder R, Hetrick S. Physiotherapy interventions for shoulder pain. *Cochrane Database Syst Rev*. 2003;(2):CD004258.
80. Miller MD, Wirth MA, Rockwood CA Jr. Thawing the frozen shoulder: the "patient" patient. *Orthopedics*. 1996;19(10):849–853.
81. Griggs SM, Ahn A, Green A. Idiopathic adhesive capsulitis: a prospective functional outcome study of nonoperative treatment. *J Bone Joint Surg Am*. 2000;82(10):1398–1407.

82. Dangoisse MJ, Wilson DJ, Glynn CJ. MRI and clinical study of an easy and safe technique of suprascapular nerve blockade. *Acta Anaesthesiol Belg*. 1994;45(2):49–54.
83. Dahan TH, Fortin L, Pelletier M, Petit M, Vadeboncoeur R, Suissa S. Double blind randomized clinical trial examining the efficacy of bupivacaine suprascapular nerve blocks in frozen shoulder. *J Rheumatol*. 2000;27(6);1464–1469.
84. Helbig B, Wagner P, Döhler R. Mobilization of frozen shoulder under general anesthesia. *Acta Orthop Belg*. 1983;49(1–2):267–274.
85. Hill JJ Jr, Bogumill H. Manipulation in the treatment of frozen shoulder. *Orthopedics*. 1988;11(9):1255–1260.
86. Parker RD, Froimson AI, Winsberg DD, Arsham NZ. Frozen shoulder. part II. Treatment by manipulation under anesthesia. *Orthopedics*. 1989;12(7):989–990.
87. Brown AR, Weiss R, Greenberg C, Flatow EL, Bigliani LU. Interscalene block for shoulder arthroscopy: comparison with general anesthesia. *Arthroscopy*. 1993;9(3):295–300.
88. Pollock RG, Duralde XA, Flatow EL, Bigliani LU. The use of arthroscopy in the treatment of resistant frozen shoulder. *Clin Orthop Relat Res*. 1994;304:30–36.
89. Magnussen RA, Taylor DC. Glenoid fracture during manipulation under anesthesia for adhesive capsulitis: a case report. *J Shoulder Elbow Surg*. 2011;20(3):e23–e26.
90. Ferrell CM, Sperling JW, Cofield RH. Manipulation for frozen shoulder: long-term results. *J Shoulder Elbow Surg*. 2005;14(5):480–484.
91. Loew M, Heichel TO, Lehner B. Intraarticular lesions in primary frozen shoulder after manipulation under general anesthesia. *J Shoulder Elbow Surg*. 2005;14(1):16–21.
92. Dodenhoff RM, Levy O, Wilson A, Copeland SA. Manipulation under anesthesia for primary frozen shoulder: effect on early recovery and return to activity. *J Shoulder Elbow Surg*. 2000;9(1):23–26.
93. Kivimäki J, Pohjolainen T, Malmivaara A, et al. Manipulation under anesthesia with home exercises versus home exercises alone in the treatment of frozen shoulder: a randomized, controlled trial with 125 patients. *J Shoulder Elbow Surg*. 2007;16(6):722–726.
94. Haggart GE, Dignam RJ, Sullivan TS. Management of the frozen shoulder. *J Am Med Assoc*. 1956;161(13):1219–1222.
95. Harmon PH. Methods and results in the treatment of 2,580 painful shoulders, with special reference to calcific tendinitis and the frozen shoulder. *Am J Surg*. 1958;95(4):527–544.
96. Conti V. Arthroscopy in rehabilitation. *Orthop Clin North Am*. 1979;10(3):709–711.
97. Rill BK, Fleckenstein CM, Levy MS, Nagesh V, Hasan SS. Predictors of outcome after nonoperative and operative treatment of adhesive capsulitis. *Am J Sports Med*. 2011;39(3):567–574.
98. Uitvlugt G, Detrisac DA, Johnson LL, Austin MD, Johnson C. Arthroscopic observations before and after manipulation of frozen shoulder. *Arthroscopy*. 1993;9(2):181–185.
99. Zanotti RM, Kuhn JE. Arthroscopic capsular release for the stiff shoulder: description of technique and anatomic considerations. *Am J Sports Med*. 1997;25(3):294–298.
100. Beaufils P, Prévot N, Boyer T, et al. Arthroscopic release of the glenohumeral joint in shoulder stiffness: a review of 26 cases. French Society for Arthroscopy. *Arthroscopy*. 1999;15(1):49–55.
101. Elhassan B, Ozbaydar M, Massimini D, Higgins L, Warner JJ. Arthroscopic capsular release for refractory shoulder stiffness: a critical analysis of effectiveness in specific etiologies. *J Shoulder Elbow Surg*. 2010;19(4):580–587.
102. Holloway GB, Schenk T, Williams GR, Ramsey ML, Iannotti JP. Arthroscopic capsular release for the treatment of refractory postoperative or post-fracture shoulder stiffness. *J Bone Joint Surg Am*. 2001;83(11):1682–1687.
103. Omari A, Bunker TD. Open surgical release for frozen shoulder: surgical findings and results of the release. *J Shoulder Elbow Surg*. 2001;10(4):353–357.

I-7

Acromioclavicular Joint and Clavicle Injuries

Joshua D. Harris, MD; Michael J. Griesser, MD; and Grant L. Jones, MD

Injuries to the acromioclavicular (AC) joint and clavicle represent a great proportion of shoulder girdle trauma prompting treatment in sports medicine clinics. Clavicle fractures represent 2.6% to 4% of fractures in adults[1–3] and 35% to 44% of fractures to the shoulder girdle.[2,4] Acromioclavicular joint separations account for 9% to 41% of shoulder girdle injuries.[3,5] Changing trends in management of these injuries have made the operative versus nonoperative decision controversial. Regardless of the treatment ultimately chosen, these injuries often result in the athlete not being able to participate in sport. Furthermore, as the athlete returns to sport participation, the rehabilitation program is vital to the success of the treatment and has the ultimate goal of returning the athlete to a pain-free, preinjury level of competition.

ACROMIOCLAVICULAR JOINT

Anatomy

The AC joint is a diarthrodial synovial joint that links the axial and appendicular skeleton via the clavicle medially and the acromion laterally (Figure 1A). Its articular surfaces can be almost vertical (sagittal-plane reference) or inclined laterally up to 50° (superior margin of the distal clavicle lies over the top of the inferior margin of the acromion) (Figure 1B).[6] An age-dependent intra-articular meniscus homologue is present in youth and early adulthood but tends to disappear by the fourth decade.[7] Although its intra-articular anatomy varies, the periarticular ligamentous structures are relatively constant. The AC joint ligaments (superior, inferior, anterior, posterior) reinforce the AC joint capsule and are the primary stabilizers to excess axial-plane (horizontal anterior-to-posterior translation) motion.[8] The superior and

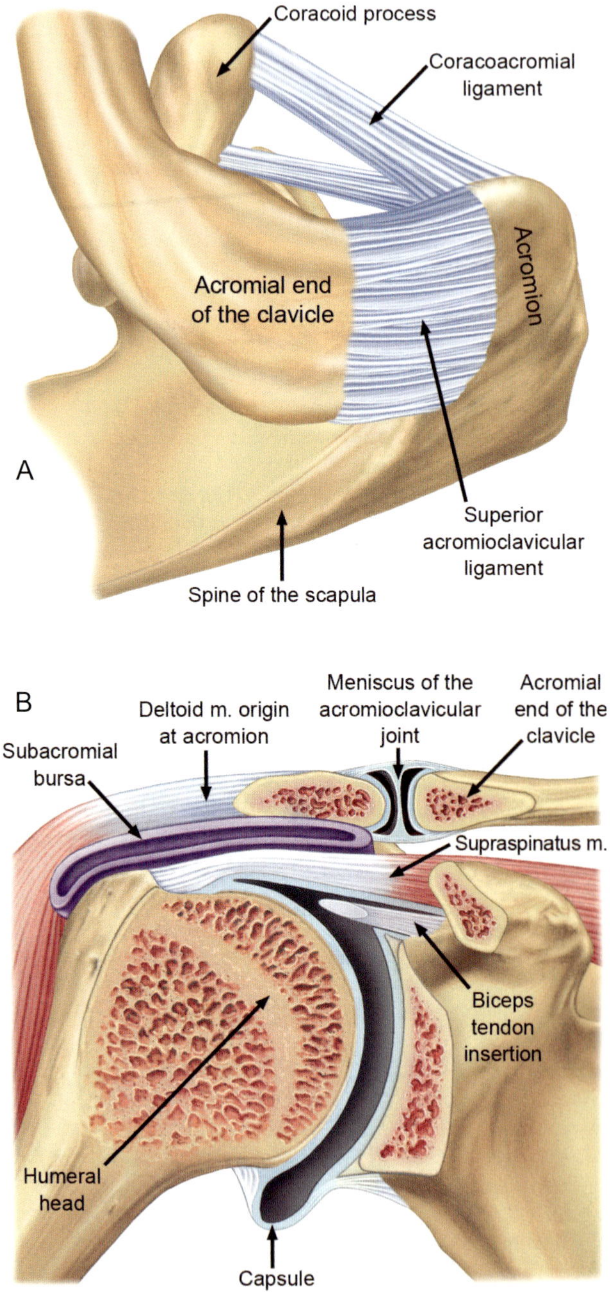

Figure 1. Acromioclavicular joint. A, Superior view. B, Coronal section. C, Anteroposterior view.

C

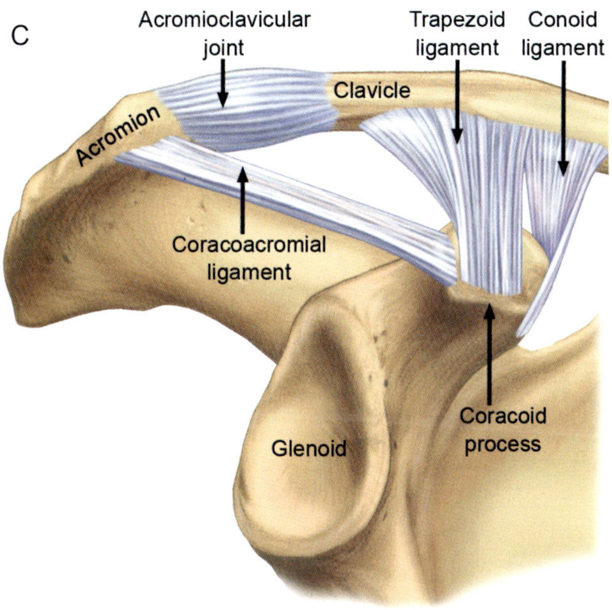

posterior AC ligaments are the principal restraints to posterior horizontal translation.[9] The coracoclavicular (CC) ligaments (conoid and trapezoid) are the primary stabilizers to excess coronal-plane (inferior-to-superior vertical translation) motion.[8] The CC ligaments, 62% of which are provided by the conoid, are the primary restraints to inferior translation of the scapulobrachial complex (ie, the weight of the upper extremity).[8] The most lateral edge of the superior AC ligament inserts anywhere from 1 to 3.5 mm medial to the edge of the joint on the distal clavicle.[10,11] The distances from the articular surface of the distal clavicle to the most lateral aspect of the trapezoid and conoid ligaments are 16.7 mm in men and 16.1 mm in women and 33.5 mm in men and 28.9 mm in women, respectively.[10] The normal CC interspace is 11 to 13 mm (Figure 1C)[12,13]; this is measured on an anteroposterior (AP) radiograph and is the distance between the superior margin of the coracoid and the inferior margin of the clavicle.

Given its morphology, the AC joint allows for translation and rotation of the clavicle relative to the acromion. This coordinated scapuloclavicular motion is coupled with elevation of the upper extremity and abduction of the shoulder via the CC ligaments. Any disruption in the AC joint or CC ligaments can alter these biomechanics and affect motion. Using fixed Kirschner wires in the acromion and distal clavicle, forward elevation of the upper extremity in the scapular plane to 180° results in 5° to 8° of clavicle rotation.[14] Because other authors have concluded that approximately 40° of clavicular rotation occurs with full elevation of the extremity,[15] the remaining 30° to 35° of clavicular rotation must occur at the sternoclavicular (SC) joint. Clinically, this can be observed after CC screw placement when compared with SC fusion; less loss of motion occurs after CC screw placement than SC fusion.[14] After CC screw placement, elevation of the upper extremity is limited to approximately 160°. After ankylosis of the SC joint, upper extremity elevation is limited to approximately 90°. Using open magnetic resonance imaging, the distal clavicle translates posteriorly 1.9 mm at 90° of abduction and anteriorly 1.6 mm at full abduction, and it concurrently translates superiorly 0.9 mm.[16] Clinically, the complex normal motion at the AC joint and the deforming forces imparted by the surrounding musculature (pectoralis major, latissimus dorsi, trapezius) must be understood and appreciated to comprehend mechanisms of injury and recommended treatments.

Injury Classification

Direct injury to the AC joint can occur with a fall onto the point of the adducted shoulder, forcing the acromion inferiorly relative to the distal clavicle. Progressive ligamentous (AC and CC) injury with greater energy accounts for the Allman[17] and Rockwood modification[18] classifications of AC joint injuries (Table). Indirect injury to the AC joint also can occur with a fall onto an outstretched hand and adducted shoulder, transmitting the energy of the fall from the hand upward through the humeral head and across to the acromion.

History and Physical Examination

A suggestive mechanism of direct or indirect injury and pain in the shoulder warrants consideration of AC joint injury. On physical examination, inspection might reveal a relative elevation of the subcutaneous distal clavicle. This prominence is due to the weight of the extremity pulling down the acromion. The area over the anterosuperior aspect of the AC joint, the anterolateral neck, and anterolateral deltoid might be tender.[19] With cross-body adduction, the AC joint is compressed and might evoke pain with AC joint injury. Furthermore, pain might be relieved with a local anesthetic

Table. Rockwood Modification of the Allman Classification of Acromioclavicular Joint Injury[a]

Type	AC Joint Status	CC Ligament Status	CC Interspace Distance	Deltotrapezial Fascia
I	Sprain	Intact	Normal	Intact
II	Complete injury	Sprain	Slightly more than normal	Intact
III	Complete injury	Complete injury	Increased <100%	Intact
IV	Complete injury	Complete injury	Variable injury	Torn
V	Complete injury	Complete injury	100–300% increase	Torn
VI	Complete injury	Intact/sprain	Less than normal	Variable injury

[a] Common to all injuries is partial or complete disruption of the acromioclavicular (AC) joint. Complete disruption of the AC joint distinguishes Type I from II. Complete disruption of the coracoclavicular (CC) ligaments (allowing for clear radiographic AC separation) distinguishes Type II from III. Greater degrees (>100% increased separation) of distal clavicle elevation (or acromial depression) with disruption of the deltotrapezial fascia and subsequent closed irreducibility of the AC joint distinguishes Type III from V. Posterior displacement of the distal clavicle through the deltotrapezial fascia identifies a Type IV injury. Type VI injuries are rare hyperabduction injuries in which the distal clavicle comes to lie under the coracoid, with inherent neurovascular injury risk.

injection into the AC joint. A high-riding, reducible distal clavicle is more suggestive of a Type III than Type V injury, which typically is irreducible because of buttonholing of the distal clavicle through the deltotrapezial fascia. The SC joint mandates assessment to identify concurrent anterior or posterior dislocation.

Imaging

Radiographic examination of traumatic shoulder pain includes a standard shoulder series consisting of true AP, scapular-Y, and axillary views (Figure 2). Further evaluation should include dedicated views of the clavicle and SC joint, given the linked strut function of the clavicle. Depending on the degree of injury, radiographic appearances are variable (Table, Figure 3). Relative elevation of the distal clavicle to the acromion can be assessed on the AP view via the CC interspace (or distance), which is normally 11 to 13 mm.[12,13] The axillary view is especially useful for evaluation of Type IV injuries, demonstrating posterior displacement of the distal clavicle with disruption of the deltotrapezial fascia. The Zanca view is a special AP image for assessing the AC joint with 10° to 20° of cephalic tilt and one-fourth to one-half the beam voltage. Normal AC joint width is 1 to 3 mm.[20] Concurrent imaging of the contralateral shoulder or weighted stress views also

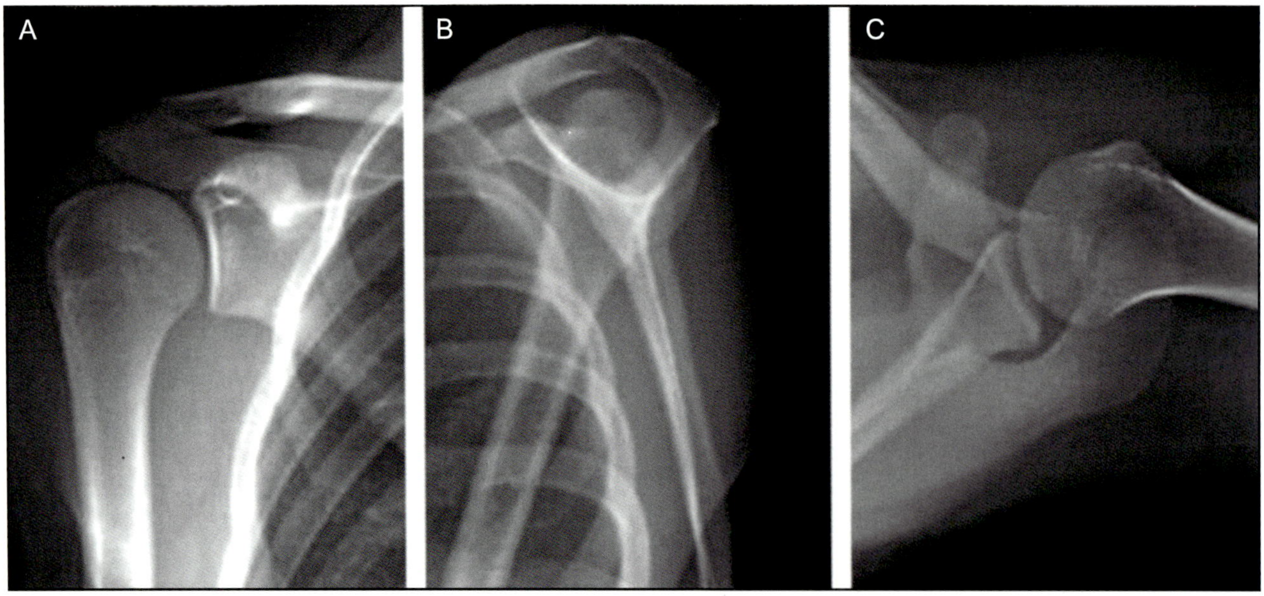

Figure 2. Standard shoulder radiograph series includes true anteroposterior, A, scapular-Y, B, and axillary, C, views.

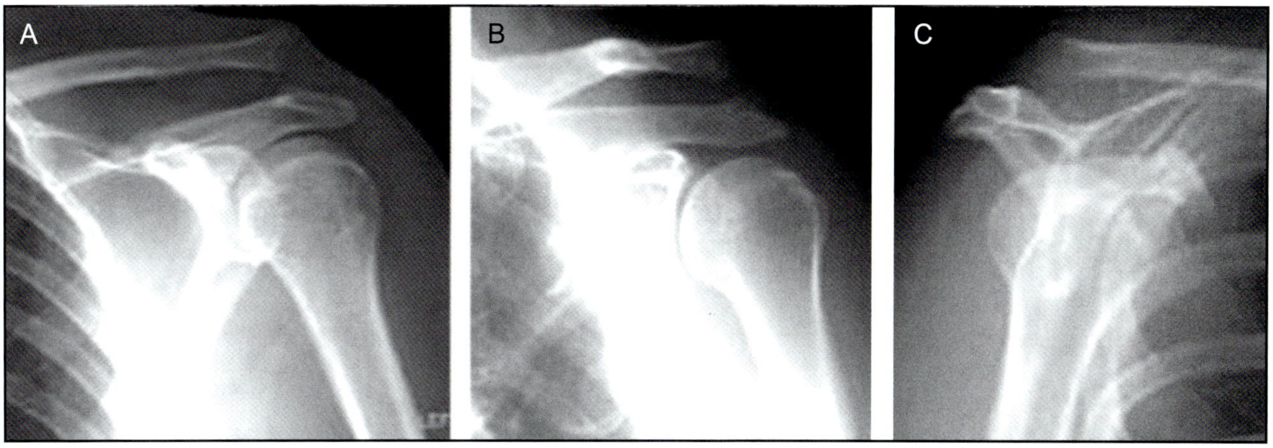

Figure 3. Type III acromioclavicular joint separation shown in anteroposterior (AP), A, true AP, B, and scapular-Y, C, views.

can be used. Computed tomography (CT) seldom is used for AC joint or clavicle injury. However, for patients with traumatic SC joint injury, the CT is mandatory to evaluate the tracheoesophageal and neurovascular structures that potentially are injured.

Nonoperative Management

General consensus exists that Types I and II AC joint injuries should be managed nonoperatively. Although controversial, most Type III injuries also can be treated nonoperatively (Figure 3).

Treatment Options. Nonoperative treatment of Types I and II and most Type III AC joint injuries involves a period of rest, immobilization with various slings or shoulder harnesses, cryotherapy, and rehabilitation. A sling supports the weight of the extremity. In Type I injuries, a sling can be used until pain subsides generally in 1 week to 10 days. Type II injuries might require use of a sling for 2 to 3 weeks. For both Type I and II injuries, the patient must avoid activities that could convert a Type I or II to at least a Type III injury or worse: a nonoperative to an operative problem. This usually takes an athlete out of sport for a variable period.

Rehabilitation. The literature is replete with low levels of evidence (IV and V) regarding the nonoperative rehabilitation programs available for the treatment of AC joint separations. No high-level evidence exists regarding the optimal program or duration of treatment time. Nevertheless, most authors agree that each case should be addressed individually without a set protocol applicable to all patients. Factors, such as age, sex, hand dominance, sport, position in sport, season timing, scholarship, bonus, and contract, contribute.

Several rehabilitative programs have been described in the literature. Common to these programs is the objective of returning to sport participation at the preinjury level of play with full range of motion and strength without pain. Acutely, this requires reduction and elimination of pain. Next, the patient begins protected motion to prevent stiffness and isometric strengthening exercises to prevent atrophy. Then, gradual strengthening with isotonic exercises can be initiated. After these have been accomplished successfully without pain, dynamic sport-specific drills can be started. Given the complex interplay of periscapular and shoulder girdle muscles and their relative contributions to glenohumeral and scapulothoracic motion, both groups must be addressed concurrently. This includes assessment for and treatment of scapular dyskinesis and of the combination of scapular malposition, inferomedial scapular winging, coracoid tenderness, and scapular dyskinesis (or the SICK scapula).

A commonly used protocol for the management of Type I and II AC separations at our institution is the 4-phase program that Gladstone et al[21] described. Phase 1 includes reduction in pain with sling immobilization, cryotherapy, limited use of nonsteroidal anti-inflammatory drugs, and immediate protected passive motion and isometric exercises. Phase 2 introduces isotonic and proprioceptive neuromuscular facilitative strengthening exercises. Phase 3 generically involves increases in strength, endurance, and control without restrictions. Phase 4 introduces sport-specific drills.

Progression of phases is stepwise, and the patient returning to competition must have documented full strength and motion without pain. Most patients with Types I and II injuries recover fully within 2 to 3 weeks.

The treatment of most Type III AC separations is similar to that described for Type I and II injuries, with the understanding that a greater degree of soft tissue disruption has occurred and an extended duration of recovery can be anticipated. Thus, sling use might be needed for up to 3 or 4 weeks. Attempts at reduction and maintenance of reduction are not only painful, but usually unsuccessful. The sling reduces the weight of the extremity and reduces the tension and subsequent insult to the AC and CC ligaments and soft tissues. Given the complete loss of static stability to the AC joint complex, rehabilitation of the dynamic stabilizers is of paramount importance. For the overhead athlete (pitchers, quarterbacks, racquet sports, swimmers, etc), this is of even greater importance. Most patients with Type III injuries recover fully within 4 to 6 weeks; however, a slower return to sport participation at up to 3 months is not uncommon.

Expected Outcomes. The long-term outcomes after nonoperative management of Type I and II AC joint separations are generally favorable and include a successful return to sport participation. In a group of 33 young athletes, more than 50% of patients remained asymptomatic at 6.3 years postinjury with a mean Constant score of 82 of 100.[22] However, in another group of athletes who were United States Naval Midshipmen (133 Midshipmen, 137 AC joint injuries), 72% (30% with Type I and 42% with Type II) of patients had mechanical clicking and pain with push-ups and dips.[23] Furthermore, pain and limitations in activities of daily living continued in 32% of patients (9% with Type I and 23% with Type II).

The most common reason a patient experiences remote pain and mechanical symptoms after the injury is posttraumatic degenerative joint disease of the AC joint. The presence of a bump on the superior aspect of the shoulder does not equate necessarily to pain or limitation of function (Figure 4). In addition, the presence of radiographic evidence of degenerative change or distal clavicle osteolysis does not equate to pain or limitation of function. Cox[24] reported that pain was present in 36% of Type I and 48% of Type II AC separations, whereas radiographic degenerative change was present in 70% and 77%, respectively. If pain or mechanical symptoms are limiting and the patient has not improved with conservative measures, distal clavicle excision might be indicated with an expectation of good to excellent results. After a distal clavicle resection in athletes at 3.7-year follow-up, Cook and Tibone[25] reported full return to preinjury level of sport participation without deficits in strength or motion.

The general consensus indicates initial nonoperative management of Type III AC joint separations, even in the throwing athlete. In the largest meta-analysis of patients with Type III injuries (1172 patients), Phillips et al[26] showed no difference in satisfactory outcomes between operative (88% satisfaction) and nonoperative (87% satisfaction) management. In this study, each treated upper extremity had its own inherent limitations, with increased risk of infection and reoperation

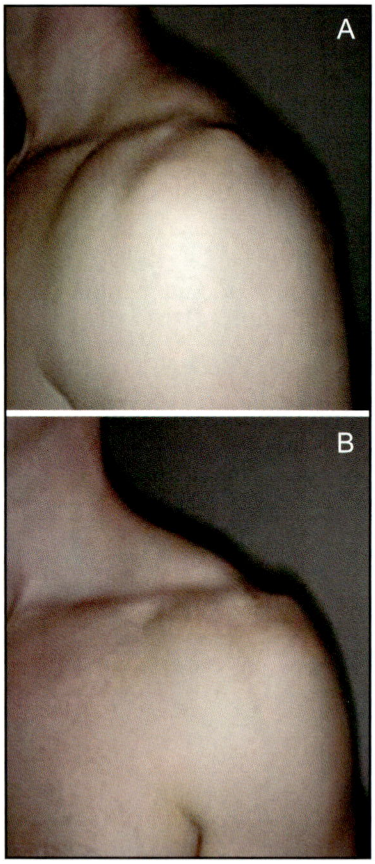

Figure 4 A and B. Patient with nonoperatively managed Type III acromioclavicular (AC) joint separation. Injury was 11 years ago. Note the presence of a bump over the AC joint. The patient had no pain at rest or with activity. Examination revealed no pain with cross-body adduction.

in those treated operatively and increased risk of deformity in those treated nonoperatively. Despite the latter and although authors of some prospective studies have demonstrated a faster return to sport participation and employment with restored motion with nonoperative treatment,[27] some surgeons have intervened operatively in the overhead athlete patient group.[28,29] The overhead throwing motion might lead to pain and mechanical symptoms in this cohort, especially baseball pitchers. This is reflected in 2 recent surveys of Major League Baseball team physicians, in which most noted they would recommend initial operative treatment for pitchers with Type III injuries.[28,29] Nevertheless, initial management of all athletes, including overhead athletes, should be nonoperative. Persistent pain and loss of function that have not improved after 3 to 6 months of nonoperative treatment indicate the need for operative intervention. However, some evidence exists that delayed reconstruction might not be as successful as early reconstruction.[22] For the management of Type III AC joint injuries, high-quality, randomized controlled trials clearly are necessary to determine if a difference exists between both early and late reconstruction and nonoperative treatment in this controversial patient group.

Operative Management

General consensus exists that Type IV, V, and VI AC joint injuries should be managed operatively. Select cases of Type III separations that have not improved with conservative measures over 3 to 6 months might be indicated for operative reconstruction.

Indications. The indications for operative intervention to treat AC joint separations include Type IV, V, VI, and select Type III injuries. The degree of soft tissue disruption with these injuries, especially the deltotrapezial fascia, typically precludes closed reduction, leaving a joint dislocated with tissue interposition. Potential acute skin compromise that is secondary to a high-riding distal clavicle might mandate operative reduction. Open injuries and those associated with neurovascular compromise also are indications for operative treatment.

Operative Techniques. More than 60 different techniques have been described in the literature to operatively treat AC joint injuries.[30] Considerable debate exists over which technique is superior, thus no criterion standard operative procedure is available at this time. Generally, 5 different categories exist: AC joint fixation, CC ligament reconstruction, CC fixation, dynamic conjoint tendon transfer, and distal clavicle excision (Mumford procedure[31]).

Acromioclavicular joint fixation is a technique that is used infrequently today. It involved metallic Kirschner wire pin fixation across the joint to allow the soft tissues to heal before hardware removal. Several complications, including pin breakage, pin migration to vital structures, infection (septic arthritis, abscess, pin-tract infection), and intentional articular cartilage damage via pin placement, preclude its use in treatment of AC joint injuries. A newer technique involves hook-plate fixation on the superior aspect of the distal clavicle and the undersurface of the acromion. This can be used to treat AC joint instability and also distal clavicle fracture. The technique requires eventual hardware removal.

Coracoclavicular fixation is a technique that is used less commonly given its technical difficulties, potential complications, and need for eventual hardware removal. Bosworth[32] initially described this technique in 1941. Although good outcomes have been reported,[33,34] the CC screw construct has high rigidity (stiffer than that of the native CC ligament complex), which can predispose the patient to early postoperative complications.[35] These complications include intraoperative iatrogenic and postoperative fracture, screw loosening, breakage, and migration.[36,37]

Dynamic muscle transfer via coracoid or conjoint tendon transfer to the undersurface of the clavicle was used in attempts to stabilize the AC joint. However, this technique did not provide any static stability to the joint and resulted in unsatisfactory long-term outcomes.[38] This technique no longer is used in clinical practice.

Isolated distal clavicle excision is a well-recognized treatment in a symptomatic degenerative AC joint. In the stable AC joint with degenerative changes, this procedure has high rates of satisfaction.[39,40] The technique has evolved from an open procedure to the option of all-arthroscopic resection. However, in the treatment of acute or chronic AC joint dislocations, this technique is not recommended as an isolated treatment because it does not address stability. Several authors have reported substantially worse outcomes after resection in the presence of instability.[41,42] Therefore, it should be combined with CC ligament reconstruction techniques in chronic AC instability with AC joint degeneration.

Coracoclavicular ligament reconstruction is a technique that attempts to recreate the conoid and trapezoid ligaments anatomically and biomechanically. The original Weaver-Dunn technique involved a transfer of the coracoacromial ligament's acromial end to the distal clavicle.[43] This technique leads to a new "CC ligament" that is only 20% of the strength of the native CC ligament.[44,45] The weaker construct with isolated coracoacromial transfer and subsequent residual subluxation and the increased risk of degenerative change at the AC joint led to the introduction of a modified Weaver-Dunn procedure that includes a distal clavicle excision and either a biologic or synthetic augmentation, increasing the strength of the construct to approach that of the native CC ligaments.

No biologic or synthetic graft consistently has shown superiority biomechanically or clinically. Biologic grafts include both autograft (semitendinosus, gracilis, toe extensor) and allograft. Synthetic grafts include wires, absorbable and nonabsorbable suture, and suture-tape constructs. The addition of a CC screw also has been used as an augment. In many situations, biologic and synthetic grafts are used together. The synthetic graft maintains reduction of the AC joint while the biologic graft incorporates and avoids creep of the tendon graft and its associated lengthening and joint instability. Several fixation techniques have been described, including high-strength, nonabsorbable suture interference screws (metallic and bioabsorbable) (Figure 5); suture anchors (metallic and bioabsorbable); bone tunnels with graft tied upon itself; and loops around the coracoid or clavicle, or both. Various complications, such as suture cut-out or pull-through, bone-tunnel widening, distal clavicle osteolysis, intraoperative or postoperative fracture, and loss of reduction have led some authors to favor certain augments over others. Nevertheless, all augment techniques increase the strength beyond that of an isolated coracoacromial transfer, and each has advantages and disadvantages. A complete review of the multitude of AC joint reconstruction and CC ligament reconstruction techniques is beyond the scope of this chapter, and we cite previous work for further information.[5,6,30]

Postoperative Rehabilitation. At our institution, the postoperative rehabilitation after anatomic CC ligament reconstruction, in which the surgeon used looped allograft around the undersurface of the coracoid and bioabsorbable interference screw fixation in the distal clavicle, requires an early period of protection for tendon graft-to-bone healing. The time for this to occur is approximately 12 weeks.[46,47] Immediately after surgery, active motion is begun at the elbow, wrist, hand, and fingers to prevent stiffness and atrophy and to

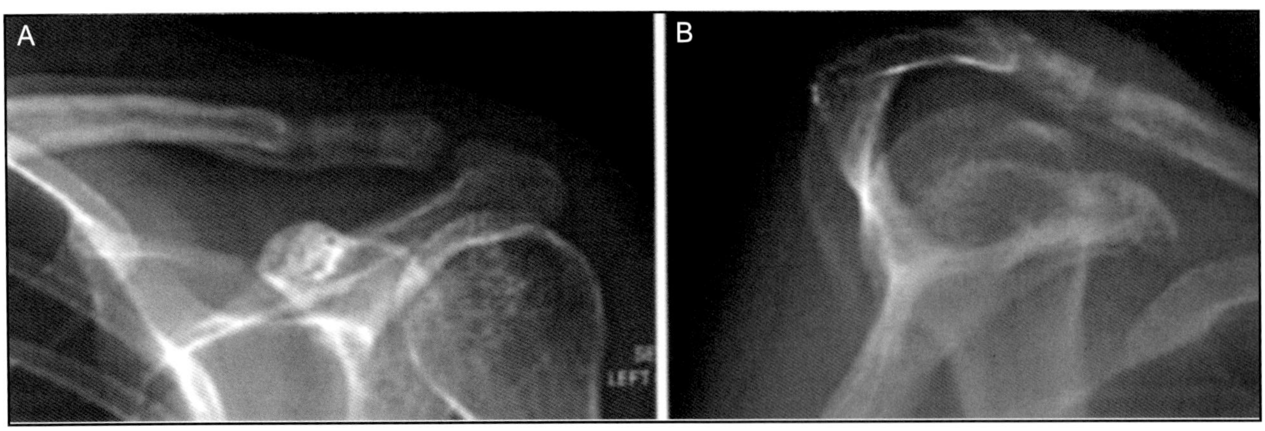

Figure 5 A and B. Postoperative radiographs taken 4 months after acromioclavicular (AC) joint reconstruction and distal clavicle excision (8-mm medial to AC joint), demonstrating maintenance of reduction and no tunnel widening or fracture. Tibialis anterior allograft was looped around the undersurface of the coracoid and was fixed into separate drill holes (6.5 mm) in the distal clavicle at anatomic insertions of the conoid and trapezoid ligaments with bioabsorbable interference screws. A 1-cm bone bridge was maintained.

promote edema control. A shoulder abduction sling or brace is used for a minimum of 6 weeks. This importantly decreases the weight of the extremity, reducing stress on the reconstruction. This sling remains on at all times except for passive therapy sessions (pendulums at 2 weeks) and bathing. If the upper extremity is removed from the sling and gravity is allowed to act on the weight of the extremity, the CC ligament graft or its fixation is stressed substantially and potentially might lead to failure.

After sling use is discontinued, active-assistive range-of-motion exercises are begun, and passive-motion exercises are continued. Shoulder stiffness is nearly universal after removal of the sling. Patients are cautioned against participating in activities that are too vigorous, including return-to-sport at this time in the rehabilitation. This also includes caution against activities that would stress the reconstruction or the AC joint itself, including carrying weights in the hand at the side or cross-body adduction motions. The safe motions include those of forward elevation, abduction, and rotation. These can be accomplished via table slides, wall slides, finger wall walks, door frame stretches, towel stretches, and supine pulleys. Active strengthening (isometric and isotonic) is not begun until the tendon graft is assumed to be healed in the bone tunnel, which occurs around 12 weeks after surgery. Continuing strengthening of the periscapular stabilizer muscles concurrently is extremely important at this point for optimal dynamic control of the shoulder girdle. Sport-specific drills generally are resumed at 4 or 5 months, and return to competitive sport participation is allowed at around 6 months. If the patient expects to participate in contact sports, waiting 9 to 12 months after surgery to return to participation might be prudent.

Expected Outcomes. The clinical outcomes after operative management of AC joint injury recently has been of great interest. Although most Type IV, V, and VI AC joint separations are treated operatively, controversy still surrounds the operative treatment of Type III AC joint injuries. Based on a meta-analysis[26] and systematic review,[48] the evidence is inconclusive on superiority of operative to nonoperative treatment of Type III separations. Nevertheless, satisfactory outcomes can be seen in high percentages of patients despite a risk of failure, which entails possible recurrent instability, infection, and longer recovery.[48]

The modified Weaver-Dunn technique is a commonly used, nonanatomic procedure with approximately 75% satisfactory outcomes.[43] However, the biomechanically weak construct leads to recurrent instability in 30% to 50% of patients.[43–45,49] Newer augmented techniques might have improved outcomes. Operatively treated patients are pain-free earlier with greater endurance and higher subjective pain, motion, functional, and cosmetic ratings, whereas nonoperatively treated patients can return to sport participation and employment earlier with less time immobilized.[50]

Patients whose jobs involve heavy manual labor and young overhead athletes might be the only patient groups to benefit from the operative treatment of Type III injuries. In the high-level throwing athlete (Major League Baseball pitchers), operative reconstruction has led to 91% of pitchers being pain-free and returning to sport participation.[29] After operative treatment, joint congruity with or without the presence of degenerative changes or development of heterotopic ossification has not been shown to be correlated with the clinical outcome.[14]

Type V AC joint injuries treated with CC reconstruction with synthetic grafts in both athletes and nonathletes have led to high percentages of patients with good to excellent outcomes, despite many patients having loss of reduction after surgery.[51,52] As in Type III operative treatment, no correlation has been noted between overall long-term clinical outcomes and the degree of residual dislocation, CC heterotopic bone, AC joint degenerative arthritis, and distal clavicle osteolysis. At 6-year follow-up, Verhaven et al[52] found that 67% of 18 athletes reported good or excellent clinical outcomes (33% fair or poor), and 44% had a loss of reduction despite initial anatomic reduction. At 5-year follow-up, Verhaven et al[51] found that 71% of 28 nonathletic patients reported good or excellent clinical outcomes (29% fair or poor) and 40% had a loss of reduction. Successful outcomes have been described in the isolated case reports of the rare Type IV[53–55] and VI[56–58] AC joint injuries.

CLAVICLE

Anatomy

The clavicle, which also is known as the *collarbone*, is one of the most unique bones in the human skeleton. It is the first bone to ossify in utero, at around the fifth week of fetal life, via intramembranous ossification; it is the only long bone in the skeleton to do so. It is the last physis to close in early adulthood at around 22 to 25 years of age (medial physis). Most of its length reached in growth (80%) is obtained from the medial physis. It is also the only long bone that lies horizontally, which is perpendicular to gravity while in the upright position.

The clavicle functions as an S-shaped, crane-like strut, linking the appendicular skeleton via the AC joint laterally and the axial skeleton via the SC joint medially (Figure 6). At the lateral end, the AC joint ligaments and capsule connect the distal clavicle and acromion. The CC ligaments connect the coracoid to the undersurface of the clavicle, with clavicular insertion (trapezoid line) of the trapezoid more lateral and anterior than its conoid insertion (conoid tubercle). The lateral curve of the clavicular S is concave anteriorly, and the medial curve of the S is concave posteriorly. Axial dimensions change from flat and wide (anterior to posterior) laterally to tubular in the middle-third and triangular medially. The junction of the lateral-third and middle-third is a unique location for the clavicle because it is unprotected by musculotendinous or ligamentous attachments and is the thinnest, weakest area of the bone where its axial geometry changes. This unique anatomy makes the junction region the most susceptible to fracture within the clavicle.

Despite its subcutaneous position, it has several musculotendinous and ligamentous attachments that become deforming forces in clavicle and AC joint injuries (Figure 6). Along the anterior aspect of the medial clavicle shaft, the clavicular head of the pectoralis major originates and then inserts on the proximal humerus. This is one of the major contributors to clavicle shortening with fracture. The clavicular head of the sternocleidomastoid inserts on the superior aspect of the medial clavicle, tending to elevate the proximal fragment with fracture. The deltoid originates on the anterior aspect of the lateral distal clavicle. When the clavicle is fractured, the weight of the upper extrem-

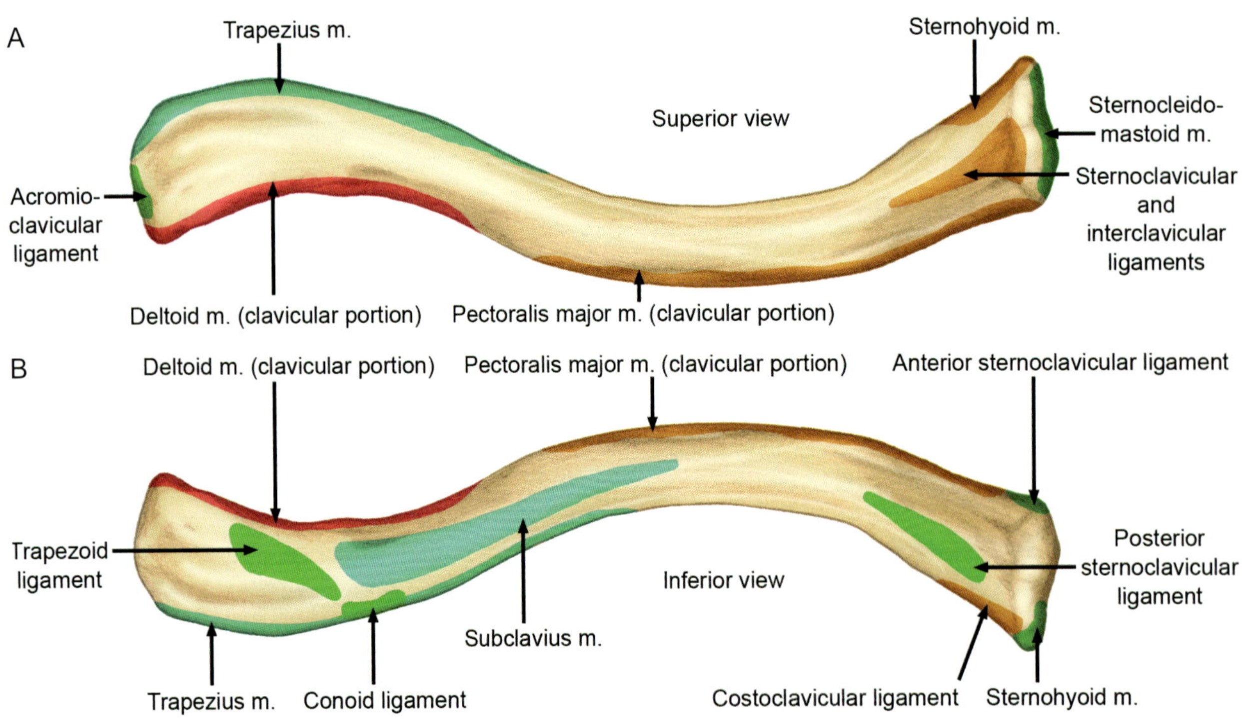

Figure 6. A, Superior view of the right clavicle. Note the S-shaped curve: convex anteromedially and concave anterolaterally. B, Inferior view of the right clavicle. On both views, note the multiple muscular attachments that become deforming forces with fracture.

ity pulls on the distal fracture fragment via the CC ligaments and deltoid muscle, accounting for the distal fragment depression relative to the proximal fragment. The trapezius inserts on the posterior aspect of the lateral distal clavicle. This muscle tends to pull the distal fragment medially and superiorly, accounting for further shortening with fracture.

Important neurovascular structures lie deep to the clavicle. The divisions of the brachial plexus lie directly underneath the clavicle; the roots and trunks are located proximal, and the cords and branches are located distal. The subclavian and axillary vessels are associated intimately with the brachial plexus at this location. Despite the anatomic proximity, plexus and vessel injuries are uncommon. The supraclavicular nerves (sensory) lie superficial to the clavicle.

Injury Classification

Several classification systems are available for clavicle fractures. The Allman[17] classification system is an easy-to-use system that groups fractures based on their anatomic location. Group I fractures are middle-third shaft fractures, accounting for approximately 80% of clavicle fractures. Group II fractures are the next most common (15%) and are located at or distal to the CC ligaments where nonunion is more common. Group III fractures are the least common (5%) and are located at the medial clavicle where nonunion and displacement are rare. Importantly, medial-third fractures should be distinguished from medial physeal injuries in patients less than 25 years of age.

Fractures of the distal clavicle are further subclassified most commonly according to the system of Neer.[59] Like the Allman classification for all clavicle fractures, the Neer system is based anatomically. Fractures are grouped according to their location relative to the CC ligaments and AC joint. Type I fractures are lateral to the CC ligaments but do not extend into the AC joint. This usually means a fracture line is less than 2 cm from the articular surface of the distal clavicle. In this fracture, intact CC ligaments stabilize the proximal fracture fragment and typically prevent substantial displacement. Type III fractures extend into the AC joint. The intra-articular nature of this fracture type accounts for a slight increase in risk of posttraumatic degenerative joint disease.

Type II fractures of the distal clavicle are the most unstable fractures of the distal clavicle. Their distinguishing trait is that the CC ligaments are no longer attached to the proximal fracture fragment. This allows for instability and much higher rates of nonunion. Type II fractures are further subclassified into IIa and IIb fractures. With Type IIa fractures, the fracture line is just medial to the conoid. This means that both CC ligaments are attached to the distal fragment and are assumed to be intact. With Type IIb fractures, the fracture line is further distal and is in between the conoid and trapezoid ligaments. The conoid is disrupted in IIb injuries, whereas the trapezoid is still intact and attached to the distal fragment.

History and Physical Examination

The mechanism of injury of most clavicle fractures is a direct blow to the point of the shoulder. This transmits the force of the fall through the acromion to the AC joint; to the distal clavicle; and then to the shaft or CC ligaments, or both. The degree of energy of the injury and the angle at which contact occurs likely determines the type of clavicle fracture. Typically, patients with displaced clavicle fractures present with an obvious bump over the shoulder that might tent the skin. Open fractures are not uncommon. A thorough physical examination of the neck and entire upper extremity is warranted to evaluate the area for associated injuries. Inspection will reveal swelling, bruising, and possibly abrasions or open lacerations. The upper extremity likely appears drooped secondary to the weight of the extremity pulling the distal fracture fragment down relative to the proximal fragment elevation. Palpation will reveal tenderness and crepitus over the fracture site. Both passive and active motion likely will be limited secondary to pain.

Imaging

The standard examination for traumatic shoulder pain includes dedicated radiographs of the shoulder (true AP, scapular-Y, and axillary views) and clavicle. Displaced middle-third clavicle shaft fractures have a characteristic appearance (Figure 7). In the Imaging section, we discussed the radiographic evaluation of clavicle and AC joint injury and variables evaluated.

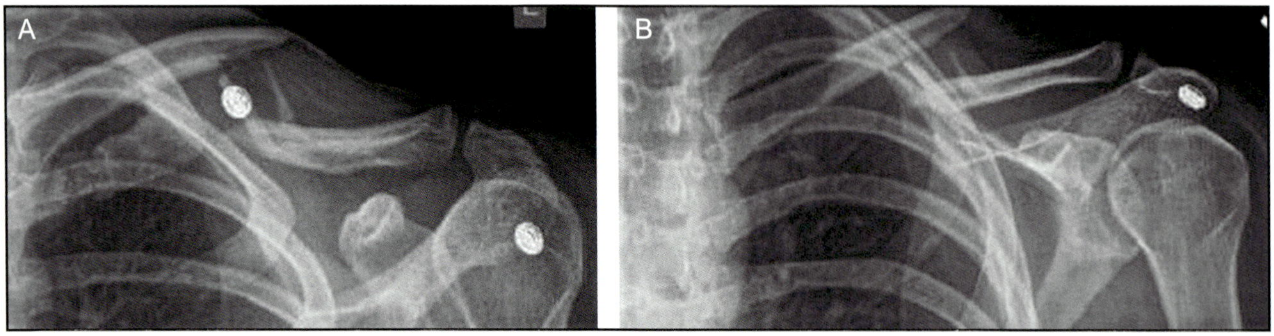

Figure 7 A and B. Anteroposterior clavicle views of the displaced middle-third left clavicle shaft fracture. Note the relative elevation of the proximal (medial) fragment and depression of the distal (lateral) fragment. The weight of the upper extremity depresses the distal fragment, whereas the sternocleidomastoid elevates the proximal fragment.

Treatment Options

Historically, middle-third clavicle fractures have been treated nonoperatively with good clinical outcomes and low rates of nonunion (Figure 8). However, more recently, researchers have shown higher rates of symptomatic malunion, nonunion, and loss of function in nonoperatively treated fractures. Thus, recent trends indicate increasing use of initial operative plate fixation of midshaft fractures (Figure 9).[60] Even displaced pediatric clavicle fractures more commonly are being treated operatively, with union shown earlier on radiographs, earlier return to activities, and low rates of complication.[61] Distal-third clavicle fractures have higher rates of nonunion than middle-third fractures have (Figure 10). Despite the higher rates of nonunion, many patients with nonunion are asymptomatic. Thus, initial nonoperative management is commonplace for most patients, and the development of a nonunion does not necessarily indicate the need for surgery. Medial

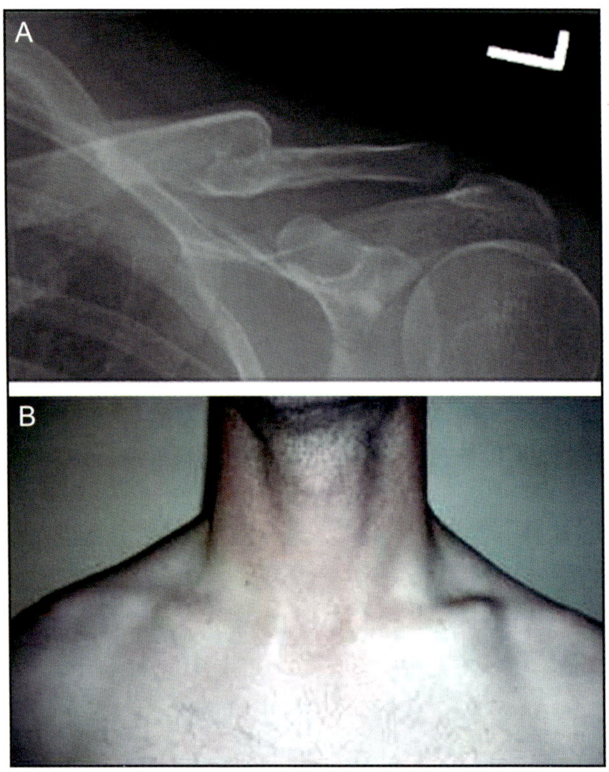

Figure 8. Healed midshaft left clavicle fracture. Patient fell from a bicycle 5 years earlier and had a closed, middle-third clavicle fracture treated with a simple sling. Note the presence of the radiographic, A, and clinical, B, bump. The patient had no pain at rest and with activity.

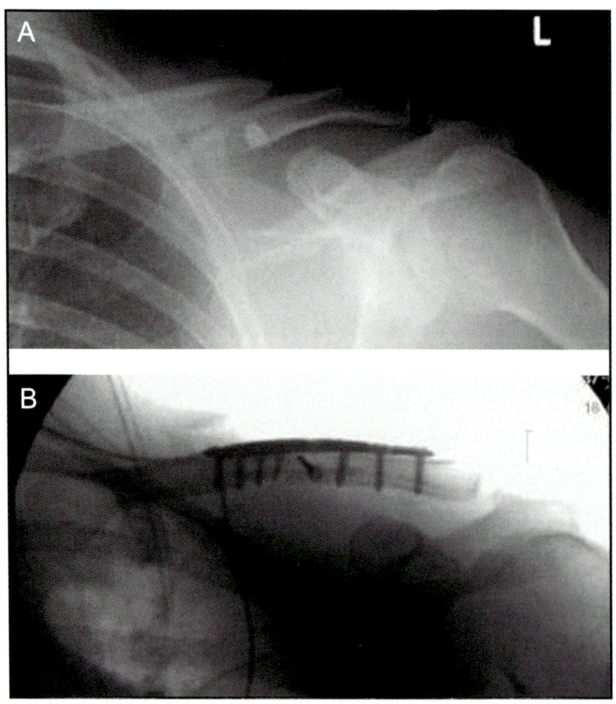

Figure 9. A, Displaced, shortened, middle-third to distal-third junction left clavicle shaft fracture. B, Open reduction and internal fixation with locking superior distal clavicle plate.

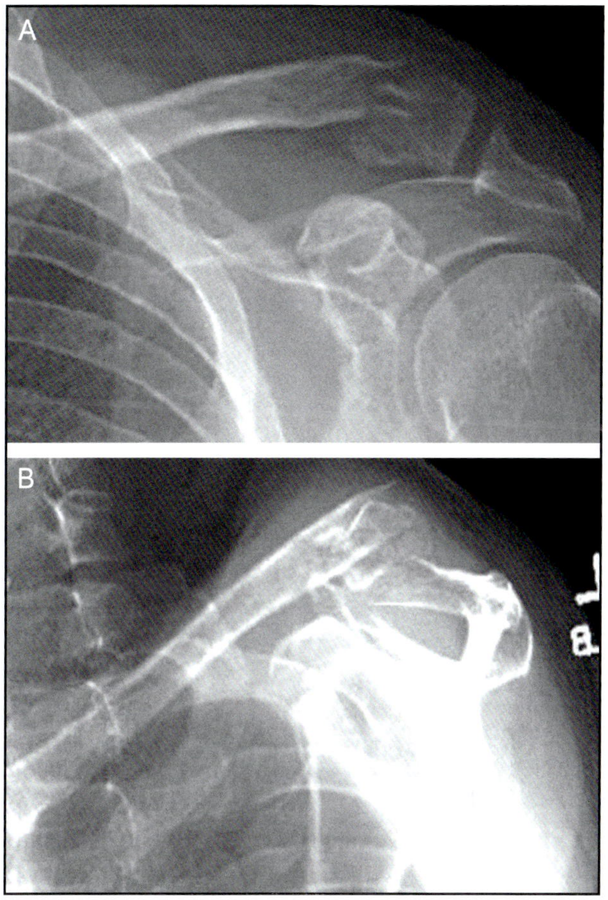

Figure 10 A and B. Minimally displaced Type I distal clavicle fracture without intra-articular extension into the acromioclavicular joint and with fracture line lateral to the coracoclavicular ligaments.

clavicle fractures are rare and rarely require operative fixation. Medial physeal injuries and SC joint dislocation should remain part of the differential diagnosis and should be treated accordingly. Medial physeal injuries are generally stable and require a brief period of immobilization. Anterior SC joint dislocations are prone to result in recurrent instability, whereas posterior SC joint dislocations are much more serious and require emergent reduction if tracheoesophageal compromise or vascular compromise ensues.

Rehabilitation

Much of the rehabilitation after both nonoperative and operative management of clavicle fractures is analogous to that of AC joint injuries. After fracture, common traditional immobilization techniques include a simple sling or figure-of-8 brace. These do not reduce the fracture but simply support the weight of the extremity and the associated droop of the extremity. Skin sores, neurovascular bundle compression, lower rates of patient satisfaction, and a slightly higher rate of nonunion with the figure-of-8 brace has led treatment providers to use the simple sling most commonly. After the pain from the injury has dissipated (usually 2 to 4 weeks), sling use is usually unnecessary, and gentle motion can begin. Throughout this time, elbow, wrist, hand, and finger motion with edema control is encouraged. Because most posterior clavicle rotation occurs above 90° of upper extremity elevation, early rehabilitation programs that stay below this level avoid the substantial rotational forces that affect stability at the site of fracture.[62] At this point, shoulder mobilization is the same as that discussed for rehabilitation after AC joint injury in the Rehabilitation subsection of the Nonoperative Management section and the Postoperative Rehabilitation subsection of the Operative Management section. After radiographic and clinical union is achieved typically from 6 to 12 weeks, a slow return to sport participation begins over the next 1 to 2 months. Refracture is not uncommon with contact sports upon early return.

After operative plate fixation, shoulder motion can begin immediately after surgery without limitations. A simple sling immobilizer generally is worn for 3 to 4 weeks. Weight bearing on the upper extremity is limited both above and below shoulder level until radiographic and clinical evidence of union is demonstrated. Operative fixation has been demonstrated to result in earlier pain relief, earlier return to work, and earlier return to sport participation.[63,64]

Expected Outcomes

Midshaft Fracture. In a recent systematic review of 22 studies (Level I to Level IV evidence) involving the treatment of midshaft clavicle fractures, Zlowodzki et al[63] concluded a relative risk (RR) reduction of 86% with plate fixation versus nonoperative treatment for displaced fractures. No nonunions occurred in plate-fixed fractures in the studies they reviewed. However, the authors reported a 15% rate of nonunion in the nonoperative group. Fracture displacement (RR = 2.3), fracture comminution (RR = 1.4), and female sex (RR = 1.4) were associated with increased risk of nonunion in nonoperatively treated patients.

Since publication of that review, the Canadian Orthopaedic Trauma Group[64] conducted a Level I evidence, multicenter, randomized controlled trial to compare clinical and radiographic outcomes in patients treated with plate fixation and those treated nonoperatively. At up to 1-year follow-up, Constant and Disabilities of the Arm, Shoulder, and Hand (DASH) scores and patient satisfaction were improved significantly in the operative group versus the nonoperative group at all time points. Furthermore, radiographic union was achieved much earlier in the operative (16 weeks) than the nonoperative (28 weeks) group. The rates of nonunion and symptomatic malunion were lower in the operative (2 and 0, respectively) than the nonoperative (7 and 9, respectively) groups. Nevertheless, in the operative group, 3 wound infections and 1 hardware failure occurred. In a separate retrospective study of 52 patients treated nonoperatively with a mean 38-month follow-up, initial fracture shortening greater than 2 cm had a highly significant association with nonunion and the chance of an unsatisfactory result.[65] In another retrospective study of 30 patients with midshaft fractures treated nonoperatively with a mean 55-month follow-up, McKee et al[66] demonstrated significant reductions in strength and endurance in flexion, abduction, internal rotation, and external rotation. In addition, the investigators found significant reductions in Constant and DASH scores. Although superior plating of midshaft fractures is substantially stronger biomechanically (tension side of fracture), anteroinferior plate positioning has been demonstrated via visual analog scale score to have fewer symptoms related to subcutaneous plate positioning.[64]

In the pediatric population, Vander Have et al[60] reviewed a consecutive patient retrospective cohort (42 patients, 43 fractures; mean age = 15 years) and reported the clinical and radiographic outcomes of operatively (plate fixation) and nonoperatively treated displaced midshaft clavicle fractures. The authors found a significant difference in the shortening of fractures at the time of diagnosis (nonoperative group = 13 mm, operative group = 28 mm). For displaced fractures, the times to radiographic union and return to activities were significantly shorter in the operative (7 and 12 weeks, respectively) than the nonoperative (10 and 16 weeks, respectively) groups. They did not find nonunions in either group. Five symptomatic malunions, 4 of which required osteotomy and internal fixation, occurred in the nonoperative group, and 0 occurred in the operative group. Three patients wanted hardware removal secondary to local irritation.

An alternative surgical option is intramedullary fixation of displaced clavicle fractures. The nomenclature of many of these devices is wide: Knowles pins, Hagie pins, Rockwood pins, Herbert screws, Steinmann pins, titanium elastic nails, cancellous screws, and Kirschner wires. Clearly, the advantage to this technique is the reduced need for soft tissue stripping around the clavicle, smaller incisions, less prominent hardware, and less reduction in strength after hardware removal. The disadvantages include the relative stability provided by this implant versus the absolute stability provided by plate fixation. Furthermore, pin migration is a risk. Although most Rockwood pins are removed in the operating room, Rockwood himself typically removes these in the office under local anesthesia. The intramedullary fixation has been demonstrated to have an RR reduction of nonunion of 87% versus that of nonoperative management of displaced midshaft fractures.[64]

Given the current evidence, we recommend initial plate fixation in patients with displaced, shortened (>2 cm), comminuted midshaft clavicle fractures. This recommendation is made within the premise of reduced risk of nonunions and symptomatic malunions and earlier return to work or sport participation. Each case must be discussed individually, and the above-mentioned potential benefits must be weighed against the risks.

Distal-Third Fracture (Lateral). Nondisplaced and minimally displaced Type I fractures of the distal clavicle, which are lateral to the CC ligaments and leave the CC ligaments intact, should be treated nonoperatively. These are stable fractures, and patients do well, with high rates of union and return to function.[59] Intra-articular fracture extension denotes a Type III distal clavicle fracture. This articular involvement portends a slightly increased risk of degenerative joint disease in the AC joint. Nevertheless, initial management should be nonoperative unless it is displaced significantly. Even if posttraumatic osteoarthritis occurs in these patients, which is still rare (5 of 33 patients), it can be treated with distal clavicle excision with excellent clinical outcomes.[67]

Most Type II distal clavicle fractures occur in middle-aged and elderly patients for whom high-level athletics and functioning are not priorities. Nonoperative management is associated with a higher risk of nonunion for these fractures than Type I and III fractures (range, 28%–44%).[68] Independent predictors of nonunion in Type II fractures include complete displacement without cortical contact and older age.[69] However, the presence of a nonunion of the distal clavicle does not necessarily indicate symptoms. Although 7 of 16 patients with a Type II distal clavicle fracture treated nonoperatively developed a nonunion (44%) in a retrospective case series, Rokito et al[70] did not find a difference in clinical outcome scores between patients treated nonoperatively and patients treated operatively. Furthermore, in their retrospective case series, Robinson and Cairns[71] compared 3 groups treated for a Type II distal clavicle fracture; 1 group was treated nonoperatively, 1 group developed a nonunion, and 1 group had nonunion or delayed union and eventually underwent operative treatment. They did not find a significant difference in clinical outcome measures among the 3 groups.

If operative treatment is chosen, many different techniques can be used and are similar to those chosen for AC joint injuries with CC ligament disruption. These include transacromial Kirschner wires, modified Weaver-Dunn techniques with distal clavicle excision, CC screw fixation, and combined plate fixation and CC ligament reconstruction with augmentation. Excellent outcomes have been reported using biological and synthetic CC ligament reconstruction.[72] Precontoured, anatomic, side-specific, locking and nonlocking plates have been developed specifically to treat distal clavicle fractures and have demonstrated success. Distal clavicle hook plates also have been used successfully.[73] However, this hardware necessitates a second operation for hardware removal and is associated with rotator cuff impingement after surgery.

Given the current evidence, we offer operative management of Type II distal clavicle fractures to patients with significantly displaced fractures. This recommendation is made based on the RR reduction of nonunion and earlier return to activities. However, each case still is approached individually, and surgery is undertaken only after an informed discussion of its risks and potential benefits. Initial nonoperative management is recommended to treat most Type I and III fractures.

Proximal-Third Fracture (Medial). Most medial-third clavicle fractures are nondisplaced or minimally displaced and usually are extra-articular. Therefore, most are stable injuries that respond well nonoperatively.[17] However, if the costoclavicular ligament is disrupted, these fractures can become unstable. Even in this situation, most are treated nonoperatively. Only the situation of tracheoesophageal or neurovascular compromise warrants closed rather than open operative reduction and internal fixation, and this usually is performed emergently. Kirschner wire fixation is fraught with the risk of migration to mediastinal structures in close proximity or even distant structures and thus should not be used.[74] Recommended techniques, which are based on very limited evidence, include Mersilene tape or high-strength braided interosseous suture, precluding a second operation for removal of hardware.[1]

CONCLUSIONS

Injuries to the AC joint and clavicle represent a major reason patients seek treatment in emergency departments and sports medicine clinics. These injuries are very common and often prevent both the athlete and nonathlete from participating in sport, activities, and work for a substantial length of time. There is a trend toward increased use of operative techniques for the management of displaced clavicle fractures. Most distal clavicle fractures can be treated successfully without surgery. Controversy still surrounds the management of Type III AC joint injuries. Type I and II AC joint injuries successfully are treated nonoperatively, whereas Type IV, V, and VI AC joint injuries are managed operatively. Common to these injuries is the paramount task of a structured, individualized rehabilitation program. Whether operative or nonoperative interventions are chosen, a delicate balance exists between early mobilization and strengthening to prevent atrophy and stiffness and the healing of bone and soft tissues because of the risk of early failure. This treatment demands communication between all health care providers and the patient to ensure the optimal outcome. The intended goal is a safe, quick, complete return to sport participation or other activities at preinjury level of function without short-term or long-term disability.

REFERENCES

1. Khan LA, Bradnock TJ, Scott C, Robinson CM. Fractures of the clavicle. *J Bone Joint Surg Am*. 2009;91(2):447–460.
2. Postacchini F, Gumina S, De Santis P, Albo F. Epidemiology of clavicle fractures. *J Shoulder Elbow Surg*. 2002;11(5):452–456.
3. Kaplan LD, Flanigan DC, Norwig J, Jost P, Bradley J. Prevalence and variance of shoulder injuries in elite collegiate football players. *Am J Sports Med*. 2005;33(8):1142–1146.
4. Nordqvist A, Petersson C. The incidence of fractures of the clavicle. *Clin Orthop Relat Res*. 1994;300:127–132.
5. Mazzocca AD, Arciero RA, Bicos J. Evaluation and treatment of acromioclavicular joint injuries. *Am J Sports Med*. 2007;35(2):316–329.
6. Simovitch R, Sanders B, Ozbaydar M, Lavery K, Warner JJ. Acromioclavicular joint injuries: diagnosis and management. *J Am Acad Orthop Surg*. 2009;17(4):207–219.
7. Depalma AF. Surgical anatomy of acromioclavicular and sternoclavicular joints. *Surg Clin North Am*. 1963;43:1541–1550.
8. Fukuda K, Craig EV, An KN, Cofield RH, Chao EY. Biomechanical study of the ligamentous system of the acromioclavicular joint. *J Bone Joint Surg Am*. 1986;68(3):434–440.
9. Klimkiewicz JJ, Williams GR, Sher JS, Karduna A, Des Jardins J, Iannotti JP. The acromioclavicular capsule as a restraint to posterior translation of the clavicle: a biomechanical analysis. *J Shoulder Elbow Surg*. 1999;8(2):119–124.
10. Renfree KJ, Riley MK, Wheeler D, Hentz JG, Wright TW. Ligamentous anatomy of the distal clavicle. *J Shoulder Elbow Surg*. 2003;12(4):355–359.
11. Stine IA, Vangsness CT Jr. Analysis of the capsule and ligament insertions about the acromioclavicular joint: a cadaveric study. *Arthroscopy*. 2009;25(9):968–974.
12. Bearden JM, Hughston JC, Whatley GS. Acromioclavicular dislocation: method of treatment. *J Sports Med*. 1973;1(4):5–17.
13. Alyas F, Curtis M, Speed C, Saifuddin A, Connell D. MR imaging appearances of acromioclavicular joint dislocation. *Radiographics*. 2008;28(2):463–479.
14. Collins DN. Disorders of the acromioclavicular joint. In: Itoi E, Morrey B, An KN, eds. *The Shoulder*. Vol 1. 4th ed. Philadelphia, PA: Saunders-Elsevier; 2009:463.
15. Inman VT, Saunders JB, Abbott LC. Observations of the function of the shoulder joint: 1944. *Clin Orthop Relat Res*. 1996;330:3–12.
16. Sahara W, Sugamoto K, Murai M, Tanaka H, Yoshikawa H. 3D kinematic analysis of the acromioclavicular joint during arm abduction using vertically open MRI. *J Orthop Res*. 2006;24(9):1823–1831.
17. Allman FL Jr. Fractures and ligamentous injuries of the clavicle and its articulation. *J Bone Joint Surg Am*. 1967;49(4):774–784.
18. Nguyen V, Williams G, Rockwood C. Radiography of acromioclavicular dislocation and associated injuries. *Crit Rev Diagn Imaging*. 1991;32(3):191–228.
19. Gerber C, Galantay RV, Hersche O. The pattern of pain produced by irritation of the acromioclavicular joint and the subacromial space. *J Shoulder Elbow Surg*. 1998;7(4):352–355.
20. Zanca P. Shoulder pain: involvement of the acromioclavicular joint. (Analysis of 1,000 cases). *Am J Roentgenol Radium Ther Nucl Med*. 1971;112(3):493–506.
21. Gladstone JN, Wilk KE, Andrews JR. Nonoperative treatment of acromioclavicular joint injuries. *Oper Tech Sports Med*. 1997;5(2):78–87.
22. Mouhsine E, Garofalo R, Crevoisier X, Farron A. Grade I and II acromioclavicular dislocations: results of conservative treatment. *J Shoulder Elbow Surg*. 2003;12(6):599–602.
23. Bergfeld JA, Andrish JT, Clancy WG. Evaluation of the acromioclavicular joint following first- and second-degree sprains. *Am J Sports Med*. 1978;6(4):153–159.
24. Cox JS. The fate of the acromioclavicular joint in athletic injuries. *Am J Sports Med*. 1981;9(1):50–53.
25. Cook FF, Tibone JE. The Mumford procedure in athletes: an objective analysis of function. *Am J Sports Med*. 1988;16(2):97–100.
26. Phillips AM, Smart C, Groom AF. Acromioclavicular dislocation: conservative or surgical therapy. *Clin Orthop Relat Res*. 1998;353:10–17.
27. Bannister GC, Wallace WA, Stableforth PG, Hutson MA. The management of acute acromioclavicular dislocation: a randomised prospective controlled trial. *J Bone Joint Surg Br*. 1989;71(5):848–850.
28. Nuber GW, Bowen MK. Acromioclavicular joint injuries and distal clavicle fractures. *J Am Acad Orthop Surg*. 1997;5(1):11–18.
29. McFarland EG, Blivin SJ, Doehring CB, Curl LA, Silberstein C. Treatment of grade III acromioclavicular separations in professional throwing athletes: results of a survey. *Am J Orthop (Belle Mead NJ)*. 1997;26(11):771–774.
30. Bishop JY, Kaeding C. Treatment of the acute traumatic acromioclavicular separation. *Sports Med Arthrosc*. 2006;14(4):237–245.
31. Mumford EB. Acromioclavicular dislocation. *J Bone Joint Surg Am*. 1941;23(4):799–802.
32. Bosworth BM. Acromioclavicular separation: new method of repair. *Surg Gynecol Obstet*. 1941;73:866–871.
33. Assaghir YM. Outcome of exact anatomic repair and coracoclavicular cortical lag screw in acute acromioclavicular dislocations. *J Trauma*. 2011;71(3):E50–E54.
34. Guy DK, Wirth MA, Griffin JL, Rockwood CA Jr. Reconstruction of chronic and complete dislocations of the acromioclavicular joint. *Clin Orthop Relat Res*. 1998;347:138–149.
35. Jari R, Costic RS, Rodosky MW, Debski RE. Biomechanical function of surgical procedures for acromioclavicular joint dislocations. *Arthroscopy*. 2004;20(3):237–245.
36. Galpin RD, Hawkins RJ, Grainger RW. A comparative analysis of operative versus nonoperative treatment of grade III acromioclavicular separations. *Clin Orthop Relat Res*. 1985;193:150–155.
37. Lowe GP, Fogarty MJ. Acute acromioclavicular joint dislocation: results of operative treatment with the Bosworth screw. *Aust N Z J Surg*. 1977;47(5):664–667.
38. Ferris BD, Bhamra M, Paton DF. Coracoid process transfer for acromioclavicular dislocations: a report of 20 cases. *Clin Orthop Relat Res*. 1989;242:184–194.

39. Levine WN, Barron OA, Yamaguchi K, Pollock RG, Flatow EL, Bigliani LU. Arthroscopic distal clavicle resection from a bursal approach. *Arthroscopy*. 1998;14(1):52–56.
40. Snyder SJ, Banas MP, Karzel RP. The arthroscopic Mumford procedure: an analysis of results. *Arthroscopy*. 1995;11(2):157–164.
41. Flatow EL, Duralde XA, Nicholson GP, Pollock RG, Bigliani LU. Arthroscopic resection of the distal clavicle with a superior approach. *J Shoulder Elbow Surg*. 1995;4(1 pt 1):41–50.
42. Eskola A, Vainionpää S, Korkala O, Rokkanen P. Acute complete acromioclavicular dislocation: a prospective randomized trial of fixation with smooth or threaded Kirschner wires or cortical screw. *Ann Chir Gynaecol*. 1987;76(6):323–326.
43. Weaver JK, Dunn HK. Treatment of acromioclavicular injuries, especially complete acromioclavicular separation. *J Bone Joint Surg Am*. 1972;54(6):1187–1194.
44. Lee SJ, Nicholas SJ, Akizuki KH, McHugh MP, Kremenic IJ, Ben-Avi S. Reconstruction of the coracoclavicular ligaments with tendon grafts: a comparative biomechanical study. *Am J Sports Med*. 2003;31(5):648–655.
45. Harris RI, Wallace AL, Harper GD, Goldberg JA, Sonnabend DH, Walsh WR. Structural properties of the intact and the reconstructed coracoclavicular ligament complex. *Am J Sports Med*. 2000;28(1):103–108.
46. Rodeo SA, Arnoczky SP, Torzilli PA, Hidaka C, Warren RF. Tendon-healing in a bone tunnel: a biomechanical and histological study in the dog. *J Bone Joint Surg Am*. 1993;75(12):1795–1803.
47. St Pierre P, Olson EJ, Elliott JJ, O'Hair KC, McKinney LA, Ryan J. Tendon-healing to cortical bone compared with healing to a cancellous trough: a biomechanical and histological evaluation in goats. *J Bone Joint Surg Am*. 1995;77(12):1858–1866.
48. Spencer EE Jr. Treatment of grade III acromioclavicular joint injuries: a systematic review. *Clin Orthop Relat Res*. 2007;455:38–44.
49. Weinstein DM, McCann PD, McIlveen SJ, Flatow EL, Bigliani LU. Surgical treatment of complete acromioclavicular dislocations. *Am J Sports Med*. 1995;23(3):324–331.
50. Press J, Zuckerman JD, Gallagher M, Cuomo F. Treatment of grade III acromioclavicular separations: operative versus nonoperative management. *Bull Hosp Jt Dis*. 1997;56(2):77–83.
51. Verhaven E, Casteleyn PP, De Boeck H, Handelberg F, Haentjens P, Opdecam P. Surgical treatment of acute type V acromioclavicular injuries: a prospective study. *Acta Orthop Belg*. 1992;58(2):176–182.
52. Verhaven E, DeBoeck H, Haentjens P, Handelberg F, Casteleyn PP, Opdecam P. Surgical treatment of acute type-V acromioclavicular injuries in athletes. *Arch Orthop Trauma Surg*. 1993;112(4):189–192.
53. Hastings DE, Horne JG. Anterior dislocation of the acromioclavicular joint. *Injury*. 1979;10(4):285–288.
54. Nieminen S, Aho AJ. Anterior dislocation of the acromioclavicular joint. *Ann Chir Gynaecol*. 1984;73(1):21–24.
55. Søndergård-Petersen P, Mikkelsen P. Posterior acromioclavicular dislocation. *J Bone Joint Surg Br*. 1982;64(1):52–53.
56. Schwarz N, Kuderna H. Inferior acromioclavicular separation: report of an unusual case. *Clin Orthop Relat Res*. 1988;234:28–30.
57. Torrens C, Mestre C, Pérez P, Marin M. Subcoracoid dislocation of the distal end of the clavicle: a case report. *Clin Orthop Relat Res*. 1998;348:121–123.
58. Patterson WR. Inferior dislocation of the distal end of the clavicle: a case report. *J Bone Joint Surg Am*. 1967;49(6):1184–1186.
59. Neer CS II. Fractures of the distal third of the clavicle. *Clin Orthop Relat Res*. 1968;58:43–50.
60. Vander Have KL, Perdue AM, Caird MS, Farley FA. Operative versus nonoperative treatment of midshaft clavicle fractures in adolescents. *J Pediatr Orthop*. 2010;30(4):307–312.
61. Fung M, Kato S, Barrance PJ, et al. Scapular and clavicular kinematics during humeral elevation: a study with cadavers. *J Shoulder Elbow Surg*. 2001;10(3):278–285.
62. Jubel A, Andemahr J, Bergmann H, Prokop A, Rehm KE. Elastic stable intramedullary nailing of midclavicular fractures in athletes. *Br J Sports Med*. 2003;37(6):480–484.
63. Zlowodzki M, Zelle BA, Cole PA, Jeray K, McKee MD; Evidence-Based Orthopaedic Trauma Working Group. Treatment of acute midshaft clavicle fractures: systematic review of 2144 fractures. On behalf of the Evidence-Based Orthopaedic Trauma Working Group. *J Orthop Trauma*. 2005;19(7):504–507.
64. Canadian Orthopaedic Trauma Group. Nonoperative treatment compared with plate fixation of displaced midshaft clavicular fractures: a multicenter, randomized clinical trial. *J Bone Joint Surg Am*. 2007;89(1):1–10.
65. Hill JM, McGuire MH, Crosby LA. Closed treatment of displaced middle-third fractures of the clavicle gives poor results. *J Bone Joint Surg Br*. 1997;79(4):537–539.
66. McKee MD, Pedersen EM, Jones C, et al. Deficits following nonoperative treatment of displaced midshaft clavicular fractures. *J Bone Joint Surg Am*. 2006;88(1):35–40.
67. Robinson CM. Fractures of the clavicle in the adult: epidemiology and classification. *J Bone Joint Surg Br*. 1998;80(3):476–484.
68. Banerjee R, Waterman B, Padalecki J, Robertson W. Management of distal clavicle fractures. *J Am Acad Orthop Surg*. 2011;19(7):392–401.
69. Robinson CM, Court-Brown CM, McQueen MM, Wakefield AE. Estimating the risk of nonunion following nonoperative treatment of a clavicular fracture. *J Bone Joint Surg Am*. 2004;86(7):1359–1365.
70. Rokito AS, Zuckerman JD, Shaari JM, Eisenberg DP, Cuomo F, Gallagher MA. A comparison of nonoperative and operative treatment of type II distal clavicle fractures. *Bull Hosp Jt Dis*. 2002;61(1–2):32–39.
71. Robinson CM, Cairns DA. Primary nonoperative treatment of displaced lateral fractures of the clavicle. *J Bone Joint Surg Am*. 2004;86(4):778–782.
72. Webber MC, Haines JF. The treatment of lateral clavicle fractures. *Injury*. 2000;31(3):175–179.
73. Kashii M, Inui H, Yamamoto K. Surgical treatment of distal clavicle fractures using the clavicular hook plate. *Clin Orthop Relat Res*. 2006;447:158–164.
74. Lyons FA, Rockwood CA Jr. Migration of pins used in operations on the shoulder. *J Bone Joint Surg Am*. 1990;72(8):1262–1267.

I-8

Proximal Humerus Fractures

Robert G. Lewis, MD

Fractures of the proximal humerus are the most common fractures of the shoulder girdle and represent 5% of all fractures.[1] They are the third most common fractures in the elderly, with only hip fractures and Colles fractures occurring more commonly.[2] They occur at approximately 70% the incidence of hip fractures,[1,3] and Palvanen et al[4] recently predicted that the incidence of proximal humerus fractures will triple over the next 3 decades. These fractures occur in women twice as often as in men.[5]

Fractures of the proximal humerus are fractures of senescence. Osteoporosis plays a large role in their cause, and the mechanism of injury is usually one of low energy. A fall directly onto the affected shoulder in patients who are 60 years of age or more is commonly reported. In contrast, proximal humerus fractures in younger patients often are caused by high-energy trauma.[5] Women who are more than 60 years of age have an 8% risk of sustaining a proximal humerus fracture during their lifetimes.[5]

Eighty percent to 85% of these fractures are non-displaced or minimally displaced and can be treated nonoperatively and with careful early motion. The remaining 15% to 20% are displaced fractures that usually require surgical intervention.[3,6,7] Although proximal humerus fractures are common, treatment of these injuries can be challenging. Defining the correct treatment guidelines is becoming increasingly important as the prevalence of these fractures increases. Knowing the anatomy and blood supply of the proximal humerus is essential in treatment.

ANATOMY

The proximal humerus consists of 4 well-defined parts: humeral head, greater tuberosity, lesser tuberosity, and proximal humeral shaft. The greater tuberosity consists of 3 facets for tendinous insertion of the supraspinatus, infraspinatus, and teres minor (Figure 1). The lesser tuberosity essentially has 1 facet for the subscapularis insertion.

As illustrated in Figure 2, the average humeral neck-shaft angle is approximately 145°. Retroversion is determined in reference to the transepicondylar axis of the elbow, and normal is 30°. Knowledge of these normal values is critical when differentiating between a fracture that can be treated operatively and a fracture that can be treated nonoperatively. It also aids in the operative restoration of normal anatomy.

With fracture, the deforming forces created by the pull of the multiple insertions on the proximal humerus result in displacement of the respective bony parts. The subscapularis muscle pulls the fractured lesser

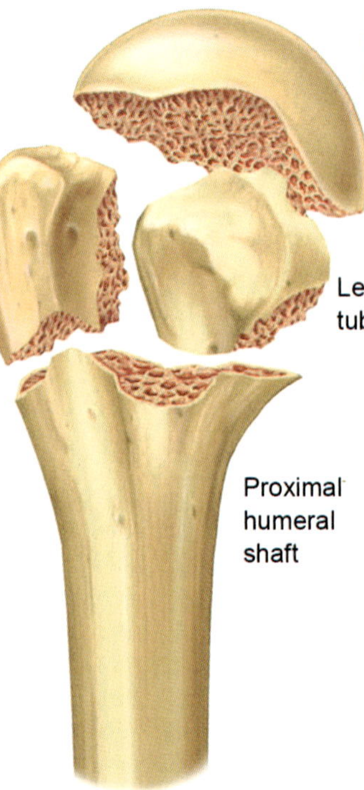

Figure 1. Four parts of the proximal humerus: humeral head, greater tuberosity, lesser tuberosity, and proximal humeral shaft.

tuberosity medially toward the scapular body. The supraspinatus and infraspinatus displace the greater tuberosity fracture fragment in a superior and posterior direction, and if comminuted, parts of the greater tuberosity can be pulled superiorly and parts can be pulled posteriorly. The pectoralis major muscle pulls the proximal humeral shaft anteromedially (Figure 3).

The main blood supply to the proximal humerus originates from the axillary artery. The anterior humeral circumflex

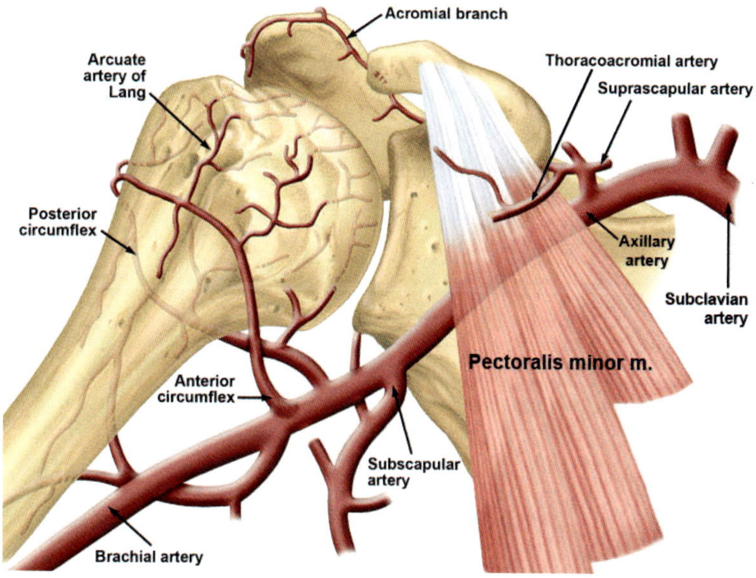

Figure 4. Blood supply to the proximal humerus.

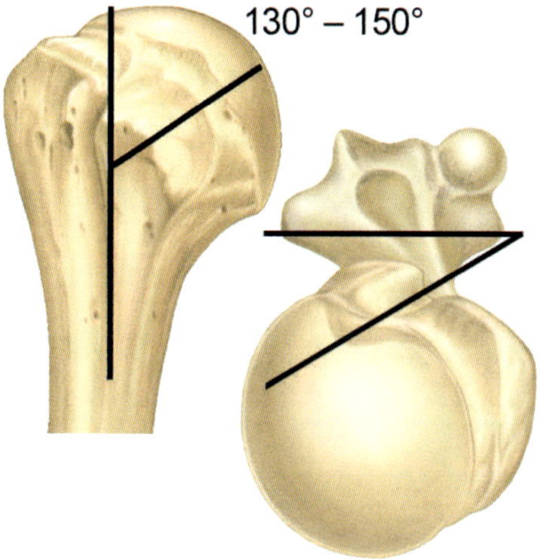

Figure 2. Normal humeral neck-shaft angle (145°) and humeral head retroversion (30°).

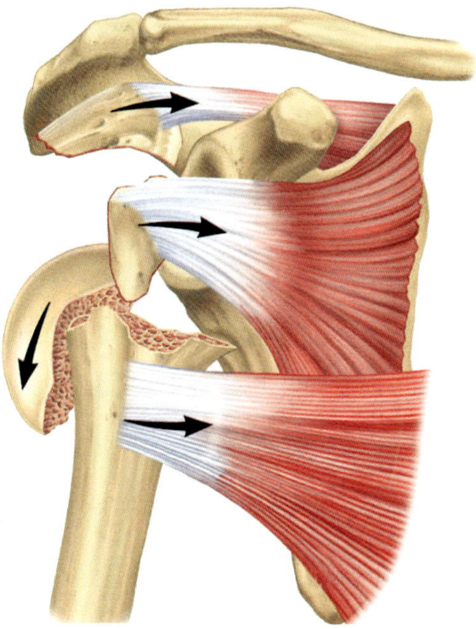

Figure 3. Deforming forces on the proximal humerus can occur with fracture.

artery branches off the axillary artery and gives rise to the ascending branch, which terminates as the arcuate artery. The arcuate artery is the most important contributor to the blood supply of the humeral head. This artery is almost always compromised with 4-part proximal humerus fractures.[8] Because the blood flow from the arcuate artery is usually disrupted, collateral circulation becomes critical to the survival of the humeral head. The posterior humeral circumflex artery and the medial periosteal vessels are 2 sources of collateral flow (Figure 4).

When blood flow from the arcuate artery and collateral sources to the humeral head are lost, avascular necrosis results. Recognizing this vascular compromise is paramount in treatment decision making. In 2004, Hertel et al[9] identified good predictors of ischemia to the humeral head based on fracture pattern. For instance, if the length of the metaphyseal neck extension, or calcar, is less than 8 mm (Figure 5) and if the medial hinge of the fracture is displaced more than 2 mm (Figure 6), then the probability is high that vascularity has been compromised and ischemia is present.[9]

ASSOCIATED INJURIES

Fractures of the proximal humerus commonly are associated with neurologic injuries. Electromyographic evaluation has revealed that approximately two-thirds (67%) of all patients with proximal humerus fractures have acute neurologic injury.[2] Axillary nerve injuries are most common (58%), followed by suprascapular nerve injuries (48%).[2] This high association of nerve injury with proximal humerus fractures stresses the importance of a thorough neurovascular examination from the evaluating health care provider.

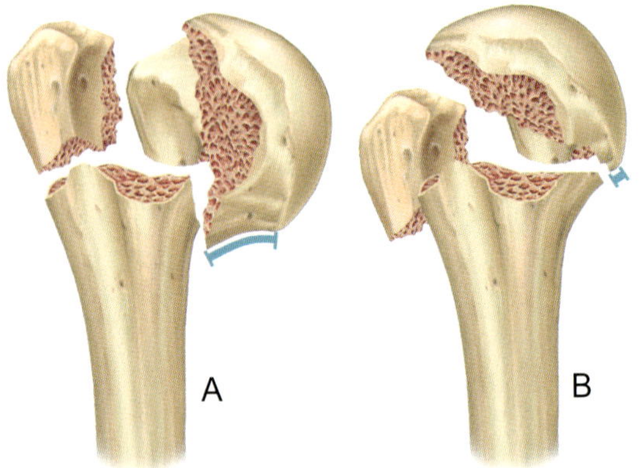

Figure 5. A, The medial calcar is maintained at more than 8 mm. B, The medial calcar is less than 8 mm and is a good predictor of ischemia to the humeral head.

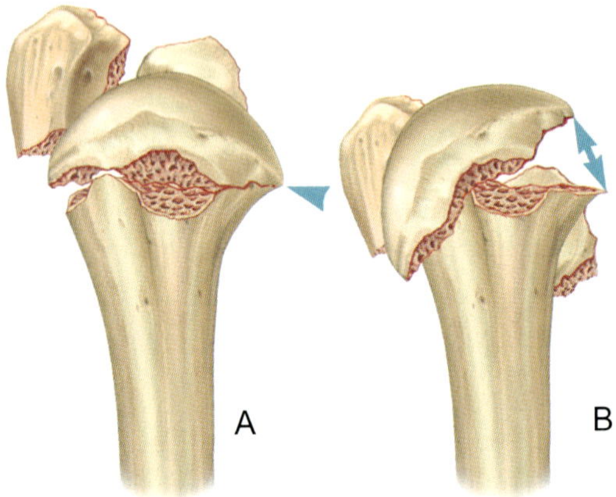

Figure 6. A, The medial hinge is intact. B, The medial hinge is gapped more than 2 mm and is a good predictor of ischemia to the humeral head.

Most of these nerve injuries result in neurapraxia or axonotmesis only, and a full recovery can be expected. Vitamin B supplementation has been shown to facilitate recovery from nerve injury.[5] When neurologic injury is suspected and persists for 3 to 4 weeks, then baseline electromyography (EMG) is recommended. Follow-up EMG is performed at 12 weeks after the injury. If the interval EMGs show no improvement, then surgery is recommended. An estimated 8% of all axillary nerve injuries occurring with proximal humerus fractures result in permanent motor loss and might require neurolysis, nerve grafting, or neurotization, which provides best results if performed within 3 to 6 months after the injury.[10]

Vascular injuries associated with proximal humerus fractures are less common than nerve injuries and occur in 5% of cases.[3] They usually involve the axillary artery or vein and occur more commonly in older patients with atherosclerotic disease and in patients who sustain fracture-dislocations of the proximal humerus. A high index of suspicion is required to diagnose this injury. In fact, 27% of patients with vascular injuries have a palpable distal pulse. An associated vascular injury must be treated as an emergency; therefore, timely evaluation with angiography is imperative[3] (Figure 7). Indications for angiography are diminished or absent distal pulses, expanding hematoma, bruit in the extremity, unexplained hypotension, pulsatile arterial bleeding, or a changing neurologic examination.[5] Vascular injuries usually are treated with reconstructive surgery.

CLASSIFICATION

Classification of proximal humerus fractures was first described by Kocher[11] in 1896. He illustrated 3 fracture lines that occur within the proximal humerus and are located at the anatomic neck, the epiphysis, and the surgical neck. Codman[12] created a new classification system in 1934 by naming the 4 commonly fractured fragments: the head, shaft, greater tuberosity, and lesser tuberosity. He described these fracture fragments as parts that fracture along the old epiphyseal lines. In 1970, Neer[13] expanded Codman's classification system by describing the parts of a proximal humerus fracture and determining the displacement criteria that establish a fracture fragment as a "part." He defined *significant displacement* as more than 1 cm of translation or more

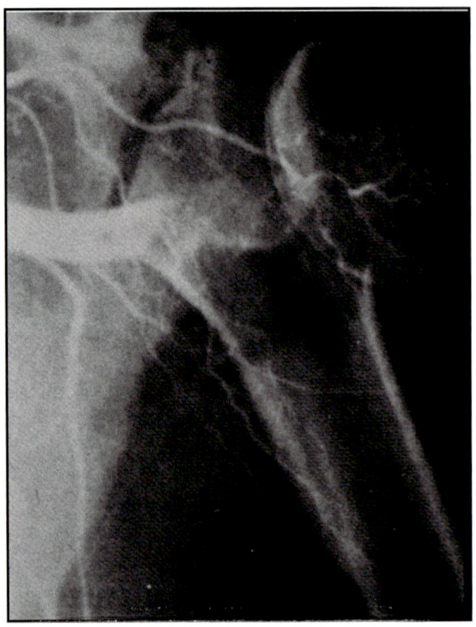

Figure 7. Angiogram shows disruption of the axillary artery associated with a proximal humerus fracture-dislocation.

than 45° of angulation in any major fracture fragment.[14] This classification system remains the simplest and most widely used for describing proximal humerus fractures.

An AO/ASIF classification system exists for proximal humerus fractures. This system involves 3 main groups and 9 subgroups, totaling 27 possible groups. The AO/ASIF system is not commonly used clinically because of its complexity. In addition, the Neer system has better interobserver and intraobserver reliability than the AO/ASIF system.[5] Even so, the reliability of the Neer system has been questioned. Using the Neer system, Bernstein et al[15] showed 64% intraobserver reliability and 52% interobserver reliability with radiographs alone. In this study, the authors demonstrated a slight increase in intraobserver reliability but no increase in interobserver reliability when basic computed tomography was used. However, when 3-dimensional computed tomography is used, interobserver reliability doubles.[16]

Three fracture patterns have been added to the Neer classification system. These patterns include valgus-impacted, head-splitting, and impression fractures (Figure 8). A true valgus-impacted fracture occurs with compression of the articular surface onto the glenoid through an abducted upper extremity. This mechanism results in a humeral head that is fractured into a valgus position on the shaft. A valgus-impacted proximal humerus fracture usually only has a small amount of displacement of the fractured parts. With this type of fracture, the blood supply of the proximal humerus is frequently maintained, resulting in a low incidence of avascular necrosis. Head-splitting and impression fractures of the humeral head are severe injuries that often must be treated with arthroplasty. Head-splitting fractures are caused by compression at the glenohumeral joint, and impression fractures occur secondary to dislocations.

EVALUATION

Clinically, patients present with pain, swelling, and tenderness to palpation over the proximal humerus. Deformity, crepitation, and ecchymosis also may be present. If minimal ecchymosis or no ecchymosis is present, the patient and his or her family should be counseled that ecchymosis usually becomes worse and can extend into the chest wall and as far distal as the elbow. A thorough neurovascular examination is very important, and the physician must maintain a high index of suspicion for these injuries.

The examiner orders a trauma series of shoulder radiographs, which includes a true anteroposterior view of the shoulder, an axillary-lateral view, and a scapular-Y view. Evaluation of the axillary-lateral view is critical for diagnosing posteriorly displaced greater tuberosity fractures and posterior fracture-dislocations, and this view provides an orthogonal view to enable the examiner to better evaluate nondisplaced and minimally displaced fractures. A nondisplaced or minimally displaced fracture of the greater tuberosity might be overlooked in 53% of initial clinical examinations.[5]

Computed tomography can help the examiner define the degree of head-splitting and impression fractures or actual displacement of a fracture fragment if any uncertainty is present after routine radiographic

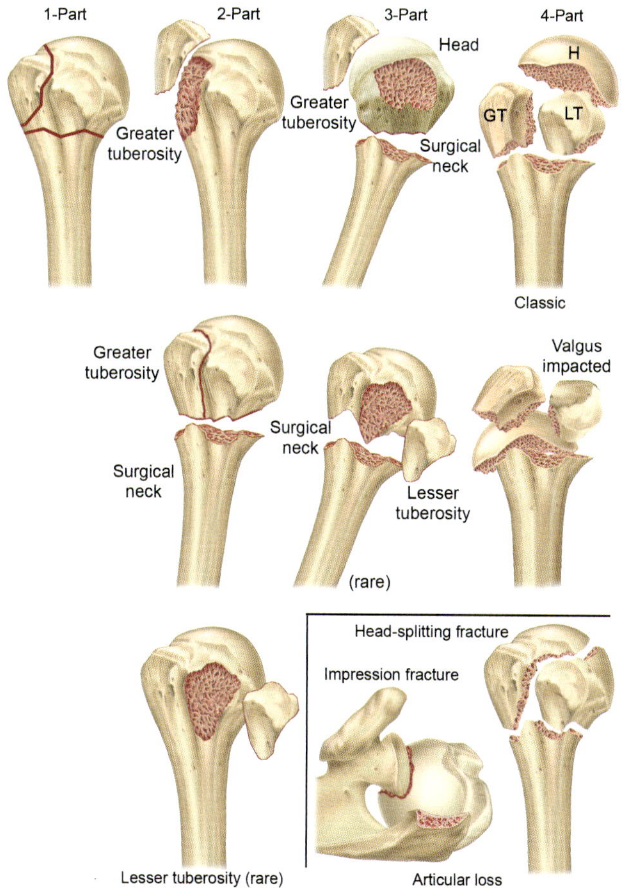

Figure 8. The Neer classification system for proximal humerus fractures. Abbreviations: H, head; GT, greater tuberosity; and LT, lesser tuberosity.

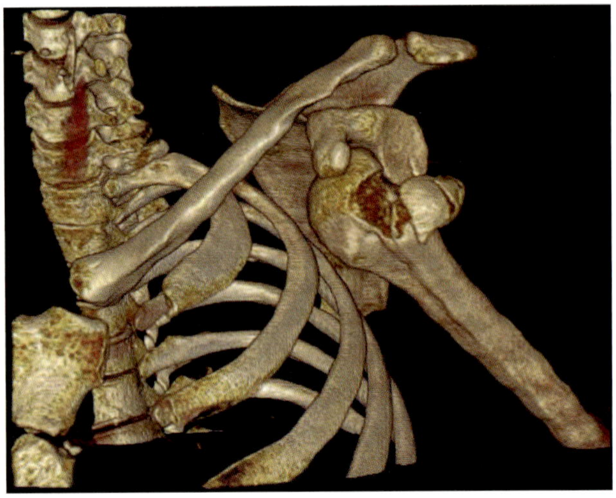

Figure 9. Three-dimensional reconstruction of an anterior glenohumeral dislocation with an associated greater tuberosity fracture.

evaluation is complete. Chronic fracture-dislocations and tuberosity displacement are depicted easily with computed tomography scans. Computed tomography reconstructions (coronal, sagittal, 3-dimensional) aid the examiner in defining the degree of displacement and increase interobserver reliability (Figure 9).[16]

Magnetic resonance imaging can help the examiner diagnose rotator cuff lesions, avascular necrosis, neurovascular injuries, occult nondisplaced fractures, or occult articular injuries. Usually, the rotator cuff is intact in patients with proximal humerus fractures. If a pre-existing rotator cuff tear is suspected, then a magnetic resonance imaging scan can help identify the extent of the tear and degree of fatty atrophy, if present. This information enables the examiner to recommend a particular procedure.

TREATMENT

Nonoperative treatment is best used for nondisplaced or minimally displaced 2-part or 3-part fractures. Most 4-part fractures should be treated operatively unless the patient is an unsuitable candidate for surgery. If nonoperative treatment is prescribed, then frequent examinations and radiographs are recommended in the early period of treatment. The position of immobilization is critical and should reflect an understanding of the pathologic anatomy and the need to "offload" the displaced fragment or fragments. For instance, an isolated greater tuberosity fracture can be treated by immobilizing the upper extremity in mild abduction and external rotation. On the other hand, an isolated lesser tuberosity fracture is treated in internal rotation. Both fracture patterns can be treated with immobilization in a sling but with instructions about maintaining the offloading position. A semi-recumbent sleeping position (recliner-chair position) is recommended during the first few weeks after injury. Liberal use of ice and edema control (edema glove and compressive stockinet) complements the initial treatment.

The period of immobilization depends on the fracture pattern and stability of fracture reduction. Hodgson et al[17] showed that immediately initiating physical therapy for minimally displaced 2-part fractures decreased the prevalence of disability 1 year after injury versus initiating physical therapy 3 weeks after immobilization. Despite these promising results, the general recommendation is immobilization in a sling for 3 to 4 weeks. The patient begins pendulum exercises during the first week after injury. In the second and third weeks after injury, the patient can begin passive forward elevation. Shoulder rotation increases the risk of tuberosity displacement; therefore, early passive rotation might exacerbate displacement with certain fracture patterns. Rotational exercises can be initiated in all proximal humerus fractures within 5 to 6 weeks after injury.[5] Full activity against gravity, isometric rotator cuff muscle activation, and passive stretching of any remaining soft tissue tightness can be started approximately 5 weeks after injury.[17]

1-Part Fractures

Nonoperative treatment is recommended for all 1-part fractures regardless of comminution (Figure 10). These fractures are treated with immobilization in a sling and early physical therapy. Koval et al[18] reported the results of 104 1-part fractures that were treated nonoperatively. At a 41-month follow-up, 77% of patients reported good or excellent results; 13%, fair results; and 10%, poor results. Ninety percent of patients had no pain or mild pain, and 94% had functional recovery.[18]

2-Part Fractures

The 4 types of 2-part proximal humerus fractures consist of anatomic-neck, greater tuberosity, lesser tuberosity, and surgical-neck fractures.

Figure 10. Radiograph demonstrates a 1-part proximal humerus fracture.

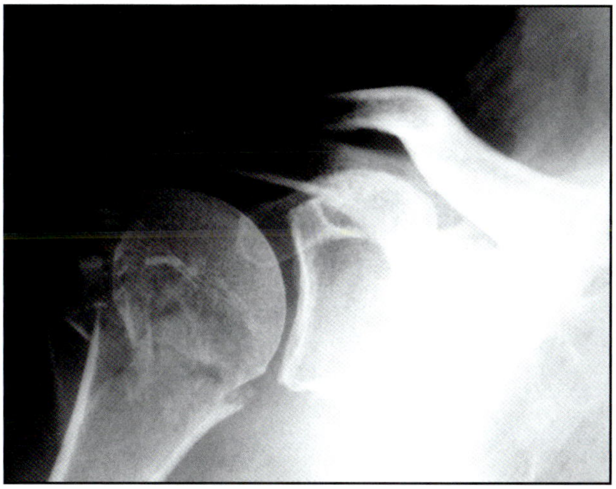

Anatomic Neck Fractures. The anatomic neck represents the old epiphyseal plate. Fractures that occur in this area are extremely rare and extremely serious. They have a high incidence of avascular necrosis because they disrupt the arcuate artery (Figure 11).

In young patients, the surgeon should try to preserve the humeral head with open reduction and internal fixation (ORIF). The difficulty with this operation is the lack of adequate bone in the small humeral head fragment to enable sufficient screw purchase.

Authors of most clinical outcome studies agree that prosthetic humeral head replacement provides the most predictable results for 2-part anatomic-neck fractures.[6] A deltopectoral approach with release of the subscapularis tendon from the lesser tuberosity provides excellent exposure and enables easy removal of the humeral head fragment. The humeral component is implanted in 30° of retroversion in relation to the transepicondylar axis of the elbow (Figure 12).

Greater Tuberosity Fractures. Two-part greater tuberosity fractures of the proximal humerus often are associated with an anterior glenohumeral dislocation. Residual displacement of the greater tuberosity fragment might be present after immediate closed reduction of the shoulder. Any displacement greater than or equal to 5 mm superior and 1 cm posterior generally is unacceptable.[7] More displacement is accepted posteriorly than superiorly because of the greater likelihood of subacromial impingement with superior displacement. In athletes, displacement in either direction is poorly tolerated, and surgical intervention is considered when displacement of 2 mm or more is found.

Many times, the greater tuberosity fragment reduces and lies in a satisfactory position after closed reduction of an anterior shoulder dislocation. Nonoperative management with a sling is indicated in this situation.

The activity level more than the age of the patient influences the decision to operatively manage the greater tuberosity fracture with borderline displacement. Active patients generally have much pain and dysfunction associated with this fracture. The operative treatment options include ORIF with heavy nonabsorbable sutures incorporated into the rotator cuff tendon and ORIF with screws and washers. Using screws and washers with greater tuberosity fractures is often difficult because of the small size of the fragment and comminution. A newer technique of arthroscopic repair with suture anchors is available to manage this injury.

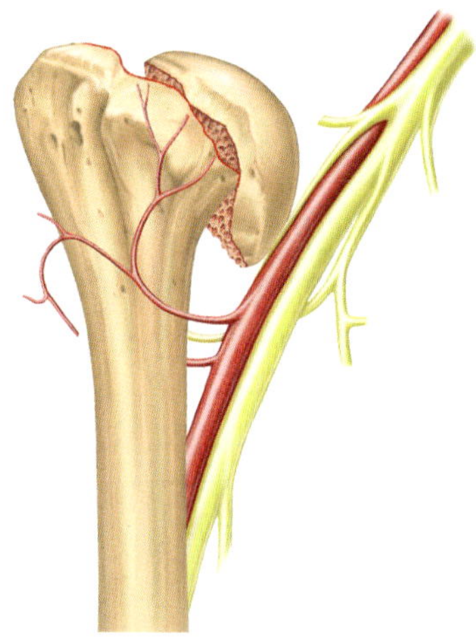

Figure 11. Two-part anatomic-neck fracture with disruption of the arcuate artery.

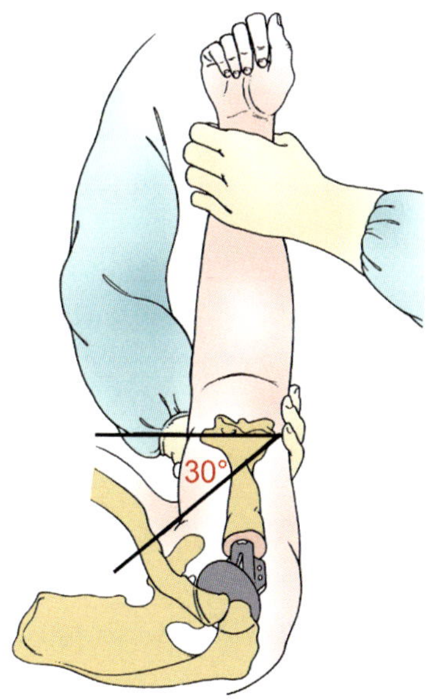

Figure 12. Implantation of a humeral head prosthesis with 30° of retroversion relative to the transepicondylar axis of the elbow.

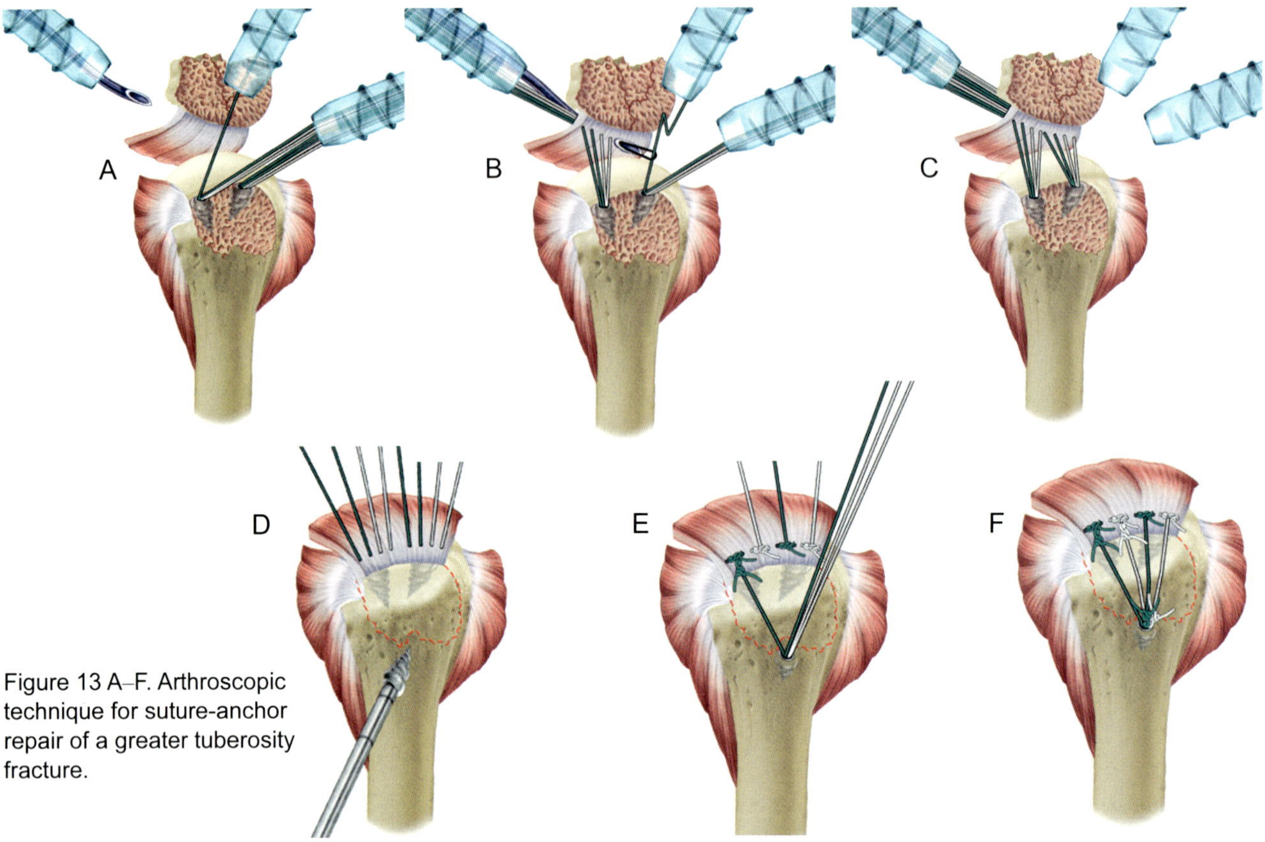

Figure 13 A–F. Arthroscopic technique for suture-anchor repair of a greater tuberosity fracture.

Arthroscopic reduction and internal fixation of greater tuberosity fractures involves fixation with suture anchors. Two anchors are placed at the superomedial aspect of the rotator cuff footprint (Figure 13A). The sutures from these anchors are passed through the greater tuberosity bone-tendon interface via arthroscopic cannulas and suture passers (Figure 13 B and C). Next, the greater tuberosity fragment is reduced, and the sutures are tied arthroscopically, creating horizontal mattress-suture configurations (Figure 13D). Only 1 suture strand is cut from each knot for later use in creating a tension band over the fracture fragments (Figure 13E). A third suture anchor is placed at the inferolateral aspect of the greater tuberosity footprint. The bone must be predrilled **and** tapped to avoid fracturing the cortical bone when placing this anchor. One strand from the third anchor is tied arthroscopically to a suture limb from the superomedial anchors (Figures 13F). This arthroscopic suture technique provides good fixation of a 2-part greater tuberosity fracture. This technique of fixation also can be used through an open approach.

Lesser Tuberosity Fractures. Two-part lesser tuberosity fractures are uncommon (Figure 14). They often are associated with posterior shoulder dislocations, which account for less than 5% of all dislocations. Muscle contraction during seizure is the most common cause of acute posterior shoulder dislocation. During physical examination, the hallmark finding for a posterior shoulder dislocation with an associated lesser tuberosity fracture is lack of passive or active external rotation. Residual displacement of the lesser tuberosity fragment might be present after immediate closed reduction of the shoulder.

The lesser tuberosity must be repaired when displacement persists after closed reduction. When no comminution and good bone stock exist, screw-and-washer fixation can be effective (Figure 15). If the surgeon notes comminution during the procedure or notes osteoporotic bone, then he or she should use heavy, nonabsorbable sutures through transosseous tunnels. Suture anchors always should be considered in tuberosity fixation (lesser or greater). Figure 16 demonstrates a very effective technique that involves suture anchors and transosseous tunnels for tuberosity fixation. Note that sutures initially are passed at the bone-tendon interface medially and tied in horizontal mattress fashion. The remaining suture limbs are

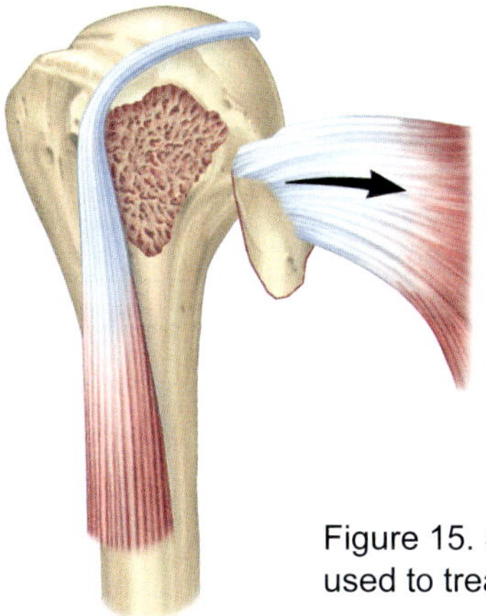

Figure 14. Two-part lesser tuberosity fracture.

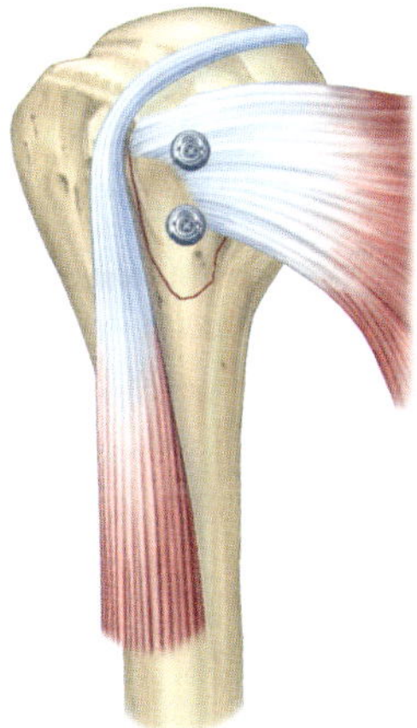

Figure 15. Screw-and-washer fixation used to treat a lesser tuberosity fracture.

passed through transosseous tunnels deep to the bicipital groove and biceps tendon and also are tied in a horizontal mattress fashion. This construct now provides medial and lateral fixation points, a "mesh" that helps capture and retain

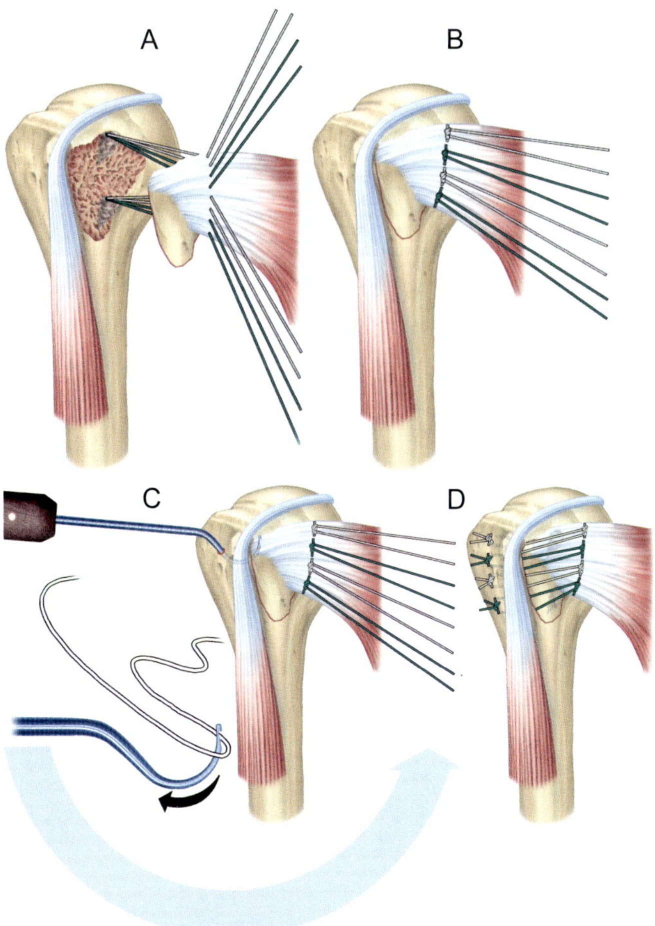

Figure 16 A–D. The technique for tuberosity fixation involves suture anchors and transosseous tunnels.

comminution, and a tension band with external rotation.

Surgical-Neck Fractures. The surgical neck of the proximal humerus represents the weakened area of bone that is below the tuberosities and humeral head and is approximately 2 cm distal to the anatomic neck.[6] The pull of the pectoralis major commonly displaces 2-part surgical-neck fractures by pulling the humeral shaft anteromedially

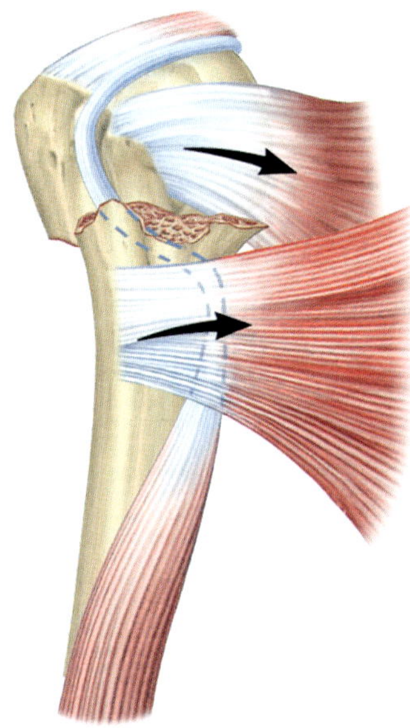

Figure 17. Two-part surgical-neck fracture with displacement of the shaft anteromedially via the pectoralis major muscle.

(Figure 17). Initial treatment of this 2-part fracture is closed reduction via distal traction and lateral displacement with simultaneous flexion of the humeral shaft. Closed reduction might be blocked by interposition of the biceps tendon, deltoid muscle, or periosteum.[6] If closed reduction is successful, then fracture stability must be determined. If the fracture is stable, then initial treatment involves immobilizing the upper extremity in a sling for 3 to 4 weeks. If the fracture is unstable, it must be stabilized with either percutaneous pin fixation or ORIF.

Percutaneous pin fixation is ideal for a 2-part surgical-neck fracture that is reducible closed but is unstable. The first 2 pins are directed from the inferolateral aspect of the humerus into the articular segment, and a third pin is inserted from the

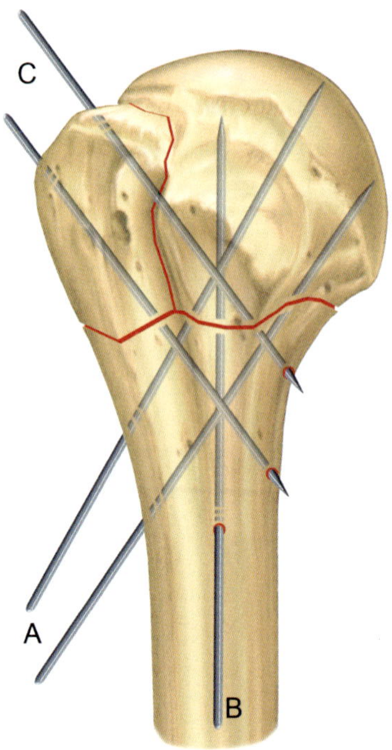

Figure 18. Percutaneous fixation of a 2-part surgical-neck fracture. A, Two pins are placed from inferior and lateral into the articular segment. B, The third pin is placed from anterior and distal into the articular segment. C, Two additional pins are placed to stabilize a greater tuberosity fragment, if present.

anterior and distal position into the articular segment. Finally, 2 more pins are added to stabilize a nondisplaced, greater tuberosity fragment, if present (Figure 18).[7]

Two-part surgical-neck fractures that are not reducible closed require ORIF that usually includes locking-plate osteosynthesis.

3-Part Fractures

Three-part proximal humerus fractures are surgical-neck fractures with 1 displaced tuberosity fragment. That fragment can be the greater or lesser tuberosity (Figure 19). Closed reduction of these fractures is difficult; therefore, surgery generally is indicated to treat this fracture pattern. The surgical options include interfragmentary fixation with sutures or wires, percutaneous pinning, ORIF with a locking plate and screws, and humeral head replacement. Rarely is humeral head replacement an option for 3-part proximal humerus fractures unless the bone is severely osteoporotic or the fractures involve the anatomic neck. Usually, humeral head replacement is reserved for 4-part fractures.

Interfragmentary fixation is an established method of treatment for 3-part fractures. Adequate fixation requires horizontal and vertical stability of the fractured parts. Heavy, nonabsorbable sutures or wires must be passed through the tendon-bone interface of the displaced tuberosity fragment. Accurate placement of the sutures or wires into the humeral head in the anteroposterior and superoinferior directions is imperative.[7] The drill holes in the humeral shaft fragment are placed medial and lateral to the bicipital groove, approximately 1 to 2 cm distal to the surgical-neck fracture site. The sutures that are passed through the drill holes and into the tuberosity and humeral head are tied in a figure-of-8 fashion.

Hawkins et al[19] demonstrated satisfactory results in 12 of 14 patients treated with interfragmentary fixation for 3-part fractures, and on average, patients obtained forward elevation to 120°. Two patients developed osteonecrosis.[19]

Percutaneous pinning is another operative treatment option for 3-part fractures, but this technique is difficult to perform. The appropriate patient has good bone stock, has minimal comminution, and is cooperative after surgery. These fractures are difficult to reduce closed, and after reducing them, the surgeon must have advanced skill to maintain the reduction for successful treatment.[7] Resch et al[20] showed good to very good functional results with percutaneous pinning for these fractures and found no radiographic evidence of avascular necrosis at 24-month follow-up.

The most commonly performed procedure for 3-part proximal humerus fractures is ORIF with a locking, anatomic proximal humeral plate. These plates have revolutionized the treatment of proximal humerus fractures. Biomechanical data have demonstrated

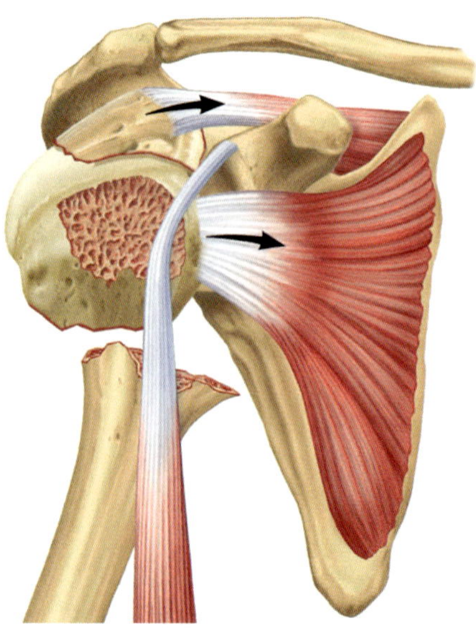

Figure 19. Three-part greater tuberosity fracture.

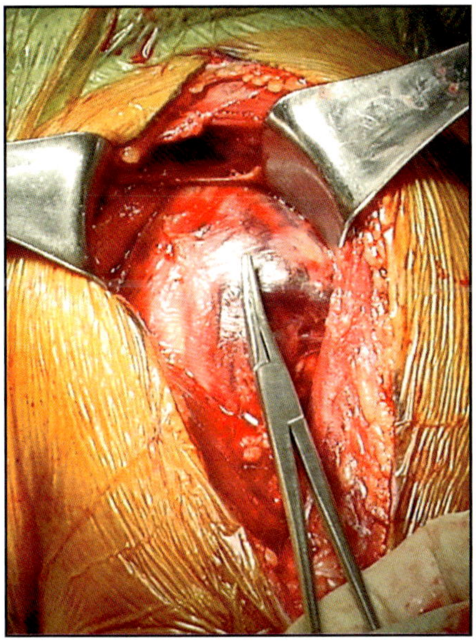

Figure 20. Deltopectoral approach.

significantly higher maximum loads to failure and significantly less loosening after torsional loading for proximal humeral locking plates than standard plates for fractures of the proximal humerus.[21–23] The indication for a proximal humeral locking plate is a displaced fracture with a viable humeral head.

The deltopectoral approach provides direct exposure of the fracture for ORIF with a proximal humeral locking plate (Figure 20). When the approach is complete, the tuberosity fragment must be reduced to the humeral head with interfragmentary sutures. After reducing the tuberosity to the humeral head and shaft, the surgeon applies the proximal humeral locking plate (Figure 21). Note that passing the sutures through the plate is a critical step in securing these fractures and creating tension bands for the abduction, external rotation, and internal rotation forces that are applied during rehabilitation. Fluoroscopy is used to confirm adequate reduction of the fracture and appropriate positioning of the plate.

Authors of early outcome studies have found good to excellent functional results when using ORIF to treat 3-part proximal humerus fractures.[24] However, Koukakis et al[25] described complications from screw displacement and cutout from the humeral head. Using good technique and leaving screws nearly 5 mm from the subchondral bone help to avoid these complications (Figure 22).

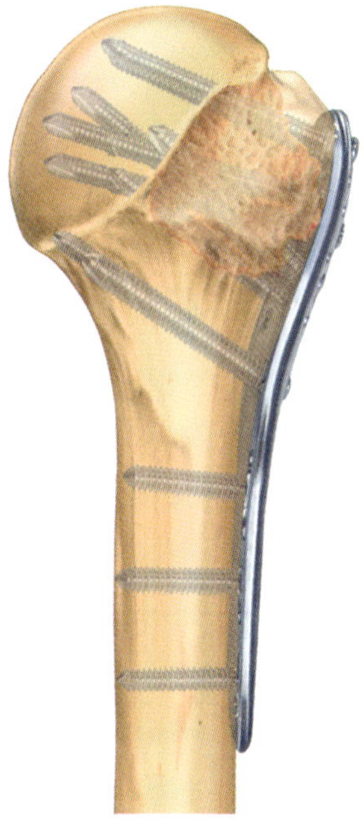

Figure 22. Proximal humeral locking plate.

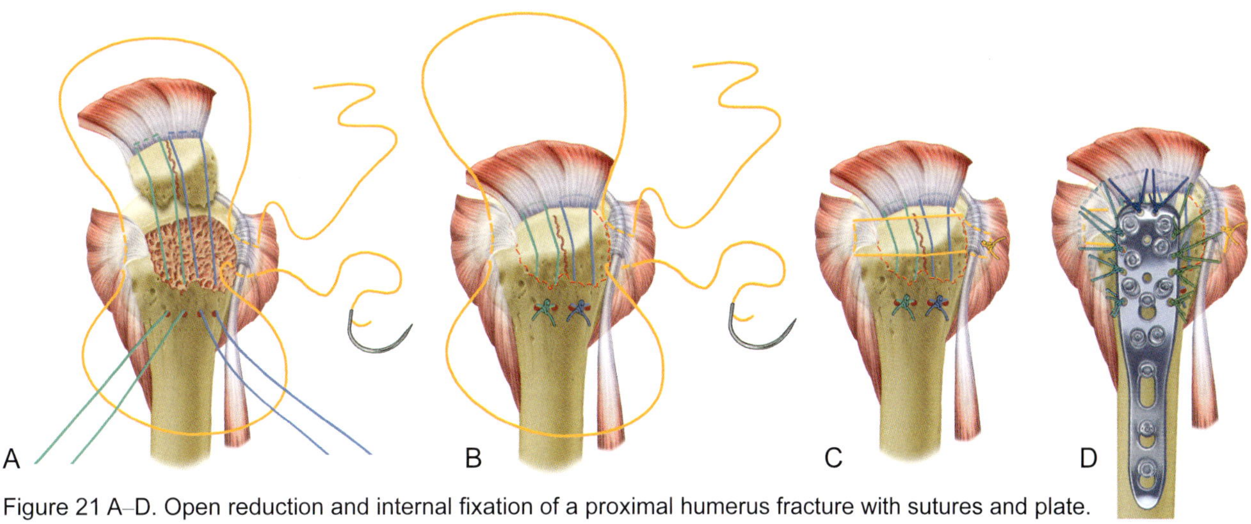

Figure 21 A–D. Open reduction and internal fixation of a proximal humerus fracture with sutures and plate.

4-Part Fractures

Four-part proximal humerus fractures include surgical-neck, greater tuberosity, and lesser tuberosity fractures with displacement of fracture fragments greater than 1 cm or with greater than 45° of angulation (Figures 23 and 24). The incidence of avascular necrosis is 90% with 4-part fractures.[6] As mentioned, good predictors of ischemia and ultimately of avascular necrosis are the length of the medial calcar and opening of the medial hinge (Figures 5 and 6). Immediate humeral head replacement is necessary when vascularity of the head is compromised.

Operative principles that must be maintained during a humeral head replacement include restoration of humeral length, restoration of retroversion, and secure fixation of the tuberosities. Length can be determined by using preoperative radiographs and by using the medial calcar as a guide to the appropriate location of the inferomedial aspect of the new humeral head. Some implants provide a "fracture jig" that also can help with length restoration. Retroversion is assessed intraoperatively and usually is restored with alignment rods from the fracture system.

The surgeon makes a standard deltopectoral approach to the proximal humerus. Usually, a vertical fracture plane exists at the intertubercular groove, and when the surgeon finds the long head of the biceps tendon, he or she finds the fracture line (Figure 25). The biceps tendon is released, and a subpectoralis tenodesis is performed with nonabsorbable sutures (Figure 26). Next, an osteotome is inserted in the groove between the tuberosities, separating them (Figure 27). Both the lesser and greater tuberosities are then tagged with heavy no. 5 suture (Figure 28). The

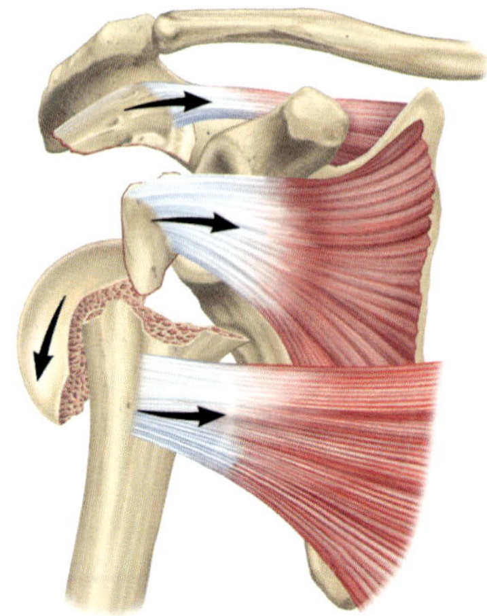

Figure 23. Four-part proximal humerus fracture.

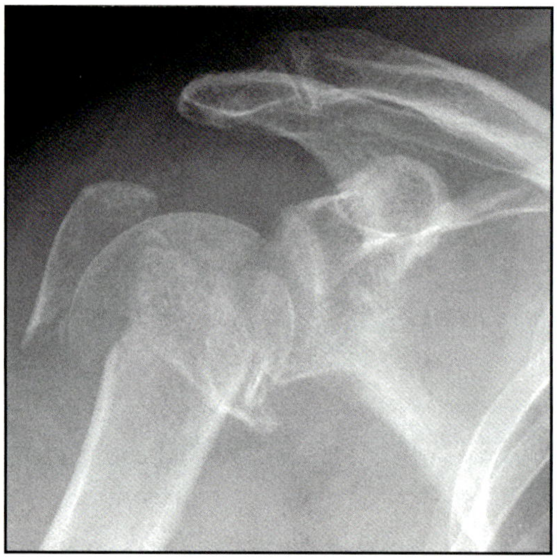

Figure 24. Radiograph shows a 4-part proximal humerus fracture.

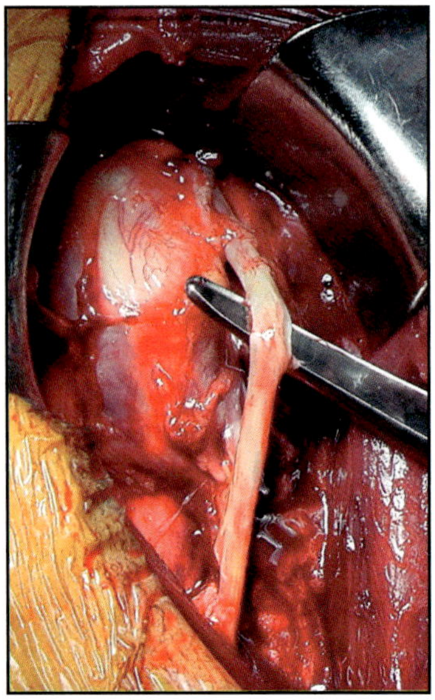

Figure 25. The long head of the biceps helps to identify the vertical fracture line.

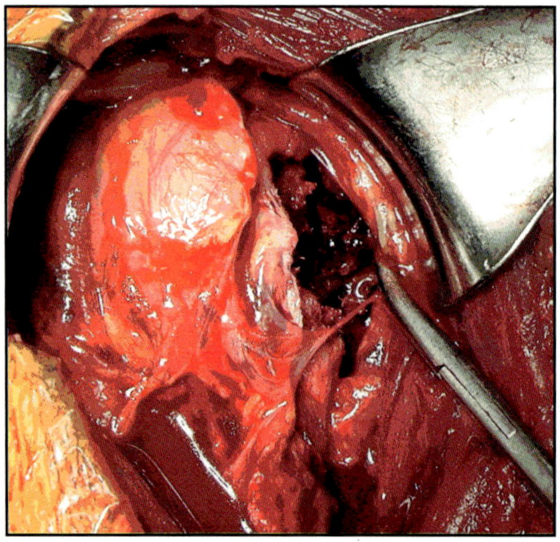

Figure 26. Subpectoralis tenodesis.

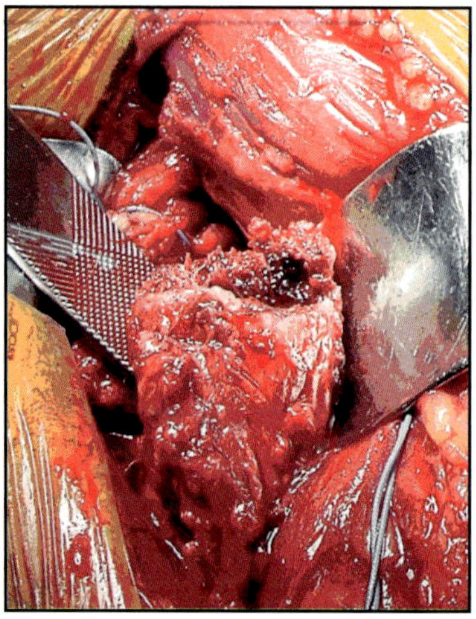

Figure 27. Osteotome separates the parts of the tuberosity fracture.

rotator interval is released to help "open" the fracture and retrieve the anatomic head (Figure 29).

The surgeon must protect the neurovascular structures if the humeral head is dislocated anteromedially. Routine inspection of the glenoid should be performed to determine if resurfacing is required.

Next, the surgeon uses the native head as a template to determine appropriate head size. The humeral shaft is delivered from the surgical wound and reamed appropriately (Figure 30). After reaming the proximal humeral shaft and determining the appropriate length, version (20°–30°), and humeral head size that is needed, the surgeon can prepare the humeral prosthesis and humeral shaft (Figure 31).

As noted, an operative principle is secure fixation of the tuberosities. Understanding the fracture planes and where postoperative forces exist helps to explain why creation of tension bands is critical to the success of tuberosity fixation. The tuberosities experience tension after surgery at the horizontal fracture lines, which exist between them and the humeral shaft, and at the vertical fracture lines, which exist between them (Figure 1). Therefore, tension-band constructs must be created to resist these tension forces and to convert them to compression. The first series of tension bands should be constructed between the tuberosities and the shaft. These vertical tension bands resist the tension of the horizontal fracture lines. Transosseous sutures placed through the humeral shaft before humeral stem insertion create these bands (Figure 32).

The prosthesis also is prepared before insertion into the shaft and includes insertion of sutures through the

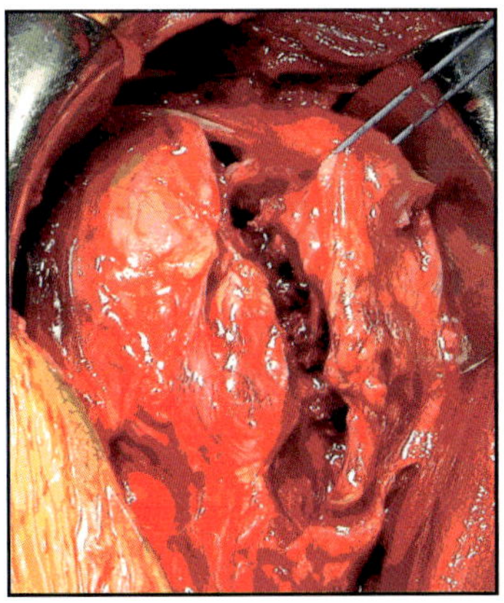

Figure 28. Lesser and greater tuberosities are tagged with sutures.

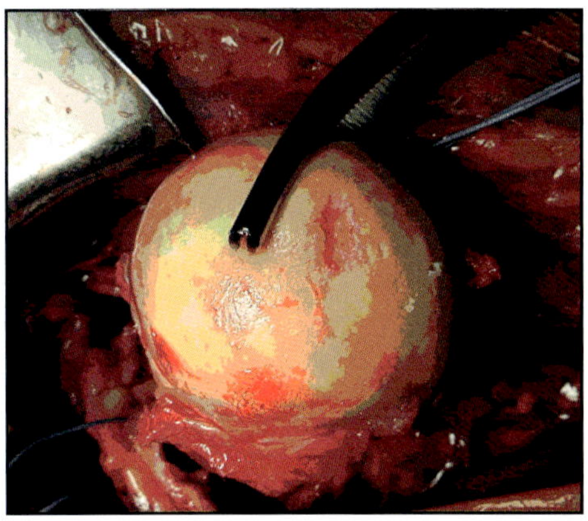

Figure 29. The humeral head is exposed and retrieved.

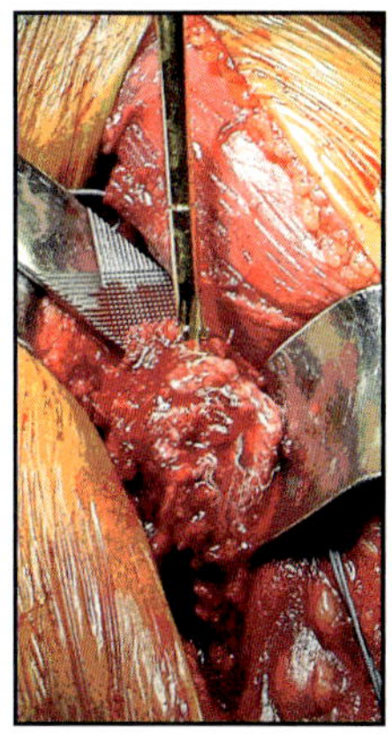

Figure 30. The humeral shaft is reamed.

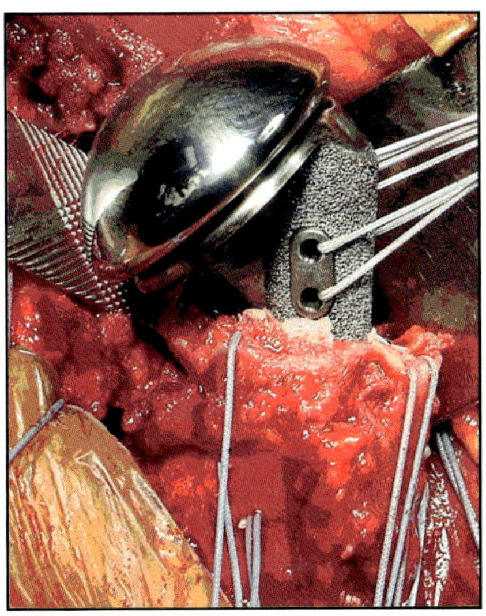

Figure 31. Placement of the humeral head prosthesis.

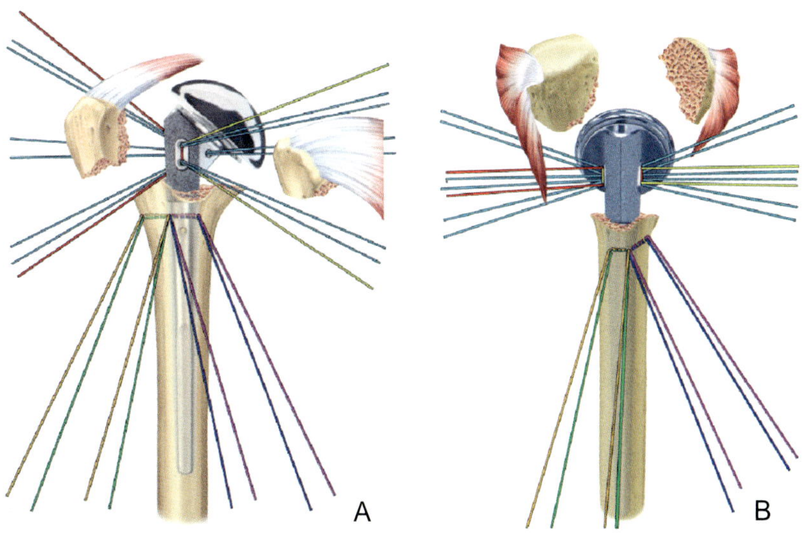

Figure 32. Transosseous suture placement through the humeral shaft. A, Anteroposterior view. B, Lateral view.

Figure 33 A and B. Cerclage sutures first are passed at the bone-tendon interface of the tuberosities.

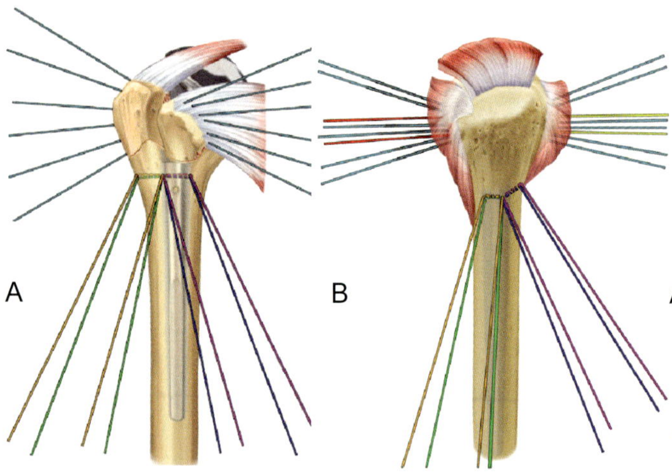

Figure 34 A and B. When tied, the cerclage sutures create the horizontal tension band.

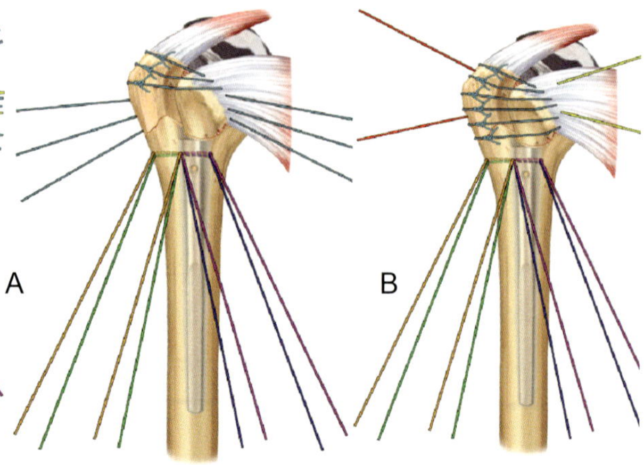

Figure 35. Completed horizontal tension bands.

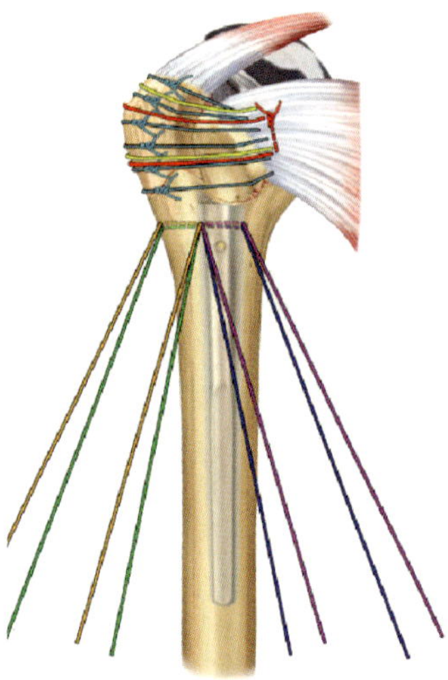

Figure 36. Vertical tension bands are created in a figure-of-8 fashion.

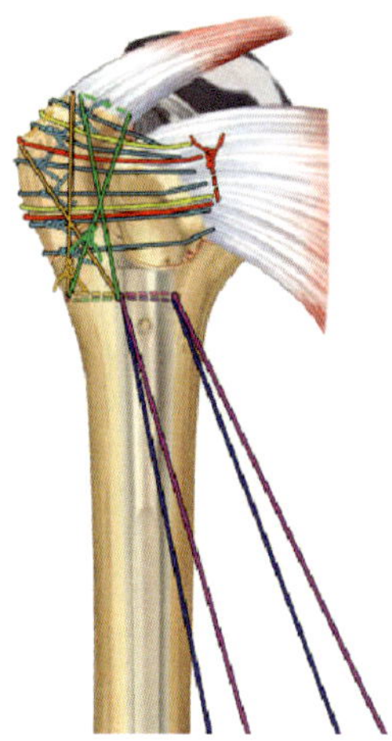

Figure 37. Completed vertical tension bands.

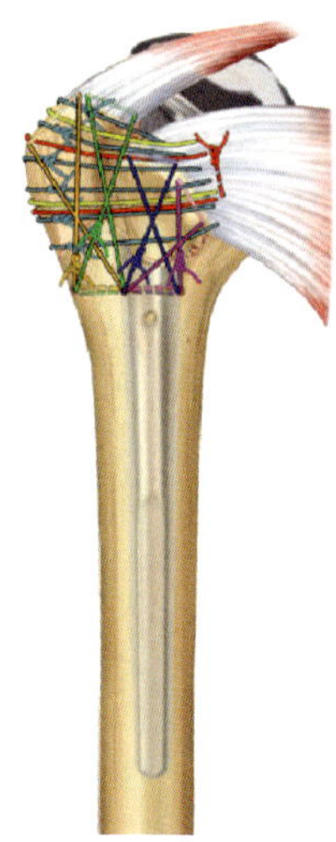

Figure 38. Lateral view shows complete fixation.

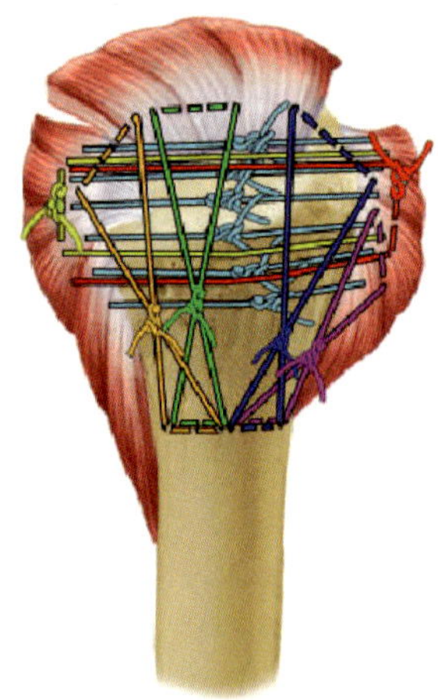

prosthetic holes or around the medial fin. These sutures serve as cerclage-type fixation and create the second series of tension bands. These horizontal tension bands resist the tension of the vertical fracture lines. Frankle et al[26] showed that the tension between the tuberosities decreases with cerclage fixation, such as this type.

After appropriate preparation of the shaft and prosthesis, the surgeon can insert the final prosthesis. The humeral stem always is cemented into the shaft when humeral head replacement is chosen for proximal humerus fractures. The cement prevents stem derotation that can occur secondary to the fractured tuberosities. A cement restrictor should be placed in the humeral shaft approximately 10 mm distal to the tip of the prosthesis to help ensure an adequate cement mantle interface. The final prosthesis is inserted while the surgeon maintains proper humeral height and version (Figure 31).

When the humeral stem is secure within the shaft, the surgeon reconstructs the tuberosities. Suture management and patience are critical throughout this step. Usually, cerclage sutures initially are passed at the bone-tendon interface of the greater tuberosity and lesser tuberosity (Figure 33). These cerclage sutures are tied, securing the tuberosities to the prothesis and creating the horizontal tension band that resists tension between the tuberosities with rotation, such as during rehabilitation (Figures 34 and 35).

With the tuberosities secured to the prosthesis, the surgeon creates the vertical tension bands. The sutures that previously were passed through the transosseous shaft tunnels are passed superiorly at the tendon-bone interface in a figure-of-8 fashion. They are distributed evenly from posterior to anterior (Figures 36–38). The surgeon completes standard closure of the shoulder (Figure 39). When anatomic positioning of the humeral head and tuberosities is performed, good and excellent functional results can be achieved.[2,27]

Malposition, malunion, or nonunion of the tuberosity results in poor functional outcomes. The success of the tuberosities healing and healing in good position initially depends on secure fixation and on implant design. The proximal aspect of the humeral component must enable maximum bone contact between the tuberosities and should be compatible with bony ongrowth or ingrowth. Krishnan et al[27] demonstrated excellent functional results in more than 80% of patients treated with humeral head replacement for proximal humerus fractures. They also presented the importance of restoring the "gothic arch" of the shoulder girdle. This arch is formed by the medial border of the proximal humeral shaft to the edge of the articular surface and is joined by the lateral border of the scapula.[27]

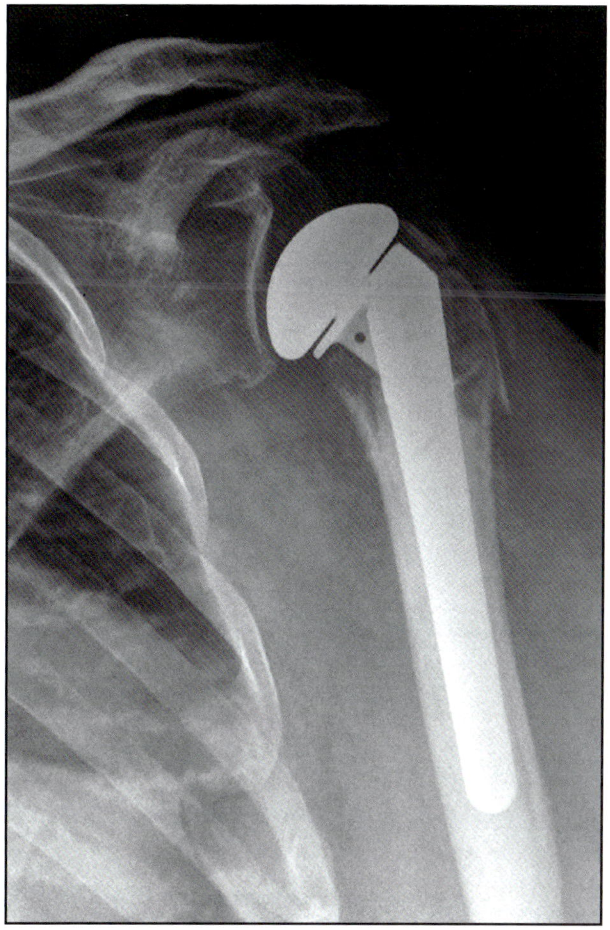

Figure 39. Radiograph shows the prosthesis in place.

Fracture-Dislocations, Articular Surface Fractures, and Epiphyseal Fractures

Fracture-Dislocations. The 6 types of proximal humerus fracture-dislocations include 2-part anterior (greater tuberosity), 2-part posterior (lesser tuberosity), 3-part anterior (surgical-neck and greater tuberosity), 3-part posterior (surgical-neck and lesser tuberosity), 4-part anterior, and 4-part posterior. The 2-part fracture-dislocations initially are treated with closed reduction. Usually, the tuberosity fragment reduces adequately, but if it does not, operative treatment is recommended. The remaining proximal humerus fracture-dislocations are treated with open reduction of the humeral head and operative management according to the fracture pattern. Care for these injuries often is complicated by neurovascular compromise. Angiography is performed immediately for any suspected case of vascular injury associated with proximal humerus fracture-dislocations.

Articular Surface Fractures. The 2 most common articular surface fractures of the proximal humerus are impression fractures and head-splitting fractures. Humeral head impression defects most often occur with posterior dislocations. The treatment of this injury depends on the size of the head defect. If the impression encompasses less than 20% of the humeral head, then these fractures are usually stable after closed reduction, and immobilization of the extremity in an external rotation sling for 6 weeks is adequate. If the defect encompasses 20% to 45% of the articular surface, then a McLaughlin transfer is indicated. This procedure consists of transferring the lesser tuberosity and subscapularis into the humeral head defect. Furthermore, a defect that encompasses more than 45% of the humeral head or a dislocation that is present for more than 6 months is treated with a humeral head replacement. A

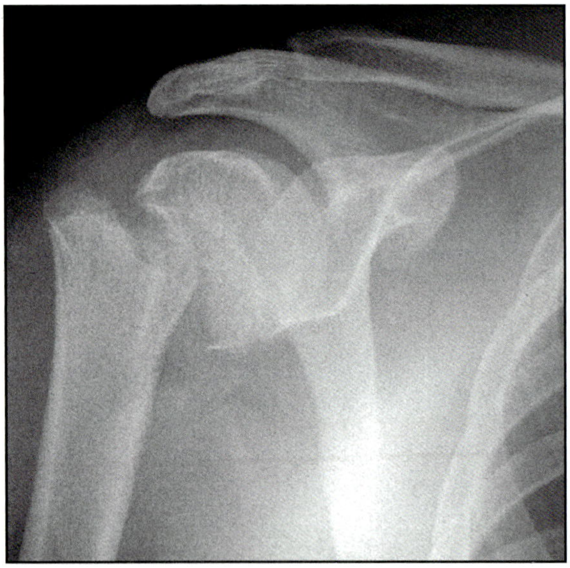

Figure 40. Radiograph depicts a humeral head-splitting fracture of the proximal humerus. Note the double-density sign of the articular surfaces.

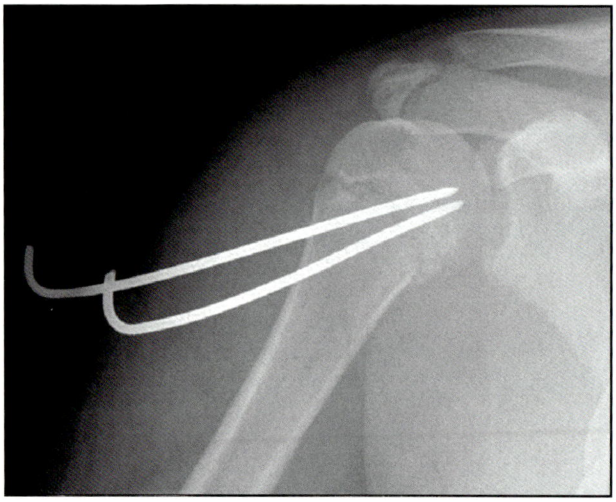

Figure 41. Prereduction radiograph shows a proximal humerus epiphyseal fracture treated with closed reduction and percuteneous pinning.

humeral head-splitting fracture is treated with humeral head replacement, as well (Figure 40).

Epiphyseal Fractures. Epiphyseal fractures occur in children who are skeletally immature. These fractures are classified according to the Salter-Harris classification system. The most common epiphyseal fracture of the proximal humerus is a Salter-Harris type 2 fracture. This injury affects both the physis and metaphysis of the proximal humerus. When these fractures are displaced substantially, they must be treated with closed reduction and percutaneous pinning, as indicated (Figures 41).

CONCLUSIONS

Proximal humerus fractures are very common injuries in the elderly population. Management of each proximal humerus fracture must be individualized. Associated injuries must be diagnosed accurately and treated appropriately. Next, the surgeon should classify the fracture and choose an appropriate treatment algorithm. When operative management is necessary, options include percutaneous pinning, ORIF, and humeral head replacement. No single technique can be applied to all proximal humerus fractures. The surgeon should be comfortable with all treatment options and should be able to convert from one to another option, as necessary.

REFERENCES

1. Nordqvist A, Petersson CJ. Incidence and causes of shoulder girdle injuries in an urban population. *J Shoulder Elbow Surg.* 1995;4(2):107–112.
2. Krishnan SG, Lin KC, Burkhead WZ. "Pins, plates, and prostheses": current concepts in treatment of fractures of the proximal humerus. *Curr Opin Orthop.* 2007;18(4):380–385.
3. Green A. Proximal humerus fractures. In: Norris TR, ed. *Orthopaedic Knowledge Update: Shoulder and Elbow 2.* Rosemont, IL: American Academy of Orthopaedic Surgeons; 2002:209–217.
4. Palvanen M, Kannus P, Niemi S, Parkkari J. Update in the epidemiology of proximal humeral fractures. *Clin Orthop Relat Res.* 2006;442:87–92.
5. Hartmann A, Resch H. Treatment of proximal humerus fractures. In: Galatz LM, ed. *Orthopaedic Knowledge Update: Shoulder and Elbow 3.* Rosemont, IL: American Academy of Orthopaedic Surgeons; 2008:405–421.
6. Schlegel TF, Hawkins RJ. Displaced proximal humeral fractures: evaluation and treatment. *J Am Acad Orthop Surg.* 1994;2(1):54–78.
7. Iannotti JP, Ramsey ML, Williams GR Jr, Warner JJP. Nonprosthetic management of proximal humeral fractures. *J Bone Joint Surg Am.* 2003;85(8):1578–1593.
8. Gerber C, Schneeberger AG, Vinh TS. The arterial vascularization of the humeral head: an anatomical study. *J Bone Joint Surg Am.* 1990;72(10):1486–1494.
9. Hertel R, Hempfing A, Stiehler M, Leunrig M. Predictors of humeral head ischemia after intracapsular fractures of the proximal humerus. *J Shoulder Elbow Surg.* 2004;13(4):427–433.

10. Steinmann SP, Moran EA. Axillary nerve injury: diagnosis and treatment. *J Am Acad Orthop Surg*. 2001;9(5):328–335.
11. Kocher T. Beitrage zur Kenntnis einiger praktisch wichtiger Fracturenformen. Basel, Switzerland: Carl Sallman Verlag; 1896.
12. Codman EA. *The Shoulder: Rupture of the Supraspinatus Tendon and Other Lesions in and About the Subacromial Bursa*. Boston, MA: T Todd; 1934.
13. Neer CS II. Displaced proximal humeral fractures, II: treatment of three-part and four-part displacement. *J Bone Joint Surg Am*. 1970;52(6):1090–1103.
14. Neer CS II. Displaced proximal humeral fractures, I: classification and evaluation. *J Bone Joint Surg Am*. 1970;52(6): 1077–1089.
15. Bernstein, J, Adler LM, Blank JE, Dalsey RM, Williams GR, Iannotti JP. Evaluation of the Neer system of classification of proximal humeral fractures with computerized tomographic scans and plain radiographs. *J Bone Joint Surg Am*. 1996;78(9): 1371–1375.
16. Edelson G, Kelly I, Vigder F, Reis ND. A three-dimensional classification for fractures of the proximal humerus. *J Bone Joint Surg Br*. 2004;86(3):413–425.
17. Hodgson SA, Mawson SJ, Saxton JM, Stanley D. Rehabilitation of two-part fractures of the neck of the humerus (two-year follow-up). *J Shoulder Elbow Surg*. 2007;16(2):143–145.
18. Koval KJ, Gallagher MA, Marsicano JG, Cuomo F, McShinawy A, Zuckerman JD. Functional outcome after minimally displaced fractures of the proximal part of the humerus. *J Bone Joint Surg Am*. 1997;79(2):203–207.
19. Hawkins RJ, Bell RH, Gurr K. The three-part fracture of the proximal part of the humerus: operative treatment. *J Bone Joint Surg Am*. 1986;68(9):1410–1414.
20. Resch H, Povacz P, Fröhlich R, Wambacher M. Percutaneous fixation of three- and four-part fractures of the proximal humerus. *J Bone Joint Surg Br*. 1997;79(2):295–300.
21. Siffri PC, Peindl RD, Coley ER, Norton J, Connor PM, Kellam JF. Biomechanical analysis of blade plate versus locking plate fixation for a proximal humerus fracture: comparison using cadaveric and synthetic humeri. *J Orthop Trauma*. 2006;20(8):547–554.
22. Walsh S, Reindl R, Harvey E, Berry G, Beckman L, Steffen T. Biomechanical comparison of a unique locking plate versus a standard plate for internal fixation of proximal humerus fractures in a cadaveric model. *Clin Biomech (Bristol, Avon)*. 2006;21(10):1027–1031.
23. Weinstein DM, Bratton DR, Ciccone WJ II, Elias JJ. Locking plates improve torsional resistance in the stabilization of three-part proximal humeral fractures. *J Shoulder Elbow Surg*. 2006;15(2):239–243.
24. Owsley KC, Gorczyca JT. Fracture displacement and screw cutout after open reduction and locked plate fixation of proximal humeral fractures. *J Bone Joint Surg Am*. 2008;90(2):233–240.
25. Koukakis A, Apostolou CD, Taneja T, Korres DS, Amini A. Fixation of proximal humerus fractures using the PHILOS plate: early experience. *Clin Orthop Relat Res*. 2006;442:115–120.
26. Frankle MA, Ondrovic LE, Markee BA, Harris ML, Lee WE III. Stability of tuberosity reattachment in proximal humeral hemiarthroplasty. *J Shoulder Elbow Surg*. 2002;11(5):413–420.
27. Krishnan SG, Pennington SD, Burkhead WZ, Boileau P. Shoulder arthroplasty for fracture: restoration of the "gothic arch." *Tech Shoulder Elbow Surg*. 2005;6(2):57–66.

RECOMMENDED READING

Beredjiklian PK, Iannotti JP, Norris TR, Williams GR. Operative treatment of malunion of a fracture of the proximal aspect of the humerus. *J Bone Joint Surg Am*. 1998;80(10):1484–1497.

Boileau P, Krishnan SG, Tinsi L, Walch G, Coste JS, Molé D. Tuberosity malposition and migration: reasons for poor outcomes after hemiarthroplasty for displaced fractures of the proximal humerus. *J Shoulder Elbow Surg*. 2002;11(5):401–412.

Kannus P, Palvanen M, Niemi S, Parkkari J, Järvinen M, Vuori I. Increasing number and incidence of osteoporotic fractures of the proximal humerus in elderly people. *BMJ*. 1996;313(7064):1051–1052.

Naranja RJ Jr, Iannotti JP. Displaced three- and four-part proximal humerus fractures: evaluation and management. *J Am Acad Orthop Surg*. 2000;8(6):373–382.

Norris TR, Green A, McGuigan FX. Late prosthetic shoulder arthroplasty for displaced proximal humerus fractures. *J Shoulder Elbow Surg*. 1995;4(4):271–280.

Pollock RG. Tissues of the shoulder and their structure. In: Norris TR, ed. *Orthopaedic Knowledge Update: Shoulder and Elbow 2*. Rosemont, IL: American Academy of Orthopaedic Surgeons; 2002:3–12.

Sidor ML, Zuckerman JD, Lyon T, Koval K, Cuomo F, Schoenberg N. The Neer classification system for proximal humeral fractures: an assessment of interobserver reliability and intraobserver reproducibility. *J Bone Joint Surg Am*. 1993;75(12):1745–1750.

Foundations of Shoulder Rehabilitation

Section II

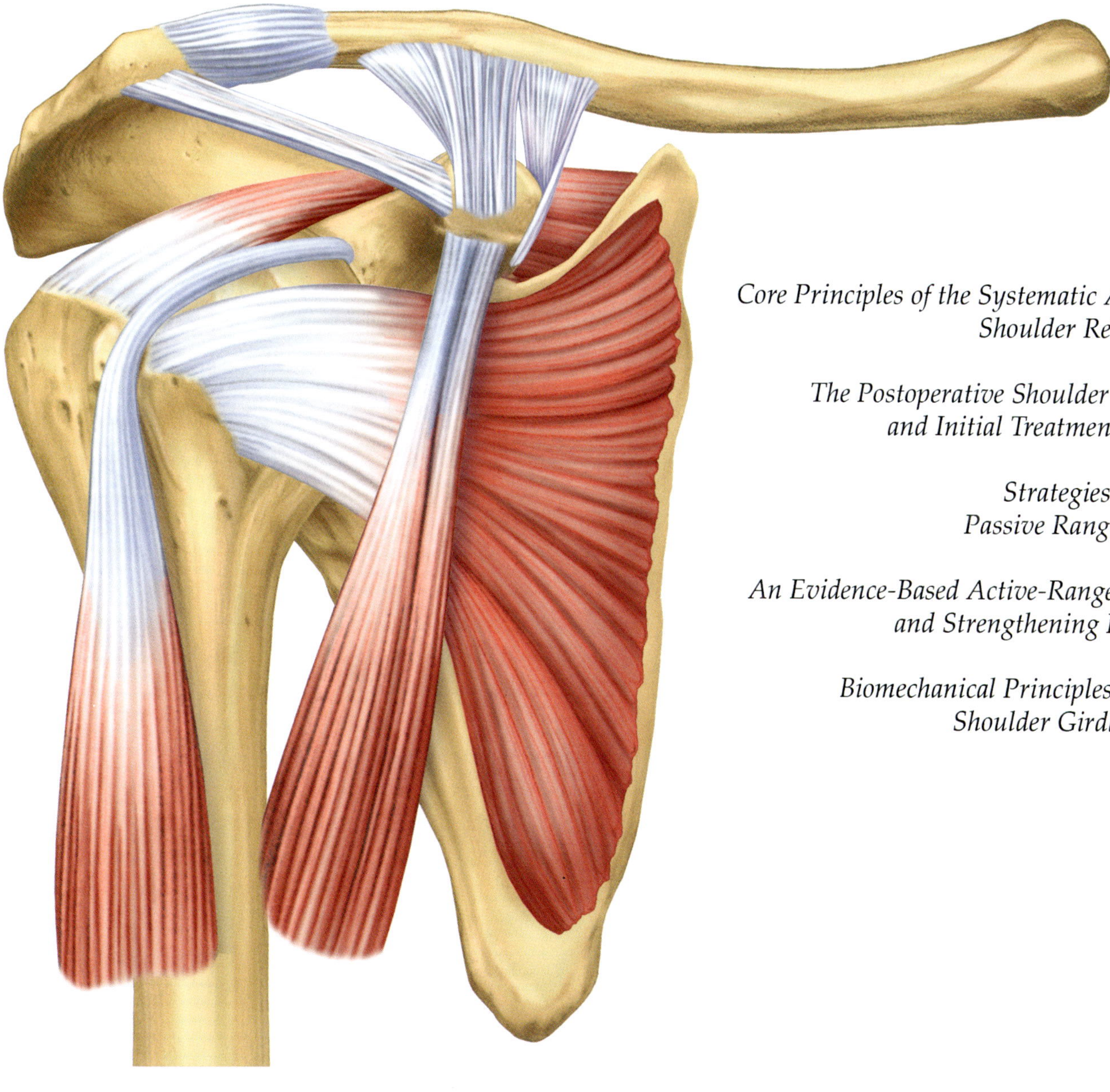

II-1

Core Principles of the Systematic Approach to Shoulder Rehabilitation

Bryce W. Gaunt, PT, SCS

CHAPTER CONTENTS

Clinical pearls are highlighted in yellow throughout the text.

In this chapter, I discuss the guiding rehabilitation principles that are specific to the system of shoulder rehabilitation used at HPRC at St. Francis Rehabilitation Center and St. Francis Orthopaedic Institute. We recognize that skilled rehabilitation is both an art and a science. As such, we recognize the need for theoretical foundations on which to base treatment. The following principles guide our clinical decision-making process as we determine the specific interventions to prescribe. The main principles specific to our approach are that we

1. are always gentle,
2. use prioritized principles of the clinical decision-making process,
3. have an "aversion" to abduction, and
4. believe that the details of rehabilitation are important.

ALWAYS GENTLE

We recognize that shoulder rehabilitation includes many levels of aggressiveness; however, this aggressiveness can be condensed to 2 rehabilitation philosophies that can be summed up as follows: (1) a sore thumb does not get better when you hit it with a hammer and (2) no pain, no gain. The first philosophy promotes an "always gentle" style of rehabilitation and conveys the point that not all rehabilitation is productive. It also recognizes that if anatomic structures are inflamed, more aggressive rehabilitation at some point will only increase the level of inflammation. On the other hand, the second philosophy (no pain, no gain) implies that aggressive rehabilitation is required for maximum effectiveness. In my experience, many rehabilitation providers who subscribe to the always gentle philosophy do not adopt it completely. However, my experience also has shown that treatment that is halfway between always gentle and no pain, no gain is not as effective as treatment that is always gentle. Maximum effectiveness in this philosophy requires that it be used consistently and completely.

Next, let us examine the attributes of each style of treatment more closely, studying the assumed positive and negative attributes of each style. The positive attributes of the always gentle philosophy are that it promotes healing of an operative repair and provides early pain relief. Positive attributes for the no pain, no gain approach are that it might promote a quicker return of range of motion (ROM) and might decrease the need for manipulation under anesthesia in a patient with shoulder stiffness. On the surface, the negative attributes of the always gentle approach seem to include an increased chance of postoperative stiffness, a delay in achievement of full ROM, and a delay in achievement of full function. The negative attributes of the no pain, no gain approach might be an increased chance of disrupting an operative repair and an elevated level of pain and inflammation during all stages of rehabilitation. Examining the positives and negatives of each approach, we believe that the negatives of the no pain, no gain approach are more detrimental than the negatives of the always gentle approach, especially in the patient who has had surgery. Later in this chapter, I discuss how rehabilitation that results in excessive pain and inflammation can be counterproductive to successful rehabilitation.[1,2] I also share evidence that suggests that gentle rehabilitation is superior to aggressive and highly painful therapy in rehabilitation of patients with shoulder stiffness.[1] Therefore, the assumed negatives of the always gentle approach likely are minimized. For these reasons, our systematic approach to shoulder rehabilitation subscribes to the always gentle style.

Although recognizing the importance of the always gentle approach is vital, the more difficult part of following this philosophy is being able to implement interventions that follow this guideline. To help us as rehabilitation providers do this, we must recognize our role in the recovery process of the patient. We need to realize that each patient whom we rehabilitate has a variable potential of ROM, strength, and function, which is demonstrated in Figure 1. The bottom of the bar signifies no functional use of the upper extremity. The top of the bar signifies perfect shoulder function. Each patient has his or her unique potential for improvement that might not include perfect shoulder function. This potential for improvement depends on many factors that include inherent patient variables, such as age, medical comorbidities, specific conditions present in the shoulder girdle, and the skill of the surgeon if an operation was performed. The presence, severity, and interaction of these factors determine the size and location of the patient's functional potential. Some patients whom we rehabilitate will have great potential for improvement (patient A, Figure 1), and some will have a small potential for improvement (patient B, Figure 1). In some patients, this potential for improvement will be shifted toward normal function (patient A, Figure 1), and in some patients, it will be shifted toward poor function (patient B, Figure 1). Given this, I believe the purpose of rehabilitation is to determine how much of this potential for improvement the patient actually will achieve. Some patients will maximize their full potential, and some will not (Figure 2). The amount of the patient's unique potential for

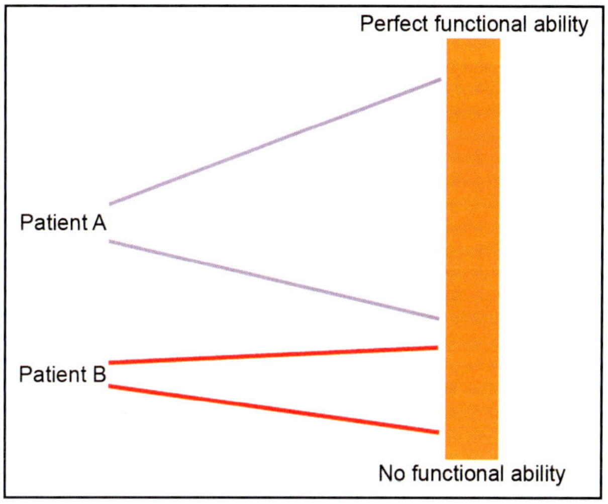

Figure 1. The gold bar demonstrates the range of shoulder function possible (from none to perfect). Patient A (purple bars) has a fairly large potential for functional improvement skewed toward a high level of function. Patient B (red bars) has a smaller potential for functional improvement that also is skewed toward a poorer level of function.

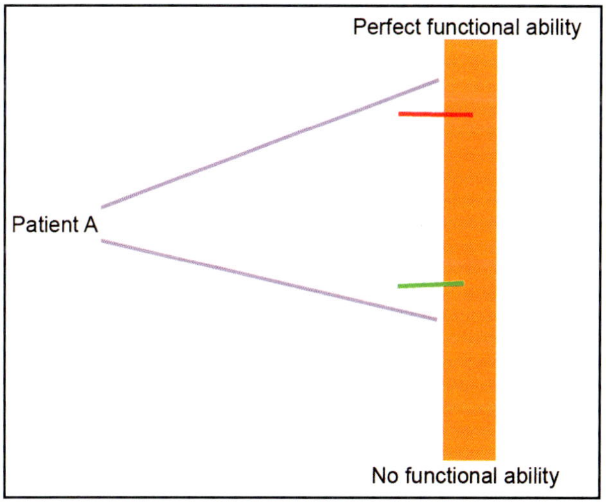

Figure 2. Ultimate patient outcome within a patient's functional potential is determined by the patient's effort during rehabilitation and the rehabilitation provider's skill. The red line demonstrates nearly optimal rehabilitation in which the patient and rehabilitation provider achieved nearly maximum functional potential. The green line demonstrates a poor rehabilitation outcome; the patient and rehabilitation provider achieved an outcome in which a patient's full functional potential was not realized.

functional improvement that is realized is a combination of the patient's effort during rehabilitation and the rehabilitation provider's skill. When considering these Figures, the most important point to understand is that appropriate rehabilitation needs to stay within each patient's unique window of functional potential during treatment. Inappropriate rehabilitation employs interventions to rehabilitate the person to a level of function significantly higher than the potential of his or her shoulder (based on the factors described) (Figure 3). Using interventions to achieve goals that are not attainable because of physiologic limits of the tissue or structural integrity of the repair is one very common way that rehabilitation providers are too aggressive in rehabilitation, and it might result in disruption of the operative repair, if present, or more commonly in excessive pain and inflammation. By being always gentle with rehabilitation, the provider recognizes the importance of rehabilitation that respects the functional potential of the patient's shoulder and the slow speed at which injured and deconditioned tissue adapts to physical stress. The challenge of rehabilitation is determining what the patient's maximum potential is and selecting interventions that maximize it but do not attempt to surpass it. This is best determined in consultation with the referring physician and is assisted by clinical experience and adherence to prioritized principles of the clinical decision-making process detailed later in this chapter.

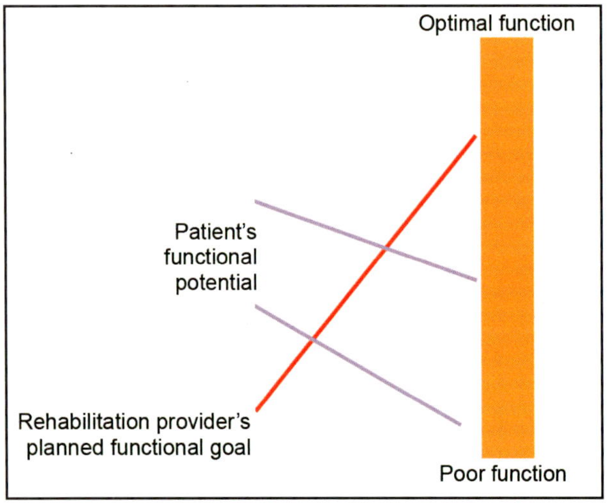

Figure 3. Inappropriate rehabilitation in which the rehabilitation provider's planned functional goals for the patient (red bar) are above the patient's functional potential (purple bars).

Always gentle rehabilitation is actually very hard to successfully accomplish because it is very easy to unknowingly overload injured or operatively repaired tissues during shoulder girdle rehabilitation. One reason that this is easy to do is because the rotator cuff muscles are very small muscles that are very mechanically disadvantaged, so fairly light external resistance can quickly overload these structures. Figures 4 and 5 provide practical illustrations of how mechanically disadvantaged the rotator cuff and deltoid are during elevation of the upper extremity, particularly with the elbow extended. In Figure 4, the way in which the child is holding the shovel is obviously not the most efficient way to hold and use it. However, in planning rehabilitation, we might not recognize that the shoulder is set up in the same mechanically disadvantaged way (Figure 5). In Figure 5, the child's right hand represents the head of the humerus. The left hand rep-

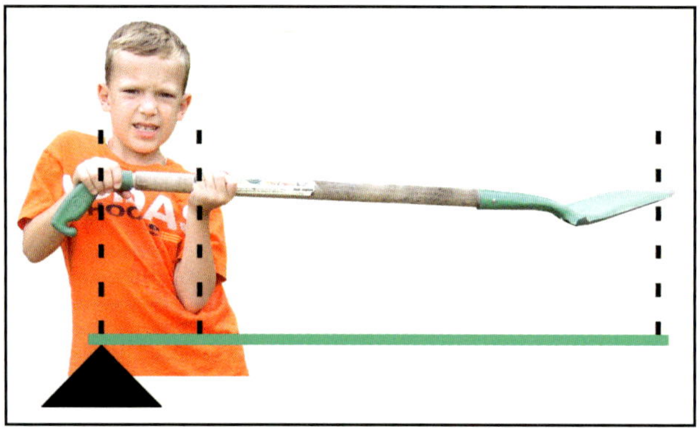

Figure 4. The inefficient use of a shovel demonstrates the disadvantaged lifting force of the left hand acting close to the fulcrum compared with the long lever resistance force of the shovel.

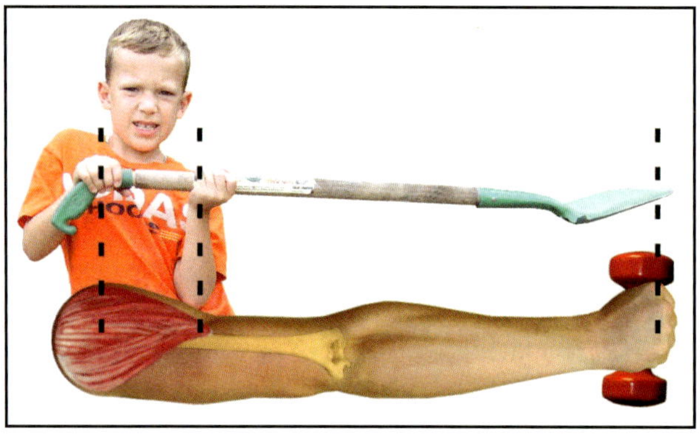

Figure 5. The similarities between using a shovel inefficiently and the mechanics of elevating the upper extremity with an extended elbow.

resents the combined resultant force of the rotator cuff and deltoid acting on the humerus and providing its force very close to the glenohumeral joint. The end of the shovel represents a patient's hand, demonstrating the long lever arm present when lifting a weight with an extended extremity compared with a short lever arm provided by the deltoid and rotator cuff muscles. Using this method to lift a heavy load with a shovel would not be wise because of the very large force needed to counter the load on the shovel. Similarly, even a very light weight lifted during rehabilitation is a significant load for the rotator cuff and deltoid to counteract when the elbow is extended. Therefore, we are very judicious in the selection of external resistance in this situation. We seldom recommend using more than 1 to 2 pounds (0.45–0.90 kg) for shoulder elevation with an extended elbow unless the patient is a skeletally mature athlete or has an occupation that requires repetitive heavy lifting above the shoulder level. In these situations, 3 to 5 pounds (1.35–2.25 kg) is generally the maximum weight used. Additionally, elastic resistance generally is not used for elevation of the extremity with the elbow extended because of the extremely high level of resistance it generates with this activity.

PRIORITIZED PRINCIPLES OF THE CLINICAL DECISION-MAKING PROCESS

Next, I will examine the prioritized principles that are used to guide the clinical decision-making process in our systematic approach to shoulder rehabilitation. These principles are the basis for all rehabilitation guidelines in our system and are the primary ways to ensure that we are always gentle during shoulder rehabilitation (Table 1).

Table 1. Prioritized Principles Used to Guide Clinical Decision Making in the Systematic Approach to Shoulder Rehabilitation

1. Protect healing tissue and the integrity of the operative repair.
2. Establish and maintain a low level of inflammation and pain.
3. Establish basic passive range of motion while decreasing pain.
4. Use progressive active range of motion and strengthening that maintains a low level of pain.
5. Use appropriate functional training.

1. Protect Healing Tissue and the Integrity of the Operative Repair.

The first and most important principle that rehabilitation providers should follow when beginning rehabilitation with every patient who has a shoulder condition and especially in patients after surgery is to determine how to protect the healing tissue and/or the integrity of the operative repair during *all rehabilitation interventions*. How this is specifically done with each disorder and operative procedure will be addressed fully in the specific rehabilitation chapters in this book. A simple way to think about this is to recognize that in all situations, rehabilitation is only safe when the strength of the operative repair or healing tissue, or both, is significantly greater than the stress that each rehabilitation exercise or intervention places on it. Adhering to this principle requires knowledge and evidence about rates of healing and strength of the operative repair, including how they change over time. Following this principle also requires that the rehabilitation provider know the general level of stress delivered by each rehabilitation intervention chosen and know how it compares with the strength of the healing tissue. A main purpose of each chapter in this book is to examine the evidence and interaction of these factors.

2. Establish and Maintain a Low Level of Inflammation and Pain.

In the systematic approach to shoulder rehabilitation, the second priority in the clinical decision-making process is that a low level of inflammation and pain should be established as quickly as possible during rehabilitation and maintained as rehabilitation advances. Inflammation obviously is required for the appropriate healing of all injured and operatively repaired tissues; however, evidence has shown that excessive inflammation might increase the chance of shoulder stiffness and also results in increased pain.[1,2] Diercks and Stevens[1] examined 77 patients with idiopathic adhesive capsulitis in a prospective, randomized study of supervised neglect versus intense physical therapy. The supervised neglect (or gentle) group performed pendulum exercises and ROM within a painless range.

The intense physical therapy (or aggressive) group performed ROM up to and beyond the threshold of pain and maximum stretching. All patients were re-examined every 3 months for 24 months. Outcomes were measured by the Constant shoulder score. For the gentle group, 64% had a Constant score greater than 80 by 12 months, and 89% had a Constant score greater than 80 at 24 months. For the aggressive group, 0% had a Constant score greater than 80 at 12 months, and 63% had a Constant score greater than 80 at 24 months. Therefore, the gentle group had vastly superior outcomes both in the short term and longer term and even long after rehabilitation had finished. The authors in part concluded, ". . . we believe that the effect of intensive passive stretching, as was done in our physical therapy group, probably had an adverse effect on the natural course of the disease process in the active phase."[1]

Looking more specifically at the negative effect that highly aggressive and painful therapy can have on shoulder rehabilitation on a microscopic level, Diercks and Stevens[1] suggested that aggressive stretching exacerbates the inflammatory process. Several authors have shown that inflammatory synovitis provokes hypervascular synovial hyperplasia, diffuse capsular fibroplasia, and contracture (Figure 6).[3–7] Figure 7 arthroscopically demonstrates a normal shoulder joint and capsule. The differences are striking and demonstrate the very high levels of inflammation, hypervascularity, and fibroplasia present in inflammatory synovitis. When this condition is present, the speed and course of rehabilitation are substantially limited. Authors of several studies have demonstrated that very gentle stretching is highly effective in restoring ROM and reducing pain over time[8–10] in patients with inflammatory synovitis and fibroplasia and is more effective than other methods of exercise.[11–13] Although most research in this area is directly related to adhesive capsulitis, we anecdotally have found that aggressive rehabilitation seems to exacerbate inflammatory synovitis, associated shoulder stiffness, and pain in other shoulder disorders and operative repairs, as well.

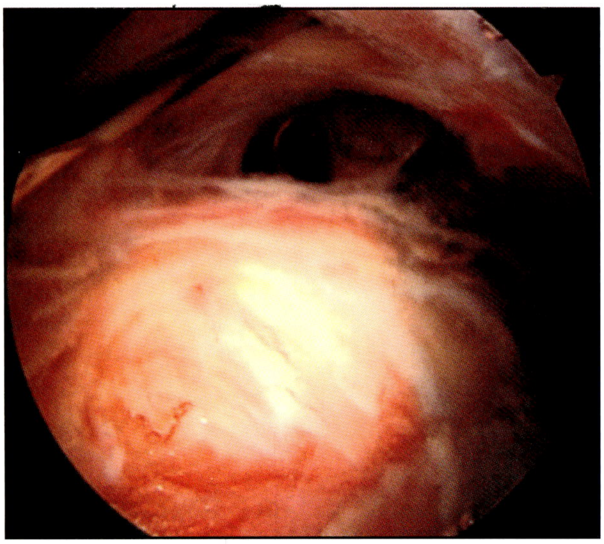

Figure 6. Inflammatory synovitis of the subacromial space.

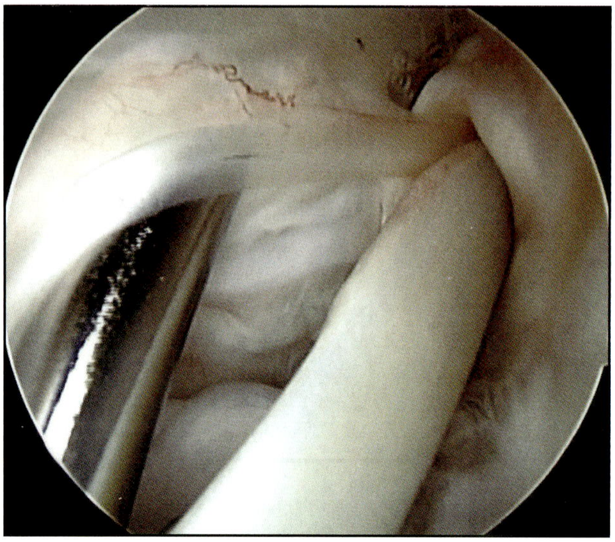

Figure 7. Normal glenohumeral joint and capsule at arthroscopy.

Even when only the level of inflammation is excessive and inflammatory synovitis is not present, aggressive and highly painful rehabilitation still negatively affects rehabilitation. This is demonstrated when the negative effect that aggressive and highly painful therapy has on shoulder rehabilitation is examined on the macroscopic level. Appropriate stretching of the glenohumeral joint moves the humerus on the glenoid with normal kinematics to the point of resistance and/or stretch of the soft tissues. Aggressive stretching goes past this point to where further movement of the humerus results in pinching of the structures in the shoulder, including structures in the subacromial space, such as the subacromial bursa and supraspinatus (Figure 8). Similarly, overly aggressive strengthening of the shoulder girdle surpasses the ability of the rotator cuff to center the humeral head in the glenoid and results in superior migration of the humeral head, which also causes pinching of the structures in the subacromial space. Repetitive pinching of these structures results in increased swelling of the subacromial bursa, increased pain, and potentially damaged tissue, which further inhibits the function of the rotator cuff.[14–17] This pain-related inhibition of the rotator cuff makes the structures of the subacromial space even easier to pinch during continued rehabilitation. This results in a vicious cycle that tends to further exacerbate signs and symptoms and that is difficult to resolve once well established.

Finally, from a clinical perspective, aggressive and highly painful therapy tends to result in increased muscle guarding by the patient, which yields a further decrease in ROM. Overly aggressive and highly painful therapy is also not pleasant to the patient and, therefore, typically negatively affects patient satisfaction and his or her attitude toward rehabilitation.

How is an appropriately low level of inflammation and pain established? The systematic approach to shoulder rehabilitation works to minimize inflammation and pain through the use of therapeutic modalities as needed but more importantly through appropriate exercise selection, volume, and intensity during both home and clinic exercises. Doing this well takes a high level of skill, diligence, and attention to detail. Appropriate use of the affected extremity with activities of daily living (ADLs), which typically involves limiting ADLs, is also a vital component of achieving a low level of pain and inflammation that frequently is overlooked. Often, it might be the most important component of achieving a low level of pain and inflammation because even the most compliant patient probably spends little more than an hour each day doing rehabilitation but might spend 23 hours each day performing ADLs. Therefore, the greater exposure to ADLs compared with rehabilitation means that what they do with their ADLs, either appropriately or probably inappropriately, has a profound effect on their levels of pain and inflammation. Many patients keep their shoulders irritated and inflamed by doing ADLs that are too difficult or too repetitive for their injured shoulders to tolerate. At our facility, we spend much time in rehabilitation talking to patients about what they are doing at home, work, and recreation and helping them to select the correct level of activity that will not inflame or exacerbate their signs and symptoms. This often requires a substantial decrease in the level of intensity and repetitiveness of their ADLs compared with their normal levels of function and what they sense is necessary, especially in patients who have had surgery or who present with acutely inflamed shoulders.

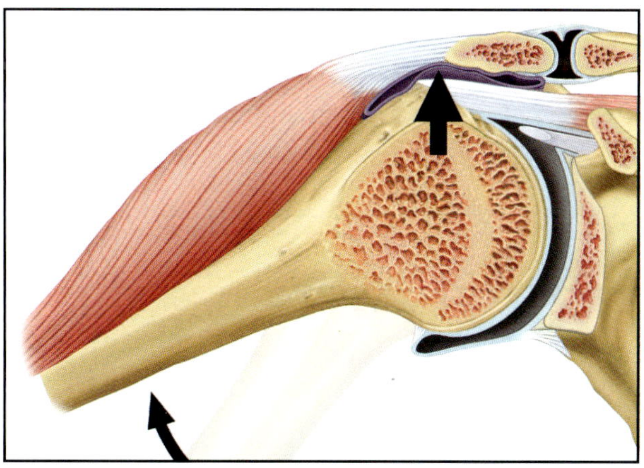

Figure 8. Overly aggressive passive range of motion results in pinching of the subacromial bursa and supraspinatus with resultant swelling, inflammation, and pain.

3. Establish Basic Passive Range of Motion While Decreasing Pain.

The third priority in the clinical decision-making process of shoulder rehabilitation is that passive ROM (PROM) should be established in a way that promotes decreased pain and inflammation. Active ROM (AROM) is not possible without at least an equivalent amount of PROM, so logically during shoulder rehabilitation, PROM should be established before AROM and strength. Even subtle limitations in ROM of the shoulder can produce altered biomechanics.[15,18,19] This yields altered movement patterns, which result in abnormal stress to structures in the shoulder joint.[19,20] The abnormal stress eventually can result in injury.[13,14,21] Specific joints that the rehabilitation provider should evaluate and subsequently treat if limitations are found include the glenohumeral joint, sternoclavicular joint, acromioclavicular joint, cervical spine, thoracic spine, and lumbar spine. Appropriate evaluation and treatment of many of these joints are discussed in other chapters. The rehabilitation provider also should consider the specific flexibility demands of the patient's functional activities, such as the functional movements required during work or sports activities. For example, a baseball pitcher needs excellent lower extremity and trunk flexibility in addition to appropriate shoulder flexibility. The rehabilitation provider should be aware that limitations in other parts of the body also can contribute to shoulder disorders.

Appropriate PROM, which moves a specific joint through the available, easily attained PROM, minimizes muscle guarding and can result in decreased stiffness, inflammation, and pain,[1] whereas we believe that overly aggressive PROM increases inflammation and pain and can promote increased shoulder stiffness,[1,3] as I have described. Gentle PROM and stretching are beneficial in many situations, especially early in rehabilitation of the patient who has had surgery. To adhere to the higher-priority rehabilitation principle of protecting healing tissues and minimizing inflammation and pain in our approach to shoulder rehabilitation, it is vitally important to select the correct stopping point during PROM and stretching. Moreover, the patient must decide where to stop ROM during PROM and stretching activities even when the rehabilitation provider is directly performing the stretching or PROM. We advise stopping stretching activities at the point where the patient senses a comfortable stretch only with a minimal amount of pain at most. If the correct stopping point is selected, the sensation of stretch that the patient feels should be equal to or greater than the sensation of pain. If the patient feels a greater amount of pain than stretch or especially if the patient feels pain before sensing a stretch, then we conclude that the patient's shoulder is too inflamed for PROM and stretching at that treatment session. Clinically, the primary problem that we see with PROM and stretching interventions is that they are performed too aggressively, often going to a maximum tolerated stretch or as far as possible.

To follow our treatment recommendations, we prompt patients to search for the "happy medium" point where the stretch is described as pleasant. It is acceptable, but not preferred, that the patient has a slight increase in pain after stretching that, at most, should not be present for longer than about an hour. We believe that promoting a low level level of inflammation and pain is a higher priority than gaining ROM; therefore, if the pain lasts longer, we conclude that the stretching was too aggressive and believe it should be performed more gently during the next treatment session. Obviously, the patient is the only person who knows the relationship between pain and stretch during these activities, so he or she is in the best position to determine the stopping point during PROM and stretching activities, even if they are being performed by the rehabilitation provider.

4. Use Progressive Active Range of Motion and Strengthening That Maintains a Low Level of Pain.

The fourth most important priority during the clinical decision-making process in the systematic approach to shoulder rehabilitation is to use progressive AROM and strengthening that promotes and maintains a low level of pain. This is accomplished by using specific principles that guide the progression of an evidence-based strengthening progression detailed in chapter II-4. The principles that guide our AROM and strengthening progression are listed in Table 2.

The first principle is for the rehabilitation provider to let AROM and strengthening come to you. This means that a specific timetable for starting certain exercises for every person should not be used. Instead, the clinician should select AROM or strengthening exercises that match or are slightly easier than the patient's comfortable use of the extremity. For example, if the patient can reach at chest level to adjust the car radio or to turn off a light switch but has pain and altered movement when attempting to comb his or her hair, then 1 step easier with rehabilitation would be to perform light elastic-band strengthening with the hand at waist level and progressive active-assistive ROM

Table 2. Principles of Progression for Active Range of Motion and Strengthening

1. Let active range of motion and strengthening come to you.
2. Pain should not increase with the advancement of exercises.
3. Exercise at a submaximal level of intensity.
4. Perform light-resistance, high-volume training.
5. Ensure a gradual stepwise progression of increased muscular demand.

at shoulder level and overhead. We term this principle *letting AROM and strengthening come to you* because instead of pushing the patient to try a more difficult intervention than his or her comfortably performed ADLs to improve AROM and strength, we recommend selecting an intervention that is equal to or slightly easier than the comfortable ADLs. Anecdotally, we have found that this method of selecting interventions allows the patient to progress through an evidence-based AROM and strengthening progression typically without altered movement patterns and without an increase in pain.

The second AROM and strengthening principle is that the patient's level of pain should not increase with the advancement of AROM and strengthening exercises if the appropriate level of exercise is chosen. This typically occurs if you follow the principle of letting AROM and strengthening come to you and follow the exercise-prescription guidelines discussed later in this section.

The third principle is that exercise should be performed at a submaximal level of intensity. The rotator cuff muscles are stabilizing muscles that primarily compress and center the humeral head in the glenoid, and as discussed, they are very mechanically disadvantaged. Therefore, they work very hard even with low levels of external resistance, so we believe that maximum-intensity training is not necessary.

Our fourth AROM and strengthening principle is that exercising at a suboptimal level allows light-resistance, high-volume training. We believe that it is usually the optimal way to rehabilitate the shoulder girdle muscles. Unlike high-resistance training, light-resistance, high-volume training theoretically promotes the ability of the rotator cuff to help center the humeral head during movement of the shoulder. With lower resistance or load, the rotator cuff is less likely to be overpowered and exceed its ability to center the humeral head during rehabilitation interventions. Light-resistance, high-volume training also promotes a high level of blood flow to the rotator cuff and surrounding tissue, which helps increase the transport of micronutrients to promote healing. Finally, anecdotal evidence suggests that light-resistance, high-volume training can result in increased tendon and ligament thickness over time.[22]

The fifth principle is to ensure that rehabilitation is progressed in a way that produces a gradual stepwise progression of increased muscular demand to the shoulder girdle. Muscle demand during shoulder rehabilitation exercises typically is evaluated by electromyography. Given the large amount of published material on the electromyographic (EMG) activity level of various rehabilitation exercises, we prefer to use exercises with known EMG activity levels. This is especially important during the early AROM and strengthening stages in patients who have been treated for rotator cuff conditions, particularly in patients with repaired rotator cuffs. The systematic approach to shoulder rehabilitation developed at HPRC at St. Francis Rehabilitation Center and St. Francis Orthopaedic Institute includes an evidence-based AROM and strengthening progression that primarily is based on EMG activity level. This progression is detailed in chapter II-4.

Ensuring that the patient appropriately tolerates AROM and strengthening exercises is vitally important to the success of rehabilitation and can be accomplished by following the AROM and strengthening principles that I have discussed, using appropriate exercise prescription and correct instructions with the patient. For most patients who have been treated with or without surgery, our typical exercise prescription is 1 set of 30 to 60 repetitions twice each day for both home AROM and strengthening exercises. More important than using the exact sets and repetitions is ensuring that the patient has the appropriate tolerance to each exercise. In our approach to rehabilitation, the patient should be able to perform every AROM and strengthening intervention ideally with no pain and ideally with fatigue only during the last 10 to 15 repetitions. In our system, fatigue that occurs during the first 5 to 10 repetitions is a sign that a little too much resistance is being used and a lighter resistance or an easier activity should be selected. If any pain beyond a minimal level is present or if a particular AROM and strengthening exercise exacerbates signs and symptoms, the rehabilitation provider also should select an easier activity. Therefore, in the systematic approach to shoulder rehabilitation, we allow slightly more pain with PROM and stretching interventions than with strengthening interventions. In addition, if abnormal movement or substitution patterns are present during

AROM and strengthening, then easier interventions are selected in most circumstances. Patients often have difficulty initially tolerating new AROM and strengthening interventions. To keep initial tolerance to new interventions within the parameters described, we use a lighter resistance and exercise volume than the clinician typically thinks is appropriate during the first week of a new exercise. Therefore, we do not aim for fatigue during the first week of a new intervention. After the patient establishes a tolerance to the new exercise, attention focuses on achieving a feeling of fatigue at the end of each set.

5. Use Appropriate Functional Training.

The fifth priority for the clinical decision-making process in shoulder rehabilitation is that appropriate functional training should be performed. Wilk and Arrigo[23] suggested that isolated movement patterns strengthen weak muscles and that combined movement patterns re-establish function. The rehabilitation provider can emphasize isolated movement patterns during the early stages of rehabilitation to address specific impairments noted during the examination. Rehabilitation should progress to integrate combined movement patterns as the patient improves, keeping a limited number of isolated rehabilitation exercises as the core components of a maintenance program. An important idea to follow regarding appropriate functional training is that the difficulty of the rehabilitation must match the integrity of the tissues and the goals of the patient. To establish this, the rehabilitation provider must understand the details of the patient's condition and/or surgery and must perform a needs analysis of the patient's functional demands. Rehabilitation should begin at a level that is appropriate for the patient's current level of impairments, injury, and tissue healing. Rehabilitation should progress in an individualized manner toward the agreed-upon specific functional goals.

Errors in the clinical decision-making process during this time occur when the level of difficulty of interventions does not accurately match the functional goals of the patient or the integrity of the healing tissues. If the interventions have not been demanding enough to meet the functional demands of the patient, then he or she is at risk of reinjury at the end of rehabilitation when resuming full functional activities because the tissues were not prepared adequately for the stress. This is most likely to occur when the patient has high functional demands, such as in the throwing athlete or heavy manual laborer. A more common problem in shoulder rehabilitation is regularly performing rehabilitation interventions that are more demanding than the regular functional activities of the patient. This problem often occurs in rehabilitation of the elderly and in rehabilitation of sedentary individual's of any age, especially those who have tendinitis or bursitis or who are recovering from surgery. Rehabilitation that is slightly more demanding than the tissue can tolerate often results in exacerbated or continued symptoms of tendinitis or bursitis. If rehabilitation places substantially more stress on injured and healing tissue than typically received during daily functional activities or if it exceeds the long-term integrity of the healing tissues, long-term tissue damage or failure of the surgical repair can occur. This is easy to do inadvertently in the shoulder; the rotator cuff muscles are small stabilizing muscles that are mechanically disadvantaged, so they are easy to overload with a fairly small amount of external resistance. Therefore, particular care should be taken to prevent overly aggressive rehabilitation of the shoulder, especially in elderly and more sedentary patients.

"AVERSION" TO ABDUCTION

The third guiding principle specific to our approach for rehabilitation is that we have an "aversion" to abduction. The primary reason that we have an aversion to abduction is elevation of the upper extremity in the scapular plane (scaption) is such a great alternative. Scaption is the preferred position for overhead PROM, AROM, and strengthening in the early and middle stages of rehabilitation because elevation in the scapular plane has been shown to provide minimal capsular stress[24]; optimal length-tension relationship for the cuff, deltoid, and scapular muscles[25]; optimal subacromial clearance[26,27]; and cuff activation equal to that provided by other standing strengthening exercises.[28] Because of biomechanics alone (compared with scaption) frontal-plane abduction produces an increased strain to the anterior aspect of the capsule and an increased likelihood for impingement. Similarly, during abduction, the rotator cuff, deltoid, and scapular muscles do not work using an optimal length-tension relationship. All of these problems are exacerbated with any limitation in PROM or strength; therefore, when straight-plane abduction is used earlier in the rehabilitation process, it is more inappropriate. Both scaption and abduction end in the same basic position (overhead elevation), and anecdotally, we have found that by the end of rehabilitation, most patients perform abduction with normal ROM and biomechanics without direct rehabilitation to restore it. Therefore, we believe the need to use straight-plane abduction during rehabilitation is limited. We do work to passively achieve abduction during the systematic approach to rehabilitation (Figures 9 and 10) but not in ways that use long-arc frontal-plane movement, especially from 80° to 120°. Active ROM and strength training using frontal-plane abduction occasionally can be used with select patients during the end phase of rehabilitation only if they have specific functional demands in their work or recreation requiring the regular use of the extremity in this position.

DETAILS OF REHABILITATION ARE IMPORTANT

The fourth and final principle of rehabilitation specific to the systematic approach to shoulder rehabilitation of the HPRC at St. Francis Rehabilitation Center and St. Francis Orthopaedic Institute is recognizing that the details of rehabilitation are important.

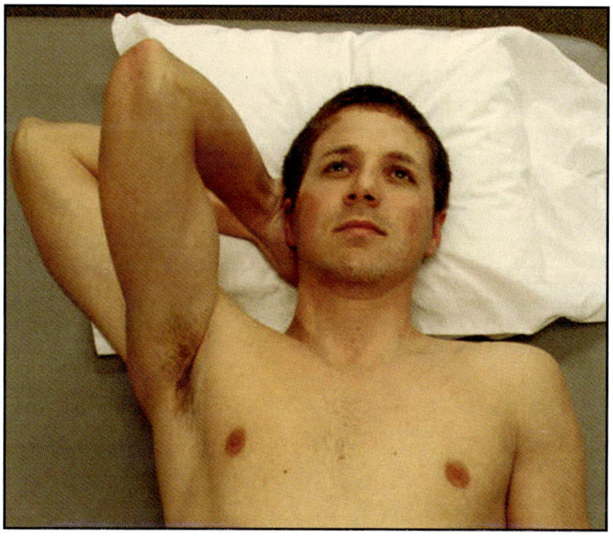

Figure 9. Supine hand-behind-head, or quadrant, stretch is an alternative means to achieve abduction.

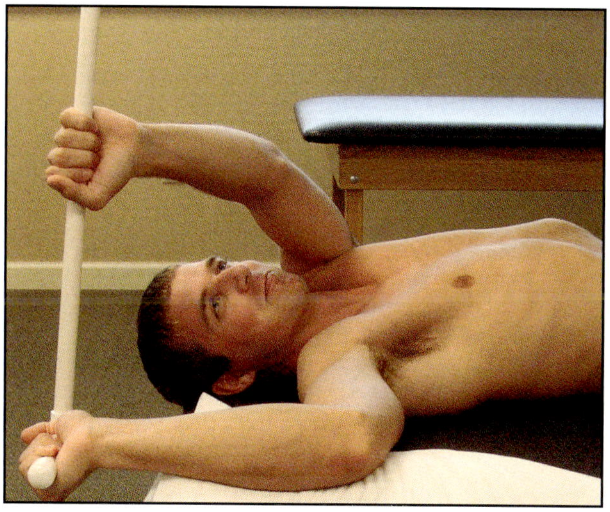

Figure 10. Supine external rotation stretching in 90° of abduction is an alternative means to help achieve abduction.

We believe that the specific details of exercise selection, exercise technique, and exercise application make a substantial difference in the effectiveness of rehabilitation, the patient's tolerance to rehabilitation, and outcomes. The skilled application of physics and biomechanical principles, close monitoring of exercise technique and tolerance, and use of current research to guide exercise progression are vitally important. Practical examples are found throughout the book and are discussed in detail in chapters II-2, II-4, and II-5.

In conclusion, we believe that the skill of the rehabilitation provider has a tremendous effect on the ease and speed of recovery, as well as on the long-term outcomes for patients with shoulder disorders. Our philosophy of shoulder rehabilitation is that it is always gentle and uses a precise priority for the clinical decision-making process that first, protects the healing tissue and operative repair. Second, it achieves a low level of inflammation and pain. Third, it establishes quality PROM while maintaining a low level of pain. Fourth, it initiates AROM and strengthening that also maintains a low level of pain. Fifth, it uses appropriate functional training. We do this in a way that de-emphasizes frontal-plane abduction and emphasizes elevation in the scapular plane. We also recognize that the details in rehabilitation are important. The rehabilitation guidelines sections of this book details how these philosophies are interrelated and are applied in specific clinical situations.

REFERENCES

1. Diercks RL, Stevens M. Gentle thawing of the frozen shoulder: a prospective study of supervised neglect versus intensive physical therapy in seventy-seven patients with frozen shoulder syndrome followed up for two years. *J Shoulder Elbow Surg*. 2004;13(5):499–502.
2. Lundberg BJ. The frozen shoulder: clinical and radiographical observations. The effect of manipulation under general anesthesia. Structure and glycosaminoglycan content of the joint capsule. Local bone metabolism. *Acta Orthop Scand*. 1969; 119(suppl):1–59.
3. Neviaser JS. Adhesive capsulitis of the shoulder: a study of the pathological findings in periarthritis of the shoulder. *J Bone Joint Surg Am*. 1945;27(2):211–222.
4. Bunker TD, Reilly J, Baird KS, Hamblen DL. Expression of growth factors, cytokines and matrix metalloproteinases in frozen shoulder. *J Bone Joint Surg Br*. 2000;82(5):768–773.
5. Bunker TD, Anthony PP. The pathology of frozen shoulder: a Dupuytren-like disease. *J Bone Joint Surg Br*. 1995;77(5):677–683.
6. Rodeo SA, Hannafin JA, Tom J, Warren RF, Wickiewica TL. Immunolocalization of cytokines in adhesive capsulitis. *J Orthop Res*. 1997;15(3):427–436.
7. Hannafin JA, DiCarlo ED, Wickiewicz TL, Warren RF. Adhesive capsulitis: capsular fibroplasia of the glenohumeral joint. *J Shoulder Elbow Surg*. 1994;3(suppl):5.
8. Parsons JL, Shepard WL, Fosdick WM. DMSO-an adjuvant to physical therapy in the chronic frozen shoulder. *Ann N Y Acad Sci*. 1967;141(1):569–571.
9. Watson-Jones R. Simple treatment of stiff shoulders [abstract]. *J Bone Joint Surg Br*. 1963;45(1):207.
10. Nicholson GG. The effects of passive joint mobilization on pain and hypomobility associated with adhesive capsulitis of the shoulder. *J Orthop Sports Phys Ther*. 1985;6(4):238–246.
11. Risk TE, Christopher RP, Pinal RS, Higgins AC, Frix R. Adhesive capsulitis (frozen shoulder): a new approach to its management. *Arch Phys Med Rehabil*. 1983;64(1):29–33.
12. Hazleman BL. The painful stiff shoulder. *Rheumatol Phys Med*. 1972;11(8):413–421.
13. Harryman DT, Lazarus MD, Rozencwaig R. The stiff shoulder. In: Rockwood CA, Matsen III FA, eds. *The Shoulder*. 2nd ed. Philadelphia, PA: WB Saunders; 1998:1064–1112.
14. Reddy AS, Mohr KJ, Pink MM, Jobe FW. Electromyographic analysis of the deltoid and rotator cuff muscles in persons with subacromial impingement. *J Shoulder Elbow Surg*. 2000;9(6):519–523.
15. Ludewig PM, Cook TM. Alterations in shoulder kinematics and associated muscle activity in people with symptoms of shoulder impingement. *Phys Ther*. 2000;80(3):276–291.
16. Sharkey NA, Marder RA. The rotator cuff opposes superior translation of the humeral head. *Am J Sports Med*. 1995;23(3): 270–275.
17. McClure PW, Michener LA, Karduna AR. Shoulder function and 3-dimensional scapular kinematics in people with and without shoulder impingement syndrome. *Phys Ther*. 2006; 86(8):1075–1090.
18. Harryman DT II, Sidles JA, Harris SL, Matsen FA III. The role of the rotator interval capsule in passive motion and stability of the shoulder. *J Bone Joint Surg Am*. 1992;74(1):53–66.
19. Harryman DT II, Sidles JA, Clark JM, McQuade KJ, Gibb TD, Matsen FA III. Translation of the humeral head on the glenoid with passive glenohumeral motion. *J Bone Joint Surg Am*. 1990;72(9):1334–1343.
20. Warner JJ, Micheli LJ, Arslanian LE, Kennedy J, Kennedy R. Patterns of flexibility, laxity, and strength in normal shoulders and shoulders with instability and impingement. *Am J Sports Med*. 1990;18(4):366–375.
21. Tyler TF, Nicholas SJ, Roy T, Gleim GW. Quantification of posterior capsule tightness and motion loss in patients with shoulder impingement. *Am J Sports Med*. 2000;28(5):668–673.
22. Hughston JC. *Knee Ligaments: Injury and Repair*. St Louis, MO: Mosby; 1993.
23. Wilk KE, Arrigo C. Current concepts in the rehabilitation of the athletic shoulder. *J Orthop Sports Phys Ther*. 1993;18(1): 365–378.
24. Doody SG, Freedman L, Waterland JC. Shoulder movements during abduction in the scapular plane. *Arch Phys Med Rehabil*. 1970;51(10):595–604.
25. Lucas DB. Biomechanics of the shoulder joint. *Arch Surg*. 1973;107(3):425–432.
26. Flatow EL, Soslowsky LJ, Ticker JB, et al. Excursion of the rotator cuff under the acromion: patterns of subacromial contact. *Am J Sports Med*. 1994;22(6):779–788.
27. Johnston TB. The movements of the shoulder-joint: a plea for the use of the "plane of the scapula" as the plane of reference for movements occuring at the humero-scapular joint. *Br J Surg*. 1937;25:252–260.
28. Blackburn TA, McLeod WD, White B, Wofford L. EMG analysis of posterior rotator cuff exercises. *Athl Train J Natl Athl Train Assoc*. 1990;25(1):41–45.

II-2

The Postoperative Shoulder Evaluation and Initial Treatment Strategies

How to Effectively Treat the Frightened and Apprehensive Patient

Bryce W. Gaunt, PT, SCS

CHAPTER CONTENTS

Clinical pearls are highlighted in yellow throughout the text.

Including a chapter on postoperative shoulder evaluation and initial treatment might seem unnecessary; however, I have found that what happens during the initial rehabilitation visits sets the stage for an easy or difficult recovery. Initially, many patients have fear and apprehension about their postoperative rehabilitation and recovery that can negatively affect the entire rehabilitation process through reactions, such as muscle guarding and a negative attitude toward the rehabilitation process. Proper initial rehabilitation can quickly minimize or negate apprehension and fear and establish a positive outlook toward rehabilitation. At my facility, the most important part of the postoperative evaluation and initial treatments is simple; the patient must have a positive initial experience with postoperative rehabilitation and establish a relaxed and trusting relationship with the rehabilitation provider. This sets the groundwork for successful initiation of shoulder girdle passive range of motion (PROM). This chapter includes the details of our methods of achieving this goal and is applicable to the management of patients after most types of shoulder surgery.

COMPONENTS OF THE POSTOPERATIVE SHOULDER EVALUATION

The evaluation component of the initial postoperative visit includes several critical parts. Most importantly, the rehabilitation provider must satisfy the legal and professional practice standards of his or her profession. Discussion of these standards is outside the scope of this article. Therefore, the points that I discuss do not compose a comprehensive list of things that should be completed during a postoperative shoulder evaluation.

Assessing the patient's neurovascular status is an important part of the evaluation because scalene nerve blocks often are used during shoulder surgery. *Scalene nerve block* describes a regional anesthetic solution injected to interrupt sensory and motor function to the surgically treated upper extremity for approximately 6 to 12 hours. If the patient is examined in the early postoperative period when the block is intact, the entire upper extremity is flaccid and numb, making proper extremity support imperative. Nerve palsy is a rare but major complication after shoulder surgery, so any motor loss that affects the muscles controlling the shoulder girdle, elbow, wrist, or hand after the effects of the scalene block have ended should be reported to the surgeon immediately. Prolonged paresthesia is a more common but less severe complication, and surgeons have different preferences for being notified about this condition. The presence or absence of excessive edema should be evaluated. Edema in the arm, forearm, wrist, and hand is occasionally a problem in the surgically treated extremity especially after open procedures, such as arthroplasty and fracture management. If edema is present, a compression glove for the hand and light compression, such as an elastic stocking with a slit in the proximal portion near the axilla, typically efficiently resolve this condition.

Assessing range of motion (ROM) of the uninvolved joints of the shoulder girdle, including active ROM (AROM) of the scapula, is also important. The ROM of these joints is detailed in the Range of Motion of the Uninvolved Joints subsection of this chapter. Similarly, when allowed by the surgeon, PROM of the glenohumeral joint should be assessed, and treatment should be started as appropriate. Assessment of glenohumeral ROM typically begins with assessment of passive external rotation (PER) and passive internal rotation with the elbow in 10° to 20° of abduction and with assessment of passive forward elevation (PFE) in the scapular plane.

Less commonly considered but just as important to assess is the patient's level of fear and apprehension and his or her attitude toward rehabilitation. We have found that a high level of fear and apprehension or a negative attitude toward rehabilitation, or both, results in patients developing a habit of muscle guarding and thus poor ROM. The rehabilitation provider usually assesses this by examining the patient's body language, facial expressions, oral comments, and muscle guarding with initial shoulder girdle ROM; however, direct questions also can be included in the evaluation that measures these attributes.

Likewise, the assessment of the patient's long-term and short-term functional goals can easily be overlooked. Long-term functional goals are important to establish because they set the ultimate destination of treatment. For example, a patient who has more demanding functional goals, such as return to throwing or to work that requires frequent heavy lifting, requires different end-stage rehabilitation than a patient whose only goal is to return to basic activities of daily living (ADLs). During the initial evaluation, *short-term functional goals*, which are defined as the functional demands the patient wants to place on the surgically treated extremity during the first 4 to 6 weeks after surgery, are more critical to assess than long-term goals. Often, patients have unrealistic expectations about the ADLs they can perform successfully with the surgically treated upper extremity during the initial postoperative period. Many patients plan to use the surgically treated extremity to perform keyboarding activities for an extended period shortly after surgery. I have found that in patients who have surgical procedures, such as rotator cuff repairs, anything more than very occasional use of the extremity in this manner tends to exacerbate pain and, therefore, limits ROM during approximately the first 6 weeks after surgery. Determination of the patient's intentions for short-term ADL use of the surgically treated extremity enables the rehabilitation provider to assess its likely effect on the recovery of the extremity and to counsel the patient regarding appropriate activities during the initial postoperative period. Appropriate patient education is detailed later in this chapter.

PURPOSE OF THE INITIAL POSTOPERATIVE TREATMENTS

The primary purpose of the initial treatments is to prevent complications, decrease the apprehension and fear of the patient, establish trust, abolish the tendency for muscle guarding at rest and with ROM, and apply some of the specific rehabilitation principles discussed in detail in chapter II-1. The specific rehabilitation principles that apply during the initial postoperative period are that we are always gentle, we protect the healing tissues and integrity of the surgical repair, we establish and maintain a low level of inflammation and pain, and we establish basic PROM while decreasing pain. The primary method to achieve these early postoperative treatment goals is to ensure that the patient has a positive experience during initial rehabilitation.

IMPORTANCE OF ENSURING A POSITIVE INITIAL EXPERIENCE DURING REHABILITATION: STRATEGIES TO REDUCE APPREHENSION AND FEAR

A positive initial experience is the primary goal of the initial postoperative evaluation. Most of us have learned that we only have 1 chance to make a good first impression. The postoperative shoulder evaluation is no different. We need to strive for the first impression to be a very positive and pleasant experience that sets the stage for the patient to relax and trust us as rehabilitation providers. We must ensure that initial treatments are not highly painful because pain promotes muscle guarding, apprehension, and distrust. Therefore, the primary objective for the end of the first treatment is to see a big smile on the patient's face and to be able to recognize that he or she is at ease. In our philosophy, the amount of ROM achieved during the first few visits is of secondary importance in almost all circumstances.

Minimizing pain, distress, and muscle guarding in early postoperative rehabilitation is important because these conditions along with inflammation, apprehension or fear, swelling, stretching of the tissues, and tension on the repair site[1–4] limit early ROM after injury and shoulder surgery. Our ideal goal during the early postoperative period is for ROM to be limited by stretching of tissue, but it is more likely limited by muscle guarding, pain, inflammation, and apprehension or fear. When the patient develops a cycle of pain, distrust, and muscle guarding, these problems are only exacerbated. Adhesions that are present preoperatively[3,5] or that have formed postoperatively in either the intra-articular or extra-articular area of the glenohumeral joint[6,7] also can limit ROM. However, we have found that if excessive muscle guarding, pain, inflammation, and/or apprehension are present, a successful stretching program to address adhesions typically cannot be completed because pain or muscle guarding limits ROM before the adhesions are stretched. In addition, overly aggressive and highly painful therapy can lead to excessive pain and inflammation, resulting in inflammatory synovitis, which can lead to capsular fibrosis and limited ROM.[8,9] This was discussed in detail in chapter II-1. Therefore, at our facility, we believe that for glenohumeral PROM to be the easiest, the rehabilitation provider should work to limit the patient's muscle guarding, pain, inflammation, apprehension, and swelling.

To limit these, the patient must have a positive initial experience on the first few postoperative visits. As noted, we have only 1 chance to make a good first impression, and we recognize that changing an established habit is difficult. Our challenge is that patients expect early postoperative shoulder rehabilitation to be painful, which results in apprehension, fear, muscle guarding, and distrust. Therefore, we have to change their minds so that they expect a pleasant experience that promotes trust between us and helps them relax.

How do we create a positive, trusting, and relaxing experience during early postoperative shoulder rehabilitation? This is accomplished through the components of the initial postoperative treatment: ROM of the uninvolved joints, extensive patient education, proper sling support, and skilled shoulder girdle ROM that abolishes the tendency for muscle guarding.

COMPONENTS OF THE INITIAL POSTOPERATIVE TREATMENTS

Range of Motion of the Uninvolved Joints

Range of motion of the uninvolved joints is the primary method that rehabilitation providers use to prevent the postoperative neurovascular complications discussed earlier in this chapter. Included are elbow, wrist, and hand active-assistive ROM to AROM and scapular AROM. Whether or not the ROM of the joints is impaired, it should be included in initial treatments to promote normal neurovascular functioning and to minimize joint stiffness. Commonly prescribed wrist and hand AROM exercises include light gripping against either no or minimal resistance and wrist flexion and extension. The primary movement included for elbow ROM is active elbow flexion and extension. We have found this most easily performed in standing with the forearm held close to the body. No weight is used for the first 6 weeks after surgery. Instead, the focus is gentle ROM to prevent joint stiffness and to promote circulation and lymphatic drainage. It is also helpful for the patient to stand with the elbow resting in extension for a few minutes at a time periodically during the day in the early postoperative period to counteract the discomfort and feelings of joint stiffness that tend to occur because so much time is spent with the elbow flexed during this time. Active-assistive ROM of the elbow is used primarily if pain or poor muscle control limits AROM. However, the surgeon might require elbow PROM or active-assistive ROM for up to 6 weeks if a biceps tenodesis or tenotomy has been performed to minimize load to the long head of the biceps tendon in these procedures. This is more fully discussed in the Special Considerations section of chapter III-1.

Supination and pronation generally are not performed after this ROM has been established as normal because these motions can irritate the long head of the biceps tendon after shoulder surgery.

Scapular elevation and retraction are vital parts of ROM of the uninvolved joints. Performing these exercises in the early postoperative period has many benefits. First, they help minimize tension to the brachial plexus. Often, before these exercises are performed, the patient's involved scapula might be positioned in excessive scapular depression, exerting unwanted traction on the brachial plexus. Second, early in the postoperative period, patients often note that the shoulder girdle feels exceptionally heavy and feels as if it is being pulled down. Scapular elevation, in particular, helps relieve this feeling and promotes the patient regaining natural support of his or her extremity. Third, these exercises begin formal scapular rehabilitation by re-establishing volitional control of basic scapular movement. Fourth, these movements help improve patient confidence because they allow the patient to see that he or she can move the shoulder girdle with minimal discomfort compared with direct glenohumeral joint movement.

Patient Education

We believe that patient education is a primary method to decrease muscle guarding, apprehension, fear, and pain while building trust. For maximum effectiveness, patient education is something we reinforce continuously with the patient. We believe that the patient needs to understand the basics of the surgical procedure so he or she can understand the necessity and importance of the tissue-healing process. For example, we want the patient with a rotator cuff repair to understand that in the long-term, the surgical repair is very strong; however, in the early postoperative period and especially during the first 6 weeks, the integrity of the repair is maintained only by sutures that can be disrupted by inappropriate rehabilitation or inappropriate use of the extremity during ADLs. Therefore, we teach the patient to think before acting and to ensure that the opportunities for reflexive motions of the surgically treated extremity are minimized. Next, we discuss the goals for the first phase of rehabilitation. For example, we teach the patient with a rotator cuff repair that during the first 6 weeks after surgery, the primary goal is to protect the surgical repair. We also discuss that secondary goals are to decrease pain and begin passive movement of the surgically treated upper extremity.

Before beginning PROM with patients, we teach them about what to expect when ROM is performed, and we teach them how to determine the correct stopping point for each exercise. This is critically important to reducing muscle guarding, apprehension, fear, and pain with shoulder girdle ROM and is discussed in detail in the Skilled Shoulder Girdle Passive Range of Motion subsection of this chapter.

We teach patients that the most comfortable way to sleep in the early postoperative period is usually in a reclined position. They should try to position the extremity in a modified neutral position, ensuring that the glenohumeral joint does not drift into extension or excessive internal or external rotation. Use of some form of physician-prescribed medication aids patients in sleeping during the early postoperative period even if medication is not needed during the day.

Education about appropriate use of the surgically treated extremity during ADLs and work is vital during the early postoperative period, especially for the first 6 weeks and especially when the active or passive stabilizers, or both, of the shoulder have been repaired. During this time, we have found that only very occasional use of the extremity for short periods successfully minimizes pain. Patients who use the surgically treated extremity even for very basic ADLs, such as keyboarding, writing, or laundry, frequently or constantly have noticeably higher levels of pain during this time. In addition, frequently using ice on the surgically treated shoulder generally results in a noticeable reduction in pain not only during all stages of postoperative recovery and rehabilitation, but especially during the early postoperative period.

The next component of patient education is ensuring that the patient understands how to appropriately use a sling, which varies depending on the surgical procedure and on surgeon preference. Proper use of the sling and positioning of the extremity can noticeably decrease pain and muscle guarding and can promote glenohumeral ROM. For example, some surgeons require nearly full-time use of the sling during the first 6 weeks after a rotator cuff repair. At our facility, we generally allow patients with "standard-sized" rotator cuff repairs to remove the sling when sitting with the upper extremity supported. We promote sitting with the extremity in various positions that are comfortable rather than just resting with the forearm against the body. Our patients generally are allowed to remove the sling when up for very short periods in the house. We instruct patients to "listen" to the extremity; if it "tells" them that it is tired of immobilization, then they can remove the sling for a few minutes. However, when they notice that the extremity is tired or starting to feel heavy, they need to either sit and support the extremity or reapply the sling. During the first 6 weeks after rotator cuff repair, our surgeons require patients to wear the sling in the community and around the house if they are performing a prolonged project. This usage is required mostly to ensure that active use of the extremity does not occur during these times, but it also is required for support. Use of the sling at night is generally at the patient's discretion, but some surgeons prefer that patients wear it but loosen it for comfort.

Proper Sling Support

During the initial postoperative visit, we ensure that the sling is properly supporting the patient's extremity because we believe this is critical to decreasing early postoperative pain and muscle guarding. During arthroscopic or open shoulder surgery, stabilization that is provided to the glenohumeral joint through the "suction-cup effect" and negative intra-articular pressure[10] is disrupted[11,12] and remains compromised throughout the early postoperative period, allowing a resulting traction force on the extremity that must be counteracted by either the active stabilizers (rotator cuff and deltoid) or passive stabilizers (glenohumeral capsule and ligaments) of the glenohumeral joint. If this traction force is not removed by properly supporting the surgically treated extremity in a sling, the counteraction to the force by the active and passive structures of the glenohumeral joint results in pain and a tendency for muscle guarding. Therefore, in the early postoperative period, the sling must support the weight of the extremity so the patient feels a slight lift through the forearm and immediate relief of the traction force at the glenohumeral joint. We have found that correcting an improperly fitted sling provides a noticeable and immediate reduction in pain and discomfort and helps establish trust between the patient and rehabilitation provider.

Skilled Shoulder Girdle Passive Range of Motion

Overview. Although important, patient education is usually the easy part of initial postoperative shoulder rehabilitation. The hard part of initial postoperative rehabilitation is establishing early PROM that limits muscle guarding, pain, apprehension, fear, and swelling in a way that is safe to the surgical repair and provides a positive experience to the patient. How do we ensure that the patient wears a smile after early PROM? As discussed, liberal use of ice, proper sling support, and instruction in appropriate use of the surgically treated extremity with ADLs are very important. In addition, before initiating the movement, the rehabilitation provider must educate the patient about what is going to occur during the ROM exercise. If the rehabilitation provider quickly begins ROM exercises for the surgically treated extremity without providing oral preparation, the result is muscle guarding, apprehension, fear, and most likely pain. Instead, before initiating ROM exercises, we discuss the importance of moving the extremity to the point at which patients feel a light pull and only minimal discomfort. We mention that if they feel like they have funny looks on their faces, they hate the exercises because they hurt so badly, they feel like they are going as far as possible, or the extremity hurts worse for hours after rehabilitation, then they have gone too far with their PROM exercises. Therefore, we discuss the importance of finding the "happy medium," where they feel a gentle stretch with no substantial delayed pain after exercise. This discussion helps patients realize that we are planning to be gentle during rehabilitation and begins to decrease the initial apprehension and fear regarding rehabilitation. The hard part for the rehabilitation provider is to ensure that this happens in practice. To find the happy medium stopping point during initial postoperative rehabilitation, **the patient must determine the stopping point** even during ROM provided by the rehabilitation provider. Although the rehabilitation provider might be able to appreciate the tissue tension associated with a given ROM, he or she has no way of knowing the pain associated with a given ROM.

The Postoperative Shoulder Evaluation and Initial Treatment Strategies

Because the patient is the one experiencing both tissue tension and the pain associated with it, he or she is in the best position to determine the point of minimal pain and light stretch. However, during the first few repetitions of the initial rehabilitation session, I prefer to stop ROM in a pain-free motion before the patient says, "Stop," to help establish a pleasant, trusting, and relaxing environment.

Other factors that need to be determined during initial postoperative shoulder girdle PROM are what planes of motion to perform, how to instruct the patient to be passive during PROM, what exercises to select, and what repetitions to choose. After most types of shoulder surgery, the only planes of motion initiated in the early postoperative period are scapular-plane elevation and PER with the extremity near the side. The rationale for choosing these planes of motion are discussed in individual chapters containing postoperative guidelines and chapter II-1. Specifically, we encourage PROM by either (1) encouraging the patient to relax and giving instructions for the patient to relax or (2) instructing the patient to "come with me" in an active-assistive manner. The most effective method is individualized for each patient. For all early PROM exercises that involve a hold, we prefer a hold of approximately 10 seconds and prefer the patient to perform approximately 6 repetitions 2 times each day initially while he or she has marked postoperative pain. We increase the volume to approximately 12 repetitions 2 times each day for each exercise after early postoperative pain subsides. If the stretching routine is well tolerated and ROM is below expected targets, we increase the frequency of stretching to 4 to 6 times each day.

Exercise Selection and Detailed Technique. At my facility, we have found that careful exercise selection and flawless exercise technique improve patient comfort and ease of ROM during initial postoperative shoulder girdle PROM. Examining exercise selection and technique, our first preferred exercise for PER with the extremity in slight abduction is sitting PER with the assistance of a rehabilitation provider or a family member (Figure 1). During this exercise, the patient's surgically treated extremity is held with the elbow in line with the midline of the body and approximately 2 to 3 inches (5.08–7.62 cm) from the side. The movement that the rehabilitation provider or

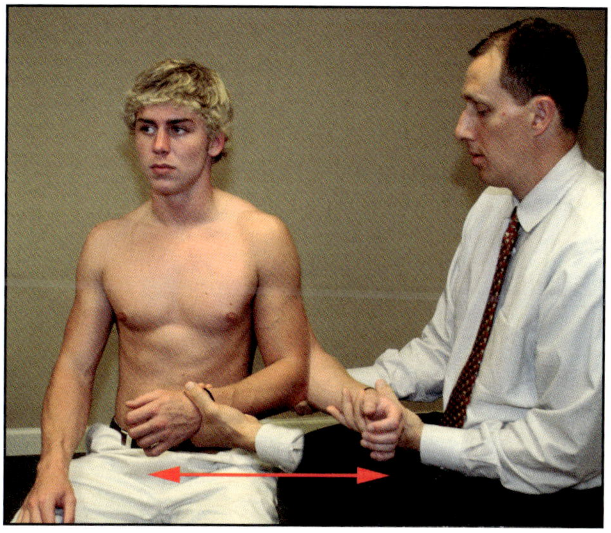

Figure 1. Passive external rotation with the assistance of a rehabilitation provider.

family member provides should be as slow as possible, moving only several degrees per second. Moving too quickly with PROM is a common error. This tends to make the patient apprehensive and muscle guard more. One reason patients tend to be apprehensive if the extremity is moved too quickly is that by the time they notice they are at the stopping point and say, "Stop," the extremity has moved 5° to 10° farther, resulting in pain. During all PER exercises, the elbow must not remain stationary and act as a pivot point; instead, it should move in a slight arc of shoulder abduction and shoulder extension to match the translation of the humeral head, which has been found to move posteriorly[13] during external rotation past early ranges because of the capsular constraint mechanism (Figure 2).[7] We

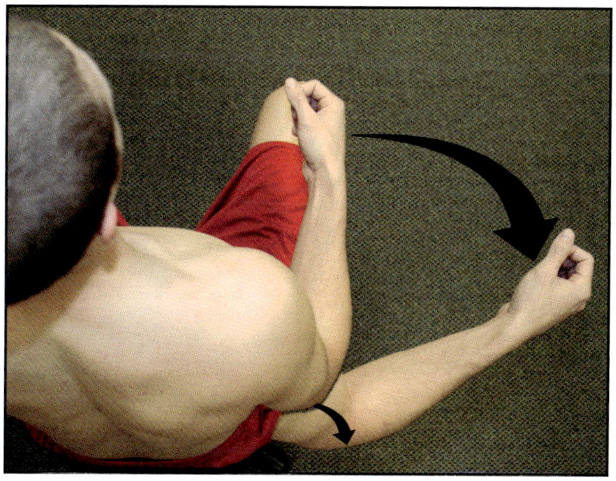

Figure 2. Biomechanically correct elbow movement during passive external rotation.

have found that PER exercises that allow the elbow to move in a slight arc are much more comfortable for patients than the more traditional supine PER exercises that do not allow the elbow to move in a slight arc during shoulder external rotation. At the first visit, PROM in patients with a rotator cuff repair, capsulolabral repair, or shoulder arthroplasty is typically from -10° of external rotation to 5° of external rotation.

Our second preferred exercise to achieve early PROM is the PER walk-around exercise during which the patient stands with the upper extremity supported on a table and rotates the body in an arc (Figure 3). This is generally the primary home method used to achieve PER by postoperative week 2 or 3. As with the assisted sitting PER exercise, the elbow is maintained about 2 to 3 inches (5.08–7.62 cm) away from the patient's side and in line with the midline of the body during the entire exercise. The patient needs to be taught how to step correctly to form an arc during the exercise. Position the patient with the surgically treated extremity supported on a corner of a table or similar object. Next, instruct the patient to step back in an arc around the corner toward the elbow while opening up the hips and shoulders. Stepping in this manner should maintain the elbow about 2 to 3 inches (5.08–7.62 cm) away from the patient's side and in line with the midline of the body. A common error is opening the shoulders and hips without stepping in an arc. This places the elbow behind the body in the finish position. A primary benefit of this exercise is that it is nearly impossible for the patient to stretch too vigorously because the forearm is not restrained during this exercise. If the patient attempts a vigorous stretch by continuing to rotate the body farther, the elbow or forearm will move on the surface supporting it, thereby preventing excessive tension on the surgical repair. This built-in safety is especially helpful after surgical procedures, such as total shoulder arthroplasty, subscapularis repair, or anterior capsulolabral repairs, during which the subscapularis or anterior glenohumeral ligaments are repaired and, therefore, require maximum protection in the early postoperative period.

During the early postoperative period, the pendulum exercise is also of primary importance to improve ROM and reduce muscle guarding, apprehension, and fear (Figure 4). In our philosophy, correct instruction of this exercise requires the rehabilitation provider to understand that the purpose of this exercise is to provide early pain relief, to improve confidence, to warm up the shoulder, and to minimize the subjective feelings of stiffness. It should not be used as a stretching exercise or to achieve maximum ROM. A crucial instruction on initial performance of this exercise during the early postoperative period is that when the patient bends at the waist, he or she must keep the surgically treated extremity very relaxed. Therefore, while leaning over, the patient should feel as if he or she is leading with the surgically treated extremity. If the patient bends at the waist then lets the surgically treated extremity relax and fall forward, he or she generally feels much more pain. In addition, the

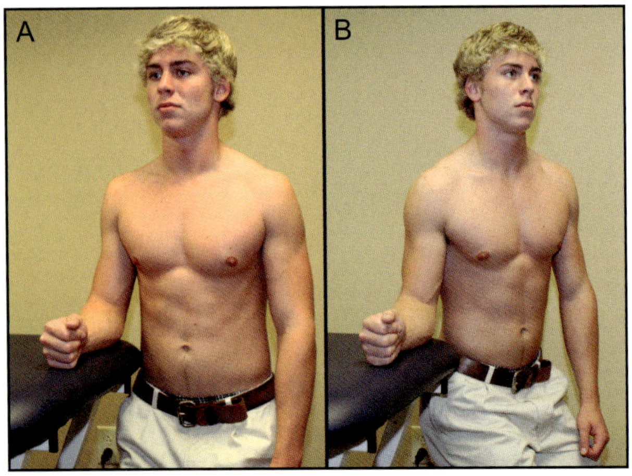

Figure 3 A and B. The passive external rotation walk-around exercise.

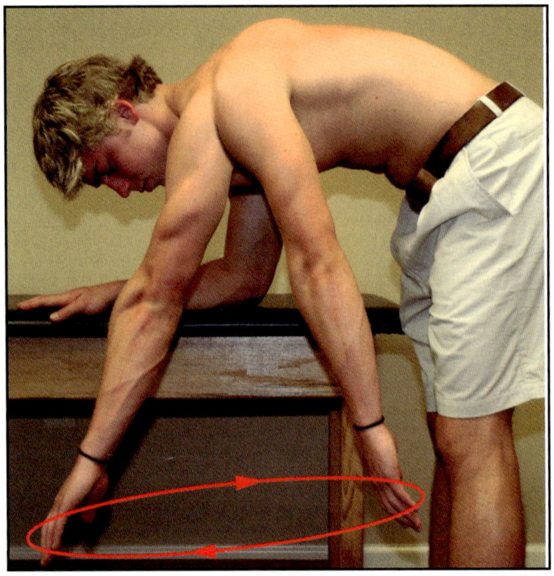

Figure 4. The pendulum exercise.

patient should only flex the trunk an amount that is very comfortable and ideally pain-free rather than to the maximum amount tolerated. Often, if this exercise is initiated the first few days after surgery, just letting the upper extremity dangle while leaning forward is more effective in reducing muscle guarding, pain, and apprehension than creating movement is. When movement is comfortable, we prefer the patient to make small active circles with the extremity, which has demonstrated very low electromyographic activity levels of the supraspinatus and anterior deltoid that are comparable with other early PROM exercises.[14,15] We prefer this method because we have found correct technique is more consistent and the exercise is more comfortable. I believe this exercise should never be performed with weight, and the motions should remain very small so they are pain-free and not strained. If performed as described, the pendulum should be the patient's favorite ROM exercise usually by around postoperative week 2. When it is very comfortable for the patient, the pendulum exercise can be performed many times each day (6 to 10 times or more each day) with very good tolerance. I have found that patients who do this exercise the most tend to feel the best in the early postoperative period.

If flawless technique is used, the easiest way to achieve early PFE in the early postoperative period is the table step-back exercise (Figure 5). The patient begins upright with the hands supported on a table and the elbows held comfortably straight. Keeping the elbows in this position, the patient slowly steps back, lets the hips shift back, and bends at the waist while looking down. The goal is for the torso to eventually become parallel to the ground while the hips are kept fairly high. One common error in technique is to primarily step back while minimally flexing at the hips. This limits the shoulder ROM that is obtained and results in a large amount of weight placed through the upper extremities. As with all early PROM exercises, the patient must stop at a point of gentle pull and, at most, minimal pain. Typical ROM on the first visit is approximately 50° to 70° in patients with rotator cuff repairs, capsulolabral reconstructions, and shoulder arthroplasties. If this exercise is extremely painful when initiated, we typically withhold starting it for about 1 week, which consistently results in improved exercise tolerance.

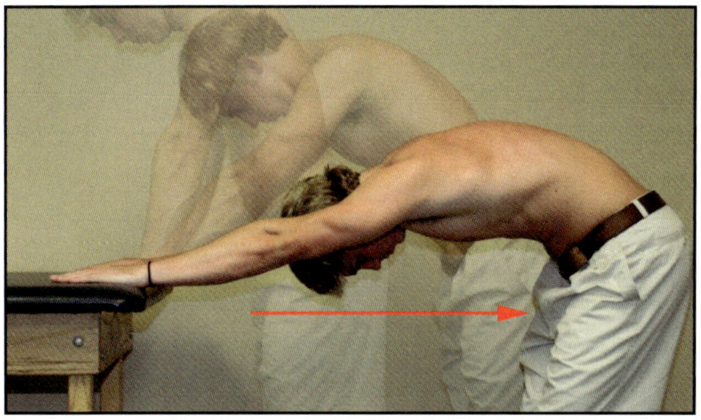

Figure 5. The table step-back exercise.

Our other preferred method for passive scapular-plane elevation in the early postoperative period is PFE in the upright position with the assistance of a rehabilitation provider or family member (Figure 6). Although this exercise is often difficult to achieve in the early postoperative period, it is very useful because we have found that a good closed chain PROM (eg, the table step-back) does not always carry over to good open chain PROM. Because it is more difficult, this exercise typically is not started until about 2 weeks after most types of shoulder surgery. Our preferred technique is for the rehabilitation provider to stand just outside the patient's involved knee oriented diagonally toward the patient. The assistant should lift the patient's involved extremity toward himself or herself in the scapular plane, maintaining the shoulder in approximately 30° of internal rotation. The patient should be instructed to keep the extremity relaxed on the way up and lightly activate the shoulder extensors

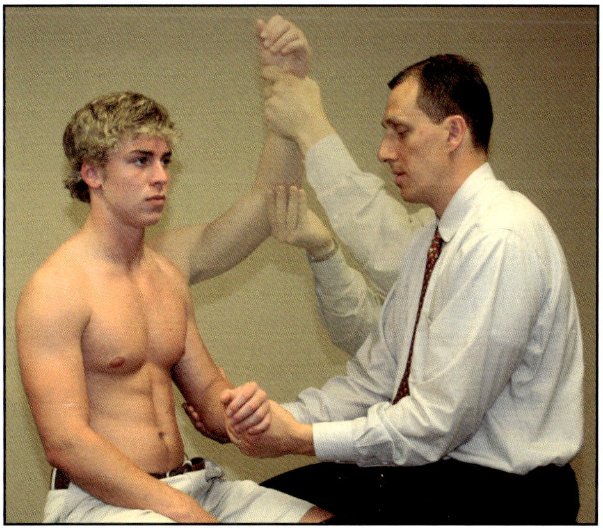

Figure 6. Upright passive forward elevation with the assistance of a rehabilitation provider.

on the way down, resulting in reciprocal inhibition of the antagonist muscles, which in this case include the rotator cuff and deltoid.[15,16]

Supine PROM by the rehabilitation provider also can be helpful in the first 6 weeks in gaining PROM; however, we believe it is an adjunctive treatment. This can be performed in a manner that is easily tolerated within the first few postoperative visits, but extreme care must be taken to ensure that the planes of motion used and ROM obtained are safe for the surgical repair. Our supine PROM techniques are detailed in chapter II-3.

CONCERNS ABOUT POOR RANGE OF MOTION

In our system of always gentle rehabilitation, when do we become worried about poor postoperative PROM? This depends on the surgical procedure and patient, so the rehabilitation provider needs to communicate with the surgeon if he or she believes that a patient is behind on the PROM goals to ensure that a consensus is reached on appropriate ROM targets and management. Generally, patients display decreased pain and increased confidence in the shoulder, which results in increased ROM, typically by week 2 or 3 after rotator cuff repairs, capsulolabral repairs, and shoulder arthroplasties. If the rehabilitation provider perceives joint tightness or a capsular end feel during ROM assessment at or after this time, we recommend increasing the frequency of stretching for patients to approximately 3 to 6 times each day as long as the stretches are performed comfortably. A slight increase in intensity can be used, but keeping stretching intensity exceptionally gentle is important. We generally do not increase repetitions, and depending on the surgical procedure and preference of the surgeon, sling use might be decreased slightly. On the other hand, if ROM is primarily pain-limited, we have found that the best course of action is to continue very light and easy ROM only to the earliest feelings of pain. This promotes a reduction in the level of inflammation that often is limiting ROM and eventually results in decreased pain. Often in the early postoperative period, excessive pain is caused by excessive use of the surgically treated extremity with ADLs, so we ensure that the patient is appropriately using it for ADLs as detailed in this chapter and often recommend a decrease in functional use of the extremity. We also recommend contacting the surgeon if the patient reports uncontrolled pain that is atypically severe. In both stiffness-limited and pain-limited ROM, we agree with others who have found that satisfactory ROM almost always comes with time and continued rehabilitation, with return of nearly normal ROM taking up to 5 to 12 months to achieve.[5,6] If necessary, we will sacrifice ROM to always protect the integrity of the surgical repair.

REFERENCES

1. Mangine B, Nuzzo G, Harrelson GL. Physiologic factors of rehabilitation. In: Andrews JR, Harrelson GL, Wilk KE, eds. *Physical Rehabilitation of the Injured Athlete*. 3rd ed. Philadelphia, PA: WB Saunders; 2004:13–33.
2. Zuckerman JD, Leblanc JM, Choueka J, Kummer F. The effect of arm position and capsular release on rotator cuff repair: a biomechanical study. *J Bone Joint Surg Br*. 1991;73(3):402–405.
3. Tauro JC. Stiffness and rotator cuff tears: incidence, arthroscopic findings, and treatment results. *Arthroscopy*. 2006;22(6):581–586.
4. Pease DG. Psychologic factors of rehabilitation. In: Andrews JR, Harrelson GL, Wilk KE, eds. *Physical Rehabilitation of the Injured Athlete*. 3rd ed. Philadelphia, PA: WB Saunders; 2004:1–7.
5. Cho NS, Rhee YG. Functional outcome of arthroscopic repair with concomitant manipulation in rotator cuff tears with stiff shoulder. *Am J Sports Med*. 2008;36(7):1323–1329.
6. Brislin KJ, Field LD, Savoie FH III. Complications after arthroscopic rotator cuff repair. *Arthroscopy*. 2007;23(2):124–128.
7. Harryman DT, Lazarus MD, Rozencwaig R. The stiff shoulder. In: Rockwood CA, Matsen FA III, eds. *The Shoulder*. 2nd ed. Philadelphia, PA: WB Saunders; 1998:1064–1112.
8. Diercks RL, Stevens M. Gentle thawing of the frozen shoulder: a prospective study of supervised neglect versus intensive physical therapy in seventy-seven patients with frozen shoulder syndrome followed up for two years. *J Shoulder Elbow Surg*. 2004;13(5):499–502.
9. Lundberg BJ. The frozen shoulder: clinical and radiographical observations. The effect of manipulation under general anesthesia. Structure and glycosaminoglycan content of the joint capsule. Local bone metabolism. *Acta Orthop Scand*. 1969; 119(suppl):1–59.
10. Matsen FA III, Thomas SC, Rockwood CA, Wirth MA. Glenohumeral instability. In: Rockwood CA, Matsen FA III, eds. *The Shoulder*. 2nd ed. Philadelphia, PA: WB Saunders; 1998:637–638.
11. Harryman DT II, Lazarus MD, Sidles JA, Matsen FA III. Pathophysiology of shoulder instability. In: McGinty JB, ed. *Operative Arthroscopy*. 2nd ed. Philadelphia, PA: Lippincott Williams & Wilkins. 1996:677–693.
12. Gibb TD, Sidles JA, Harryman DT II, McQuade KJ, Matsen FA III. The effect of capsular venting on glenohumeral laxity. *Clin Orthop Relat Res*. 1991;268:120–127.

13. Novotny JE, Nichols CE, Beynnon BD. Normal kinematics of the unconstrained glenohumeral joint under coupled moment loads. *J Shoulder Elbow Surg*. 1998;7(6):629–639.
14. Dockery ML, Wright TW, LaStayo PC. Electromyography of the shoulder: an analysis of passive modes of exercise. *Orthopedics*. 1998;21(11):1181–1184.
15. McCann PD, Wootten ME, Kadaba MP, Bigliani LU. A kinematic and electromyographic study of shoulder rehabilitation exercises. *Clin Orthop Relat Res*. 1993;288:179–188.
16. Kisner C, Colby LA. *Therapeutic Exercise: Foundations and Techniques*. 2nd ed. Philadelphia, PA: FA Davis; 1990:109–146.

II-3

Strategies to Improve Passive Range of Motion

Joseph H. Kostuch, PT, SCS

CHAPTER CONTENTS

Clinical pearls are highlighted in yellow throughout the text.

Establishing and restoring normal passive range of motion (PROM) for patients treated nonoperatively or operatively should be one of the rehabilitation provider's primary goals in developing the treatment plan. This is a primary and invaluable skill that rehabilitation providers claim to have expertise in evaluating and treating. Whether in a postoperative progression or conservative management of a shoulder disorder, the inability for the glenohumeral (GH) and scapulothoracic (ST) joints to move though a pain-free and nonrestricted range of motion (ROM) often is a primary hurdle to cross for a full recovery. After surgery, PROM is restricted primarily by postoperative pain and apprehension early then by any subsequent operative tensioning or repair along with normal scarring and adhesions that occur. Nonoperatively treated patients whose shoulders are in a highly reactive state have similar PROM limitations due to pain and apprehension, but they also present with much different capsular restrictions underlying the initial painful apprehension. Each condition requires a thorough evaluation to identify the specific limitation, and varying treatment approaches are applied based on the findings. Although the techniques and instructions for achieving PROM differ based on the specific diagnosis and presentation, we at St. Francis Rehabilitation Center (SFRC) always strive to maintain a pain-free approach to PROM stretching and mobilization. We base this recommendation on the work of Diercks and Stevens[1] who illustrated that aggressive stretching or mobilization negatively affects the patient's tolerance to stretching and increases his or her overall level of reactivity.

POSTOPERATIVE PROM

The operatively treated patient requires a much different approach for gaining PROM because of the combination of operative pain and inflammation along with the absolute necessity of protecting the repaired bone or tissue. As described in chapter II-2, although PROM appears straightforward, the rehabilitation provider must convey the correct details of the PROM technique for home-exercise-program (HEP) stretching along with specific and thorough patient education on the factors that affect healing. The patient's ability to successfully balance his or her pain with his or her PROM progression is a critical phase of the recovery. This can set the stage for a smooth recovery that is limited only by tissue-healing precautions or, for a longer, more difficult recovery, is limited by the level of inflammation and shoulder stiffness rather than the landmarks of healing.

Excluding special circumstances in which the surgeon values protection of the soft tissue or fracture healing over potential stiffness, PROM is begun within postoperative week (POW) 1. We believe that gentle, graded PROM within the constraints of the operative repair works successfully to negate the detrimental effects of immobilization, including formation of adhesions, muscle atrophy with sarcomere loss, and articular cartilage degradation.[2–6] These initial planes of motion are passive forward elevation (PFE) in the plane of the scapula and passive external rotation (PER) with the elbow at the side. These planes of motion are sufficient to gain the positive effects of early PROM and are appropriate to protect surgically repaired tissue. These motions are gained through a combination of clinic PROM with the rehabilitation provider and stretching that is part of the patient's HEP.

Phase 1 Rehabilitation Provider PROM

The primary limitation to gaining postoperative PROM in the first 1 to 3 POWs is pain, which leads to apprehension and guarding in the patient with PROM. As described in chapter II-2, great care is taken to teach the patient that during these first POWs, he or she should endure little to no pain with the HEP stretching presented in Figure 1. The rehabilitation provider also must adhere to these guidelines. Patient communication along with skilled stretching by the rehabilitation provider ensures a positive session in which pain is minimized and comfortable PROM is achieved while the patient's apprehension is minimized and his or her confidence is gained.

At SFRC, we perform PROM with the assistance of the rehabilitation provider in both seated and supine positions (Figures 2 and 3). The interaction of gravity and the body position of the patient differently affect how easily and comfortably the GH joint moves. A comfortable range is achieved with slow and smooth movement and is held for 10 to 15 seconds for 6 to 10 repetitions. The hold time at a comfortable end range helps establish the patient's confidence and allows the tissue to accommodate to the newly gained ROM.

Figure 1. Phase 1 passive range-of-motion checklist.

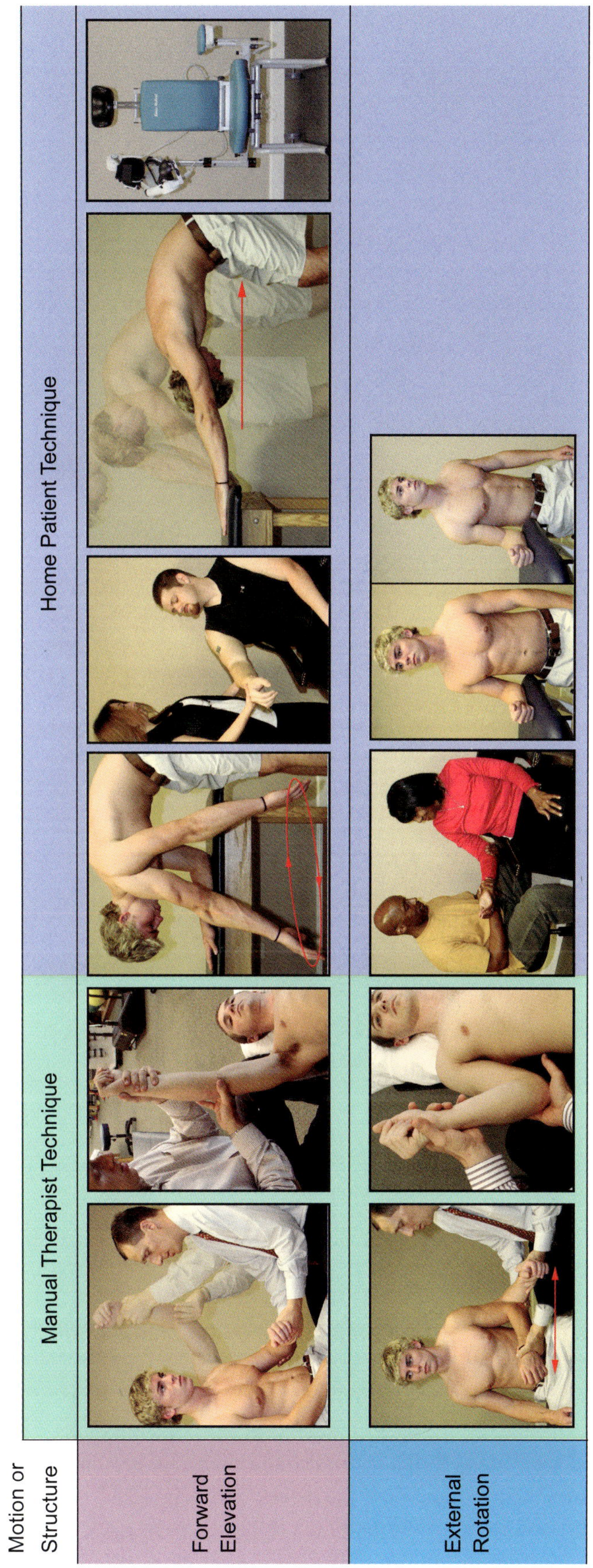

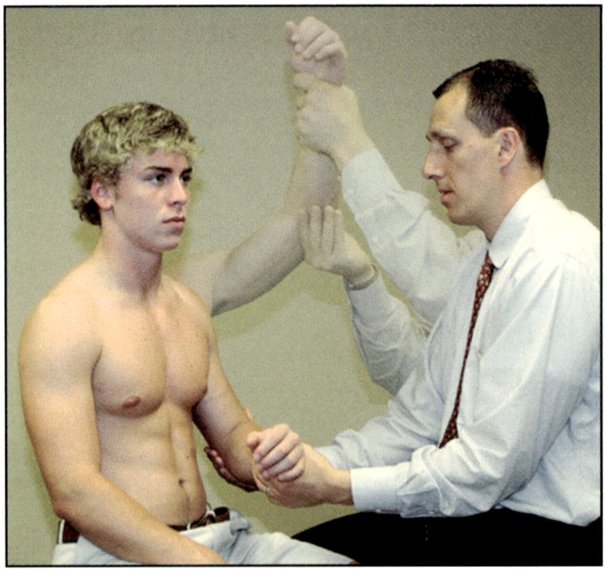

Figure 2. Upright passive forward elevation with the assistance of a rehabilitation provider.

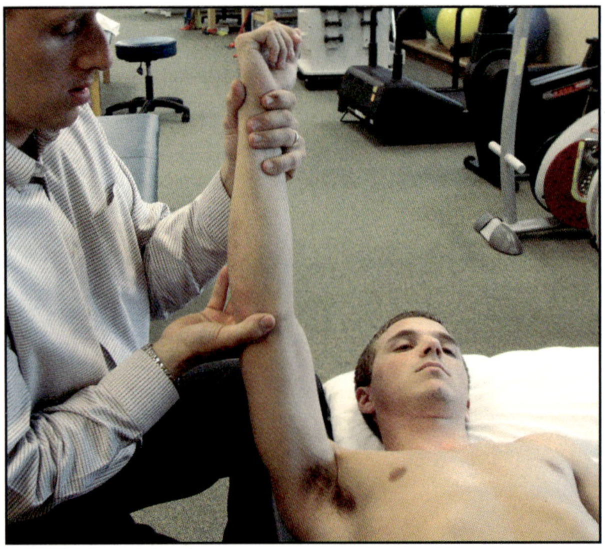

Figure 3. Therapist-assisted passive range of motion in the supine position.

This comfortable, progressive, "building-blocks" approach promotes gradual and comfortable gains in PROM over the initial POWs. The rehabilitation provider takes care to move slowly and communicate with the patient while stretching him or her to ensure that the end feel of the rehabilitation provider matches a comfortable stopping point for the patient. These points carry over to both the seated and supine PROM stretching by the rehabilitation provider. One measure that we use at SFRC to guide our intensity of PROM stretching is to monitor the patient's response during our sessions and the time to return to a baseline level of soreness after our sessions. Ideally, we want patients to be at or near their baseline levels of pain after stretching and icing for 20 minutes. If they return to our clinic describing hours or days of soreness after our stretching sessions, then we decrease our intensity.

No GH joint mobilizations are performed during this phase of recovery because we are not working into any true capsular restriction but specifically are moving the joint through a small comfortable arc. The rehabilitation provider who chooses to perform grades I to II mobilizations during this early postoperative phase should take great care to not stress the repaired tissue.

Infrequently, active ROM (AROM) or PROM of the ST joint is limited postoperatively. The rehabilitation provider must be able to identify early and evaluate this specific situation. Causes can range from limitation or apprehension due to pain to pre-existing thoracic kyphosis with a hypomobile scapula or more serious cervical nerve issues. Often, the muscles supporting the scapula simply are overloaded initially. When the operatively treated upper extremity is supported by the opposite hand to eliminate gravity, the scapular elevators can fire more efficiently, and this allows for the scapula to move into a more natural AROM in upcoming visits. Correctly working with the patient to eliminate this scapular ROM or positioning deficit helps ensure more comfortable and appropriate GH joint PROM progression.

Phase 1 Home PROM

After surgery, the patient also is instructed in an HEP for graded PROM stretching, including home versions of both PFE and PER stretching. We have had the most success and fewest complications teaching PFE with Codman and table step-back exercises and PER with the table walk-around exercise (Figures 4–6). Because the patient remains in full control of the range, he or she has less apprehension and more relaxation, creating the optimum "happy medium" stretch point.

The principles of a comfortable stopping point with a hold of 10 to 15 seconds are emphasized along with the concept of progressive gains within the stretching session. As established, pain more than true capsular tightness is the primary restriction for early PROM, and the rehabilitation provider ensures the patient begins the session at approximately a 75% point of

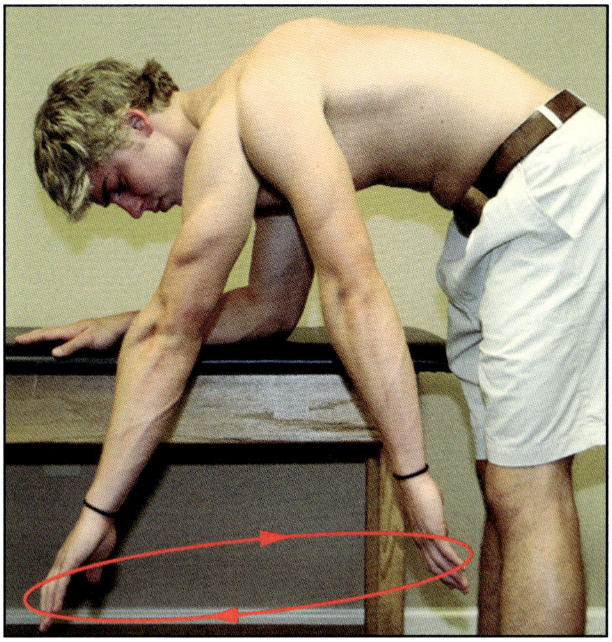

Figure 4. The pendulum exercise.

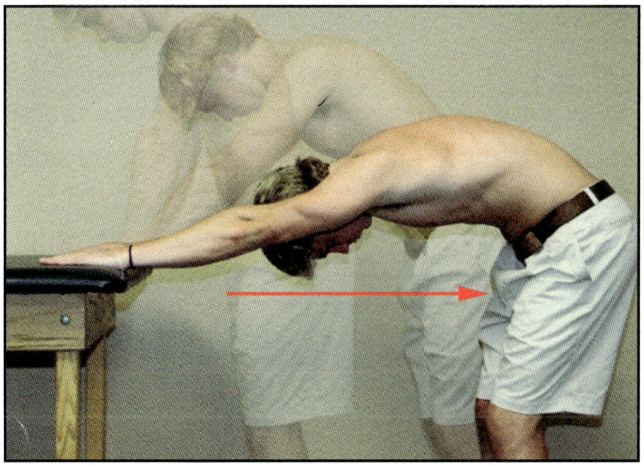

Figure 5. The table step-back exercise.

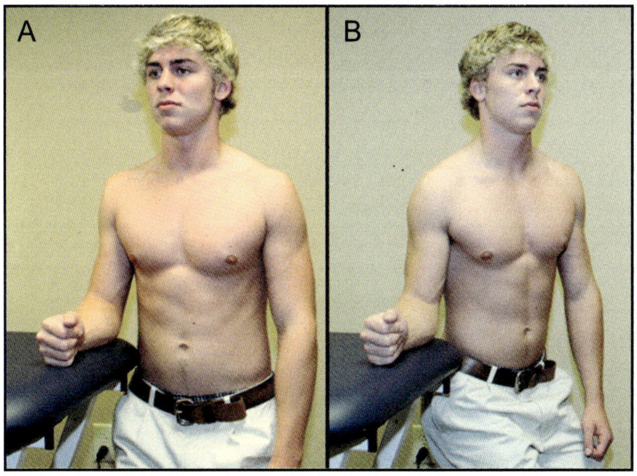

Figure 6 A and B. The passive external rotation walk-around exercise.

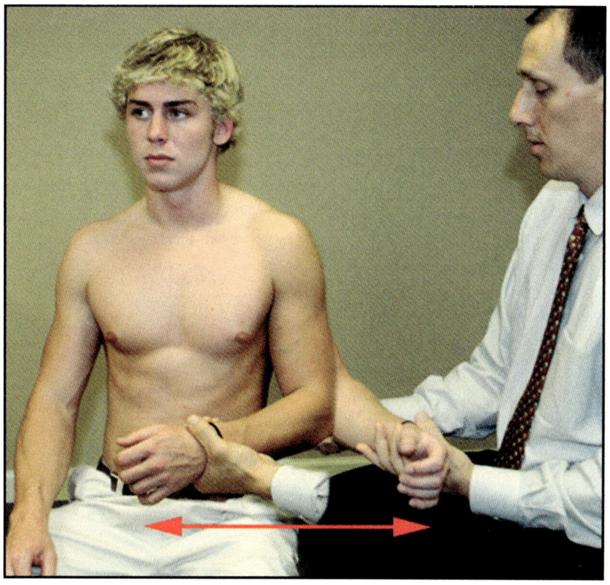

Figure 7. Passive external rotation with the assistance of a rehabilitation provider.

stretch, progressively working to 100% over several repetitions. By beginning with a submaximal stretch, patients can keep pain at a low level or gone while working into their limited PROMs over 3 to 5 repetitions. Total repetitions range from 6 to 12, depending on the patient. Two to 3 sessions of table-assisted PROM are instructed during the first few weeks of recovery as the surgical pain resolves. After resting pain has decreased and tolerance to the HEP has improved, the patient can be instructed to participate in 5 to 6 sessions per day, depending on his or her progress toward the graded ROM goals. In addition, the patient can increase to performing 8 to 10 seconds of the Codman exercise each day because this submaximal stretch

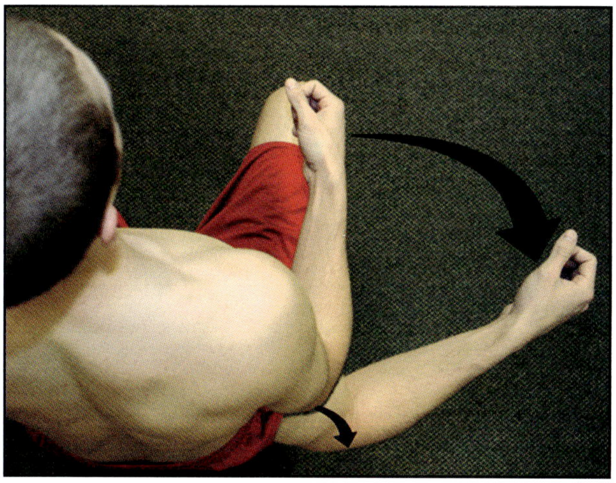

Figure 8. Seated passive external rotation.

allows a measure of relief of pain or ache and safely moves the upper extremity away from the body.

Some patients have reliable family members who can be instructed appropriately in performing seated PFE (Figure 2) and PER (Figure 7) similar to the sessions in physical therapy with the rehabilitation provider. This is often the best scenario if the patient cannot bend or lean forward to perform table step-back PFE because of back or hip issues. In this case, we do not recommend instruction of seated PFE until POW 2 and the patient has had several sessions with the rehabilitation provider to be able to appropriately relax and benefit from the exercise. Seated PER also must be instructed properly to prevent locking the elbow at the patient's side and to allow it to gently rotate around the torso while the forearm is rotated (Figure 8). These pearls will provide the most beneficial HEP experience.

Several researchers[7–12] have studied the safest techniques to gain GH joint PROM while allowing the surrounding musculature to remain relaxed so repaired tissue will not be strained during the healing phase. For early PROM to be safe, the rehabilitation provider not only must choose planes of motion that provide low stress to the repair, but also must use specific exercises that have been documented as having low electromyographic (EMG) activity in the rotator cuff and deltoid.

The Table summarizes the documented EMG activity levels of the supraspinatus (SSP) and anterior deltoid (AD) for common passive elevation exercises performed in the plane of the scapula. Researchers have demonstrated that PFE performed in the supine or upright position with the assistance of the rehabilitation provider or PFE performed in the supine position with the patient assisting himself or herself has much less EMG activity in the SSP and AD than the rope-and-pulley PFE has.[13,14] The pendulum, the table step-back, and aquatic exercises also demonstrate very low EMG activity. We have found that the pendulum, table step-back, and sitting exercises with the assistance of a rehabilitation provider or family member are the most effective and well-tolerated exercises to achieve PFE during the first few weeks after surgery (Figures 2, 4, and 5). In addition, Long et al[10] found that the pendulum exercise elicited percentages of muscle activation that are considered safe when it is performed correctly. We have found that small, active circles not only provide a safe option for PFE, but also have the highest degree of reproducibility and provide the most comfortable option for our patients.

Table. Common Passive Elevation Exercises in the Plane of the Scapula and the Associated Electromyographic Activity Levels of the Supraspinatus and Anterior Deltoid

Exercise	Electromyographic Activity
Therapist-assisted forward elevation	Average supraspinatus 4%, anterior deltoid 8%[7] Average supraspinatus 5%, anterior deltoid 7% supine[8] Average supraspinatus 12%, anterior deltoid 4% upright[8]
Self-assisted forward elevation supine	Average supraspinatus 3%, anterior deltoid 11%[8]
Pulley forward elevation	Average supraspinatus 17%, anterior deltoid 25%[7] Average supraspinatus 13%, anterior deltoid 21%[8] Maximum supraspinatus 17%, anterior deltoid 31%[9]
Pendulum	Average supraspinatus 9%, anterior deltoid 3%[8] Average supraspinatus 6%[7] Maximum supraspinatus (small 10-cm diameter circle) 8–8.7%[10] Maximum supraspinatus (large 51-cm diameter circle) 13.7–18.8%[10]
Specific aquatic exercises	Average supraspinatus 1–5%, anterior deltoid 1–8%[11]
Closed chain (table step-back)	Average supraspinatus 5%, anterior deltoid 2%[12]
Continuous passive motion machine	Average supraspinatus 5%, average anterior deltoid 3%[7]

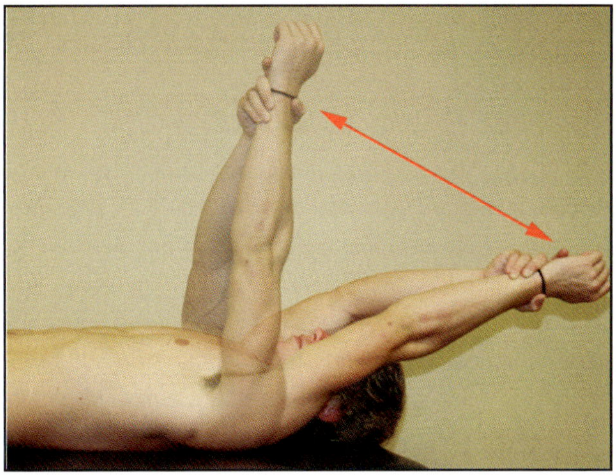

Figure 9. Self-assisted supine passive range of motion.

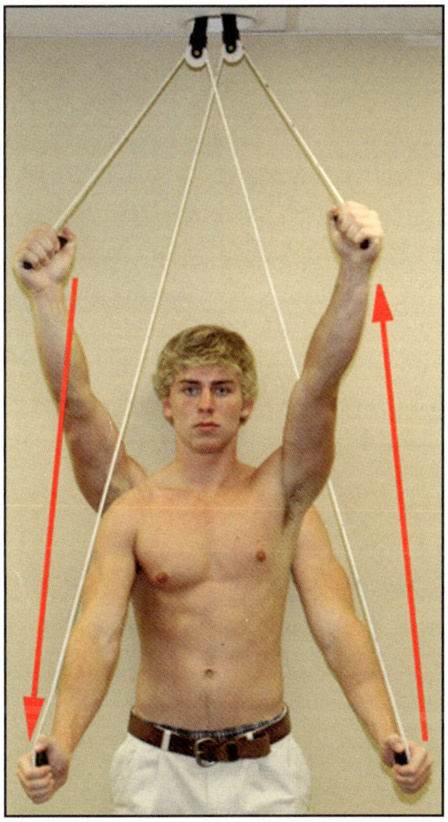

Figure 10. Rope-and-pulley active-assistive forward elevation exercise.

We have found that although self-assisted PROM in the supine position (Figure 9) is safe to start immediately after surgery, it typically is not well tolerated until the patient achieves about 110° of PFE. As the Table demonstrates, the rope-and-pulley exercise (Figure 10) has a noticeably higher EMG activity level in the SSP than the other exercises listed, so we do not recommend starting this exercise until POW 6 for the typical patient after arthroscopic soft tissue repair. Because of the theorized increased mechanical stress to the SSP with end-range PFE, we also restrict the end ranges of this motion during the first 6 weeks of recovery.

For PER, McCann et al[8] and Dockery et al[7] demonstrated very low levels of EMG activity in the SSP, AD, and infraspinatus with all exercises tested. However, neither group of investigators evaluated the EMG activity in the subscapularis, which is likely the muscle most at risk of injury with these exercises, so extreme caution must be used when prescribing PER exercises for patients with subscapularis repairs. Clinically, we have found that PER performed while sitting and with the assistance of a family member or rehabilitation provider and the PER walk-around are the most gentle, effective, and well-tolerated exercises in the early postoperative period (Figures 6 and 7).

At SFRC, we have tracked thousands of patients after surgery and have determined a critical phase of recovery occurs between the third and seventh weeks of recovery. During this timeframe, the patients whom we tracked (primarily patients who have had rotator cuff repairs) and who could achieve smooth PFE up to the range of 140° to 150° had substantially faster and easier recoveries with less therapy visits required than those who were still struggling for their smooth PROM into their second or third month of recovery. During the first several weeks, patients still have moderate postoperative pain that limits their overall tolerance to PROM stretching. Between POWs 2 and 3, pain has decreased in most patients, allowing an increased stretching program. During this time, we advance their programs to include increased frequency of HEP between 4 and 6 sessions per day with up to 10 repetitions and with each stretch held for a slow count to 10. Increased frequency of stretching does NOT mean increased intensity. In addition, we emphasize regular attendance in physical therapy to maximize rehabilitation provider PROM with up to 3 visits per week. Modalites, specifically cryotherapy, remain crucial to help manage any stretching soreness that occurs. With these findings, we recommend increasing HEP stretching during this crucial phase to help provide the safest, fastest recovery. Patients who do not achieve these PROM goals during their first 2 months of recovery should still expect full recovery after their procedures, but they might need to expend additional time and energy stretching into recovery.

Continuous Passive Motion

At SFRC, we have been working with Kinex Medical Company, LLC, (Waukesha, WI) and using its Kinex KS2 continuous passive motion (CPM) chair for specific postoperative conditions. With rehabilitation provider adjustment and fitting of the CPM, we successfully have replicated seated rehabilitation-provider-assisted PFE in the CPM chair (Figure 11). This option has worked well for improving PFE in all of our patients after surgery and specifically in those who might be at higher risk for postoperative stiffness. In addition, patients who do not have a family member available for home PFE stretching or cannot tolerate the table step-back PFE exercise have benefitted from this technique.

The PFE in the CPM machine is begun during POW 1 after specific instruction from the rehabilitation provider and initial home fitting from the chair representative. We instruct patients to spend 15 to 20 minutes in the chair 3 to 4 times per day. The movement arm is set to a slow speed of 25%, which patients typically tolerate very well after surgery. Our patients keep full control over their machines and are instructed to stop their PFE stretches at the point where they feel a mild stretch or any degree of pain and to hold this position for 10 seconds. We discourage patients from focusing too much on the PFE measurement and encourage them to concentrate on the happy medium feel that we have described. The movement arm then cycles down, relieving the stretch, and begins the process again. Patients often can substantially progress their PFE ROM during their sessions.

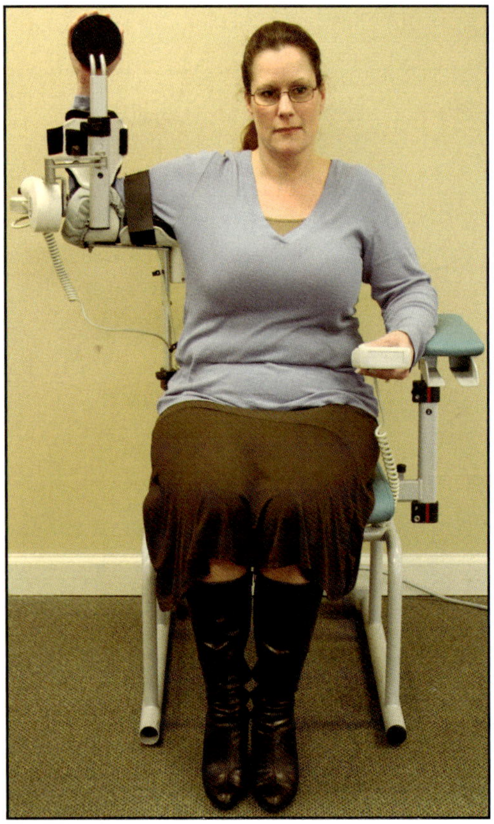

Figure 11. Seated passive forward elevation in the continuous passive motion chair.

A CPM machine, or CPM unit, is used to help achieve greater flexibility of a joint. Often after injury or surgery, the muscles and other surrounding tissues of a joint can stiffen or shorten because the joint has been immobile for an extended period. Potential causes of joint immobility include increased pain, inflammation, swelling, and apprehension to using the affected extremity. A CPM unit can assist in restoring ROM in a slow and controlled manner that will make moving the joint easier and less painful.

Numerous investigators have evaluated the effectiveness of a CPM machine in helping to restore ROM and reduce pain after an injury or surgery of the shoulder. After rotator cuff repair, the use of a CPM unit has been shown to provide earlier ROM when used with physical therapy compared with therapy alone,[15] has been shown to be a source of pain relief,[16] and also might help to prevent secondary complications after surgery.[17] A CPM unit can be used regardless of the size of the rotator cuff tear (small, medium, or large),[14] and because it is a passive form of motion, it might increase the safety margin for obtaining early PROM without disrupting a rotator cuff repair.[7] The use of a shoulder CPM unit also has been shown to provide greater reduction in pain at rest, with movement of the upper extremity, and at night in patients with adhesive capsulitis.[18]

ADVANCED PROM

Phase 2 Rehabilitation Provider PROM

Progression to an advanced stretching program with either a nonoperatively or operatively treated patient must be defined clearly by several factors upon which the rehabilitation provider and referring surgeon decide. Note that our

Figure 12. Phase 2 passive range-of-motion checklist.

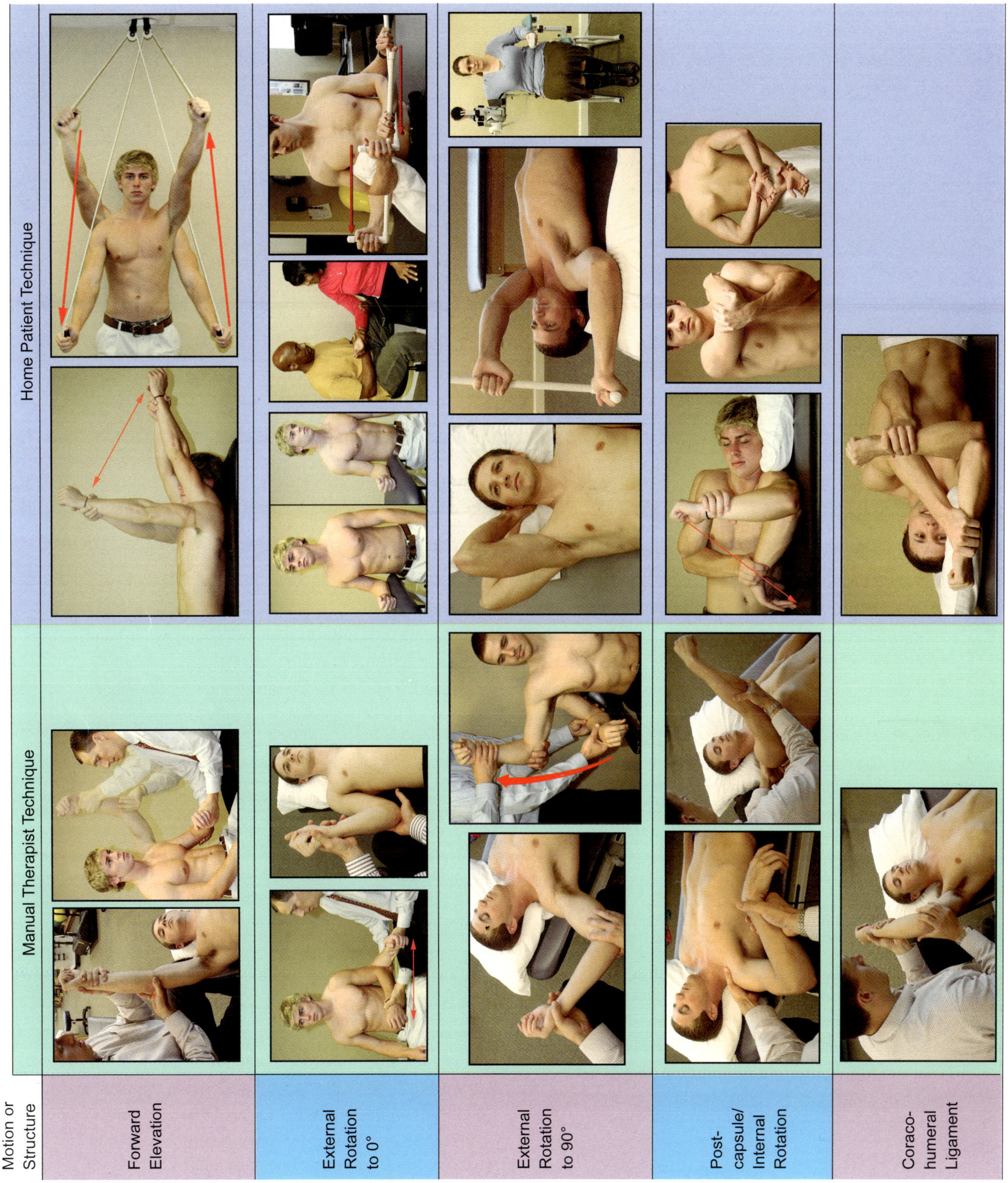

phase 2 stretching program is an all-planes stretching program but is NOT a more intense stretching program. Because so many degrees of freedom exist about the GH joint, a full recovery of function that specifically addresses all planes of motion is crucial. The phase 2 program will work to maintain and advance PER at 0° and PFE while adding progression to PER at 45° and 90° of abduction, passive internal rotation at 45° and 90°, horizontal adduction, functional internal rotation, diagonal PFE, and a specific coracohumeral ligament stretch. The order in which these additional planes of movement are incorporated into each patient's treatment plan varies depending on the diagnosis and individual presentation.

Postoperatively, there is a critical combination of postoperative healing time, specific structures repaired, patient's overall level of pain, and patient's tolerance to the current forward elevation and external rotation stretching program. The rehabilitation provider and surgeon must address all of these factors before progressing to a more advanced PROM program. By specifically addressing each of these factors, the order in which the new planes of motion are added can be determined and safely implemented into the patient's stretching program. The addition of multiple planes of stretching must not increase the risk to the healing tissues or substantially increase the patient's overall level of pain. In most postoperative situations, these additional planes of motion are not initiated for rehabilitation provider or home stretching until POW 6 or later.

Patients who have not had surgery must be evaluated in a similar manner. Combining their diagnoses and evaluations along with assessing their levels of reactivity, the rehabilitation provider can determine more specifically a safe PROM stretching program. Because no specific structures require protection, patients treated nonoperatively often move from the phase 1 to phase 2 stretching program almost immediately, addressing almost all the PROM deficits from the start. The exception to this approach is a patient presenting with a moderately to highly reactive shoulder in great pain, such as someone in the first phase of idiopathic adhesive capulitis, active synovitis, or calcific tendinitis. I further address this situation in the Special Considerations section.

Phase 2 Home PROM

At SFRC we use a specific checklist of PROM directions to evaluate and determine the patient's need for a manual or home stretch to address this deficit (Figure 12). By following this checklist, we can fully appreciate the "circle theory" of the shoulder capsule as described by Levine and Flatow,[19] which allows us to achieve unrestricted PROM for our patients. Appropriate screening of all directions listed enables us to make progress with a more difficult or stiff plane of motion by simply addressing the entire "circle" of capsular tissue and stretching where needed. For example, limited PFE can be improved with passive internal rotation stretching at 90°.[20]

TERMINAL PROM

Phase 3 Rehabilitation Provider PROM

Terminal PROM stretching only should be used long after any postoperative healing timeframes have expired. Typically, we use these stretches at postoperative month 3 at the earliest and most often closer to postoperative month 4 and later. Patients should have no lasting pain after stretching and subjectively should report tightness as a greater limitation than pain. Terminal stretching is instructed as a means to achieve the final 10% to 15% of any remaining PROM deficit. Inclusion of these terminal stretches before this point of recovery nearly always creates pain and substitution patterns and promotes excess scapular rather than GH joint PROM. Therefore, specific care is taken in prescribing these home stretches only to a specific population that fits the given criteria. The rehabilitation provider continues the manual stretching in the clinic as described in phase 2, advancing ROM based on the patient's tolerance.

Phase 3 Home PROM

The advantage of many of the terminal stretches described for the HEP is that the patient uses his or her body position to perform them. With no special equipment or supine positioning, this makes frequent stretching easier to achieve during the day. Because the patient is using his or her body mass to counter the stretch position, great care must be taken in instructing him or her to maintain an upright body position where the mass is balanced under the feet rather than to lean into the stretch. With the increased intensity of these stretches, patients are instructed to perform only 3 to 5 repetitions with a 10- to 15-second hold for each stretch 3 to 4 times each day.

The checklist presented in Figure 13 is not intended to provide an order for introducing new stretches but simply is intended as a screening tool to ensure full coverage of the capsule. New stretches must be introduced in an appropriate manner as discussed earlier. A large population of patients will not require the advanced terminal stretching techniques and will gain full PROM with the phase 2 program or possibly just a select few terminal stretches to reach their maximum ROMs.

Figure 13. Phase 3 terminal passive range-of-motion checklist.

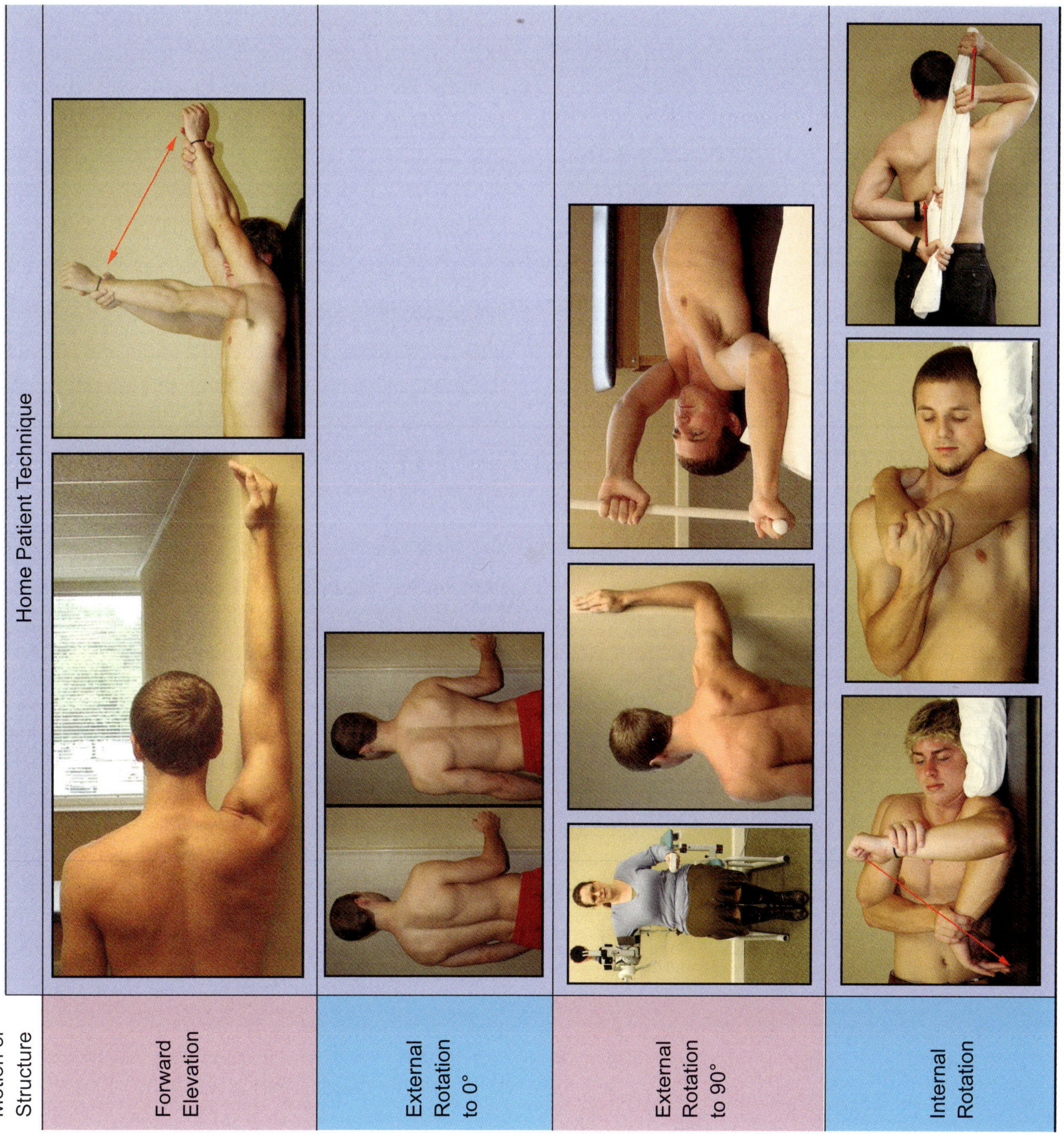

SPECIAL CONSIDERATIONS

Idiopathic Adhesive Capsulitis and Synovitis

With certain diagnoses and situations, simply evaluating PROM and addressing deficits with the appropriate stretch is too aggressive. Both the physician and rehabilitation provider need to identify this patient subgroup as an outlier and to alter their treatment approach. The physician helps the rehabilitation provider when he or she identifies this group at the evaluation and might provide either an injection or medication to help reduce the inflammatory response. These specific PROM interventions might not always be appropriate, but the oral communication from the physician that teaches the patient about the importance of modalities and comfortable therapy can be invaluable in our treatment of his or her problem. With these cases, the rehabilitation provider must base the exercise prescription entirely on the patient's comfortable tolerance to a simplified stretching program. Simplifying the approach can be challenging for the provider, knowing that multiple deficits need to be addressed but that trying to implement a comprehensive phase 2 stretching program too early will only make the problem worse and slow progress. More specific interventions for these diagnoses are presented in chapters III-10 and III-15.

Mobilizations

Glenohumeral Joint. At SFRC, we implement an anatomic approach to our joint mobilizations by following the normal shoulder joint arthrokinematics best described and referenced through the International Academy of Orthopedic Medicine technique.[21] By having a complete understanding of how the GH joint rolls, glides, and slides, we simply mobilize the joint in these same triplanar accessory motions to complement the associated plane of motion. These mobilizations typically are performed at or near end ROMs to better appreciate the restriction. Because the upper extremity is positioned near end range, visualizing and appreciating the orientation of the glenoid when mobilizing the joint is crucial to achieving the desired plane of pressure. Although technique varies among rehabilitation providers, these are typically grade II or III mobilizations that are held for 10 to 20 seconds and a gentle oscillation into the capsular restriction. Because these are performed near the end ranges, we keep our repetitions low (between 3 and 6 repetitions). We also employ the unifying technique of providing slight compression with our arthrokinematic mobilization. Because our mobilization philosophy is based on normal physiologic joint movement, compression is a constant component with any active joint movement. As discussed, we discourage the use of GH joint mobilizations during the first phase of recovery after surgery because these might compromise healing tissue or create unneeded pain for the patient.

Johnson et al[13] specifically demonstrated the necessity and advantages of mobilizing the GH joint in a posterior direction to help achieve not only greater internal rotation, but also more forward elevation and external rotation. We employ this technique by again placing the upper extremity in a nearly maximum stretch position then employing a posteriorly guided force with the described intensity and repetitions. The rehabilitation provider must orient himself or herself appropriately to the correct direction of the mobilization. As the upper extremity is positioned in end range, the scapula also rotates and creates an altered direction of mobilization needed to address the desired tissue.

Acromioclavicular and Sternoclavicular Joints. A population of both nonoperatively and operatively treated patients has a specific limitation in elevation created by the sternoclavicular or acromioclavicular joint not moving properly. If the patient is not examined thoroughly, this limitation can be missed and, therefore, will not allow full return of active forward elevation and PFE. Several techniques of evaluation can be used to screen for this hypermobility, but the combination of pain at either the acromioclavicular or sternoclavicular joint along with the presence of either GH or scapular hypomobility into all planes of motion is the primary indicator. At SFRC, we mobilize and treat this condition similar to that described in the International Academy of Orthopedic Medicine[21] literature, and our patients have appreciated excellent short-term relief, with lasting return to full overhead function (Figure 14).

Scapula. Because scapular upward rotation is crucial for achieving normal AROM and PROM, treatment of

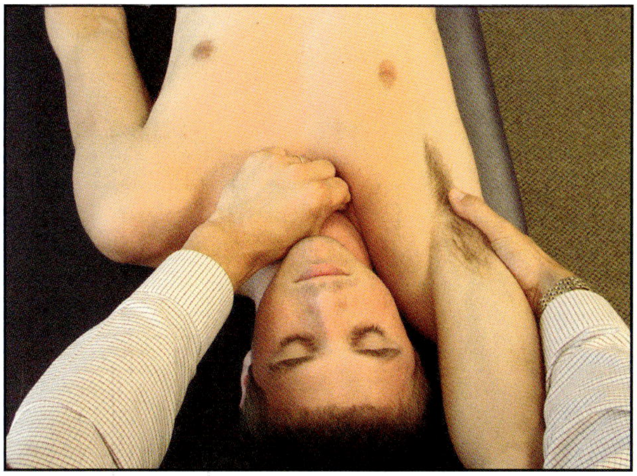

Figure 14. Sternoclavicular joint mobilization.

hypomobility of the ST joint should be included in the assessment of PFE limitation. Scapular rotation does not occur in a discernable amount until the patient has achieved more than 90° of forward elevation. It then contributes as much as 50% of the total arc of motion up to full elevation. Most scapular hypomobility issues are identified early in postoperative recovery and can be addressed appropriately and safely with a combination of seated and side-lying, manual passive and active techniques meant to increase the patient's awareness of this motion. As mentioned, scapular hypomobility might be a direct result of poor sternoclavicular and acromioclavicular mobility and should be examined thoroughly.

REFERENCES

1. Diercks RL, Stevens M. Gentle thawing of the frozen shoulder: a prospective study of supervised neglect versus intensive physical therapy in seventy-seven patients with frozen shoulder syndrome followed up for two years. *J Shoulder Elbow Surg*. 2004;13(5):499–502.
2. Dehne E, Torp RP. Treatment of joint injuries by immediate mobilization: based upon the spinal adaptation concept. *Clin Orthop Relat Res*. 1971;77:218–232.
3. Namba RS, Kabo JM, Dorey FJ, Meals RA. Continuous passive motion versus immobilization: the effect on posttraumatic joint stiffness. *Clin Orthop Relat Res*. 1991;267:218–223.
4. Williams PE. Use of intermittent stretch in the prevention of serial sarcomere loss in immobilized muscle. *Ann Rheum Dis*. 1990;49(5):316–317.
5. Williams PE. Effect of intermittent stretch on immobilised muscle. *Ann Rheum Dis*. 1988;47(12):1014–1016.
6. Salter RB, Simmonds DF, Malcolm BW, Rumble EJ, MacMichael D, Clements ND. The biological effect of continuous passive motion on the healing of full-thickness defects in articular cartilage: an experimental investigation in the rabbit. *J Bone Joint Surg Am*. 1980;62(8):1232–1251.
7. Dockery ML, Wright TW, LaStayo PC. Electromyography of the shoulder: an analysis of passive modes of exercise. *Orthopedics*. 1998;21(11):1181–1184.
8. McCann PD, Wootten ME, Kadaba MP, Bigliani LU. A kinematic and electromyographic study of shoulder rehabilitation exercises. *Clin Orthop Relat Res*. 1993;288:179–188.
9. Gaunt BW, McCluskey GM, Uhl TL. Electromyographic evaluation of subdividing active-assistive shoulder exercises. *Sports Health*. 2010;2(5):424–432.
10. Long JL, Ruberte Thiele RA, Skendzel JG, et al. Activation of the shoulder musculature during pendulum exercises and light activities. *J Orthop Sports Phys Ther*. 2010;40(4):230–237.
11. Fujisawa H, Suenaga N, Minami A. Electromyographic study during isometric exercise of the shoulder in head-out water immersion. *J Shoulder Elbow Surg*. 1998;7(5):491–494.
12. Uhl TL, Muir TA, Lawson L. Electromyographical assessment of passive, active assistive, and active shoulder rehabilitation exercises. *PM R*. 2010;2(2):132–141.
13. Johnson AJ, Godges JJ, Zimmerman GJ, Ounanian LL. The effect of anterior versus posterior glide joint mobilization on external rotation range of motion in patients with shoulder adhesive capsulitis. *J Orthop Sports Phys Ther*. 2007;37(3):88–99.
14. Lastayo PC, Wright T, Jaffe R, Hartzel J. Continuous passive motion after repair of the rotator cuff: a prospective outcome study. *J Bone Joint Surg Am*. 1998;80(7):1002–1011.
15. Michael JW, König DP, Imhoff AB, et al. Efficiency of a postoperative treatment after rotator cuff repair with a continuous passive motion device (CPM) [in German]. *Z Orthop Ihre Grenzgeb*. 2005;143(4):438–445.
16. Raab MG, Rzeszutko D, O'Connor W, Greatting MD. Early results of continuous passive motion after rotator cuff repair: a prospective, randomized, blinded, controlled study. *Am J Orthop (Belle Meade NJ)*. 1996;25(3):214–220.
17. Du Plessis M, Eksteen E, Jenneker A, et al. The effectiveness of continuous passive motion on range of motion, pain and muscle strength following rotator cuff repair: a systematic review. *Clin Rehabil*. 2011;25(4):291–302.
18. Dundar U, Toktas H, Cakir T, Evcik D, Kavuncu V. Continuous passive motion provides good pain control in patients with adhesive capsulitis. *Int J Rehabil Res*. 2009;32(3):193–198.
19. Levine WN, Flatow EL. The pathophysiology of shoulder instability. *Am J Sports Med*. 2000;28(6):910–917.
20. Gerber C, Werner CM, Macy JC, Jacob HA, Nyffeler RW. Effect of selective capsulorrhaphy on the passive range of motion of the glenohumeral joint. *J Bone Joint Surg Am*. 2003;85(1):48–55.
21. Winkel D, Matthijs O, Phelps V, Vleeming A. *Diagnosis and Treatment of the Upper Extremities: Nonoperative Orthopaedic Medicine and Manual Therapy*. Gaithersburg, MD: Aspen Publishers; 1997.

II-4

An Evidence-Based Active-Range-of-Motion and Strengthening Progression

Bryce W. Gaunt, PT, SCS

CHAPTER CONTENTS

- Elevation progression
- Elastic-resistance training below shoulder level
- Static closed kinetic chain exercise progression
- Advanced strengthening exercises and exercises with maximum EMG activity

Clinical pearls are highlighted in yellow throughout the text.

Skillful exercise progression that is based on evidence, is well tolerated by the patient, and is effective is one of the most challenging aspects of shoulder rehabilitation. The ability to order exercises correctly to help protect healing tissues, reduce pain during rehabilitation, and assist clinical decision making also is crucial. Exercise progression can be based on several factors, including the muscle demand, biomechanical principles, pain level, and range of motion (ROM) required. A combination of these factors is important to consider in all situations when developing an exercise progression; however, for certain shoulder disorders, some factors are more important. For example, for patients who are being rehabilitated either nonoperatively or postoperatively for rotator cuff disorders, ordering exercises based on muscle demand or activity level as measured by electromyography takes priority over all other factors. Exercising within a precise ROM limit is of primary importance in the early postoperative rehabilitation of a patient after a capsulolabral repair.

In this chapter, I detail the evidence-based active-ROM (AROM) and strengthening progression we use for shoulder girdle rehabilitation at St. Francis Rehabilitation Center and the St. Francis Orthopaedic Institute. It is largely an electromyography-based progression that progressively exercises the entire shoulder girdle and incorporates the sound physics and biomechanical principles detailed in chapter II-5. Various ROMs can be used for most exercises based on the needs of each patient. Our evidenced-based shoulder girdle exercise progression is outlined in Figure 1. Low electromyographic (EMG), passive ROM (PROM) exercises are the first level of our shoulder girdle exercise progression. This evidence-based PROM exercise progression is detailed in chapter II-3. Our AROM and strengthening progression begins with 3 interrelated tracts that often are used simultaneously. Patients who want to return to activities requiring heavy lifting, explosive movements, or repetitive overhead activities eventually are progressed to our advanced strengthening phase, which generally is not needed for other patient populations.

Although I will detail discrete levels of exercise progression, great overlap and intermixing between levels occurs in clinical practice. Therefore, this chapter is best used as a tool to assist clinical decision making; the rehabilitation provider must realize the specific exercises that are best for each patient are individualized based on each patient's diagnosis and response to each exercise and must be particularly watchful to minimize pain and abnormal movement patterns during exercise prescription. The initial AROM and strengthening progression for most patients includes using at least 2 of the initial 3 tracts shown in Figure 1, which typically are performed at the same time. The elevation progression focuses on achieving full-motion, overhead, active elevation of the upper extremity in the plane of the scapula and then strengthening that motion. Because the elastic-resistance program provides light to moderate strengthening to the entire rotator cuff

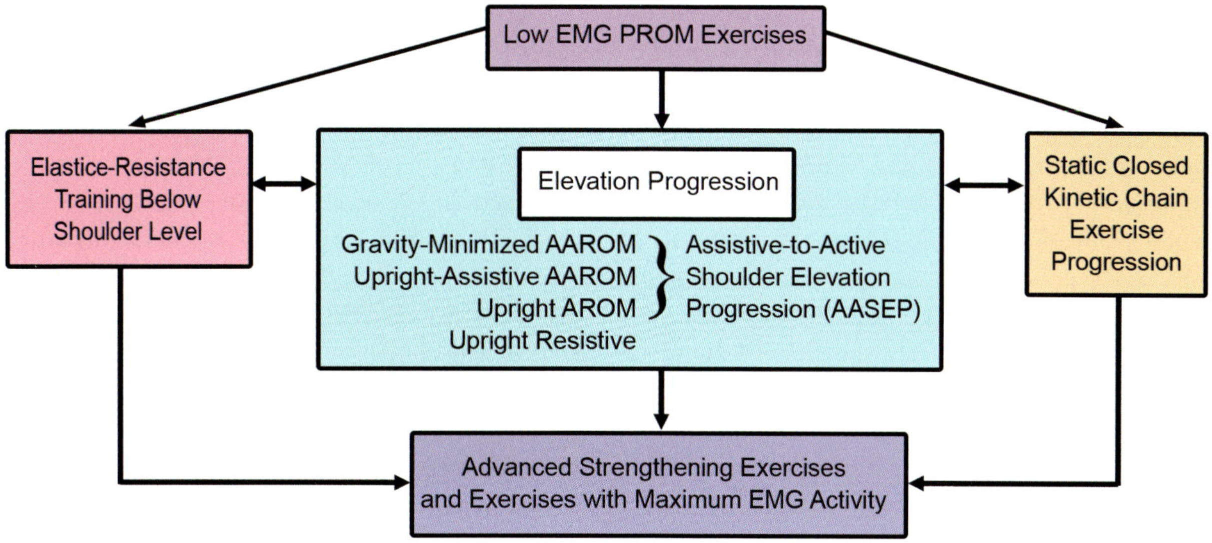

Figure 1. The St. Francis Rehabilitation Center and St. Francis Orthopaedic Institute Evidence-Based Shoulder Girdle Exercise Progression flowsheet. The active range of motion (AROM) and strengthening progression comprises all components other than the low-electromyographic (EMG) passive-range-of-motion (PROM) exercises. Abbreviation: AAROM, active-assistive range of motion.

and scapular muscles in nonprovocative positions, this program is ideal to be used both in the early stages of strengthening and for long-term maintenance of rotator cuff and scapular strengthening. The static closed chain progression is another light to moderate rotator cuff strengthening program that activates the shoulder girdle and improves weight-bearing tolerance through the affected extremity without movement. Because each tract has a different emphasis, the tracts can be used concurrently to help patients achieve individual goals.

ELEVATION PROGRESSION

The elevation progression is one of the initial AROM and strengthening tracts. The purpose of this progression is to provide an organized stepwise manner for patients to progress from passive forward elevation of the upper extremity overhead to full-motion active forward elevation (AFE) of the extremity overhead without then with light resistance (Figure 2). Forward elevation is the natural plane of motion in which a person lifts his or her extremity overhead. It typically is lateral to the sagittal plane and anterior to the plane of the scapula. Achieving AFE is often one of the most difficult steps in rehabilitation and is frustrating for both patients and rehabilitation providers.

This progression emphasizes training the rotator cuff, deltoid, and scapular upward rotation force couple for the forward elevation motion. Rotational strengthening of the external and internal rotators is not part of this progression. The elevation progression has 4 levels:

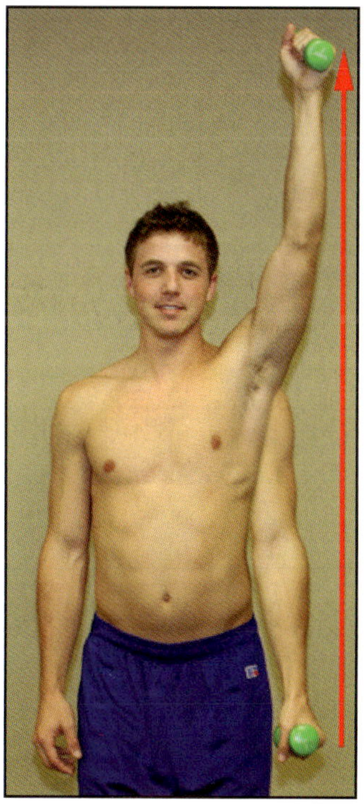

Figure 2. Active forward elevation with light weight is the goal of the elevation progression.

gravity-minimized active-assistive ROM (AAROM), upright assistive AAROM, upright AROM, and upright resistive elevation.

The first 3 levels are termed the *assistive-to-active shoulder elevation progression* (AASEP),[1] and depending on the patient, they can constitute a very small part of rehabilitation or might take several months to complete. The philosophy of the AASEP is to manipulate lever arms and the effect of gravity on the forward elevation movement for patients who cannot perform full-range AFE without pain or substitution (Figure 2). At first during gravity-minimized AAROM exercises, the load to the muscles that contribute to the forward-elevation movement is minimized then gradually increased during upright assistive AAROM exercises and upright AROM exercises. Minimizing the load during the early stages of the AASEP by creative patient positioning or upper extremity support allows the patient to perform "strengthening" exercises that use a larger ROM than the ROM used to perform the same motion upright and unassisted against gravity (Figure 3). We use this progression to facilitate muscle activation and dynamic motor control through a large ROM that we believe speeds achievement of upright AROM overhead against gravity. We also have found this progression helpful for retraining abnormal movement and substitution patterns during active elevation of the extremity. This style of progression has both biomechanical[2,3] and EMG[4,5] evidence supporting its use.

In the AASEP, *gravity-minimized AAROM* has been defined as any exercise in which gravity provides assistance to complete the concentric portion of the exercise or any exercise in which the primary movement is perpendicular to gravity while the weight of the extremity is supported.[4] Gravity-minimized exercises include activities, such as horizontal dusting, side-lying active elevation, supine forward elevation with elastic resistance from 90°, and the supine reaching progression (Figures 4–7). *Upright assistive AAROM*

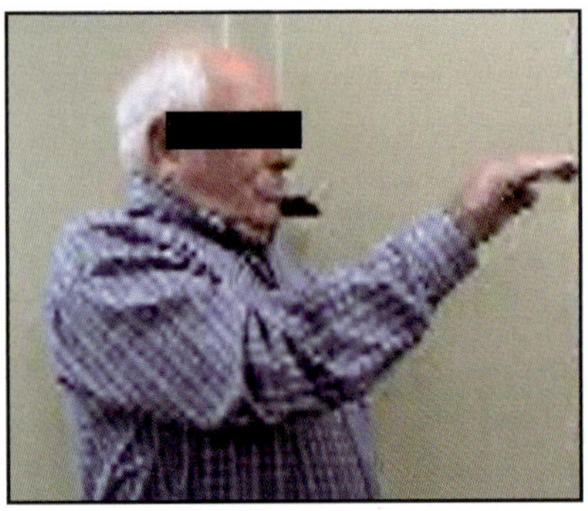

Figure 3A. A patient demonstrates maximum upright active elevation 5 months after a massive rotator cuff repair of the supraspinatus and infraspinatus.

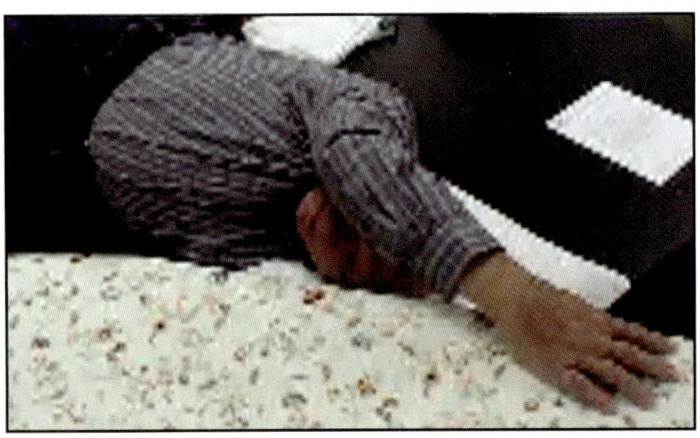

Figure 3B. On the same day, he demonstrates maximum active elevation in a gravity-minimized position.

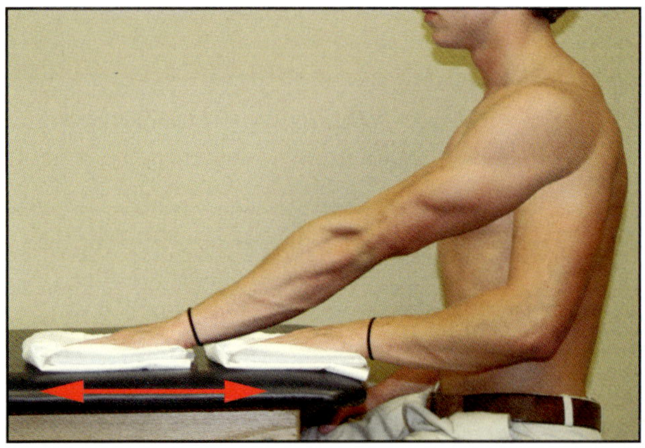

Figure 4. Horizontal dusting.

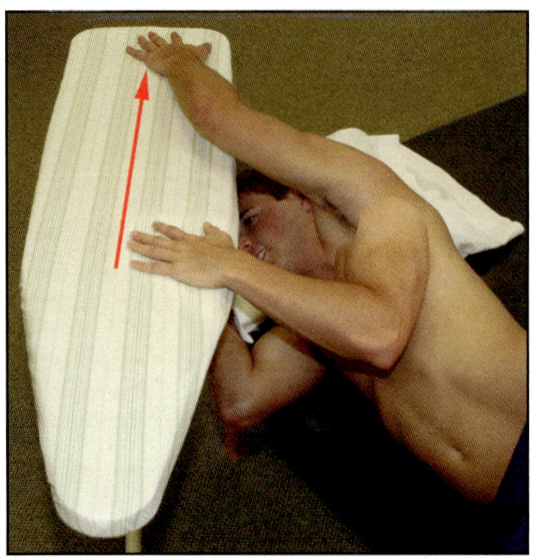

Figure 5. Side-lying active elevation.

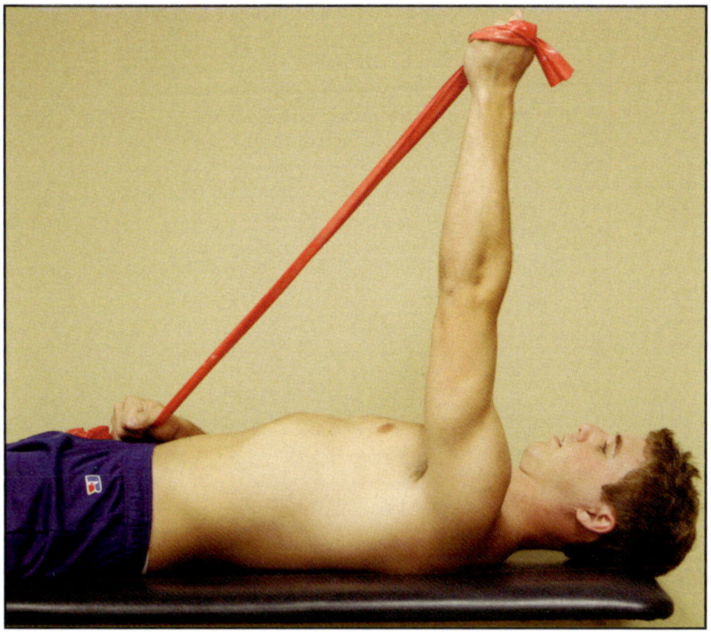

Figure 6. Supine forward elevation with elastic resistance from 90°.

exercise has been defined as any exercise during which the patient is in the upright position and elevating the extremity against gravity during the concentric phase of motion with assistance.[4] Assistance to the involved extremity is provided by the hand being supported by an object during movement or by the hand moving on an object, which lessens the weight of the upper extremity. Examples of upright assistive elevation exercises include rope-and-pulley forward elevation, incline dusting, wall slides, ball roll, standing T-bar active-assistive forward elevation, and standing T-bar assistive elevation with active lowering (Figures

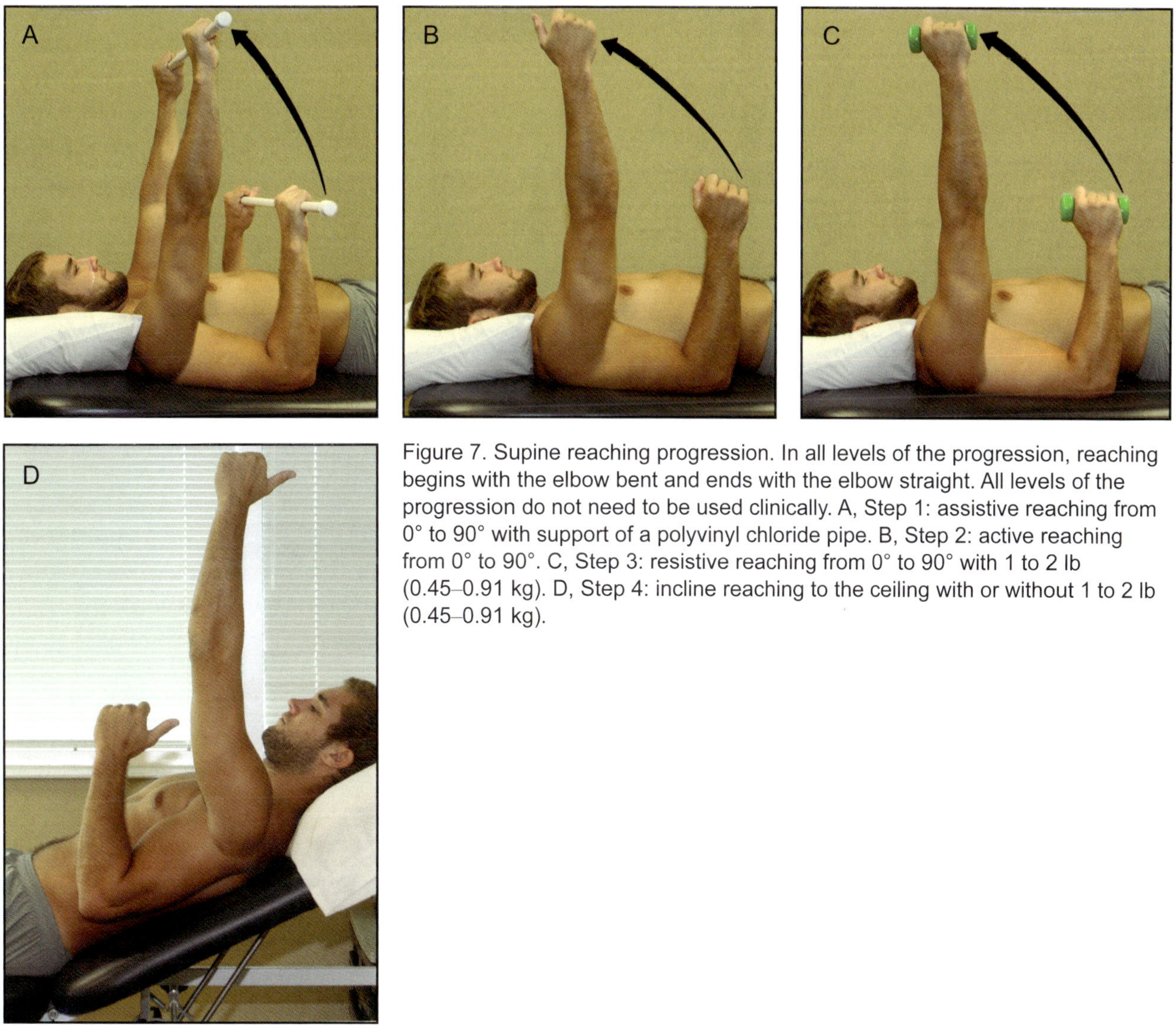

Figure 7. Supine reaching progression. In all levels of the progression, reaching begins with the elbow bent and ends with the elbow straight. All levels of the progression do not need to be used clinically. A, Step 1: assistive reaching from 0° to 90° with support of a polyvinyl chloride pipe. B, Step 2: active reaching from 0° to 90°. C, Step 3: resistive reaching from 0° to 90° with 1 to 2 lb (0.45–0.91 kg). D, Step 4: incline reaching to the ceiling with or without 1 to 2 lb (0.45–0.91 kg).

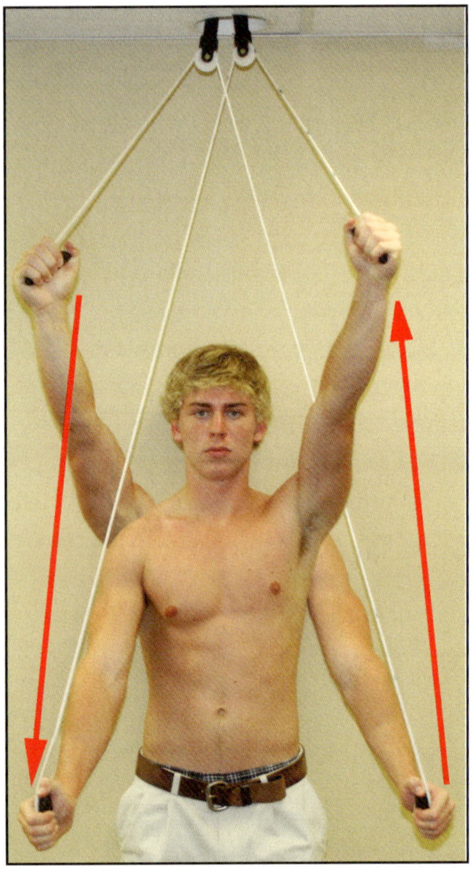

Figure 8. Rope-and-pulley assistive forward elevation.

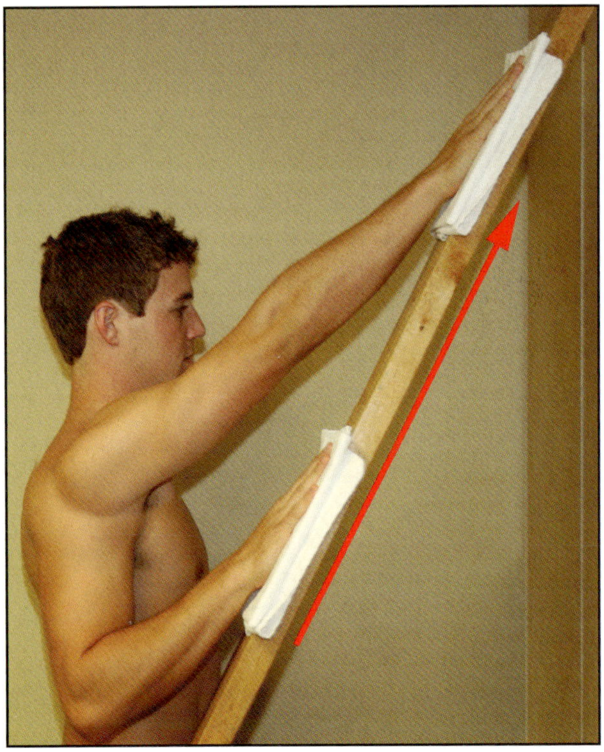

Figure 9. Incline dusting.

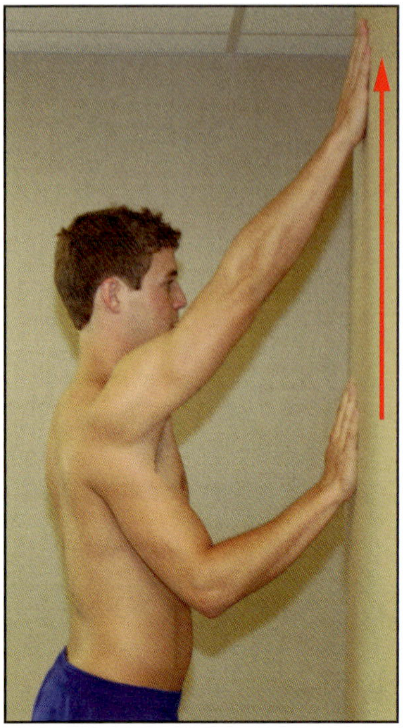

Figure 10.
Wall slides are preferred over wall walk or finger ladder.

8–13). Upright AFE unsupported against gravity is the third level of the AASEP and the goal of the program (Figure 14).

In clinical use of the AASEP, not all the exercises I listed are used with each patient. The list is a menu of choices for which EMG evidence to document muscle demand is available. The rehabilitation provider should choose exercises for each patient that are biomechanically sound, performed without pain, and can be completed naturally without substitution but are

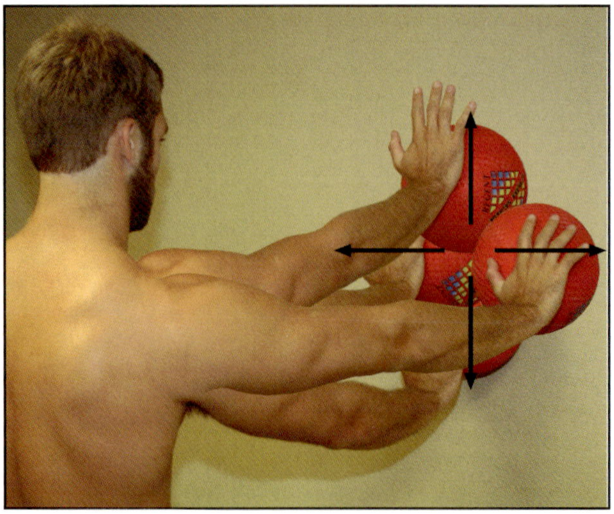

Figure 11. Ball roll on a wall. The elbow remains straight throughtout the exercise.

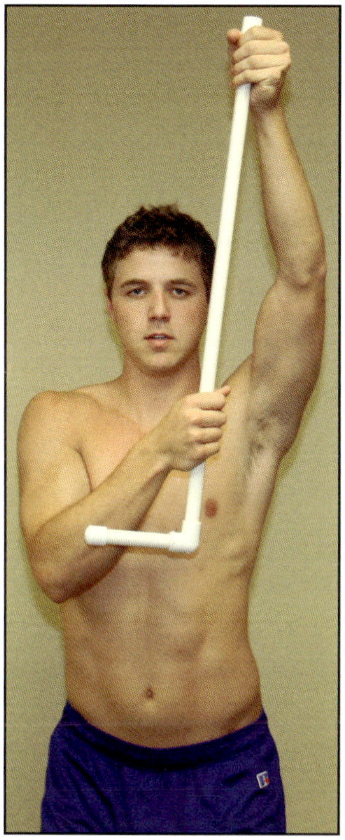

Figure 12. Standing T-bar active-assistive range-of-motion elevation and lowering.

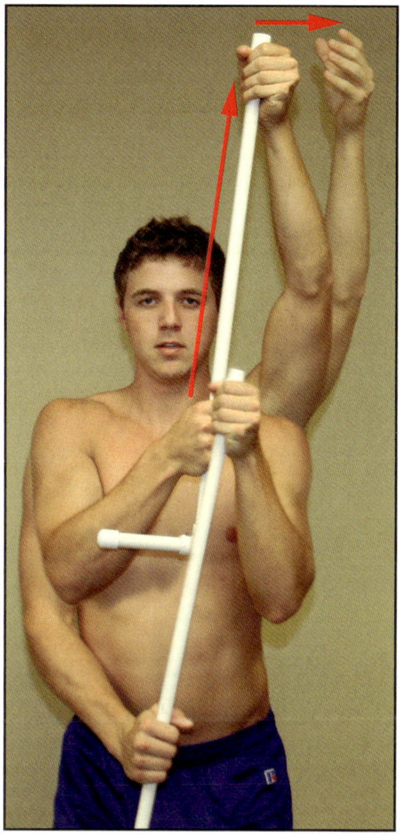

Figure 13. Standing T-bar assistive elevation and active lowering. Support also can be provided by the unaffected hand instead of the T-bar.

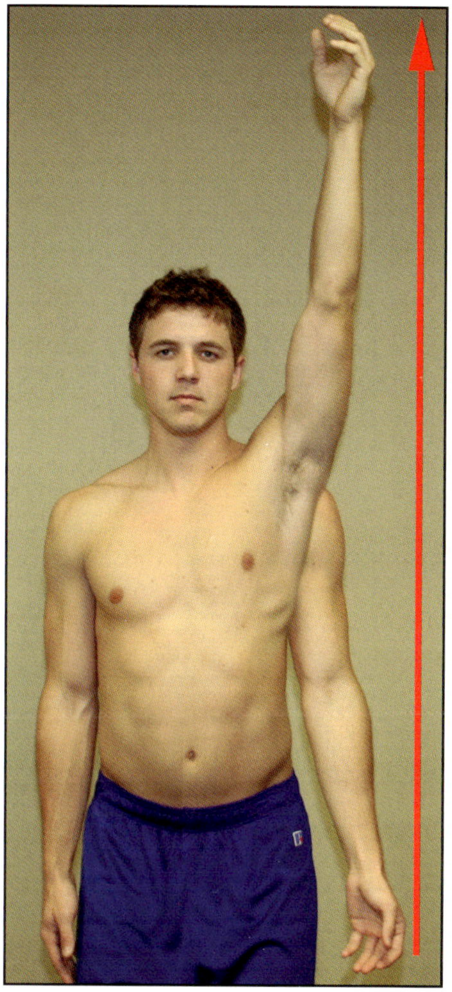

Figure 14. Upright active forward elevation.

fatiguing between about 15 and 30 repetitions. Usually, only 1 or 2 exercises from the progression at a time are used, and new exercises are chosen as the patient improves. Correct selection often requires educated trial and error to find exercises that fatigue the shoulder girdle but that do not cause pain or abnormal movement patterns. For a discussion of why we do not perform strengthening exercises through pain, see chapter II-1. A typical AASEP progression used with some patients is horizontal dusting (Figure 4) progressing to incline dusting (Figure 9), to wall slides (Figure 10), and to AFE (Figure 14). Another example of a clinical progression of the AASEP is supine reaching with polyvinyl chloride piping (Figure 7A) progressing to supine reaching AROM (Figure 7B), to supine forward elevation with an elastic band (Figure 6), to standing T-bar active-assistive forward elevation (Figure 12), and to AFE (Figure 14).

Research in which investigators have evaluated the EMG activity level of various shoulder exercises can be very helpful in determining the relative difficulty of clinical exercises. Results commonly are reported as percentages of maximal voluntary isometric contractions (MVICs), meaning EMG activity level of the muscle being studied is expressed as a percentage of the maximum value of that muscle during isometric manual muscle testing. Relative muscular demand has been classified into 4 categories based on EMG activity: low (<20%), moderate (20–40%), high (41–60%), and very high (>60%). In situations such as rehabilitation of patients with rotator cuff repairs, initial rehabilitation should include exercises with only low EMG activity level then should progress gradually to higher levels of EMG activity during the later stages of rehabilitation.

In several electromyography studies,[4–6] researchers have documented the progressive muscle demand of the forward elevation exercises included in our overall

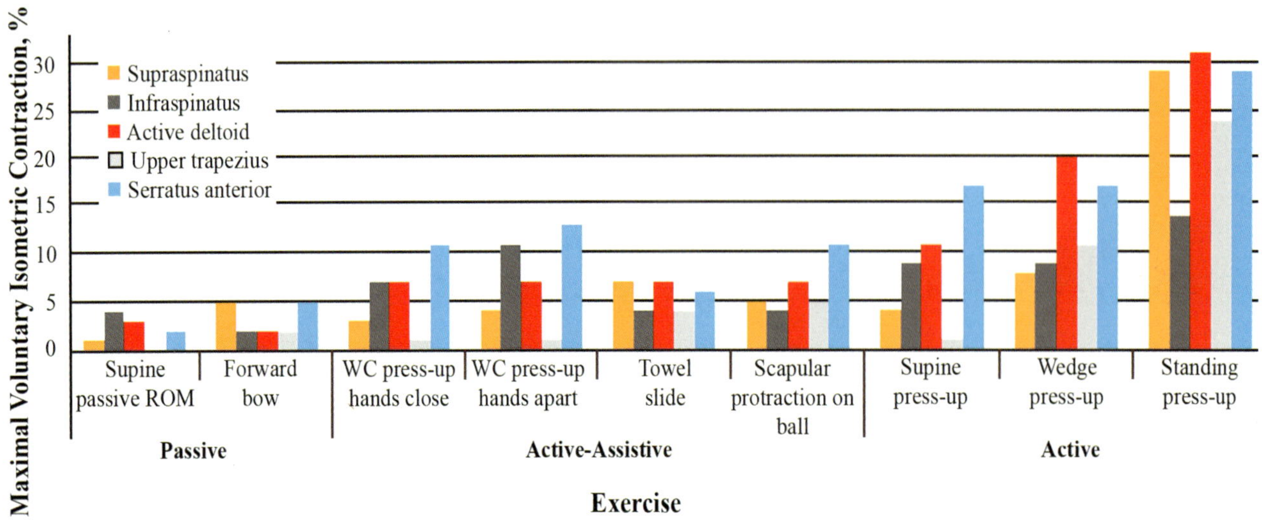

Figure 15. Mean electromyographic activity of selected muscles demonstrating increasing electromyographic activity level as exercises progress from passive to active-assistive range of motion and to active.[5] Abbreviations: ROM, range of motion; WC, wash cloth.

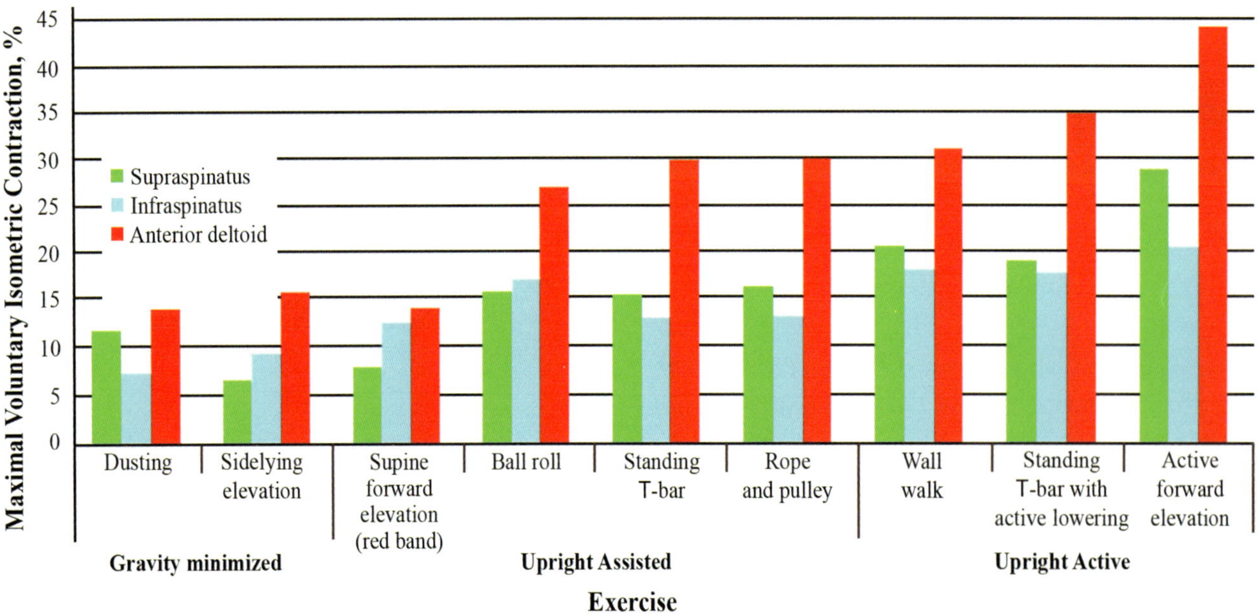

Figure 16. Maximum electromyographic activity of the supraspinatus, infraspinatus, and anterior deltoid during gravity-minimized exercises, upright assistive exercises, and active forward elevation evaluated in Gaunt et al.[4]

exercise progression, advancing from passive to gravity-minimized AAROM, to upright AAROM, to upright active, and to upright resistive exercise (Figures 15 and 16; Table 1).[4,5] In addition, Wise et al[7] demonstrated that performing both inclined and vertical reaching with support resulted in significantly less supraspinatus activity than performing the same activity without support. This supports the use of upright assistive exercise as a precursor to upright active exercise in the AASEP. However, this does not mean that vertical reaching with support, such as the wall slide, wall walking, or finger ladder, is a beginning rehabilitation activity. Electomyographic evidence has demonstrated that out of a wide range of upright AAROM exercises, wall walking was the most demanding exercise for the supraspinatus, which suggests it should be used in the later stages of an upper extremity elevation progression just before the patient can achieve AFE and after almost all other gravity-minimized and upright assistive exercises.[1] Clinically, we believe this is the appropriate

An Evidence-Based Active-Range-of-Motion and Strengthening Progression

Table 1. Mean (± SD)[a] of Relative Electromyographic Activity Level of Selected Muscles Demonstrating Increasing Electromyographic Activity Level as Exercises Progress From Supine Passive Forward Elevation to Upright Active-Assistive Forward Elevation, to Upright Active Forward Elevation, and to Upright Resistive Forward Elevation

Exercise	Supraspinatus	Infraspinatus
Supine assistive elevation (low electromyographic passive range of motion)	0.05 (0.09)	0.05 (0.01)
Pulley active-assistive range of motion (upright active-assistive range of motion)	0.13 (0.17)	0.20 (0.31)
Active forward elevation (upright active range of motion)	0.24 (0.29)	0.29 (0.16)
Forward elevation with 5 lb (2.25 kg) (upright resistive)	0.46 (0.30)	0.57 (0.40)

[a] Indicates values are mean (± SD) electromyographic activity relative to maximum electromyographic activity for that muscle during abduction with 5 lb (2.25 kg).[6]

Table 2. Summary of Mean (± SD) Percentage of Maximal Voluntary Isometric Contraction From Researchers Evaluating Active Forward Elevation With and Without Weight

Active Forward Elevation	Study	Elbow Position	Resistance Used	Supraspinatus
No weight	Gaunt et al, 2010[4]	Straight	None	29 (13)
	Uhl et al, 2010[5]	Bent to straight	None	15 (18)
	Wise et al, 2004[7]	Bent to straight	None	16 (11)
With weight	Uhl et al, 2010[5]	Bent to straight	Aerosol can	29 (18)
	Reinold et al, 2007[8]	Straight	10 rm[a]	62 (40)
	Townsend et al, 1991[9]	Straight	Light weight	64 (28)

[a] Indicates mean is 4 lb (1.81 kg).

timing of these exercises. We have found the wall-walk exercise and its variations are detrimental to rehabilitation if used to improve PROM or flexibility or if used during the early stages of an elevation strengthening progression.

The last stages of the elevation progression are upright AFE without weight and upright AFE with weight. Several researchers have evaluated the EMG activity level of these exercises performed various ways (Table 2).[4–9] Results have demonstrated that depending on the resistance used, AFE without weight requires light to moderate EMG activity level of the supraspinatus and deltoid and that AFE with weight requires moderate to very high EMG activity level of these muscles.

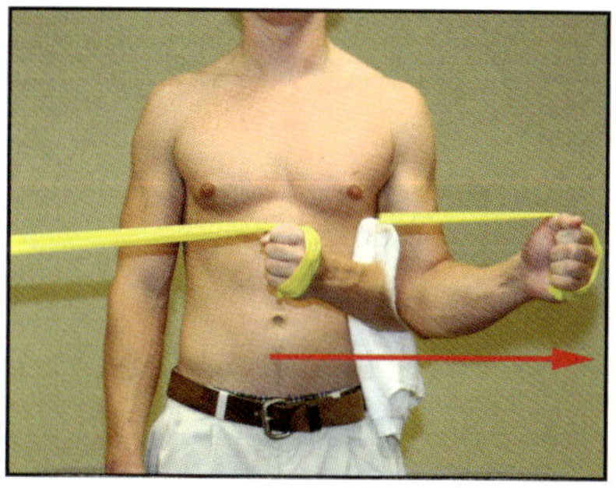

Figure 17. External rotation with an elastic band.

ELASTIC-RESISTANCE TRAINING BELOW SHOULDER LEVEL

Elastic-resistance training below shoulder level is one of the main strengthening tracts used in the early stages of the AROM and strengthening progression of the St. Francis Rehabilitation Center and St. Francis Orthopaedic Institute. The purpose of this tract is to provide light to moderate strengthening to the entire rotator cuff and scapular muscles in nonprovocative, easy-to-tolerate positions. Therefore, this program is ideal to be used both in the early stages of strengthening and for long-term maintenance of rotator cuff and scapular strengthening in

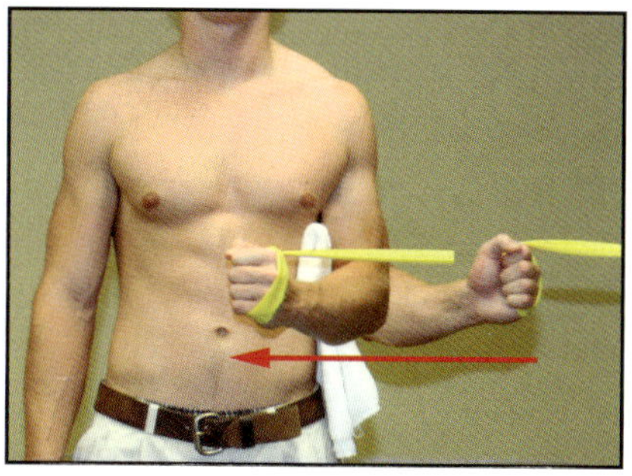

Figure 18. Internal rotation with an elastic band.

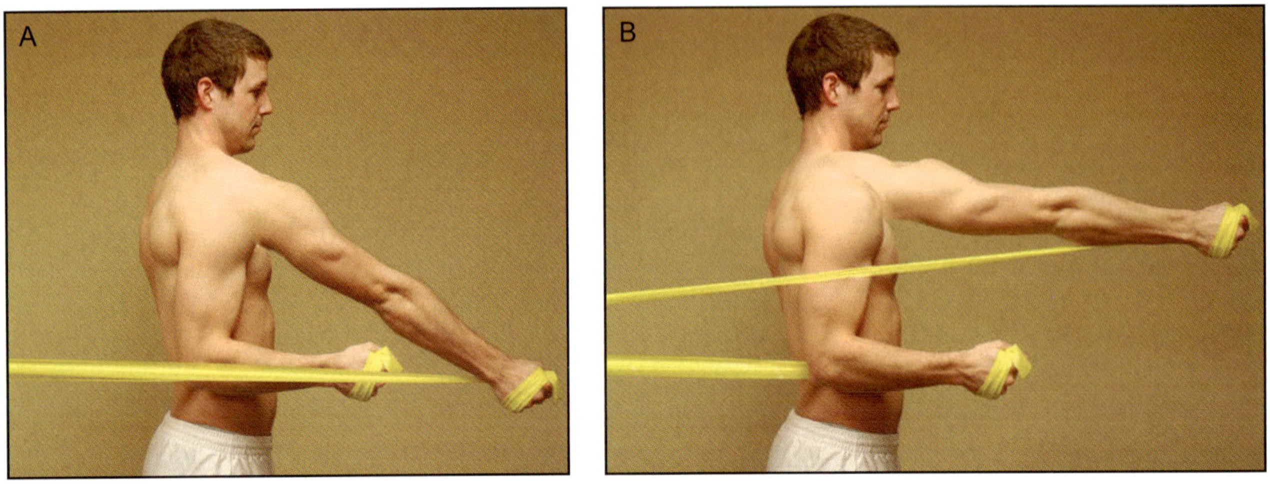

Figure 19. Forward reaching with an elastic band at waist level, A, and at chest level, B, which is more difficult

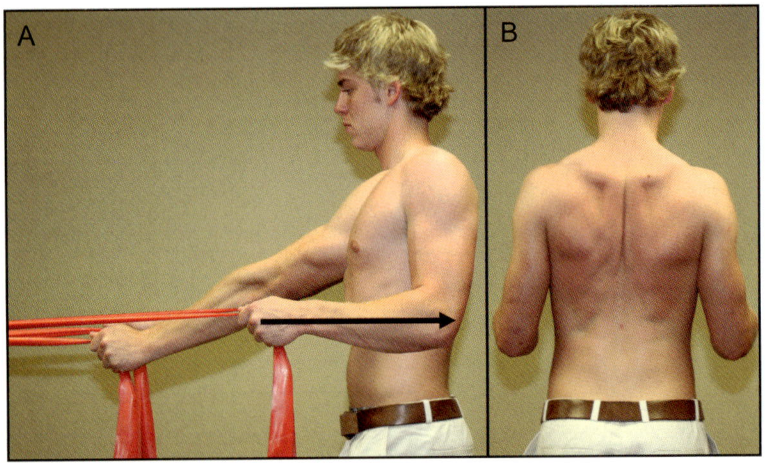

Figure 20 A and B. Scapular retraction with an elastic band. Care is taken to start the exercise in a forward-reaching position with scapular protraction and to finish the exercise with scapular retraction and the shoulder positioned in neutral and not extension.

patients with a variety of nonoperative and postoperative conditions. The "base" exercises of this program are external and internal rotation with the elbow near the side, forward reaching at waist level progressing to chest level, and scapular retraction, each performed with elastic resistance (Figure 17–20).

Investigators evaluating the EMG activity level of these exercises have reported a very wide range of values (Tables 3–5).[10–12] For example, average EMG values for internal rotation with elastic resistance for the subscapularis range from 10% MVIC[10] to 74% MVIC.[11] As detailed in chapter II-5, the specific exercise technique used has a very large bearing on the difficulty of elastic-resistance exercise. Factors, such as elasticity of the band or tubing, length, pretension, size of the motion, and band-to-arm angle make great differences in the final difficulty of these exercises. During clinical practice, rehabilitation professionals must understand that these basic exercises can be performed in a way that requires very low muscle demand or in

Table 3. Summary of Results of Average (± SD) Electromyographic Activity of the Infraspinatus During External Rotation at 0° of Abduction With an Elastic Band

External Rotation at 0° With an Elastic Band	Maximal Voluntary Isometric Contraction of the Infraspinatus, %
Hintermeister et al, 1998[10]	7 (3)
Myers et al, 2005[11]	46 (20)

Table 4. Summary of Results of Average (± SD) Electromyographic Activity of the Supraspinatus During Forward Punching or Reaching With an Elastic Band

Forward Punch	Maximal Voluntary Isometric Contraction of the Supraspinatus, %
Hintermeister et al, 1998[10]	6.5 (2.6)[a]
Myers et al, 2005[11]	46.0 (31.0)[a]
Decker et al, 2003[12]	43.0 (23.0)[a]
Decker et al, 2003[12]	71.0 (43.0)[b]

[a] Indicates average amplitude.
[b] Indicates peak amplitude.

Table 5. Summary of Results of the Average (± SD) Electromyographic Activity of the Subscapularis During Internal Rotation With an Elastic Band

Internal Rotation	Maximal Voluntary Isometric Contraction of the Subscapularis, %
Hintermeister et al, 1998[10]	10 (5)[a]
Myers et al, 2005[11]	74 (47)[a]
Decker et al, 2003[12]	36 (23)[a]
Decker et al, 2003[12]	61 (27)[b]

[a] Indicates average amplitude.
[b] Indicates peak amplitude.

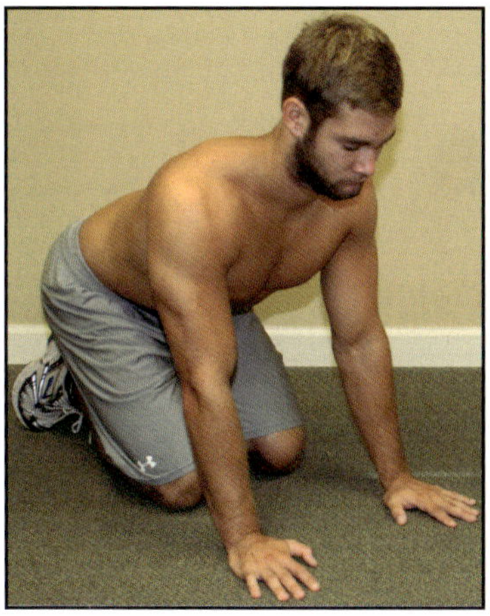

Figure 21. The prayer exercise position. Weight-bearing force is 6 ± 3% of body mass. Normalized electromyographic activity is 2 ± 2% maximal voluntary isometric contraction (MVIC) for the supraspinatus and 4 ± 3% MVIC for the infraspinatus.[13]

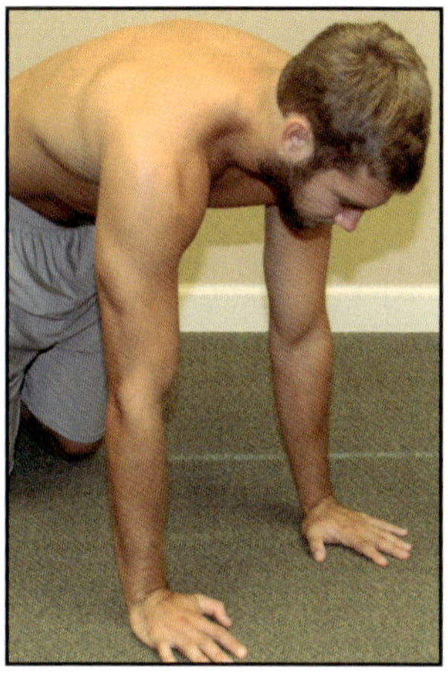

Figure 22. The quadruped exercise position. Weight-bearing force is 19 ± 2% of body mass. Normalized electromyographic activity is 6 ± 10% maximal voluntary isometric contraction (MVIC) for the supraspinatus and 11 ± 8% MVIC for the infraspinatus.[13]

a way that requires very high muscle demand. Therefore, the details of exercise prescription are especially important for these exercises. When used in the beginning phases of the AROM and strengthening progression, I ensure that the lightest resistance is used, the patient holds the end of a band or tube approximately 6 feet (1.8 m) long, no pretension is used, and a small ROM is used in a nonprovocative position so only minimal muscle demand is required. As the patient progresses, these factors can be modified systematically as described in chapter II-5 to increase the muscle demand required up to a very high level.

STATIC CLOSED KINETIC CHAIN EXERCISE PROGRESSION

The static closed chain progression is our final strengthening tract used in the early stages of the St. Francis Rehabilitation Center and St. Francis Orthopaedic Institute AROM and strengthening progression. The purpose of this tract is to provide light to moderate activation of the rotator cuff and shoulder girdle muscles. It also improves weight-bearing tolerance through the affected extremity without movement of the affected extremity, which might be helpful in patients with certain diagnoses, such as instability, or in patients who are active in sports requiring weight bearing through the upper body, such as wrestling or football. Anecdotally, I also have noticed that in patients recovering from various shoulder girdle injuries, good open chain stability and functional

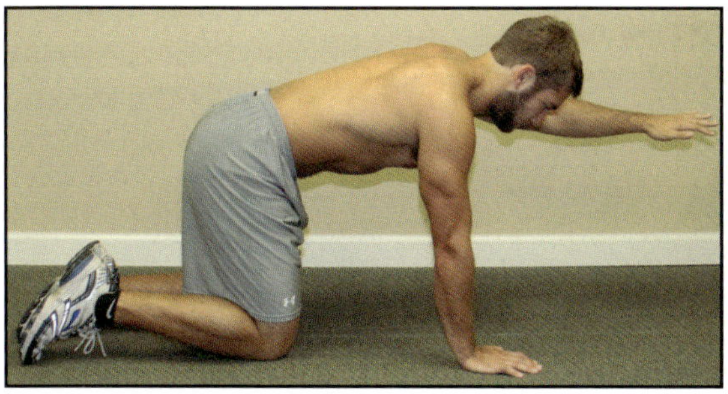

Figure 23. The tripod exercise position. Weight-bearing force is 32 ± 3% of body mass. Normalized electromyographic activity is 10 ± 11% maximal voluntary isometric contraction (MVIC) for the supraspinatus and 37 ± 26% MVIC for the infraspinatus.[13]

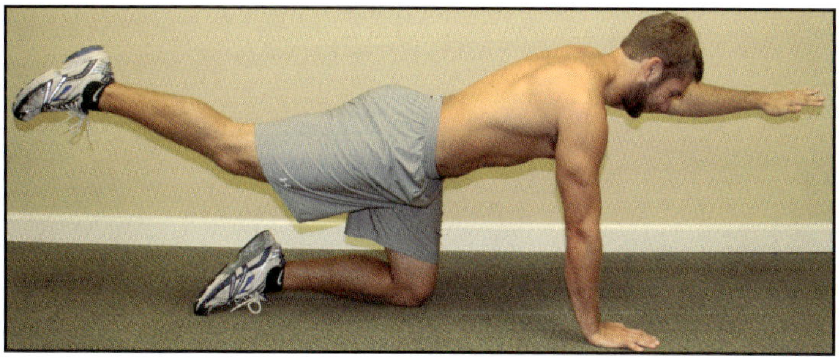

Figure 24. The pointer exercise position. Weight-bearing force is 34 ± 4% of body mass. Normalized electromyographic activity is 12 ± 13% maximal voluntary isometric contraction (MVIC) for the supraspinatus and 42 ± 33% MVIC for the infraspinatus.[13]

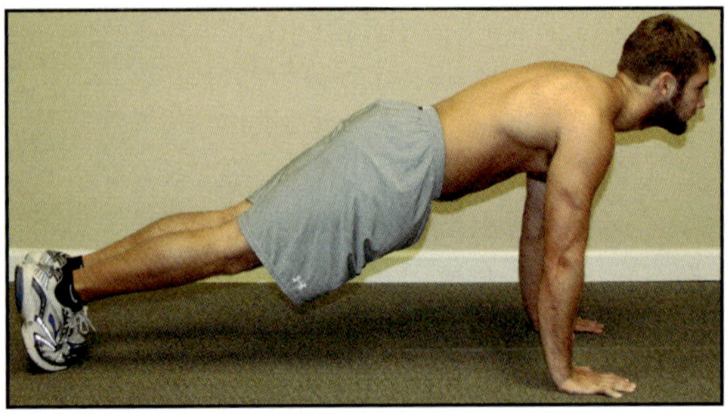

Figure 25. The push-up exercise position. Weight-bearing force is 34 ± 3% of body mass. Normalized electromyographic activity is 14 ± 14% maximal voluntary isometric contraction (MVIC) for the supraspinatus and 44 ± 31% MVIC for the infraspinatus.[13]

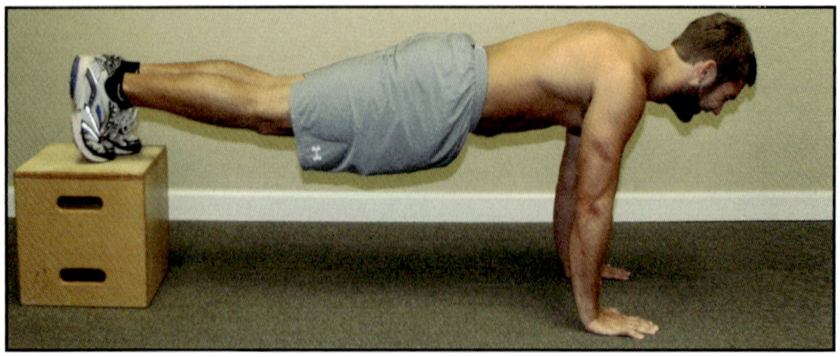

Figure 26. The push-up with feet elevated exercise position. Weight-bearing force is 39 ± 5% of body mass. Normalized electromyographic activity is 18 ± 16% maximal voluntary isometric contraction (MVIC) for the supraspinatus and 52 ± 32% MVIC for the infraspinatus.[13]

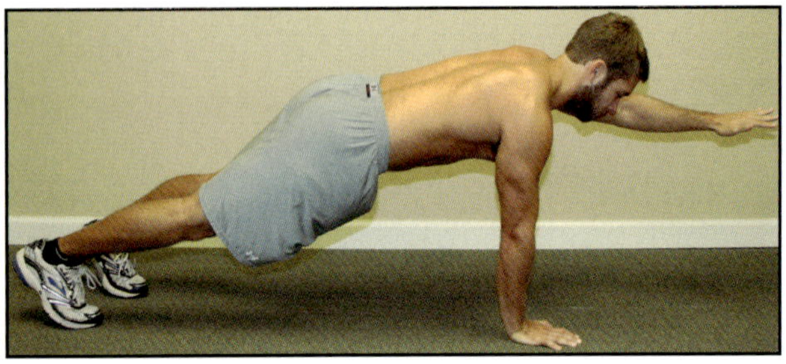

Figure 27. The 1-arm push-up exercise position. Weight-bearing force is 60 ± 6% of body mass. Normalized electromyographic activity is 29 ± 20% maximal voluntary isometric contraction (MVIC) for the supraspinatus and 86 ± 56% MVIC for the infraspinatus.[13]

strength does not translate necessarily to good stability and functional strength in a weight-bearing position.

Researchers have examined the EMG activity level of shoulder musculature during weight-bearing exercises and the relationship between increasing weight-bearing posture and shoulder muscle activation during a series of static closed chain exercises (Figures 21–27).[13] Their results have demonstrated a high correlation between increasing weight-bearing posture and muscular activity ($r = 0.97$, $P = .01$).[13] Average EMG activity ranged from very low (4 ± 3% MVIC) to very high (86 ± 56% MVIC) for the infraspinatus during the exercise progression, whereas average EMG activity ranged from very low (2 ± 2% MVIC) to only moderate (29 ± 20% MVIC) for the supraspinatus. Figures 21–27 also include the weight-bearing force (mean ± SD) represented as a percentage of the participant's body mass and the normalized EMG activity for the supraspinatus and infraspinatus.[13] These findings suggest that low-load, static, weight-bearing exercises produce low-level muscle coactivation.

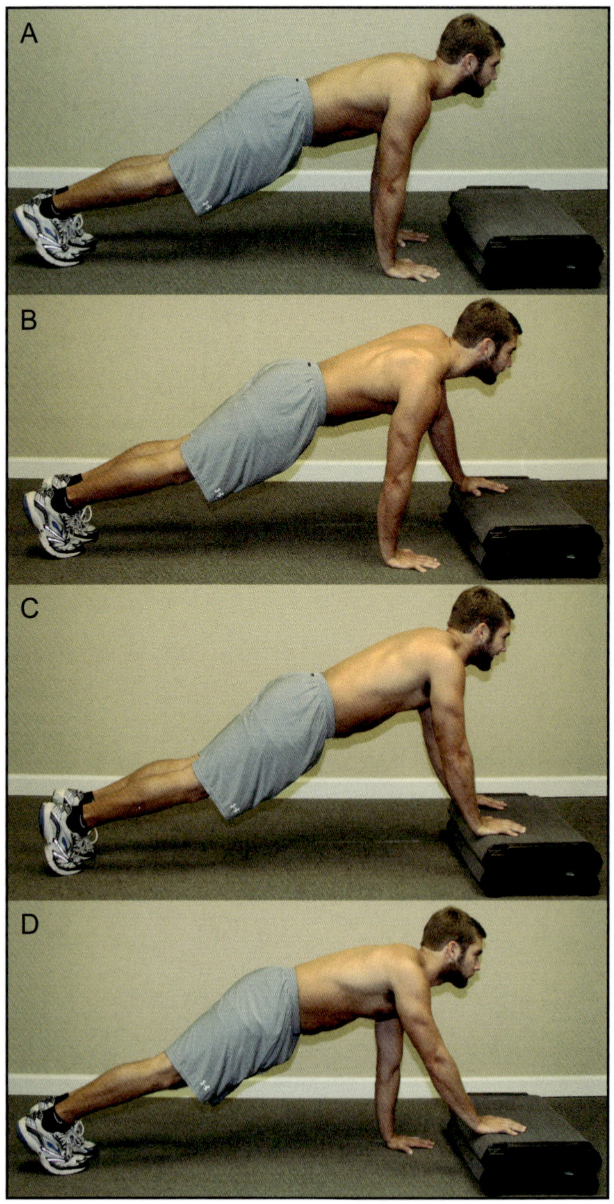

Figure 28 A–D. The upper extremity step-up exercise.

These researchers who examined weight-bearing exercises near 90° of flexion demonstrated that progressing to higher-load exercises increased activity of the infraspinatus, 1-handed activities increased activation of the posterior deltoid, and 2-handed activities tended to increase activity levels of the anterior deltoid and pectoralis major. Because the correlation between increased weight bearing and muscular activity was so strong, one might be able to generally estimate the difficulty level of other weight-bearing exercises that were not examined in this study, such as upper extremity step-ups (Figure 28).

ADVANCED STRENGTHENING EXERCISES AND EXERCISES WITH MAXIMUM EMG ACTIVITY

The advanced strengthening exercises are exercises with the purpose of maximally activating one or more shoulder girdle muscles, strengthening the shoulder girdle in end ranges of motion, or providing high-speed strength training. The purpose of this final level of the St. Francis Rehabilitation Center and St. Francis Orthopaedic Institute AROM and strengthening progression is to bridge the gap between the lower-level strengthening exercises I have described and the demands placed on the shoulder girdle during heavy lifting, repetitive or heavy overhead activities, or high-velocity powerful activities. Overhead throwing athletes, swimmers, and heavy laborers are examples of patients who benefit from advanced strengthening exercises.

This level encompasses many exercises that are familiar to most rehabilitation professionals and are used frequently. However, rehabilitation professionals must take care that these exercises are sequenced appropriately in the rehabilitation plan of each patient. Exercises in this category have high to very high EMG activity; therefore, I believe they are most appropriate to use in the middle to late stages of rehabilitation for young, healthy, and athletic individuals with high demands on the shoulder girdle. These exercises might not be appropriate for patients with extensive rotator cuff damage, patients with only basic demands on the shoulder girdle, and elderly patients.

At our facility, the patient meets certain criteria before starting advanced strengthening exercises. He or she should demonstrate manual muscle testing strength of the rotator cuff muscles of at least 4+/5. The patient must have full, pain-free, active use of the extremity overhead; must be asymptomatic with basic activities of daily living; and must have good tolerance to easier levels of our AROM and strengthening progression. Finally, he or she must have the goal of returning to sport participation, heavy labor, repetitive overhead work, or heavy overhead work. If the patient has only lower functional demands, then the elevation

Table 6. The Top 4 Exercises of Selected Rotator Cuff Muscles From Townsend et al[9] by Mean (± SD) Percentage of Maximal Voluntary Isometric Contraction in the Peak 30° Arc and Peak Arc Range in Degrees

Muscle	Maximal Voluntary Isometric Contraction, %	Peak Arc, °
Supraspinatus		
Military press	80 (48)	0–30
Empty can	74 (33)	90–120
Flexion	67 (14)	90–120
Scaption with external rotation	64 (28)	90–120
Infraspinatus		
Prone horizontal abduction with external rotation	88 (25)	90–120
Side-lying external rotation	85 (26)	60–90
Prone horizontal abduction with internal rotation	74 (32)	90–120
Upright abduction	74 (23)	90–120
Subscapularis		
Empty can	62 (33)	120–180
Military press	56 (48)	60–90
Flexion	52 (42)	120–150
Abduction	50 (44)	120–150

progression, elastic-resistance training below shoulder level, and the static closed chain progression usually are sufficient to return the patient to his or her desired level of function.

In several electromyography studies, investigators have examined which dumbbell exercises best activate the rotator cuff and deltoid. Townsend et al[9] examined 15 healthy male participants performing 16 dumbbell exercises plus the press-up using light weight and low speeds. They calculated and analyzed the average EMG activity per 30° arc. Their top 4 exercises for the supraspinatus, infraspinatus, and subscapularis are shown in Table 6. Reinold et al[14] examined 10 healthy participants performing 7 common dumbbell external rotation strengthening exercises with a variable weight to accomplish a 10-repetition-maximum set. The average percentage MVIC was calculated and analyzed. Selected results are shown in Tables 7 and 8. In a separate study, Reinold et al[8] examined 22 healthy participants performing the full-can exercise with 4 pounds (1.8 kg), the empty-can exercise with 4 pounds (1.8 kg), and prone horizontal abduction at 100° with 3.3 pounds (1.5 kg). The average percentage MVIC was calculated and analyzed (Table 9).

High to very high EMG activity levels for a variety of rotator cuff and deltoid muscles were found for almost all exercises examined in these studies. Prone horizontal abduction at 100°, prone external rotation at 90°, the military press, and side-lying external rotation at 0° are electromyography-supported dumbbell exercises I commonly use during the advanced strengthening phase for maximum rotator cuff and deltoid recruitment (Figures 29–32). Along with other people, I advocate using the thumb-up (full-can) position for active and resisted elevation activities because it provides better subacromial clearance,[15] better scapular mechanics,[16] and equal rotator cuff activation[8] compared with the empty-can position.

Myers et al[11] examined the EMG activity level of 15 active male participants performing 12 tubing exercises commonly used by throwing athletes. The average percentage MVIC was calculated and analyzed for 13 shoulder girdle muscles, including all 4 rotator cuff muscles and the anterior and middle deltoid. Results of selected exercises and selected muscles are shown in Tables 3–5 and 10. As mentioned earlier in this chapter and detailed in chapter II-5, the specific exercise technique used during elastic-resistance exercise has a very large bearing on the difficulty of the exercise. Although throwing acceleration, throwing deceleration, external rotation at 90°, and internal rotation at 90° have EMG values similar to more basic elastic-resistance exercises, these exercises are included in our advanced phase of rehabilitation because they allow incorporation of many principles used in the progression of

Table 7. Mean (± SD) Electromyographic Activation of the Infraspinatus Expressed as a Percentage of Maximal Voluntary Isometric Contraction From Reinold et al[14]

Infraspinatus	Maximal Voluntary Isometric Contraction, %
Side-lying external rotation at 0°	62 (13)
Standing external roation with scaption	53 (25)
Prone external rotation at 90°	50 (23)
Standing external rotation at 90°	50 (25)
Standing external rotation at 0° with a towel	50 (14)
Standing external rotation at 0° without a towel	40 (14)
Prone horizontal abduction at 100° of full external rotation	39 (17)

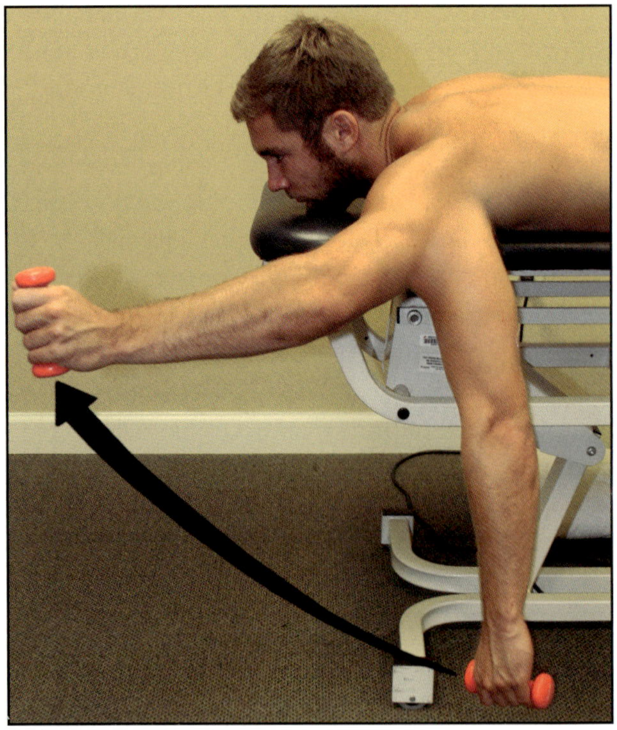

Figure 29. Prone horizontal abduction at 100° with full external rotation.

Table 8. Mean (± SD) Electromyographic Activation of the Supraspinatus Expressed as a Percentage of Maximal Voluntary Isometric Contraction From Reinold et al[14]

Supraspinatus	Maximal Voluntary Isometric Contraction, %
Prone horizontal abduction at 100° of full external rotation	82 (37)
Prone external rotation at 90°	68 (33)
Standing external rotation at 90°	57 (32)
Side-lying external rotation at 0°	51 (47)
Standing external rotation at 0° with a towel	41 (37)
Standing external rotation at 0° without a towel	41 (38)
Standing external rotation with scaption	32 (24)

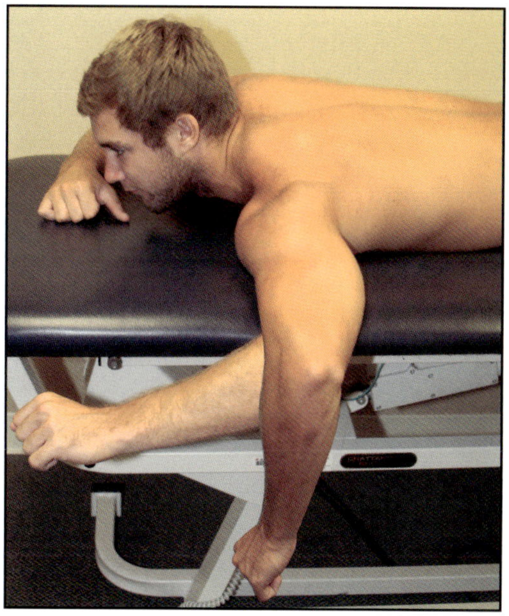

Figure 30. Prone external rotation at 90° of abduction.

Table 9. Mean (± SD) Electromyographic Activity Level Expressed as a Percentage of Maximal Voluntary Isometric Contraction for Each Exercise From Reinold et al[8]

Muscle	Full Can to 90° With Weight	Empty Can With Weight	Prone Horizontal Abduction With Weight
Supraspinatus	62 (40)	63 (45)	67 (50)
Middle deltoid	52 (27)	77 (44)[a]	63 (31)[a]
Posterior deltoid	38 (32)	54 (28)	87 (53)[a]

[a] Indicates exercise has greater activity level ($P < .05$).

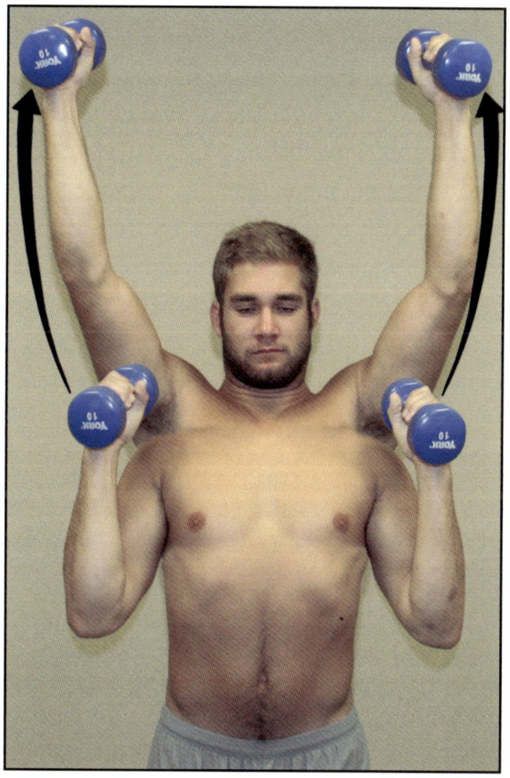

Figure 31. Dumbbell military press.

Table 10. Mean (± SD) Maximal Voluntary Isometric Contraction of the Supraspinatus, Infraspinatus, and Subscapularis of Elastic-Resistance Exercises Requiring Positioning in Abduction With External Rotation From Myers et al[11]

Exercise	Supraspinatus	Infraspinatus	Subscapularis
Throwing			
Accelerate	36 (31)	33 (22)	93 (51)
Decelerate	63 (32)	44 (21)	68 (48)
External rotation at 90°	50 (21)	50 (29)	56 (50)
Internal rotation at 90°	41 (29)	23 (21)	71 (43)

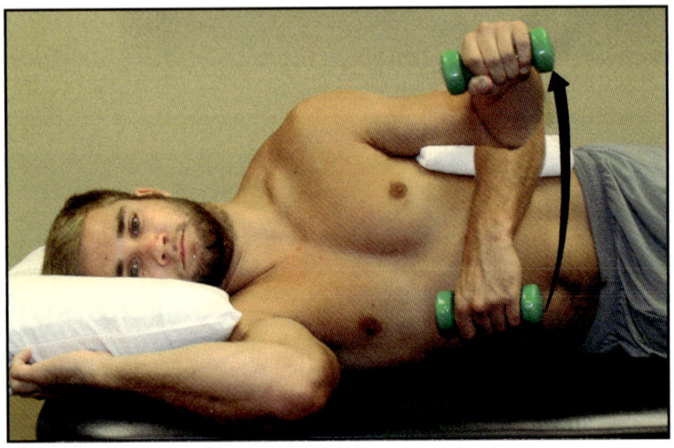

Figure 32. Side-lying external rotation at 0°.

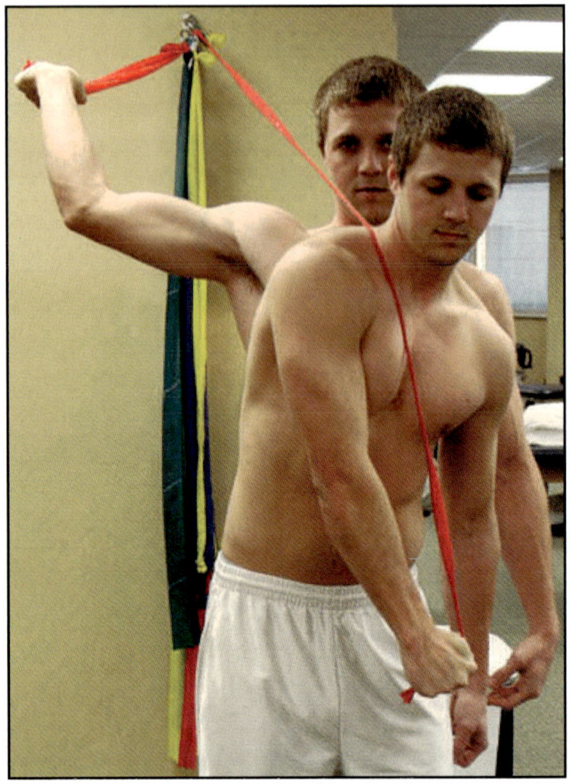

Figure 33. Throwing acceleration or diagonal resisting extension and internal rotation with an elastic band.

advanced strengthening activities (Figures 33–36; Tables 3–5, 10, and 11). They require positioning the shoulder in more provocative and functional positions for overhead athletes; they challenge the neuromuscular control of the shoulder girdle; and if done at higher speeds, they are a step toward speed-specific training for overhead athletes compared with dumbbell or basic elastic-resistance exercises.

Although EMG activity level is a main factor used in exercise selection during the advanced strengthening phase, it is not the only criterion. The rehabilitation program is individualized based on each patient's unique situation to help him or her progress from the current levels of ROM, strength, endurance, power, and neuromuscular control to the levels needed to participate in heavy or repetitive work, high-speed activities, or sports. This is accomplished by formulating a step-by-step rehabilitation plan to systematically progress patients from their current levels of performance to the levels required to complete their desired activities. Therefore, this stage of rehabilitation is different for each patient because patients begin advanced strengthening with different levels of current function and different functional goals. Chapter III-4 contains 2 case studies that clarify how advanced strengthening and functional progressions can differ and how a needs analysis is used to guide advanced rehabilitation.

Table 11. Principles for Progression of Advanced Strengthening Exercises

- Use exercises with increasing electromyographic activity levels.
- Decrease the amount of support provided to the shoulder girdle.
- Integrate functional patterns, including abduction with external rotation.
- Increase the speed of movements.
- Integrate kinesthetic awareness drills into strengthening activities.
- Include the entire kinetic chain.
- Decrease rest time to improve endurance.
- Train larger upper extremity muscles wisely.

Although this level of rehabilitation is individualized, certain general principles for progression are used during clinical decision making (Table 11). Rehabilitation activities requiring heavy lifting and power training, such as plyometrics, typically are implemented 3 to 6 weeks later after more basic exercises. Return-to-sports and modified weight-training programs are essential if the patient wants to participate regularly in these activities. The appropriate use of the programs varies greatly depending on the diagnosis of the patient, and these programs are discussed in detail in chapters IV-4 through IV-8; however, they typically are initiated after 3 to 8 weeks of advanced strengthening exercises.

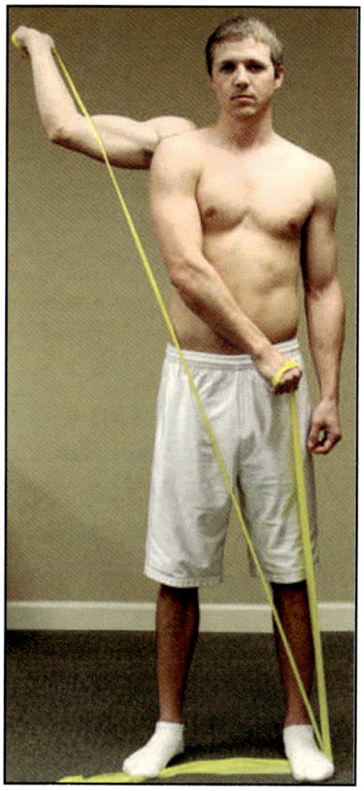

Figure 34. Throwing deceleration or diagonal resisting extension and external rotation with an elastic band.

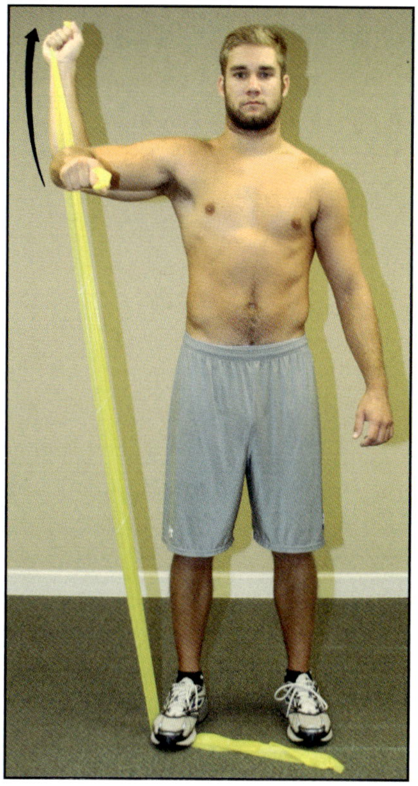

Figure 35. External rotation at 90° of abduction with elastic resistance.

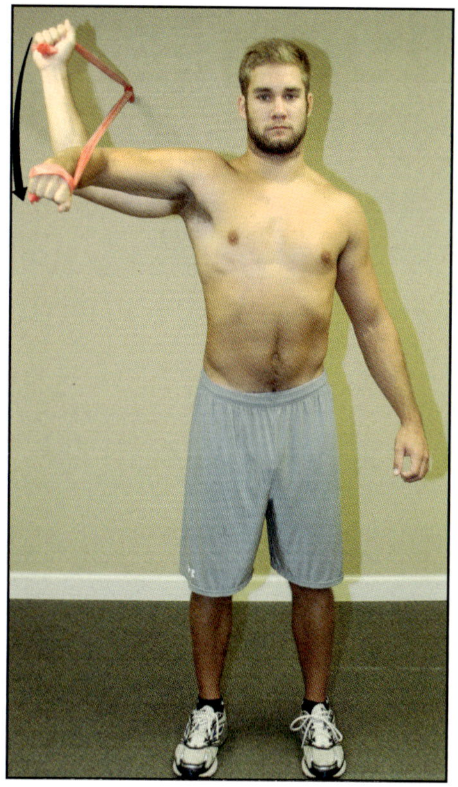

Figure 36. Internal rotation at 90° of abduction with elastic resistance.

REFERENCES

1. Gaunt B, Shaffer M, Sauers E, Michener L, McCluskey G, Thigpen C. The American Society of Shoulder and Elbow Therapists' consensus rehabilitation guideline for arthroscopic anterior capsulolabral repair of the shoulder. *J Orthop Sports Phys Ther*. 2010;40(3):155–168.
2. Levy O, Mullett H, Roberts S, Copeland S. The role of anterior deltoid reeducation in patients with massive irreparable degenerative rotator cuff tears. *J Shoulder Elbow Surg*. 2008;17(6):863–870.
3. Krupp RJ, Kevern MA, Gaines MD, Kotara S, Singleton SB. Long head of the biceps tendon pain: differential diagnosis and treament. *J Orthop Sports Phys Ther*. 2009;39(2):55–70.
4. Gaunt BW, McCluskey GM, Uhl TL. An electromyographic evaluation of subdividing active-assistive shoulder elevation exercises. *Sports Health*. 2010;2(5):424–432.
5. Uhl TL, Muir TA, Lawson L. Electromyographical assessment of passive, active assistive, and active shoulder rehabilitation exercises. *Am Acad Phys Med Rehabil*. 2010;2(2):132–141.
6. McCann PD, Wooten ME, Kadaba MP, Bigliani LU. A kinematic electromyographic study of shoulder rehabilitation exercises. *Clin Orthop Relat Res*. 1993;288:179–188.
7. Wise MB, Uhl TL, Mattacola CG, Nitz AJ, Kibler WB. The effect of limb support on muscle activation during shoulder exercises. *J Shoulder Elbow Surg*. 2004;13(6):614–620.
8. Reinold MM, Macrina LC, Wilk KE, et al. Electromyographic analysis of the supraspinatus and deltoid muscles during 3 common rehabilitation exercises. *J Athl Train*. 2007;42(4):464–469.
9. Townsend H, Jobe FW, Pink M, Perry J. Electromyographic analysis of the glenohumeral muscles during a baseball rehabilitation program. *Am J Sports Med*. 1991;19(3):264–272.
10. Hintermeister RA, Lange GW, Shultheis JM, Bey MJ, Hawkins RJ. Electromyographic activity and applied load during shoulder rehabilitation exercises using elastic resistance. *Am J Sports Med*. 1998;26(2):210–220.
11. Myers JB, Pasquale MR, Laudner KG, Sell TC, Bradley JP, Lephart SM. On-the-field resistance-tubing exercises for throwers: an electromyographic analysis. *J Athl Train*. 2005;40(1):15–22.
12. Decker MJ, Tokish JM, Ellis HB, Torry MR, Hawkins RJ. Subscapularis muscle activity during selected rehabilitation exercises. *Am J Sports Med*. 2003;31(1):126–134.
13. Uhl TL, Carver TJ, Mattacola CG, Mair SD, Nitz AJ. Shoulder musculature activation during upper extremity weight-bearing exercise. *J Orthop Sports Phys Ther*. 2003;33(3):109–117.
14. Reinold MM, Wilk KE, Fleisig GS, et al. Electromyographic analysis of the rotator cuff and deltoid musculature during common shoulder external rotation exercises. *J Orthop Sports Phys Ther*. 2004;34(7):385–394.
15. Flatow EL, Soslowsky LJ, Ticker JB, et al. Excursion of the rotator cuff under the acromion: patterns of subacromial contact. *Am J Sports Med*. 1994;22(6):779–788.
16. Thigpen CA, Padua DA, Morgan N, Kreps C, Karas SG. Scapular kinematics during supraspinatus rehabilitation exercise: a comparison of full-can versus empty-can techniques. *Am J Sports Med*. 2006;34(4):644–652.

II-5

Biomechanical Principles of Selected Shoulder Girdle Exercises

How Physics and Exercise-Resistance Properties Influence the Effectiveness of Therapeutic Exercises

Brian J. Phillips, PT, DPT, and Shannon B. Lucas, PTA

CHAPTER CONTENTS

- Elastic-band resistance properties: the details matter!
- The biomechanics of active elevation and the 1 physics equation you must know
- Isotonic dumbbell versus elastic resistance in supine
- Isotonic dumbbell versus elastic resistance in standing
- Supine versus standing versus prone isotonic strengthening

Clinical pearls are highlighted in yellow throughout the text.

One of the most challenging aspects of shoulder rehabilitation is the skillful exercise progression that is based on scientific evidence, is well tolerated by the patient, and most importantly is effective. The ability to order exercises correctly is crucial to helping protect healing tissues, prevent substitution patterns, reduce pain during rehabilitation, and provide a framework for clinical decision making. Exercise progression can be based on several factors, including muscle demand, biomechanical principles, and the range of motion (ROM) required. A combination of these factors is important to consider in all situations when developing an exercise progression. Chapters II-3 and II-4 detail exercise progressions of passive ROM, active ROM, and strengthening that are based primarily on muscle demand measured by electromyography (EMG). In this chapter, we detail the biomechanical principles we believe are vital to understand and apply to make skilled clinical decisions regarding appropriate exercise selection and progression in patients with shoulder girdle disorders. We highlight practical examples that demonstrate how changing small details of exercises, such as body position, the size of the motion, or the type of resistance, can make a meaningful change in the difficulty of the exercise or even the muscles activated.

ELASTIC-BAND RESISTANCE PROPERTIES: THE DETAILS MATTER!

Rehabilitation providers use many different types of exercises to strengthen the muscles of the shoulder girdle. These include isotonic, isokinetic, and isometric exercises.[1] Resistance for isotonic and isokinetic exercises typically is provided by the use of free weights, resistance bands, weight machines, or the weight of the patient's upper extremity. Elastic-resistance bands commonly are used for training in both the rehabilitation clinic and on the athletic field because they are lightweight, easy to transport, easy to use, and inexpensive. Elastic-resistance band exercises can be performed with various amounts of tension and at various speeds of motion and can be used for both concentric (muscle-shortening) and eccentric (muscle-lengthening) forms of strengthening.

Hintermeister et al[2] showed that the use of both concentric and eccentric muscle strengthening can be incorporated as part of a rehabilitation protocol for the shoulder to help a patient achieve full functional use of his or her upper extremity. The speed at which an exercise is performed can have a profound effect on the difficulty of a specific exercise. During concentric strengthening exercises, the exercise becomes more challenging as the patient's upper extremity moves faster within an arc of motion. When using eccentric training as part of a strengthening program, the opposite effect is noted, with slower speeds of movement causing the exercise to become more difficult and challenging to the targeted muscles.

These characteristics of strength training are important for the rehabilitation provider to consider because they can greatly affect the amount of muscle activity generated during an exercise. For example, in EMG studies of the maximal voluntary isometric contraction (MVIC) of the infraspinatus during external rotation at 0° of abduction using elastic-resistance tubing, researchers have demonstrated a range from 9% to 46% MVIC.[2,3] Observing such a wide range of MVIC values from similarly performed exercises might be a result of the resistance that the elastic band provides during performance of the exercise. Many important, but often overlooked, characteristics of elastic-resistance bands can greatly influence their effectiveness during rehabilitation exercises. When considering the use of resistance bands as part of an exercise program, the rehabilitation provider must consider the physical characteristics of elastic-resistance bands, including the elasticity of the band (band thickness), percentage of elongation, resting length, and pretension. Modifications to any of these variables can substantially alter the degree of difficulty of the exercise, the amount of ROM that can be achieved during the exercise, and the number of repetitions that can be performed before the initiation of muscle fatigue. If the initial physical characteristics of an exercise using elastic-resistance bands are not appropriate for the patient or if the wrong modification to the characteristics of an exercise is made, incorrect form and poor tolerance to the exercise can result. When this occurs, there is a risk of causing increased pain and possibly injury to the patient. Therefore, the details of exercise prescription are especially important for these types of resistance exercises.

The physical characteristic of elastic-resistance bands with which rehabilitation providers are most familiar is the elasticity of the band. The amount of elasticity is based on the thickness of the band. The different colors represent the various levels of thickness and tensile strength that the band provides. Thera-Band (The Hygenic Corporation, Akron, OH) resistance bands, which commonly are used in rehabilitation clinics and athletic training rooms, are available in 8 colors, ranging from tan (extra-thin resistance) to gold (maximum resistance).[4] Yellow, red, green, and blue Thera-Bands are the most commonly used resistance levels during shoulder-strengthening exercises. We believe that a large percentage of rehabilitation providers are not aware of how much resistance these bands provide. Because of the extensive use of the bands in rehabilitation settings, rehabilitation providers need to understand the approximate amount of resistance that each piece of elastic band provides to the patient so they can prevent overstressing the muscle.

Researchers have shown that the yellow Thera-Band provides from 2 pounds (0.9 kg) to nearly 6 pounds (2.7 kg) of resistance.[5,6] The red Thera-Band provides from 2 pounds (0.9 kg) to 7 pounds (3.15 kg) of resistance, and the green Thera-Band provides from 2.4 pounds (1.08 kg) to more than 9 pounds (4.05) of resistance.[5,6] A piece of gold Thera-Band, which is the strongest of these elastic bands, can provide from 7.9 pounds (3.56 kg) to more than 40 pounds (18 kg) of resistance.[6] The variation in the amount of resistance each color of band provides is due to the different physical properties of elastic bands (percentage of elongation, resting length, and pretension).

Another physical characteristic of elastic-resistance bands that needs to be considered when implementing an exercise program is the percentage of elongation of the band during the exercise. Moving the upper extremity through a larger arc of motion during an exercise will result in a larger percentage of elongation of the resistance band, leading to an increase in the amount of resistance that the band provides (Table).[4-6] Researchers have shown a strong linear

Table. Thera-Band[a] Resistance Levels Based on Percentage of Elongation During External Rotation at 0° of Abduction[5]

Color	Neutral Begins Tension, lb	30° of ER = 6-in Elongation, lb	45° of ER = 9-in Elongation, lb
Yellow	<2.2	<2.2	2.2
Red	1.9	2.8	3.3
Green	2.4	3.5	4.4
Blue	2.8	4.4	5.3
Silver	4.4	7.9	9.2

[a] The Hygenic Corporation, Akron, OH. Abbreviation: ER, external rotation.

relationship exists between the tension of the band and the percentage of elongation.[1,7] Therefore, to reduce the amount of resistance that an elastic band provides, the patient should perform the exercise in a smaller arc of motion, and to increase the amount of resistance, he or she should perform the exercise in a larger arc of motion.

Modifying the resting length of the elastic band is another variable that will determine the amount of resistance that the band provides. The *resting length* of a band is defined as the overall length of a band with all of the slack removed from it before the initiation of movement or stretch.[7] When a longer length of band is used, the resting length of the band naturally increases, that is, the patient will need to move farther away from where the band is anchored to remove all slack from the band. The inverse principle applies if a shorter band is used. We have observed clinically that when the same overall ROM is performed, using a band with a shorter resting length provides a larger amount of resistance than a band with a longer resting length.

For example, a patient starts by holding the end of an elastic band across her chest in approximately 45° of internal rotation and with all slack removed from the band (Figure 1). The initial resting length of the band is 0.6 m. She then rotates her upper extremity to approximately 45° of external rotation, elongating the band to 1.0 m. Based on the amount of elongation (0.4 m) in relation to the resting length of the band, the percentage of band deformation is approximately 67%. If she detaches the end of the band from the door and holds both ends of the band in her hands, the resting length of the band decreases to 0.3 m (Figure 2). Assuming the same starting position and same amount of rotation (to 45° of external rotation), she now elongates the band to 0.7 m. Based on the amount of elongation (again 0.4 m) in relation to the initial resting length of the band (0.3 m), the percentage of band deformation is now approximately 133%, increasing the amount of resistance from the band to nearly twice as much as that provided by a band with a longer resting length.[7] The amount of resistance generated is determined by the change in length of the band as a percentage of its resting length as opposed to only the actual change in length (elongation) of the band.[7]

Similar to the resting length of a band, the amount of pretension of an elastic band is another variable that can be manipulated to determine the amount of resistance that the band provides. Whereas the *resting length* of a band is defined as the length of band that is used when all slack has been removed before the initiation of movement, *pretension* simply describes the amount of tension of a band before initiation of movement regardless of whether the band has any slack.

In general, a band with an increased amount of pretension will produce a greater amount of resistance than a band with a small amount of pretension. For example, if the patient in Figure 1 positions her upper extremity in a more internally rotated starting position or if she stands closer to where the band is inserted into the door, she will create some slack in the band, causing it to dip. Thus, the band will have a lower amount of pretension and will provide less resistance as she externally rotates her upper extremity. In contrast, if she either wraps the band around her hand or steps out away from the door, she causes the band to stretch out

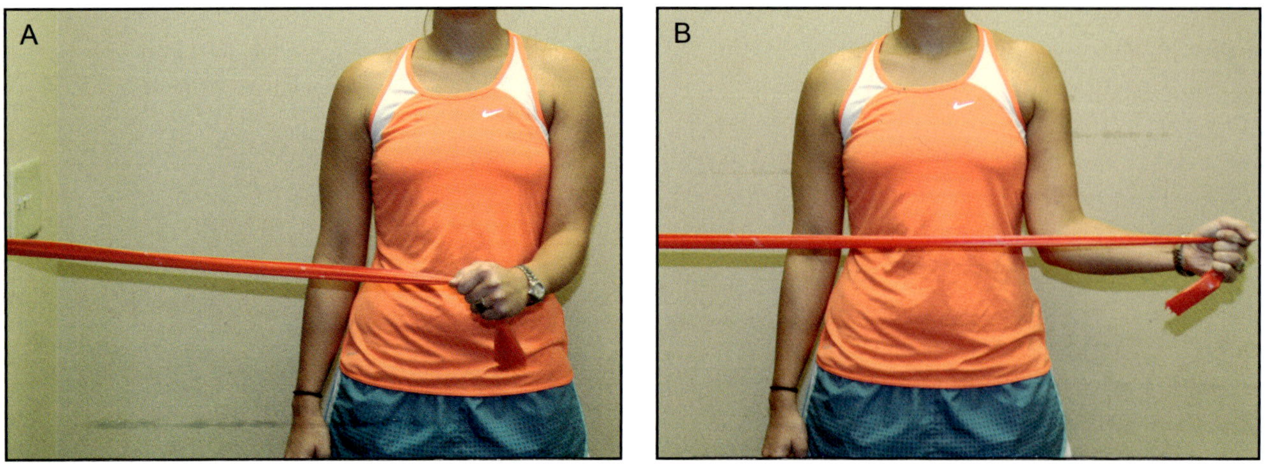

Figure 1. Start, A, and finish, B, positions for the elastic-band external rotation exercise with an initial band length of 0.6 m.

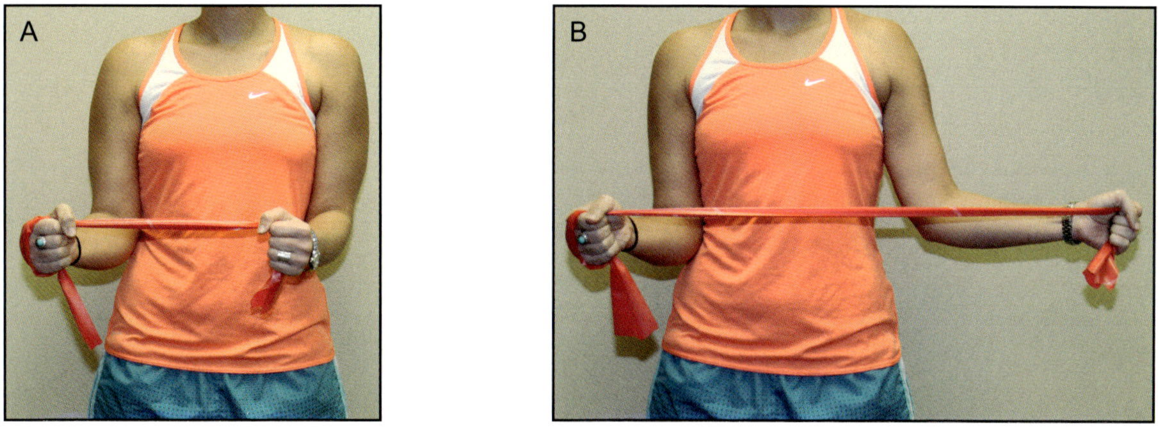

Figure 2. Start, A, and finish, B, positions for the elastic-band external rotation exercise with an initial band length of 0.3 m.

and become more taut, increasing the pretension and consequently the amount of resistance from the band.

By understanding the different physical attributes of elastic-resistance bands, one can easily see how small changes in the various aspects of resistance training can play a big role in the physical characteristics of an exercise. These characteristics can be manipulated by the rehabilitation provider to provide progressive resistance to the rotator cuff, deltoid, scapular stabilizers, and other muscles of the shoulder girdle via elastic-resistance bands. By having a greater understanding of the physical characteristics of elastic-resistance bands, rehabilitation providers can ensure that the specific exercises performed in an exercise program for the shoulder are appropriate, efficient, and safe for their patients.

THE BIOMECHANICS OF ACTIVE ELEVATION AND THE 1 PHYSICS EQUATION YOU MUST KNOW

Open kinetic chain (OKC) exercises are performed more frequently than closed kinetic chain exercises during shoulder rehabilitation because many functional activities of the upper extremity are performed in an OKC (ie, washing hair, reaching into a cabinet to get dishes). Another benefit of performing OKC exercises is that the sequential muscle activation of the upper extremity is from proximal to distal, allowing rapid acceleration and speed of the distal segment.[8] Such dynamic principles are important during the rehabilitation of an overhead athlete, such as returning a baseball player to pitching or a tennis player to a competitive level of participation after shoulder injury.

One of the primary goals of shoulder rehabilitation after a shoulder injury is for the patient to be able to actively raise the injured upper extremity overhead easily and comfortably. Active forward elevation is essential for activities ranging from combing one's hair to hanging up clothes in a closet and to more dynamic activities, such as shooting a basketball. Strengthening the rotator cuff, the deltoid, and scapular rotators is essential in helping the patient overcome the weight of the upper extremity against the force of gravity and any external weight the patient has in his or her hands while trying to raise the extremity overhead.

Selection of the appropriate exercises during progressive resistance training is critical to prevent overstraining the muscles of the shoulder girdle. When considering specific exercises to include as part of an elevation strengthening progression, we believe 1 equation regarding the biomechanics of active forward elevation is critical to understand. The rehabilitation provider must have a fundamental understanding that the amount of torque required to actively elevate the upper extremity varies based on the specific ROM of the shoulder, the lever arm produced as the shoulder moves through the ROM, and the effect gravity has on this lever arm.

Torque (T) is defined as the product of the magnitude of a force (F) and the perpendicular distance ($\perp$ d) that force lies from the axis of rotation ($T = F \cdot \perp d$).[9] The *perpendicular distance* is defined as the length of a line drawn perpendicular to the line of action of the force and the axis of rotation

(Figure 3).[9] This is a crucial concept that all rehabilitation providers must understand and use as they formulate exercise programs. Changes can be made to the amount of force applied (ie, using a weight) and to the distance or length of the lever arm (ie, shoulder abduction with the elbow flexed to 90° or the elbow fully extended) to make an exercise easier or harder for a patient.

Figure 3 demonstrates how a change in the perpendicular length of the lever arm alters the amount of resistance that the muscles of the shoulder girdle must overcome as the upper extremity is moved through a ROM (in this example, abduction). With the upper extremity resting by the side, no effective lever arm is created between the center of rotation of the shoulder and the center of mass of the extremity, thus no torque is generated. As the upper extremity begins to move away from the side, the length of the lever arm that is created by the perpendicular distance of the line of action around the shoulder joint increases. This increases the amount of torque that the shoulder musculature must generate to overcome the downward resistance force to raise the upper extremity. At 90° of abduction, the extremity is at a perpendicular angle to the downward force of gravity, creating the greatest distance between the center of mass of the upper extremity and the axis of rotation. This increase in distance makes 90° of shoulder elevation the angle producing the longest lever arm and consequently the largest amount of resistance torque acting on the glenohumeral joint (Figure 4). As the upper extremity continues into abduction above shoulder level, the length of the lever arm acting perpendicular to the downward force of gravity begins to decrease, leading to a decrease in the resistance torque generated. This decrease in torque continues as the upper extremity continues toward terminal elevation (Figure 5). Therefore, if the desire were to strengthen the supraspinatus, having the patient stop at shoulder level rather than abducting the upper extremity through a full ROM when performing an active elevation exercise would be more challenging to the muscle.

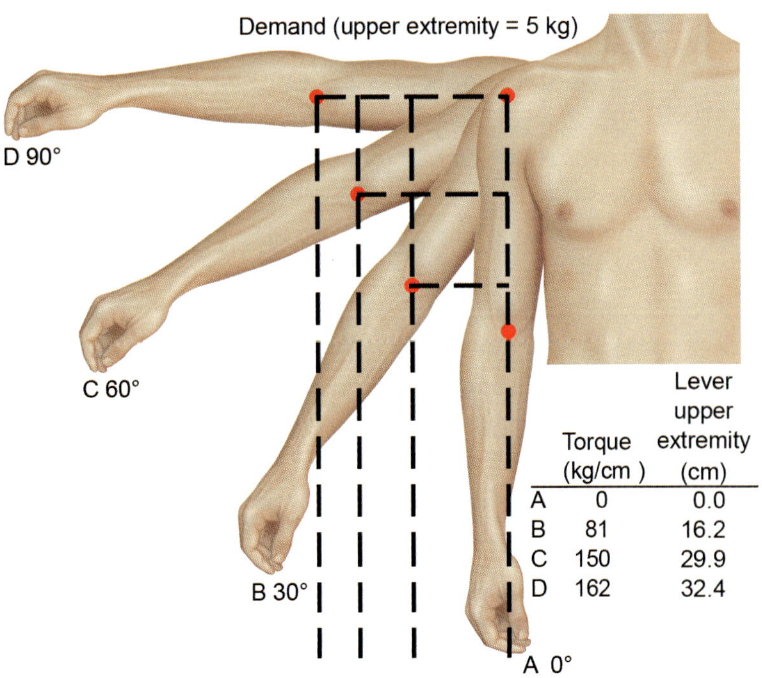

Figure 3. The effect of increasing the lever arm of the upper extremity during shoulder abduction.

ISOTONIC DUMBBELL VERSUS ELASTIC RESISTANCE IN SUPINE

Rehabilitation providers commonly use both elastic-resistance bands and free weights during strengthening exercises for the shoulder girdle. A common misconception regarding the use of free weights and resistance bands is that they both provide the same amount of resistance to the patient throughout an exercise. Hughes et al[1] showed the amount of resistance that free weights and resistance bands provide varies as the extremity moves through a given ROM. Examining the differences in the amount of resistance provided by these 2 types of resistance exercises during overhead strengthening in the supine and upright positions will better explain this concept.

For the patient who cannot actively elevate his or her upper extremity against gravity while standing or for the patient who has substantial pain when lifting the upper extremity, the use of gravity-minimized strengthening exercises is appropriate to reduce the resistance effect of gravity on elevating the extremity overhead. Supine forward elevation exercises can be used to strengthen the anterior deltoid muscle to enable a patient to raise his or her upper extremity overhead.

When using free weights during overhead strengthening exercises in the

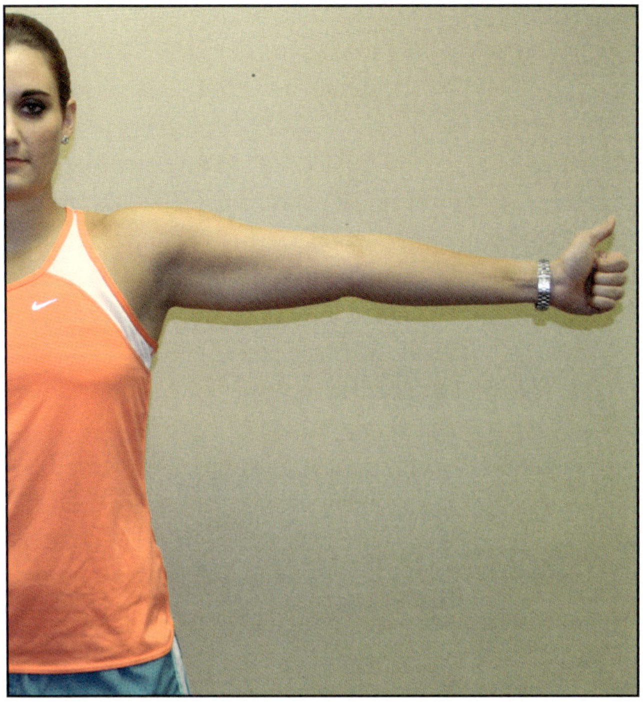

Figure 4. Shoulder abduction at 90° of elevation.

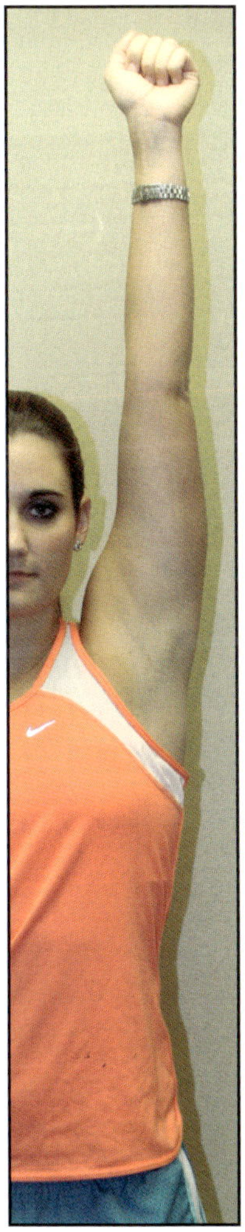

Figure 5. Shoulder abduction at terminal elevation.

supine position, the force of gravity against the upper extremity plays an important role in both the amount of resistance and the direction in which the resistance is applied to the shoulder girdle muscles. To perform the exercise, the patient begins by resting the upper extremity at the side while holding a hand weight. As the patient lifts the extremity off the table, the downward force of gravity on the long lever arm of the extended extremity produces a substantial amount of resistance to the extremity (Figure 6). This requires the shoulder muscles to generate a large amount of torque to continue to lift the upper extremity upward against this downward resistive force.

As the upper extremity reaches shoulder level (90° of forward elevation), the activity of the anterior shoulder muscles decreases as the perpendicular distance from the line of action to the center of rotation of the shoulder decreases the length of the lever arm in relation to the downward resistance of gravity.[10] This point of upper extremity elevation (approximately 90°–115° of forward elevation) is considered to be a "balance point" for the shoulder because of the minimal muscle activation needed by the rotator cuff to keep the humeral head centered in the glenoid. This is accomplished by the downward axial compressive force of

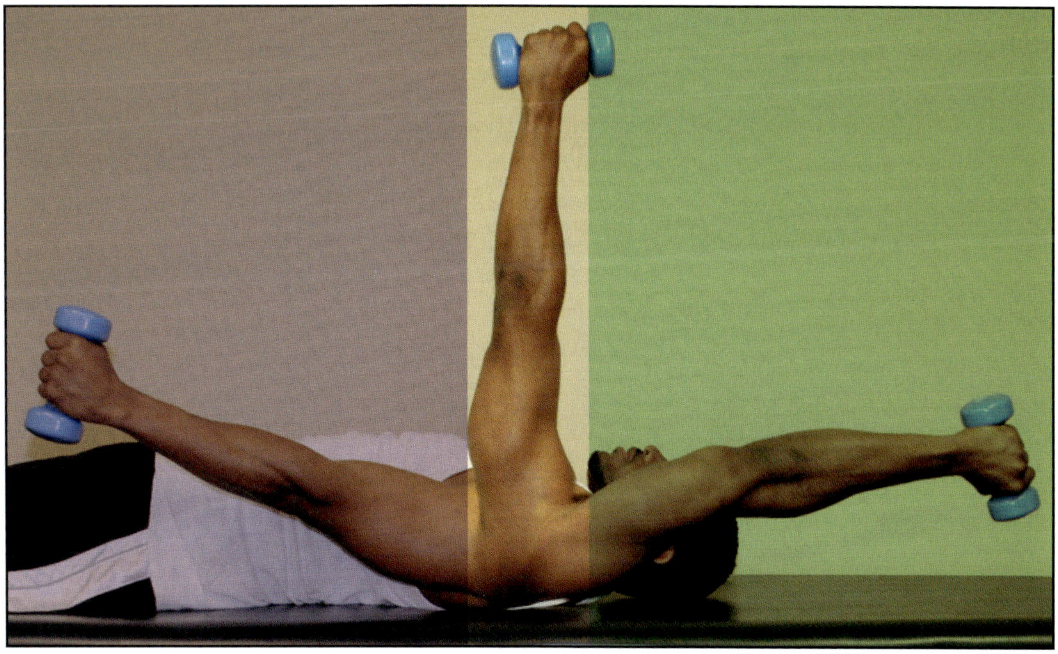

Figure 6. Supine forward elevation with dumbbell resistance. The region shaded in purple represents arc of motion requiring activation of the shoulder flexors. The nonshaded region represents the balance point of the shoulder where minimal muscle activation is needed to stabilize the shoulder. The region shaded in green represents the arc of motion requiring activation of the shoulder extensors.

gravity on the glenohumeral joint and a medially directed force vector of the deltoid on the humerus.[11]

As the upper extremity continues to travel overhead, the amount of downward force from gravity on the extremity again increases, but the direction of the force from gravity is now on the posterior aspect of the extremity. The weight of the patient's upper extremity, the downward force of gravity, and the resistance from the free weight are no longer providing resistance to the muscles that flex the shoulder, such as the anterior deltoid and supraspinatus, but instead are assisting in forward elevation of the extremity. If this force is large because of the weight of the upper extremity or a heavier dumbbell, then the shoulder extensors, such as the latissimus dorsi and the long head of the triceps, would become active to resist the torque that is moving the extremity into flexion. Therefore, supine isotonic strengthening from approximately 100° to the overhead position is not a biomechanically advantageous way to strengthen the muscles that actively elevate the upper extremity in standing.

The use of resistance bands for overhead strengthening in the supine position provides both a different amount and direction of resistance to the anterior shoulder muscles compared with a free weight. In the starting position with the upper extremity by the side, the band initially provides no resistance. As the extremity is lifted away from the body, the band tightens and begins to exert resistance to the shoulder muscles (Figure 7). As the extremity reaches 90° of forward elevation, the band applies its largest amount of resistance to the anterior shoulder muscles.[1] This is the opposite of the resistance provided by the free weight at this same position. As with the free weight when the upper extremity moves beyond 90° of elevation, the direction of resistance from gravity changes from pulling the extremity into extension to assisting the extremity into flexion. With the upper extremity now above shoulder level, the amount of resistance to the shoulder flexors decreases somewhat because of the change in the resistance from gravity and a decrease in the band-to-arm angle; however, the resultant force of this exercise still pulls the upper extremity into extension throughout the entire ROM. The *band-to-arm angle* is defined as the angle created by the long axis of the resistance band and the longitudinal axis of the upper extremity (Figure 8).[1] As the upper extremity moves away from the body, the angle at the glenohumeral joint between the trunk of the patient and the extended extremity constantly increases as the extremity continues in an overhead direction. This change in the angle of motion at the shoulder causes a simultaneous change in the band-to-arm angle at the hand. As the angle of motion at the shoulder increases, the band-to-arm angle at the hand simultaneously decreases. This decrease in the band-to-arm angle contributes to the slight decrease in the amount of resistance that the band provides in the supine position after the upper extremity moves above 90° of flexion. Despite this slight decrease in resistance from the band, the tension of the band continues to increase as the upper extremity moves overhead. The band continues

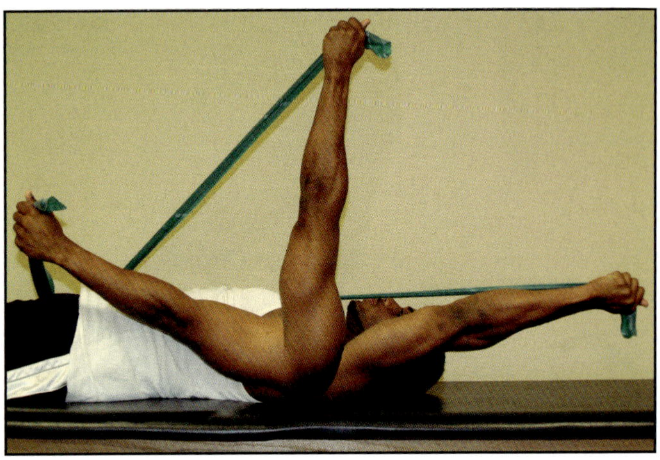

Figure 7. Supine forward elevation with elastic-band resistance.

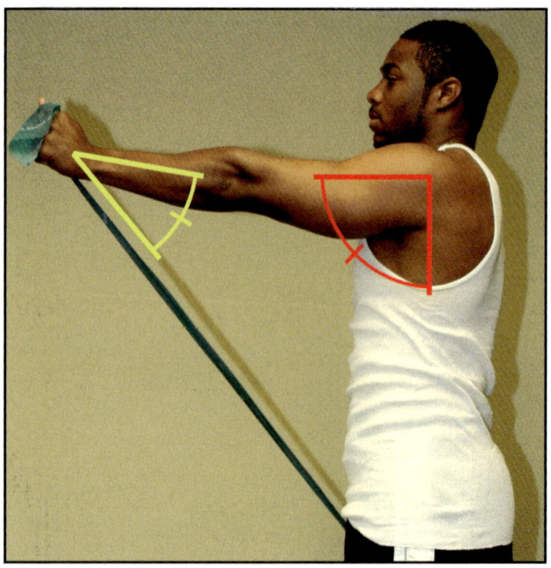

Figure 8. Band-to-arm angle during shoulder flexion. The yellow angle represents the band-to-arm angle. The red angle represents the range of motion of the glenohumeral joint.

to provide a force pulling the extremity into extension and requiring the shoulder flexors to be active as the extremity moves through its full ROM, but the amount of resistance is less than it was when the extremity was at 90° of forward elevation and the amount of resistance from the band was at its largest.[1] The amount of rotator cuff and deltoid activation required to perform this exercise is also much less than that required to perform standing active elevation of the upper extremity.[12] The continued resistance from the band into extension beyond 90° of elevation is vastly different from what is seen when using the free weights above shoulder level in the supine position, where the resistance provides a force assisting the upper extremity into flexion. Therefore, when using resistance to strengthen the shoulder flexors in the supine position, the rehabilitation provider must consider that the use of resistance bands can provide resistance throughout the full ROM of the upper extremity, whereas the use of free weights cannot.

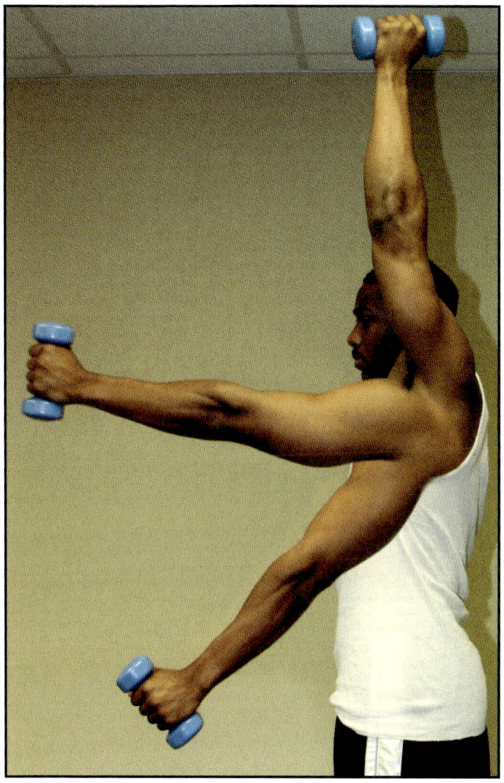

Figure 9. Standing forward elevation with dumbbell resistance.

ISOTONIC DUMBBELL VERSUS ELASTIC RESISTANCE IN STANDING

The effect of gravity on the shoulder changes the biomechanics of overhead strengthening as the patient progresses from supine to standing exercises. When using a dumbbell for overhead strengthening in the standing position, the patient begins the exercise with the upper extremity at the side. As the upper extremity is lifted away from the body, the downward resistance from gravity steadily increases until the extremity is at 90° of flexion (Figure 9). At this point in the exercise, the resistance from gravity and from the dumbbell is at its largest because of the long lever arm created by the perpendicular distance between the downward resistive force and the center of rotation at the glenohumeral joint (Figure 3). This is a sharp contrast to the amount of resistance noted with the extremity at shoulder level in the supine position when using the free weight. The torque required to elevate the upper extremity begins to decrease as the extremity continues to move overhead and the effective lever arm begins to decrease, as we discussed in this chapter. When the extremity is completely overhead, the torque required to maintain that position is smallest because of the small lever arm of the extended extremity. If plotted on a graph, the

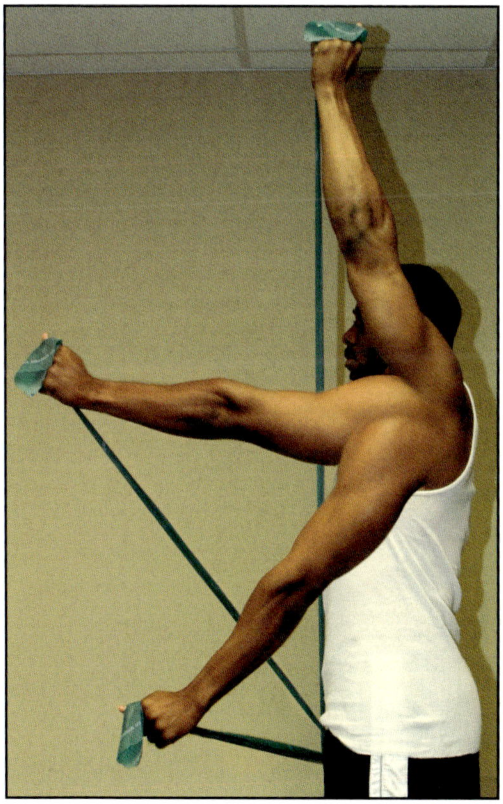

Figure 10. Standing forward elevation with elastic-band resistance.

amount of resistance from using free weights in the standing position would create a bell-shaped curve, with the smallest amounts of resistance occurring at the beginning and ending points in the motion and the largest amount of resistance occurring at the midpoint of the motion.

Resistance from the elastic-resistance band in the standing position follows a pattern similar to that of the free weight in the standing position with only minor differences noted. In the standing position, the band provides a minimal amount of resistance as the upper extremity initially moves away from the patient's side (Figure 10). As the patient continues to lift the upper extremity upward, the amount of resistance from the band increases. The largest amount of resistance from the band is noted when the upper extremity is at shoulder level. This is the same position in which the largest amount of resistance is noted when using free weights in the standing position. It is also the same position of the upper extremity in which the elastic band provides the largest amount of resistance in the supine position.

Similar to what is noted in the supine position, as the upper extremity continues to move above shoulder level in the standing position, the amount of resistance from the elastic band slightly decreases despite the amount of tension from the band continuing to increase. Hughes et al[1] showed that as the upper extremity moves from its initial starting position next to the body to a position of terminal elevation, the resistive torque of the elastic band is minimal at the extreme ROMs and is maximum at 90° of flexion. Again, this occurs because the band-to-arm angle decreases as the angle of overhead shoulder motion increases, reducing the amount of resistance from the resistance noted at 90° of flexion.

SUPINE VERSUS STANDING VERSUS PRONE ISOTONIC STRENGTHENING

As we have explained throughout this chapter, the specific exercise technique used during resistive training has a very large bearing on the direction and amount of resistance applied during an exercise and thus the level of difficulty of the exercise. Understanding the physics and biomechanics of isotonic exercises performed with the body in varying positions will assist the rehabilitation provider in formulating a progressive-resistive exercise program for the shoulder girdle. In this final section, we briefly examine the differences among supine, standing, and prone strengthening exercises.

One can now appreciate how the downward force of gravity at varying degrees of motion, changes in the band-to-arm angle during elastic-resistance band training, and the biomechanics of free weights as resistance play an important role during supine strengthening exercises. Further examination of isotonic overhead strengthening with either a dumbbell or an elastic-resistance band in the supine position provides some intriguing insight into the biomechanics of these exercises.

As mentioned, from 0° to 90° of elevation, the downward force of gravity and the resistance from the dumbbell provide resistance to forward flexion and attempt to assist the upper extremity into extension. From 90° to 180° of elevation, the downward forces of gravity and of the dumbbell assist the upper extremity into further flexion. We also noted that the use of elastic bands in the supine position provides resistance into extension throughout the entire ROM and not simply from 0° to 90° of elevation as with the free weight. Because of this difference in resistance between these 2 exercises, assumptions can be made about the recruitment patterns of the shoulder girdle muscles during supine overhead elevation. Because the downward forces of gravity and of the dumbbell are assisting the upper extremity into further elevation from 90° to 180°, the activity of the deltoid muscles to advance the extremity into terminal elevation decreases, and increased eccentric activity occurs in the shoulder extensors to help control the extremity as it travels overhead. The assumption then is that supine isotonic elevation strengthening with the use of free weights from 0° to 90° and the use of elastic-resistance bands throughout the entire overhead ROM biomechanically will promote the same pattern of recruitment as standing overhead strengthening exercises using either free weights or elastic-resistance bands, whereas supine isotonic elevation strengthening with the use of free weights from 90° to 180° promotes a different pattern of muscle recruitment.

Biomechanical Principles of Selected Shoulder Girdle Exercises

To help advance the patient along a continuum of progressive-resistive exercises, the rehabilitation provider should advance from using gravity-minimized strengthening exercises in supine to standing exercises. By advancing to standing strengthening exercises, the effects of the increased downward force of gravity on longer lever arms will permit greater resistance than that permitted with supine exercise. Standing activities also provide a more functional pattern of movement to simulate activities of daily living better than supine exercises.

One of the more common strengthening exercises in the upright position is overhead strengthening in the plane of flexion, abduction, or scaption. As noted in the previous section of this chapter, the largest amount of resistance during standing overhead strengthening with the elbow fully extended occurs when the upper extremity is at shoulder level (90° of elevation), with decreased amounts of resistance at terminal elevation. Therefore, for optimal strengthening of the shoulder (particularly the deltoids) in standing, the rehabilitation provider should consider strengthening within a 0° to 90° arc of motion. This arc of motion can be used for functional strengthening for the patient with work demands at or below shoulder level. For the overhead worker, this limited arc of motion is good for optimally strengthening the shoulder, but strengthening exercises also should be performed within a full ROM because these exercises are also essential for functional overhead strengthening to mimic work-related activities.

Elastic-resistance bands routinely are used in gymnasiums and rehabilitation clinics during standing overhead strengthening exercises. Again, the physical characteristics of elastic-resistance training and the biomechanics of overhead strengthening play an important role in determining the progressive resistance of these types of exercises. We examine 2 different exercises for overhead strengthening using an elastic-resistance band: forward overhead press with elastic resistance (Figure 11) and active forward elevation with elastic resistance (Figure 12).

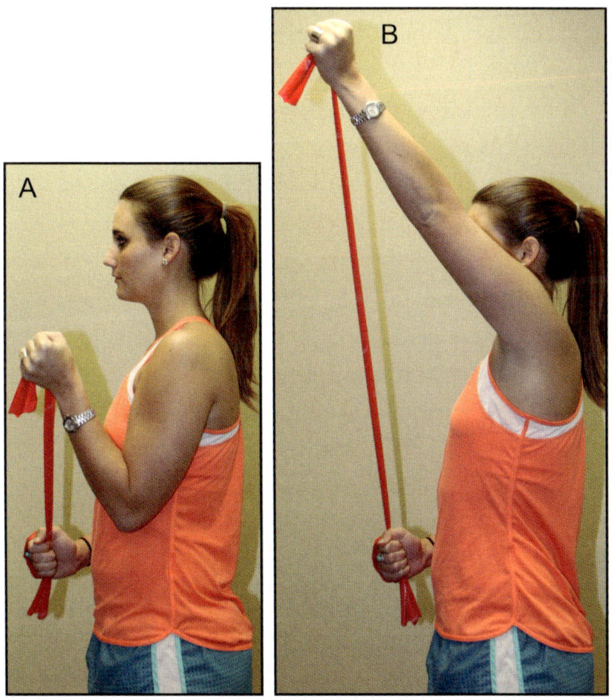

Figure 11. Start, A, and finish, B, positions of the overhead press exercise with elastic-band resistance.

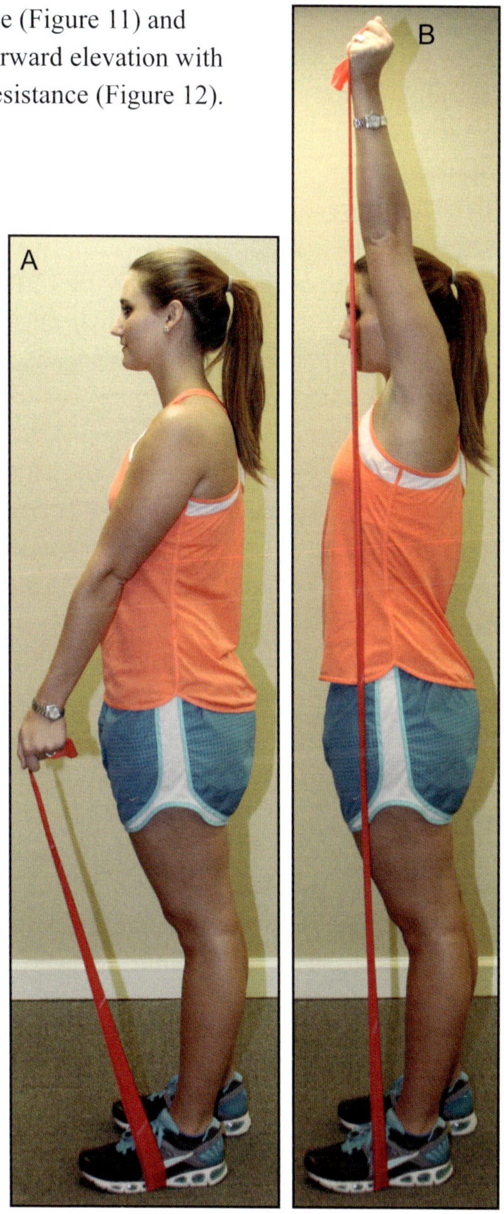

Figure 12. Start, A, and finish, B, positions of the active forward elevation exercise with elastic-band resistance.

For the forward overhead press with elastic-resistance exercise, the patient begins with one hand placed at waist level to anchor the band against the body and the upper extremity to be strengthened resting at her side with the elbow fully flexed (Figure 11A). To perform this exercise, the patient pushes the upper extremity upward until it is elevated overhead with the elbow now fully extended (Figure 11B).

The active forward elevation with elastic-resistance exercise begins with the patient standing on one end of the band with the ipsilateral foot and the upper extremity to be strengthened resting at her side with the elbow fully extended (Figure 12A). This is similar to the standing elevation exercise with elastic-resistance described in the previous section of this chapter (Figure 10). The only difference between that exercise and this one is the band is now anchored at the patient's foot and not in the hand at waist level. Keeping the elbow fully extended throughout the entire ROM of the exercise, the patient raises the upper extremity overhead into terminal elevation (Figure 12B).

Analysis of these 2 exercises will help the reader appreciate the differences between them and will help to appropriately place them in the continuum of progressive resistance exercises. Biomechanical characteristics of the forward overhead press with elastic-resistance exercise include a shorter lever arm, smaller overall ROM, and a shorter length of resistance band used. The biomechanical characteristics of the active forward elevation with elastic-resistance exercise are opposite to these characteristics; a longer lever arm is used, a larger overall ROM is used, and the length of the resistance band is much longer.

The shorter lever arm means that less downward force from gravity is encountered and also creates a smaller band-to-arm angle, reducing the resistance of the band as the upper extremity moves upward. The amount of ROM spanned during the arc of motion affects the percentage of elongation of the resistance band. As noted in the Elastic-Band Resistance Properties: The Details Matter! section, moving the upper extremity through a larger arc of motion during an exercise will result in a larger percentage of elongation of the resistance band, leading to an increase in the amount of resistance that the band provides.[4,6] Finally, the use of a short resistance band means the initial resistance to initiate movement of the band will be greater than when a longer band is used because of the initial resting length of each band, respectively. This is indicated by the increased tautness of the shorter band at its initial resting position compared with the increased amount of slack noted with a longer band. With all of these characteristics taken as a whole, the active forward elevation with elastic-resistance exercise is a more challenging exercise than the forward overhead press with elastic resistance.

As the patient continues to gain overhead strength of the shoulder, the rehabilitation provider needs to advance to more demanding exercises to further challenge the shoulder. Advancing from standing to prone strengthening exercises will allow for a continued progression of shoulder strength because of the increased muscle demand of the shoulder in the prone position. In EMG studies, researchers have demonstrated increased activity of the rotator cuff and deltoid during prone flexion and abduction exercises compared with standing flexion and abduction exercises.[13,14] We compare 2 exercises, standing forward elevation and prone forward elevation, to examine how the biomechanics of these exercises contribute to the differences in electromyographic activity levels reported in the literature.

As we have noted, the biomechanics of standing forward elevation strengthening produces the largest amount of torque at shoulder level (90° of elevation), with decreased amounts noted at terminal elevation. This pattern of resistance obviously changes as the patient assumes a prone position. For the prone forward elevation exercise, the patient begins with the upper extremity hanging down toward the floor at 90° of elevation. The patient completes the exercise by raising the extremity into terminal elevation. This can be performed in true flexion, in the plane of the scapula, or in horizontal abduction. In the prone position, the largest amount of resistance to forward elevation now is seen at terminal elevation, and no resistance is noted at 90° of elevation, which is the starting position of the exercise. In the overhead position, the shoulder creates a large perpendicular lever arm, resulting in increased downward resistance from gravity and thus increasing the difficulty of the exercise in this position. In the prone position, the compensatory use of trunk extension to assist in elevation of the upper extremity also is minimized compared with when overhead strengthening is performed in the standing position.

This decrease in trunk extension can contribute to the increased EMG data of the scapula and rotator cuff muscles noted during prone elevation because these muscles are working harder in this position to stabilize the scapula to allow for adequate force production to achieve overhead elevation.

Another explanation for the increased electromyographic activity and increased difficulty of prone forward elevation is the change in the length-tension relationship of the rotator cuff muscles at terminal elevation. During prone terminal elevation, the muscles of the rotator cuff are placed in a mechanically disadvantaged, shortened position, causing an increase in the force production of the rotator cuff muscles to achieve and maintain the shoulder in this position. In contrast, during standing forward elevation where 90° of elevation creates the largest amount of resistance to shoulder elevation, the length-tension relationship of the rotator cuff muscles is in a better position at that point in the arc of motion, and less activity of the cuff is needed to overcome the large level of resistance. Overall, prone isotonic strengthening into elevation or horizontal abduction requires greater muscle activation of the rotator cuff and deltoid muscles than standing elevation. During these prone exercises, minimum resistance is provided at 90°, and maximum resistance is provided in the overhead or horizontally abducted position.

In summary, when formulating an exercise routine to help a patient return to full function after an injury to the shoulder, the rehabilitation provider must have a thorough understanding of the specific exercises that he or she instructs the patient to perform. A detailed understanding of the physical characteristics of elastic-resistance bands; how lever arms influence the amount of resistance produced by an exercise; and the biomechanical differences among supine, standing, and prone exercises is essential to help advance the patient along a continuum of progressive-resistive exercises. By using sound judgment and an evidence-based strengthening progression for the muscles of the shoulder girdle, the rehabilitation provider can ensure that each patient is progressed properly in a safe and effective manner.

REFERENCES

1. Hughes CJ, Hurd K, Jones A, Sprigle S. Resistance properties of Thera-Band tubing during shoulder abduction exercise. *J Orthop Sports Phys Ther*. 1999;29(7):413–420.
2. Hintermeister RA, Lange GW, Schultheis JM, Bey MJ, Hawkins RJ. Electromyographic activity and applied load during shoulder rehabilitation exercises using elastic resistance. *Am J Sports Med*. 1998;26(2):210–220.
3. Myers JB, Pasquale MR, Laudner KG, Sell TC, Bradley JP, Lephart SM. On-the-field resistance-tubing exercises for throwers: an electromyographic analysis. *J Athl Train*. 2005;40(1):15–22.
4. Thera-Band Academy. *Thera-Band Resistance Band & Tubing Instruction Manual*. Vol 4. Akron, OH: The Hygenic Corporation; 2006. http://www.thera-bandacademy.com/exercises/prodManuals.asp. Accessed October 27, 2009.
5. Leggin BG, Neuman RM, Williams GR, Iannotti JP. Qualification of resistance provided by Thera-Band during shoulder exercise. Poster presented at: Combined Sections Meeting of the American Physical Therapy Association; February 1995; Reno, NV.
6. Page P, Labbe A, Topp RV. Clinical force production of Thera-Band elastic bands. *J Orthop Sports Phys Ther*. 2000;30(1):A47–A48.
7. Simoneau GG, Bereda SM, Sobush DC, Starsky AJ. Biomechanics of elastic resistance in therapeutic exercise programs. *J Orthop Sports Phys Ther*. 2001;31(1):16–24.
8. Rogol IM, Ernst G, Perrin DH. Open and closed kinetic chain exercises improve shoulder joint reposition sense equally in healthy subjects. *J Athl Train*. 1998;33(4):315–318.
9. Levangie PK, Norkin CC. *Joint Structure and Function: A Comprehensive Analysis*. 3rd ed. Philadelphia, PA: FA Davis Co; 2001:1–48.
10. Uhl TL, Muir TA, Lawson, L. Electromyographical assessment of passive, active assistive, and active shoulder rehabilitation exercises. *PM R*. 2010;2(2):132–141.
11. Poppen NK, Walker PS. Forces at the glenohumeral joint. *Clin Orthop Relat Res*. 1978;135:165–170.
12. Gaunt BW, McCluskey GM, Uhl TL. An electromyographic evaluation of subdividing active-assistive shoulder elevation exercises. *Sports Health*. 2010;2(5):424–432.
13. Blackburn TA, McLeod WD, White B, Wofford L. EMG analysis of posterior rotator cuff exercises. *Athl Train J Natl Athl Train Assoc*. 1990;25(1):40–45.
14. Reinold MM, Macrina LC, Wilk KE, et al. Electromyographic analysis of the supraspinatus and deltoid muscles during 3 common rehabilitation exercises. *J Athl Train*. 2007;42(4):464–469.

Specific Shoulder Girdle Rehabilitation Guidelines

Section III

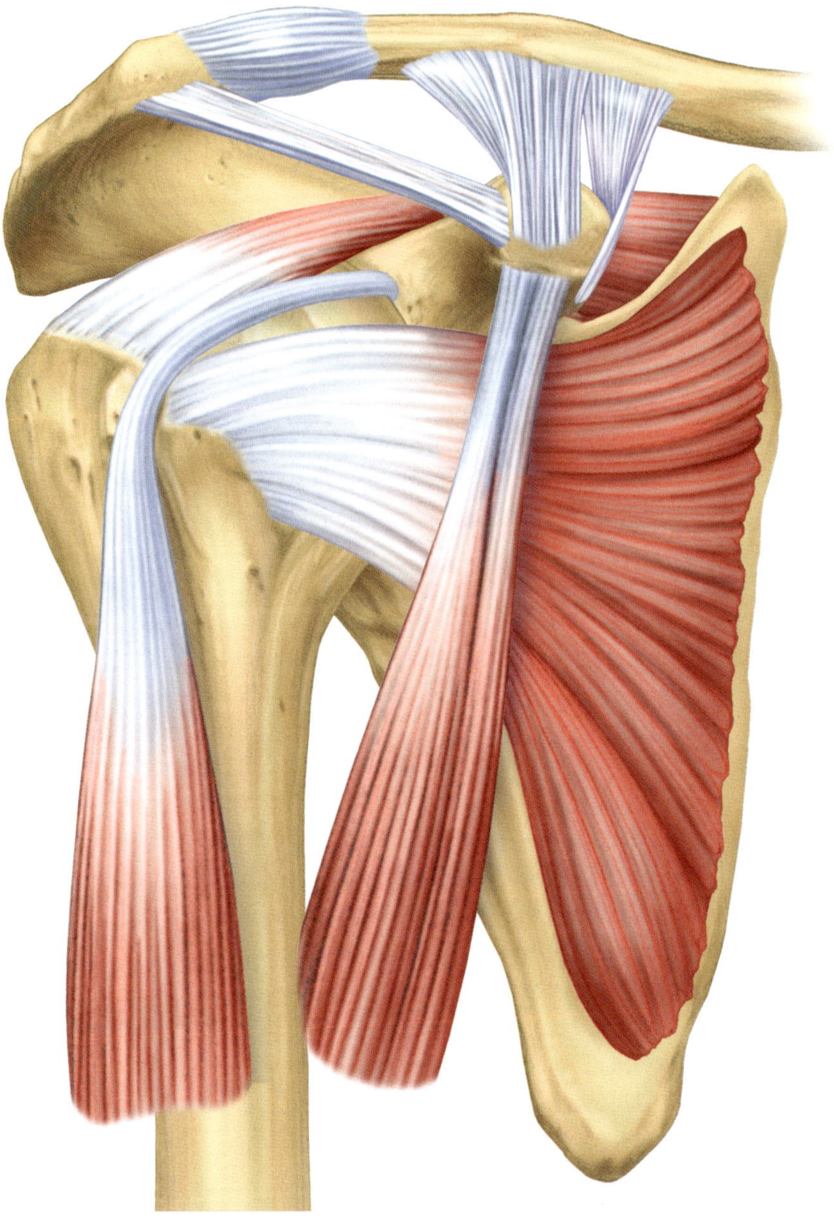

Routine Rotator Cuff Repair

Massive Rotator Cuff Repair

Partial Repair of the Massive Rotator Cuff Tear

Arthroscopic Capsular Plication With or Without Bankart Repair

Superior Labrum Anterior-Posterior (SLAP) Lesion Repair

Rehabilitation After Subacromial Decompression, Excision of the Distal Clavicle, or Acromioplasty

Traditional Shoulder Arthroplasty

Reverse Shoulder Arthroplasty

Manipulation Under Anesthesia, Lysis of Adhesions, and Capsular Release

Synovectomy

Postoperative and Nonoperative Rehabilitation of Proximal Humerus Fractures

Conservative Rehabilitation of Subacromial Impingement and Internal Impingement

Conservative Rehabilitation of Rotator Cuff Disorders

Conservative Rehabilitation of Glenohumeral Instability

Conservative Rehabilitation of Adhesive Capsulitis

Conservative Rehabilitation of Glenohumeral Arthritis

Rehabilitation of Scapular Nerve Palsies

Limited-Goals Rehabilitation

III-1

Routine Rotator Cuff Repair

Bryce W. Gaunt, PT, SCS

CHAPTER CONTENTS

WHAT PATIENTS ARE APPROPRIATE FOR THE USE OF THIS GUIDELINE?

- Patients with arthroscopic and mini-open repairs
- Patients with small, medium, and large tears
- Patients with good-quality or fair-quality tissue
- Patients with or without concomitant subacromial decompression, excision of the distal clavicle, bursectomy, or debridement of the labrum or glenohumeral joint

Clinical pearls are highlighted in yellow throughout the text.

THE MOST IMPORTANT FACTOR THAT SHOULD GUIDE CLINICAL DECISION MAKING

The strength of the surgical repair always should be much greater than the mechanical stress that is placed on the repaired tendon during rehabilitation. For every rehabilitation activity, this stress is determined by (1) the amount of muscle activation of the repaired musculotendon unit, (2) the plane of motion that is used, (3) the specific glenohumeral joint range of motion (ROM) and (4) the number of times the tissue is loaded (the number of repetitions prescribed). The stress on the repaired tendon must be considered for all rehabilitation activities (home exercises, clinic exercises, and manual therapy).

KEY PRINCIPLES IN REHABILITATION OF THIS PROBLEM

For optimal rehabilitation of the patient after rotator cuff repair, the rehabilitation provider must know the details of the surgical procedure; be aware of key factors that affect healing of the repaired tendon or tendons; know the stresses that each rehabilitation intervention places on the surgical repair; apply a precise priority for clinical decision making; maintain close communication among the patient, physician, and himself or herself; and carefully consider how these diverse issues affect each other.

Knowledge Gained From the Surgical Procedure

The size and number of tendons torn and repaired, the quality of the soft tissue, and the presence of associated lesions significantly affect rehabilitation. In many clinical studies, investigators have demonstrated the effect that the size of the rotator cuff tear and the subsequent repair has on both short-term and long-term outcomes. Patients with larger tears and repairs historically demonstrate slower gains in passive ROM (PROM) and active ROM (AROM), more limited

AROM, more limited rotator cuff strength, more modest functional outcomes, and a higher rate of retear.[1–5] At my institution, we use the same rehabilitation guidelines for patients with repairs of small to large rotator cuff tears, but we realize that patients with repairs of large cuff tears likely will progress through rehabilitation at a slower pace, especially during the AROM and strengthening phases, and that the physician might lower expectations on an individual basis. Because our standard rehabilitation is gentle and our progression is based on successful completion of staged ROM goals and comfortable participation in lower-stress activities before progression to higher-stress activities, patients with repairs of larger cuff tears are advanced as rehabilitation milestones are met and are not arbitrarily held back or arbitrarily advanced. Often, a patient with a repair of a large cuff tear needs an extended length of rehabilitation compared with a patient with a repair of a small tear. The clinician must note that patients with repairs of massive cuff tears follow an alternate protocol, which is discussed in chapter III-2.

Tissue quality is another factor that affects the potential of cuff repair healing and rehabilitation.[3] Better-quality tissue is healthier and thicker and has greater structural strength. Therefore, it provides a stronger construct to securely hold suture material and provides a better medium to facilitate the process of tissue repair. Clinically, tissue quality is expressed several ways. A subjective rating of good, fair, or poor by the surgeon at the time of repair is common. Rotator cuff tears also can be classified as acute (repair typically performed within the first 6 weeks after injury) or chronic. Chronic tears generally have poorer-quality tissue than acute tears have.

Rating the amount of fatty degeneration is another clinical way to grade the quality of the musculotendon unit. Numerous researchers have demonstrated that when a rotator cuff tendon is torn completely from its insertion, associated muscle tissue dies and is replaced by fat over time. This change might be irreversible and negatively affects muscle performance, even if the tendon is repaired. The presence of a large amount of atrophy or fatty infiltration also negatively influences healing and outcomes after repair.[5–7] Note that the quality of the other soft tissues in the shoulder that are not repaired also affects the speed of rehabilitation and the long-term outcome. When writing our standard rotator cuff repair rehabilitation guideline, we generally considered the patient who has a chronic cuff tear, fair-quality to good-quality tissue, and no significant fatty degeneration. However, it can be applied to patients with a broad spectrum of tissue quality by varying the speed of progression. Although we always ensure that a patient tolerates a particular exercise routine well before adding repetitions, resistance, or a new exercise, we typically attempt an advancement in rehabilitation and a larger advancement more quickly in patients with better-quality tissue. For a patient with poorer-quality tissue, we might wait until the patient demonstrates several weeks of good tolerance to a particular exercise before making a very small advancement because we know that the tissues are structurally weaker and more prone to overload. Therefore, patients with poor-quality tissue often are given a more conservative rehabilitation program and often take longer to complete their rehabilitation. If a muscle unit has a documented large amount of fatty infiltration and clinically presents with poor recruitment during middle-stage and late-stage rehabilitation, isolated strengthening is de-emphasized, and muscle training that targets coordinated recruitment of many muscles, cocontraction, and training the synergist muscles to have a larger role are emphasized instead.

Associated lesions in the shoulder girdle also can affect rehabilitation after rotator cuff repair. Patients undergoing concomitant subacromial decompression; excision of the distal clavicle; bursectomy; or debridement of the labrum, glenohumeral joint, or another rotator cuff tendon do not require any changes to the standard rehabilitation program. Because of the increased tissue trauma associated with these surgeries, the patients typically experience some increase in the level of pain and inflammation, as well as a potential for increased stiffness, that can make the first 4 to 6 weeks of rehabilitation more difficult. An increased focus on controlling inflammation and establishing quality, early PROM in a gentle way is emphasized.

Another surgical variable that does not significantly affect rehabilitation after rotator cuff repair is whether a repair is performed arthroscopically or via a mini-open technique in which the deltoid is split in line with its fibers and not removed from the acromion. Both techniques are commonly used and yield excellent results when used by surgeons familiar with the surgical technique. The procedures look different on the outside, but the same surgical steps and principles are used inside to repair the rotator cuff. In the mini-open procedure, the tissue that limits the speed of rehabilitation is the cuff repair rather than the morbidity of the deltoid during exposure through that muscle. For these reasons, the rate and method of healing is the same for arthroscopic and mini-open repairs; therefore, the same rehabilitation guideline applies. However, compared with an arthroscopic repair, the mini-open repair violates the deltoid more extensively, especially if the surgeon aggressively retracts the muscle during repair of medium and large tears that require tendon mobilization. This might affect rehabilitation by initially causing increased pain, which might make early PROM more difficult.

Other Factors That Affect Rehabilitation

Certain coexisting conditions, such as previous shoulder surgeries, advanced age, smoking, and the presence of systemic diseases that compromise the immune system (eg, rheumatoid arthritis), affect the speed of healing or quality of the associated soft tissue and, therefore, affect rehabilitation. Similarly, conditions, such as fibromyalgia and lupus, typically negatively affect exercise tolerance. In planning rehabilitation, the clinician must identify these coexisting conditions. For coexisting conditions that delay healing, increase inflammation, and negatively affect exercise tolerance, the rehabilitation provider uses a program that (1) is slightly to moderately more gentle in intensity and progression of both stretching and strengthening; (2) emphasizes passive and assistive motion over AROM and strengthening; (3) is more conservative in the initiation, exercise selection, and advancement of AROM and strengthening activities; and (4) includes a smaller volume of exercise. Coexisting conditions resulting in preoperative shoulder stiffness, such as adhesive capsulitis and osteoarthritis, require slightly different management and are addressed in the Special Considerations section of this chapter.

The patient's preoperative functional use of the involved extremity and the weight of the involved extremity also affect rehabilitation after rotator cuff repair. Both issues give clues about the likely speed of progression through rehabilitation. A patient who has had limited or no preoperative functional use of the involved extremity at and above shoulder level for many months or years cannot be expected to progress through rehabilitation at the same pace as someone who had nearly normal AROM and PROM immediately before surgery. The patient with longstanding functional limitation can be expected to have a slower recovery of PROM and especially AROM overhead, so a more gradual progression should be planned. The weight of the upper extremity affects rehabilitation because it is the resistance against which the shoulder girdle muscles act. This effect is magnified because the shoulder girdle muscles are mechanically disadvantaged in elevating the extremity. Therefore, a patient with disproportionately heavy extremities typically requires extended rehabilitation to achieve active elevation of the extremity.

Knowledge of Stress Placed on the Surgical Repair During Rehabilitation Versus the Strength of the Repair

Before starting rehabilitation after any surgical procedure, the rehabilitation provider must ensure that rehabilitation activities will not damage the surgical repair. How can we ensure that this does not happen? To put it very simply, a postoperative exercise is safe when the strength of a given surgery is **much greater** than the mechanical stress that each exercise places on the surgical repair. During rehabilitation of the repaired rotator cuff, the rehabilitation provider must have basic knowledge about the strength of the surgical repair and about the mechanical stress that **each** exercise during the entire course of rehabilitation places on the surgical repair. The strength of the rotator cuff repair depends on many factors, including the quality of the patient's tissue, the strength of the sutures, the strength of the suture knots, the fixation strength of the surgical anchors in the bone, and the frequency of upper extremity movement. Investigators have shown that rotator cuff failure strength in control groups is close to 2400 N.[8] During the first 6 weeks after surgery, failure strength is about 200 to 400 N.[8–11] At 12 weeks after surgery, failure strength is about 700 N,[8] and it returns to normal levels about 6 months after repair.[12] Therefore, significant protection of the repaired tendon or tendons by minimizing the mechanical stress placed on them is required, especially during the first 6 to 12 weeks of rehabilitation.

The mechanical stress that rehabilitation places on the repaired rotator cuff tendon depends on the muscle activation that each exercise (both passive and active) generates, the plane of motion that is used, the specific ROM that is achieved, and the number of repetitions that are performed. These issues are discussed in detail in the next section of this chapter. However, the clinician must always be aware that the failure strength of the surgical construct and the stress applied by exercise cannot be compared directly. Failure strength of the surgical repair typically is measured in newtons. Although the force in newtons that is placed on the rotator cuff tendons is known for movement in certain planes, exercise demand in the shoulder largely has been evaluated by researchers examining the relative electromyographic (EMG) activity level in muscles, which is expressed as a percentage of maximum muscle activation. No direct relationship between dynamic EMG activity level and tension in muscle and tendon has been established. Electromyography measures muscle activity but does not measure stress to the tendon. The exact stress in newtons that specific shoulder rehabilitation exercises place on the repaired rotator cuff tendon is unknown. However, a progressive order of difficulty (muscular demand) in exercises can be established. Therefore, we recommend using rehabilitation exercises that have low demands in planes of motion demonstrated to minimally stress the repair during the time when the surgical repair is the weakest and gradually increasing exercise demand as the surgical repair strength increases. In addition, we obviously do not know the exact failure strength of the surgical repair in each patient with whom we work. For these reasons, rehabilitation providers need to proceed with caution and to keep the exercise demands much less than the estimated failure strength of the surgical repair.

Priority for Clinical Decision Making

To aid in the selection of exercises, we use a precise priority for clinical decision making for all patients after shoulder surgery. First, rehabilitation must protect the healing tissues and the integrity of the surgical repair. Second, it must establish and maintain a low level of inflammation and pain. Third, rehabilitation must establish basic PROM while maintaining a low level of pain. Fourth, it must include a progressive strategy for AROM and strengthening that maintains a low level of pain. Fifth, rehabilitation must include appropriate and progressive functional training. This progression dictates the order of activities that are added and the order of importance in clinical decision making. Earlier principles always take precedence over later principles. For example, if PROM, the level of inflammation, or the integrity of the surgical repair is affected negatively during advancement of strengthening activities, then a lower level of strengthening activities should be used. We believe that appropriate rehabilitation after rotator cuff repair is never forceful. A detailed description and rationale for these principles can be found in chapter II-1.

Interaction of These Factors and Communication

Finally, all of the factors that I have discussed do not exist in isolation. Their interaction must be taken into account to determine the appropriate speed of rehabilitation. Most patients have a balance of factors; some factors enable a more aggressive approach to rehabilitation to be used, and others necessitate that a much more gentle and conservative approach be used. For most patients, this balance means that the "routine" guideline can be used, so the speed of progression can vary with individual tolerance. However, if a preponderance of factors necessitates that a much more conservative approach must be used, then a patient with a "routine-sized" rotator cuff repair might rehabilitate using a noticeably different progression. This example is detailed in the Special Considerations: Multiple Coexisting Conditions section of this chapter. Because the interaction of these issues is complex, communication among the physician, patient, and rehabilitation provider is vital to determine the best initial course to take as led by the surgeon. All parties must understand the issues described, and the patient's tolerance to the rehabilitation program must be re-evaluated at each visit to the rehabilitation provider and must be modified as appropriate. Therefore, although the rehabilitation provider uses standard rehabilitation guidelines, the actual rehabilitation program used for each patient is highly individualized based on the unique situation and his or her tolerance of the rehabilitation program. Extensive and regular patient education is also vital during the entire course of rehabilitation. Often, the patient needs help understanding that the repair must be significantly protected for an extended period and needs instruction in how to protect the upper extremity during rehabilitation and daily functional activities.

SPECIFIC REHABILITATION GUIDELINE

The Appendix specifies our complete routine rotator cuff repair rehabilitation guideline. In this section, I explain the rationale for selected components of the guideline. It is divided into 3 phases based on general timeframes of healing and staged ROM targets. To advance from one rehabilitation phase to the next, the patient must gain approval from the physician to advance, successfully complete the core components of the previous rehabilitation activities, and meet the time criteria.

Phase 1

The primary focus of phase 1 rehabilitation, which constitutes the first 6 postoperative weeks, is to maximally protect the surgical repair, and the secondary focus is to achieve, but not significantly exceed, the staged ROM goals that the referring physician helps establish. As mentioned, for a rehabilitation activity to be safe after a rotator cuff repair, the strength of the surgical repair always should be much more than the stress that is placed on the repaired tendon during each rehabilitation exercise. During rehabilitation after rotator cuff repair, this stress is determined for all rehabilitation activities (home exercises, clinic exercises, and manual therapy) by (1) the amount of muscle activation of the repaired musculotendon unit, (2) the plane of motion that is used, (3) the specific glenohumeral joint ROM, and (4) the number of times the tissue is loaded (the number of repetitions). Appropriate exercise selection cannot occur without understanding these factors.

Hatakeyama et al[13] and Zuckerman et al[14] evaluated the mechanical stress that specific glenohumeral PROM placed on the supraspinatus (SSP) in cadavers. Hatakeyama et al[13] found that passive external rotation (PER) with the extremity in slight abduction (20°–30°) resulted in very low stress (<5 N) to the SSP from 60° of internal rotation to 60° of external rotation. Zuckerman et al[14] found very low stress in the SSP (<5 N) with PROM from 0° to 120° of elevation performed in the plane of the scapula (passive forward elevation [PFE]). Therefore, these motions appear safe to use during the immediate postoperative period. These investigators did not test motion at more than 120°, but they theorized that tension on the rotator cuff likely increases with end-range PFE.

Orthopaedic surgeons and rehabilitation providers are almost in universal consensus that elevation in the plane of the scapula with the thumb oriented up (humeral external rotation) is **the** preferred plane of movement to use during early overhead motion of the shoulder. It provides minimal capsular stress; optimal length-tension relationship to the rotator cuff, deltoid, and scapular muscles to enable efficient function; and optimal subacromial clearance to minimize impingement. Therefore, for PROM during phase 1 rehabilitation after rotator cuff repair, the only planes of motion that the patient performs at home are PER with the upper extremity in slight abduction and PFE.

However, for early PROM after rotator cuff repair to be safe, the rehabilitation provider not only must choose planes of motion that provide low stress to the repair, but also must use specific exercises that have documented low EMG activity in the repaired rotator cuff. The Table lists the documented EMG activity levels of the SSP and anterior deltoid (AD) for common passive elevation exercises performed in the plane of the scapula. In studies, researchers have demonstrated that PFE performed in the supine or upright position with the assistance of the rehabilitation provider or PFE performed in the supine position with the patient assisting himself or herself has much less EMG activity in the SSP and AD than the rope-and-pulley PFE has.[15,16] The pendulum, the table step-back, continuous passive motion (CPM) machine, and aquatic exercises also have demonstrated very low EMG activity. We have found that the pendulum, table step-back, Kinex KS2 (Kinex Medical Company, LLC, Waukesha, WI) shoulder CPM machine, and rehabilitation-provider-assisted or family-assisted sitting exercises are the most effective and well-tolerated exercises to achieve PFE during the first few weeks after surgery (Figures 1–3). We also have found that although self-assisted

Routine Rotator Cuff Repair

Table. Common Passive Elevation Exercises in the Scapular Plane and the Associated Electromyographic Activity Levels of the Supraspinatus and Anterior Deltoid

Exercise	Electromyographic Activity
Therapist-assisted forward elevation	Average supraspinatus 4%, anterior deltoid 8%[15] Average supraspinatus 5%, anterior deltoid 7% supine[16] Average supraspinatus 12%, anterior deltoid 4% upright[16]
Self-assisted forward elevation supine	Average supraspinatus 3%, anterior deltoid 11%[16]
Pulley forward elevation	Average supraspinatus 17%, anterior deltoid 25%[15] Average supraspinatus 13%, anterior deltoid 21%[16] Maximum supraspinatus 17%, anterior deltoid 31%[17]
Pendulum	Average supraspinatus 9%, anterior deltoid 3%[16] Average supraspinatus 6%[15] Maximum supraspinatus (small 10-cm diameter circle) 8–8.7%[18] Maximum supraspinatus (large 51-cm diameter circle) 13.7–18.8%[18]
Specific aquatic exercises	Average supraspinatus 1–5%, anterior deltoid 1–8%[19]
Closed chain (table step-back)	Average supraspinatus 5%, anterior deltoid 2%[20]
Continuous passive motion machine	Average supraspinatus 5%, average anterior deltoid 3%[15]

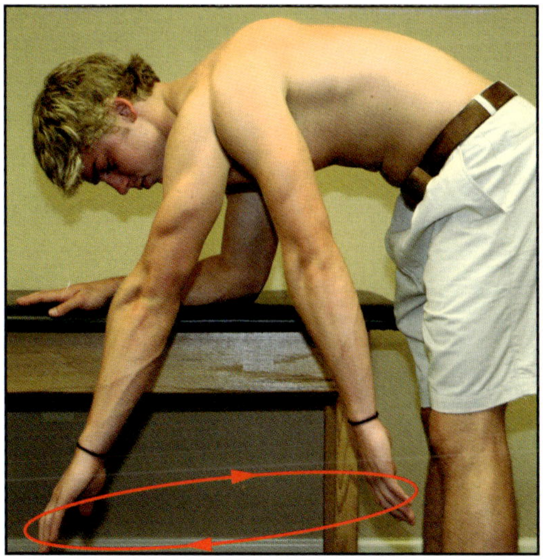

Figure 1. Pendulum exercise initially is performed with small circles.

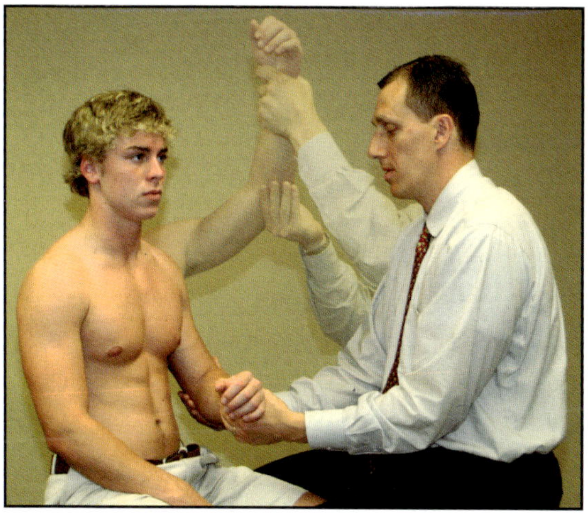

Figure 3. Assisted passive forward elevation. The assistant typically stands diagonally in front of patient.

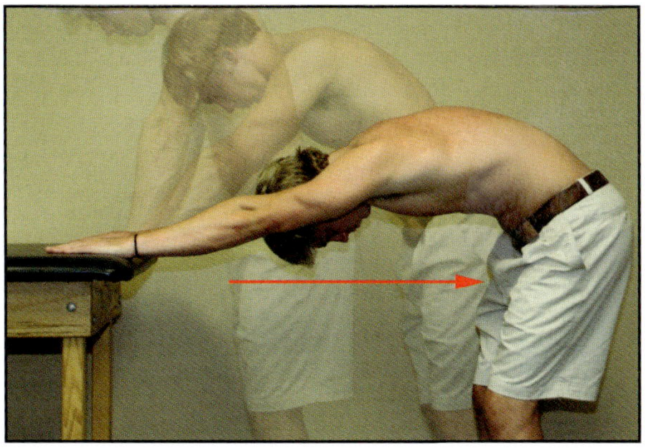

Figure 2. Table step-back exercise for passive forward elevation.

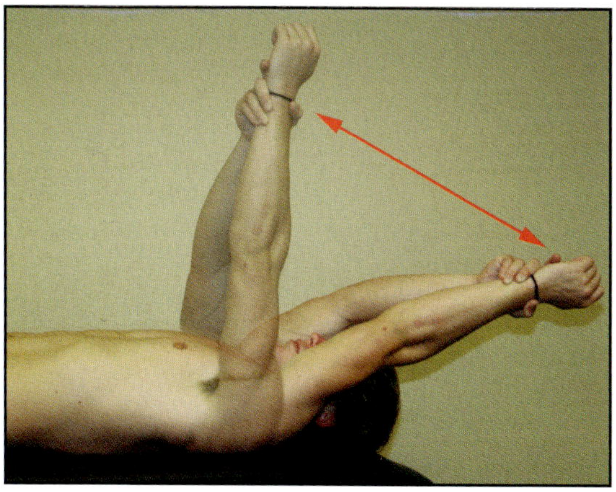

Figure 4. Self-assisted supine active-assisted forward elevation. The hand-assisted exercise is preferred.

PROM in the supine position (Figure 4) is safe to start immediately after surgery, it typically is not well tolerated until the patient achieves about 110° of PFE. More detailed information about the benefits and safety of shoulder CPM machine use and how we specifically use the Kinex KS2 with our patients after rotator cuff repair can be found in chapter II-3. As the Table demonstrates, the rope-and-pulley exercise has a noticeably higher EMG activity level in the SSP than the other exercises listed, so we do not recommend starting this exercise until postoperative week 6 for the typical patient after arthroscopic rotator cuff repair. Because of the theorized increased mechanical stress to the SSP with end-range PFE, we also restrict the end ranges of this motion during the first 6 weeks of recovery.

For PER, McCann et al[16] and Dockery et al[15] demonstrated very low EMG activity levels in the SSP, AD, and infraspinatus with all exercises tested. However, neither group of investigators evaluated the EMG activity in the subscapularis, which is likely the muscle most at risk of injury with these exercises, so extreme caution must be used when prescribing PER exercises for patients with subscapularis repairs. Clinically, we have found that PER performed while sitting and with the assistance of a family member or rehabilitation provider and the PER walk-around are the most gentle, most effective, and most well-tolerated exercises in the early postoperative period (Figures 5 and 6).

The number of times a rotator cuff repair is stressed or loaded, even in a submaximal manner, is an important, but often overlooked, rehabilitation variable that has important implications regarding the length of immobilization and the number of repetitions performed during early exercise. Much in the same way micromotion prevents bony union during fracture healing, submaximal tissue loading or cyclic loading potentially can disrupt the tenuous tissue-healing bonds between the rotator cuff tendon and its bony insertion. In human cadavers, cyclic loading has been shown to increase the gap between the repaired tendon and the bone to which it is repaired.[21,22] This increased gap, at some point, is believed detrimental to healing of the repair.[21] Although the exact effect of submaximal loading during various rehabilitation interventions is unknown, the rehabilitation provider should keep in mind that repeated and excessive submaximal tensioning of the repair during the early phases of tissue healing might be detrimental to the clinical healing of the repaired rotator cuff to its humeral insertion. Therefore, repetitive submaximal stresses should be carefully controlled during phase 1 rehabilitation.

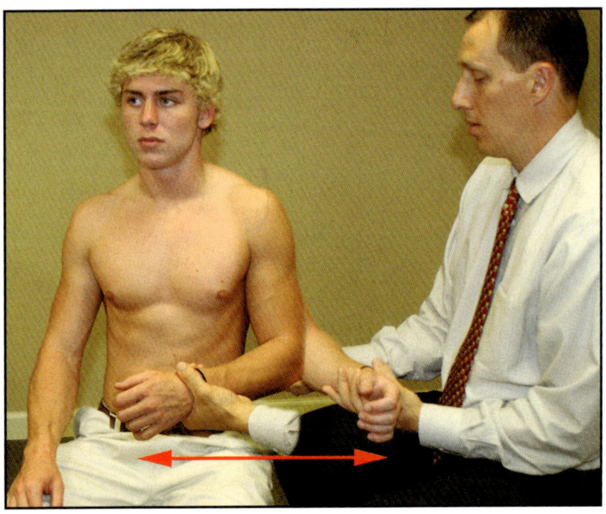

Figure 5. Assisted sitting passive external rotation.

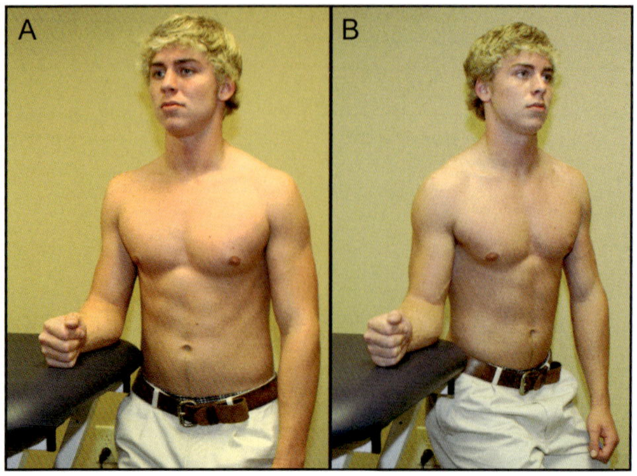

Figure 6 A and B. Passive external rotation walk-around exercise.

Clinically, this has implications for both exercise volume and immobilization. This research suggests that during phase 1 rehabilitation, as able both AROM and PROM should be minimized during exercise and functional activities. Therefore, although enough PROM needs to be prescribed to achieve staged ROM goals and prevent excessive joint stiffness, we recommend keeping both the number of exercises performed and total repetitions fairly low during this timeframe. We also emphasize educating patients about the importance of minimizing active use of the upper extremity during the first 6 postoperative weeks.

Routine Rotator Cuff Repair

Based on the cyclic loading studies discussed, the results of basic science research on tendon healing in animal models,[23–26] and recent ultrasound evidence suggesting that a moderate percentage of arthroscopic rotator cuff repairs might not heal completely to bone,[27,28] surgeons are re-evaluating the concept of immediate PROM after rotator cuff repair. Rehabilitation providers at a few facilities delay the initiation of traditional glenohumeral PROM up to 6 weeks even after routine-sized rotator cuff repairs in an attempt to maximize early healing. Parsons et al[29] retrospectively reviewed 43 patients who had undergone arthroscopic rotator cuff repair and were immobilized 6 weeks before glenohumeral ROM was initiated. They grouped these patients into a stiff group and a nonstiff group at the time ROM was initiated. Patients were considered *stiff* if their PFE was less than 100° and their PER was less than 30° at the time ROM was initiated. Ten (23%) patients were considered *stiff* at postoperative week 6. At 1 year, they found no difference in ROM, the American Shoulder and Elbow Surgeons score, or the Constant score. However, they reported a trend toward a lower retear rate in the stiff group (70% versus 36%). In nonpublished work, Leggin et al[30] evaluated the effect of delayed rehabilitation on PROM, AROM, and function by comparing PROM starting at an average of 4.5 weeks after surgery and starting at an average of 1 week after surgery in a group of patients after arthroscopic rotator cuff repair. At 12 weeks, they found only a 4° difference in PFE and an 8° difference in PER between groups. They also found the delayed rehabilitation group had 32° less active forward elevation (AFE) and scored 9 points lower on the Penn Shoulder Scale than the early PROM group. Overall, they found that delayed rehabilitation seemed to shift the recovery back a few weeks but did not impede recovery. In the next few years, I believe the concept of delaying the initiation of rehabilitation after rotator cuff repair will be evaluated more extensively to determine its effectiveness for improving healing rates while minimizing recurrent stiffness. If successful in both of these areas, then this practice likely will become more widespread.

Even given this possibility, we believe that early PROM (initiated in the first 1 to 5 postoperative days) is beneficial, and if only exercises demonstrating very low EMG activity are used and performed correctly, it is not detrimental to healing after the routine rotator cuff repair. Early glenohumeral PROM traditionally has been a well-accepted technique for rehabilitation after shoulder surgery because it helps minimize the negative effects of immobilization, such as formation of adhesions and joint contracture, muscle atrophy and serial sarcomere loss, and articular cartilage degradation.

Merely choosing the appropriate exercises is not sufficient to successfully achieve early rehabilitation goals. Helping the patient to maximally relax the extremity, paying attention to detail with exercise technique, stopping the PROM at a point of mild stretch and slight discomfort, and thoroughly educating the patient play enormous roles in the success of rehabilitation during the early stage of rehabilitation. These issues are outlined in the Appendix and are addressed extensively in chapter II-2. Supplementary PROM that is performed very gently by the rehabilitation provider is helpful, especially if the patient is behind in achieving staged ROM goals. Directions of motion used during phase 1, which are performed as comfortable, include abduction with neutral rotation to less than 90º, external and internal rotation in middle ranges of abduction, PFE, and external rotation at 80º to 90º of forward elevation to stretch the coracohumeral ligament. Detailed descriptions of these motions are presented in chapter II-3.

Although every attempt is made to help the patient achieve his or her staged PROM goals in forward elevation and external rotation as outlined in the Appendix through early PROM, careful exercise selection, and flawless exercise technique, some patients will fall behind our staged ROM targets. In these situations, we typically increase the frequency of the home exercise program to 4 to 6 times each day and increase the frequency of clinic visits. We do not increase the intensity of clinic or home exercise stretching, so we do not impede healing of the repair. Therefore, if necessary, it is better for the patient to be behind targeted PROM goals than to meet these goals but undermine healing of the repair.

Phase 2

The focus of phase 2, which typically constitutes postoperative weeks 6 through 12, is to continue to protect the surgical repair that while getting stronger, is still weak; to gently normalize PROM; to begin a well-structured AROM and strengthening progression that gradually increases demand to the musculature of the shoulder girdle while protecting the repair; and to minimize inflammation and pain. The rehabilitation provider still must ensure that the stress of the activities in the rehabilitation program is less than the strength of the surgical repair.

Obtaining adequate flexibility while keeping the level of pain and inflammation low should be the first priority of phase 2 rehabilitation. A variable amount of stretching is needed to achieve this goal. If the ROM of the patient is much less than staged goals, then the initiation of AROM and strengthening should be delayed until PROM is improved. To effectively improve PROM, the rehabilitation provider must recognize the influence that multiple structures have on a single glenohumeral motion. For example, a limitation in forward elevation of the upper extremity might be associated with limited mobility of any portion of the glenohumeral capsule, especially the posterior capsule, surrounding soft tissues, acromioclavicular joint, sternoclavicular joint, scapulothoracic joint, cervical spine, thoracic spine, or lumbar spine. These factors are addressed in chapters II-3, IV-2, and IV-3. Therefore, a thorough assessment of the entire upper extremity is warranted.

For PROM at the beginning of phase 2, the patient gradually starts gentle stretching in planes of motion other than PFE and PER in slight abduction. This stretching might include external rotation in increasing degrees of abduction, posterior shoulder stretching, and functional internal rotation (Figures 7–10). The last 2 directions place direct stress on an SSP repair, so the clinician needs to take extra care in prescribing and properly teaching the patient how to perform these exercises. For example, initiation of these 2 directions typically is delayed in repairs of larger cuff tears and in patients with poor-quality tissue.

The failure strength of the repaired rotator cuff during phase 2 rehabilitation is much less than that of a healthy shoulder and varies widely based on many factors. Therefore, when starting the AROM and strengthening phase of rehabilitation, the rehabilitation provider must use great care to select exercises that start with very low stress to the healing tissue and progress in a gradual and measured way. When beginning AROM and strengthening, selecting exercises that have a very low documented EMG activity and ordering them so that the activity level in the rotator cuff slowly increases should be the primary criteria

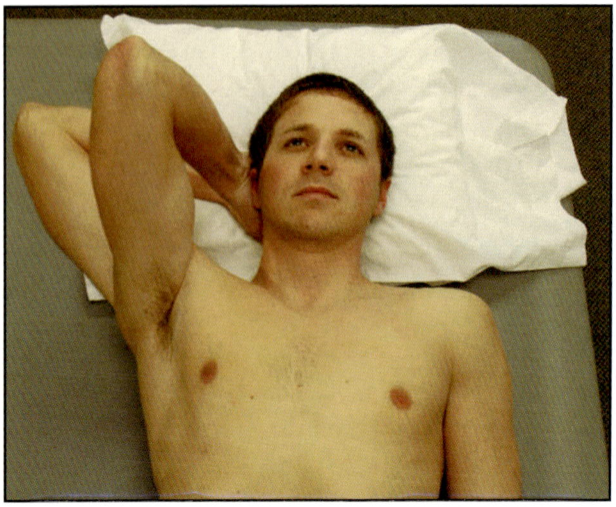

Figure 7. Supine hand-behind-head stretch to increase abduction and external rotation.

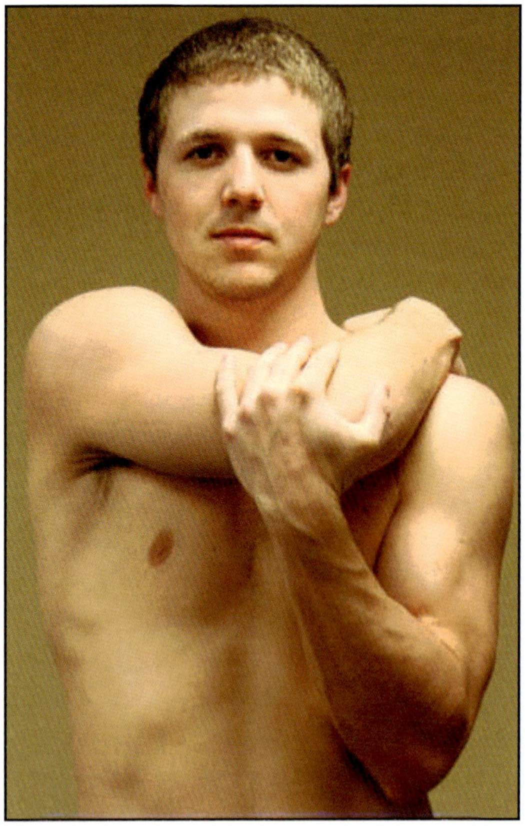

Figure 8. Horizontal adduction stretch.

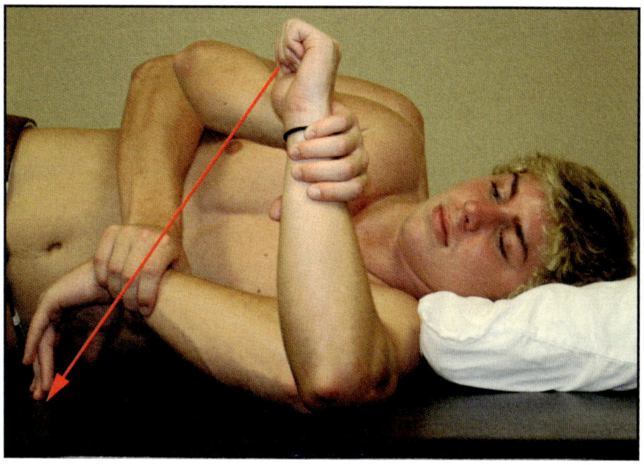

Figure 9. Sleeper stretch.

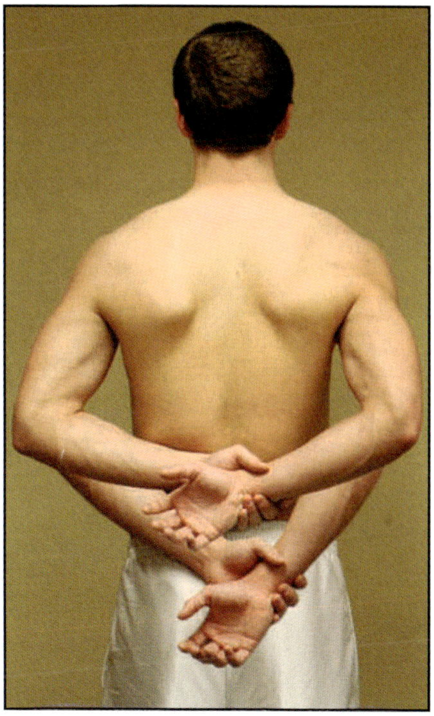

Figure 10. Functional internal rotation active-assistive range of motion.

for advancing exercises along with selecting planes of movement that do not place excessive tension on the repair. An evidence-based AROM and strengthening progression is incorporated and outlined in our rehabilitation guideline and detailed in chapter II-4.

The rehabilitation provider also should remember several clinical hints that help in the appropriate selection of AROM and strengthening exercises. First, during appropriate advancement of these exercises, the patient's level of pain should not increase, and substitution patterns should not occur. A reliable way to achieve this is to choose rehabilitation exercises that are at or below the patient's comfortable use of the extremity. For example, a patient who cannot reach the top of his or her head without pain should perform an assistive exercise in the overhead position rather than an active exercise. Second, because of the physics of the shoulder girdle, a little resistance to the shoulder provides a very large stress to the rotator cuff. Therefore, 1 to 2 pounds (0.45–0.90 kg) of resistance is usually all that is necessary until the late stages of rehabilitation, and no external resistance is used early in overhead AROM and strengthening. Third, most patients should perform AROM and strengthening exercises below shoulder level for several weeks before starting overhead AROM or strengthening exercises. Fourth, AROM and strengthening exercises should be progressed slower and performed more gently in the elderly patient, in the patient with repair of a larger tear, and in the patient who describes longstanding limited functional use of the extremity before surgery.

Several researchers have demonstrated that an exercise performed with the extremity supported places less demand on activated muscles than the same exercise performed without support.[17,31] Supported horizontal AROM, such as dusting, is an example of this type of activity (Figure 11). This activity and gentle weight-bearing activities have demonstrated very low EMG activity in the SSP of 6% to 9% of

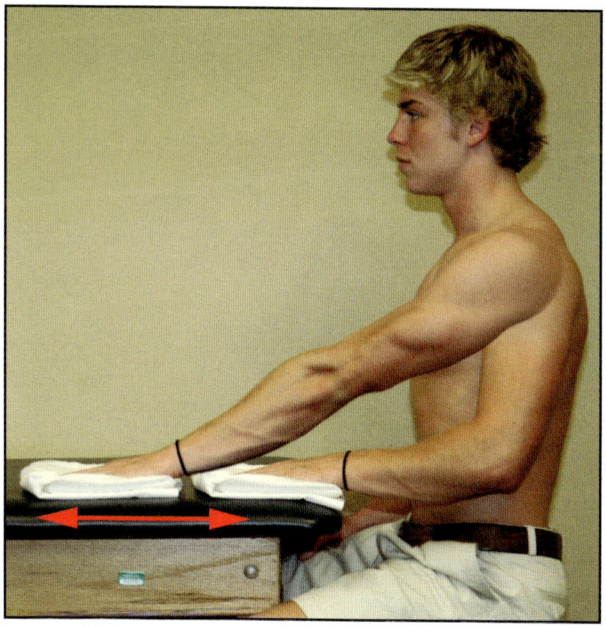

Figure 11. Horizontal dusting.

maximal voluntary isometric contraction (MVIC) (Figure 12),[17,32] which makes these exercises very good choices for initial "strengthening" exercises. Initiation of the next level of our strengthening progression (base strengthening) occurs when the patient comfortably can reach forward at waist level (eg, shaking hands motion). Our preferred exercises during this step are light strengthening with elastic-band resistance (Figures 13–15). Proper technique is critical for these activities because the resistance that elastic resistance provides varies greatly depending on the technique used. Arm elevation progressions complement the previous level and are initiated at either the same time as base strengthening or a few weeks later. The purpose of arm elevation progressions is to provide an organized method to help patients achieve full overhead active elevation of their extremities, which is often one of the most difficult steps in rehabilitation after rotator cuff repair. This progression is outlined in the Appendix and is described in detail in chapter II-4. After the patient comfortably masters AFE, which has a maximum of 29+/-13% MVIC in the SSP,[17] this exercise is progressed by gradually adding 1 to 3 pounds (0.45–1.35 kg) of weight, depending on the body mass of the patient. This constitutes our next level of resistive strengthening. When this level is achieved, the patient might be able to progress to more vigorous rehabilitation. However, many patients who have rotator cuff repairs and who lead relatively sedentary lifestyles have returned to their preinjury levels of function at this point and can be discharged. Therefore, more vigorous rehabilitation after rotator cuff repair is only appropriate in patients returning to demanding physical work or consistently demanding recreational activities. These patients constitute a small percentage of patients who have had rotator cuff repairs.

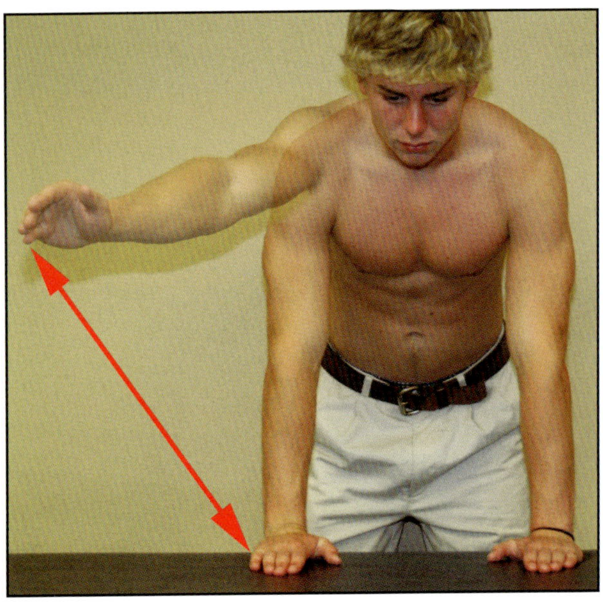

Figure 12. Quadruped weight-bearing exercise.

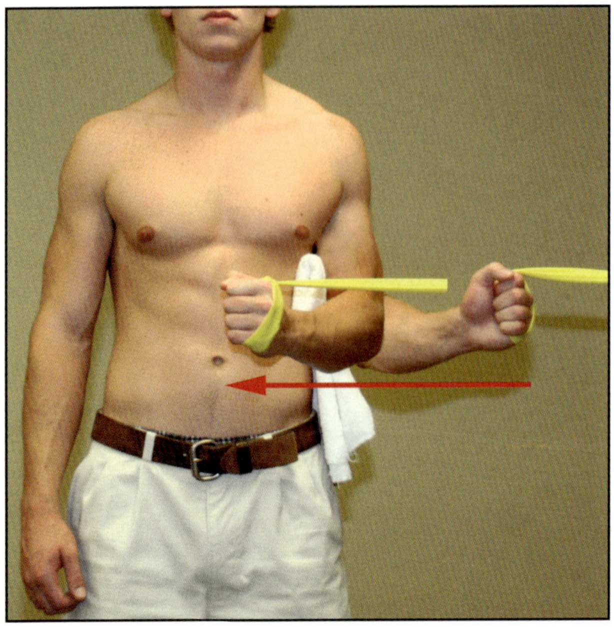

Figure 13. Internal rotation with an elastic band.

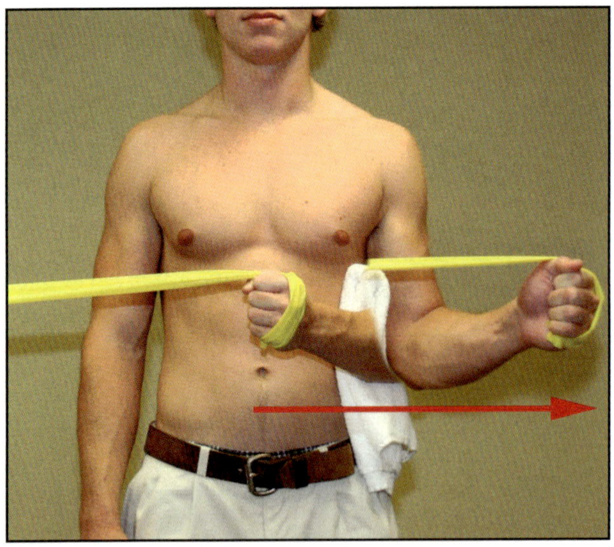

Figure 14. External rotation with an elastic band.

Phase 3

The focus of phase 3 rehabilitation, which might begin as early as postoperative week 12, is to normalize

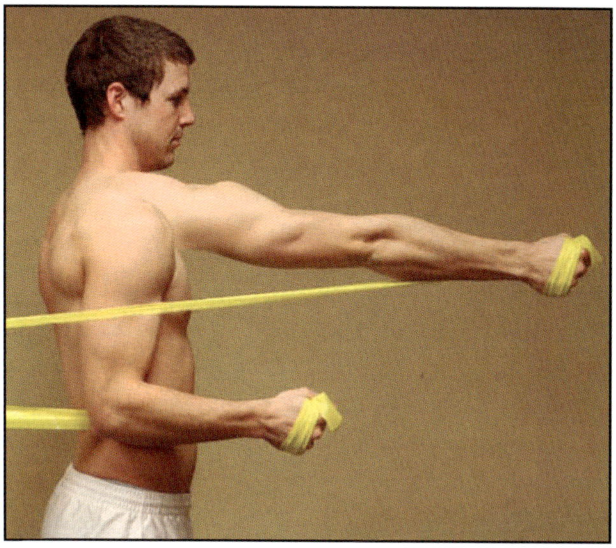

Figure 15. Forward reaching with an elastic band.

PROM, AROM, strength, endurance, and power and to help the patient return to demanding activities of daily living, work, and recreation. The necessity, extent, and makeup of phase 3 rehabilitation is highly individualized based on the patient's functional demands and on the factors discussed in the Key Principles in Rehabilitation of This Problem section of this chapter. Often, initial phase 3 rehabilitation is the completion or continuation of phase 2 activities.

For PROM, attempting to regain full flexibility is not appropriate for all patients with a rotator cuff repair. Other joint disorders or degeneration, poor-quality tissue, repair of a large cuff tear, or limited functional demand might be reasons to settle for functional ROM instead of full ROM. In addition, further increases in ROM over time tend to occur even without direct stretching. Finally, the general pain level of the patient often improves when terminal stretching has stopped. Therefore, the surgeon, patient, and rehabilitation provider should reach a consensus about the appropriate time to discontinue passive stretching.

Before beginning more advanced AROM and strengthening activities, the patient should achieve normal AFE by completing the AROM and strengthening progression that was outlined in phase 2 then should advance to AFE with 1 to 3 pounds (0.45–1.35 kg) of weight, depending on body size and functional demands. In addition, for the patient with a rotator cuff repair, advanced strengthening should be used to restore a specific functional deficit. The functional demand might be a return to demanding and repetitive work activities or a return to vigorous recreational activities, such as competitive tennis. Therefore, this level of rehabilitation is highly individualized to help the patient meet functional demands without overloading the surgical repair. The typical patient who has had a rotator cuff repair and who wants to return to basic activities of daily living and to light to moderate work and recreational activities usually does not need this level of advanced strengthening. Other criteria to start advanced strengthening are detailed in the Appendix.

Included in our advanced strengthening program are core exercises for the rotator cuff, deltoid, and scapula from phase 2 rehabilitation, such as base strengthening activities and AFE with light weight. We believe that a beginning point for advanced strengthening activities includes the historically standard rotator cuff and scapula exercises, such as prone forward elevation and prone horizontal abduction.[33–35] These exercises were developed to optimally activate the rotator cuff (60–80% MVIC in the SSP), so they should **not** be used as early strengthening exercises for the patient with a rotator cuff repair. Advanced strengthening progressions at this stage should provide a gradual buildup in stress to meet more demanding functional, work, and recreational activities of the patient. Higher-speed activities, functional movements, functional resistance through multiple planes of motion, heavier lifting, and training larger upper extremity muscles should be introduced and progressed gradually during this stage of rehabilitation. Although plyometrics are listed, they are seldom used in this patient population. Return-to-sport and modified weight-training programs are essential if the patient wants to regularly participate in these activities but are used only as needed.

SPECIAL CONSIDERATIONS

In this section, I describe some situations that require varying amounts of modification to our standard rotator cuff repair rehabilitation guideline.

Multiple Coexisting Conditions

A noticeably slower progression should be used in patients who have both surgical findings and multiple coexisting conditions that negatively affect healing and, therefore, necessitate a more conservative approach. An 80-year-old patient with rheumatoid arthritis, a large rotator cuff repair, and poor-quality tissue is an example. For these patients, the speed of progression is highly individualized and is determined by the referring physician, but it likely would include delaying AROM and strengthening for 3 to 6 weeks, progressing AROM and strengthening at a slower pace, keeping PROM and stretching more gentle, or incorporating a combination of these approaches.

Revision Rotator Cuff Repair

Rehabilitating a patient after a revision rotator cuff repair is another highly individualized situation. The speed of progression should be determined by the referring physician and depends on the number of previous failed repairs, quality of tissue, size of the repair, and other coexisting conditions. A slower rehabilitation program usually is warranted if the tissues already have shown the tendency to fail. Appropriate modifications can include initiating limited-goals rehabilitation (chapter III-18), initiating a rehabilitation program typically used for patients with repair of a massive rotator cuff tear (chapter III-2), delaying the start of strengthening for 2 to 4 weeks, or using the routine guideline but following a more conservative progression of PROM and AROM.

Biceps Tenodesis

Biceps tenodesis is a procedure in which the long head of the biceps tendon is detached from its origin spanning the glenohumeral joint and is reattached to the humeral head near the bicipital groove (Figure 16). It is indicated for symptomatic tears of the long head of the biceps tendon and is performed to relieve pain. The tendon is stabilized by various soft tissue or bone tenodesis methods, all of which provide secure fixation for early protected motion. Occasionally, a physician might prefer passive elbow flexion only for 3 to 6 weeks; however, generally, assistive elbow flexion that progresses to active elbow flexion as comfortable is allowed immediately after surgery. Note that the patient usually needs from 4 to 7 days to achieve comfortable active motion. Refraining from resistive biceps activity for a minimum of 6 weeks is vitally important. Patients must receive extensive and repeated education that emphasizes the prohibition against lifting anything of consequential weight in the hand during this period. This weight depends on many factors, including the age, mass, and tendon quality of the patient, and should be determined on an individual basis. No other change to the standard rehabilitation guideline is needed.

Biceps Tenotomy

Biceps tenotomy is a procedure in which the long head of the biceps tendon is released from its origin and is not reattached. The goal is for the released tendon to scar to an area near the bicipital grove, maintaining a relatively normal looking biceps. It is indicated to relieve pain in patients who have symptomatic tears of the long head of the biceps tendon. Typically, it is performed instead of tenodesis in patients who are elderly and who do not use their biceps for regular heavy lifting. To give the released tendon the best chance to scar to the proximal humerus and to prevent retraction that would result in a "Popeye" deformity, active flexion of the elbow should be minimized during the first 6 weeks after surgery. Elbow PROM is allowed, and resistive biceps activity is not suggested.

Rotator Cuff Repair Combined With Repair of a Superior Labrum Anterior-Posterior Lesion or Glenohumeral Instability

The patient who has had a rotator cuff repair combined with a glenohumeral ligament plication with or without Bankart repair, superior labrum anterior-

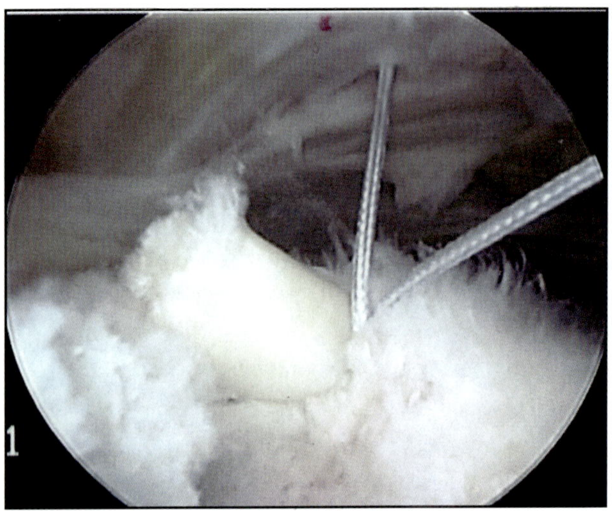

Figure 16. Arthroscopic view of the biceps tendon reattached to the humeral head near the bicipital groove.

posterior (SLAP) repair, or other procedure to address instability of the glenohumeral joint is difficult to rehabilitate because of extensive procedures involving both the passive and active restraints of the glenohumeral joint. This combined surgical procedure generally results in increased pain during the first 4 to 6 weeks after surgery and a more difficult time achieving ROM goals, especially PROM. Because 2 completely different surgeries are performed at once and each has its own specific rehabilitation guideline, 1 guideline must be chosen as the primary guideline for the patient. The rotator cuff repair guideline takes priority; however, the chosen rehabilitation variable influences this decision. For PROM, a ROM that is detrimental to any of the surgical procedures is not safe during rehabilitation. The staged ROM goals for routine rotator cuff, instability, Bankart, and SLAP repairs are roughly the same. Note that early horizontal adduction excessively stresses an SSP repair; early functional internal rotation excessively stresses an SSP and SLAP repair; and excessive PER, especially in increasing degrees of abduction, excessively stresses an anterior capsular plication or Bankart repair during phase 1 and early phase 2 rehabilitation. However, as mentioned, limited PROM is often a greater problem with these patients compared with excessive PROM beyond allowed limits.

For AROM, the rotator cuff repair guideline always is used to ensure adequate protection of the cuff repair. The instability repair is not affected negatively by the AROM and strengthening activities during the timeframes used in the rotator cuff repair guideline. Delaying the initiation of AROM and strengthening often is indicated if the patient is delayed in achieving the PROM goals or if the level of pain or inflammation appears elevated.

For advanced rehabilitation, a gradual increase in stress to all repaired structures is required. However, for almost all rehabilitation activities in phase 3, the rotator cuff repair needs the greatest protection. Therefore, the rotator cuff repair guideline is given priority at this time, and the rehabilitation provider keeps in mind that a gradual progression of activities should be accomplished in the throwing position to appropriately apply a gradual increase in load to an anterior instability, Bankart, or SLAP repair. Compared with patients who have had repairs of more isolated lesions, these patients generally progress through all phases of rehabilitation much slower, and they typically need at least 6 to 8 weeks longer to complete rehabilitation.

Supraspinatus Repair Combined With Shoulder Arthroplasty

For the patient who has had an SSP repair with a shoulder arthroplasty, the shoulder arthroplasty guideline is used as the base guideline. Often, the initiation of AROM and strengthening progressions is delayed about 2 weeks. This patient generally progresses through all phases of rehabilitation slower than the patient who has had arthroplasty without an SSP repair and typically needs from 6 to 8 weeks longer to complete rehabilitation.

Rotator Cuff Repair and Preoperative Adhesive Capsulitis or Synovitis

Preoperative stiffness is important to identify and address before rotator cuff repair because significant preoperative stiffness usually translates into postoperative stiffness and pain. Therefore, the preferred modification to the routine rotator cuff repair guideline is to address significant shoulder stiffness before surgery with a structured and comprehensive rehabilitation program (chapter III-15). Every effort should be made to maximize ROM and control inflammation before a rotator cuff repair is performed.

Perhaps even more important than normalizing PROM before surgery is timing the cuff repair surgery so that it is performed at the appropriate stage of adhesive capsulitis. The pathogenesis of adhesive capsulitis is now better understood. In what is classically termed the *freezing phase*, vascular inflammatory synovitis is present, and it progresses to hypervascular synovial hyperplasia. During the freezing and thawing phases, the inflammation in the synovium decreases, and resulting capsular fibroplasia and scar formation limit ROM.

Performing a rotator cuff repair when capsular fibroplasia and scarring are present is better than when substantial inflammatory synovitis is present. The surgeon can use a capsular release to address the stiffness associated with capsular fibroplasia. In addition, because the level of inflammation with this condition is usually relatively low, PROM is easier to maintain.

These patients typically tolerate rehabilitation after normal cuff repair fairly well. Although the typical cuff repair guideline must be used to enable the repair to heal, a slightly more aggressive approach to PROM is used. These patients typically do not experience much more pain than normal. Initiation of AROM and strengthening might or might not need to be delayed to ensure that acceptable early PROM is achieved.

If possible, the surgeon should avoid performing a rotator cuff repair in a patient with vascular inflammatory synovitis or hypervascular synovial hyperplasia due to early adhesive capsulitis or isolated synovitis. Even if the synovitis is addressed during the surgery, the cascade of events resulting in great shoulder stiffness is still present and often results in much long-term postoperative pain and stiffness.

Therefore, the signs and symptoms of early adhesive capsulitis must be identified, and the rotator cuff repair must be delayed, if at all possible. This is challenging to determine preoperatively because the signs and symptoms of early adhesive capsulitis often overlap with those of a rotator cuff tear or impingement. However, if not caught preoperatively, inflammatory synovitis is easy to identify at time of surgery (Figure 17), so modifications to the standard rehabilitation program can be initiated immediately.

Patients who have had a rotator cuff repair and have active inflammatory synovitis or synovectomy present a great rehabilitation challenge. We have observed that overly aggressive PROM appears to exacerbate the inflammatory response and results in a large increase in long-term stiffness and pain. This observation is supported by work from Diercks and Stevens.[36] Overly aggressive early PROM also might be detrimental to the healing of the rotator cuff repair, which is still the first priority in this situation. On the other hand, ROM that is too conservative also results in stiffness. Our preferred management is to start PROM (still only in PFE and PER in slight abduction) on the day of surgery or postoperative day 1, striving for the same ROM targets as the typical rotator cuff repair but realizing that ROM likely will be limited. We realize that compared with the standard patient with a cuff repair, these individuals usually have much more pain both at rest and with PROM exercises; therefore, patients are encouraged to take appropriate pain medications, especially in conjunction with their exercises, and to ice their shoulders more often. Because the pain level is higher, patients typically cannot achieve the desired ROM on their own. Therefore, we prefer an increased frequency of clinic treatments, especially the first month after surgery, to enable more regular manual PROM by the rehabilitation provider. He or she continues gentle PROM but attempts to achieve normal staged PROM goals **as concisely as possible** in the early weeks, realizing that the patient will experience increased pain due to the synovitis or synovectomy. Increased daily frequency of exercises appears to help some patients and limit others. During phase 2 to 3 rehabilitation, we have found that after a comfortable amount of PROM is established, an exacerbation in inflammation and subsequent stiffness results if terminal PROM is aggressively attempted. Therefore, we prefer gentle stretching to minimal discomfort only during middle-stage to later-stage rehabilitation. This preference often means settling for functional ROM, but it empirically appears to achieve joint homeostasis quicker. Because PROM is almost always painful and difficult to achieve, the initiation of AROM and strengthening also is delayed until the overall level of inflammation is low and a functional amount of PROM is well established. A 1- to 2-month delay in AROM and strengthening is common.

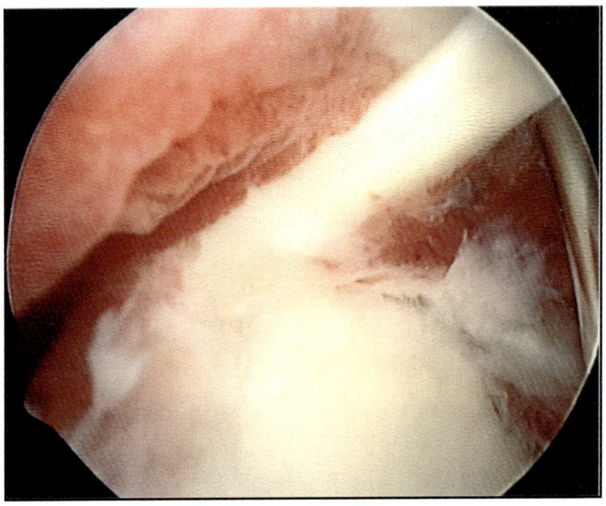

Figure 17. Arthroscopic view of inflammatory synovitis.

Rotator Cuff Repair and Significant Preoperative Degenerative Arthritis

Significant preoperative osteoarthritis or posttraumatic arthritis minimally affects rehabilitation after a rotator cuff repair. The ROM limitations caused by osteophytes, degeneration, and/or malposition of the humeral head or glenoid must be respected during rehabilitation. Although the rehabilitation provider should still work to increase PROM and AROM beyond preoperative ROM, a more gentle approach to PROM should be used, and the clinician should discontinue activities that are associated with a hard end feel or are highly painful, especially when working toward end-range motions. These patients also tend to be less tolerant to PROM and AROM in both isolated and combined abduction and external rotation. Functional ROM, rather than full ROM, is often the goal for these patients.

REFERENCES

1. Nho SJ, Shindle MK, Adler RS, Warren RF, Altchek DW, MacGillivray JD. Prospective analysis of arthroscopic rotator cuff repair: subgroup analysis. *J Shoulder Elbow Surg*. 2009;18(5):697–704.
2. Nho SJ, Adler RS, Tomlinson DP, et al. Arthroscopic rotator cuff repair: prospective evaluation with sequential ultrasonography. *Am J Sports Med*. 2009;37(10):1938–1945.
3. Nho SJ, Brown BS, Lyman S, Adler RS, Altchek DW, MacGillivray JD. Prospective analysis of arthroscopic rotator cuff repair: prognostic factors affecting clinical and ultrasound outcome. *J Shoulder Elbow Surg*. 2009;18(1):13–20.
4. Oh JH, Kim SH, Ji HM, Jo KH, Bin SW, Gong HS. Prognostic factors affecting anatomic outcome of rotator cuff repair and correlation with functional outcome. *Arthroscopy*. 2009;25(1):30–39.
5. Chung SW, Oh JH, Gong HS, Kim JY, Kim SH. Factors affecting rotator cuff healing after arthroscopic repair: osteoporosis as one of the independent risk factors. *Am J Sports Med*. 2011;39(10):2099–2107.
6. Gerber C, Schneeberger AG, Hoppeler H, Meyer DC. Correlation of atrophy and fatty infiltration on strength and integrity of rotator cuff repairs: a study in thirteen patients. *J Shoulder Elbow Surg*. 2007;16(6):691–696.
7. Goutallier D, Postel JM, Radier C, Bernageau J, Zilber S. Long-term functional and structural outcome in patients with intact repairs 1 year after open transosseous rotator cuff repair. *J Shoulder Elbow Surg*. 2009;18(4):521–528.
8. St Pierre P, Olson EJ, Elliott JJ, O'Hair KC, McKinney LA, Ryan J. Tendon-healing to cortical bone compared with healing to a cancellous trough: a biomechanical and histological evaluation in goats. *J Bone Joint Surg Am*. 1995;77(12):1858–1866.
9. Reed SC, Glossop N, Ogilvie-Harris DJ. Full-thickness rotator cuff tears: a biomechanical comparison of suture versus bone anchor techniques. *Am J Sports Med*. 1996;24(1):46–48.
10. Schneeberger AG, von Roll A, Kalberer F, Jacob HA, Gerber C. Mechanical strength of arthroscopic rotator cuff repair techniques: an in vitro study. *J Bone Joint Surg Am*. 2002;84(12):2152–2160.
11. Gerber C, Schneeberger AG, Beck M, Schlegel U. Mechanical strength of repairs of the rotator cuff. *J Bone Joint Surg Br*. 1994;76(3):371–380.
12. Lewis CW, Schlegel TF, Hawkins RJ, James SP, Turner AS. The effect of immobilization on rotator cuff healing using modified Mason-Allen stitches: a biomechanical study in sheep. *Biomed Sci Instrum*. 2001;37:263–268.
13. Hatakeyama Y, Itoi E, Pradhan RL, Urayama M, Sato K. Effect of arm elevation and rotation on the strain in the repaired rotator cuff tendon: a cadaveric study. *Am J Sports Med*. 2001;29(6):788–794.
14. Zuckerman JD, Leblanc JM, Choueka J, Kummer F. The effect of arm position and capsular release on rotator cuff repair: a biomechanical study. *J Bone Joint Surg Br*. 1991;73(3):402–405.
15. Dockery ML, Wright TW, La Stayo PC. Electromyography of the shoulder: an analysis of passive modes of exercise. *Orthopedics*. 1998;21(11):1181–1184.
16. McCann PD, Wootten ME, Kadaba MP, Bigliani LU. A kinematic and electromyographic study of shoulder rehabilitation exercises. *Clin Orthop Relat Res*. 1993;288:179–188.
17. Gaunt BW, McCluskey GM, Uhl TL. Electromyographic evaluation of subdividing active-assistive shoulder exercises. *Sports Health*. 2010;2(5):424–432.
18. Long JL, Ruberte Thiele RA, Skendzel J, et al. Activation of the shoulder musculature during pendulum exercises and light activities. *J Orthop Sports Phys Ther*. 2010;40(4):230–237.
19. Fujisawa H, Suenaga N, Minami A. Electromyographic study during isometric exercise of the shoulder in head-out water immersion. *J Shoulder Elbow Surg*. 1998;7(5):491–494.
20. Uhl TL, Muir TA, Lawson L. Electromyographical assessment of passive, active assistive, and active shoulder rehabilitation exercises. *PM R*. 2010;2(2):132–141.
21. Ahmad CS, Kleweno C, Jacir AM, et al. Biomechanical performance of rotator cuff repairs with humeral rotation: a new rotator cuff repair failure model. *Am J Sports Med*. 2008;36(5):888–892.
22. Waltrip RL, Zheng N, Dugas JR, Andrews JR. Rotator cuff repair: a biomechanical comparison of three techniques. *Am J Sports Med*. 2003;31(4):493–497.
23. Gimbel JA, Van Kleunen JP, Williams GR, Thomopoulos S, Soslowsky LJ. Long durations of immobilization in the rat result in enhanced mechanical properties of the healing supraspinatus tendon insertion site. *J Biomech Eng*. 2007;129(3):400–404.
24. Gimbel JA, Van Kleunen JP, Lake SP, Williams GR, Soslowsky LJ. The role of repair tension on tendon to bone healing in an animal model of chronic rotator cuff tears. *J Biomech*. 2007;40(3):561–568.
25. Peltz CD, Sarver JJ, Dourte LM, Würgler-Hauri CC, Williams GR, Soslowsky LJ. Exercise following a short immobilization period is detrimental to tendon properties and joint mechanics in a rat rotator cuff injury model. *J Orthop Res*. 2010;28(7):841–845.
26. Peltz CD, Dourte LM, Kuntz AF, et al. The effect of postoperative passive motion on rotator cuff healing in a rat model. *J Bone Joint Surg Am*. 2009;91(10):2421–2429.
27. Sugaya H, Maeda K, Matsuki K, Moriishi J. Repair integrity and functional outcome after arthroscopic double-row rotator cuff repair: a prospective outcome study. *J Bone Joint Surg Am*. 2007;89(5):953–960.

28. Bishop J, Klepps S, Lo IK, Bird J, Gladstone JN, Flatow EL. Cuff integrity after arthroscopic versus open rotator cuff repair: a prospective study. *J Shoulder Elbow Surg*. 2006;15(3):290–299.
29. Parsons BO, Gruson KI, Chen DD, Harrison AK, Gladstone J, Flatow EL. Does slower rehabilitation after arthroscopic rotator cuff repair lead to long-term stiffness? *J Shoulder Elbow Surg*. 2010;19(7):1034–1039.
30. Leggin BG, Kelley MJ, Glasser DL. Short term outcome of rehabilitation following rotator cuff repair: standard vs. delayed protocol. Paper presented at: 3rd International Congress of Shoulder & Elbow Therapists; September 2010; Edinburgh, UK.
31. Wise MB, Uhl TL, Mattacola CG, Nitz AJ, Kibler WB. The effect of limb support on muscle activation during shoulder exercises. *J Shoulder Elbow Surg*. 2004;13(6):614–620.
32. Uhl TL, Carver TJ, Mattacola CG, Mair SD, Nitz AJ. Shoulder musculature activation during upper extremity weight-bearing exercise. *J Orthop Sports Phys Ther*. 2003;33(3):109–117.
33. Townsend H, Jobe FW, Pink M, Perry J. Electromyographic analysis of the glenohumeral muscles during a baseball rehabilitation program. *Am J Sports Med*. 1991;19(3):264–272.
34. Reinold MM, Wilk KE, Fleisig GS, et al. Electromyographic analysis of the rotator cuff and deltoid musculature during common shoulder external rotation exercises. *J Orthop Sports Phys Ther*. 2004;34(7):385–394.
35. Blackburn TA, McLeod WD, White B, Wofford L. EMG analysis of posterior rotator cuff exercises. *Athl Train J Natl Athl Train Assoc*. 1990;25(1):41–45.
36. Diercks RL, Stevens M. Gentle thawing of the frozen shoulder: a prospective study of supervised neglect versus intensive physical therapy in seventy-seven patients with frozen shoulder syndrome followed up for two years. *J Shoulder Elbow Surg*. 2004;13(5):499–502.

Appendix.

ROTATOR CUFF REPAIR (ARTHROSCOPIC, MINI-OPEN WITH FAIR-QUALITY OR GOOD-QUALITY TISSUE) WITH OR WITHOUT SUBACROMIAL DECOMPRESSION AND/OR EXCISION OF THE DISTAL CLAVICLE REHABILITATION GUIDELINE

St. Francis Orthopaedic Institute and St. Francis Rehabilitation Center

All information contained in this protocol is to be used as a general guideline only. Specific variations might be appropriate for each patient and might be specified by the physician. In all cases, it is acceptable to advance the program more slowly than stated. If the patient experiences excessive pain, discontinue exercise until the physician is contacted. ***Achieving and maintaining a low level of pain and inflammation and protecting the surgical repair are the guiding principles in all stages of rehabilitation, even if less passive and active range of motion are accomplished.***

SYMBOLS AND ABBREVIATIONS

AAFE, active-assistive forward elevation
AAROM, active-assistive range of motion
AASEP, assistive-to-active shoulder elevation progression
ADLs, activities of daily living
AFE, active forward elevation
AROM, active range of motion
EMG, electromyography
ER, external rotation
FE, forward elevation
IR, internal rotation
MMT, manual muscle testing
NA, not applicable
PER, passive external rotation
PFE, passive forward elevation
PNF, proprioceptive neuromuscular facilitation
POD, postoperative day
POM, postoperative month
POW, postoperative week
PRN, as needed
PROM, passive range of motion
ROM, range of motion
T-Band, Thera-Band (The Hygenic Corporation, Akron, OH)
WNL, within normal limits

Forward elevation, either active or passive, is the plane of motion in which an individual naturally lifts his or her arm that is anterior to the plane of the scapula and lateral to flexion.

STAGED GOALS FOR RANGE OF MOTION

These are approximate targets for range of motion. Specific limits might be specified by the physician, especially if a subscapularis repair was performed.

Time	PFE	PER at 20° of Abduction	PER at 90° of Abduction	AFE
POD 1	60°	0°–20°	NA	NA
POW 1	80°–100°	10°–30°	NA	NA
POW 3	115°–130°	30°–45°	NA	NA
POW 6	130°–150°	45°–60°	45°–60°	45°–120°
POW 9	140°–165°	WNL	60°–80°	75°–145°
POW 12+	145°–WNL	WNL	WNL	115°–155°+

PHASE 1

Goals

°Minimize pain and inflammatory response
°Maximally protect the surgical repair
°Achieve staged ROM goals
°Educate the patient about postoperative precautions
°Establish a stable scapula

POD 1 to POW 6

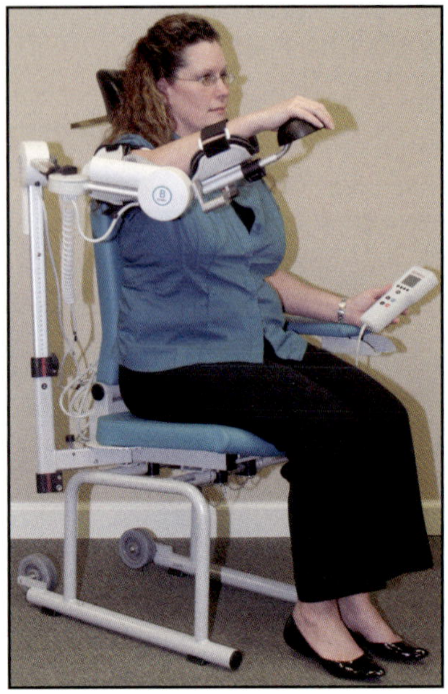

Figure 18. Passive forward elevation performed by the Kinex KS2 (Kinex Medical Company, LLC, Waukesha, WI) shoulder continuous passive motion machine.

°Elbow, wrist, and hand AROM with no weight
°Scapular elevations and retractions (no weight) in or out of sling
°Pendulum exercises
- °Lean over the table a comfortable amount
- °Let the arm hang down relaxed
- °Keep the body still
- °As able, move the arm in small comfortable circles only

°Upright PER in slight abduction until mild stretch and discomfort
- °7 to 12 repetitions 2 times per day
- °Preferred exercises
  - °Sit with family member or therapist rotating the arm (Figure 5)
  - °PER walk-around (stand with the arm supported on a table and rotate the body) (Figure 6)

°PFE until mild stretch and discomfort
- °7 to 12 repetitions 2 times per day
- °Preferred exercises
  - °Sit with family member or therapist lifting the arm (Figure 3)
  - °Kinex KS2 (Kinex Medical Company, LLC, Waukesha, WI) continuous passive motion machine 10 to 20 minutes 2 to 4 times per day (Figure 18)
  - °Table step-back exercise (Figure 2)
  - °After achieving more than 110° of PFE, progress to self-assisted AAFE in the supine position, as tolerated (Figure 4)

°Ice for pain reduction
°Fit sling properly
- °Ensure sling provides slight lift to the shoulder girdle and supports the wrist

°Patient education
- °Primary focus of phase 1: encourage initial healing of the surgical repair
- °Use of sling as instructed by physician; typically, full time in community and when up for more than 5 to 10 minutes at home
- °Minimal use of the arm for light waist-level activities, as comfortable
  - °Ensure level of pain is not increasing because of excessive use of the arm for ADLs or work
- °Sleep in a recliner
  - °3 weeks (required)
  - °6 weeks (preferred)

Adjunctive Exercises

°Therapist-assisted supine PROM within comfortable ROM to
- °Decrease muscle guarding
- °Gain patient confidence
- °Achieve staged PROM goals (no mobilizations)

°Cervical spine AROM
°Pain-control agents PRN
°Aquatic therapy for gentle pain-free AAROM (no swimming strokes) after the incision has healed completely

Interventions to Avoid

°Home exercise glenohumeral PROM in planes other than PFE and PER
°Exercises that result in moderate or severe pain
°Exercises that result in excessive guarding or splinting of muscles
°Weighted exercises
°Cross-body adduction, reaching behind the back, and active elevation of the arm above waist level
°Repetitive activity with the affected extremity

PHASE 2

Goals

°Achieve staged ROM goals
°Minimize shoulder pain
°Begin to increase AROM, strength, and endurance
°Increase functional activities

POW 6 to 9

°Achieve staged ROM goals in FE
  °Preferred exercises
    °Rope-and-pulley exercise (elbows remain straight)
    °Patient-assisted supine AAFE exercise (use the unaffected arm for assistance) (Figure 4)
°Achieve staged ROM goals in ER at 20° of abduction using upright exercises
°Initiate horizontal adduction (Figure 8) or sleeper stretch (Figure 9), or both, PRN
°Initiate supine hand-behind-head stretch (Figure 7)
  °Progress to gentle ER stretching in 70° to 90° of abduction
°Therapist-assisted PROM to achieve staged ROM goals with mobilizations PRN
°Initiate base strengthening progression
  °Includes standard rotator cuff, deltoid, and scapular strengthening program
  °2 times per day, at most, with light resistance and increasing repetitions
  °Yellow T-Band for ER and IR
    °5- to 6-foot band length and light or no pretension
    °Can use side-lying ER instead of T-Band
  °Yellow T-Band forward reach (Figure 15)
    °Initially, 5- to 6-foot band length and light or no pretension in a 3- to 6-inch arc of motion
    °Start with the elbow bent and by the side and the band tied behind the patient
    °Reach **forward** with the hand at waist level, progressing to reaching **forward** at chest level
    °**Do not initiate until forward reach at waist level without resistance is pain-free**
    °If forward reach is painful or difficult, replace with a "gravity-minimized" exercise from the AASEP (described below) until the forward reach can be done comfortably
  °Scapular strengthening emphasizing scapular retractions and scapular upward rotators (chapter IV-2)
  °Low-level closed chain strengthening (chapter II-4)
  ° **No prone FE, abduction, or ER**
°Initiate the AASEP as comfortable (chapter II-4)
  °A stepwise progression in difficulty of strengthening exercises from PFE to AFE against gravity
  °The goal of the progression is to achieve pain-free, full AFE

°EMG demonstrates progressive activation of the cuff and deltoid during the progression[17]
°If scapular or glenohumeral substitutions or pain are present, choose an easier exercise in the progression
°The order of the exercise sequence has some variability
°Usually not all exercises need to be performed
°Progression might not be completed until after POW 12
°**Do not perform the base strengthening program or overhead strengthening progression until the overall level of pain is low. Ensure that these exercises do not increase signs and symptoms.**
°Exercises are divided into 3 levels of difficulty

1. Gravity-minimized exercises
    °Horizontal dusting (Figure 11)
        °Perform straight ahead and perform at 20° angles medially and laterally if comfortable
    °T-Band supine FE (Figure 19)
        °Must start involved arm at 90° of elevation
        °Pull the arm into FE
    °Side-lying, gravity-eliminated AFE (Figure 20)
        °Lie on the uninvolved side
        °Place the involved arm on an ironing board
        °Slide the hand on the board
    °Jackins supine reaching progression
        °Begin at 0° with the elbow bent and end at 90° of elevation with the elbow extended
        °Start with the assistance of a cane or wand (Figure 21)
        °Progress to active motion (Figure 22)
        °Can progress to using 1 to 2 pounds of weight
        °Can progress to inclined position, continuing to reach to the ceiling (Figure 23)
2. Assistive elevation exercises
    °Rope-and-pulley AAFE
    °Incline dusting (Figure 24)
    °Standing AAFE (assistive elevation and descent via T-bar or unaffected arm)
    °Standing assistive elevation and active independent eccentric lowering

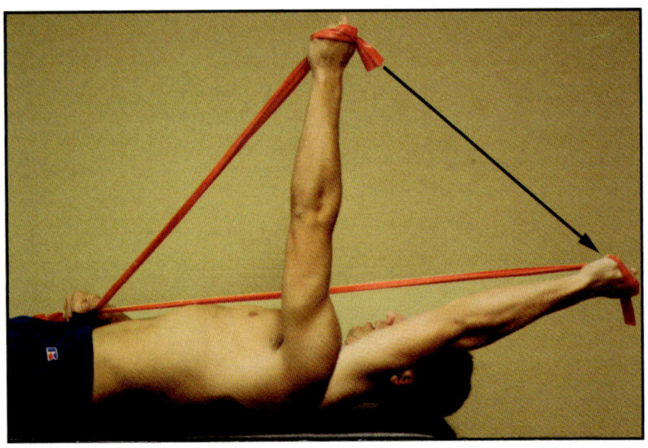

Figure 19. Supine forward elevation with an elastic band.

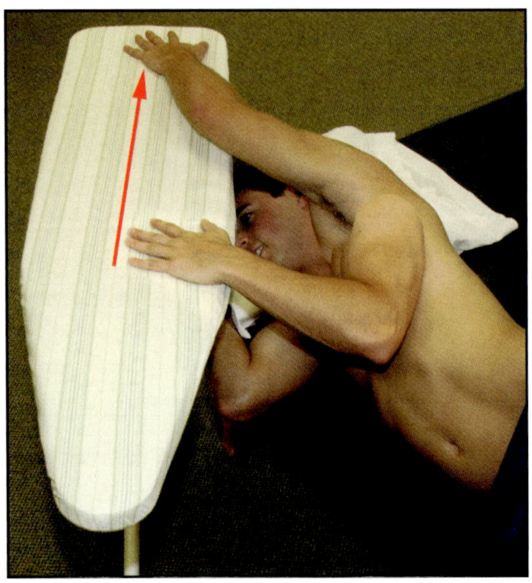

Figure 20. Side-lying, gravity-eliminated active forward elevation.

°Wall slide AAFE
  °Ensure that the patient is in FE and is not in flexion
  °Must be pain-free and natural when performing
3. Unsupported elevation exercises
  °Overhead wall taps
  °AFE (Figure 25)

Adjunctive Exercises

°Moist heat or ice
°Modalities PRN
°Aquatic exercises (chapter IV-9)
  °AAROM
  °AROM
  °Light strengthening
°Spine therapy assessment and mobilization if
  °Nonneurogenic cervical or scapular pain or
  °Limitation in end-range shoulder FE
°Trunk stabilization and strengthening

POW 9 to POM 3

°Continue the previously described exercises, including completion of the AASEP progression, as comfortable
°Initiate functional IR AAROM and stretching as tolerated (Figure 10)
°Initiate AFE when the AASEP is complete
  °Only perform if full or nearly full AROM is possible and comfortable
  °Eventually progress to 1 to 3 pounds for resistance, depending on body size

Adjunctive Exercises

°Light PNF of the cuff, deltoid, and scapula (rhythmic stabilization or slow reversal hold)
°Open chain kinesthetic awareness drills (eg, ROM replication)

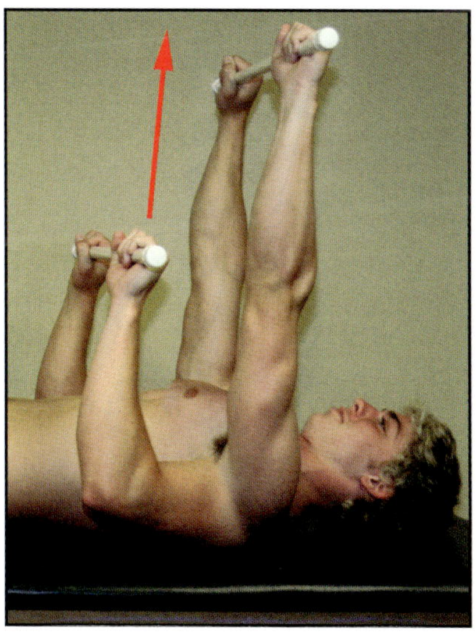

Figure 21. Jackins supine assistive reach.

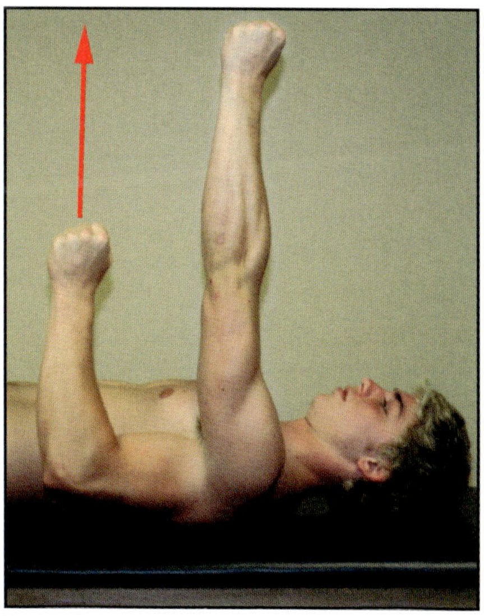

Figure 22. Jackins supine active reach.

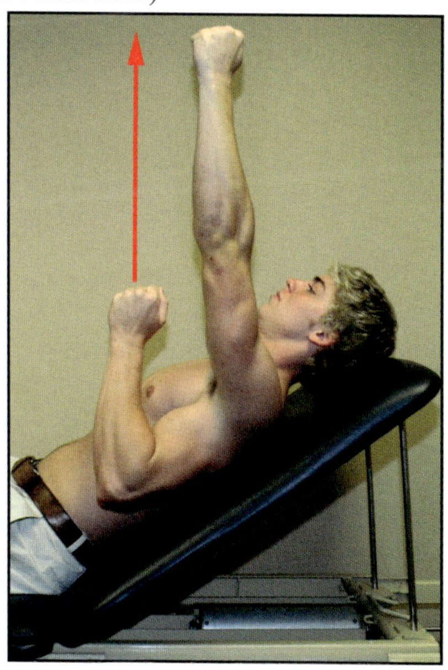

Figure 23. Jackins incline reach.

°Golf chipping and putting
°Aquatic therapy, adding light breast stroke

Interventions to Avoid

°Initiating base strengthening program or overhead strengthening progression before overall level of pain is low
°Exercises that greatly increase signs and symptoms
°Strengthening if PROM is substantially below staged ROM
°Heavy lifting with elbows away from the body
°Any forceful jerking motions with the involved arm
°Highly repetitive rehabilitation activities with the elbow at or above chest level, including upper extremity ergometer
°Strengthening into straight-plane abduction

PHASE 3

Goals

°Normalize AROM and PROM
°Normalize strength, endurance, and power
°Return to full ADLs, work, and recreation

POM 3 to 5

°PROM, stretching as needed, and warm-up stretching
°Continue base strengthening program
  °Progress T-Band color very gradually
  °Continue progressive AFE as previously described
°Discharge when functional goals are met

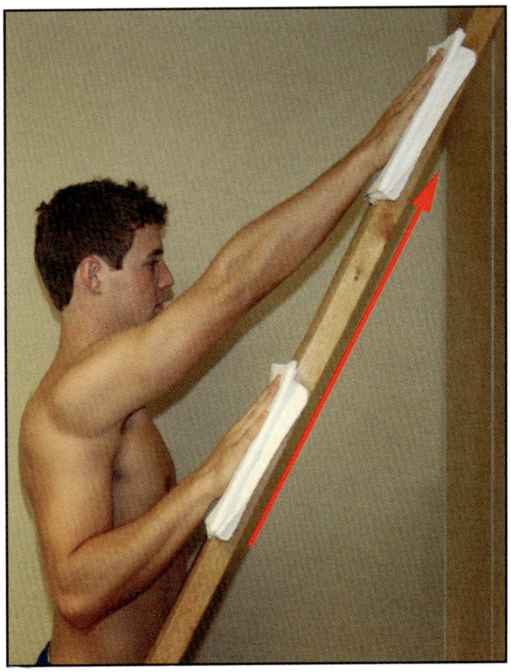

Figure 24. Incline dusting.

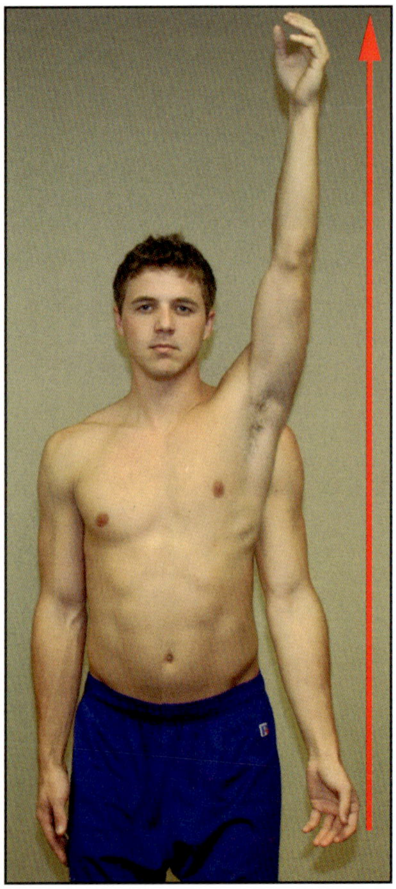

Figure 25. Active forward elevation.

- °**Many patients, especially those who are elderly or have lower demands, do not progress to any of the rehabilitation described below**
- °Participate in dumbbell overhead shoulder press **PRN**
  - °Must meet the criteria to start the advanced strengthening progression (described below)
  - °Place hands in front of the shoulder with the elbows bent and naturally reach overhead
  - °Sets of 15 to 20 repetitions with 3 pounds or more 3 to 7 times per week
- °Initiate the advanced strengthening progression **PRN** (chapter II-4)
  - °**Strict criteria to start program**
    - °MMT at least 4+/5 of the shoulder girdle
    - °Pain-free with basic ADLs and all phase 2 strengthening activities
    - °Full AFE
    - °Goals of returning to sports, heavy labor, or repetitive or heavy overhead work
    - °**Approval of physician**
    - °Use of the following principles to develop exercises to gradually progress the patient from the current level of functioning to desired goals
  - °**Exercise principles**
    - °Decrease the amount of external stabilization provided to the shoulder girdle
    - °Integrate functional patterns
    - °Increase speed of movements
    - °Integrate kinesthetic awareness drills into strengthening activities
    - °Decrease rest time to improve endurance
    - °Initiate prone strengthening PRN
    - °Train larger upper extremity muscles wisely
  - °**Sample exercises**
    - °T-Band standing PNF-type patterns (Figures 26 and 27)
    - °T-Band 90° of ER and 90° of IR with or without arm support
    - °T-Band simulation of batting, golf, or tennis forehand and backhand
    - °Weighted shoulder shrugs
- °Initiate progressive replication of moderate-intensity ADLs and work

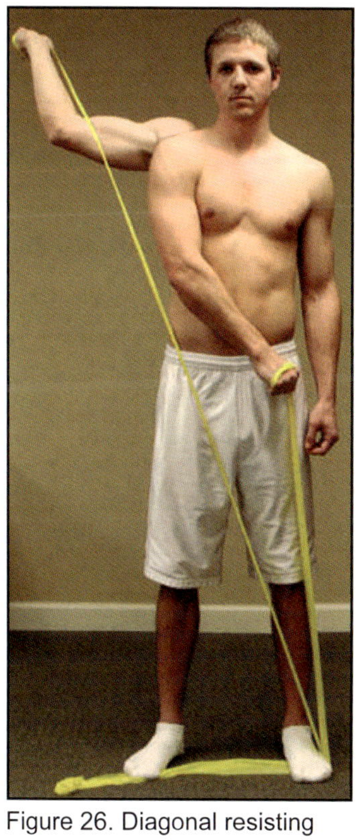

Figure 26. Diagonal resisting elevation and external rotation with an elastic band.

Adjunctive Exercises

- °Return to golf progression (advanced strengthening progression not needed)
- °Modalities PRN
- °Therapist-assisted stretching and mobilizations PRN
- °Isokinetic strengthening
- °Trunk stabilization and strengthening

POM 5 to 8

- °Use the same exercises as described and add the following as appropriate
- °Transition to a maintenance strengthening program
- °Initiate plyometric program (**PRN and if approved by physician**)
  - °Can begin after 3 to 6 weeks of the advanced strengthening program
  - °Do not begin until 5/5 MMT for the rotator cuff and scapula
  - °Use only 2 to 3 times per week
  - °Begin with a beach ball or tennis ball and progress to weighted balls

°Progressions

1. 2-handed tosses
    - °Waist level
    - °Overhead
    - °Diagonally
2. 1-handed drop-and-catch drills
3. 1-handed tosses, varying the amount of
    - °Abduction
    - °Arm support
    - °Protected ER

°Can begin interval throwing program after 3 to 6 weeks of plyometrics (**when approved by physician**) (chapter IV-6)

°Initiate progressive replication of demanding ADLs and work

°Initiate modified return to weight-training program (**when approved by physician**) (chapter IV-4)

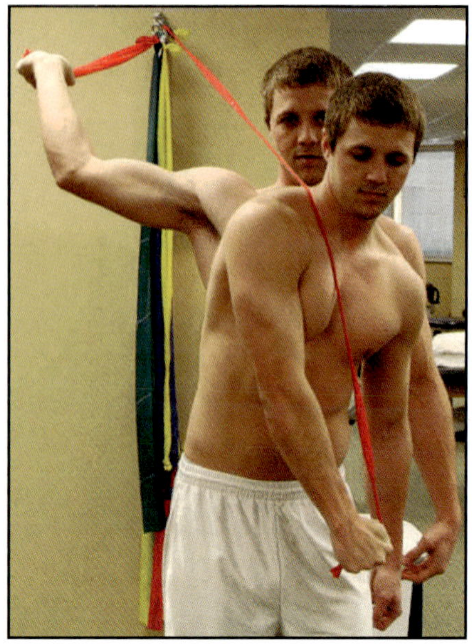

Figure 27. Diagonal resisting extension and internal rotation with an elastic band.

Interventions to Avoid

°Any rehabilitation activity that is much more demanding than daily or expected activities

°Any rehabilitation activity that is a moderate to large increase in demand compared with previous rehabilitation

°Any rehabilitation activity that results in level of pain high enough for the patient to need modalities

III-2

Massive Rotator Cuff Repair

Bryce W. Gaunt, PT, SCS

CHAPTER CONTENTS

WHAT PATIENTS ARE APPROPRIATE FOR THE USE OF THIS GUIDELINE?

- Patients with arthroscopic or mini-open repairs of massive rotator cuff tears. A *massive tear of the rotator cuff* is determined by the physician at surgery and is classically defined as either a (1) complete disinsertion of at least 2 rotator cuff tendons or (2) a rotator cuff tear that is more than 5 cm in area.
- Patients with good-quality, fair-quality, or poor-quality tissue.
- Patients with or without concomitant subacromial decompression, excision of the distal clavicle, bursectomy, or debridement of the labrum or glenohumeral joint.

Clinical pearls are highlighted in yellow throughout the text.

THE MOST IMPORTANT FACTOR THAT SHOULD GUIDE CLINICAL DECISION MAKING

The strength of the surgical repair always should be much greater than the mechanical stress that is placed on the repaired tendon during rehabilitation. For every rehabilitation activity, this stress is determined by (1) the amount of muscle activation of the repaired musculotendon unit, (2) the plane of motion that is used, (3) the specific glenohumeral joint range of motion (ROM), and (4) the number of times the tissue is loaded (the number of repetitions prescribed). The stress on the repaired tendon must be considered for all rehabilitation activities (home exercises, clinic exercises, and manual therapy).

KEY PRINCIPLES IN REHABILITATION OF THIS PROBLEM

As with rehabilitation after repair of a "routine-sized" tear of the rotator cuff, optimal rehabilitation of the patient after repair of a massive tear of the rotator cuff requires the rehabilitation provider to know the details of the surgical procedure; to be aware of key factors that affect healing of the repaired tendon or tendons; to know the stresses that each rehabilitation intervention places on the surgical repair; to apply a precise priority for clinical decision making; to maintain close communication among the patient, physician, and himself or herself; and to carefully consider how these diverse issues affect each other.

Knowledge Gained From the Surgical Procedure

The size and number of tendons torn and repaired, the quality of the soft tissue, and the presence of associated lesions significantly affect rehabilitation. In many clinical studies, investigators have demonstrated the effect that the size of the rotator cuff tear and the subsequent repair have on both short-term and long-term outcomes.[1–4] Compared with patients who have had repairs of smaller tears, patients with repairs of massive tears historically have demonstrated a much larger rate of retear, slower gains in active ROM (AROM), more limited AROM, more limited rotator cuff strength, and more modest functional outcomes.[5–9] Given the published larger long-term retear rates after massive repair,[1,10,11] we, at my institution, progress rehabilitation much slower after this repair than after the routine rotator cuff repair at all phases, and we emphasize delaying the initiation of AROM and strengthening. Typically, a patient with a repair of a massive rotator cuff tear needs a longer rehabilitation than a patient with a smaller tear.

Tissue quality is another factor that affects the potential healing and rehabilitation of the rotator cuff repair.[7] Better-quality tissue is healthier and thicker and has greater structural strength. Therefore, it provides a stronger construct to securely hold suture material and provides a better medium to facilitate the process of tissue repair. Clinically, tissue quality is expressed several ways. A subjective rating of good, fair, or poor by the surgeon at the time of repair is common. Rotator cuff tears also can be classified as acute (repair typically performed within the first 6 weeks after injury) or chronic. Chronic tears generally have poorer-quality tissue than acute tears have.

Rating the amount of fatty degeneration is another clinical way to grade the quality of the musculotendon unit. Numerous researchers have demonstrated that when a rotator cuff tendon is torn completely from its insertion, associated muscle tissue dies and is replaced by fat over time. This change might be irreversible and negatively affects muscle performance, even if the tendon is repaired. The presence of a large amount of atrophy or fatty infiltration also has a negative influence on healing and outcomes after repair.[9,12,13] Note that the quality of the other soft tissues in the shoulder that are not repaired also affects the speed of rehabilitation and the long-term outcome.

Patients undergoing massive rotator cuff repairs typically present with fair-quality or poor-quality tissue and are more likely to have fatty degeneration than patients with smaller tears. Because multiple rotator cuff tendons are torn and repaired, fewer uninvolved tendons are available to share the load of rehabilitation. These are the primary reasons that a much slower and gentler approach is needed throughout the entire rehabilitation process. One example of this slower progression is that in patients with massive rotator cuff repairs, we often wait until they demonstrate several weeks of good tolerance to a particular exercise before making a very small advancement because we know that the tissues are structurally weaker and more prone to overload.

Associated lesions in the shoulder girdle also can affect rehabilitation after rotator cuff repair. Patients undergoing concomitant subacromial decompression; excision of the distal clavicle; bursectomy; or debridement of the labrum, glenohumeral joint, or another rotator cuff tendon do not require any changes to the standard rehabilitation program. Because of the increased tissue trauma associated with these surgeries, these patients typically experience some increase in pain, inflammation, and potentially stiffness that can make the first 4 to 6 weeks of rehabilitation more difficult. An increased focus on controlling inflammation and establishing quality, early passive ROM (PROM) in a gentle way is emphasized.

Other Factors That Affect Rehabilitation

Certain coexisting conditions (previous shoulder surgeries, advanced age, smoking, and the presence of systemic diseases that compromise the immune system), the patient's preoperative functional use of the involved extremity, and the weight of the involved extremity affect rehabilitation after massive rotator cuff repair. The effect of these factors is the same in massive rotator cuff repairs and in routine rotator cuff repairs; therefore, please refer to this section in chapter III-1 for a full discussion of these issues.

Knowledge of Stress Placed on the Surgical Repair During Rehabilitation Versus the Strength of the Repair

Before starting rehabilitation after any surgical procedure, the rehabilitation provider must ensure that rehabilitation activities will not damage the surgical repair. How can we ensure this? To put it very simply, a postoperative exercise is safe when the strength of a given surgery is **much greater** than the mechanical stress that each exercise places on the surgical repair. During rehabilitation after the rotator cuff repair, the rehabilitation provider must have basic knowledge about the strength of the surgical repair and about the stress that **each** exercise during the entire course of rehabilitation places on the surgical repair. The strength of the rotator cuff repair depends on many factors, including the quality of the patient's tissue, the strength of the sutures, the strength of the suture knots, the fixation strength of the surgical anchors in the bone, and the frequency of upper extremity movement. Investigators have shown that failure strength of the rotator cuff in control groups is close to 2400 N.[14] During the first 6 weeks after repair of a routine tear, failure strength is about 200 to 400 N.[14–17] At 12 weeks after surgery, failure strength is about 700 N,[14] and it returns to normal levels about 6 months after a typical repair.[18] However, the failure strength of massive rotator cuff repairs is generally less than that of smaller repairs. In addition, authors of many clinical studies have demonstrated a significantly larger rate of retear after massive rotator cuff repairs than after repairs of smaller tears.[1,10,11] Therefore, significant protection of the repaired tendon or tendons by minimizing the mechanical stress placed on them is required, especially during the first 12 weeks of rehabilitation after the massive rotator cuff repair. Rehabilitation **must** be significantly slower and gentler during its entire course compared with rehabilitation after the routine repair. The initiation of AROM and strengthening especially must be delayed and then progressed very gradually.

The mechanical stress that rehabilitation places on the repaired rotator cuff tendon depends on the muscle activation that each exercise (both passive and active) generates, the plane of motion that is used, the specific ROM that is achieved, and the number of repetitions that are performed. These issues are discussed in detail in the next section of this chapter. However, the clinician must always be aware that the failure strength of the surgical construct and the stress applied by exercise cannot be compared directly. Failure strength of the surgical repair typically is measured in newtons. Although the force in newtons that is placed on the rotator cuff tendons is known for movement in certain planes, exercise demand in the shoulder largely has been evaluated by researchers examining the relative electromyographic (EMG) activity level in muscles, which is expressed as a percentage of maximum muscle activation. No direct relationship between dynamic EMG activity level and tension in muscle and tendon has been established. Electromyography measures muscle activity but does not measure stress to the tendon. The exact stress in newtons that specific shoulder rehabilitation exercises place on the repaired rotator cuff tendon is unknown. However, a progressive order of difficulty (muscular demand) in exercises can be established. Therefore, we recommend using rehabilitation exercises that are known to have very low demands in planes of motion demonstrated to minimally stress the repair during the first 12 weeks after repair of a massive tear and then gradually increasing the exercise demand as the strength of the surgical repair increases. In addition, we obviously do not know the exact failure strength of the surgical repair in each patient with whom we work. For these reasons, rehabilitation providers need to proceed with caution and to keep the exercise demands much less than the estimated failure strength of the surgical repair.

Priority for Clinical Decision Making

To aid in the selection of exercises, we use a precise priority for clinical decision making for all patients after shoulder surgery. First, rehabilitation must protect the healing tissues and the integrity of the surgical repair. Second, it must establish and maintain a low level of inflammation and pain. Third, rehabilitation must establish basic PROM while maintaining a low level of pain. Fourth, it must include a progressive strategy for AROM and strengthening that maintains a low level of pain. Fifth, rehabilitation must include appropriate and progressive functional training. This progression dictates the order of activities that are added and the order of importance in clinical decision making. Earlier principles always take precedence over later principles. For example, if PROM, the level of inflammation, or the integrity of the surgical repair is affected negatively during advancement of strengthening activities, then a lower level of strengthening activities should be used. We believe that appropriate rehabilitation after rotator cuff repair is never forceful. A detailed description and rationale for these principles can be found in chapter II-1.

Interaction of These Factors and Communication

Finally, all of the factors that I have discussed do not exist in isolation. Their interaction must be taken into account to determine the appropriate speed of rehabilitation. Most patients have a balance of factors; some factors enable a more accelerated approach to rehabilitation to be used, and others necessitate use of a much gentler and conservative approach. Because the interaction of these issues in the patient with a massive rotator cuff repair is complex, communication among the physician, patient, and rehabilitation provider is vital to determine the best initial course to take as led by the surgeon. All parties must understand the issues described, and the patient's tolerance to the rehabilitation program must be re-evaluated at each visit to the rehabilitation provider and must be modified as appropriate. Therefore, although the rehabilitation provider uses standard rehabilitation guidelines, the actual rehabilitation program used for each patient is based on the unique situation and his or her tolerance of the rehabilitation program. Extensive and regular patient education is also vital during the entire course of rehabilitation. Often, the patient needs help understanding that the repair must be significantly protected for an extended period and needs instruction in how to protect the extremity during rehabilitation and daily functional activities.

SPECIFIC REHABILITATION GUIDELINE

The Appendix specifies our complete Massive Rotator Cuff Repair Rehabilitation Guideline. In this section, I explain the rationale for selected components of the guideline. It is divided into 3 phases based on general timeframes of healing and staged ROM targets. To advance from one rehabilitation phase to the next, the patient must gain approval from the physician, successfully complete the core components of the previous rehabilitation activities, and meet the time criteria.

Phase 1

The primary focus of phase 1 rehabilitation, which constitutes the first 6 postoperative weeks, is to maximally protect the surgical repair, and the secondary focus is to achieve, but not significantly exceed, the staged ROM goals that the referring physician helps establish. As mentioned, for a rehabilitation activity to be safe after a rotator cuff repair, the strength of the surgical repair always should be much more than the stress that is placed on the repaired tendon during each rehabilitation exercise. During rehabilitation after massive rotator cuff repair, this stress is determined for all rehabilitation activities (home exercises, clinic exercises, and manual therapy) by (1) the amount of muscle activation of the repaired musculotendon unit, (2) the plane of motion that is used, (3) the specific glenohumeral joint ROM, and (4) the number of times the tissue is loaded (the number of repetitions). Appropriate exercise selection cannot occur without understanding these factors.

Hatakeyama et al[19] and Zuckerman et al[20] evaluated the mechanical stress that specific glenohumeral PROM places on the supraspinatus (SSP) in cadavers. Hatakeyama et al[19] found that passive external rotation (PER) with the extremity in slight abduction (20°–30°) resulted in very low stress (<5 N) to the SSP from 60° of internal rotation to 60° of external rotation. Zuckerman et al[20] found very low stress (<5 N) in the SSP with PROM from 0° to 120° of upper extremity elevation performed in the plane of the scapula (passive forward elevation [PFE]). Therefore, these motions appear safe to use during the immediate postoperative period. These investigators did not test motion at more than 120° of upper extremity elevation, but they theorized that tension on the rotator cuff likely increases with end-range PFE. Because of this research, our 6-week staged ROM goals are not significantly more than these known safe limits for forward elevation.

Orthopaedic surgeons and rehabilitation providers are almost in universal consensus that elevation in the plane of the scapula with the thumb oriented up (humeral external rotation) is **the** preferred plane of movement to use during early overhead motion of the shoulder. It provides minimal capsular stress; optimal length-tension relationship to the rotator cuff, deltoid, and scapular muscles to enable efficient function; and optimal subacromial clearance to minimize impingement. Therefore, for PROM during phase 1 rehabilitation after massive rotator cuff repair, the only planes of motion that the patient performs at home are PER with the upper extremity in slight abduction and PFE.

However, for early PROM after rotator cuff repair to be safe, the rehabilitation provider not only must choose planes of motion that provide low stress to the repair, but also must use specific exercises that have documented low EMG activity in the repaired rotator cuff in these planes of motion. The Table lists the documented EMG activity levels of the SSP and anterior deltoid (AD) for common passive elevation exercises performed in the plane of the scapula. Researchers have demonstrated that PFE performed in the supine or upright position with the assistance of the rehabilitation provider or PFE performed in the supine position with the patient assisting himself or herself has much less EMG activity in the SSP and AD than the rope-and-pulley PFE has.[21,22] The pendulum, the table step-back, continuous passive motion (CPM) machine, and aquatic exercises also demonstrate very low EMG activity. We have found that the pendulum, table step-back, Kinex KS2 (Kinex Medical Company, LLC, Waukesha, WI) shoulder CPM machine, and rehabilitation-provider-assisted or family-assisted sitting exercises are the most effective and well-tolerated exercises to achieve PFE during the first few weeks after surgery (Figures 1–3). More detailed information about the benefits and safety of using shoulder CPM and how we specifically use the Kinex KS2 with our patients after rotator cuff surgery can be found in chapter II-3. We have found that although self-assisted PROM in the supine position is safe to start immediately after surgery, it typically is not well tolerated during the first 6 weeks after repair of a massive tear and,

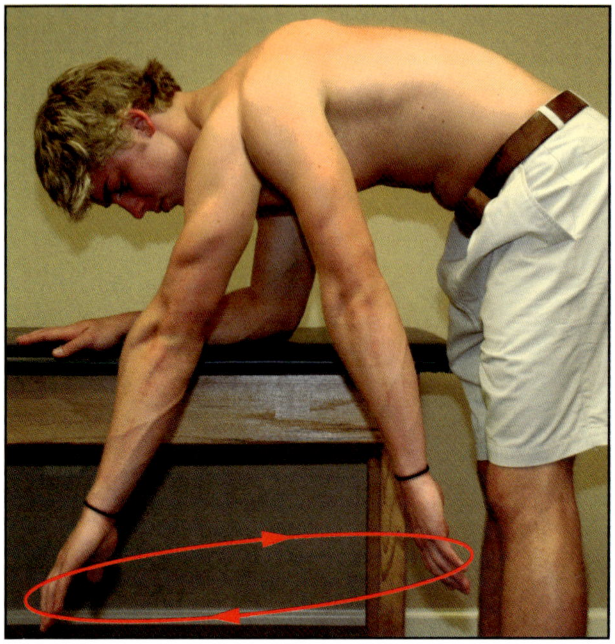

Figure 1. Pendulum exercise initially uses smaller circles.

Table. Common Passive Elevation Exercises in the Plane of the Scapula and the Associated Electromyographic Activity Levels of the Supraspinatus and Anterior Deltoid

Exercise	Electromyographic Activity
Therapist-assisted forward elevation	Average supraspinatus 4%, anterior deltoid 8%[21] Average supraspinatus 5%, anterior deltoid 7% supine[22] Average supraspinatus 12%, anterior deltoid 4% upright[22]
Self-assisted forward elevation supine	Average supraspinatus 3%, anterior deltoid 11%[22]
Pulley forward elevation	Average supraspinatus 17%, anterior deltoid 25%[21] Average supraspinatus 13%, anterior deltoid 21%[22] Maximum supraspinatus 17%, anterior deltoid 31%[23]
Pendulum	Average supraspinatus 9%, anterior deltoid 3%[22] Average supraspinatus 6%[21] Maximum supraspinatus (small 10-cm diameter circle) 8–8.7%[24] Maximum supraspinatus (large 51-cm diameter circle) 13.7–18.8%[24]
Specific aquatic exercises	Average supraspinatus 1–5%, anterior deltoid 1–8%[25]
Closed chain (table step-back)	Average supraspinatus 5%, anterior deltoid 2%[26]
Continuous passive motion machine	Average supraspinatus 5%, average anterior deltoid 3%[21]

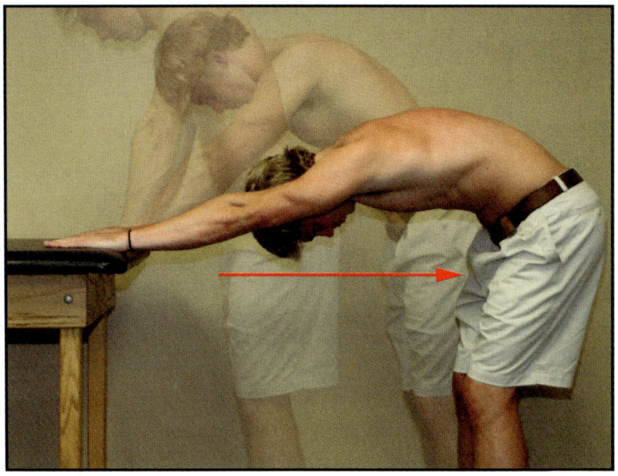

Figure 2. Table step-back exercise for passive forward elevation.

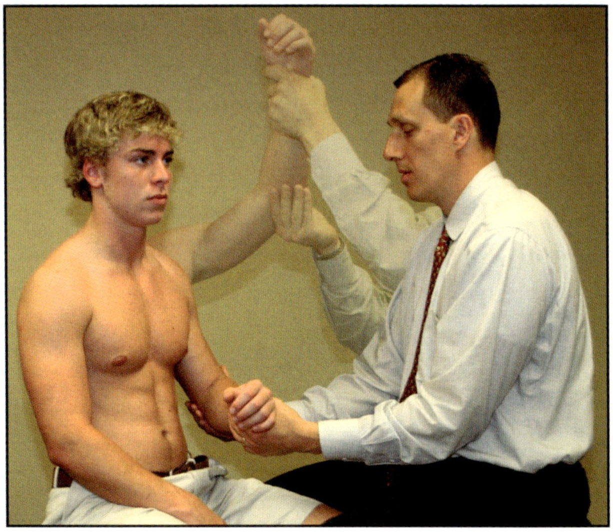

Figure 3. Assisted passive forward elevation. The assistant typically stands diagonally in front of the patient.

therefore, is withheld from our guideline during phase 1 (Figure 4). As the Table demonstrates, the rope-and-pulley exercise has a noticeably higher EMG activity level in the SSP than the other exercises listed, so we do not recommend using this exercise during phase 1 rehabilitation after the massive rotator cuff repair.

For PER, McCann et al[22] and Dockery et al[21] demonstrated very low EMG activity levels in the SSP, AD, and infraspinatus with all exercises tested. However, neither group of investigators evaluated the EMG activity in the subscapularis, which is likely the muscle most at risk of injury with these exercises because it stretches passively with external rotation and is actively contracted when muscle guarding occurs against PER. Because of this, minimizing stress to the subscapularis with PER in massive rotator cuff repairs that involve a subscapularis repair is vitally important because the subscapularis is at high risk for rupture with overly aggressive PER. Clinically, we have found that PER performed while sitting and with the assistance of a family member or rehabilitation provider and the PER walk-around are the gentlest, most effective, and most well-tolerated exercises in the early postoperative period (Figures 5 and 6). In particular, the PER walk-around is very safe in this situation because it provides no direct counterforce to PER. If the patient tries to stretch too aggressively, the forearm simply rotates on its support surface. Other exercises to achieve PER that use an L-bar or wall to provide a counterforce to the forearm have much greater potential for placing excessive stress on the subscapularis. We believe that

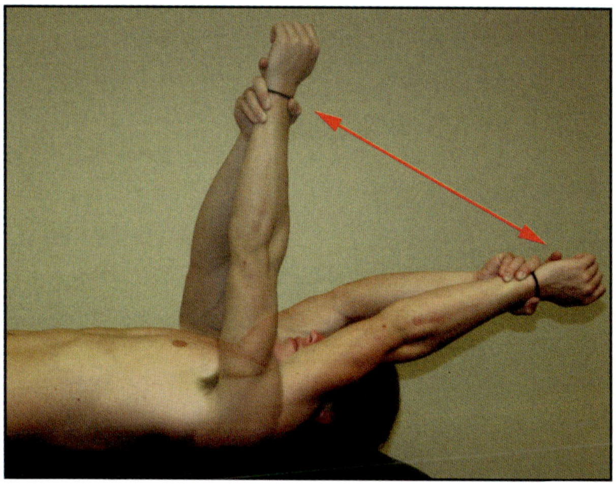

Figure 4. Self-assisted supine active-assistive forward elevation. The hand-assisted exercise is preferred.

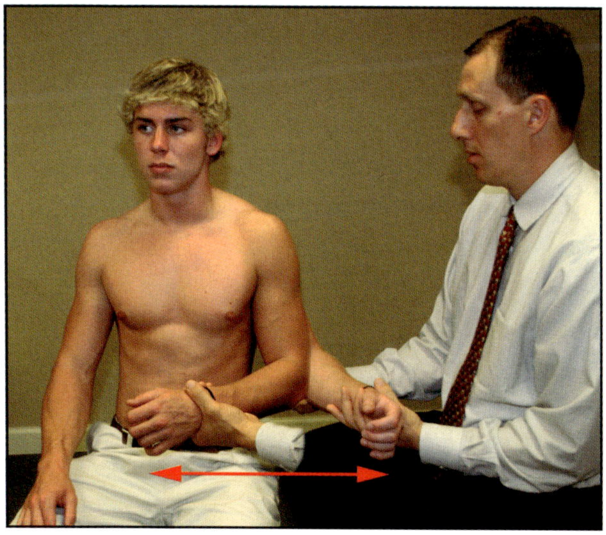

Figure 5. Assisted sitting passive external rotation.

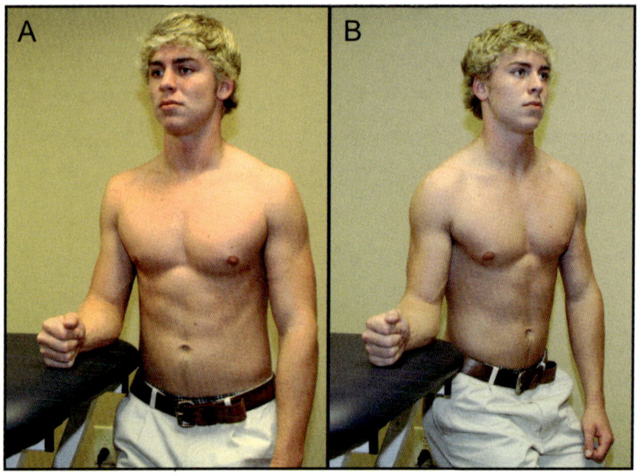

Figure 6 A and B. Passive external rotation walk-around exercise.

these exercises are generally inappropriate for phase 1 rehabilitation after a massive rotator cuff repair that involves a subscapularis repair because of the risk of excessive stress to the subscapularis with incorrect exercise technique.

The number of times a rotator cuff repair is stressed or loaded, even in a submaximal manner, is an important, but often overlooked, rehabilitation variable that has important implications regarding the length of immobilization and the number of repetitions performed during early exercise. Much in the same way micromotion prevents bony union during fracture healing, submaximal tissue loading or cyclic loading potentially can disrupt the tenuous tissue healing bonds between the rotator cuff tendon and its bony insertion. In human cadavers, cyclic loading has been shown to increase the gap between the repaired tendon and the bone to which it is repaired.[27,28] This increased gap, at some point, is believed detrimental to healing of the repair.[16] Although the exact effect of submaximal loading during various rehabilitation interventions is unknown, the rehabilitation provider should keep in mind that repeated and excessive submaximal tensioning of the repair during the early phases of tissue healing might be detrimental to the clinical healing of the repaired rotator cuff to its humeral insertion. Therefore, repetitive submaximal stresses should be carefully controlled during phase 1 rehabilitation.

Clinically, this has implications for both exercise volume and immobilization. This research suggests that during phase 1 rehabilitation, both AROM and PROM as able should be minimized during exercise and functional activities. Therefore, although enough PROM needs to be prescribed to achieve staged ROM goals and prevent excessive joint stiffness, we recommend keeping both the number of exercises performed and total repetitions fairly low during this timeframe. We also emphasize educating patients about the importance of minimizing active use of the upper extremity during the first 6 postoperative weeks.

Based on the cyclic loading studies discussed, the results of basic science research on tendon healing in animal models,[29–32] and recent ultrasound evidence suggesting that a moderate percentage of repaired massive rotator cuff tears might not heal completely to bone,[14,15,33] surgeons are re-evaluating the concept of immediate PROM after massive rotator cuff repair. Rehabilitation providers at a few facilities delay the initiation of traditional glenohumeral PROM for up to 6 weeks in an attempt to maximize early healing. Parsons et al[34] retrospectively reviewed 43 patients after arthroscopic rotator cuff repair who were immobilized 6 weeks before glenohumeral ROM was initiated. They grouped these patients into stiff and nonstiff groups at the time ROM was initiated. Patients were considered *stiff* if their PFE was less than 100° and their PER was less than 30° at the time ROM was initiated. Ten (23%) patients were considered *stiff* at postoperative week 6. At 1-year follow-up, the authors found no difference in ROM, American Shoulder and Elbow Surgeons score, or Constant score.[34] However, they found a trend toward a lower retear rate in the stiff group (70% versus 36%).

Leggin et al[35] evaluated the effect of delayed rehabilitation on PROM, AROM, and function by comparing PROM starting at an average of 4.5 weeks after surgery and PROM starting at an average of 1 week after surgery in a group of patients after arthroscopic rotator cuff repairs. At 12 weeks, they found only a 4° difference in PFE and an 8° difference in PER between groups. They also found the delayed rehabilitation group had 32° less active forward elevation (AFE) and scored 9 points lower on the Penn Shoulder Scale than the early PROM group. Overall, they found that delayed rehabilitation seemed to shift the recovery back a few weeks but did not impede recovery. In the next few years, I believe the concept of delaying the initiation of rehabilitation after rotator cuff repair will be evaluated more extensively to determine its effectiveness for improving rates of healing while minimizing recurrent stiffness. If successful in both of these areas, then this practice likely will become more widespread.

Even given this possibility, we believe that early PROM (initiated in the first 1 to 5 postoperative days) is beneficial, and if only exercises demonstrating very low EMG activity are used and performed correctly, it is not detrimental to healing of most repairs of massive tears. Early glenohumeral PROM traditionally has been a well-accepted technique for rehabilitation after shoulder surgery because it helps minimize the negative effects of immobilization, such as formation of adhesions and joint contracture, muscle atrophy and serial sarcomere loss, and articular cartilage degradation.

Merely choosing the appropriate exercises is not sufficient to successfully achieve early rehabilitation goals. Helping the patient to maximally relax the upper extremity, paying attention to detail with exercise technique, stopping the PROM at a point of mild stretch and slight discomfort, and thoroughly educating the patient play enormous roles in the success of rehabilitation during the early stage of rehabilitation. These issues are outlined in the Appendix and are addressed extensively in chapter II-2. Supplementary PROM that is performed very gently by the rehabilitation provider is helpful, especially if the patient is behind in achieving staged ROM goals. Directions of motion used during phase 1, which are performed as comfortable, include abduction with neutral rotation to less than 90°, external and internal rotation in the middle ranges of abduction, PFE, and external rotation at 80° to 90° of forward elevation to stretch the coracohumeral ligament. Detailed descriptions of these motions are presented in chapter II-3.

Although every attempt is made to help the patient achieve his or her staged PROM goals in forward elevation and external rotation as outlined in the Appendix through early PROM, careful exercise selection, and flawless exercise technique, some patients will fall behind our staged ROM targets. In these situations, we typically increase the frequency of the home exercise program to 4 to 6 times per day and increase the frequency of clinic visits. We do not increase the intensity of clinic or home exercise stretching, so we do not impede healing of the repair. Therefore, if necessary, it is better for the patient to be behind targeted PROM goals than to meet these goals but undermine healing of the repair.

Phase 2

The focus of phase 2, which typically constitutes postoperative weeks 6 through 12, is to continue to maximally protect the surgical repair that while getting stronger, is still very weak; to achieve staged PROM goals; to minimize shoulder pain; and to work toward achieving active forward reaching at waist level. The rehabilitation provider still must ensure that the stress of the activities in the rehabilitation program is significantly less than the strength of the surgical repair. The interpretation of results from biomechanical studies and from studies in which long-term clinical healing rates were analyzed[29,30,32] shows that continued minimization of stress to the massive rotator cuff repair during rehabilitation and activities of daily living during phase 2 is prudent. Therefore, phase 2 of rehabilitation after this repair is only a minimal advancement from phase 1 rehabilitation and is substantially different from phase 2 rehabilitation after routine rotator cuff repair.

For PROM, home exercises continue to include only exercises to achieve staged ROM goals in forward elevation and external rotation in 20° of abduction. For forward elevation, rope-and-pulley elevation (Figure 7) and self-assisted supine active-assistive forward elevation (Figure 4) as tolerated replace the PFE exercises of phase 1. Instruct the patient to perform these exercises as passively as possible but recognize that some rotator cuff activity occurs in all situations.

If the subscapularis has been repaired, it is vital that only very gentle exercises continue to be used to increase PER. This still means that the PER walk-around (Figure 6) or family-assisted external rotation (Figure 5) is the preferred method. In addition, if PER is easily meeting or exceeding staged ROM goals, then exercises that increase PER must be discontinued because detrimental stress can occur if end-range stretching is performed during this time. If the subscapularis has not been repaired, then any PER exercise is safe to perform, but anecdotally, I have found that upright stretching exercises are very well tolerated and very effective during this time.

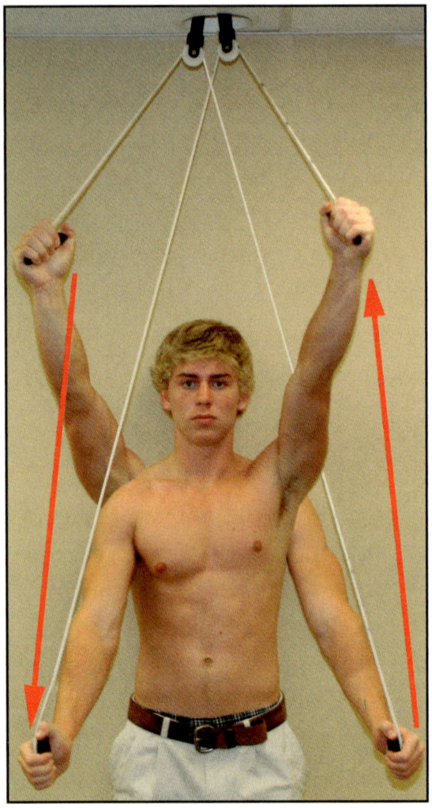

Figure 7. Rope-and-pulley active-assistive forward elevation exercise.

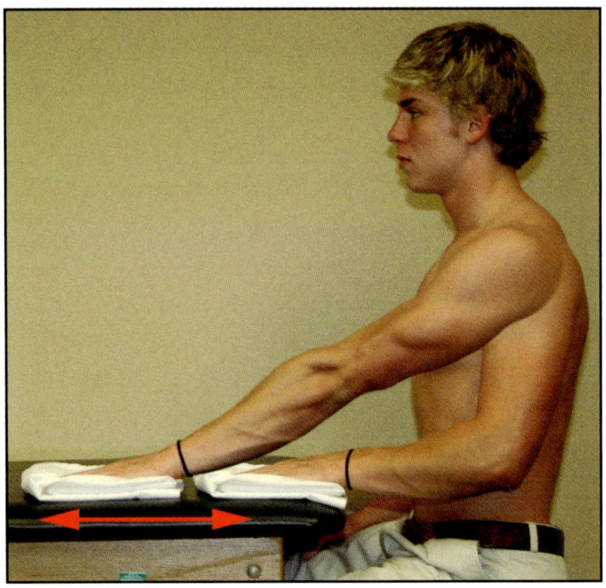

Figure 8. Horizontal dusting exercise.

Comfortable active use of the upper extremity at this time is quite variable among patients. Many patients struggle to actively reach the hand fully forward at waist level. However, a few patients are comfortable actively lifting the extremity to 90º or more. For most patients who have difficulty actively reaching forward at waist level, horizontal dusting is initiated (Figure 8). The inability to actively reach the hand forward at waist level signifies that the shoulder girdle muscles cannot counteract the weight of the extremity against gravity in this position without assistance. Horizontal dusting provides assistance to the recently repaired shoulder girdle muscles by decreasing the weight that the muscles must work against because the hand is resting on the table. The load of the surgically repaired upper extremity is effectively decreased, so the muscle force required to actively move the extremity is correspondingly diminished. Patients who cannot actively move the elbow away from the side without support almost always will be able to completely extend the elbow by sliding the hand back and forth on the table. We prefer that this exercise involve a forward and backward motion at very slight angles and never extend the elbow past the midline of the body. We want to primarily train the muscles that are active during the functional task of forward reaching rather than the muscles that are active during circular motions or reaching at wide angles. Electromyographic data are also available for the muscle activity level of horizontal dusting at 30º.[23] To our knowledge, no EMG data are available on circular dusting or dusting at larger angles.

A large part of phase 2 rehabilitation after massive rotator cuff repair is educating the patient about the necessity of continuing to minimize active use of the upper extremity during activities of daily living at this time to promote long-term clinical healing of the repair. Nonrepetitive waist-level reaching for objects of negligible weight (less than 1 to 2 pounds [0.45–0.90 kg]) is allowed as long as it can be done comfortably. Use of the surgically repaired extremity at waist level with weight and active use of the extremity with the elbow at chest level or higher are discouraged during phase 2, even if these activities do not cause pain, because they place stress on the repair. The physicians and rehabilitation providers at our facility believe that frequent use of the upper extremity for these types of activities theoretically might diminish the chance and quality of healing of the repaired tendons. Although these activities are not clearly detrimental, we believe that the short-term benefit derived from using the extremity for these activities during this time is not worth the potential risk of disturbing the one chance that the repair has to heal. Therefore, some patients are held back from activities that they have the physical ability to perform. For patients who achieve their staged ROM and functional goals easily, regular therapy sessions with the rehabilitation provider are not needed. These patients continue very limited exercises at home. A very occasional clinical follow-up can be used to determine compliance with restrictions on activity and to reinforce that adhering to these restrictions is important.

Phase 3

Phase 3 rehabilitation after massive rotator cuff repair closely resembles phase 2 rehabilitation after routine rotator cuff repair with some slight adjustments because realistically, all patients will not achieve full PROM, full AROM, or full strength. The focus of phase 3, which typically constitutes postoperative week 12 and beyond, is to gently normalize PROM, to begin a well-structured AROM and strengthening progression that gradually increases demand to the musculature of the shoulder girdle while protecting the repair, and to minimize inflammation and pain. The later part of phase 3 focuses on increasing strength, endurance, and functional use of the upper extremity to a realistic level. The rehabilitation provider still must always ensure that the stress of the activities in the rehabilitation program is less than the strength of the surgical repair.

Obtaining realistic flexibility while keeping the level of pain and inflammation low should be an early priority of phase 3 rehabilitation. A variable amount of stretching is needed to achieve this goal. If the ROM of the patient is significantly less than staged goals but the physician expects nearly normal flexibility, then PROM should be emphasized. During home-based exercise, the patient with a massive rotator cuff repair is allowed to initiate gentle stretching in planes of motion other than PFE and PER in slight abduction. This stretching might include the supine hand-behind-head stretch, posterior shoulder stretching, and functional internal rotation (Figures 9–12). During rehabilitation of a patient with a massive rotator cuff repair, almost all passive stretching might place direct stress on the repair. Whether this is advantageous depends on the details of the repair, the quality of repaired tissues, the

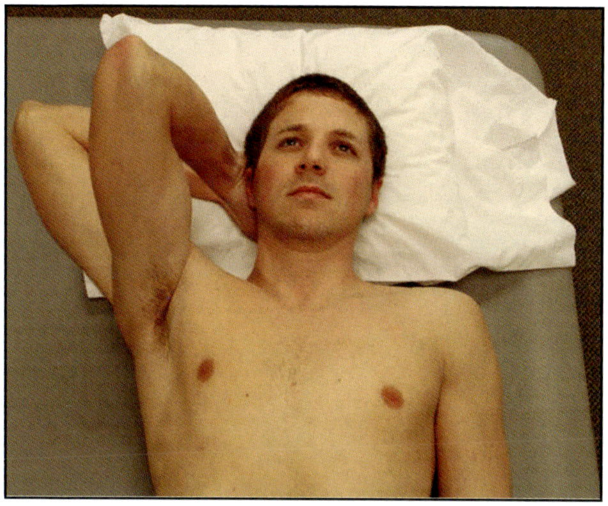

Figure 9. Supine hand-behind-head stretch to increase abduction and external rotation.

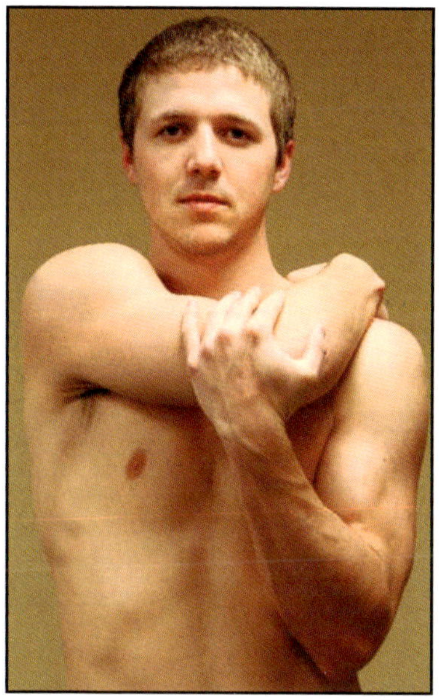

Figure 10. Horizontal adduction stretch.

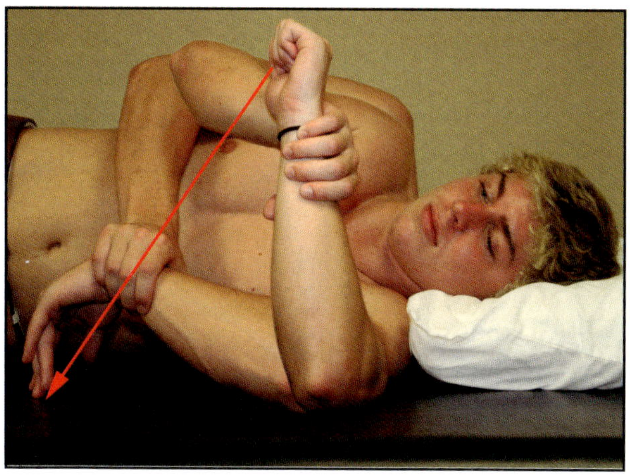

Figure 11. Sleeper stretch.

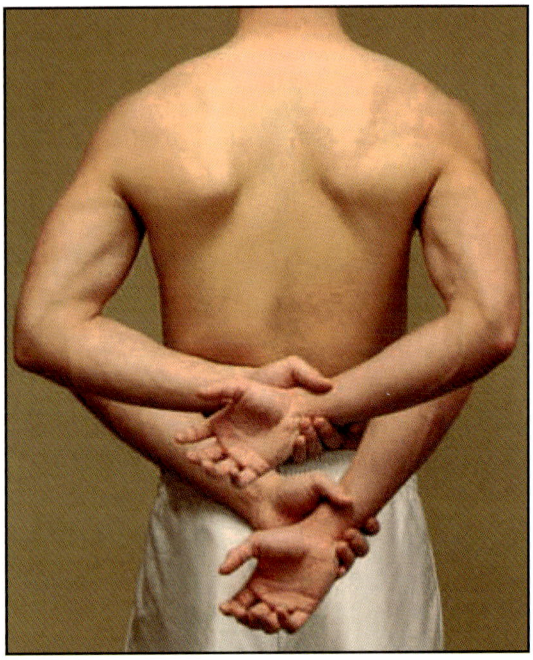

Figure 12. Functional internal rotation active-assistive range of motion.

severity of the ROM limitation, and the desired functional goals of the patient. The patient, physician, and rehabilitation provider must jointly decide specific and realistic ROM goals for planes of motion other than PFE and PER on an individual basis.

The failure strength of the massive rotator cuff repair during phase 3 rehabilitation is much less than that of a healthy shoulder and varies widely based on many factors. In addition, because a large portion of the rotator cuff has been repaired, the patient's ability to achieve AROM against gravity, especially overhead, is often a very long and difficult process, occasionally taking from 6 to 9 months or longer to achieve. Therefore, when starting the AROM and strengthening phase of rehabilitation, the rehabilitation provider must carefully select exercises that start with very low stress to the healing tissue and progress in a gradual and measured way. When beginning AROM and strengthening, selecting exercises that have a very low documented EMG activity and ordering them so that the activity level in the rotator cuff slowly increases should be the primary criteria for advancing exercises and for selecting planes of movement that do not place excessive tension on the repair. An evidence-based AROM and strengthening progression is incorporated and outlined in the Appendix and detailed in chapter II-4.

The rehabilitation provider also should remember several clinical hints that help in the appropriate selection of AROM and strengthening exercises. First, during appropriate advancement of these exercises, the patient's level of pain should not increase, and substitution patterns should not occur. A reliable way to achieve this is to choose rehabilitation exercises that are at or below the patient's comfortable use of the upper extremity. For example, a patient who cannot reach the top of his or her head without pain should perform an assistive exercise in the overhead position rather than an active exercise. Second, because of the physics of the shoulder girdle, a little resistance to the shoulder provides a very large stress to the rotator cuff. Therefore, 1 to 2 pounds (0.45–0.90 kg) of resistance is usually the maximum resistance used, and no external resistance is used early in overhead AROM and strengthening during rehabilitation after the massive rotator cuff repair. Third, most patients should perform AROM and strengthening exercises below shoulder level for several weeks before starting overhead AROM or strengthening exercises. Fourth, AROM and strengthening exercises should be progressed slower and performed more gently in the elderly patient, in the patient with a repair of a larger tear, and in the patient who describes longstanding limited functional use of the upper extremity before surgery.

Several researchers have demonstrated that an exercise performed with the extremity supported places less demand on activated muscles than the same exercise performed without support.[23,36] Supported horizontal AROM, such as dusting, is an example of this type of activity (Figure 8). This activity and gentle weight-bearing activities have demonstrated a very low EMG activity in the SSP of 6% to 9% of maximal voluntary isometric contraction (MVIC),[23,37] which makes these

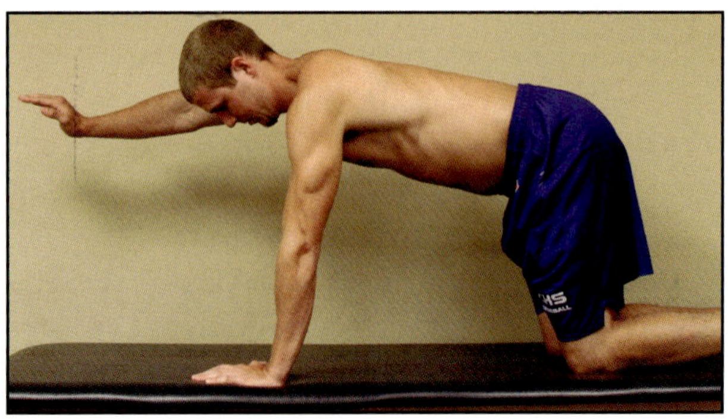

Figure 13. Quadruped weight-bearing exercise.

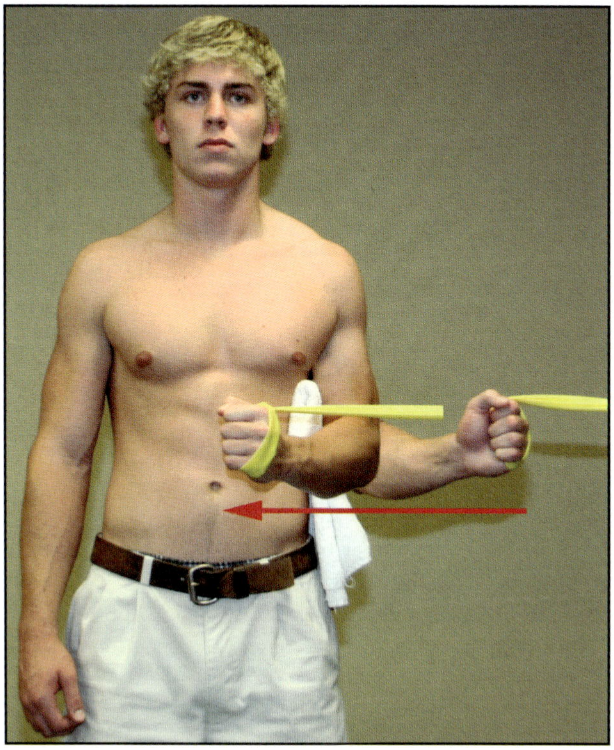

Figure 14. Internal rotation with an elastic band.

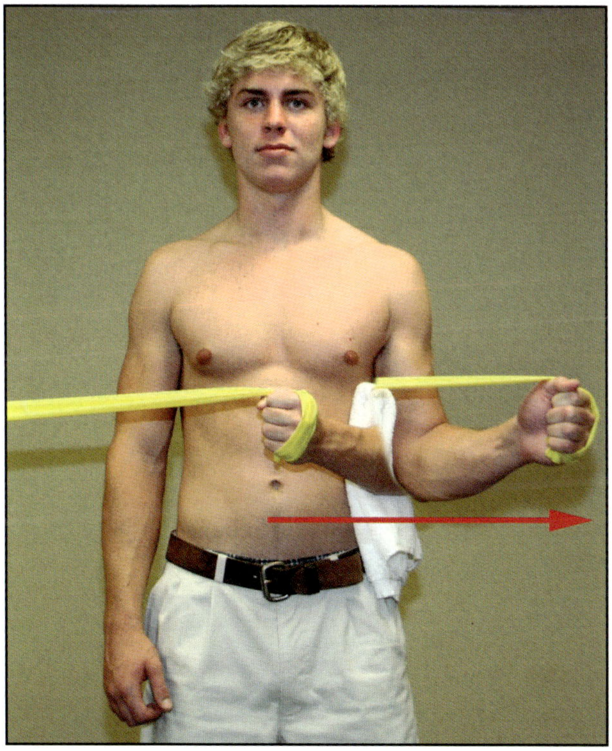

Figure 15. External rotation with an elastic band.

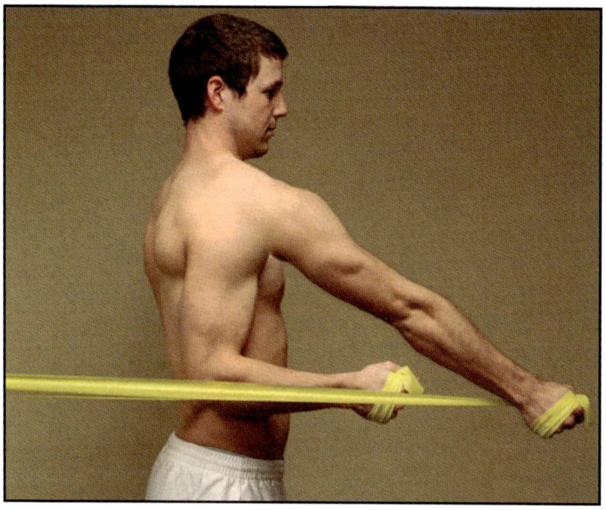

Figure 16. Forward reaching with an elastic band.

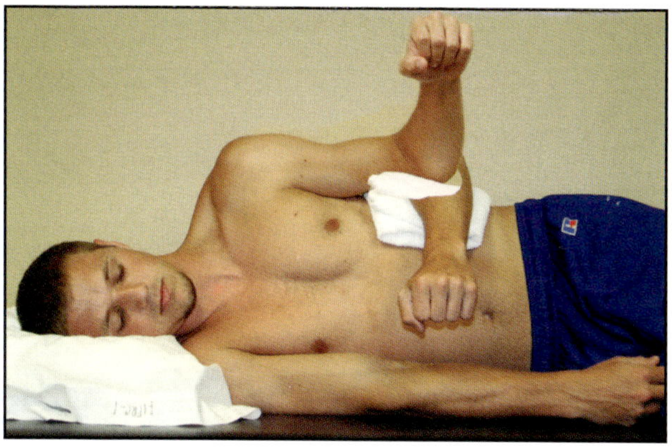

Figure 17. Side-lying external rotation exercise.

exercises very good choices for initial "strengthening" exercises in the patient with a massive rotator cuff repair (Figure 13). Initiation of the next level of our strengthening progression (base strengthening and arm elevation progressions) occurs when the patient comfortably can reach forward at waist level (eg, shaking hands motion). Our preferred base strengthening exercises during this step are light strengthening with elastic-band resistance using the technique described in the Appendix to ensure that resistance is minimal (Figures 14–16). If the patient is not able to easily overcome the external resistance of the band, which is common after massive rotator cuff repair, then he or she can perform an easier activity, such as side-lying external rotation or upright small-arc active external and internal rotation, or a gravity-minimized exercise, such as the Jackins supine assistive reach or side-lying, gravity-eliminated forward elevation (Figures 17–20). Arm elevation progressions provide an organized method to help patients achieve full overhead active elevation of the upper extremity, which is often the most difficult step in rehabilitation after massive rotator cuff repair.

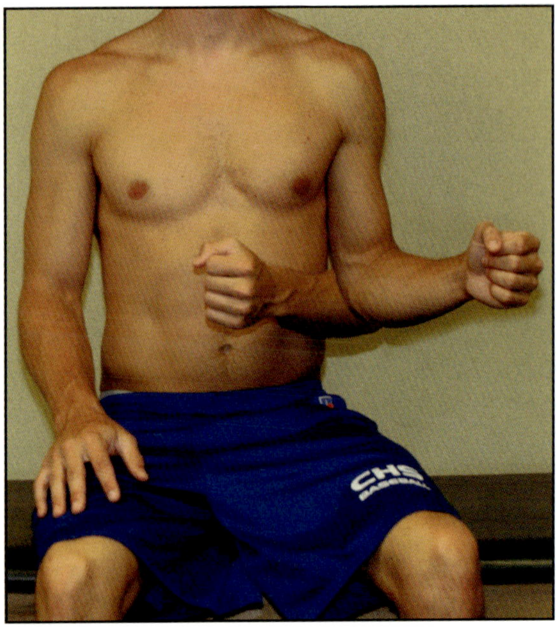

Figure 18. Active external and internal rotation.

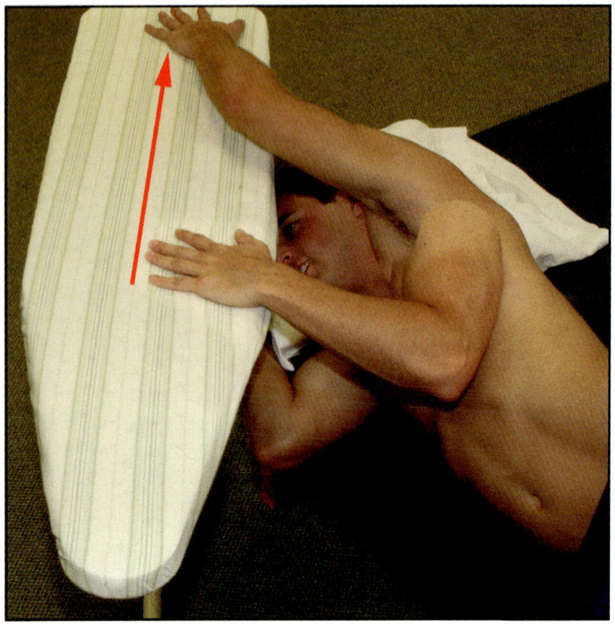

Figure 20. Side-lying, gravity-eliminated active forward elevation.

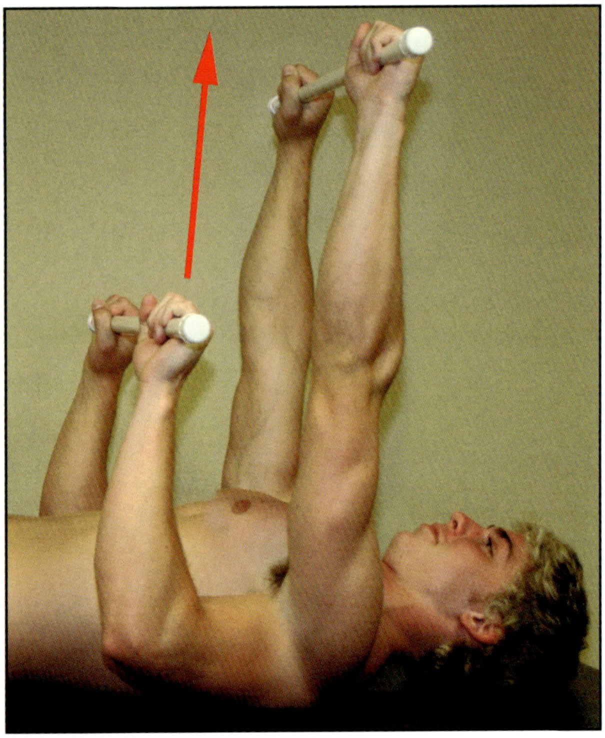

Figure 19. Jackins supine assistive reach.

This progression is outlined in the Appendix and is described in detail in chapter II-4. The time needed to complete this progression can vary from 3 weeks to 4 months or longer. After patients comfortably master AFE, which has a maximum of 29+/-13% MVIC in the SSP,[23] they progress this exercise by gradually adding very light weight (typically, 0.5 to 2.0 pounds [0.225–0.90 kg]), the amount of which depends on the details of the repair, the quality of repaired tissues, the desired functional goals, and the body mass of the patient. Together, the rehabilitation provider and the physician should determine the maximum advisable weight for AFE. This constitutes our next, and typically last, level of resistive strengthening. Most patients who have had a massive rotator cuff repair have returned to their preinjury level of function at this point and can be discharged with a basic maintenance home exercise program. The historically standard rotator cuff and scapula exercises, such as prone forward elevation, prone horizontal abduction, and press-ups,[38–40] are not used during typical rehabilitation after massive rotator cuff repair at my facility. These exercises were developed to optimally activate the rotator cuff (60–80% MVIC in the SSP), so we believe that they are too demanding to be included in standard rehabilitation after this procedure.

More vigorous rehabilitation after massive rotator cuff repair, such as inclusion of exercises that maximally activate the rotator cuff, replication of demanding work activities, or return to vigorous weight training, is only appropriate in very few patients, such as those returning to demanding physical work or consistently demanding recreational activities. This level of rehabilitation after a massive rotator cuff repair **only** should be initiated if the physician **specifically approves it** after counseling the patient about the potential advantages and disadvantages of consistent use of the repaired shoulder for this level of activity.

SPECIAL CONSIDERATIONS

In this section, I describe some situations that require varying amounts of modification to our standard massive rotator cuff repair rehabilitation guideline.

Repair of the Supraspinatus and Subscapularis

Rehabilitation of the patient with a massive rotator cuff repair that includes repair of the SSP and subscapularis must focus on protecting the subscapularis repair, especially during the first 2 to 3 months after surgery. As discussed in the Specific Rehabilitation Guideline section of this chapter, early PROM into external rotation, while necessary, can provide a direct stress to the repair that easily can surpass the integrity of the repair if the rehabilitation provider is not careful. The amount of protection only can be determined by the surgeon but commonly takes the form of limiting PROM (eg, PER to a maximum of 30º until postoperative week 6), delaying initiation of PER as an exercise, delaying internal rotation strengthening until postoperative month 3, and/or ensuring that the patient does not guard or reflexively contract the subscapularis during PER exercises. In the typical patient, the subscapularis typically is well healed by postoperative month 3 and tolerates progressive stretching and strengthening well with a small chance of damaging the subscapularis. In addition, patients with this type of repair often gain AFE easier than patients with other types of massive rotator cuff repairs and, after the early phases of rehabilitation, might not present much differently from a patient with a large SSP repair.

Repair of the Supraspinatus and Infraspinatus

Rehabilitation of the patient with a massive rotator cuff repair that involves repair of the SSP and infraspinatus requires specific attention to protecting the infraspinatus repair during the entire rehabilitation process, especially during the AROM and strengthening phase. During phases 1 and 2 of rehabilitation, using horizontal adduction stretching and the sleeper stretch for direct passive stretching of the infraspinatus generally is not appropriate. However, typical sling immobilization, in which the extremity often is positioned in prolonged internal rotation with the forearm near the stomach, is not detrimental to the usual repair of this type of massive rotator cuff tear. Researchers have demonstrated that the SSP and infraspinatus consistently work together with complementary levels of activation during rehabilitation exercises[41] and likely during activities of daily living. These muscles are innervated by the same nerve and appear to work together to control positioning of the upper extremity. We believe that when they are both repaired, extra care is needed during the entire AROM and strengthening process because limited direct help is available from other muscles to assist with the specific functions that these muscles perform. This protection is reflected in our standard Massive Rotator Cuff Repair Rehabilitation Guideline (Appendix). Patients with this type of repair might need 6 months or longer to achieve nearly normal active elevation of the extremity, and they might present with long-term diminished strength during overhead activities compared with patients with isolated SSP repairs or combined SSP and subscapularis repairs. Long-term vigorous rehabilitation is seldom advisable for these patients.

Repair of the Supraspinatus, Subscapularis, and Infraspinatus

Rehabilitation of the patient with a massive rotator cuff repair that includes repair of the SSP, subscapularis, and infraspinatus must focus on protecting all of the repaired structures in the ways described for each scenario. During phase 1 rehabilitation, the subscapularis must be protected, especially during PER exercises. During phases 2 and 3 rehabilitation, the rehabilitation provider must prevent overloading of the healing tendons, especially the SSP and infraspinatus during active-assistive ROM, AROM, and strengthening. Because of the extensive nature of repairs of this type, increased stiffness might be present throughout rehabilitation and results in a slower return of ROM. In addition, full ROM often cannot be attained, especially in patients with longstanding limited ROM before surgery. Some patients with this type of repair do gain PROM very easily, however. In all patients with a subscapularis, SSP, and infraspinatus repair, very simple and gentle rehabilitation typically is preferred. The rehabilitation provider must realize that achieving maximum AFE can take at least 6 months, so longer-term occasional therapy sessions with the provider (1 to 2 times per month) is often helpful during the late stages of rehabilitation.

Other Concomitant Surgical Procedures of the Shoulder

Other procedures, such as a biceps tenodesis, instability repair, or shoulder arthroplasty, that are performed at the same time as repair of a massive rotator cuff tear require slight modification to the standard Massive Rotator Cuff Repair Rehabilitation Guideline. Generally, this guideline is used with the modifications that are described in chapter III-1.

Is a Quicker Rehabilitation Progression Ever Warranted?

Whether a quicker rehabilitation progression is indicated is highly dependent on the preference of the physician and should be considered on a case-by-case basis. Examples of patients for whom a quicker rehabilitation progression might be considered include patients who are less than 50 years of age, patients with repairs of acute injuries, patients with combined SSP and subscapularis repairs, and patients with good-quality tissue. For these patients, the physician might choose to advance rehabilitation to the same speed as rehabilitation after repair of a routine rotator cuff tear, might choose a normal PROM progression at 6 weeks but delayed initiation of AROM and strengthening until postoperative week 12, might choose to initiate typical phase 2 routine cuff repair activities around postoperative week 9, or might choose another progression.

REFERENCES

1. Bishop J, Klepps S, Lo IK, Bird J, Gladstone JN, Flatow EL. Cuff integrity after arthroscopic versus open rotator cuff repair: a prospective study. *J Shoulder Elbow Surg*. 2006;15(3):290–299.
2. DeFranco MJ, Bershadsky B, Ciccone J, Yum JK, Iannotti JP. Functional outcome of arthrscopic rotator cuff repairs: a correlation of anatomic and clinical results. *J Shoulder Elbow Surg*. 2007;16(6):759–765.
3. Harryman DT II, Mack LA, Wang KY, Jackins SE, Richardson ML, Matsen FA III. Repairs of the rotator cuff: correlation of functional results with integrity of the cuff. *J Bone Joint Surg Am*. 1991;73(7):982–989.
4. Iannotti JP, Bernot MP, Kuhlman JR, Kelley MJ, Williams GR. Postoperative assessment of shoulder function: a prospective study of full-thickness rotator cuff tears. *J Shoulder Elbow Surg*. 1996;5(6):449–457.
5. Nho SJ, Shindle MK, Adler RS, Warren RF, Altchek DW, MacGillivray JD. Prospective analysis of arthroscopic rotator cuff repair: subgroup analysis. *J Shoulder Elbow Surg*. 2009;18(5):697–704.
6. Nho SJ, Adler RS, Tomlinson DP, et al. Arthroscopic rotator cuff repair: prospective evaluation with sequential ultrasonography. *Am J Sports Med*. 2009;37(10):1938–1945.
7. Nho SJ, Brown BS, Lyman S, Adler RS, Altchek DW, MacGillivray JD. Prospective analysis of arthroscopic rotator cuff repair: prognostic factors affecting clinical and ultrasound outcome. *J Shoulder Elbow Surg*. 2009;18(1):13–20.
8. Oh JH, Kim SH, Ji HM, Jo KH, Bin SW, Gong HS. Prognostic factors affecting anatomic outcome of rotator cuff repair and correlation with functional outcome. *Arthroscopy*. 2009;25(1):30–39.
9. Chung SW, Oh JH, Gong HS, Kim JY, Kim SH. Factors affecting rotator cuff healing after arthroscopic repair: osteoporosis as one of the independent risk factors. *Am J Sports Med*. 2011;39(10):2099–2107.
10. Galatz LM, Ball CM, Teefey SA, Middleton WD, Yamaguchi K. The outcome and repair integrity of completely arthroscopically repaired large and massive rotator cuff tears. *J Bone Joint Surg Am*. 2004;86(2):219–224.
11. Lee E, Bishop JY, Braman JP, Langford J, Gelber J, Flatow EL. Outcomes after arthroscopic rotator cuff repairs. *J Shoulder Elbow Surg*. 2007;16(1):1–5.
12. Gerber C, Schneeberger AG, Hoppeler H, Meyer DC. Correlation of atrophy and fatty infiltration on strength and integrity of rotator cuff repairs: a study in thirteen patients. *J Shoulder Elbow Surg*. 2007;16(6):691–696.
13. Goutallier D, Postel JM, Radier C, Bernageau J, Zilber S. Long-term functional and structural outcome in patients with intact repairs 1 year after open transosseous rotator cuff repair. *J Shoulder Elbow Surg*. 2009;18(4):521–528.
14. St Pierre P, Olson EJ, Elliott JJ, O'Hair KC, McKinney LA, Ryan J. Tendon-healing to cortical bone compared with healing to a cancellous trough: a biomechanical and histological evaluation in goats. *J Bone Joint Surg Am*. 1995;77(12):1858–1866.

15. Reed SC, Glossop N, Ogilvie-Harris DJ. Full-thickness rotator cuff tears: a biomechanical comparison of suture versus bone anchor techniques. *Am J Sports Med.* 1996;24(1):46–48.
16. Schneeberger AG, von Roll A, Kalberer F, Jacob HA, Gerber C. Mechanical strength of arthroscopic rotator cuff repair techniques: an in vitro study. *J Bone Joint Surg Am.* 2002; 84(12):2152–2160.
17. Gerber C, Schneeberger AG, Beck M, Schlegel U. Mechanical strength of repairs of the rotator cuff. *J Bone Joint Surg Br.* 1994;76(3):371–380.
18. Lewis CW, Schlegel TF, Hawkins RJ, James SP, Turner AS. The effect of immobilization on rotator cuff healing using modified Mason-Allen stitches: a biomechanical study in sheep. *Biomed Sci Instrum.* 2001;37:263–268.
19. Hatakeyama Y, Itoi E, Pradhan RL, Urayama M, Sato K. Effect of arm elevation and rotation on the strain in the repaired rotator cuff tendon: a cadaveric study. *Am J Sports Med.* 2001;29(6):788–794.
20. Zuckerman JD, Leblanc JM, Choueka J, Kummer F. The effect of arm position and capsular release on rotator cuff repair: a biomechanical study. *J Bone Joint Surg Br.* 1991;73(3):402–405.
21. Dockery ML, Wright TW, La Stayo PC. Electromyography of the shoulder: an analysis of passive modes of exercise. *Orthopedics.* 1998;21(11):1181–1184.
22. McCann PD, Wootten ME, Kadaba MP, Bigliani LU. A kinematic and electromyographic study of shoulder rehabilitation exercises. *Clin Orthop Relat Res.* 1993;288:179–188.
23. Gaunt BW, McCluskey GM, Uhl TL. Electromyographic evaluation of subdividing active-assistive shoulder exercises. *Sports Health.* 2010;2(5):424–432.
24. Long JL, Ruberte Thiele RA, Skendzel J, et al. Activation of the shoulder musculature during pendulum exercises and light activities. *J Orthop Sports Phys Ther.* 2010;40(4):230–237.
25. Fujisawa H, Suenaga N, Minami A. Electromyographic study during isometric exercise of the shoulder in head-out water immersion. *J Shoulder Elbow Surg.* 1998;7(5):491–494.
26. Uhl TL, Muir TA, Lawson L. Electromyographical assessment of passive, active assistive, and active shoulder rehabilitation exercises. *PM R.* 2010;2(2):132–141.
27. Ahmad CS, Kleweno C, Jacir AM, et al. Biomechanical performance of rotator cuff repairs with humeral rotation: a new rotator cuff repair failure model. *Am J Sports Med.* 2008;36(5):888–892.
28. Waltrip RL, Zheng N, Dugas JR, Andrews JR. Rotator cuff repair: a biomechanical comparison of three techniques. *Am J Sports Med.* 2003;31(4):493–497.
29. Gimbel JA, Van Kleunen JP, Williams GR, Thomopoulos S, Soslowsky LJ. Long durations of immobilization in the rat result in enhanced mechanical properties of the healing supraspinatus tendon insertion site. *J Biomech Eng.* 2007;129(3): 400–404.
30. Gimbel JA, Van Kleunen JP, Lake SP, Williams GR, Soslowsky LJ. The role of repair tension on tendon to bone healing in an animal model of chronic rotator cuff tears. *J Biomech.* 2007;40(3):561–568.
31. Peltz CD, Sarver JJ, Dourte LM, Würgler-Hauri CC, Williams GR, Soslowsky LJ. Exercise following a short immobilization period is detrimental to tendon properties and joint mechanics in a rat rotator cuff injury model. *J Orthop Res.* 2010;28(7):841–845.
32. Peltz CD, Dourte LM, Kuntz AF, et al. The effect of postopertive passive motion on rotator cuff healing in a rat model. *J Bone Joint Surg Am.* 2009;91(10):2421–2429.
33. Sugaya H, Maeda K, Matsuki K, Moriishi J. Repair integrity and functional outcome after arthroscopic double-row rotator cuff repair: a prospective outcome study. *J Bone Joint Surg Am.* 2007;89(5):953–960.
34. Parsons BO, Gruson KI, Chen DD, Harrison AK, Gladstone J, Flatow EL. Does slower rehabilitation after arthroscopic rotator cuff repair lead to long-term stiffness? *J Shoulder Elbow Surg.* 2010;19(7):1034–1039.
35. Leggin BG, Kelley MJ, Glasser DL. Short term outcome of rehabilitation following rotator cuff repair: standard vs. delayed protocol. Paper presented at: 3rd International Congress of Shoulder & Elbow Therapists; September 2010; Edinburgh, UK.
36. Wise MB, Uhl TL, Mattacola CG, Nitz AJ, Kibler WB. The effect of limb support on muscle activation during shoulder exercises. *J Shoulder Elbow Surg.* 2004;13(6):614–620.
37. Uhl TL, Carver TJ, Mattacola CG, Mair SD, Nitz AJ. Shoulder musculature activation during upper extremity weight-bearing exercise. *J Orthop Sports Phys Ther.* 2003;33(3):109–117.
38. Townsend H, Jobe FW, Pink M, Perry J. Electromyographic analysis of the glenohumeral muscles during a baseball rehabilitation program. *Am J Sports Med.* 1991;19(3):264–272.
39. Reinold MM, Wilk KE, Fleisig GS, et al. Electromyographic analysis of the rotator cuff and deltoid musculature during common shoulder external rotation exercises. *J Orthop Sports Phys Ther.* 2004;34(7):385–394.
40. Blackburn TA, McLeod WD, White B, Wofford L. EMG analysis of posterior rotator cuff exercises. *Athl Train J Natl Athl Train Assoc.* 1990;25(1):41–45.
41. Dark A, Ginn KA, Halaki ML. Shoulder muscle recruitment patterns during commonly used rotator cuff exercises: an electromyographic study. *Phys Ther.* 2007;87(8):1039–1046.

MASSIVE ROTATOR CUFF REPAIR REHABILITATION GUIDELINE

St. Francis Orthopaedic Institute and St. Francis Rehabilitation Center

All information contained in this protocol is to be used as a general guideline only. Specific variations might be appropriate for each patient and might be specified by the physician. In all cases, it is acceptable to advance the program more slowly than stated. If the patient experiences excessive pain, discontinue exercise until the physician is contacted. ***Achieving and maintaining a low level of pain and inflammation and protecting the surgical repair are the guiding principles in all stages of rehabilitation, even if less passive and active range of motion are accomplished.***

SYMBOLS AND ABBREVIATIONS

AAFE, active-assistive forward elevation
AAROM, active-assistive range of motion
AASEP, assistive-to-active shoulder elevation progression
ADLs, activities of daily living
AFE, active forward elevation
AROM, active range of motion
EMG, electromyography
ER, external rotation
FE, forward elevation
IR, internal rotation
NA, not applicable
PER, passive external rotation
PFE, passive forward elevation
POD, postoperative day
POM, postoperative month
POW, postoperative week
PRN, as needed
PROM, passive range of motion
ROM, range of motion
T-Band, Thera-Band
(The Hygenic Corporation, Akron, OH)
WFL, within functional limits
WNL, within normal limits

Forward elevation, either active or passive, is the plane of motion in which an individual naturally lifts his or her arm that is anterior to the plane of the scapula and lateral to flexion.

STAGED GOALS FOR RANGE OF MOTION

These are approximate targets for range of motion. Specific limits might be specified by the physician, especially if a subscapularis repair was performed.

Time	PFE	PER at 20° of Abduction	PER at 90° of Abduction	AFE
POD 1	50°	0°	NA	NA
POW 1	70°–100°	0°–20°	NA	NA
POW 3	90°–120°	15°–35°	NA	NA
POW 6	120°–145°	40°–50°	45°–60°	NA
POW 12	140°–155°	WFL	60°–90°	60°–90°
POM 5	WNL	WFL	WFL	120°–155°

PHASE 1

Goals

°Minimize pain and inflammatory response
°Maximally protect the surgical repair
°Achieve staged ROM goals
°Educate the patient about postoperative precautions
°Establish a stable scapula

POD 1 to POW 6

- °Elbow, wrist, and hand AROM with no weight
- °Scapular elevations and retractions (no weight) in or out of the sling
- °Pendulum exercises
  - °Lean over the table a comfortable amount
  - °Let the arm hang down relaxed
  - °Keep the body still
  - °As able, move the arm in small comfortable circles only
- °Upright PER in slight abduction until mild stretch and discomfort
  - °7 to 12 repetitions 2 times per day
  - °Preferred exercises
    - °Sit with family member or therapist rotating the arm (Figure 5)
    - °PER walk-around (stand with the arm supported on a table and rotate the body) (Figure 6)
- °PFE until mild stretch and discomfort
  - °7 to 12 repetitions 2 times per day
  - °Preferred exercises
    - °Sit with family member or therapist lifting the arm (Figure 3)
    - °Table step-back exercise (Figure 2).
    - °Kinex KS2 (Kinex Medical Company, LLC, Waukesha, WI) continous passive motion machine for 10 to 20 minutes 2 to 4 times per day (Figure 21)
- °Ice for pain reduction
- °Fit sling properly
  - °Ensure the sling provides slight lift to the shoulder girdle and supports the wrist
- °Patient education
  - °Primary focus of phase 1: encourage initial healing of the surgical repair
  - °Use of sling and as instructed by the physician; typically, full time in the community and if up at home for more than 5 to 10 minutes
  - °Minimal use of the arm for light waist-level activities as comfortable
  - °Ensure the level of pain is not increasing because of excessive use of the arm for ADLs or work
  - °Sleep in a recliner
    - °3 weeks (required)
    - °6 weeks (preferred)

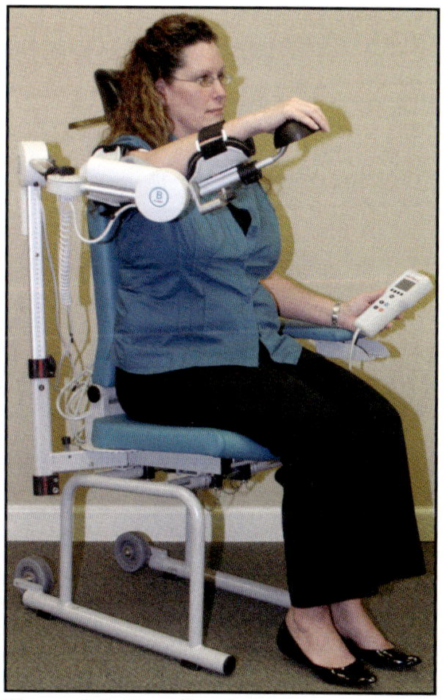

Figure 21. Passive forward elevation performed by the Kinex KS2 (Kinex Medical Company, LLC, Waukesha, WI) shoulder continuous passive motion machine.

Adjunctive Exercises

- °Therapist-assisted supine PROM within comfortable ROM to
  - °Decrease muscle guarding
  - °Gain patient confidence
  - °Achieve staged PROM goals (no mobilizations)
- °Cervical spine AROM
- °Pain-control agents PRN
- °Aquatic therapy for gentle, pain-free AAROM (no swimming strokes) after the incision has healed completely

Interventions to Avoid

- °Home exercise glenohumeral PROM in planes other then PFE and PER
- °Exercises that result in moderate or severe pain
- °Exercises that result in excessive guarding or splinting of muscles
- °Weighted exercises
- °Cross-body adduction, reaching behind the back, rope-and-pulley for elevation, and active elevation of the arm above waist level
- °Repetitive activity with the affected extremity

PHASE 2

Goals

- °Continue to maximally protect the surgical repair
- °Achieve staged PROM goals
- °Minimize shoulder pain
- °Work toward active forward reaching to waist level

POW 6 to 12

- °Achieve staged ROM goals in FE
  - °Preferred exercises
    - °Rope-and-pulley exercise (elbows remain straight)
    - °Patient-assisted supine AAFE exercise (use unaffected arm for assistance) (Figure 4)
    - °Continue table step-back exercise if above exercises are not tolerated
- °Achieve staged ROM goals in ER at 20° using upright exercises
- °Initiate horizontal dusting (Figure 8)
  - °Perform straight ahead
  - °Perform at 20° angles medially and laterally, if comfortable

Adjunctive Exercises

- °Therapist-assisted supine PROM and light stretching
  - °Can include ER and IR in increased angles of abduction, diagonal elevation, and horizontal adduction if ROM is below staged goals
- °Modalities PRN
- °Aquatic exercises (chapter IV-9)
  - °AAROM
  - °AROM
- °Spine therapy assessment and mobilization if
  - °Nonneurogenic cervical or scapular pain or
  - °Limitation in end-range shoulder FE
- °Golf chipping and putting if approved by the physician

Interventions to Avoid

- °Any AROM exercise into elevation or strengthening exercise with resistance
- °Exercises that greatly increase signs and symptoms

PHASE 3

Goals

- °Achieve staged ROM goals
- °Minimize shoulder pain
- °Normalize AROM
- °Increase strength and endurance
- °Return to realistic functional activities

POM 3 to 6 and Longer

- °Achieve staged ROM goals in FE
- °Achieve staged ROM goals in ER at 20° using upright exercises
- °Initiate horizontal adduction (Figure 10) and sleeper stretch (Figure 11), or both, PRN
- °Initiate supine hand-behind-head stretch PRN (Figure 9)
- °Initiate functional IR AAROM and stretching PRN (Figure 12)
- °Therapist-assisted PROM to achieve staged ROM goals with mobilizations PRN
- °Initiate base strengthening progression
  - °Includes beginning rotator cuff, deltoid, and scapular strengthening program
  - °2 times per day at most with light resistance and increasing repetitions
  - °Yellow T-Band for ER and IR
    - °5- to 6-foot band length and light or no pretension in a 3- to 6-inch arc of motion
    - °Can use side-lying ER instead of T-Band
  - °Yellow T-Band forward reach (Figure 16)
    - °Initially, 5- to 6-foot band length and light or no pretension
    - °Start with the elbow bent and by the side and the band tied behind the patient
    - °Reach **forward** with the hand at waist level, progressing to reaching **forward** at chest level
    - **°Do not initiate until forward reach at waist level without resistance is pain-free**
    - °If forward reach is painful or difficult, replace with a gravity-minimized exercise from the AASEP described below until it is comfortable
  - °Scapular strengthening emphasizing scapular retractions and scapular upward rotators (chapter IV-2)
  - °Low-level closed chain strengthening PRN (chapter II-4)
  - **°No prone FE, abduction, or ER**
- °Initiate the AASEP as comfortable (chapter II-4)
  - °A stepwise progression in difficulty of strengthening exercises from PFE to AFE against gravity
  - °Goal of the progression is to achieve pain-free full AFE
  - °EMG demonstrates progressive activation of the cuff and deltoid during the progression[23]
  - °If scapular or glenohumeral substitutions or pain are present, choose an easier exercise in the progression
  - °The order of the exercise sequence has some variability
  - °Usually not all exercises need to be performed
  - °The patient might advance through this progression exceptionally slowly, so this might constitute a very large portion of phase 3 rehabilitation
  - **°Do not perform the base strengthening program or overhead strengthening progression until the overall level of pain is low**
  - **°Ensure that these exercises do not increase signs and symptoms**

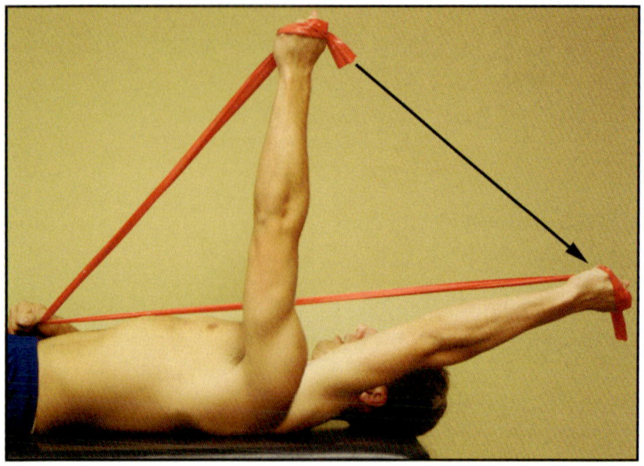
Figure 22. Supine forward elevation with an elastic band.

- °Exercises are divided into 3 levels of difficulty
  1. Gravity-minimized exercises
     - °Horizontal dusting (Figure 8)
       - °Perform straight ahead and perform at 20° angles medially and laterally if comfortable
     - °T-Band supine FE (Figure 22)
       - °Must start involved arm at 90° of elevation
       - °Pull the arm into FE
     - °Side-lying, gravity-eliminated AFE (Figure 20)
       - °Lie on the uninvolved side
       - °Place the involved arm on an ironing board
       - °Slide the hand on the board
     - °Jackins supine reaching progression
       - °Begin at 0° with the elbow bent and end at 90° of elevation with the elbow extended
       - °Start with the assistance of a cane or wand (Figure 19)
       - °Progress to active motion (Figure 23)
       - °Can progress to using 1- to 2-pound weight
       - °Can progress to the inclined position, continuing to reach to the ceiling (Figure 24)
  2. Assistive elevation exercises
     - °Rope-and-pulley AAFE
     - °Incline dusting (Figure 25)
     - °Standing AAFE (assistive elevation and descent via a T-bar or the unaffected arm)
     - °Standing assistive elevation and active independent eccentric lowering
     - °Wall-slide AAFE
       - °Ensure that the patient is in FE and is not in flexion
       - °Must be pain-free and natural when performed

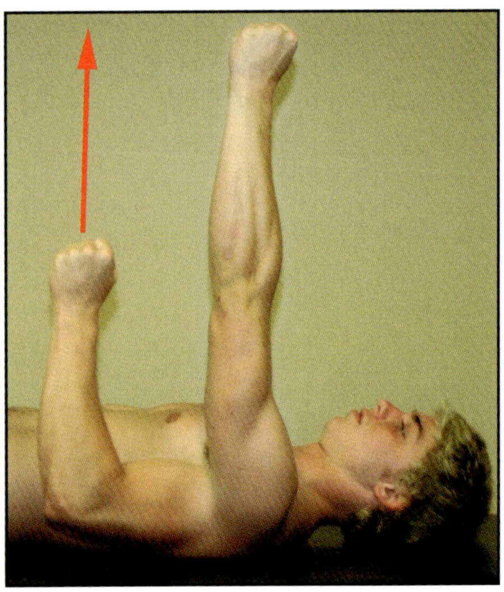
Figure 23. Jackins supine active reach.

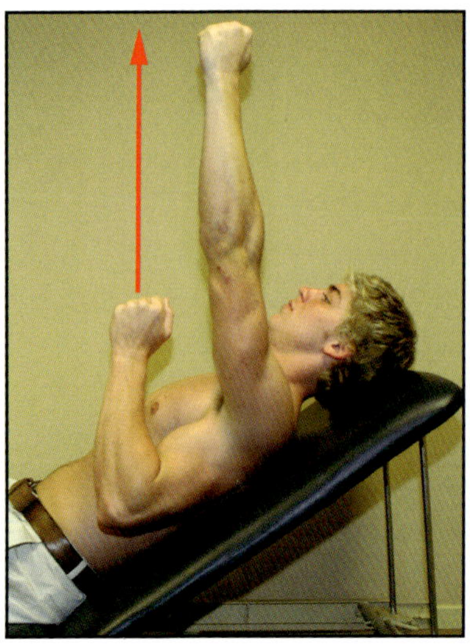
Figure 24. Jackins incline reach.

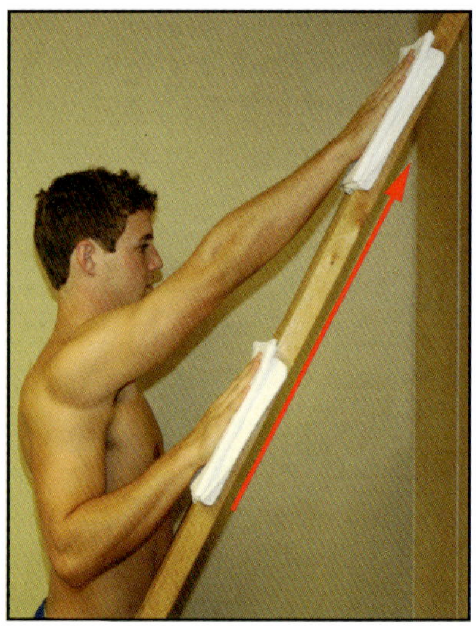
Figure 25. Incline dusting.

3. Unsupported elevation exercises
   - °Overhead wall taps
   - °AFE (Figure 26)
   - °Initiate AFE after the AASEP is complete
   - °Only perform if full or nearly full AROM is possible and comfortable
   - °Consider progressing to very light resistance (typically, 0.5 to 2 pounds for resistance, depending on body size and coexisting conditions of the patient, tissue quality of the repair, and typical functional demands)

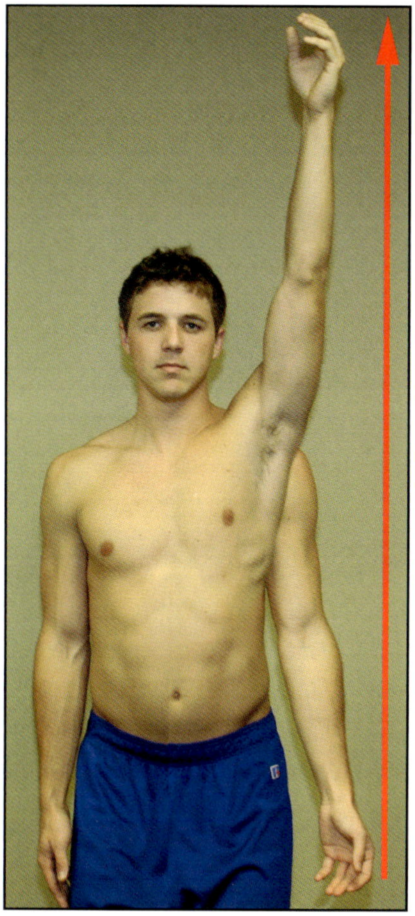

Figure 26. Active forward elevation.

Adjunctive Exercises

- °Therapist-assisted stretching and mobilizations PRN
- °Modalities PRN
- °Aquatic exercises (chapter IV-9)
- °Trunk stabilization and strengthening PRN
- °Progressive replication of demanding ADLs and work (if applicable for ADLs or occupation and **only when approved by physician**)
- °Initiate modified return to weight-training program (**only when approved by physician**)
- °Return-to-golf progression

Interventions to Avoid

- °Initiating base strengthening program or overhead strengthening progression before overall level of pain is low
- °Exercises that significantly increase signs and symptoms
- °Any forceful jerking motions with the involved arm
- °Highly repetitive rehabilitation activities with the elbow at or above chest level, including upper extremity ergometer
- °Strengthening into straight-plane abduction
- °Any rehabilitation activity that is significantly more demanding than daily or expected activities

III-3

Partial Repair of the Massive Rotator Cuff Tear

Bryce W. Gaunt, PT, SCS

CHAPTER CONTENTS

WHAT PATIENTS ARE APPROPRIATE FOR THE USE OF THIS GUIDELINE?

- Patients with a multitendon rotator cuff tear in which the supraspinatus is irreparable but the subscapularis or infraspinatus, or both, are completely or partially repaired if torn.
- Patients with a multitendon rotator cuff tear in which all damaged tendons are irreparable. Use this guideline with modifications discussed in the Special Considerations section.

Clinical pearls are highlighted in yellow throughout the text.

THE MOST IMPORTANT FACTOR THAT SHOULD GUIDE CLINICAL DECISION MAKING

The most important factor that should guide clinical decision making in the patient with a partial repair of a massive rotator cuff tear is understanding that because the normal anatomy of the rotator cuff cannot be restored, the ability of the rotator cuff (both repaired and native tissue) to function normally is compromised. Therefore, extra protection of the repair and a more gentle rehabilitation program are prudent during all phases of recovery. The rehabilitation provider must pay special attention to notice if rehabilitation is being advanced too quickly by watching for and teaching the patient to watch for signs of rotator cuff overload and by adjusting and teaching the patient to adjust interventions and activities of daily living (ADLs) accordingly.

KEY PRINCIPLES IN REHABILITATION OF THIS PROBLEM

As with rehabilitation after repair of a routine or massive tear of the rotator cuff, optimal rehabilitation of the patient after partial repair of a massive rotator cuff tear requires that the rehabilitation provider know the details of the surgical procedure; be aware of key factors that affect healing of the repaired tendon or tendons; know the stresses that each rehabilitation intervention places on the surgical repair; apply a precise priority for clinical decision making; maintain close communication among the patient, physician, and himself or herself; and carefully consider how these diverse issues affect each other. Refer to chapters III-1 and III-2 for in-depth discussions of these topics.

Biomechanics of the Uninjured, Torn, and Partially Repaired Rotator Cuff

To appreciate why extra care is needed during rehabilitation of patients after a partial repair of a massive rotator cuff tear, one must understand the anatomy, biomechanics, and basic function of the uninjured shoulder, the shoulder with a multitendon rotator cuff tear, and the partially repaired rotator cuff. Normal function of the glenohumeral joint depends on the coordinated muscle forces of the deltoid and rotator cuff acting together to create essential force couples in which the rotator cuff provides anterior and posterior stability to the humeral head and provides an inferiorly directed force against the superior pull of the deltoid.[1,2] Investigators believe that with the upper extremity at the side, the supraspinatus initiates abduction of the shoulder, and the deltoid muscle with its dominant force directed vertically provides most of the remaining force required to bring the extremity to and above shoulder level.[3] This pull of the deltoid creates a vertical shear force at the glenohumeral joint that is offset by an inferiorly directed stabilizing force generated by the rotator cuff (Figure 1).

Although often considered by their individual functions (ie, external rotation, internal rotation), the rotator cuff tendons primarily function as a cohesive unit to dynamically stabilize the humeral head, keeping it centered in the glenoid throughout shoulder motion. Due in large part to the force couple between the deltoid and rotator cuff in uninjured shoulders, the geometric center of the humeral head moves less than 1 mm during scapular-plane abduction (Figures 1 and 2).[4,5] Excessive superior migration of the humeral head (Figure 3) has been shown to be present in individuals with a variety of conditions, such as rotator cuff tears,[4,5] impingement,[6] and rotator cuff fatigue.[7]

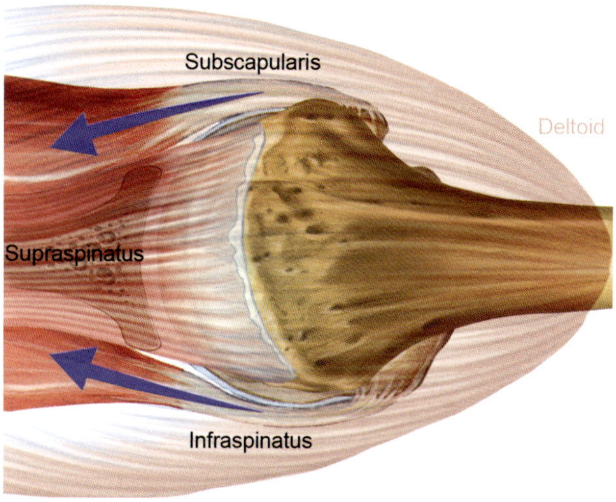

Figure 2. The force couple of the transverse plane balances the anterior rotator cuff against the posterior rotator cuff. This balance is needed to create a fulcrum for overhead movement in combination with the superior pull of the deltoid shown in Figure 1.

In patients with multitendon rotator cuff tears, reestablishing the rotator cuff's ability to stabilize the humeral head against the superior pull of the deltoid is essential for successful rehabilitation of this problem.[2]

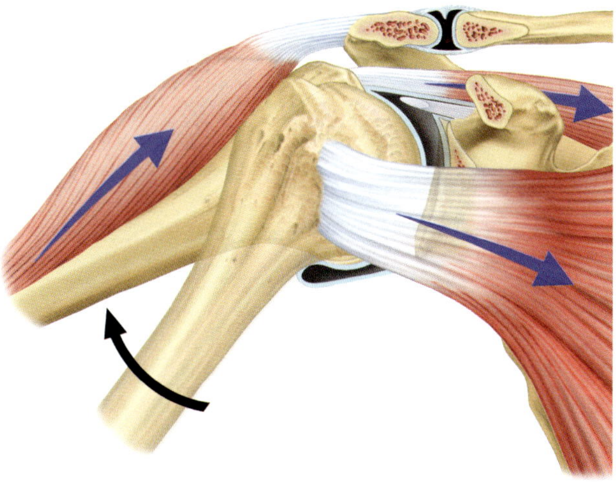
Figure 1. The rotator cuff stabilizes the superior pull of the deltoid by providing a fulcrum for rotation and elevation of the extremity, resulting in only about 1 mm of humeral head migration during scapular-plane elevation.

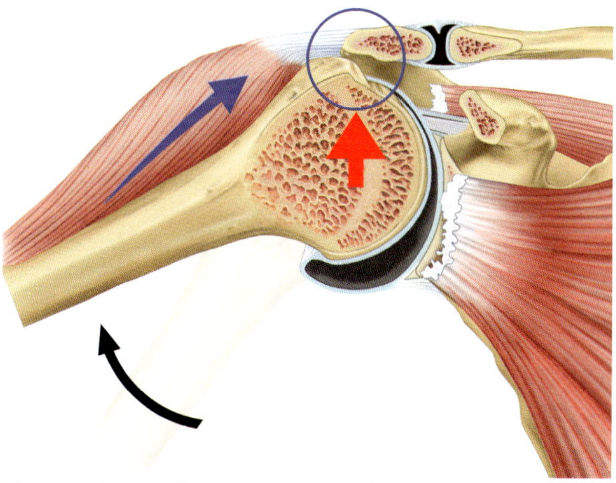
Figure 3. Excessive superior migration of the humeral head, which is shown by the red arrow and blue circle, occurs due to some multitendon rotator cuff tears where the rotator cuff does not adequately stabilize the superior pull of the deltoid.

It requires the combined efforts of the surgeon, rehabilitation provider, and patient. In cadaveric models, activation of the infraspinatus consistently has been shown to be necessary to prevent excessive superior migration of the humerus either alone[8] or in conjunction with the subscapularis[2,9,10] and teres minor.[2,10] Conversely, in this model, activation of the deltoid muscle alone results in substantial superior migration of the humeral head.[2,9,10] Whereas one function of the supraspinatus is to assist in depression of the humeral head, it has not been shown to be effective in this role during elevation of the shoulder in a cadaveric model without activation of the other rotator cuff muscles.[2,8,9,11] This is likely because the vector of pull of the supraspinatus has a minimal inferior component compared with the subscapularis and infraspinatus, which have a much larger inferiorly directed force (Figure 4).[12] Therefore, in a cadaveric model, evidence has been found that the humeral head can be stabilized effectively during elevation of the shoulder with a deficient supraspinatus as long as the remaining rotator cuff is intact.[2,8–11]

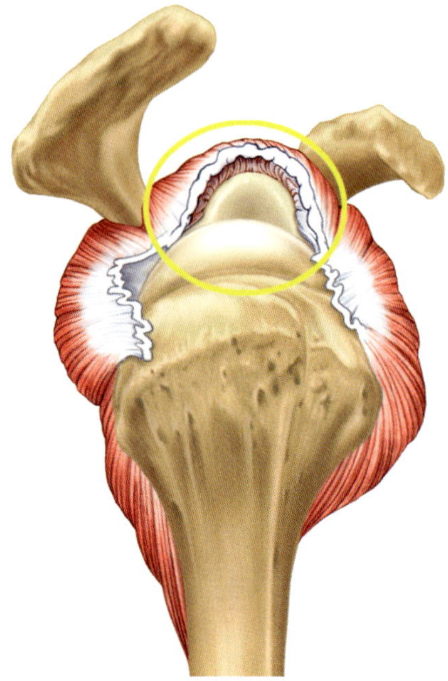

Figure 5. A rotator cuff tear of the supraspinatus, infraspinatus, and subscapularis demonstrates tendon loss and irreparableness of the supraspinatus tendon, which is circled in yellow.

In some patients, multitendon rotator cuff tears might not be amenable to complete anatomic repair of all torn tendons. In these patients, the less retracted edges of the tear near the anterior and posterior margins usually are reparable, but the central portion of the tear with the greatest retraction might be irreparable due to tendon loss (Figure 5). Researchers have shown that in the patient with an irreparable suprapinatus, the intact or reparable subscapularis and infraspinatus together can provide a stable fulcrum during active motion of the upper extremity[13] with very little increased superior humeral head migration compared with a uninjured shoulder in a cadaveric

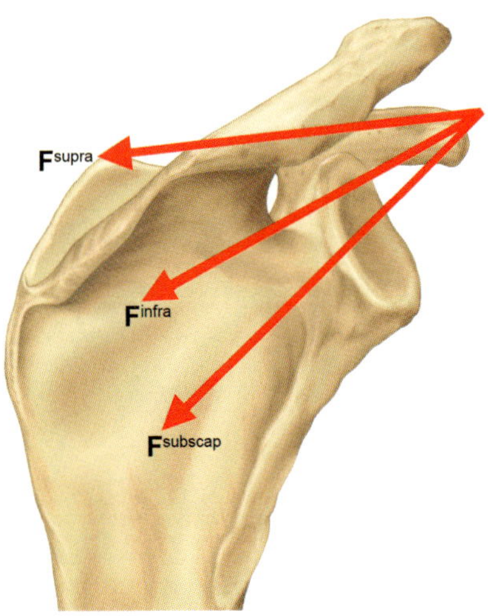

Figure 4. The resultant force vectors of the supraspinatus (F^{supra}), infraspinatus (F^{infra}), and subscapularis ($F^{subscap}$) are illustrated. Note that the infraspinatus and subscapularis have a much larger inferiorly directed force than the supraspinatus and thus are thought to play a more important role in humeral head stability.

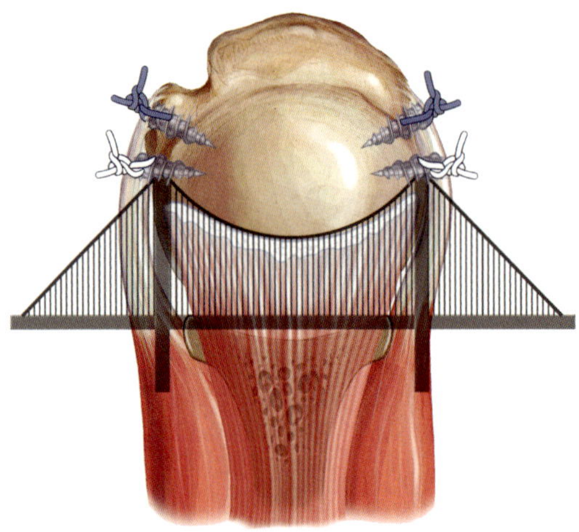

Figure 6. A rotator cuff repair of the subscapularis and infraspinatus with an irreparable supraspinatus has a configuration similar to a suspension bridge. The free margin of the tear corresponds to the cable, and the anterior and posterior attachments of the repair correspond to the supports at each end of the cable's span.

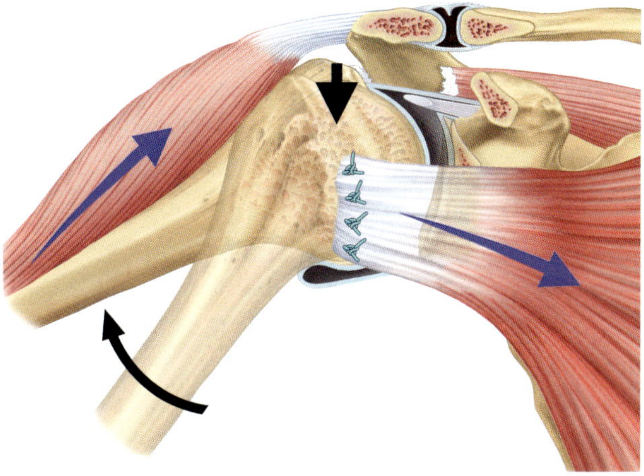

Figure 7. A stable fulcrum for elevation of the extremity is achieved with a repaired subscapularis but an irreparable supraspinatus.

model.[2] Burkart[13] described this as a *functional rotator cuff tear* and likened it to a suspension bridge in which the free margin of the tear corresponds to the cable and the anterior and posterior attachments of the tear correspond to the supports at each end of the cable's span (Figure 6). As long as both supports (subscapularis and infraspinatus) are present, the biomechanical integrity of the suspension bridge and force couple is restored. In the shoulder, this means the combination of an intact or repaired subscapularis and infraspinatus provide anteroposterior stability in the transverse plane, allowing a stable fulcrum for movement against the pull of the deltoid even if the supraspinatus is irreparably torn (Figures 6 and 7). In patients with multitendon rotator cuff tears involving the supraspinatus and large tears of the subscapularis or infraspinatus, the suspension bride is disrupted, unbalancing the essential anteroposterior force couple and resulting in the inability to create a stable fulcrum against the force of the deltoid (Figure 8). In other words, when 1 or both sides of the bridge are unattached, it cannot function properly.[13]

In summary, partial repair of a massive multitendon rotator cuff tear is an attempt to restore the biomechanical integrity of the rotator cuff through repair of the infraspinatus or subascapularis, or both, if restoring the complete anatomic integrity is not possible due to loss of the supraspinatus tendon.[14] Repairing the suspension bridge and rotator cuff cable re-establishes a stable fulcrum to restore normal force couples (Figures 6 and 7). This can result in a large improvement in active range of motion (AROM) and function in select patients.[14,15]

Burkhart et al[14] evaluated a group of 14 patients with partial repairs of massive rotator cuff tears. Active forward elevation (AFE) improved from 60° to 150°, the University of California-Los Angeles shoulder score improved from 9.8 to 27.6, and 13 patients were satisfied with their results.[14]

Why Extra Care Is Needed

Whereas the same general mechanisms of how the repaired rotator cuff heals and how it is protected during rehabilitation applies when rehabilitating the patient with a partial repair of a massive tear and when working with a patient who has a repair of a routine rotator cuff tear, the rehabilitation provider must recognize that extra protection of the repair and more gentle rehabilitation are needed in this situation because the ability of the rotator cuff to perform its job is compromised. Why are modifications needed in these patients? Whereas the rotator cuff force couples might be re-established due to the presence or repair of the subscapularis and infraspinatus tendons, evidence exists that when the supraspinatus is irreparable, (1) the remaining rotator cuff has some decreased ability to provide stabilization of the humeral head with simulated elevation of the extremity[16]; (2) the remaining rotator cuff tendons have increased strain[17] with movement of the extremity and decreased material, structural, and viscoelastic properties that progressively decline over time[18]; and (3) the glenohumeral joint can have altered biomechanics if the remaining rotator cuff lacks suf-

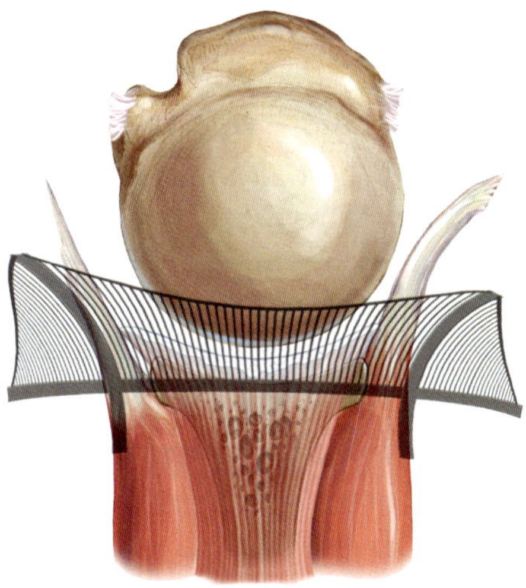

Figure 8. Tears of the infraspinatus and subscapularis disrupt the suspension bridge and force couples of the rotator cuff.

ficient strength.[13,19] In addition, the outcomes tend to be more modest, and clinical healing rates tend to be lower because patients with massive rotator cuff tears tend to have larger tears and poorer-quality tissue and are more likely to have fatty degeneration than patients with smaller tears.[20–23]

Hallmarks of Our Approach to Rehabilitation

Because of these factors, the progression used at my facility during rehabilitation of patients with a partial repair of a massive rotator cuff tear is similar to the one used for patients with a complete repair of a massive rotator cuff tear and is much slower and more gentle than the progression used for patients with a repair of a routine rotator cuff tear. The primary differences between this progression and the typical massive rotator cuff rehabilitation guideline detailed in chapter III-2 are that we individualize the rehabilitation plan more than normal and that we use an especially careful, well-monitored, and thoughtful progression of active-assistive range of motion (AAROM), AROM, and strengthening exercises.

An individualized rehabilitation plan is necessary, especially after progressive AAROM and strengthening are allowed, because a wide variety of outcomes are common after this procedure. Some patients achieve normal to nearly normal AROM, good shoulder-level and overhead strength, and normal to nearly normal function. Other patients might achieve normal to nearly normal AROM but have noticeable deficits in strength and some deficits in overhead function. Patients also might achieve AROM only to shoulder level or below, with marked deficits in strength and function that are limited substantially. We do not know what outcome the patient eventually will achieve during the rehabilitation process, so rehabilitation cannot be prescribed to achieve a given outcome. Instead, rehabilitation must match the patient's current level of impairment and function, taking into account passive range of motion (PROM), pain, and the functioning of the muscles of the shoulder girdle individually and as a synergistic group.

Properly progressing the rehabilitation plan after an AAROM to AROM to strengthening progression is allowed requires great skill, close observation, patience, and adaptability because normal functioning of the rotator cuff is impaired in this patient population with an irreparable supraspinatus. Even if not torn or repaired, the remaining rotator cuff muscles and tendons might have a low capacity to generate substantial force due to atrophy, degeneration, or fatty infiltration.[20] Therefore, modifications to our typical strengthening programs often are needed. These will be discussed in more detail in the next section; however, in these patients, we emphasize rehabilitation of the scapula, perform light isolated strengthening of the remaining rotator cuff and deltoid muscles, and especially emphasize training the remaining muscles to work together to create a successful force couple and fulcrum for elevation of the upper extremity.

As rehabilitation progresses, especially into AAROM and strengthening, I am especially vigilant to ensure that I am not overloading the rotator cuff and affecting its ability to successfully center the humeral head. Whereas this evaluation most accurately is accomplished with imaging equipment, such as radiography or 3-dimensional motion analysis, it can be performed crudely by careful palpation or visual inspection, or both (Figure 9), to determine if excess superior migration of the humeral head is occurring during ADLs or rehabilitation activities. If so, this is a sign

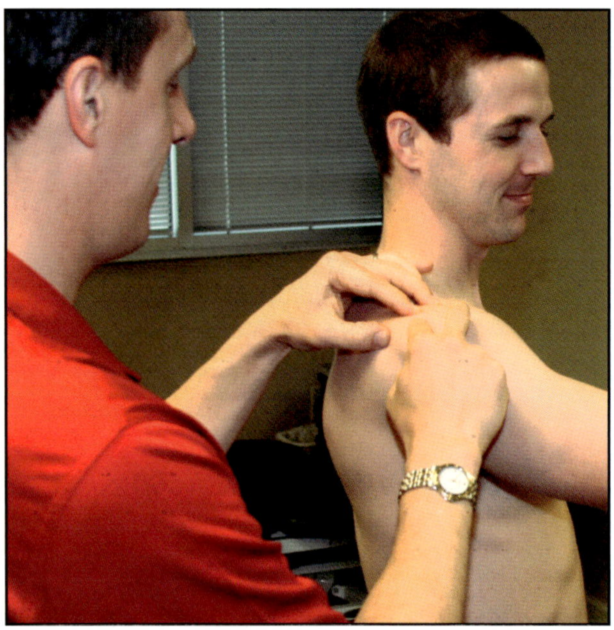

Figure 9. Evaluation of excessive migration of the humeral head by visual inspection and palpation of the humeral head and acromion during active elevation of the shoulder.

that the load to the rotator cuff is greater than what it can stabilize and control. I believe patients should try and perform only rehabilitation activities and ADLs that they can accomplish with good centering of the humeral head to facilitate correct activation of the rotator cuff force couples and minimize abnormal strain to the remaining tissues. Anecdotally, I also have found that patients' AROM seems to progress quicker if abnormal biomechanics are minimized. How I do this will be discussed in more detail in the next section. Finally, it is especially important in this patient population to remember that the first goal of rehabilitation besides protecting the repair is to establish appropriate PROM and a low level of pain and to maintain the low level of pain as rehabilitation progresses.

SPECIFIC REHABILITATION GUIDELINE

The Appendix specifies our complete Partial Repair of the Massive Rotator Cuff Tear Rehabilitation Guideline, which is very similar to our Massive Rotator Cuff Repair Rehabilitation Guideline detailed in chapter III-2. In this section, I highlight the differences between the 2 guidelines and explain the rationale for selected components of the partial repair guideline. See chapter III-2 for details on the rationale and clinical decision making of our more conservative approach to rehabilitation of all repairs of massive rotator cuff tears. The current guideline is divided into 3 phases based on general timeframes of healing and staged range-of-motion (ROM) targets. To advance from one rehabilitation phase to the next, the patient must gain approval from the physician, successfully complete the core components of the previous rehabilitation activities, and meet the time criteria.

Phase 1

The primary focus of phase 1 rehabilitation, which constitutes the first 6 postoperative weeks, is to maximally protect the surgical repair, and the secondary focus is to achieve, but not substantially exceed, the staged ROM goals that the referring physician helps establish. As detailed in chapters III-1 and III-2, a rehabilitation activity is safe after a rotator cuff repair only if the strength of the surgical repair is always much more than the stress that is placed on the repaired tendon during each rehabilitation exercise. During rehabilitation after a repair of a massive rotator cuff tear, this stress is determined for all rehabilitation activities (home exercises, clinic exercises, and manual therapy) by (1) the amount of muscle activation of the repaired musculotendon unit, (2) the plane of motion

Table. Common Passive Elevation Exercises in the Plane of the Scapula and the Associated Electromyographic Activity Levels of the Supraspinatus and Anterior Deltoid

Exercise	Electromyographic Activity
Therapist-assisted forward elevation	Average supraspinatus 4%, anterior deltoid 8%[24] Average supraspinatus 5%, anterior deltoid 7% supine[25] Average supraspinatus 12%, anterior deltoid 4% upright[25]
Self-assisted forward elevation supine	Average supraspinatus 3%, anterior deltoid 11%[25]
Pulley forward elevation	Average supraspinatus 17%, anterior deltoid 25%[24] Average supraspinatus 13%, anterior deltoid 21%[25] Maximum supraspinatus 17%, anterior deltoid 31%[26]
Pendulum	Average supraspinatus 9%, anterior deltoid 3%[25] Average supraspinatus 6%[24] Maximum supraspinatus (small 10-cm diameter circle) 8–8.7%[27] Maximum supraspinatus (large 51-cm diameter circle) 13.7–18.8%[27]
Specific aquatic exercises	Average supraspinatus 1–5%, anterior deltoid 1–8%[28]
Closed chain (table step-back)	Average supraspinatus 5%, anterior deltoid 2%[29]
Continuous passive motion machine	Average supraspinatus 5%, average anterior deltoid 3%[24]

that is used, (3) the specific glenohumeral joint ROM, and (4) the number of times the tissue is loaded (the number of repetitions). Appropriate exercise selection cannot occur without understanding these factors.

Patients with a partial repair of a massive rotator cuff tear almost always obtain their PROM goals very easily after the initial postoperative pain and apprehension have subsided. Although not detailed in this chapter, all phase 1 ROM interventions need to provide a low stress to the rotator cuff, especially regarding electromyographic (EMG) activity. The Table demonstrates common passive elevation exercises in

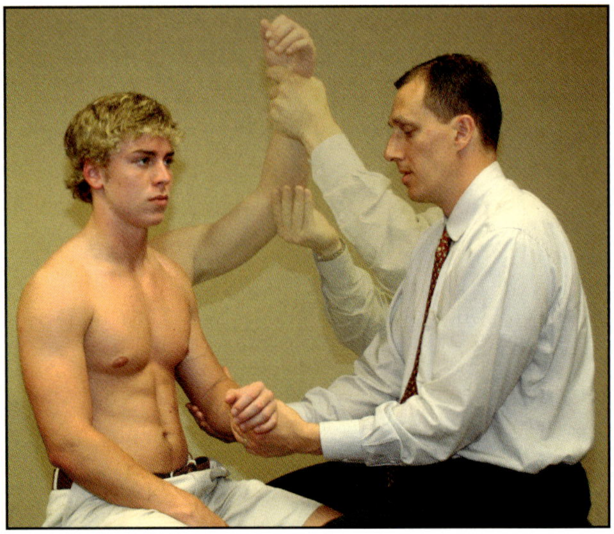

Figure 12. Assisted passive forward elevation. The assistant typically stands diagonally in front of the patient.

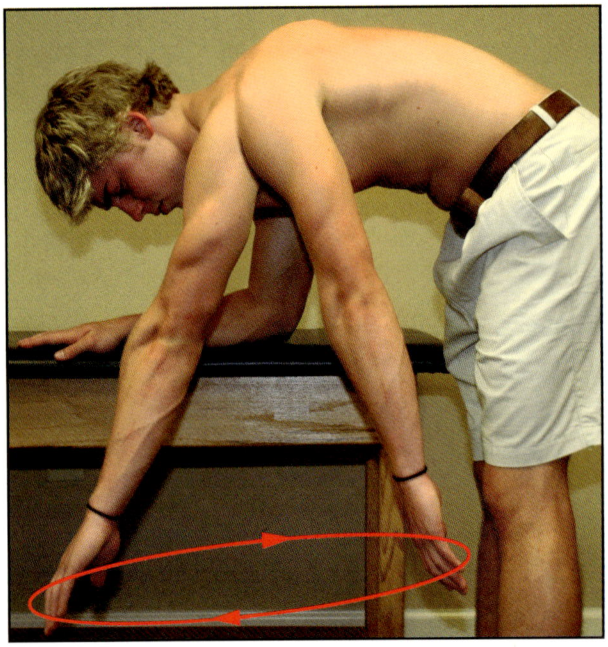

Figures 10. The pendulum exercise initially uses smaller circles.

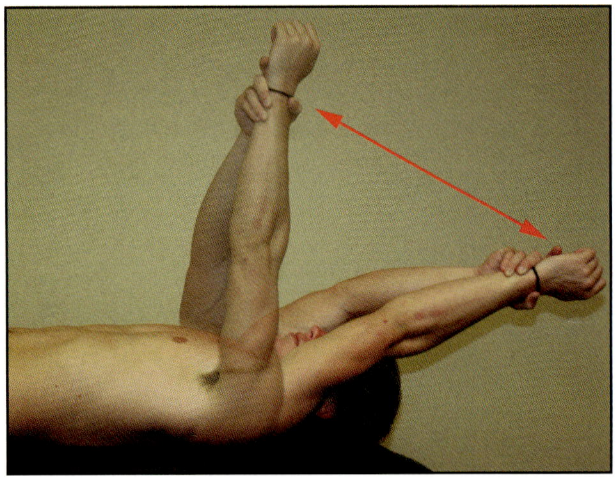

Figure 13. Self-assisted supine active-assisted forward elevation. The hand-assisted exercise is preferred.

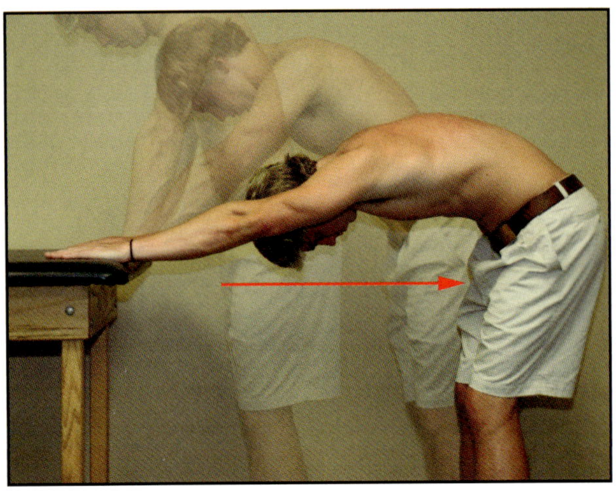

Figure 11. Table step-back exercise for passive forward elevation.

the plane of the scapula and the associated EMG activity of the supraspinatus and deltoid. We have found that the pendulum, table step-back, and rehabilitation-provider-assisted or family-assisted sitting exercises are the most effective and well-tolerated exercises to achieve passive forward elevation (PFE) during the first few weeks after surgery (Figures 10–12). We have found that although self-assisted PROM in the supine position is safe to start immediately after surgery based on EMG activity, it typically is not well-tolerated until at least the late stages of phase 1 (Figure 13). Because PROM goals usually are achieved easily in these patients, a continuous passive motion machine rarely is needed. As the Table demonstrates, the rope-and-pulley exercise has a noticeably higher EMG activity level in the supraspinatus than the other exercises listed, so we do not recommend using this exercise during phase 1 rehabilitation of these patients.

For passive external rotation (PER), McCann et al[25] and Dockery et al[24] demonstrated very low EMG activity levels in the supraspinatus, anterior deltoid, and infraspinatus with all exercises tested. However, neither group of investigators evaluated the EMG activity in the subscapularis, which is likely the muscle most at risk of injury with these exercises because it stretches passively with external rotation and is actively contracted when muscle guarding occurs against PER. Because of this, minimizing stress to the subscapularis with PER in partial repairs of massive rotator cuff tears that involve subscapularis repair is vitally

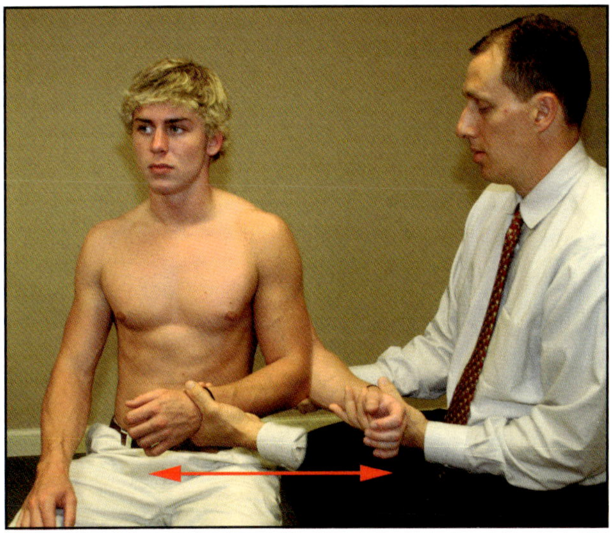

Figure 14. Assisted sitting passive external rotation.

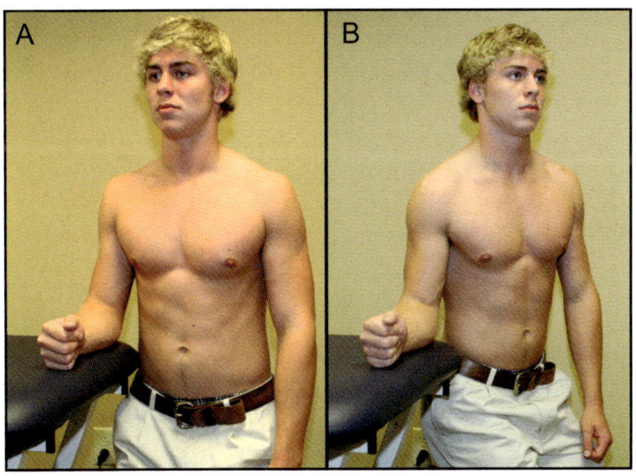

Figure 15 A and B. Passive external rotation walk-around exercise.

important because the subscapularis is at high risk for rupture with overly aggressive PER. Clinically, we have found that PER performed while sitting and with the assistance of a family member or rehabilitation provider and the PER walk-around are the gentlest, the most effective, and the most well-tolerated exercises in the early postoperative period (Figures 14 and 15). In particular, the PER walk-around is very safe in this situation because it provides no direct counterforce to PER. If the patient tries to stretch too aggressively, the forearm simply rotates on its support surface. Other exercises to achieve PER that use an L-bar or wall to provide a counterforce to the forearm have much greater potential for placing excessive stress on the subscapularis. We believe that these exercises are generally inappropriate for phase 1 rehabilitation after a partial repair of a massive rotator cuff tear that involves a subscapularis repair because of the risk of placing excessive stress on the subscapularis with incorrect exercise technique.

Although not in our base rehabilitation guideline for this problem, other modifications might be made more often than with a typical massive rotator cuff repair guideline. The physician might prescribe PROM limits for forward elevation or external rotation especially during phase 1 to protect the repair. Because patients usually do not have recurrent stiffness with this procedure, the surgeon might be more likely to delay the start of rehabilitation until postoperative weeks 4 to 6 because authors of basic science research on tendon healing in animal models have suggested this might improve healing of the rotator cuff.[30–33]

Phase 2

The focus of phase 2, which typically constitutes postoperative weeks 6 through 12, is to continue to maximally protect the surgical repair that while getting stronger, is still very weak; to achieve staged PROM goals; to minimize shoulder pain; and to work toward achieving active forward reaching at waist level. The rehabilitation provider still must ensure that the stress of the activities in the rehabilitation program is substantially less than the strength of the surgical repair. The interpretation of results from biomechanical studies and from studies in which long-term clinical healing rates were analyzed[30,31,33] shows that continued

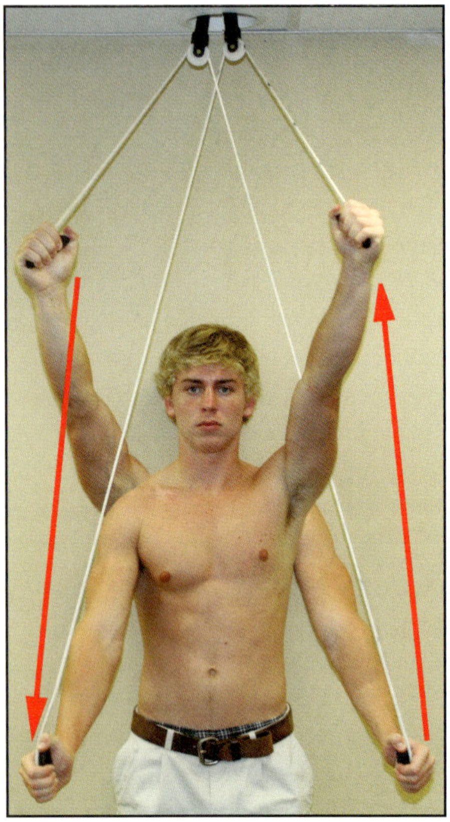

Figure 16. Rope-and-pulley active-assistive forward elevation exercise.

minimization of stress to the repair of the massive rotator cuff tear during rehabilitation and ADLs during phase 2 is prudent. Therefore, phase 2 of rehabilitation after this repair is only a minimal advancement from phase 1 rehabilitation and is substantially different from phase 2 rehabilitation after repair of a routine rotator cuff tear. It is essentially the same as the rehabilitation after a standard repair of a massive rotator cuff tear.

For PROM, home exercises continue to include only exercises to achieve staged ROM goals in forward elevation and external rotation in 20° of abduction. For forward elevation, rope-and-pulley elevation (Figure 16) and self-assisted supine active-assistive forward elevation (AAFE) (Figure 13), as tolerated, usually replace the PFE exercises of phase 1.

If the subscapularis has been repaired, it is vital that only very gentle exercises continue to be used to increase PER. This still means that the PER walk-around (Figure 15) or family-assisted external rotation (Figure 14) is the preferred method. In addition, if PER is easily meeting or exceeding staged ROM goals, then exercises that increase PER must be discontinued because detrimental stress can occur if end-range stretching is performed during this time. If the subscapularis has not been repaired, then any PER exercise is safe to perform, but anecdotally, I have found that upright stretching exercises are very well tolerated and very effective during this time.

Comfortable active use of the upper extremity at this time is quite variable among patients. Many of them struggle to actively reach the hand fully forward at waist level. However, a few patients are comfortable actively lifting the extremity to 90° or more. For most patients who have difficulty actively reaching forward at waist level, horizontal dusting is initiated (Figure 17). The inability to actively reach the hand forward at waist level signifies that the shoulder girdle muscles and rotator cuff force couples cannot counteract the weight of the extremity against gravity in this position without assistance. Horizontal dusting provides assistance to the recently repaired shoulder girdle muscles by decreasing the weight that the muscles must work against because the hand is resting on the table. The load of the surgically repaired upper extremity is effectively decreased, so the muscle force required to actively move the extremity correspondingly is diminished. Patients who cannot actively move the elbow away from the side without support almost always will be able to completely extend the elbow by sliding the hand back and forth on the table. We prefer

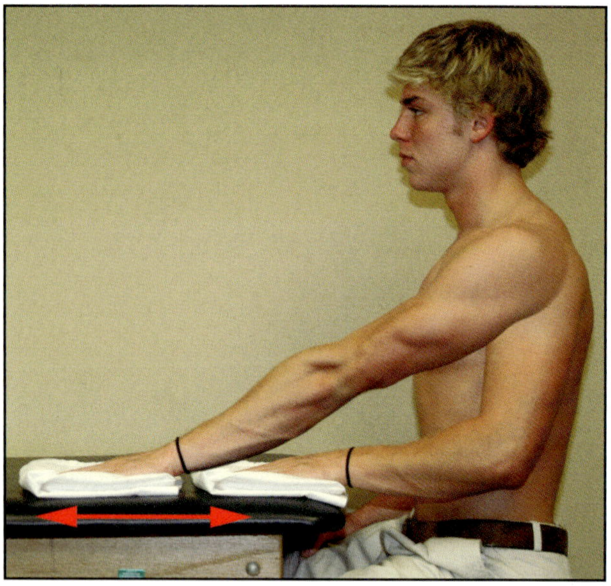

Figure 17. Horizontal dusting exercise.

that this exercise involve a forward and backward motion at very slight angles and never extend the elbow past the midline of the body. We primarily want to train the muscles that are active during the functional task of forward reaching rather than the muscles that are active during circular motions or reaching at wide angles. Electromyographic data are also available for the muscle activity level of horizontal dusting at 30°.[26] To our knowledge, no EMG data are available on circular dusting or dusting at larger angles.

Submaximal isometric exercises sometimes are allowed by the surgeon during phase 2, as well. A combination of flexion, external rotation, internal rotation, and abduction are used always with the elbow in 90° of flexion to shorten the lever arm and always with instructions to push with only 1 to 2 pounds (0.45–0.90 kg) of pressure in a pain-free manner. Note that if a long lever arm or a large pushing force is used, then an unsafe strain might occur on the repair even if it is not directly activated by the isometric exercise. Depending on the preference of the physician and the security of the repair, sometimes isometric exercises that activate the repaired tendon might be allowed during phase 2 rehabilitation, and at other times, they might be withheld. In certain situations, the physician might allow light strengthening into directions that do not stress the repair (eg, external rotation strengthening if only the subscapularis is repaired). Only light force should be used with limited repetitions in this situation during phase 2 if these activities are included.

A large part of phase 2 rehabilitation after repair of a massive rotator cuff tear is educating the patient about the necessity of continuing to minimize active use of the upper extremity during ADLs at this time to promote long-term clinical healing of the repair. Nonrepetitive waist-level reaching for objects of negligible weight (<1–2 pounds [0.45–0.90 kg]) is allowed as long as it can be done comfortably. Use of the surgically repaired extremity at waist level with weight and active use of the extremity with the elbow at chest level or higher are discouraged during phase 2, even if these activities do not cause pain, because they place stress on the repair. The physicians and rehabilitation providers at our facility believe that frequent use of the upper extremity for these types of activities theoretically might diminish the chance and quality of healing of the repaired tendons. Although these activities are not clearly detrimental, we believe that the short-term benefit derived from using the extremity for these activities during this time is not worth the potential risk of disturbing the one chance that the repair has to heal. Therefore, some patients are held back from activities that they have the physical ability to perform. For patients who achieve their staged ROMs and functional goals easily, regular therapy sessions with the rehabilitation provider are not needed. These patients continue very limited exercises at home. A very occasional clinical follow-up can be used to determine compliance with restrictions of activity and to reinforce that adhering to these restrictions is important.

Phase 3

Phase 3 rehabilitation after partial repair of the massive rotator cuff tear is similar to phase 2 rehabilitation after repair of a routine rotator cuff tear but has moderate adjustments because, realistically, all patients will not achieve full PROM, full AROM, or full strength and the patient in this situation does not have an anatomically normal shoulder. The focus of phase 3, which typically constitutes postoperative week 12 and later, is to achieve functional PROM, to begin a well-structured AROM and strengthening progression that gradually increases demand to the musculature of the shoulder girdle while protecting the repair and not overloading the rotator cuff force couples, and to minimize inflammation and pain. The later part of phase 3 focuses on strengthening within reason and improving endurance and functional use of the upper extremity. The rehabilitation provider still always must ensure that the stress of the activities in the rehabilitation program is less than the strength of the surgical repair.

Obtaining realistic functional flexibility while keeping the levels of pain and inflammation low should be an early priority of phase 3 rehabilitation if this has not already been achieved in phase 2. A variable amount of stretching is needed to achieve this goal. Typically, these patients gain PROM very easily in phase 2 and phase 3, so often they do not need advanced stretching or need only very minimal selected stretching that does not directly stress repaired tissues unless substantial tightness is present because the supraspinatus is absent. If the ROM of the patient is substantially less

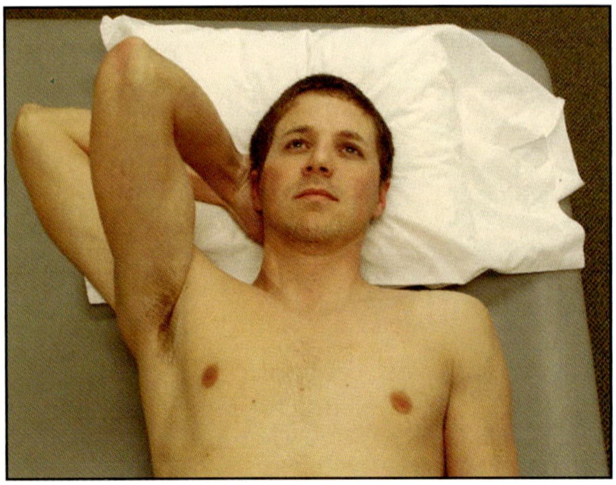

Figure 18. Supine hand-behind-head stretch to increase abduction and external rotation.

than staged goals but the physician expects nearly normal flexibility, then PROM might be emphasized. During home-based exercise at this time, the patient with a partial repair of a massive rotator cuff tear is allowed to initiate gentle stretching in planes of motion other than PFE and PER in slight abduction. This stretching most commonly includes the supine hand-behind-head stretch and functional internal rotation (Figures 18 and 19). Posterior shoulder stretching, such as the horizontal adduction stretch or sleeper stretch, is rarely appropriate in these patients. These motions place a moderate direct stress on the infraspinatus, which must be protected because it is the posterior pillar of the suspension bridge. The quality of the repaired or native tissue of this tendon is frequently fair to poor; its failure strength is usually fairly low; and because the supraspinatus is irreparable, few structures are available to shield it from stress during these interventions. Therefore, protecting the integrity of the infraspinatus is of the utmost importance during all aspects of phase 3 rehabilitation. This is an example that during rehabilitation of these patients, almost all passive stretching might place direct stress on the repair. Whether this is advantageous depends on the details of the repair, the quality of repaired tissues, the severity of the ROM limitation, and the desired functional goals of the patient. The patient, physician, and rehabilitation provider jointly must decide specific and realistic ROM goals for planes of motion other than PFE and PER on an individual basis.

For the reasons discussed, the failure strength of the repair in the patient with a partial repair of a massive

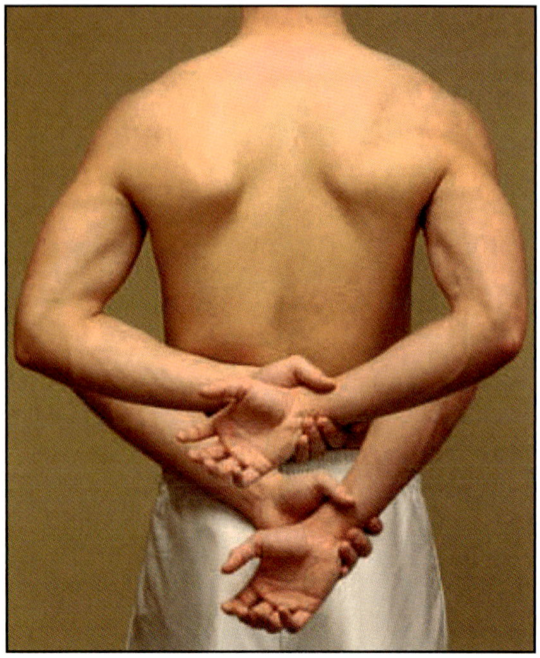

Figure 19. Functional internal rotation active-assistive range of motion.

rotator cuff tear during phase 3 rehabilitation is much less than that of a repair of a routine-sized tear and usually less than that of a repair of a massive-sized tear. Failure strength varies widely based on many factors. In addition, because part of the rotator cuff is irreparable and a portion of the remaining rotator cuff has been repaired, the patient's ability to achieve AROM against gravity, especially overhead, might not be realistic, or it is often a very long and difficult process, occasionally taking from 6 to 9 months or longer to achieve. Therefore, when starting the AROM and strengthening phase of rehabilitation, the rehabilitation provider carefully must select exercises that start with very low stress to the healing tissue and must progress in a gradual and measured way that does not overload the rotator cuff force couple. When beginning AROM and strengthening, selecting exercises that have a very low documented EMG activity and ordering them so that the activity level in the rotator cuff slowly increases should be the primary criteria for advancing exercises and selecting planes of movement that do not place excessive tension on the repair. Our base AROM to strengthening progression, which is outlined in the Appendix and detailed in chapter II-4, incorporates these principles.

Modifications to the base program often are needed in this patient population because the force-generating

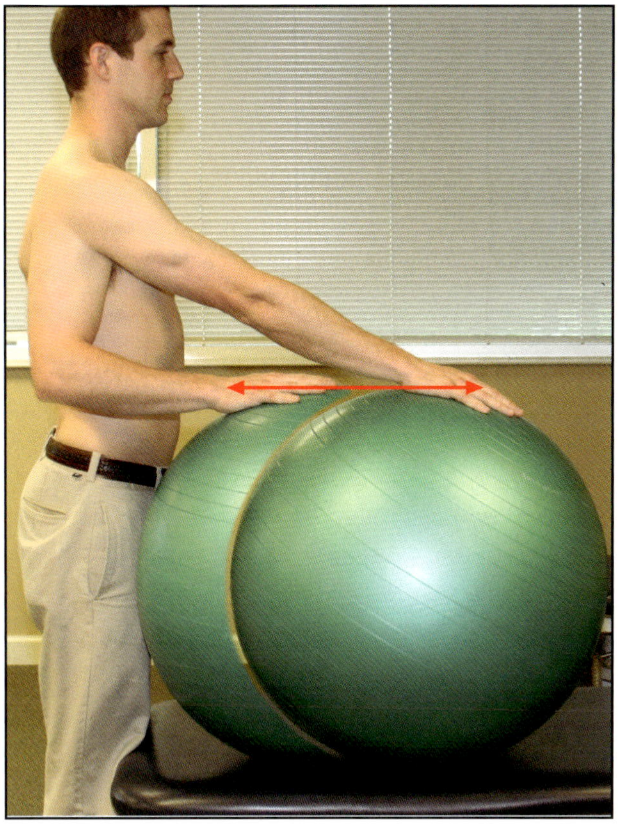

Figure 20. Horizontal dusting on a Swiss ball.

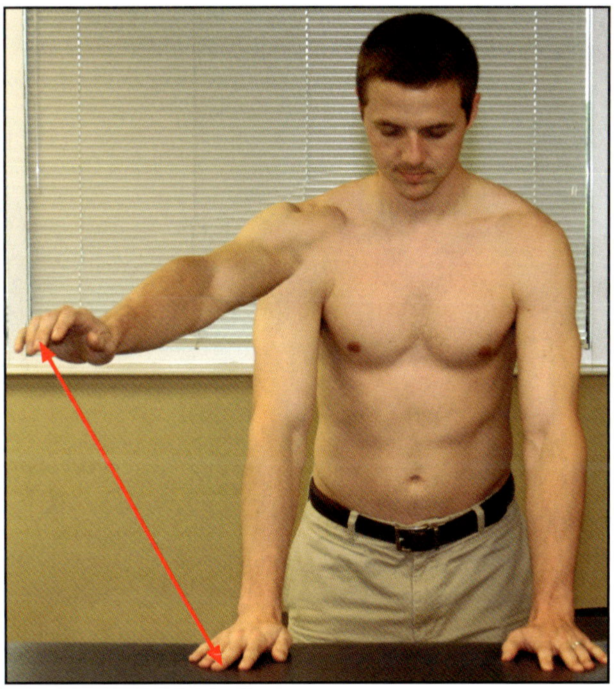

Figure 21. Static closed chain stabilization of the affected (left) extremity with reaching of the right hand to provide a minimal perturbation. Ensure that only minimal weight bearing is present through the affected extremity and no excessive superior humeral head migration occurs.

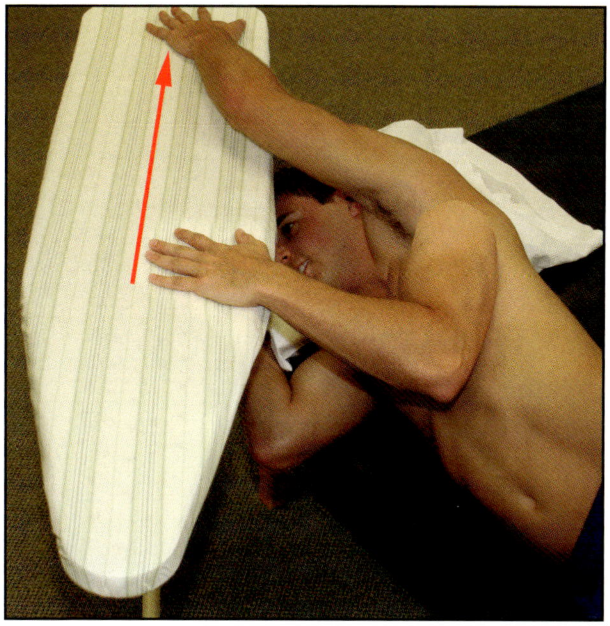

Figure 22. Side-lying, gravity-minimized forward elevation.

and stabilizing capacity of the rotator cuff might be very minimal at this time. Although our AROM and strengthening progression begins at a very low level and progresses slowly, adjustments often need to be made to the Appendix to help ensure that the rotator cuff force couple is not overloaded. This means that the load to the rotator cuff is greater than what it can stabilize and control. These adjustments are discussed in the following paragraphs. As mentioned, I believe it is important to use only rehabilitation activities and ADLs that the patient can perform with good centering of the humeral head to help facilitate correct activation of the rotator cuff force couples and minimize abnormal strain to the remaining tissues.

The beginning phase 3 AROM and strengthening program for these patients often includes interventions, such as horizontal dusting on a table top (Figure 17) or on a Swiss ball (Figure 20); gentle static closed chain activities in which the involved hand does not move with minimal weight bearing (Figure 21); more frequent use of the side-lying, gravity-minimized AFE exercise (Figure 22); and use of supine exercises in the shoulder's "balance position." To exercise in the balance position of the shoulder, the patient is positioned supine with the elbow extended and the shoulder flexed to 90° (Figure 23A). In this position, the perpendicular distance from the line of action to the center of rotation of the shoulder is minimal or zero. The length of this lever arm in relation to the downward

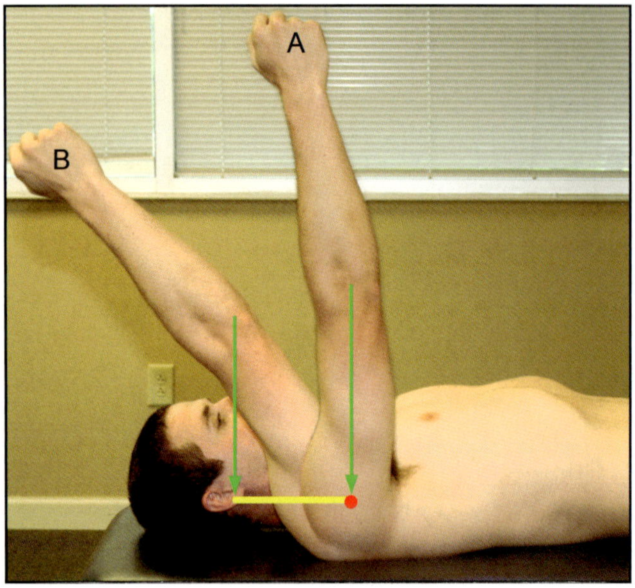

Figure 23. A, The balance position of the shoulder in the supine position. The perpendicular distance from the line of action (green arrow) to the center of rotation of the shoulder (red dot) is zero. B, Outside of the balance position. The perpendicular distance from the line of action (green arrow) to the center of rotation of the shoulder (red dot) has increased greatly and is illustrated by the yellow line.

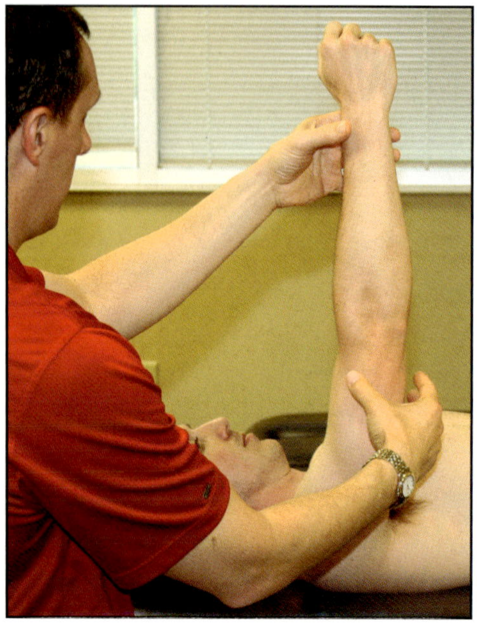

Figure 24. The rehabilitation provider assists the patient to the balance point. The assistance is then removed, and the patient must maintain a stationary position independently. The support is close by in case the patient cannot maintain this position.

resistance of gravity also is minimal or zero (Figure 23A).[29] In this position, the rotator cuff needs minimal muscle activation to keep the humeral head centered in the glenoid. Instead, it mainly is accomplished by the downward axial compressive force of gravity on the glenohumeral joint and a medially directed force vector of the deltoid on the humerus.[34] As the shoulder moves away from this balance point in any direction, the muscle activity needed to stabilize the shoulder progressively increases as the effective lever arm increases (Figure 23B). The specific muscles that are most active vary depending on the direction of movement. Chapter II-5 provides a more detailed discussion of these concepts. Figures 24–26 illustrate the balance point exercises that I commonly use in the early part of phase 3 rehabilitation.

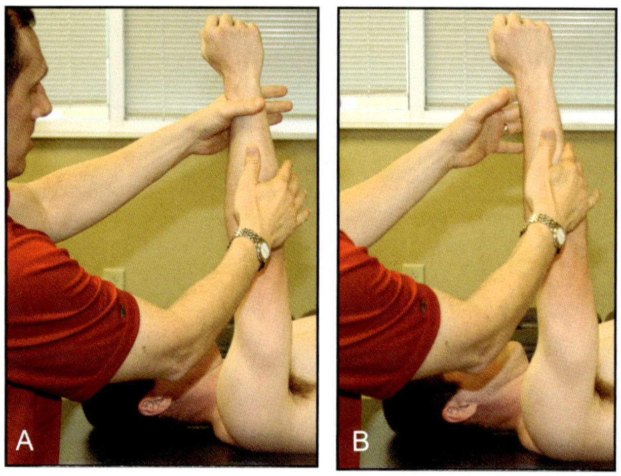

Figure 25 A and B. The patient begins in and must maintain the balance point while the rehabilitation provider applies gentle, manual perturbations in multiple planes.

After the patient can easily perform these types of exercises, active forward reaching at waist to chest level typically can be performed with minimal to no excessive superior humeral head migration. At this point, selected exercises in the base strengthening progression and assistive-to-active shoulder elevation progression (AASEP) are initiated. Typically, forward reaching with an elastic band is too difficult due to pain, weakness, or abnormal movement. Internal rotation with an elastic band and scapular strengthening with elastic resistance commonly are prescribed. External rotation with an elastic band is often too difficult, so side-lying external rotation (Figure 27) can be used at this stage without weight. The AASEP exercises that I commonly use at this stage include supine forward elevation with an elastic band (Figure 28), supine reaching progression (Figure 29), rope-and-pulley AAROM in the plane of the scapula, and

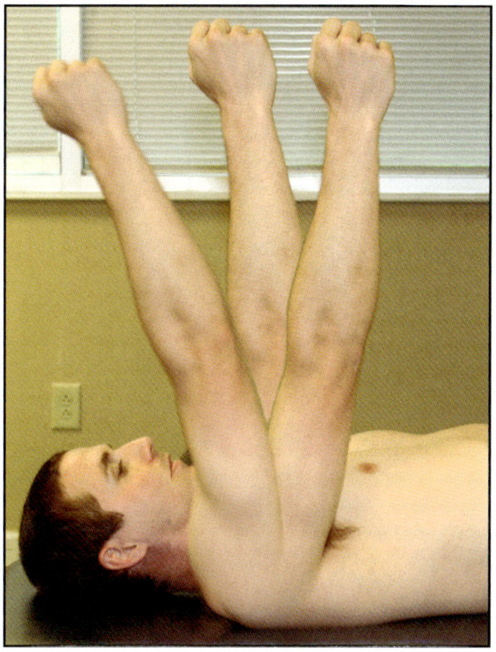

Figure 26. The patient begins in the balance point then actively moves outside this position into flexion and extension. He keeps the motion fairly small to actively control the extremity because larger range of motion requires more muscle activation.

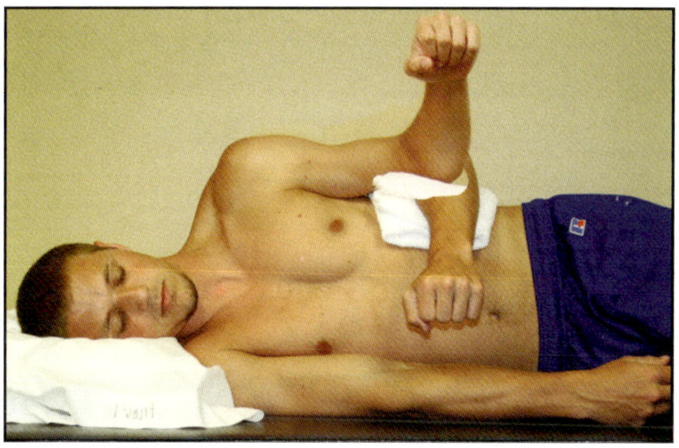

Figure 27. Side-lying external rotation exercise.

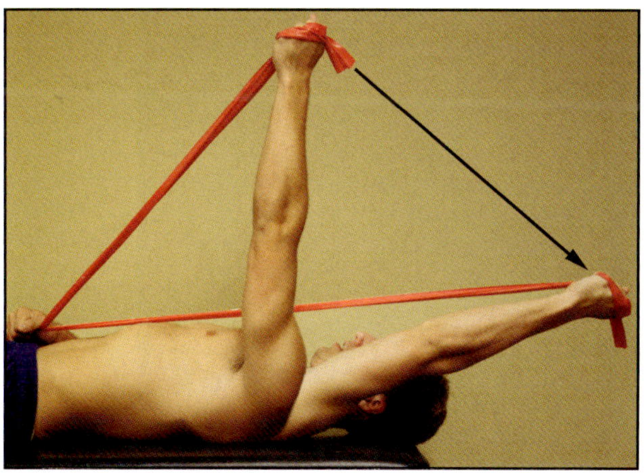

Figure 28. Supine forward elevation with an elastic band.

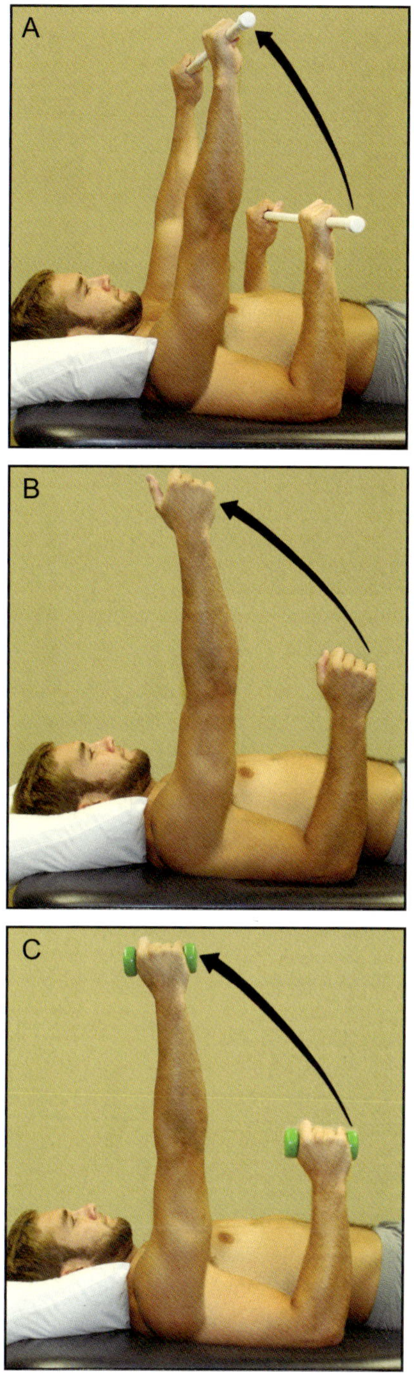

Figure 29 A–C. Supine reaching progression. In all levels of the progression, reaching begins with the elbow bent and ends with the elbow straight. All levels of the progression do not need to be used clinically. A, Step 1: assistive reaching from 0° to 90° with support via a polyvinyl chloride pipe. B, Step 2: active reaching from 0° to 90°. C, Step 3: resistive reaching from 0° to 90° with 1 to 2 lb (0.45–0.90 kg).

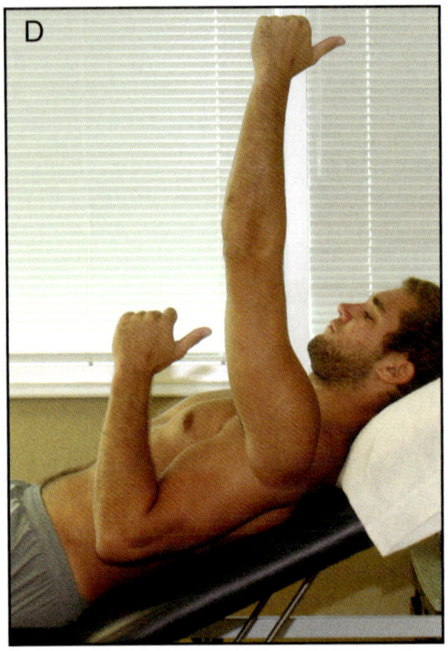

Figure 29 D. Step 4: incline reaching to the ceiling with or without 1 to 2 lb (0.45–0.90 kg).

ball roll on a wall (Figure 30). I carefully evaluate all interventions to make sure moderate ROM can be used without deviation and that the humeral head remains visually centered.

When the patient can easily perform these types of exercise, AFE is typically between 80° and 120°. The base strengthening program that is outlined in the Appendix and detailed in chapter II-4 is still emphasized, and external rotation and forward reaching exercises with an elastic band (Figure 31) are more likely to be used. However, some patients never have enough strength to properly perform these exercises, so they are not used for all patients. To maximize the patient's active overhead use of the upper extremity, I commonly employ the AASEP, such as incline dusting (Figure 32), upright AAFE and assisted lowering, progressing to AAFE with independent active lowering (Figure 33), and eventually upper extremity wall slides.

A long-term maintenance home exercise program is established after the physician and rehabilitation provider agree that the patient has maximized his or her functional potential for overhead AROM. At our center, we believe it is vitally important for these patients to keep their remaining rotator cuff optimally functional because the irreparable supraspinatus leaves an anatomic deficit. We believe the maintenance program for this patient population should not be a high-intensity program but instead should be a

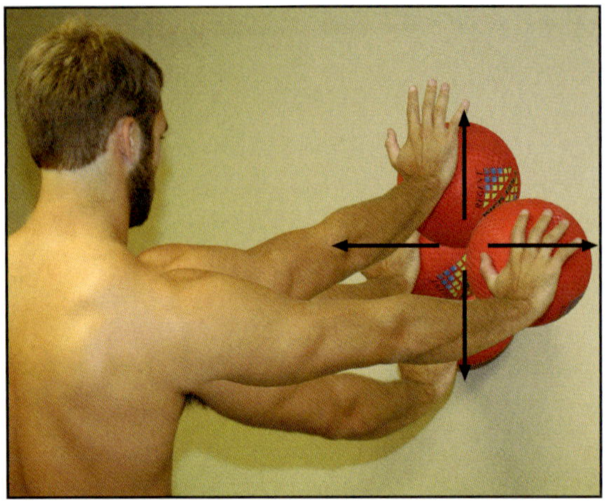

Figure 30. Ball roll on a wall. The elbow remains straight throughout the entire exercise.

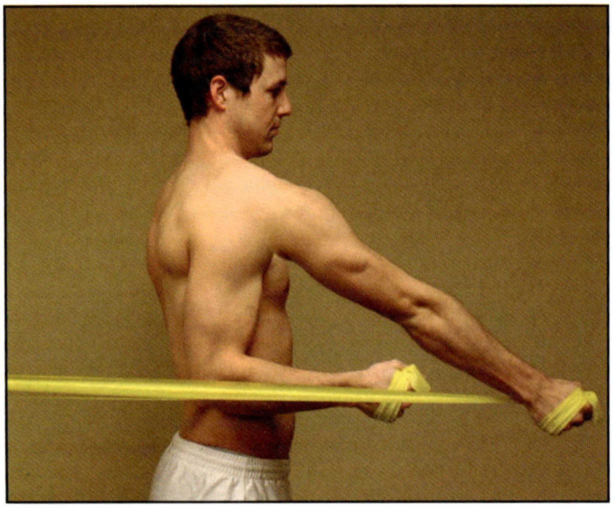

Figure 31. Forward reaching with an elastic band.

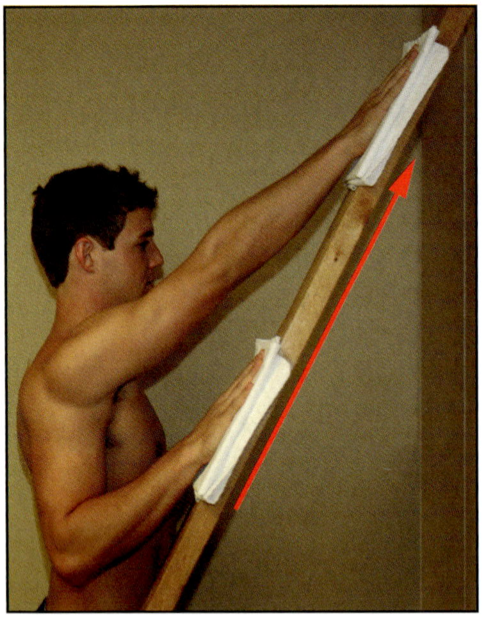

Figure 32. Incline dusting.

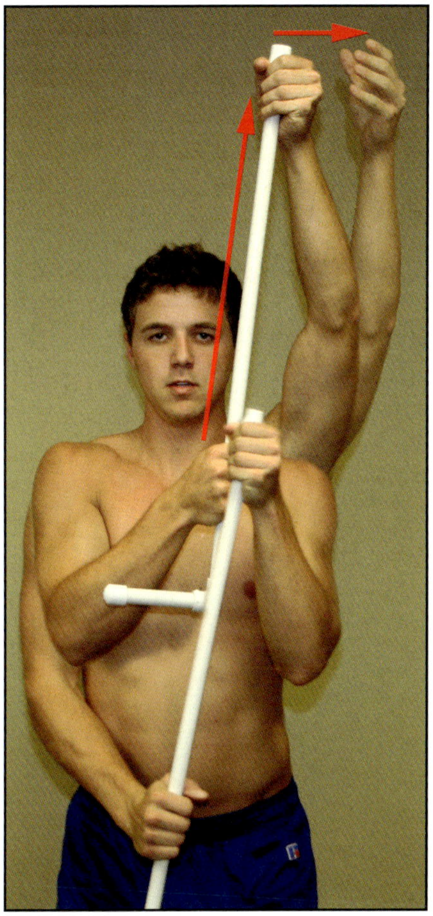

Figure 33. Standing L-bar assistive elevation and active lowering. Support also can be provided by the unaffected hand instead of the L-bar.

program that includes light resistance and moderate to large numbers of repetitions, with the rehabilitation provider choosing basic interventions that are of low risk for overloading the rotator cuff force couple. Typically, it includes internal rotation with an elastic band, either side-lying external rotation or external rotation with an elastic band, and resisted scapular retraction. It might include forward reaching with an elastic band if the exercise can be performed easily without excessive superior migration of the humeral head. Finally, it usually includes 1 or 2 AASEP exercises to help facilitate proper functioning of the rotator cuff and deltoid force couple without overloading it. In a patient with nearly normal function, AFE with either a 0.5-pound (0.225-kg) or 1-pound (0.45-kg) weight might be appropriate. In a patient with more limited overhead AROM, incline dusting or supine forward elevation with elastic resistance might be appropriate. In a patient who cannot actively reach above shoulder level, rope-and-pulley AAROM might be appropriate. This program typically is prescribed to be performed for 30 to 40 repetitions 3 to 7 times each week.

Finally, general rehabilitation guidelines, principles for progression, and hints for proper exercise selection that are detailed in phase 3 of the text of chapter III-2 are critically important to understand and follow. The reader is encouraged to review that chapter to fully understand the clinical decision-making process for patients with a partial repair of a massive rotator cuff tear.

SPECIAL CONSIDERATIONS

Infraspinatus or Subscapularis Repaired and the Opposing Tendon Intact

In this situation, one side of the theoretical suspension bridge is damaged preoperatively and restored during surgery. For these patients, the base protocol is used, ensuring that the strengthening progression targeting the repaired tendon is very gentle and realizing that direct stretching to the repair is not performed unless substantial tightness is present. The surgeon might allow initiation of strengthening to unrepaired tendons sooner than postoperative week 12, especially if the subscapularis is repaired and the infraspinatus is intact; however, great care must be used so that the rotator cuff force couples stay balanced and the repaired tissues are protected from repetitive stress.

Infraspinatus or Subscapularis Repaired and the Opposing Tendon Torn and Not Reparable

In this situation, both sides of the suspension bridge are damaged preoperatively, and only 1 side can be repaired or restored during surgery, so proper functioning of the rotator cuff force couples in the transverse or coronal planes is not expected. Often, a part of the irreparable subscapularis or infraspinatus tendon still is attached to its insertion and might provide some dynamic stability. In this scenario, PROM usually is achieved easily, so basic stretching exercises are typically all that are ever used. Active ROM and function usually return slowly and might be very limited, and poor active use of the extremity overhead is not uncommon. The patient often uses a slower and more limited version of our standard rehabilitation guideline, focusing on training the remaining muscles to work together as a unit to improve force coupling during the AROM and strengthening phase. Occasionally, the physician determines that the patient might be more appropriate for a limited-goals rehabilitation program that is detailed in chapter III-18.

Debridement of the Completely Irreparable Massive Rotator Cuff Tear

In this situation, no rotator cuff repair is performed. If the subscapularis and infraspinatus are intact and only the supraspinatus is irreparably torn, then the normal rehabilitation guideline is used except the surgeon typically allows the patient to begin isometric exercises at postoperative weeks 3 to 4 and also allows the patient to begin base strengthening and the AASEP at postoperative week 6 instead of postoperative week 12. If the subscapularis or infraspinatus is irreparably torn in addition to the supraspinatus, the quicker initiation of isometric exercises and dynamic strengthening still might be allowed, but a much slower and more limited progression is prudent because much more limited AROM and function are expected. A limited-goals rehabilitation program commonly is used especially if the infraspinatus, supraspinatus, and subscapularis are irreparable.

Is a Faster Progression Ever Warranted?

If the patient had only debridement of an irreparable single-tendon or multitendon rotator cuff tear (ie, no repair), isometric exercises can be started as early as postoperative weeks 3 to 4, and strengthening of the remaining shoulder girdle muscles can begin at postoperative week 6 in the manner discussed. In some younger patients with a partial repair of a massive rotator cuff tear and good-quality tissue, some surgeons might allow isometric exercises to begin between postoperative weeks 3 to 6 and base strengthening and the AASEP progression to begin at postoperative weeks 6 to 9. In this situation, the rehabilitation provider must be especially careful and use a slow exercise progression so the rotator cuff force couples are not overloaded and no excessive superior migration of the humeral head occurs.

REFERENCES

1. Inman VT, Saunders JBDM, Abbot LC. Observations of the function of the shoulder joint. *J Bone Joint Surg Am.* 1944;26(1):1–30.
2. Sharkey NA, Marder RA. The rotator cuff opposes superior translation of the humeral head. *Am J Sports Med.* 1995;23(3):270–275.
3. Colachis SC Jr, Strohm BR. Effect of suprascapular and axillary nerve blocks on muscle force in upper extremity. *Arch Phys Med Rehabil.* 1971;52(1):22–29.
4. Poppen NK, Walker PS. Normal and abnormal motion of the shoulder. *J Bone Joint Surg Am.* 1976;58(2):195–201.
5. Yamaguchi K, Sher JS, Andersen WK, et al. Glenohumeral motion in patients with rotator cuff tears: a comparison of asymptomatic and symptomatic shoulders. *J Shoulder Elbow Surg.* 2000;9(1):6–11.
6. Deutsch A, Altchek DW, Schwartz E, Otis JC, Warren RF. Radiologic measurement of superior displacement of the humeral head in impingement syndrome. *J Shoulder Elbow Surg.* 1996;5(3):186–193.
7. Chen SK, Simonian PT, Wickiewicz TL, Otis JC, Warren RF. Radiographic evaluation of glenohumeral kinematics: a muscle fatigue model. *J Shoulder Elbow Surg.* 1999;8(1):49–52.
8. Mura N, O'Driscoll SW, Zobitz ME, et al. The effect of infraspinatus disruption on glenohumeral torque and superior migration of the humeral head: a biomechanical study. *J Shoulder Elbow Surg.* 2003;12(2):179–184.
9. Halder AM, Zhao KD, O'Driscoll SW, Morrey BF, An KN. Dynamic contributions to superior shoulder stability. *J Orthop Res.* 2001;19(2):206–212.
10. Thompson WO, Debski RE, Boardman ND III, et al. A biomechanical analysis of rotator cuff deficiency in a cadaveric model. *Am J Sports Med.* 1996;24(3):286–292.
11. Apreleva M, Parsons IM IV, Warner JJP, Fu FH, Woo SLY. Experimental investigation of reaction forces at the glenohumeral joint during active abduction. *J Shoulder Elbow Surg.* 2000;9(5):409–417.
12. Klein AH, McKernan DJ, Harner CD, Davis PL, Fu FH. A study of rotator cuff force vectors across the glenohumeral joint using magnetic resonance imaging. *Trans Orthop Res Soc.* 1989;14:230.
13. Burkhart SS. Fluoroscopic comparison of kinematic patterns in massive rotator cuff tears: a suspension bridge model. *Clin Orthop Relat Res.* 1992;284:144–152.
14. Burkhart SS, Nottage WM, Ogilvie-Harris DJ, Kohn HS, Pachelli A. Partial repair of irreparable rotator cuff tears. *Arthroscopy.* 1994;10(4):363–370.
15. Duralde XA, Bair B. Massive rotator cuff tears: the result of partial rotator cuff repair. *J Shoulder Elbow Surg.* 2005;14(2):121–127.
16. Yu J, McGarry MH, Lee YS, Duong LV, Lee TQ. Biomechanical effects of supraspinatus repair on the glenohumeral joint. *J Shoulder Elbow Surg.* 2005;14(1 suppl S):65S–71S.
17. Andarawis-Puri N, Ricchetti ET, Soslowsky LJ. Interaction between the supraspinatus and infraspinatus tendons: effect of anterior supraspinatus tendon full-thickness tears on infraspinatus tendon strain. *Am J Sports Med.* 2009;37(9):1831–1839.

18. Perry SM, Getz CL, Soslowsky LJ. After rotator cuff tears, the remaining (intact) tendons are mechanically altered. *J Shoulder Elbow Surg*. 2009;18(1):52–57.
19. Levy O, Mullett H, Roberts S, Copeland S. The role of anterior deltoid reeducation in patients with massive irreparable degenerative rotator cuff tears. *J Shoulder Elbow Surg*. 2008;17(6):863–870.
20. Gerber C, Schneeberger AG, Hoppeler H, Meyer DC. Correlation of atrophy and fatty infiltration on strength and integrity of rotator cuff repairs: a study in thirteen patients. *J Shoulder Elbow Surg*. 2007;16(6):691–696.
21. Goutallier D, Postel JM, Radier C, Bernageau J, Zilber S. Long-term functional and structural outcome in patients with intact repairs 1 year after open transosseous rotator cuff repair. *J Shoulder Elbow Surg*. 2009;18(4):521–528.
22. Galatz LM, Ball CM, Teefey SA, Middleton WD, Yamaguchi K. The outcome and repair integrity of completely arthroscopically repaired large and massive rotator cuff tears. *J Bone Joint Surg Am*. 2004;86(2):219–224.
23. Nho SJ, Brown BS, Lyman S, Adler RS, Altchek DW, MacGillivray JD. Prospective analysis of arthroscopic rotator cuff repair: prognostic factors affecting clinical and ultrasound outcome. *J Shoulder Elbow Surg*. 2009;18(1):13–20.
24. Dockery ML, Wright TW, La Stayo PC. Electromyography of the shoulder: an analysis of passive modes of exercise. *Orthopedics*. 1998;21(11):1181–1184.
25. McCann PD, Wootten ME, Kadaba MP, Bigliani LU. A kinematic and electromyographic study of shoulder rehabilitation exercises. *Clin Orthop Relat Res*. 1993;288:179–188.
26. Gaunt BW, McCluskey GM, Uhl TL. Electromyographic evaluation of subdividing active-assistive shoulder exercises. *Sports Health*. 2010;2(5):424–432.
27. Long JL, Ruberte Thiele RA, Skendzel J, et al. Activation of the shoulder musculature during pendulum exercises and light activities. *J Orthop Sports Phys Ther*. 2010;40(4):230–237.
28. Fujisawa H, Suenaga N, Minami A. Electromyographic study during isometric exercises of the shoulder in head-out water immersion. *J Shoulder Elbow Surg*. 1998;7(5):491–494.
29. Uhl TL, Muir TA, Lawson L. Electromyographic assessment of passive, active assistive, and active shoulder rehabilitation exercises. *PM R*. 2010;2(2):132–141.
30. Gimbel JA, Van Kleunen JP, Williams GR, Thomopoulos S, Soslowsky LJ. Long durations of immobilization in the rat result in enhanced mechanical properties of the healing supraspinatus tendon insertion site. *J Biomech Eng*. 2007;129(3):400–404.
31. Gimbel JA, Van Kleunen JP, Lake SP, Williams GR, Soslowsky LJ. The role of repair tension on tendon to bone healing in an animal model of chronic rotator cuff tears. *J Biomech*. 2007;40(3):561–568.
32. Peltz CD, Sarver JJ, Dourte LM, Würgler-Hauri CC, Williams GR, Soslowsky LJ. Exercise following a short immobilization period is detrimental to tendon properties and joint mechanics in a rat rotator cuff injury model. *J Orthop Res*. 2010;28(7):841–845.
33. Peltz CD, Dourte LM, Kuntz AF, et al. The effect of postoperative passive motion on rotator cuff healing in a rat model. *J Bone Joint Surg Am*. 2009;91(10):2421–2429.
34. Poppen NK, Walker PS. Forces at the glenohumeral joint in abduction. *Clin Orthop Relat Res*. 1978;135:165–170.

PARTIAL REPAIR OF THE MASSIVE ROTATOR CUFF TEAR REHABILITATION GUIDELINE

St. Francis Orthopaedic Institute and St. Francis Rehabilitation Center

All information contained in this protocol is to be used as a general guideline only. Specific variations might be appropriate for each patient and might be specified by the physician. In all cases, it is acceptable to advance the program more slowly than stated. If the patient experiences excessive pain, discontinue exercise until the physician is contacted. ***Achieving and maintaining a low level of pain and inflammation and protecting the surgical repair are the guiding principles in all stages of rehabilitation, even if less passive and active range of motion are accomplished.***

SYMBOLS AND ABBREVIATIONS

AAFE, active-assistive forward elevation
AAROM, active-assistive range of motion
AASEP, assistive-to-active shoulder elevation progression
ADLs, activities of daily living
AFE, active forward elevation
AROM, active range of motion
EMG, electromyography
ER, external rotation
FE, forward elevation
IR, internal rotation
NA, not applicable
PER, passive external rotation
PFE, passive forward elevation
POD, postoperative day
POM, postoperative month
POW, postoperative week
PRN, as needed
PROM, passive range of motion
ROM, range of motion
T-Band (Thera-Band, The Hygenic Corporation, Akron, OH)
WFL, within functional limits
WNL, within normal limits

Forward elevation, either active or passive, is the plane of motion in which an individual naturally lifts his or her arm that is anterior to the plane of the scapula and lateral to flexion.

STAGED GOALS FOR RANGE OF MOTION

These are approximate targets for range of motion. Specific limits might be specified by the physician, especially if a subscapularis repair was performed.

Time	PFE	PER at 20° of Abduction	PER at 90° of Abduction	AFE
POD 1	50°	0°	NA	NA
POW 1	70°–100°	0°–20°	NA	NA
POW 3	90°–120°	15°–35°	NA	NA
POW 6	120°–145°	40°–50°	45°–60°	NA
POW 12	140°–160°	WFL	60°–80°	50°–90°
POM 5	WNL	WFL	WFL	90°–155°

PHASE 1

Goals

°Minimize pain and inflammatory response
°Maximally protect the surgical repair
°Achieve staged ROM goals
°Educate the patient about postoperative precautions
°Establish a stable scapula

HPRC at St. Francis Rehabilitation Center

POD 1 to POW 6

- °Elbow, wrist, and hand AROM with no weight
- °Scapular elevations and retractions (no weight) in or out of the sling
- °Pendulum exercises
  - °Lean over the table a comfortable amount
  - °Let the arm hang down relaxed
  - °Keep the body still
  - °As able, move the arm in small comfortable circles only
- °Upright PER in slight abduction until mild stretch and discomfort
  - °7 to 12 repetitions 2 times per day
  - °Preferred exercises
    - °Sit with family member or therapist rotating the arm (Figure 14)
    - °PER walk-around (stand with the arm supported on a table and rotate the body) (Figure 15)
- °PFE until mild stretch and discomfort
  - °7 to 12 repetitions 2 times per day
  - °Preferred exercises
    - °Sit with family member or therapist lifting the arm (Figure 12)
    - °Table step-back exercise (Figure 11)
    - °Kinex KS2 (Kinex Medical Company, LLC, Waukesha, WI) continous passive motion machine for 10 to 20 minutes 2 to 4 times per day
    - °Patient-assisted supine AAFE exercise (usually not before POW 4 and use the unaffected arm for assistance) (Figure 13)
- °Ice for pain reduction
- °Fit the sling properly
  - °Ensure the sling provides a slight lift to the shoulder girdle and supports the wrist
- °Patient education
  - °Primary focus of phase 1: encourage initial healing of the surgical repair
  - °Use of a sling and as instructed by physician; typically, full time in community and if up at home for more than 5 to 10 minutes
  - °Minimal use of the arm for light waist-level activities as comfortable
  - °Ensure the level of pain is not increasing because of excessive use of the arm for ADLs or work
  - °Sleep in a recliner
    - °3 weeks (required)
    - °6 weeks (preferred)

Adjunctive Exercises

- °Therapist-assisted supine PROM within comfortable ROM to
  - °Decrease muscle guarding
  - °Gain patient confidence
  - °Achieve staged PROM goals (no mobilizations)
- °Cervical spine AROM
- °Pain-control agents PRN
- °Aquatic therapy for gentle, pain-free AAROM (no swimming strokes) after the incision has healed completely

Interventions to Avoid

- °Home exercise glenohumeral PROM in planes other then PFE and PER
- °Exercises that result in moderate or severe pain
- °Exercises that result in excessive guarding or splinting of muscles
- °Weighted exercises
- °Cross-body adduction, reaching behind the back, rope-and-pulley for elevation, and active elevation of the arm above waist level
- °Repetitive activity with the affected extremity

PHASE 2

Goals

- °Continue to maximally protect the surgical repair
- °Achieve staged PROM goals
- °Minimize shoulder pain
- °Work toward active forward reaching to waist level

POW 6 to 12

- °Achieve staged ROM goals in FE
- °Preferred exercises
  - °Rope-and-pulley exercise (elbows remain straight) (Figure 16)
  - °Patient-assisted supine AAFE exercise (use unaffected arm for assistance) (Figure 13)
  - °Continue table step-back exercise if above exercises are not tolerated
- °Achieve staged ROM goals in ER at 20° using upright exercises
- °Initiate horizontal dusting (Figure 17)
  - °Perform straight ahead
  - °Perform at 20° angles medially and laterally if comfortable
- °Submaximal pain-free isometrics **(if approved by physician)**
  - °Perform with elbow flexed and instruct the patient to press with a 1- to 2-pound force only
  - °Flexion, ER, IR, and abduction might be allowed

Adjunctive Exercises

- °Therapist-assisted supine PROM and light stretching
  - °Can include ER and IR in increased angles of abduction, diagonal elevation, and horizontal adduction if ROM is below staged goals
- °Modalities PRN
- °Aquatic exercises (chapter IV-9)
  - °AAROM
  - °AROM
- °Spine therapy assessment and mobilization if
  - °Nonneurogenic cervical or scapular pain or
  - °Limitation in end-range shoulder FE
- °Golf chipping and putting if approved by the physician

Interventions to Avoid

- °Any AROM exercise into elevation or strengthening exercise with resistance
- °Exercises that greatly increase signs and symptoms

PHASE 3

Goals

- °Achieve staged ROM goals
- °Minimize shoulder pain
- °Maximize AROM
- °Increase strength and endurance
- °Return to realistic functional activities

POM 3 to 6 and Longer

- °Achieve staged ROM goals in FE
- °Achieve staged ROM goals in ER at 20° using upright exercises
- °Initiate home exercise PROM into expanded directions judiciously **only if a large deficit is present**
  - °Supine hand-behind-head stretch PRN (Figure 18)
  - °Functional IR AAROM and stretching PRN (Figure 19)
  - °Horizontal adduction or sleeper stretch, or both, is seldom used
- °Initiate base strengthening progression
  - °Includes beginning rotator cuff, deltoid, and scapular strengthening program
  - °2 times per day at most with light resistance and increasing repetitions
  - °Yellow T-Band for ER and IR
    - °5- to 6-foot band length and light or no pretension in a 3- to 6-inch arc of motion
    - °Often use side-lying ER (Figure 27) instead of T-Band due to ER weakness
  - °Yellow T-Band forward reach (Figure 31) PRN
    - **°Do not initiate until most assistive elevation exercises from the AASEP described below can be performed easily and ensure that this exercise can be performed without excessive superior humeral head migration. Often, this is later than POM 4.**
    - °Initially, 5- to 6-foot band length and light or no pretension
    - °Start with the elbow bent and by the side and the band tied behind the patient
    - °Reach forward with the hand at waist level, progressing to reaching **forward** at chest level
    - °If forward reach is painful or difficult, replace with a gravity-minimized exercise from the AASEP described below until it is comfortable
  - °Scapular strengthening emphasizing scapular retractions and scapular upward rotators (chapter IV-2)
  - °Low-level closed chain strengthening PRN (chapter II-4)
  - **°No prone FE, abduction, or ER**
- °Initiate the AASEP as comfortable (chapter II-4)
  - °A stepwise progression in difficulty of strengthening exercises from PFE to AFE against gravity
  - °Goal of the progression is to achieve pain-free full AFE
  - °EMG demonstrates progressive activation of the cuff and deltoid during the progression
  - °If scapular or glenohumeral substitutions or pain are present, choose an easier exercise in the progression
  - °The order of the exercise sequence has some variability
  - °Usually not all exercises need to be performed

°The patient might advance through this progression exceptionally slowly, so this might constitute a very large portion of phase 3 rehabilitation

°Do not perform the base strengthening program or overhead strengthening progression until overall level of pain is low

°Ensure that these exercises do not increase signs and symptoms

°Exercises are divided into 3 levels of difficulty

1. Gravity-minimized exercises
    - °Horizontal dusting (Figure 17)
        - °Perform straight ahead and perform at 20° angles medially and laterally if comfortable
    - °T-Band supine FE (Figure 28)
        - °Must start the involved arm at 90° of elevation
        - °Pull the arm into FE
    - °Side-lying, gravity-minimized AFE (Figure 22)
        - °Lie on the uninvolved side
        - °Place the involved arm on an ironing board
        - °Slide the hand on the board
    - °Jackins supine reaching progression
        - °Begin at 0° with the elbow bent and end at 90° of elevation with the elbow extended
        - °Start with the assistance of a cane or wand (Figure 29A)
        - °Progress to active motion (Figure 29B)
        - °Can progress to using a 1- to 2-pound weight (Figure 29C)
        - °Can progress to the inclined position, continuing to reach to the ceiling (Figure 29D)
2. Assistive elevation exercises
    - °Rope-and-pulley AAFE (Figure 16)
    - °Incline dusting (Figure 32)
        - °Standing AAFE (assistive elevation and descent via T-bar or unaffected arm)
        - °Standing assistive elevation and active independent eccentric lowering (Figure 33)
        - °Wall-slide AAFE
            - °Ensure that the patient is in FE and is not in flexion
            - °Must be pain-free and natural when performed
3. Unsupported elevation exercises
    - °Overhead wall taps
    - °AFE (Figure 34)
    - °Initiate AFE after the AASEP is complete
    - °Only perform if full or nearly full AROM is possible and comfortable
    - °Consider progressing to very light resistance (typically, 0.5 to 1 pound for resistance, depending on body size and ability to perform without substitution, tissue quality of the repair, and typical functional demands)

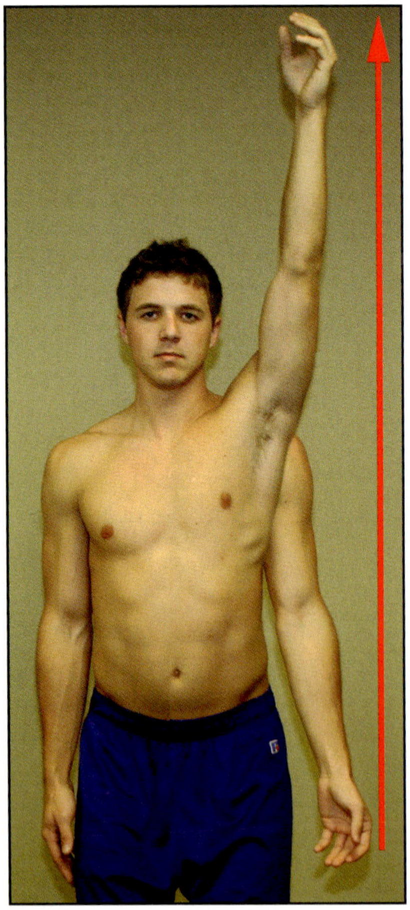

Figure 34. Active forward elevation.

Adjunctive Exercises

°Supine balance point exercises (Figures 24–26)
°Therapist-assisted PROM to achieve staged ROM goals with mobilizations PRN
°Modalities PRN
°Aquatic exercises (chapter IV-9)
°Trunk stabilization and strengthening PRN
°Progressive replication of demanding ADLs and work (if applicable for ADLs or occupation and **only if approved by physician**)
°Initiate modified return to weight-training program (**only if approved by physician**)
°Return-to-golf progression

Interventions to Avoid

°Initiating base strengthening program or overhead strengthening progression before overall level of pain is low
°Exercises that significantly increase signs and symptoms
°Any forceful jerking motions with the involved arm
°Highly repetitive rehabilitation activities with the elbow at or above chest level, including upper extremity ergometer
°Strengthening into straight-plane abduction
°Any rehabilitation activity that is significantly more demanding than daily or expected activities

III-4

Arthroscopic Capsular Plication With or Without Bankart Repair

Bryce W. Gaunt, PT, SCS

CHAPTER CONTENTS

WHAT PATIENTS ARE APPROPRIATE FOR THE USE OF THIS GUIDELINE?

- Patients with a suture or suture-anchor repair to the capsule and/or labrum complex
- Patients with preoperative anterior instability
- Patients with preoperative multidirectional instability
- Patients with traumatic, acquired, or atraumatic instability
- Patients with or without concomitant bursectomy or debridement of the labrum, rotator cuff, or glenohumeral joint

Clinical pearls are highlighted in yellow throughout the text.

THE MOST IMPORTANT FACTOR THAT SHOULD GUIDE CLINICAL DECISION MAKING

The strength of the surgical repair always should be much greater than the mechanical stress that is placed on the repaired capsulolabral structures during rehabilitation. Rehabilitation providers can manipulate and apply stress to a capsulolabral repair in 3 ways to positively affect patient outcome during rehabilitation activities: (1) through controlling the amount of range of motion (ROM) used, (2) by controlling submaximal tissue loading, and (3) through dynamic stabilization.[1] The stress on the repaired capsulolabral structures must be considered for all rehabilitation activities (home exercises, clinic exercises, and manual therapy).

KEY PRINCIPLES IN REHABILITATION OF THIS PROBLEM

A *successful outcome* after shoulder surgery for instability is defined as a pain-free and stable shoulder that has enough mobility, strength, and muscle control for a patient's desired level of work, recreation, and activities of daily living (ADLs). The American Society of Shoulder and Elbow Therapists (ASSET) has identified 4 principles that are critically important to follow so the rehabilitation professional successfully can apply controlled stress to the shoulder and optimize patient outcome in this patient population: (1) an understanding of the surgical procedure; (2) an understanding of the anatomic structures that must be protected, how they are stressed, and the rate at which they heal; (3) the identification and skilled application of techniques to impart varying levels of stress to the healing tissues; and (4) management of the initial immobilization period and the rate of ROM progression.[1]

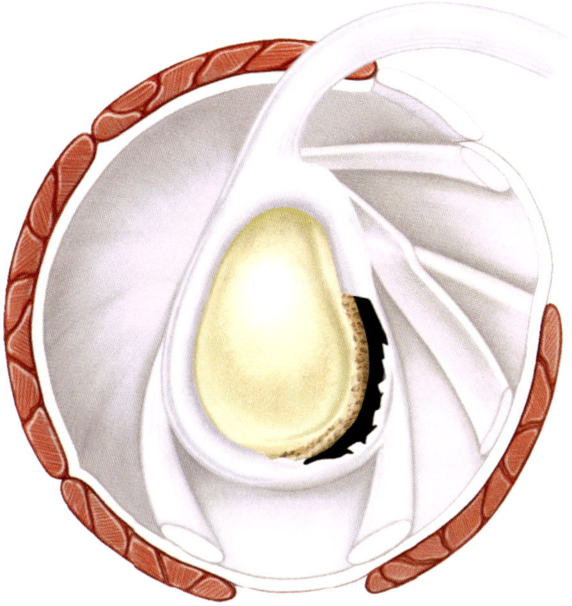

Figure 1. A Bankart lesion.

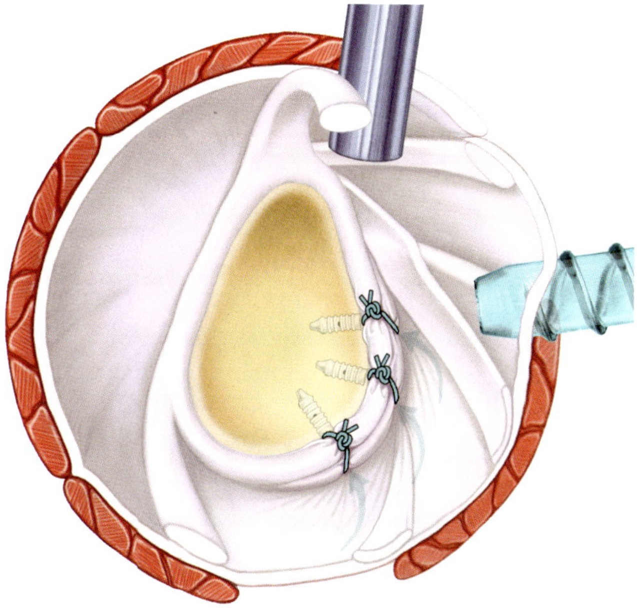

Figure 2. A completed Bankart repair and capsular shift showing the labrum has been stabilized and the capsule has been shifted 5 to 10 mm superiorly with each suture limb.

Knowledge Gained From the Surgical Procedure

Understanding the surgical procedure is important for the rehabilitation provider because it provides knowledge about the extent of tissue damage and the method of surgical repair, both of which guide the speed and specific activities of rehabilitation. Arthroscopic repairs for instability often are described as capsulolabral repairs (designating that both the capsule and labrum are repaired) or capsular plications (tensioning) either with or without a repair of the labrum. These general descriptions do not designate which part of the capsule and/or labrum was repaired (anterior, inferior, posterior, or a combination of these). Knowing which part of the capsule and/or labrum was repaired is vital because the repaired capsulolabral structures need protection from undue stress during rehabilitation and because the various parts of the capsulolabral complex are stressed by different planes of ROM.

Arthroscopic anterior capsulolabral repair addresses anterior shoulder instability by repairing an unstable anteroinferior labrum, which is known as a Bankart lesion, back to the glenoid through the use of sutures or suture anchors (Figure 1). In addition to a Bankart repair, capsular plication, which describes folding and suturing the capsule onto itself and/or stabilizing it to the labrum (Figure 2), is added as necessary to address permanent plastic deformation of the glenohumeral joint capsule that often accompanies recurrent anteroinferior dislocations. Similar procedures that restore normal tension to the capsule and labrum are performed in patients with inferior, posterior, and multidirectional instability. More detailed information about these surgical procedures and associated pathologic conditions can be found in chapter I-7.

Understanding the Structures That Require Protection During Rehabilitation, How They Are Stressed, and the Rate at Which They Heal

Understanding the anatomic structures that must be protected, how they are stressed, and the rate at which they heal is also important before rehabilitation begins. Arthroscopic capsulolabral repair involves a direct repair of damaged capsular and labral structures via suture and/or suture-anchor reattachment that requires protection from excessive stresses to facilitate appropriate tissue healing.[2,3] Investigators have well documented that specific portions of the capsule and labrum are tensioned selectively with specific glenohumeral motions.[4–6] An anterior capsulolabral repair that addresses attenuation of the anteroinferior capsule most directly is stressed by external rotation (ER), particularly above 90° of abduction.[4,6] However, in a cadaveric model, Itoi et al[7] demonstrated that with the upper extremity by the side, ER to 30° could be applied safely to the shoulder without separating a simulated Bankart lesion. Therefore, controlling the rate at which ER is gained during rehabilitation is important.

During the classic open Bankart repair, the subscapularis is either detached or split to access the capsule and then subsequently is reattached or closed with sutures, necessitating protection from active internal rotation (IR) during the early postoperative period. However, during the standard arthroscopic anterior capsulolabral repair, the subscapularis is not detached or split; therefore, it does not need specific protection from excessive stress during the rehabilitation program.

Activities need to be limited to those that produce less stress to the healing tissues than the failure strength of the repair. The challenge for guiding rehabilitation based on the tissue healing is the limited ability for clinicians to measure tissue healing. The amount of stress imparted by many rehabilitation activities remains unknown.

At our center, the rehabilitation process is divided into 3 phases of 6- to 12-week duration because we believe these timeframes coincide with healing and clinical milestones. The first 6 weeks after surgery include the inflammatory and the proliferative (fibroplasia and wound contraction) phases and the beginning of the scar-maturation phase of tissue healing.[8] Scar maturation and remodeling of the tissue likely continues throughout the rehabilitation process and might not be complete until 40 to 50 weeks after surgery.[9,10]

Other factors, such as the patient's age, history of upper extremity and spine surgery, and the presence of comorbidities, might affect tissue healing and should be considered when deciding how quickly to progress a patient. Diabetes mellitus, peripheral vascular disease, and connective tissue disorders might impair healing; therefore, patients with these diseases might have or require a slower rehabilitation progression. No researchers have examined the influence of comorbidities on shoulder function after capsulolabral repair. Comorbidities negatively influence outcome after rotator cuff repair and shoulder arthroplasty[11,12]; therefore, comorbidities might negatively affect rehabilitation and outcomes after capsulolabral repair.

The Identification and Skilled Application of Techniques to Impart Varying Levels of Stress to the Healing Tissues

Perhaps the single most important rehabilitation concept after arthroscopic capsulolabral repair is that the healing capsulolabral structures must receive a gradual, measured, and well-planned increase in stress to stimulate optimal healing while protecting the repair from excessive tension. The gradual application of stress is a stimulus for further proliferation and differentiation of fibroblasts.[8,12] A gradual increase in applied stress, in a process analogous to Wolff's Law of bone healing,[10] results in enhanced structural integrity of the capsulolabral complex as additional collagen fibers are laid down in response to controlled stresses. However, equally important is understanding that with excessive stress to the capsulolabral complex in terms of magnitude or timing, the tissues will be unable to adequately adapt[13,14] and damage to the healing tissues or to the stabilizing material (sutures, anchors) will result. During rehabilitation, rehabilitation providers apply stress to the surgical repair with 3 mechanisms to positively affect patient outcome: (1) absolute ROM, (2) controlled submaximal tissue loading, and (3) dynamic stabilization.[1]

Initially after surgery, the integrity of the repair is based solely on the mechanical strength of the sutures or suture anchors, or both. Therefore, the absolute ROM limit that initially is deemed safe is based on the surgical fixation and structural integrity of the repair. As time passes, the repaired tissues begin to heal through fibrous scar formation and gradually increase in tensile strength. With a Bankart lesion, the labrum develops immature connective tissue links to the glenoid rim, and with a capsular plication, the plicated layers of the capsule initiate formation of immature connective tissue links to one another. Excessive stretching during ROM activities might overload the structural integrity of these immature cross-links in the healing tissues.[4-6,15]

In a way similar to the way micromotion prevents bony union during fracture healing, submaximal tissue loading potentially can disrupt the tissue-healing bonds between the labrum and bone and between the plicated layers of the capsule.[13,14] Repeated submaximal stress on a ligament plication in an animal model has been shown to negatively affect mechanical resistance properties as late as postoperative week (POW) 12.[13] Although similar work has not been completed on a pathologic human condition, these findings are similar to the effects of submaximal loading in human cadavers. Repetitive submaximal loading has been shown to increase the length and decrease the subsequent load to failure of the anteroinferior glenohumeral ligament.[16] The exact effect of submaximal loading during various rehabilitation interventions on patients after capsulolabral repair is unknown. However, clinicians should keep in mind that repeated and excessive submaximal tensioning of the repair during the remodeling phases of tissue healing theoretically might cause the capsule to heal at a longer length. Thus, although they are below the failure strength of the capsulolabral tissues, repetitive submaximal stresses should be controlled carefully in all phases of rehabilitation because they pose a potential threat to capsuloligamentous integrity.

On the other hand, dynamic stabilization or active stabilization of a joint by the muscles directly surrounding it protects the surgical repair[17–20] by supporting the joint capsule,[21] increasing joint compression forces,[19,22] and resisting joint displacement.[22] Understanding that these 3 factors (absolute ROM, submaximal tissue loading, and dynamic stabilization) do not occur in isolation but are interrelated in all rehabilitation activities is vital and should be the primary consideration when selecting interventions during rehabilitation of patients after arthroscopic repair for instability.

Managing the Initial Immobilization Period and the Rate of ROM Progression

Appropriate management of the initial immobilization period and ROM progression is important for rehabilitation specialists because the tensile strength of the arthroscopic capsulolabral repairs is reduced through the first 12 POWs.[13] Therefore, protecting the surgical repair from undue stress is important during the early and middle postoperative periods (about 12 weeks total), which compose the first 2 phases of rehabilitation, by controlling the rate at which ROM is regained. Gaining ROM too quickly can limit the normal tissue-healing process and might lead to recurrent laxity.[23,24] Therefore, an initial period of controlled ROM is common after arthroscopic anterior capsulolabral repair to facilitate healing of the surgically repaired tissues,[25–28] theoretically allowing time for the surgically reattached labrum to bind to the glenoid and the plicated layers of capsule to heal to each other.

Absolute immobilization (no glenohumeral ROM exercises and constant sling use) in the first 6 weeks after arthroscopic capsulolabral repair of the shoulder was advocated during the infancy of these procedures[25,28] when operative techniques were evolving rapidly and failure rates were high.[29] However, researchers advocating absolute immobilization as a means to decrease long-term failure rates used operative procedures, such as transglenoid sutures or staple repair, which are no longer common. Current operative methods typically employ sutures and suture anchors to repair the labrum and retension the glenohumeral ligaments,[26,27,30] producing outcomes similar to open repair for instability.[31–33] Therefore, the need for absolute immobilization after arthroscopic Bankart repair also has been re-examined.

Researchers have shown periods of short or no absolute immobilization result in no greater recurrence of shoulder instability and have demonstrated improved ROM over the course of recovery.[31,34] In a randomized controlled trial in which they compared 3 weeks of absolute immobilization with immediate staged ROM in a select group of patients undergoing Bankart repair, Kim et al[34] found that immediate ROM yielded no greater recurrence rate in dislocation or difference in pain or functional scores. These results were in patients with recurrent (nonacute) instability due to trauma and with Bankart lesions without the presence of bony fragments (bony Bankart lesions). These investigators did not include other groups of patients, but authors of case series employing staged ROM beginning at POW 1 have demonstrated low rates of failure and high outcome scores for contact athletes[31] and patients with posterior capsular plication.[35] In addition, considering that the capsulolabral complex appears to be within the safe boundaries of stress with the upper extremity in adduction and up to 30° of ER,[7] immediate postoperative ROM in this range typically is considered safe.[1]

Based largely on this evidence, the ASSET rehabilitation guideline recommends a variable period of absolute immobilization between 0 and 4 weeks after an arthroscopic anterior capsulolabral repair in which sutures or suture anchors are used.[1] It recommends relative immobilization (out of the sling only for ROM exercises or short periods of sitting or standing) for 6 weeks followed by use of a sling for comfort. My facility's guideline for arthroscopic capsulolabral repair for instability uses the same period of relative immobilization, but we standardly use less than 1 week of absolute immobilization. A longer period of absolute immobilization is used only occasionally as determined by the surgeon and depends on factors, such as the extent of the pathologic lesion, the quality of the capsuloligamentous structures, the patient's goals, the patient's age, and comorbidities. Some examples that might warrant longer periods of absolute immobilization include repairs in a patient who has had exceptional laxity, has had a posterior repair for instability, or has had a revision repair for instability. These scenarios are discussed in more detail in the Special Considerations section of this chapter.

Regardless of the period of absolute and relative immobilization, controlling the rate of ROM progression is vitally important. The integrity of the surgical repair is thought to be affected negatively by the patient regaining ROM too quickly during the first 8 to 12 POWs.[2,3,13] Staged ROM goals are an effective tool to guide the rate of ROM progression.[27,34] We use a general guideline for staged ROM that is very similar to the staged ROM goals (Appendix and Table 1) in the ASSET guideline.[1] As with the specific period of immobilization, ROM goals might be modified by the surgeon or rehabilitation provider based on the patient. The ROM goals have the patient comfortably progressing ROM to the specified angle. If the patient's ROM is less than the targeted range, gentle stretching should be implemented to facilitate ROM gains to the targeted range and to prevent the development of contractures and adhesions. On the other hand, if the targeted ROM is obtained easily, then stretching in the directions in which the target motions have been met should be avoided to prevent overstressing the healing tissues.[8]

SPECIFIC REHABILITATION GUIDELINE

The Appendix contains our complete Arthroscopic Capsular Plication With or Without Bankart Repair Rehabilitation Guideline. In this section, I explain the rationale for selected components of the guideline. It is divided into 3 phases based on general timeframes of healing and staged ROM targets. To advance from one rehabilitation phase to the next, the patient must gain approval from the physician, successfully complete the core components of the previous rehabilitation activities, and meet the time criteria.

Phase 1

The primary focus of phase 1 rehabilitation, which constitutes the first 6 POWs, is to maximally protect the surgical repair; to facilitate tissue healing; and to achieve, but not significantly exceed, the staged ROM goals (Table 1), being especially careful to not greatly exceed ER limits. Because of the minimally invasive nature of the surgical procedure, some patients experience little pain and might be able to use their surgically treated upper extremity more than is advisable during this phase. Therefore, for most patients, phase 1 rehabilitation is fairly limited and often can be accomplished with very few clinic visits, and staged

Table 1. The Staged Range-of-Motion Goals[a]

Postoperative Week	Passive Forward Elevation	Passive External Rotation at 20° of Abduction	Passive External Rotation at 90° of Abduction	Active Forward Elevation
1	100°	10°–30°	Not applicable	Not applicable
3	130°	20°–40°	Not applicable	Not applicable
6	150°	45°–55°	45°	115°
9	165°	50°–65°	75°	145°
12	Within normal limits	Within normal limits	Within normal limits	Within normal limits

[a] These are approximate targets for range of motion. Specific limits might be specified by the physician. These range-of-motion goals **should not** be greatly exceeded.

ROM goals are achieved fairly easily with minimal stretching. However, patient education is critical to repeatedly convey the importance of staying within the prescribed ROM limits and the importance of minimizing use of the upper extremity during ADLs to protect the healing tissues from excessive submaximal forces and excessive load. Potentially injurious forces can be avoided during phase 1 rehabilitation by slowly progressing through staged ROM goals, by limiting repetitive activity of the upper extremity during rehabilitation activities and during ADLs, and by counseling the patient not to lift objects weighing greater than 3 to 5 pounds (1.35–2.25 kg) with the affected extremity.

Because the rotator cuff muscles are not detached during this procedure, both passive and active-assistive ROM exercises are appropriate in the early stages of postoperative rehabilitation. Therefore, unlike with rehabilitation of the patient after rotator cuff repair, active-assistive exercises can be performed immediately for the patient after arthroscopic capsulolabral repair.

Forward elevation and ER in slight abduction within the prescribed ROM limits are the glenohumeral motions performed during phase 1. Although active-assistive ROM activities are safe to the healing tissues, I prefer to use the specific passive exercises described in phase 1 of the Appendix. I have found these exercises are more comfortable to the patient in the first 3 to 4 POWs, and they facilitate achieving without greatly exceeding the staged ROM goals compared with other exercises we have used.

To protect the surgical repair, ROM should never be forceful during phase 1. Stretching exercises should stop at the point when the patient experiences a sensation of a light stretch as long as ROM is less than the staged ROM goals. If it significantly exceeds the staged goals without any sensation of stretch, the patient no longer has a ROM deficit, and ROM exercises in this plane are discontinued until it is consistent with the staged goals. During this phase, ROM exercises that stretch into end-range ER, particularly at 90° of abduction, or that position the patient in shoulder extension should not be used because they directly stress the anterior or anteroinferior glenohumeral capsule.

Although the rotator cuff does not specifically require protection after arthroscopic stabilization, glenohumeral active ROM (AROM) and rotator cuff strengthening purposefully are de-emphasized in our rehabilitation guideline during the early postoperative period. Light strengthening and AROM within the staged ROM goals likely would not result in excessive loading on healing tissue; however, other authors and I believe it sends an inconsistent message to the patient during this early postoperative period that some strengthening is approved yet significant restrictions of ADLs and immobilization are necessary.[1] At our center, we believe this inconsistency can lead to excessive use of the upper extremity by the patient in terms of both loading and ROM, resulting in too much stress to the surgical repair. During phase 1, we allow limited active use of the upper extremity for waist-level ADLs as comfortable and consider this our AROM and dynamic stabilization exercises for this phase. The ASSET guideline[1] recommends submaximal isometric strengthening during phase 1, and although not included in our guideline, I support the use of isometrics in this phase if desired.

Phase 2

The focus of phase 2 rehabilitation, which typically constitutes POWs 6 through 12, is continued patient education about postoperative activity limitations; the initiation and subsequent progression of rotator cuff and scapular neuromuscular control activities to improve strength and dynamic stability; and achievement of, without greatly exceeding, staged ROM goals (Table 1). The rehabilitation provider still must ensure that the stress of the rehabilitation activities is lower than the strength of the surgical repair, which relatively speaking, is still in the early stages of healing during this period.[10,13,15] During phase 2, choosing appropriate rehabilitation activities means selecting activities that (1) appropriately control the ROM used, (2) minimize then gradually progress the submaximal loads to the capsulolabral structures, and (3) improve the dynamic stability of the shoulder girdle. During this phase, activities that place a large load on the capsulolabral structures, high-intensity strengthening, and strengthening activities performed at the extremes of motion are not appropriate. Rehabilitation interventions of low-intensity exercise progressing to moderate-intensity exercise performed primarily in the middle ranges of motion are emphasized.

The goal of our ROM and flexibility progression in phase 2 is to achieve full ROM in all planes at about 12 POWs. Whereas forward elevation and ER in slight abduction are important motions to monitor during this phase, measuring and, if limited, beginning interventions to increase horizontal adduction, ER in abduction, and IR of the glenohumeral joint also is important. For motions that do not have specific staged goals, such as horizontal adduction, ROM of the operatively treated side can be compared with ROM of the nonoperately treated side. For instance, to attain nearly normal ROM at 12 weeks after surgery in a gradual way, about 50% of the motion of the uninvolved side would be expected at 6 POWs and about 75% of normal motion should be attained at 9 POWs with a normal joint end feel. A variable amount of stretching is needed to achieve these ROM goals in patients with capsulolabral repairs based on the number of directions that are behind staged ROM goals, the size of the deficit, and the joint end feel that is noted during ROM assessment. Often, only very little and very gentle stretching is necessary to achieve the desired ROM. Occasionally, no PROM or stretching is needed to achieve ROM goals in phase 2, whereas a comprehensive stretching program occasionally is appropriate. Therefore, phase 2 ROM exercises require a selective and individualized approach. The Appendix contains typical examples of stretches we consider using during this stage. For patients with an anterior or multidirectional capsulolabral repair, the rehabilitation provider must not perform passive stretching to gain end-range ER or ER at 90° of abduction unless significant restriction in ROM or an overly tight end feel is present because these motions impart the greatest stress to the healing capsulolabral repair.[4,6]

At the same time that ROM targets are being met, the focus of phase 2 rehabilitation begins: progressive rotator cuff, deltoid, and scapular neuromuscular control and strengthening activities. Certain guidelines and principles for progression are used. Chosen neuromuscular retraining and strengthening activities must be performed within the staged ROM goals and should provide a stepwise increase in muscular demand. Rehabilitation activities should train the entire shoulder girdle and can incorporate the entire kinetic chain, such as the trunk and lower body.

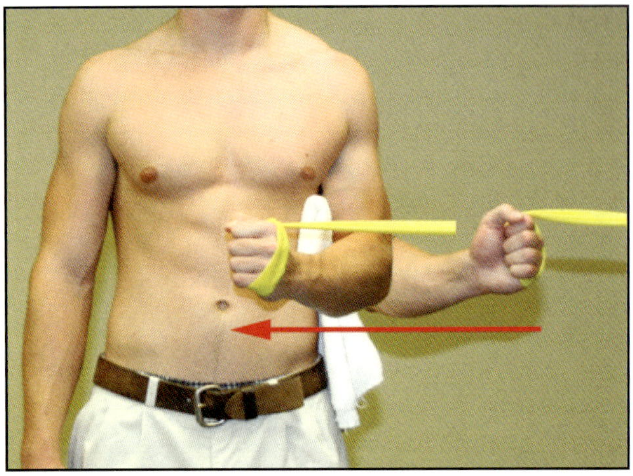

Figure 3. Internal rotation with an elastic band.

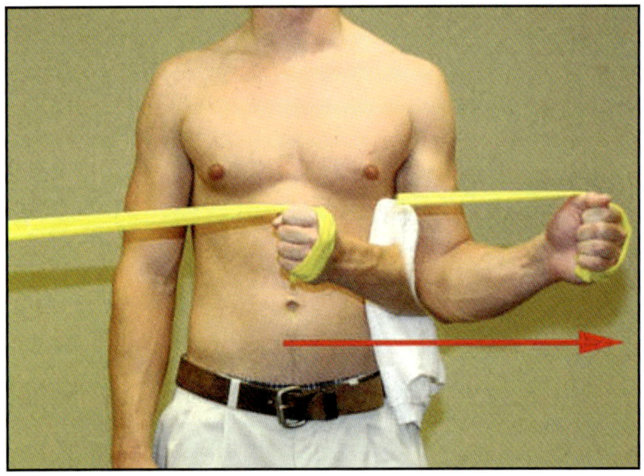

Figure 4. External rotation with an elastic band.

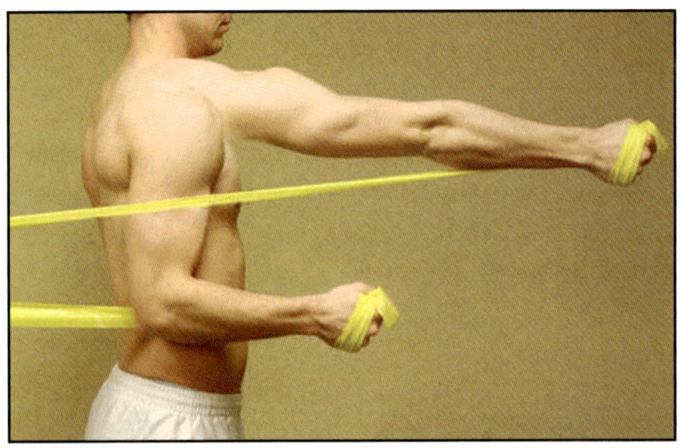

Figure 5. Forward reaching with an elastic band at chest level.

At our facility, phase 2 neuromuscular training and strengthening progression, which is detailed in the Appendix, begins with light- to moderate-resistance activities with elastic-resistance activities (Figures

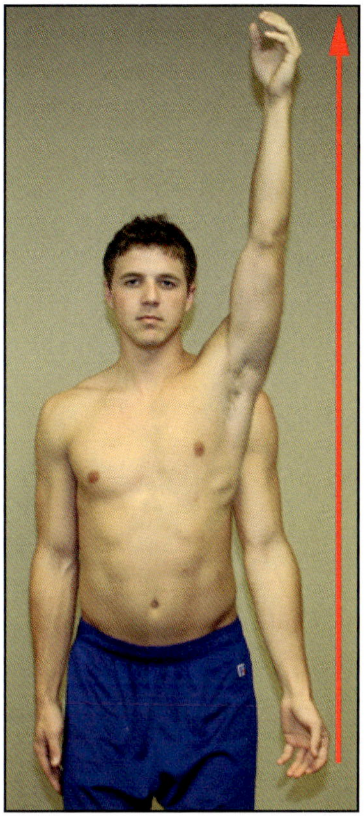

Figure 6. Active forward elevation.

3–5) performed below the shoulder level, emphasizing a controlled ROM and relatively high repetitions (range, 30–60). Active elevation of the upper extremity overhead in or near the scapular plane (Figure 6) performed through the patient's available ROM with progressive resistance is also an early emphasis of the phase 2 neuromuscular retraining progression. If substitution or pain is present, then the assistive-to-active shoulder elevation progression (Appendix and chapter II-4) is used as a precursor to active elevation (Figure 7). In the later stages of phase 2 when the patient can complete the basic strengthening exercises with moderate resistance and without difficulty or pain, more advanced activities can thoughtfully be added. Exercises with higher documented electromyographic activity levels (eg, prone horizontal abduction and prone ER), medium-speed activities, activities with less stabilization of the operated extremity by external means, and multiplanar activities can begin to be used with careful visual and hands-on monitoring to ensure the humeral head maintains a centralized position within the glenoid fossa. Late phase 2 activities

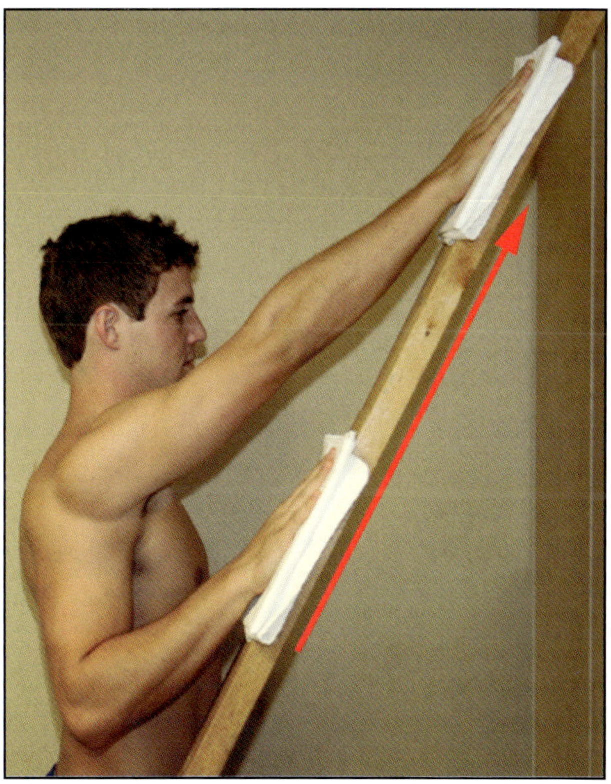

Figure 7. Incline dusting is an example of an assistive-to-active shoulder elevation progression exercise.

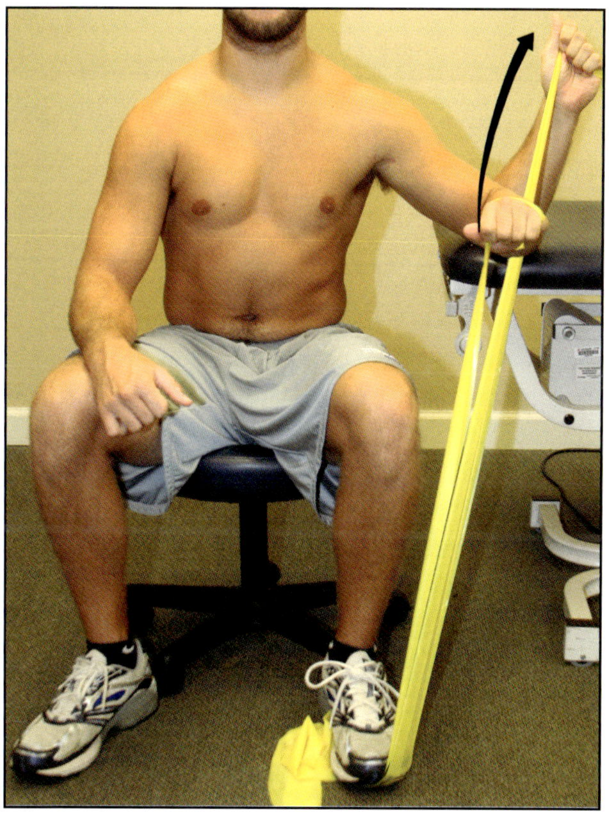

Figure 8. External rotation at 45° of abduction with support and an elastic band.

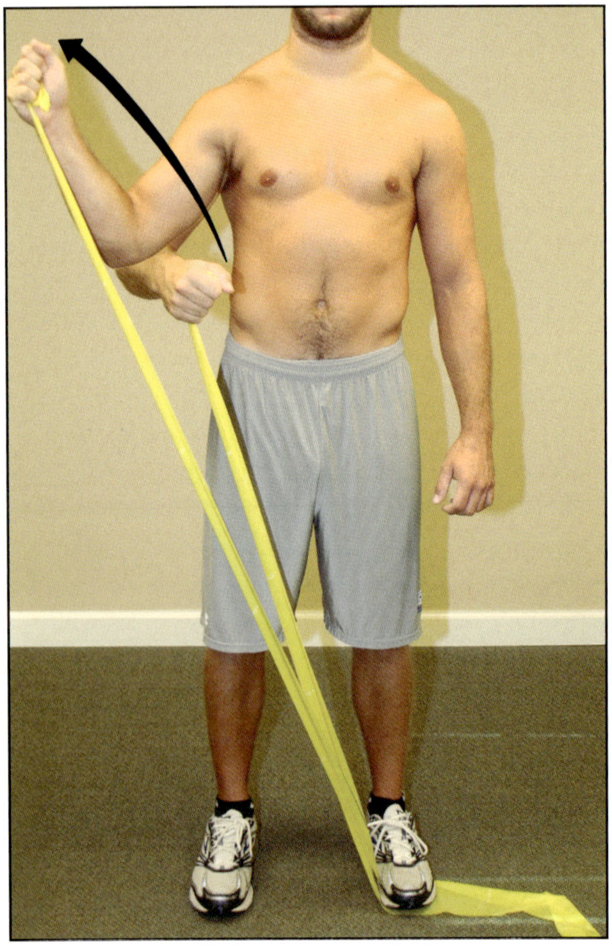

Figure 9. External rotation at 45° of abduction without support and with an elastic band.

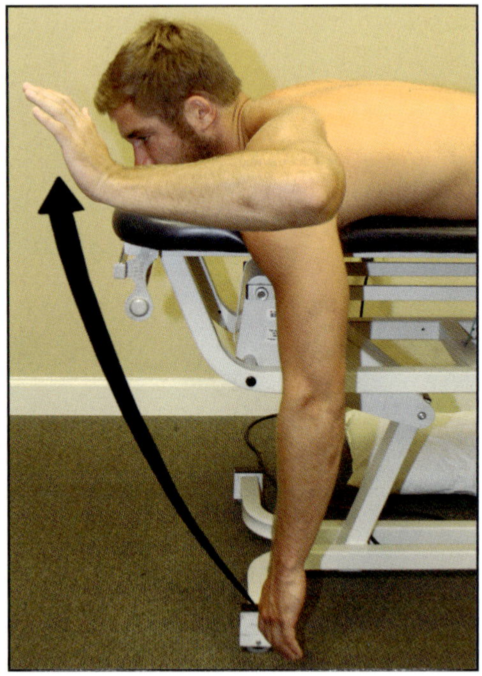

Figure 10. Prone hang to external rotation near 90° of abduction without support.

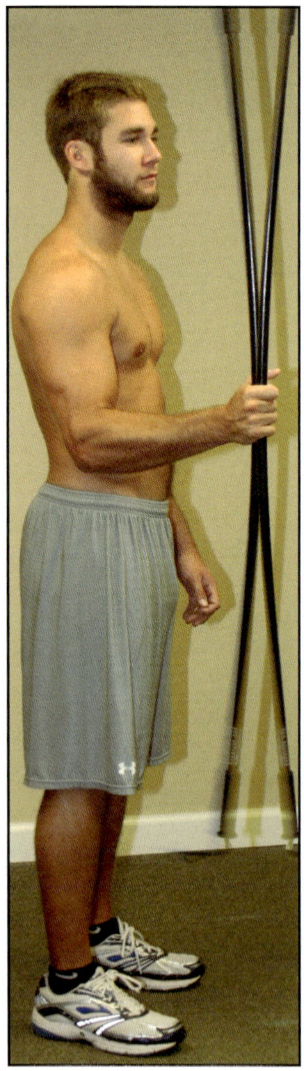

Figure 11. Oscillations with a flexible wand.

must not be performed in the extremes of ROM, must not be painful, must not be powerful, and must not be uncontrolled. In addition, the goal of the progression eventually should be replicating an activity that the patient needs for daily life, work, or recreation. Figures 8 through 10 show an example of a late stage 2 strengthening progression for a throwing athlete.

Use of equipment, such as a flexible rod (Figure 11), also can be of great value during this timeframe as long as activities are performed within the staged ROM goals, substitution patterns are not allowed, and other rehabilitation progression principles are followed. In all phase 2 AROM and strengthening activities, our center's philosophy is that performing or advancing activities should not be painful and should not increase the patient's resting pain level. If any of these things occur, easier interventions should be selected.

Exercises with weight bearing applied through the upper extremities can help improve neuromuscular control and dynamic stability of the shoulder girdle; however, the stresses that these exercises place on the surgical repair can be high. Appropriate weight-bearing scapular exercises during phase 2 include maintaining correct scapular and humerus position in the quadruped position and progressing to 3-point and finally 2-point position (Figure 12). This can be implemented early in phase 2 for a patient with an anterior capsulolabral repair. For patients with a posterior or multidirectional capsulolabral repair, this progression is appropriate to start only at the very end stage of phase 2 rehabilitation after good rotator cuff strength, endurance, and neuromuscular control have been achieved. The rehabilitation provider must ensure good static positioning of the humerus is maintained while these exercises are performed and must ensure no posterior movement occurs at the glenohumeral joint. Although extrapolating this information to a true push-up exercise is tempting, other authors and I believe traditional push-ups are not appropriate during phase 2 for an anterior, multidirectional, or posterior repair because they produce relatively high loads on the shoulder and stress the anterior capsule when the upper extremity is brought into horizontal abduction (down position).[1] However, push-ups performed in standing with the hands placed on the wall (ie, wall push-ups) would be appropriate at this time.

Patient education regarding appropriate upper extremity positions and loading is crucial during this phase so the patient understands that although the shoulder might be starting to feel much better, he or she should not perform uncontrolled end-range stretching, heavy lifting, or quick motions with the operated upper extremity during rehabilitation or ADLs. The importance of this cannot be overstated because the patient will spend more time performing ADLs than directly performing rehabilitation exercises. Patient education should stress that tissue healing is incomplete through POW 12[13] and might not be complete until POWs 40 to 50.[10,15]

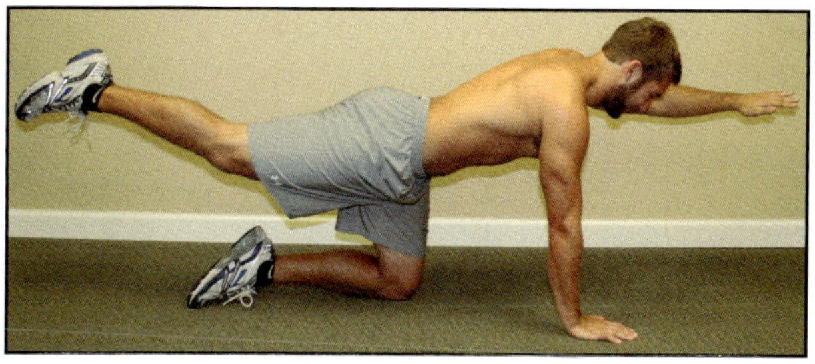

Figure 12. The quadruped position alternating with 2-point stabilization. The operatively repaired upper extremity remains weight bearing.

Phase 3

The focus of phase 3 rehabilitation, which might begin as early as POW 12, is to normalize AROM, strength, endurance, power, and passive ROM (PROM) and to complete a functional progression to facilitate the patient returning to his or her desired level of function. The necessity, extent, and makeup of phase 3 rehabilitation are highly individualized based on the patient's ADLs, work, and recreation. For patients with sedentary work and limited recreational demands, phase 3 rehabilitation might be only the completion or continuation of phase 2 rehabilitation activities. However, for patients who want to return to strenuous work or recreational activities requiring throwing, heavy lifting, or powerful upper extremity movements, phase 3 rehabilitation can be very extensive.

Typically, PROM is normal or nearly normal when beginning phase 3 rehabilitation. In these cases, PROM or stretching exercises might not be necessary. If a patient's PROM is moderately limited in any plane of motion, phase 2 stretching is continued. In addition, if restricted end-range motion is present in the direction that directly stresses the capsulolabral repair (eg, limited abduction with ER in an anterior capsulolabral repair), a stretching program can be initiated to address these specific deficits at this time.

To improve AROM, strength, and endurance, many strengthening exercises from phase 2 are continued during phase 3 rehabilitation. External rotation and IR strengthening in adduction (Figures 3 and 4), active forward elevation (Figure 6) with weight, prone horizontal abduction, prone forward elevation, prone ER (Figure 10), and resisted scapular retraction are examples of common strengthening exercises that are important to include in phase 3 rehabilitation. Before beginning advanced AROM and strengthening activities, the patient should have strength of at least 4+/5 on manual muscle testing of all rotator cuff muscles and should be asymptomatic during ADLs. Other criteria to start advanced strengthening are detailed in the Appendix.

Advanced strengthening and functional progressions should provide a gradual buildup in stress to eventually meet all functional, work, and recreational demands of the patient. High-speed activities, movements that progressively simulate functional activities, activities performed in extremes of ROM, activities with functional resistance through multiple planes of motion, and activities that train larger upper extremity muscles should be introduced as needed and progressed gradually during this stage of rehabilitation. Rehabilitation activities requiring heavy lifting and power training, such as plyometrics, typically are added 3 to 6 weeks later. Return-to-sport and modified weight-training programs are essential if the patient wants to participate regularly in these activities, but they are used only as needed at the end of phase 3 rehabilitation. The rehabilitation provider must remember that the capsulolabral repair will not have normal biomechanical properties or strength at the time of functional training or early return to vigorous activities.[9,10,13] However, ligaments and tendons do adapt in response to exercise stress,[8] which is why a gradual functional progression is essential before return to vigorous work or recreational activities.

Determining the appropriate phase 3 functional progression requires the rehabilitation provider to complete a needs analysis of the patient's functional activity to which he or she wants to return. A needs analysis involves assessing the AROM, PROM, strength, neuromuscular control, functional movements, endurance, speed, and power required to complete the patient's desired functional activity and comparing the analysis with the patient's current levels of these factors. A step-by-step rehabilitation plan then is created to systematically progress the patient from the current level of performance to the level required to complete the desired activity. Therefore, this stage of rehabilitation is different for each patient because patients begin phase 3 with different levels of current function and different functional goals. Two case studies will clarify how phase 3 advanced strengthening and functional progressions can differ and how needs analysis is used to guide phase 3 rehabilitation.

Case 1. Case 1 involves a 17-year-old male baseball shortstop whose conservative treatment of anteroinferior instability, bursitis, and a small partial-thickness rotator cuff tear failed. This patient underwent an anterior capsulorrhaphy, which required 3 suture anchors and debridement of the rotator cuff and bursa. The patient had no other important medical comorbidities and was cleared by the physician to begin phase 3 rehabilitation at POW 12. At this time, the patient displayed normal PROM of the involved extremity, except passive ER at 90° of abduction was limited to 90°. Manual muscle testing strength of the infraspinatus, subscapularis, lateral deltoid, and supraspinatus was 5/5.

In addition to basic phase 2 rehabilitation exercises, late phase 2 rehabilitation progressed from the type of activity shown in Figure 8 to the types of activities shown in Figures 9 and 10. The results of the needs analysis for this high school baseball player are shown in Table 2. From the needs analysis, the patient continued phase 2 basic rotator cuff, deltoid, and scapular strengthening and also began stretching to achieve end-range passive ER ROM in 90° of abduction (Figure 13). I initiated advanced strengthening and his functional progression by increasing the speed of exercises performed in abduction with ER and during activities that progressively mimicked the throwing and batting motions. Figures 14 through 17 show activities that I believe are important to use dur-

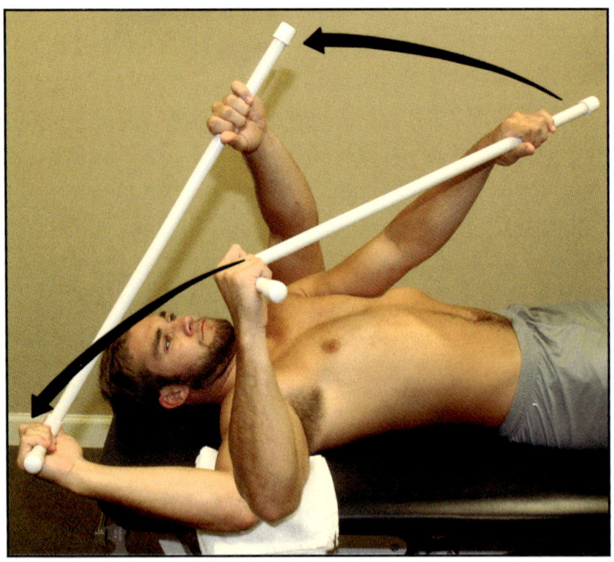

Figure 13. Passive external rotation stretching at 90° of abduction.

Table 2. Needs Analysis for Patient Case 1: 17-Year-Old High School Shortstop

Rehabilitation Variable	Current Level	Requirements of Sport	Rehabilitation Needs
Shoulder girdle active and passive range of motion	WNL except external rotation at 90° of abduction = 90°	External rotation at 90° of abduction = 100°–115°	Increase external rotation at 90° of abduction
Strength	Manual muscle testing rotator cuff: all 5/5	Manual muscle testing rotator cuff: all 5/5	Continue basic strengthening Emphasize strengthening in abduction with external and internal rotation Initiate resistance activities in throwing motion Initiate and/or continue resistance training in muscles used in batting
Functional movements	Basic reaching and activities of daily living	End-range abduction with external rotation moving to horizontal adduction with internal rotation as in throwing	Include end-range abduction with with external rotation as passive range of motion improves
	Limited external rotation at 90° of abduction done only at slow speed	Batting motion	Include throwing motion in rehabilitation activities Include batting motion in rehabilitation activities
Speed of movement	Fairly slow	Very high: up to 7000°/s	Initiate medium progressing to high speed in activities, such as internal and external rotation in abduction Progress to throwing motion at medium to high speed Progress to batting motion at medium to high speed Eventually progress to interval throwing program and return to batting
Neuromuscular control	Good control with current level of rehabilitation	Good control with high-speed powerful movements	Ensure good control with advancing rehabilitation If poor control during rehabilitationor functional activity, return to more basic activity
Power	Not included in phase 2 rehabilitation	Very high	Gradually increase through structured resistance training and increasing speed of activities

Abbreviation: Within normal limits.

ing this stage of rehabilitation for throwing athletes. In this patient, these exercises were initiated on POW 12 using a medium speed and nearly full ROM. Over 2 to 4 weeks, the patient was advanced using full ROM and high speed during these activities as long as he had no pain during them and had good neuromuscular control. Relatively light resistance was used throughout rehabilitation to better replicate the functional demands of throwing and to ensure the speed of the exercises remained high. To improve endurance, these 4 exercises usually were performed for time, with a goal of completing 2 to 3 sets of 30 to 45 seconds for each set of either the exercises shown in Figures 14 and 15 or the exercises shown in Figures 16 and 17.

At POW 14, a batting progression began. For 2 weeks, the patient performed light- to moderate-intensity swings with a polyvinyl chloride pipe that was 32 inches (81.28 cm) long. The patient progressed to hitting with a bat off a tee and soft tosses 3 times per week for 2 weeks. The patient then was allowed to return to hitting pitches.

At POW 16 while the patient continued the high-speed activities shown in Figures 14 through 17, he was allowed to throw a balled up pillowcase to a partner or wall at a distance of 10 feet (3 m). This was used as progressive motion and speed-specific training before a formal throwing program was initiated at POW 18 using the principles discussed in chapter IV-

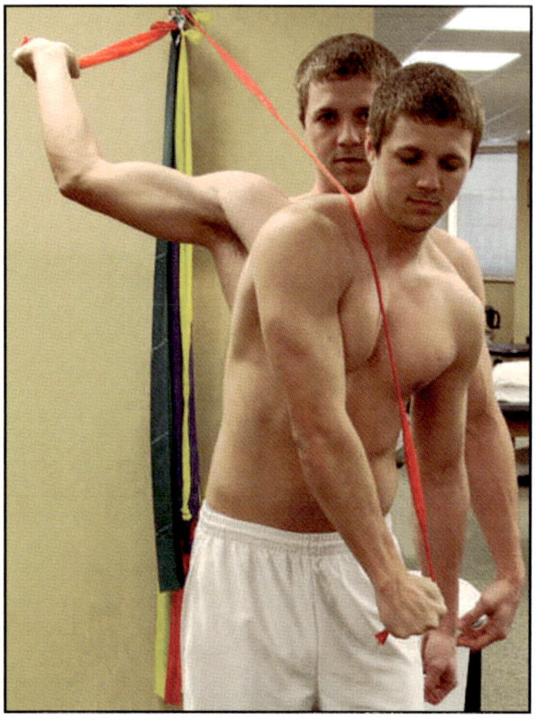

Figure 14. Diagonal resisting extension and internal rotation with an elastic band.

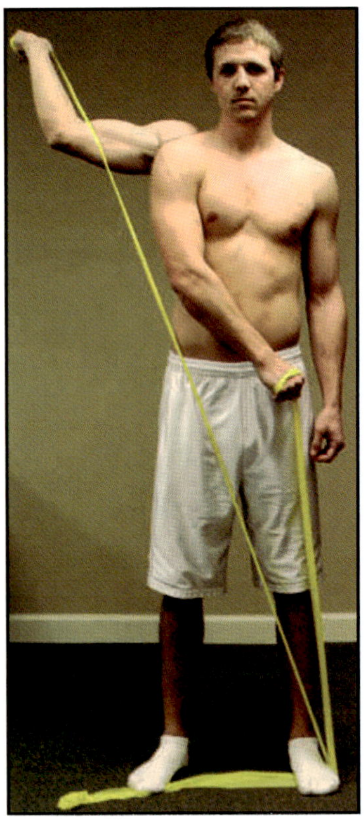

Figure 15. Diagonal resisting elevation and external rotation with an elastic band.

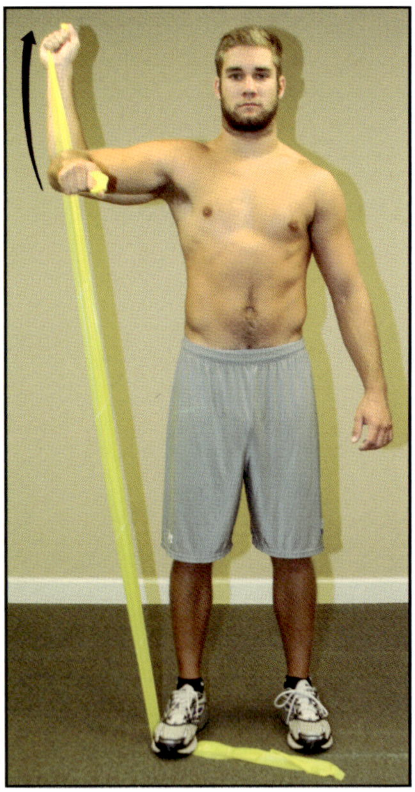

Figure 16. External rotation at 90° of abduction with an elastic band.

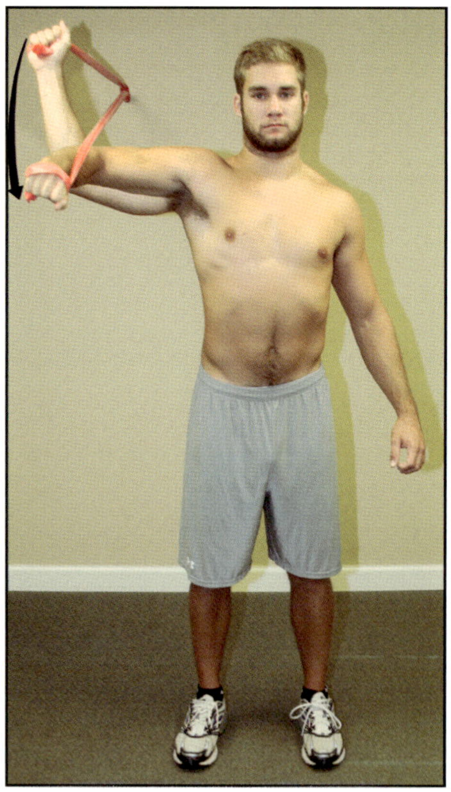

Figure 17. Internal rotation at 90° of abduction with an elastic band.

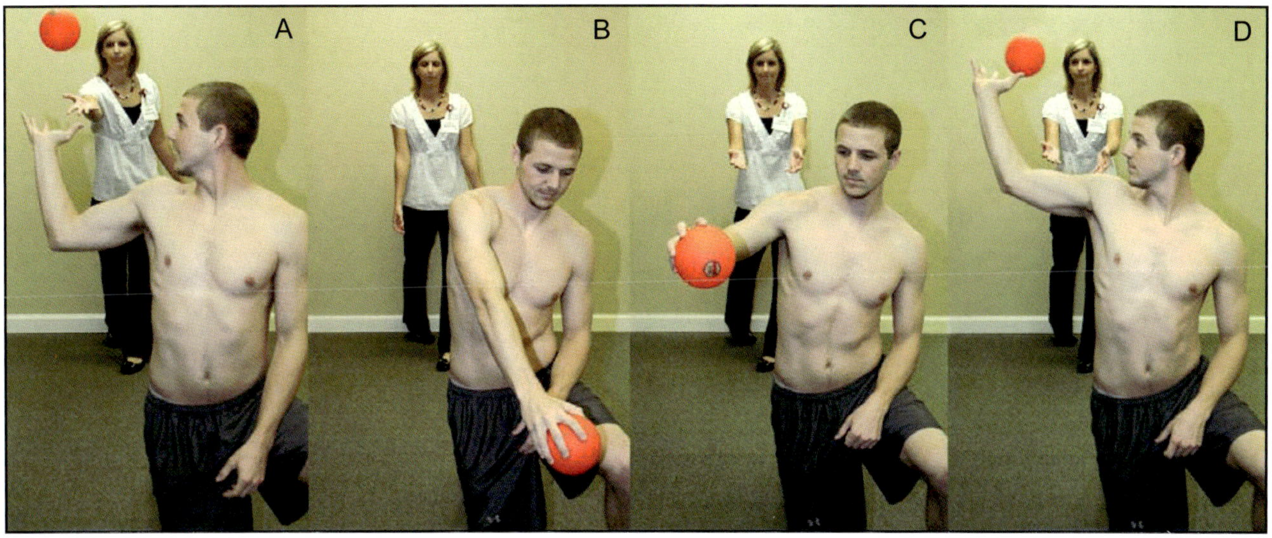

Figure 18. Plyometric proprioceptive neuromuscular facilitation diagonal 2 reverse throws. The rehabilitation provider throws the ball over the patient's shoulder, A, and the patient catches the ball and decelerates it down to the foot, B, begins to accelerate the ball, C, and throws it back over the shoulder to the rehabilitation provider, D.

6. Plyometric exercises, such as those shown in Figure 18, were not used with this patient because clinic visits occurred only 1 time every 2 weeks at this stage, and I did not want the patient performing these exercises without supervision. However, if regular skilled supervision had been available, plyometrics would have been used appropriately between POWs 16 and 20. This patient completed his throwing program at 24 POWs and successfully returned to sport in the middle of his fall season.

Case 2. Case 2 involves a 17-year-old male high school football offensive lineman whose conservative treatment for anteroinferior instability with a labral tear and a partial-thickness rotator cuff tear caused by acute subluxation failed. This patient underwent a Bankart repair with anterior capsulorrhaphy, which required 3 suture anchors and debridement of the rotator cuff. The patient had no other significant medical comorbidities and was cleared by the physician to begin phase 3 rehabilitation at POW 12. At this time, the patient displayed normal PROM of the involved extremity, including passive ER at 90° of abduction equal to 95°. Manual muscle testing strength of the infraspinatus, subscapularis, lateral deltoid, and supraspinatus was 5/5.

In addition to basic phase 2 rehabilitation exercises, late phase 2 rehabilitation included weight-bearing activities, such as those shown in Figures 12 and 19. The results of the needs analysis for this high school football player are shown in Table 3. Although this patient's level of function upon entering phase 3 was very similar to that of the patient in case 1, the requirements of their sports and thus the rehabilitation needs were different.

From the needs analysis, this patient continued basic rotator cuff, deltoid, and scapular strengthening from phase 2 and began phase 3 advanced strengthening and functional progression at POW 12 by progressing upper extremity weight-bearing exercises with the hands in front of the body, beginning limited upper extremity weight-training activities, and progressing multiplanar activities while continuing to avoid activities that placed a large load on the shoulder in the position of horizontal abduction or the combined position of abduction with ER. Upper extremity weight-bearing

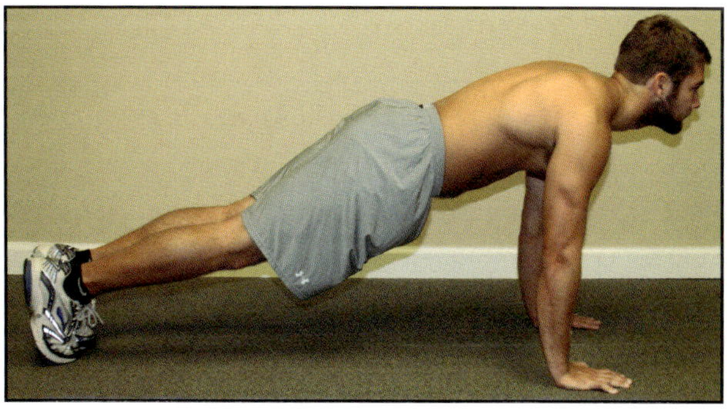

Figure 19. The plank position.

Table 3. Needs Analysis for Patient Case 2: 17-Year-Old High School Offensive Lineman

Rehabilitation Variable	Current Level	Requirements of Sport	Rehabilitation Needs
Shoulder girdle active and passive range of motion	Within normal limits	Met	Not applicable
Strength	Manual muscle testing rotator cuff: all 5/5	High level of strength of large upper extremity muscles, such as pectoralis major, trapezius, and latissimus dorsi	Continue rotator cuff and deltoid strengthening
	Strength of large upper extremity muscle groups not assessed Support upper extremity body mass in plank position	Support large amounts of weight through upper extremity	Progressive upper extremity weight-bearing exercises with hands in front of body Initiate resistance activities emphasizing large upper extremity muscle groups
Functional movements	Basic reaching and activities of daily living	Horizontal abduction nearing end ranges needed for weight training	Continue weight-bearing activities with arms in front of body
	Restricted from end-range horizontal abduction	Use of hands and upper extremities in front of body	Include multiplanar activities including abduction with external rotation
		Ability to use hands and upper extremities in all planes of motion	Progress to activities that require functional horizontal abduction
Speed of movement	Fairly slow	Medium- and high-speed with upper extremities in front of body	Initiate medium-speed progressing to high-speed activities in multiple planes of motion
Neuromuscular control	Good control with current level of rehabilitation	Good control with high-speed powerful movements in all planes of motion	Ensure good control with advancing rehabilitation If poor control during rehabilitation or functional activity, return to more basic activity
Power	Not included in phase 2	Very high	Gradually increase through advancing rehabilitation resistance training and increasing speed of activities

exercises were progressed to activities that required increased neuromuscular control but maintained a similar amount of weight bearing through the upper extremities with the hands in front of the body and the elbows relatively extended (Figures 20–22). I avoided loading the capsulolabral repair in abduction with ER or horizontal abduction during this phase of the progression. A complete weight-training program was not started at this time to allow maturation of the surgical repair, but biceps curls, triceps push-downs (Figure 23), low cable rows (Figure 24), "V" raises

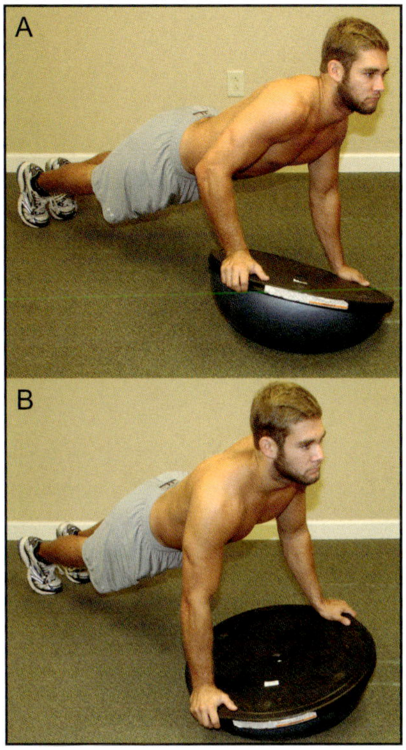

Figure 20 A and B. BOSU (BOSU, Canton, OH) ball rocking.

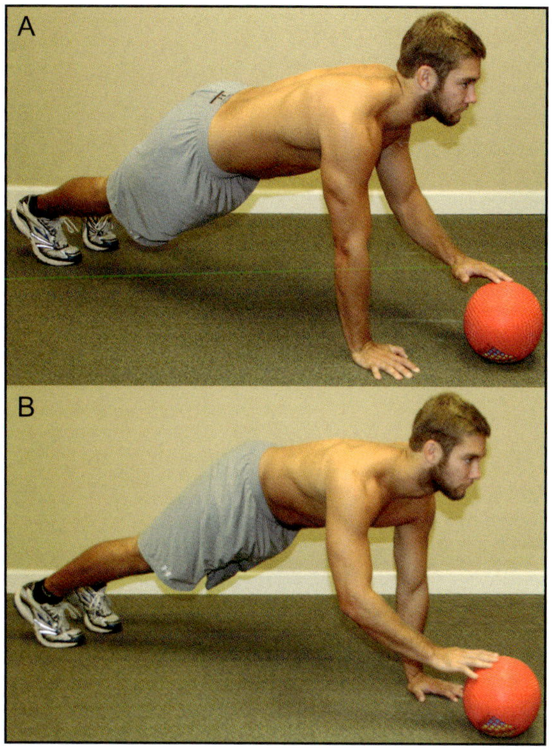

Figure 22 A and B. Ball taps.

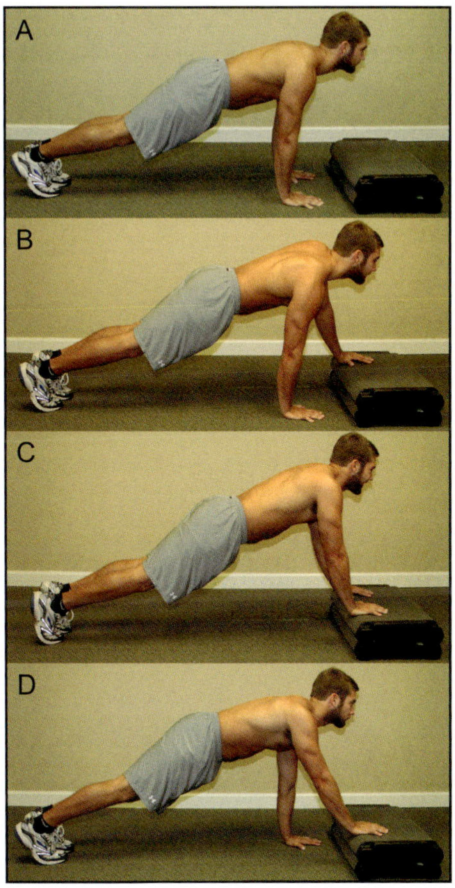

Figure 21 A–D. Upper extremity step-ups.

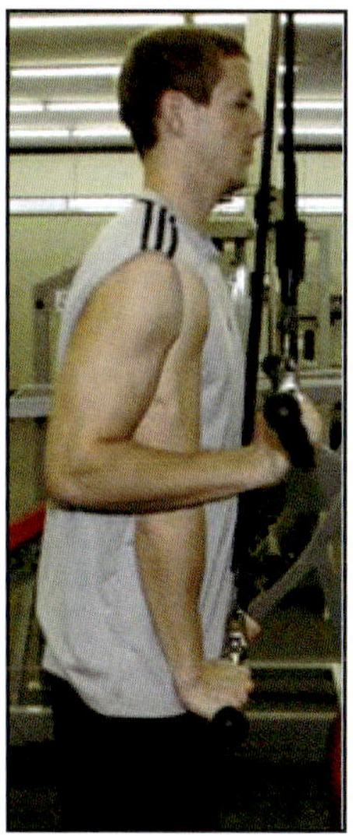

Figure 23. The triceps push-down exercise.

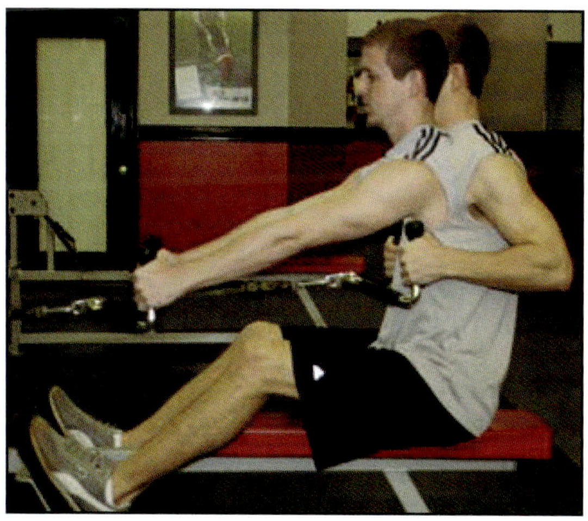

Figure 24. The low cable row exercise.

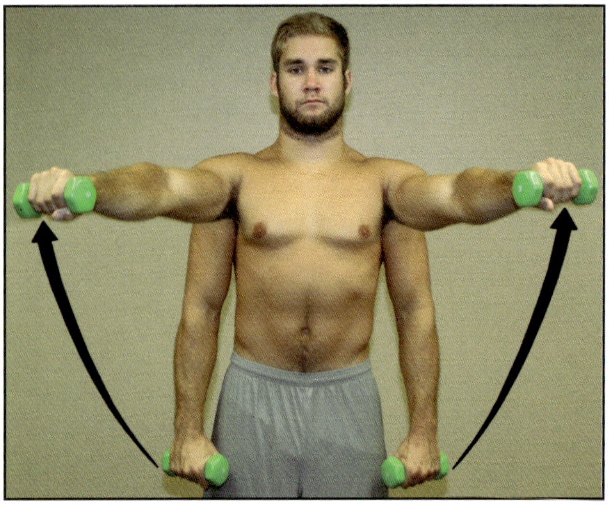

Figure 25. The "V" raise exercise.

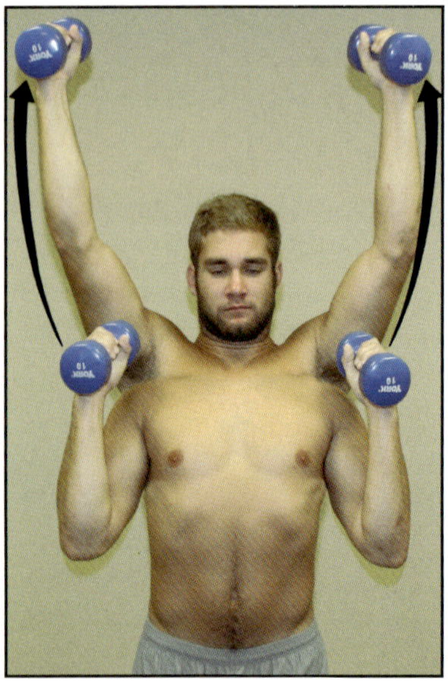

Figure 26. Dumbbell overhead press with hands starting in front of the shoulders.

(Figure 25), and a modified dumbbell overhead press (Figure 26) that was done in a way to minimize stress to the capsulolabral repair were performed with light to moderate weight for sets of 15 to 25 repetitions. Medium-speed progressing to high-speed modified proprioceptive neuromuscular facilitation diagonal 2 patterns using elastic bands for resistance were chosen for multiplanar activities (Figures 16 and 17). Plyometric chest passes, 2-hand overhead throws, 2-hand side throws, and 2-hand diagonal throws also were used first with a basketball and second with a weighted ball as part of the progression of multiplanar, high-speed, and power activities from POW 12 through POW 18.

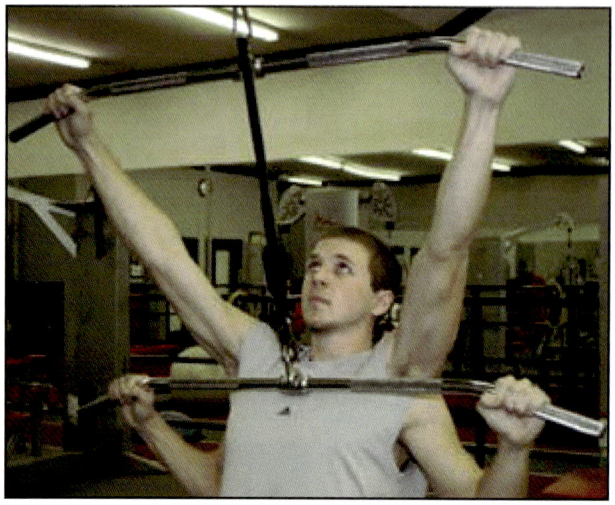

Figure 27. Pull-downs in front of the head.

At POW 18, the patient received clearance to begin a more comprehensive modified weight-training progression (chapter IV-4), including exercises with a gradual increase in stress to the anterior capsulolabral structures. Lateral bar pull-downs with the bar in front of the head (Figure 27), weighted shoulder shrugs, and partial-range push-ups in which the elbows were not allowed to pass behind the plane of the glenohumeral joint were initiated at this time. Full-range push-ups began 2 weeks later, and partial-range machine chest press and barbell press were begun at postoperative month (POM) 5.5. During this time, the amount of weight was kept light by requiring the patient to perform sets of 15 to 25 repetitions with all exercises. At POM 6, full-range chest presses and deadlifting were allowed with gradually progressing weight. The patient was allowed to begin power cleans and dumbbell chest presses at POM 7. He was counseled to always avoid weight-training exercises that place a stretch on the anterior portion of the shoulder, such as dips, shoulder presses with a barbell behind the head, and full-range pectoralis flys.

Regarding football-specific conditioning and training drills, the patient was allowed to begin jogging at POM 2. Sprinting and lower body agility drills began at POM 3. Activities requiring modest upper body weight bearing, such as bear crawls, began at POM 5. Individual football drills that impart high levels of stress to the shoulder, such as hitting a blocking sled, were begun at POM 6. The patient was fully released to participation at POM 7.

SPECIAL CONSIDERATIONS

In this section, I describe some situations that require varying amounts of modification to our standard rehabilitation guideline for arthroscopic plication with or without Bankart repair.

Open Repair for Instability

Open repair for instability has demonstrated very good long-term results with a low rate of recurrence.[36] Rehabilitation of patients after primary open repair for anterior or multidirectional instability is different from rehabilitation after arthroscopic repair in the early postoperative period but is essentially the same in the later stages of rehabilitation. Differences in early rehabilitation are needed to protect the subscapularis and to minimize the loss of ROM, which can occur after these procedures. Revision open repair for instability requires different modifications and is addressed later in the Special Considerations section.

Open repair of a Bankart lesion or open anterior or inferior capsular shift of the glenohumeral ligaments requires either splitting or detaching the subscapularis during the procedure to gain access to the capsulolabral complex. If the surgeon detaches the subscapularis, which is repaired anatomically at the end of the surgical procedure, it is an additional structure that requires protection for appropriate healing. No active or resistive IR, including isometrics, is appropriate during the first 6 POWs, and gentle measured strengthening is important for the next 3 to 4 weeks. The subscapularis also must be protected during ER PROM exercises during the first 6 weeks to avoid excessive stress to the healing suture line. Generally, the same staged ROM goals for ER that are shown in Table 1 are appropriate in this situation, but some physicians might limit the maximum ER to be obtained during phase 1 rehabilitation to a greater degree. Just as important is ensuring the patient relaxes to prevent muscle guarding of the subscapularis during ER PROM exercises. To avoid muscle guarding, the early passive ER exercises I prefer are seated passive ER with the assistance of the rehabilitation provider or family member (Figure 28) or the passive ER table walk-around (Figure 29). If the surgeon splits the subscapularis then sutures it closed instead of detaching the tendon, these modifications are used until the acute postoperative pain subsides.

Likely due to the increased tissue dissection required with open repair for instability compared with arthroscopic repair, the staged ROM goals shown in Table 1 are often more difficult to achieve. Therefore, most surgeons start PROM within the first week after open repairs. A bigger emphasis on PROM usually is required during phase 1 and often during phase 2 and phase 3 rehabilitation. In addition, the rehabilitation provider must ensure the patient stretches frequently and must closely monitor PROM gains to ensure staged goals are met. With a rehabilitation emphasis on frequent gentle stretching to achieve staged PROM goals, long-term PROM loss has been shown to be

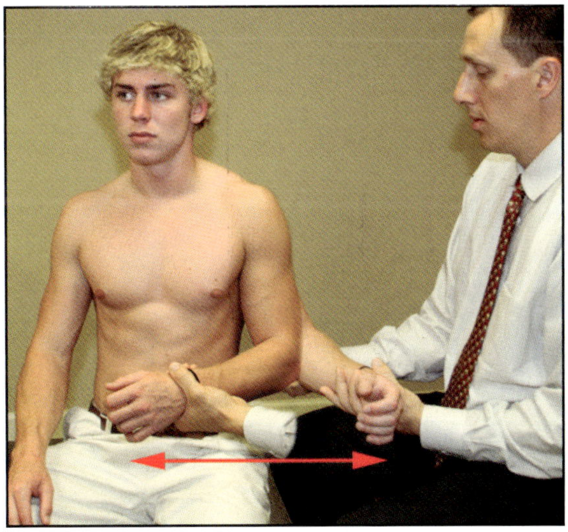

Figure 28. Assisted sitting passive external rotation.

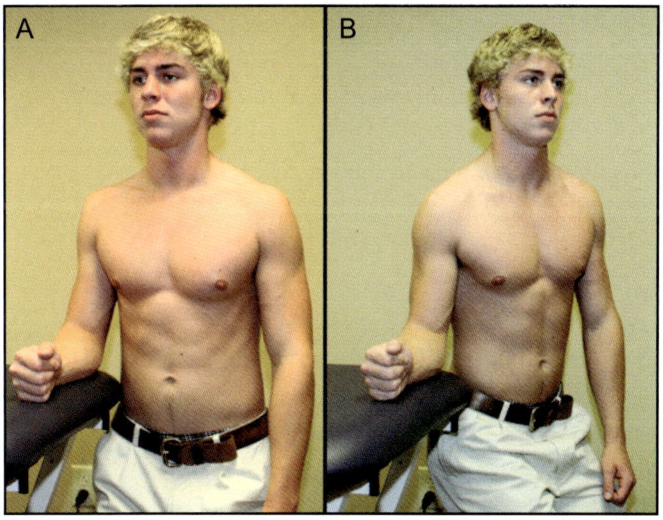

Figure 29 A and B. Passive external rotation walk-around exercise.

very minimal in these procedures.[32,37,38] After POW 6, the AROM, strengthening, neuromuscular control, and dynamic stability progression for open repair to treat instability is not different from arthroscopic repair. Return-to-sport time also is similar.

The Patient With Hyperlaxity

The patient with generalized hyperlaxity who undergoes an arthroscopic repair for instability requires a different rehabilitation emphasis and modifications to the base rehabilitation guideline. Generally, the surgeon is more concerned about recurrent instability in these patients than in typical patients, so changes to rehabilitation are individualized but often are made to slow the ROM progression, promote healing, and place extra emphasis on dynamic stability. Patients with hyperlaxity typically present with atraumatic multidirectional instability and are managed with an arthroscopic capsular shift that addresses the instability in multiple areas of the capsule. Labral tears and subsequent repairs are uncommon in this patient population.

At our center, the most important change made to phase 1 rehabilitation is strict adherence to not exceeding the staged ROM goals, especially ER. In addition, when a range of staged ROM is given in Table 1, the more conservative measure generally is used as the stopping point. Therefore, the ROM limit for passive ER that we use at POW 3 in the patient with hyperlaxity is typically 20°. To promote the slower ROM progression, the physician might delay the initiation of glenohumeral PROM until POWs 2 to 6. During this time, the patient only performs elbow, wrist, hand, and scapular AROM. When ROM is initiated, the patient might have more available PROM than the ROM limit. If this occurs, then no PROM is given to the patient for a home exercise in that direction. Therefore, phase 1 rehabilitation often is quite limited. Because dynamic stability provides protection to the repair, patients with hyperlaxity often are allowed to initiate some low-level, dynamic-stability exercises during the latter half of phase 1 rehabilitation. Submaximal isometrics and protected ER and IR ROM exercises with an elastic band might be used. Often, these patients also present with significant scapular dyskinesia, so scapular interventions that do not provide stress through the glenohumeral joint, such as manual pectoralis minor stretching and active scapular positioning, also can be used. Whereas closed chain activities are good dynamic-stability exercises, those that require any substantial weight bearing through the upper extremity are not advised during this stage of rehabilitation.

During phase 2 rehabilitation, stretching and PROM exercises still are de-emphasized, and AROM, strengthening, and dynamic-control exercises are emphasized. Passive ROM and stretching are not used for patients with preoperative hyperlaxity unless their ROMs are moderately behind staged ROM goals. We have found that small deficits in PROM can be corrected with active-assistive or active strengthening into the restricted ROM in the late stages of phase 2. Exercises included in the assistive-to-active elevation progression, such as that shown in Figure 30, often are used for this purpose. The standard AROM and strengthening progression is used with increased emphasis on improving active control of the upper extremity, generalized muscle tone, and proprioception. Less emphasis is placed on activities with moderate to high resistance, and a slower progression to strengthening in end ranges of abduction with ER is employed. Closed chain exercises, such as that shown in Figure 12, are important to improve dynamic stability; however, careful monitoring is required to ensure that the patient is strong enough to maintain the humeral head centered in the glenoid because most patients with hyperlaxity present with preoperative multidirectional instability.

Differences in phase 3 are mainly changes to timing and aggressiveness of rehabilitation. Because patients with hyperlaxity are thought to have to rely on dynamic stability to maintain stability in the shoulder more

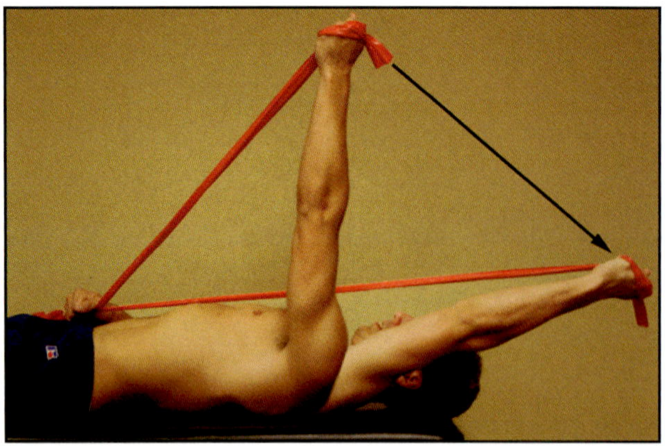

Figure 30. Supine forward elevation with an elastic band.

Arthroscopic Capsular Plication With or Without Bankart Repair

Table 4. General Rehabilitation Guideline for Arthroscopic or Open Posterior Instability Repair

Phase (Postoperative Weeks)	Rehabilitation Guideline
Phase 1 (0–6)	
Bracing and sling options	Rigid brace or sling with abduction pillow to limit or prevent internal rotation and worn at all times except bathing and dressing Standard sling for support and positioning of forearm near abdomen allowed
Range of motion	Begin passive range of motion sometime between postoperative day 1 and postoperative week 6, depending on physician preference and patient Passive range of motion in the true scapular plane (more abduction than normal) with or without range of motion limits Passive range of motion into external rotation at 20° of abduction with or without range of motion limits
Motions to avoid	Horizontal adduction Functional internal rotation
Phase 2 (6–12)	Passive range of motion and stretching as needed to achieve full range of motion at postoperative week 12 No horizontal adduction, functional internal rotation, or sleeper stretch unless range of motion is at least moderately behind range of motion targets Begin phase 2 active range of motion and strengthening progression same as Appendix At postoperative weeks 9–12, allowed to begin closed-chain stability exercises, such as quadruped positioning and quadruped to biped (Figure 12), if open chain strengthening exercises are going well and overhead active range of motion is full and painless No large posteriorly directed forces
Phase 3 (12–24)	Passive range of motion and stretching as needed to address any remaining deficits. Often little to no stretching is required. Continue phase 2 strengthening Initiate advanced strengthening progression as needed as in the Appendix Gradually advance activities requiring upper extremity weight bearing and posterior load as needed Must obtain clearance from physician to begin activities with large posteriorly directed forces (eg, push-ups, bench press, football blocking)

than other patients, we typically use a slower and more judicious return to advanced rehabilitation activities, such as multiplanar, high-speed exercises, at our facility. A slower return to participation in sport activities and activities that require heavy lifting often is used, as well.

Revision Repair for Instability

Rehabilitating a patient after either arthroscopic or open revision repair to treat instability is another highly individualized situation. The speed of progression should be determined by the referring physician and depends on factors, such as the number of previous failed repairs, quality of tissue, bone loss of the humeral head and glenoid, whether bone grafting was necessary, and other coexisting conditions. A slower rehabilitation program is warranted because the tissues already have shown the tendency to fail. Appropriate modifications might include one or more of the following: using limited-goals rehabilitation (chapter III-18), placing PROM limits on ER or forward elevation during the first 6 to 12 weeks, delaying the initiation of PROM exercises up to 6 weeks, or delaying the start of strengthening for 2 to 6 weeks. Depending on the patient, return to advanced strengthening activities, such as high-speed multiplanar exercises that require end-range abduction with ER and return-to-sport activities, are delayed or might never be appropriate. The surgeon always determines these modifications. The rehabilitation provider plays a vital role in repeated patient education throughout the rehabilitation process so patients understand the importance of complying with this slower-paced rehabilitation program.

Repair for Posterior Instability

Rehabilitation of either arthroscopic or open repair for posterior instability uses the same guiding rehabilitation principles and the same methods to manipulate stress to the surgical repair as anterior and multidirectional capsulolabral repair. However, the part of the capsule that requires protection is obviously different; therefore, whereas the timing of rehabilitation is the same, somewhat different interventions are needed. The posterior capsule is thinner and weaker than the anterior capsule, which is thickened by the glenohumeral ligament complex. Repairs for posterior instability, therefore, require more protection and gentle rehabilitation than other repairs for instability, especially during phase 1 and the early part of phase 2 rehabilitation. The motions that are most stressful to the posterior repair are horizontal adduction, functional IR, and IR in both adduction and abduction.

Rehabilitation of these patients, especially during phase 1, varies widely based on preference of the surgeon and on the patient. Table 4 outlines general rehabilitation guidelines for arthroscopic or open repair for posterior instability. The initial timeframe and extent of immobilization varies widely in these patients, as described in Table 4. Gaining staged PROM overhead in the true plane of the scapula is important to prevent a posteriorly directed force on the posterior capsule. Passive ER with the upper extremity near the side usually is achieved fairly easily with gentle stretching during this time. The amount of IR allowed in the first 6 weeks is restricted. The amount of restriction varies by the surgeon and patient and will be determined by the surgeon, but it typically is between 0° and 30° of IR.

Variable PROM and stretching generally is needed during phase 2 rehabilitation because full ROM in all planes, including IR, horizontal adduction, and functional IR, is not targeted before 12 POWs. Often, limited stretching is needed, but more regular stretching is required if a particular motion is moderately restricted. Discretion should be used when issuing direct posterior capsule stretches, such as cross-body adduction or the sleeper stretch, as part of a home program. The rehabilitation provider only should give them when a moderate restriction in motion is present and should monitor progress closely to ensure ROM is not gained too quickly.

Active ROM and strengthening principles and interventions for patients with a repair for posterior instability are very similar to that with repair for anterior instability, but the amount of load to the posterior capsule needs to be controlled. This mainly is done by delaying exercises that require a moderate body weight or external load through the repaired extremity. For example, exercises in the quadruped position are not begun until at least POW 9 and then are advanced slowly. Return to exercises or sports that require large amounts of posteriorly directed force through the shoulder girdle, such as bench pressing, football, and wrestling, are highly variable depending on preference of the surgeon and on the patient but usually are not allowed before POM 6.

Rotator Cuff Repair Combined With Arthroscopic Capsulolabral Repairs

The patient who has had a rotator cuff repair at the same time as a glenohumeral ligament plication with or without a Bankart repair is difficult to rehabilitate because the surgeon has performed extensive procedures involving both the passive and active restraints of the glenohumeral joint. This combined surgical procedure generally results in increased pain during the first 4 to 6 POWs and a more difficult time achieving ROM goals, especially PROM. Because 2 completely different operations are performed at once and each has its own specific rehabilitation guideline, 1 guideline must be chosen as the primary guideline for these patients. The rotator cuff repair guideline takes priority; however, the chosen rehabilitation variable influences this decision. For PROM, a ROM that is detrimental to any of the surgical procedures is not safe during rehabilitation. The staged ROM goals for both procedures are roughly the same. Early horizontal adduction excessively stresses a supraspinatus repair, and excessive passive ER, especially in increasing degrees of abduction, excessively stresses an anterior capsular plication or Bankart repair during phase 1 and early phase 2 rehabilitation. As mentioned, limited PROM is often a greater problem with these patients compared with excessive PROM beyond allowed limits.

For AROM, the rotator cuff repair guideline always is used to ensure adequate protection of the cuff repair. The instability repair is not affected negatively by the AROM and strengthening activities in the rotator cuff repair guideline. Delaying the initiation of AROM and strengthening often is indicated if the patient is behind in achieving the PROM goals or if the level of pain or inflammation appears elevated.

For advanced rehabilitation, a gradual increase in stress to all repaired structures is required. However, for almost all rehabilitation activities in phase 3, the rotator cuff repair needs the greatest protection. Therefore, the rotator cuff repair guideline is given priority at this time, and the rehabilitation provider keeps in mind that a gradual progression of activities should be accomplished in the throwing position to appropriately apply a gradual increase in load to a capsulolabral repair. Compared with patients who have had either a rotator cuff repair or a capsulolabral repair, these patients generally progress through all phases of rehabilitation much slower, and they typically need at least 6 to 8 weeks longer to complete rehabilitation.

Arthroscopic Capsulolabral Repair Combined With Repair of a Superior Labrum Anterior-Posterior Lesion

Rehabilitation guidelines for these 2 procedures are complimentary, so very few changes to the base rehabilitation program are needed when these 2 procedures are combined. Although performed for slightly different reasons, staged ROM goals, time to initiate AROM, strengthening, advanced rehabilitation activities, and return-to-sport timeframes are nearly identical. Where differences do exist, the more conservative guideline always should be used. I have found that the patient who has both procedures performed at the same time might have more pain in the early postoperative period and might have a harder time gaining PROM during all stages of rehabilitation. Therefore, a greater emphasis often is placed on PROM and stretching in these patients, avoiding end-range abduction with ER until POW 12 to protect both the superior labrum anterior-posterior lesion repair and capsulolabral repair. I have found these patients also tend to progress 2 to 6 weeks slower through phase 3 strengthening and return-to-sport progressions than patients with isolated procedures.

Other Associated Anatomic Injuries

Several specific types of soft tissue and bony injuries require modification to the standard rehabilitation guideline. An anterior labroligamentous periosteal sleeve avulsion (or ALPSA) lesion is an avulsion of the inferior glenohumeral ligament and anterior labrum with an intact scapular periosteum that allows the labrum and ligaments to displace medially and rotate inferiorly on the scapular neck (Figure 31). Repair of

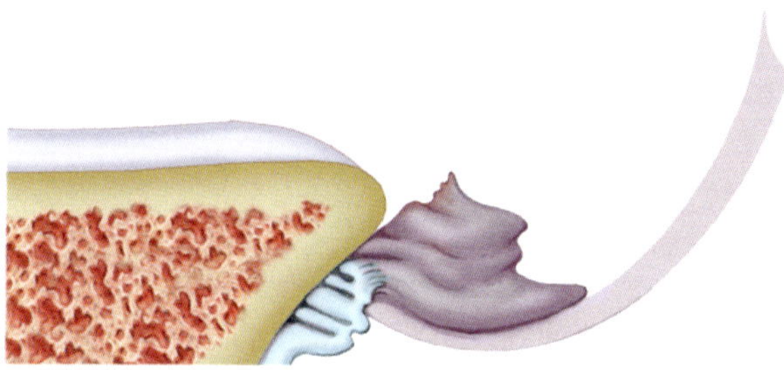

Figure 31. An anterior labroligamentous periosteal sleeve avulsion lesion shows displacement of the labrum and ligaments from their anatomic positions on the scapular neck.

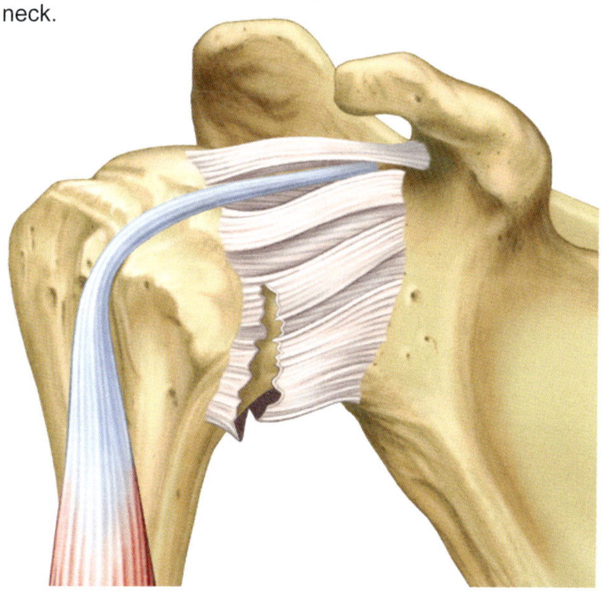

Figure 32. A humeral avulsion of the glenohumeral ligament lesion.

this injury usually warrants extra ROM limitations during the first 6 POWs. Stiffness in ER also might occur. Patients with repair of a humeral avulsion of the glenohumeral ligament (or HAGL) lesion, which is a tearing of the anatomic humeral neck attachment of the inferior glenohumeral ligament (Figure 32), also might have extra ROM limitations into ER for the first 6 POWs.

In addition to capsule and labral injuries, other associated injuries can be present in patients with repairs for glenohumeral instability, such as partial-thickness rotator cuff tears, and injuries to the humeral head and glenoid, such as Hill-Sachs lesions or glenoid fractures. A Hill-Sachs lesion is an impression fracture of the posterolateral humeral head caused by contact against the anterior rim of the glenoid during an anterior shoulder dislocation (Figure 33). It commonly is seen in patients with their first dislocations and patients with recurrent instability; however, it generally does not affect rehabilitation, and modifications do not need to be made because of it unless bone grafting is performed. Glenoid erosion, compression fractures, or avulsion fractures occasionally affect rehabilitation. If any of these associated injuries is managed by open reduction and internal fixation or by bone grafting, then the physician might delay initiation of ROM activities or dictate a slower ROM progression with strict ROM limits during the first 6 to 8 POWs. If debridement of a partial-thickness rotator cuff tear is performed, no modification to the standard program is needed; however, we realize these patients might have increased pain in the early postoperative period and they typically need longer to regain normal rotator cuff strength than other patients.

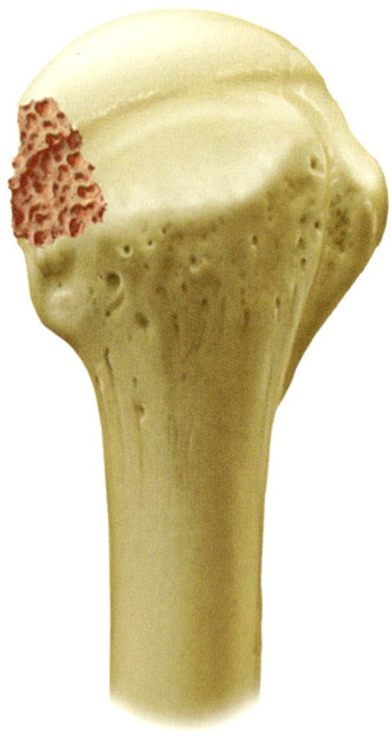

Figure 33. A Hill-Sachs lesion.

REFERENCES

1. Gaunt B, Shaffer M, Sauers E, Michener L, McCluskey G, Thigpen C. The American Society of Shoulder and Elbow Therapists' consensus rehabilitation guideline for arthroscopic anterior capsulolabral repair of the shoulder. *J Orthop Sports Phys Ther*. 2010;40(3):155–168.
2. McEleney ET, Donovan MJ, Shea KP, Nowak MD. Initial failure strength of open and arthroscopic Bankart repairs. *Arthroscopy*. 1995;11(4):426–431.
3. Roth CA, Bartolozzi AR, Ciccotti MG, et al. Failure properties of suture anchors in the glenoid and the effects of cortical thickness. *Arthroscopy*. 1998;14(2):186–191.
4. O'Connell PW, Nuber GW, Mileski RA, Lautenschlager E. The contribution of the glenohumeral ligaments to anterior stability of the shoulder joint. *Am J Sports Med*. 1990;18(6):579–584.
5. Terry GC, Hammon D, France P, Norwood LA. The stabilizing function of passive shoulder restraints. *Am J Sports Med*. 1991;19(1):26–34.
6. Turkel SJ, Panion MW, Marshall JL, Girgis FG. Stabilizing mechanisms preventing anterior dislocation of the glenohumeral joint. *J Bone Joint Surg Am*. 1981;63(8):1208–1217.
7. Itoi E, Hatakeyama Y, Urayama M, Pradhan RL, Kido T, Sato K. Position of immobilization after dislocation of the shoulder: a cadaveric study. *J Bone Joint Surg Am*. 1999;81(3):385–390.
8. Delforge G. *Musculoskeletal Trauma: Implications for Sports Injury Management*. Champaign, IL: Human Kinetics; 2002.
9. Lin TW, Cardenas L, Soslowsky LJ. Biomechanics of tendon injury and repair. *J Biomech*. 2004;37(6):865–877.
10. Woo SLY, Chan SS, Yamaji T. Biomechanics of knee ligament healing, repair and reconstruction. *J Biomech*. 1997;30(5):431–439.
11. Boissonnault WG, Badke MB, Wooden MJ, Ekedahl S, Fly K. Patient outcome following rehabilitation for rotator cuff repair surgery: the impact of selected medical comorbidities. *J Orthop Sports Phys Ther*. 2007;37(6):312–319.
12. Humphries W, Jain N, Pietrobon R, Socolowski F, Cook C, Higgins L. Effect of the Deyo score on outcomes and costs in shoulder arthroplasty patients. *J Orthop Surg (Hong Kong)*. 2008;16(2):186–191.
13. Hill AM, Jones IT, Hansen U, et al. Treatment of ligament laxity by electrothermal shrinkage or surgical plication: a morphologic and mechanical comparison. *J Shoulder Elbow Surg*. 2007;16(1):95–100.
14. Wetzler MJ, Bartolozzi AR, Gillespie MJ, et al. Fatigue properties of suture anchors in anterior shoulder reconstructions: Mitek GII. *Arthroscopy*. 1996;12(6):687–693.

15. Hiemstra LA, Sasyniuk TM, Mohtadi NG, Fick GH. Shoulder strength after open versus arthroscopic stabilization. *Am J Sports Med*. 2008;36(5):861–867.
16. Pollock RG, Wang VM, Bucchieri JS, et al. Effects of repetitive subfailure strains on the mechanical behavior of the inferior glenohumeral ligament. *J Shoulder Elbow Surg*. 2000;9(5):427–435.
17. Blasier RB, Guldberg RE, Rothman ED. Anterior shoulder instability: contributions of rotator cuff forces and the capsular ligaments in a cadaver model. *J Shoulder Elbow Surg*. 1992;1(3):140–150.
18. Cain PR, Mutschler TA, Fu FH, Lee SK. Anterior stability of the glenohumeral joint: a dynamic model. *Am J Sports Med*. 1987;15(2):144–148.
19. Labriola JE, Lee TQ, Debski RE, McMahon PJ. Stability and instability of the glenohumeral joint: the role of shoulder muscles. *J Shoulder Elbow Surg*. 2005;14(1 suppl S):32S–38S.
20. Lee SB, Kim KJ, O'Driscoll SW, Morrey BF, An KN. Dynamic glenohumeral stability provided by the rotator cuff muscles in the mid-range and end-range of motion: a study in cadavera. *J Bone Joint Surg Am*. 2000;82(6):849–857.
21. Cleland J. On the actions of muscles passing over more than one joint. *J Anat Physiol*. 1867;1(1):85–93.
22. Karduna AR, Williams GR, Williams JL, Iannotti JP. Kinematics of the glenohumeral joint: influences of muscle forces, ligamentous constraints, and articular geometry. *J Orthop Res*. 1996;14(6):986–993.
23. Louie JK, Mote CD Jr. Contribution of the musculature to rotatory laxity and torsional stiffness at the knee. *J Biomech*. 1987;20(3):281–300.
24. Wilk KE. Rehabilitation after shoulder stabilization surgery. In: Warren RF, Craig EV, Altchek DW, eds. *The Unstable Shoulder*. Philadelphia, PA: Lippincott-Raven; 1999:367–402.
25. Johnson LL. The shoulder joint: an arthroscopist's perspective of anatomy and pathology. *Clin Orthop Relat Res*. 1987;233:113–125.
26. Kim SH, Ha KI, Cho YB, Ryu BD, Oh I. Arthroscopic anterior stabilization of the shoulder: two to six-year follow-up. *J Bone Joint Surg Am*. 2003;85(8):1511–1518.
27. Levine WN, Rieger K, McCluskey GM III. Arthroscopic treatment of anterior shoulder instability. *Instr Course Lect*. 2005;54:87–96.
28. Morgan CD, Bodenstab AB. Arthroscopic Bankart suture repair: technique and early results. *Arthroscopy*. 1987;3(2):111–122.
29. Grana WA, Buckley PD, Yates CK. Arthroscopic Bankart suture repair. *Am J Sports Med*. 1993;21(3):348–353.
30. Boileau P, Villalba M, Héry JY, Balg F, Ahrens P, Neyton L. Risk factors for recurrence of shoulder instability after arthroscopic Bankart repair. *J Bone Joint Surg Am*. 2006;88(8):1755–1763.
31. Bacilla P, Field LD, Savoie FH III. Arthroscopic Bankart repair in a high demand patient population. *Arthroscopy*. 1997;13(1):51–60.
32. Fabbriciani C, Milano G, Demontis A, Fadda S, Ziranu F, Mulas PD. Arthroscopic versus open treatment of Bankart lesion of the shoulder: a prospective randomized study. *Arthroscopy*. 2004;20(5):456–462.
33. Kim SH, Ha KI, Kim SH. Bankart repair in traumatic anterior shoulder instability: open versus arthroscopic technique. *Arthroscopy*. 2002;18(7):755–763.
34. Kim SH, Ha KI, Jung MW, Lim MS, Kim YM, Park JH. Accelerated rehabilitation after arthroscopic Bankart repair for selected cases: a prospective randomized clinical study. *Arthroscopy*. 2003;19(7):722–731.
35. Radkowski CA, Chhabra A, Baker CL III, Tejwani SG, Bradley JP. Arthroscopic capsulolabral repair for posterior shoulder instability in throwing athletes compared with nonthrowing athletes. *Am J Sports Med*. 2008;36(4):693–699.
36. Lenters TR, Franta AK, Wolf FM, Leopold SS, Matsen FA III. Arthroscopic compared with open repairs for recurrent anterior shoulder instability: a systematic review and meta-analysis of the literature. *J Bone Joint Surg Am*. 2007;89(2):244–254.
37. Hubbell JD, Ahmad S, Bezenoff LS, Fond J, Pettrone FA. Comparison of shoulder stabilization using arthroscopic transglenoid sutures versus open capsulolabral repairs: a 5-year minimum follow-up. *Am J Sports Med*. 2004;32(3):650–654.
38. Bigliani LU, Kurzweil PR, Schwartzbach CC, Wolfe IN, Flatow EL. Inferior capsular shift procedure for anterior-inferior shoulder instability in athletes. *Am J Sports Med*. 1994;22(5):578–584.

ARTHROSCOPIC CAPSULAR PLICATION WITH OR WITHOUT BANKART REPAIR REHABILITATION GUIDELINE

St. Francis Orthopaedic Institute and St. Francis Rehabilitation Center

All information contained in this protocol is to be used as a general guideline only. Specific variations might be appropriate for each patient and might be specified by the physician. In all cases, it is acceptable to advance the program more slowly than stated. If the patient experiences excessive pain, discontinue exercise until the physician is contacted. ***Achieving and maintaining a low level of pain and inflammation and protecting the surgical repair are the guiding principles in all stages of rehabilitation, even if less passive and active range of motion are accomplished.***

SYMBOLS AND ABBREVIATIONS

AAFE, active-assistive forward elevation
AAROM, active-assistive range of motion
AASEP, assistive-to-active shoulder elevation progression
ADL, activity of daily living
AFE, active forward elevation
AROM, active range of motion
ER, external rotation
FE, forward elevation
IR, internal rotation
MMT, manual muscle testing
NA, not applicable
PER, passive external rotation
PFE, passive forward elevation
PNF, proprioceptive neuromuscular facilitation
POD, postoperative day
POM, postoperative month
POW, postoperative week
PRN, as needed
PROM, passive range of motion
ROM, range of motion
T-Band, Thera-Band (The Hygenic Corporation, Akron, OH)
WNL, within normal limits

Forward elevation, either active or passive, is the plane of motion in which an individual naturally lifts his or her arm that is anterior to the plane of the scapula and lateral to flexion.

STAGED GOALS FOR RANGE OF MOTION

These are approximate targets for range of motion. Specific limits might be specified by the physician. These ROMs should not be greatly exceeded.

Time	PFE	PER at 20° of Abduction	PER at 90° of Abduction	AFE
POW 1	100°	10°–30°	NA	NA
POW 3	130°	20°–40°	NA	NA
POW 6	150°	45°–55°	45°	115°
POW 9	165°	50°–65°	75°	145°
POW 12	WNL	WNL	WNL	WNL

PHASE 1

Goals

°Maximally protect surgical repair (capsule, ligaments, labrum, and sutures)
°Achieve staged ROM goals but DO NOT greatly exceed them
°Educate the patient about postoperative precautions
°Minimize pain and inflammatory response
°Ensure adequate scapular function

POD 3 to POW 6

- °Elbow, wrist, and hand AROM with no weight
- °Scapular elevations and retractions (no weight) in or out of sling
- °Pendulum exercises
  - °Lean over the table a comfortable amount
  - °Let the arm hang down relaxed
  - °Keep the body still
  - °As able, move the arm in small comfortable circles only
  - °Discontinue if the patient describes feelings of instability
- °Upright PER in slight abduction until mild stretch and mild discomfort at most
  - °7 to 12 repetitions 2 times per day
  - °Do not exceed staged ROM goals
  - °Preferred exercises
    - °Sit with family member or therapist rotating the arm (Figure 28)
    - °PER walk-around (stand with the arm supported on a table and rotate the body) (Figure 29)
- °PFE until mild stretch and mild discomfort at most
  - °7 to 12 repetitions 2 times per day
  - °Do not greatly exceed staged ROM goals
  - °Preferred exercises
    - °Sit with family member or therapist lifting the arm (Figure 34)
    - °Table step-back exercise (Figure 35)
    - °After achieving more than 110° of PFE, progress to self-assisted AAFE in the supine position as tolerated (Figure 36)
- °Ice for pain reduction
- °Fit sling properly
  - °Ensure the sling provides a slight lift to the shoulder girdle and supports the wrist
- °Patient education
  - °Primary focus of phase 1: encourage initial healing of the surgical repair
  - °Use of sling as instructed by physician
    - °Typically, full time in community and when up for more than 5 to 10 minutes at home
  - °Minimal use of the arm for light waist-level activities as comfortable

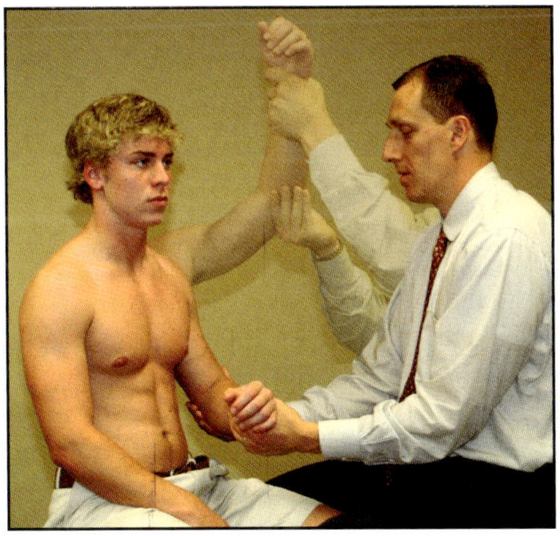

Figure 34. Assisted PFE. The assistant typically stands diagonally in front of patient.

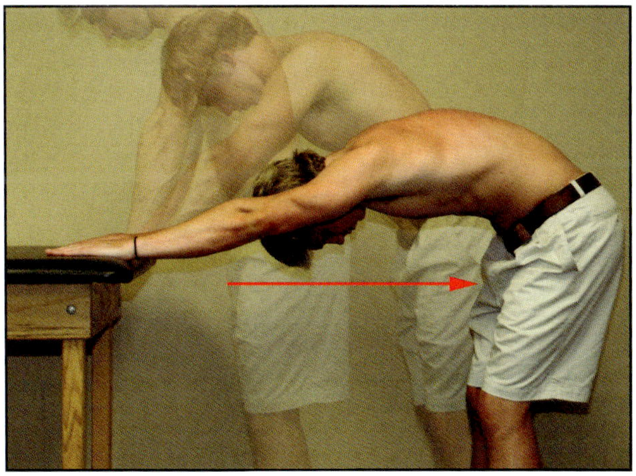

Figure 35. Table step-back exercise.

°Ensure level of pain is not increasing because of excessive use of the arm for ADLs or work

°Sleep in a recliner

°3 weeks (required)

°6 weeks (preferred)

Adjunctive Exercises

°Therapist-assisted supine PROM within comfortable ROM to

°Decrease muscle guarding

°Gain patient confidence

°Achieve but NOT EXCEED staged PROM goals (no mobilizations)

°Cervical spine AROM

°Pain-control agents PRN

°Aquatic therapy for gentle pain-free AAROM (no swimming strokes) after incision has healed completely

Interventions to Avoid

°Home exercise glenohumeral PROM except PFE and PER

°Do not allow or perform ROM or stretching greatly exceeding staged ROM goals, especially ER both by the side and in abduction

°Do not allow the patient to use the arm for heavy lifting or any activity that requires ROM greater than the staged ROM goals

°Weighted exercises

°Repetitive activity with affected extremity

PHASE 2

Goals

°Achieve staged ROM goals to normalize PROM and AROM at end of phase but DO NOT greatly exceed them

°Minimize shoulder pain

°Begin to increase strength and endurance

°Increase functional activities

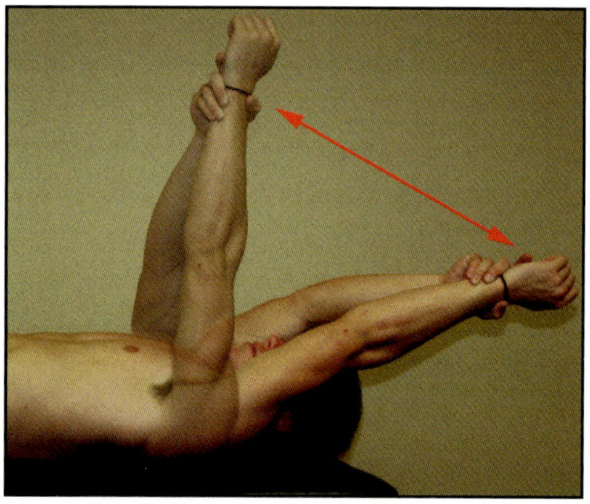

Figure 36. Self-assisted supine active-assisted forward elevation. The hand-assisted exercise is preferred.

POW 6 to 9

°Progress PROM and AAROM exercises PRN to achieve staged ROM goals in all planes. Many times only light stretching or no stretching is needed.

°Achieve staged ROM goals in FE but do not exceed them

°Preferred exercises

°Rope-and-pulley AAROM in FE (elbows remain straight)

°Patient-assisted supine AAFE exercise (use the unaffected arm for assistance) (Figure 36)

°Achieve staged ROM goals in ER at 20° abduction but do not greatly exceed them

°Use upright exercises

°Initiate horizontal adduction (Figure 37) and/or sleeper stretch PRN

°Goal of obtaining flexibility WNL at about POM 3

°Initiate supine hand-behind-head stretch (Figure 38) PRN

- °Progress to gentle ER stretching in 70° to 90° of abduction ONLY IF ROM is behind staged goals
- °Initiate functional IR AAROM and stretching as tolerated
- °Therapist-assisted PROM to achieve staged ROM goals if ROM is moderately behind staged goals with mobilizations PRN
- °Initiate base strengthening progression
    - °Includes standard rotator cuff, deltoid, and scapular strengthening program
    - °2 times per day at most with light resistance and increasing repetitions (generally 40–50 repetitions)
    - °Yellow T-Band for ER and IR
        - °Initially 5- to 6-foot band length and light or no pretension in a 3- to 6-inch arc of motion, with progressive tension as tolerated
        - °Can use side-lying ER instead of T-Band
    - °Yellow T-Band forward reach (Figure 5)
        - °Initially, 5- to 6-foot band length and light or no pretension with progressive tension as tolerated
        - °Start with the elbow bent and by the side and the band tied behind the patient
        - °Reach **forward** with the hand at waist level, progressing to reaching **forward** at chest level
        - °Do not initiate until forward reach at waist level without resistance is pain-free
        - °If forward reach is painful or difficult, replace with a "gravity-minimized" exercise from the AASEP (described below) until the forward reach can be done comfortably
        - °Scapular strengthening emphasizing scapular retractions and scapular upward rotators (chapter IV-2)
        - °**No prone FE, abduction, or ER**
- °Initiate the AASEP as comfortable (chapter II-4)
    - °A stepwise progression in difficulty of strengthening exercises from PFE to AFE against gravity
    - °Goal of the progression is to achieve pain-free full AFE
    - °Electromyography demonstrates progressive activation of cuff, deltoid, and scapular upward rotators during the progression
    - °If scapular or glenohumeral substitutions or pain are present, choose an easier exercise in the progression
    - °The order of the exercise sequence has some variability

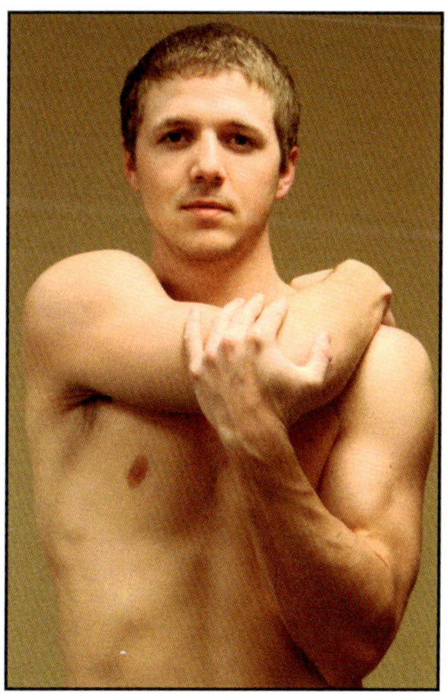

Figure 37. Horizontal adduction stretch.

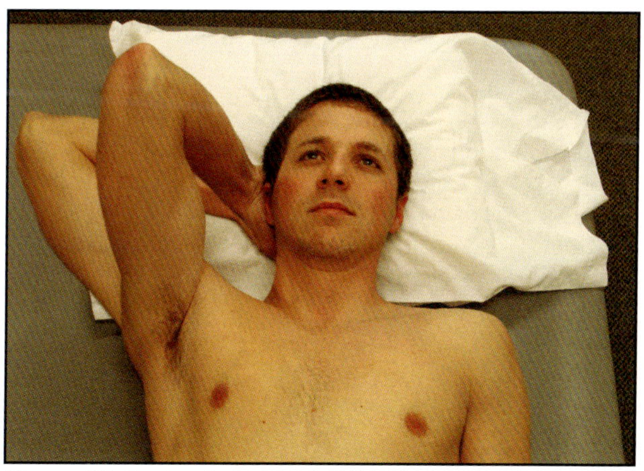

Figure 38. Supine hand-behind-head stretch to increase abduction and external rotation.

°Usually not all exercises need to be performed. Choose an exercise that is comfortable and can be performed without deviations but that is fatiguing.

°Exercises are divided into 3 levels of difficulty

1. Gravity-minimized exercises
    - °Horizontal dusting (Figure 39)
        - °Perform straight ahead
        - °Perform at 20° angles medially and laterally if comfortable
    - °T-Band supine FE (Figure 30)
        - °Must start involved arm at 90° of elevation
        - °Pull arm into FE
    - °Side-lying, gravity-eliminated AFE
        - °Lie on the uninvolved side
        - °Place the involved the arm on an ironing board
        - °Slide the hand on the board
    - °Jackins supine reaching progression
        - °Begin at 0° with the elbow bent and end at 90° of elevation with the elbow extended
            - °Start with the assistance of a cane or wand
            - °Progress to active motion
            - °Can progress to using 1 to 2 pounds of weight
        - °Can progress to inclined position, continuing to reach to ceiling
2. Assistive elevation exercises
    - °Rope-and-pulley AAFE
    - °Incline dusting (Figure 7)
    - °Standing AAFE (assistive elevation and descent via T-bar or unaffected arm)
    - °Standing assistive elevation and active independent eccentric lowering
    - °Wall-slide AAFE (Slide the hand on the surface. Do not walk with the fingers.)
        - °Ensure that the patient is in FE and is not in flexion
        - °Must be pain-free and natural when performing
3. Unsupported elevation exercises
    - °Overhead wall taps
    - °AFE (Figure 6)

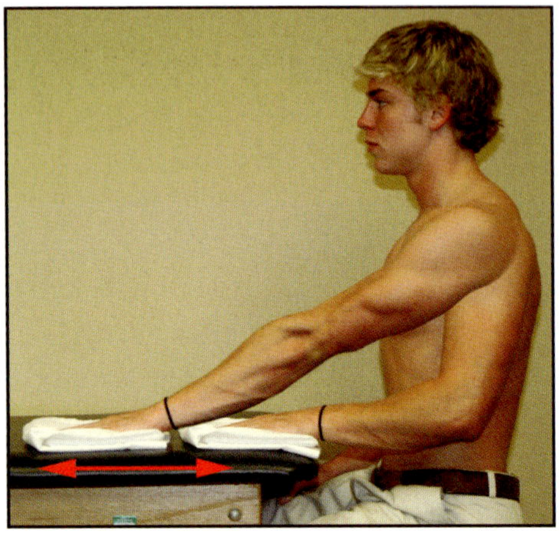

Figure 39. Horizontal dusting.

°Initiate AFE when the AASEP is complete
- °Only perform if full or nearly full AROM is possible and comfortable
- °Eventually progress to 1 to 3 pounds for resistance, depending on body size

°Closed chain exercises that do not place a large load on the shoulder in the position of horizontal abduction or the combined position of abduction with ER (chapter II-4)

Adjunctive Exercises

°Cryotherapy

°Modalities PRN

°Aquatic exercises (chapter IV-9)
- °AAROM
- °AROM
- °Light strengthening

- °Spine therapy assessment and mobilization if
  - °Nonneurogenic cervical or scapular pain or
  - °Limitation in end-range shoulder FE
- °Trunk stabilization and strengthening

POW 9 to POM 3

- °Continue the previously described PROM and stretching exercises PRN to achieve staged ROM goals, realizing sometimes very little or no stretching is needed to reach staged goals
- °Continue the previously described strengthening and neuromuscular control exercises
  - °Completion of the AASEP, progressing to AFE with light weight
  - °Progress elastic-resistance color with base strengthening as appropriate
- °When AFE with light weight and base strengthening are easy, can include exercises that gradually work toward increasing abduction with ER if the patient's functional goals require this position (Figures 8–10)
- °Rehabilitation activities also can be progressive in terms of speed when the patient demonstrates proficiency at slower speeds

Adjunctive Exercises

- °Light PNF
- °Open chain kinesthetic awareness drills (eg, ROM replication)
- °Begin return to golf progression: chipping and putting and progressing to half swings
- °Aquatic therapy, adding light breaststroke

Interventions to Avoid

- °Do not perform stretching significantly beyond staged ROM goals
- °Do not perform any stretch to gain end range ER or ER at 90° of abduction unless significant tightness is present
- °Do not allow the patient to use the arm for heavy lifting or any activities that require ROM beyond the staged goals
- °Do not perform any strengthening exercises that place a large load on the shoulder in the position of horizontal abduction or the combined position of abduction with ER (eg, NO push-ups, bench presses, or pectoralis flys)
- °Do not perform strengthening into straight-plane abduction

PHASE 3

Goals

- °Normalize AROM and PROM
- °Normalize strength, endurance, neuromuscular control, and power
- °Gradual and planned buildup of stress to capsulolabral tissues
- °Return to full ADLs, work, and recreation

POM 3 to 4.5

- °PROM and stretching PRN to address any remaining deficits, realizing that often very little or no stretching is needed at this time
- °Continue base strengthening program
  - °Continue to progress color of elastic resistance
  - °Continue progressive AFE, advancing up to 5 pounds depending on body size and functional goals

- °**Discharge when functional goals are met**
  - °**Many patients, especially those who have lower demands, do not progress to any of the rehabilitation described below**
- °Initiate the advanced strengthening progression **PRN** (chapter II-4)
  - °**Strict criteria to start program**
    - °MMT at least 4+/5 of shoulder girdle
    - °Pain-free with basic ADLs and all phase 2 strengthening activities
    - °Full AFE
    - °Goals of returning to sport participation, heavy labor, or repetitive or heavy overhead work
    - °Approval of physician
    - °Use of the following principles to develop exercises to gradually progress patient from current level of functioning to desired goals
  - °**Exercise principles**
    - °Decrease amount of external stabilization provided to shoulder girdle
    - °Integrate functional patterns, including abduction and ER
    - °Increase speed of movements
    - °Integrate kinesthetic awareness drills into strengthening activities
    - °Include the entire kinetic chain
    - °Decrease rest time to improve endurance
    - °Initiate prone strengthening PRN
    - °Train larger upper extremity muscles wisely
  - °**Sample exercises**
    - °T-Band standing PNF-type patterns (Figures 14 and 15)
    - °T-Band 90°/90° ER and IR with or without arm support (Figures 16 and 17)
    - °T-Band simulation of batting, golf, or tennis forehand and backhand
    - °Weighted shoulder shrugs
- °Participate in dumbbell overhead shoulder press **PRN** (Figure 26)
  - °Must meet the criteria to start the advanced strengthening progression (described above)
  - °Place hands in front of the shoulder with the elbows bent and naturally reach overhead
  - °Sets of 15 to 20 repetitions with 3 pounds or more 3 to 7 times a week
- °Initiate progressive replication of moderate-intensity ADLs and work
- °Initiate plyometric program **(PRN and if approved by physician)**
  - °Can begin after 3 to 6 weeks of advanced strengthening program
  - °Do not begin until 5/5 MMT for the rotator cuff and scapula
  - °Use only 2 to 3 times per week
  - °Begin with a beach ball or tennis ball and progress to weighted balls
  - °**Progressions**
    1. 2-handed tosses
       - °Waist level
       - °Overhead
       - °Diagonally
    2. 1-handed drop-and-catch drills
    3. 1-handed tosses, varying the amount of
       - °Abduction
       - °Arm support
       - °Protected ER

Adjunctive Exercises

°Complete return-to-golf progression (chapter IV-7) (advanced strengthening progression not needed)
°Modalities PRN
°Therapist-assisted stretching and mobilizations PRN
°Spine therapy assessment and mobilization if
  °Nonneurogenic cervical or scapular pain or
  °Limitation in end-range shoulder FE
°Isokinetic strengthening
°Trunk stabilization and strengthening

POM 4.5 to 8

°Use same exercises as described and add the following as appropriate
°Transition to maintenance strengthening program
°Can begin interval throwing program **(when approved by physician)** (chapter IV-6)
°Initiate progressive replication of demanding ADLs and work
°Initiate modified return to weight-training program **(when approved by physician)** (chapter IV-4)

Interventions to Avoid

°Any rehabilitation activity that is much more demanding than daily or expected activities
°Any rehabilitation activity that is a moderate to large increase in demand compared with previous rehabilitation
°Any rehabilitation activity that results in level of pain is high enough that the patient needs to use modalities

III-5

Superior Labrum Anterior-Posterior (SLAP) Lesion Repair

Timothy F. Tyler, MS, PT, ATC, and
Stephanie M. Squitieri, PT, DPT, CSCS

CHAPTER CONTENTS

- What patients are appropriate for the use of this guideline
- The most important factors that should guide clinical decison making
- Key principles in rehabilitation of this problem
- Specific rehabilitation guideline

WHAT PATIENTS ARE APPROPRIATE FOR THE USE OF THIS GUIDELINE?

- Patients who have undergone superior labrum anterior-posterior (SLAP) lesion repairs (types I–IV)
- Patients with combined lesions (SLAP tear and rotator cuff repair or subacromial decompression)

Clinical pearls are highlighted in yellow throughout the text.

Superior labrum anterior-posterior (SLAP) lesions were not realized until the advent of shoulder arthroscopy. Andrews et al[1] first described labral tears of the biceps anchor; however, Synder et al[2] first classified them, outlined their treatment, and described 4 basic types of lesions (Figure 1). Since then, several variants have been described. Superior labrum anterior-posterior lesions can best be understood by how they are treated and by the patient's symptoms. The 2 major ways that SLAP lesions can be treated are by debridement and repair. These lesions are seen in patients who either have instability or impingement, and the rehabilitation of patients is determined by which factors they have.

Overall, nonoperative management has been unsuccessful for many patients with unstable SLAP lesions.[1,3,4] Many researchers have reported that patients undergo diagnostic arthroscopy at an average of 12 to 30 months from the onset of their initial symptoms. In 1 study, patients participated in an extended trial of activity modification and rehabilitation exercises.[5] Most patients had been treated with rest, physical therapy, steroid injections, and nonsteroidal anti-inflammatory drugs without relief of their symptoms before diagnostic arthroscopy. As the surgical equipment and our

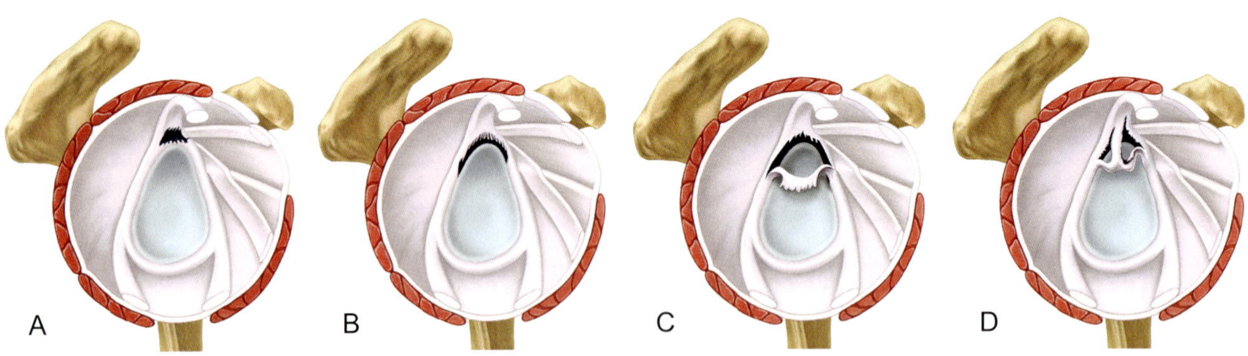

Figure 1. Classification of superior labrum anterior-posterior lesions. A, Type I; B, Type II; C, Type III; D, Type IV.[2]

understanding of SLAP lesions have evolved, a more effective operative treatment has become available.[6–10] The lesion is treated according to its type. In general, types I and III lesions are debrided, whereas type II and many type IV lesions are repaired.[4,11] Rehabilitation plays an integral part in the patient's outcome after all SLAP repairs.[12]

CAUSE

The superior labrum is part of the attachment of the long head of the biceps.[3,8,10,13] The role of the long head of the biceps is humeral head depressor and anterior stabilizer.[6,9] The SLAP area is in continuity with the anterior and posterior labrum. Therefore, a tear in the superior labrum can affect the entire labrum, and conversely, a tear in the anterior or posterior labrum can disrupt the superior labrum. The classic mechanism of injury is force, which either pushes the humeral head over or pulls the humeral head away from the superior labrum.[7] The humeral head pulls on the superior labrum and the biceps anchor, tearing them away from the glenoid. In addition, a tear of the anterior or posterior labrum due to a dislocation can extend into the superior labrum. Repetitive overhead lifting, which can pinch the superior labrum and pull downward on it, also can cause degenerative SLAP tears. In the late cocking phase of pitching, the biceps tendon winds upon itself, creating a peel-back mechanism that places a force across the superior labrum. This repetitive action is thought to cause SLAP lesions in pitchers.

CLINICAL EVALUATION

The rehabilitation provider should take the patient's history to discover whether he or she had an injury that placed an upward shear force across the shoulder. For example, the patient might describe falling on the upper extremity that was outstretched and overhead, placing a traction force across the extremity, suddenly grabbing and pulling on something, or experiencing a forceful pull on the extremity (eg, the shoulder being pulled on while walking dog). He or she also might describe mild instability in the shoulder with the repetitive throwing motion. Some patients can develop SLAP lesions with no apparent cause. In questioning the patient to discover the cause, it is important to ask about repetitive overhead lifting and throwing activities. The patient's response can range from instability to a vague ache in the shoulder. Many patients can show signs of impingement, and some have symptoms of locking, popping, and catching. No classic symptom pinpoints a SLAP lesion, but many baseball pitchers report having a "dead" arm. Many physical examination tests have been described to help diagnose a SLAP lesion.[4,11,12,14] The 2 most common tests are the Speed test and O'Brien test. These modified supraspinatus isolation tests can be positive if the patient has impingment.[15] Diagnosing a SLAP lesion can be difficult because it is usually found in combination with either impingement or instability.

CONCOMITANT INJURIES

Superior labrum anterior-posterior lesions occur with anterior and posterior labrum tears, impingement, or rotator cuff tears. Kim et al[16] reported 123 of 139 (88.5%) SLAP lesions were found with other intra-articular lesions during arthroscopy. They concluded that an isolated SLAP lesion is uncommon.

All concomitant lesions should be treated when the SLAP lesion is repaired. Rehabilitation providers usually treat patients who have had multiple procedures. To design a proper treatment plan, the rehabilitation provider needs to understand the type of SLAP lesion, what concomitant lesions were present, and the procedure or procedures used to treat the lesions.

OUTCOMES

Overall, the operative treatment of SLAP lesions has been successful, but as noted, nonoperative care has been unsuccessful.[17] Short-term improvement has been reported in patients with simple debridement, but at long-term follow-up, these patients had a high rate of failure,[18] which probably resulted from the surgeon not addressing the underlying instability. Yoneda et al[17] reported that early treatment with staple fixation yielded good to excellent results in 80% of patients. The first investigators to study suture anchor repair reported 100% success.[14] Later studies, in which various techniques of fixation were used, yielded a success rate of about 85%.[11,12] Stetson et al[4] reported an 82% rate of success in patients who only had SLAP repairs. When properly performed, repair of a SLAP lesion is a reliable procedure.

THE MOST IMPORTANT FACTORS THAT SHOULD GUIDE CLINICAL DECISION MAKING

After surgery, protecting the repair and decreasing the amount of stress placed upon the repair are important. Understanding the type of SLAP tear (I, II, III, and IV) and the operative procedure used enables the rehabilitation provider to develop a rehabilitation program that does not place the repaired tissue in a stressed position. Avoid early winding of the biceps tendon (peel-back mechanism) by restricting stretching of the glenohumeral (GH) joint into internal rotation (IR) and external rotation (ER) in 90° of abduction.

KEY PRINCIPLES IN REHABILITATION OF THIS PROBLEM

Postoperatively, the shoulder is placed in a sling without a swathe for 2 to 4 weeks to minimize biceps muscular activity and protect any other structures treated during surgery. The position of the upper extremity is in IR slightly anterior to the frontal plane. Because the early tensile strength of the labrum is weak, the early rehabilitation program after this repair is more conservative than after other open stabilization procedures.[14,17,19] The main focus of the early protective postoperative period (weeks 0 to 4) is to maintain proximal and distal strength and mobility, provide pain relief, and prevent selective hypomobility of sections of the capsule caused by iatrogenic change from the surgery. During this period, elbow range of motion (ROM) and gripping exercises are encouraged. We have found that instructing the patient to sleep with a pillow under the elbow to support the shoulder can take stress off the labrum and reduce discomfort. Modalities can relieve pain. The level of pain, postoperative swelling, and type of SLAP tear that was surgically treated determines progression of the patient through rehabilitation.[20,21] Good communication between the treating clinician and the surgeon is essential to proper care.[20] Understanding the specific procedure, concomitant injuries, and tissue quality also might affect the level of progression.

The rehabilitation process focuses on 4 keys to success. They include (1) regaining ROM, (2) providing scapular stabilization, (3) restoring posterior shoulder extensibility, and (4) returning rotator cuff strength.

SPECIFIC REHABILITATION GUIDELINE

In this section, we discuss each phase of rehabilitation. Our rehabilitation guidelines are outlined in the Appendix.

Phase 1 (Early Protective Phase)

Time: Weeks 0 to 4 after surgery

Goals: Protect the repair, educate the patient about the procedure and therapeutic progression, regulate pain and control inflammation, initiate ROM and dynamic stabilization, and initiate neuromuscular re-education of external rotators and scapulothoracic muscles

Initial Postoperative Examination. Outpatient physical therapy can begin as early as 3 days after a SLAP repair. At this time, the mobility of the sternoclavicular (SC), acromioclavicular (AC), and scapulothoracic joints are addressed, and they are mobilized, if indicated. Documentation of the initial evaluation should include the observation of the portal sites, atrophy, swelling, posture, and functional difficulties. The patient's ROM and general willingness to move the shoulder and his or her neurovascular measurements should be observed and documented. The patient must avoid contracting the biceps (active elbow flexion) until week 4. Tests to assess shoulder instability or labral disorders are inappropriate at this point.

Early Protective Postoperative Rehabilitation. When the milestone of mobility of the proximal joints is reached, manual scapular stabilization is initiated. In the side-lying position, manual resistance can be applied to the scapula to resist elevation, depression, protraction, and retraction (Figure 2). Pain can limit initiation of stabilization and rotator cuff isometrics; however, submaximal pain-free alternating isometrics for IR and ER may begin as early as 7 days after surgery (Figure 3). Because the rotator cuff muscles are not violated, this exercise can begin with the upper extremity at the side. Early mobilization exercises, such as pendulum exercises, are recommended for pain relief and could prevent adhesions from forming.

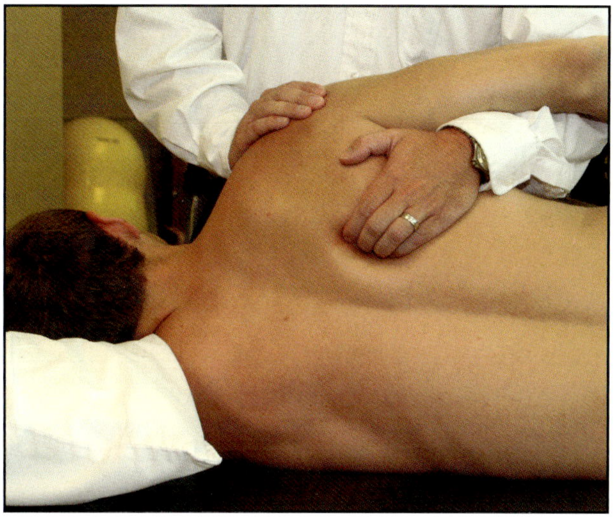

Figure 2. Mobilization and rhythmic stabilization position for the scapula.

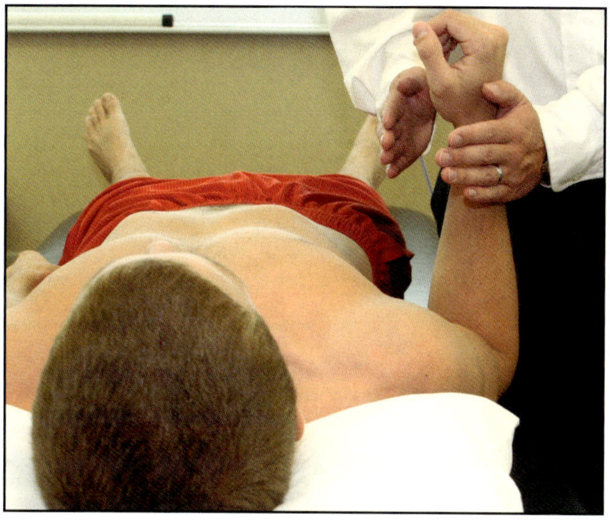

Figure 3. Rhythmic stabilization exercise for internal rotation and external rotation in 0° of abduction.

Pendulum exercises have been shown to produce little muscular activity and are considered to be safe during this period after most shoulder procedures.[22] However, some surgeons believe that the extremity hanging in a dependent position might put unwanted stress on the repaired labrum. We advise initiating active-assistive range of motion (AAROM) using a pulley for sagittal-plane flexion and scapular-plane elevation. In addition, a cane, golf club, or umbrella can be used to assist with regaining flexion, abduction, adduction, and ER at 0° and 30° of abduction (or where the surgeon sets the shoulder during surgery). Gentle mobilization (grades I and II) consisting of posterior glides can be performed at this time for pain relief.

Contraindications. Contraindications include the following:

- No ER past the set point for 3 weeks
- No ER in the 90°/90° position for 6 weeks to avoid the peel-back mechanism
- No active biceps contraction for 4 weeks

Early strengthening of the serratus anterior muscle also is encouraged if it is maintained slightly below 90° of shoulder flexion and is pain-free. Subsequent atrophy of the serratus anterior muscle, which results from immobilization, might allow the scapula to rest in a downwardly rotated position, causing inferior border prominence. Decker et al[23] used electromyography to determine which exercises consistently elicited the greatest maximal voluntary isometric contraction (MVIC) of the serratus anterior. They found that the serratus anterior punch, scaption, dynamic hug, knee push-up with a plus, and push-up with a plus exercises consistently elicited more than 20% MVIC. Most importantly, they determined that the push-up with a plus and the dynamic hug exercises maintained the greatest MVIC and maintained the scapula in an upwardly rotated position (Figure 4). Although it would be too early in the rehabilitation process to perform the push-up with a plus and dynamic hug exercises, Decker et al[23] highlighted the serratus anterior punch as a valuable exercise. Performed in a controlled, supervised setting, this is an excellent choice to initiate early

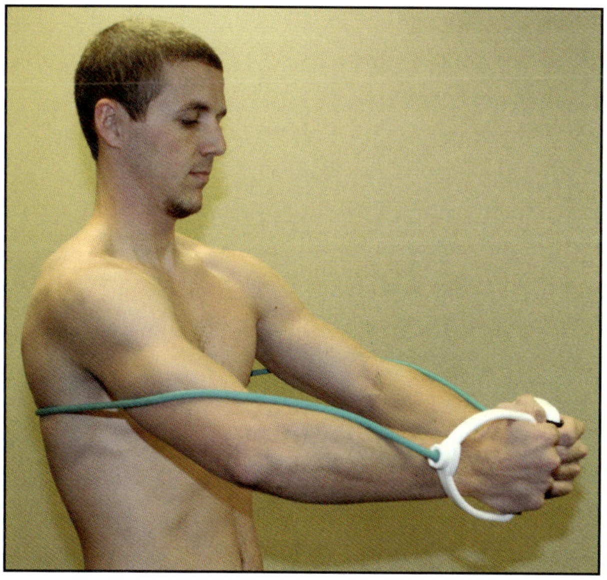

Figure 4. Dynamic hug exercise.

serratus anterior strengthening. Transition to the more challenging serratus anterior exercises should occur after 8 weeks and should be based on logical exercise progression.

A fine line exists between pushing patients too hard and progressing them as planned. Often, patients might feel better than expected during this early protective phase; therefore, rehabilitation providers must always respect the laws of tissue healing. Three milestones to achieve for progression to the next phase of rehabilitation are (1) to educate the patient about the procedure he or she had and what to expect during the rehabilitation; (2) to provide some pain relief so the patient can tolerate submaximal isometrics of the rotator cuff muscles at 0° of abduction; and (3) to attain symmetrical mobility of the SC, AC, and scapulothoracic joints, as well as the ability to protract, retract, elevate, and depress the scapula against submaximal manual resistance. The AAROM goals include achieving flexion to 110° to 130°, abduction to 70°, scapular-plane IR to 60°, and scapular-plane ER to a set point.

Phase 2 (Intermediate Phase)

Time: Weeks 5 to 8 after surgery

Goals: Normalization of arthrokinematics, gains in neuromuscular control, and normalization of posterior shoulder flexibility

During weeks 5 to 8, the rehabilitation provider should focus 3 visits per week on the return of scapular stability and GH ROM. Later in this period, rotator cuff isotonic strengthening is initiated. During this period, the patient removes the sling, and more aggressive AAROM exercises are initiated. These exercises might include the use of a pulley or cane to assist in forward elevation in the scapular plane and IR. External rotation stretching initially is performed in the guarded neutral position with the extremity at the side, then it is progressed into the scapular plane. While progressing through rehabilitation, the rehabilitation provider always should consider the patients' conditions, understanding if they naturally have joint hypermobility and motion is returning more quickly and easily than expected; if so, they do not need to be pushed. Patients with excessive joint laxity or generalized joint hypermobility must be progressed with caution.[24] Excessive ER stretching in the 90°/90° position in these patients too early during their postoperative care may jeopardize the end result. One problem that can occur is the peel-back mechanism. This phenomenon occurs when the biceps-labrum complex is abducted and externally rotated, causing a posterior biceps vector and shearing the biceps anchor repair off its origin. Burkhart and Morgan[25] discovered the peel-back mechanism, which can occur during rehabilitation when ER is forced passively in the 90°/90° position before healing has occurred. Kuhn et al[26] demonstrated failure of the biceps–superior-labrum complex in 9 of 10 cadaveric shoulders when the biceps was tensioned in the cocking position.

One therapeutic intervention that can assist in decreasing tension in the biceps-labrum complex is restoring posterior extensibility. When extensibility of the posterior capsule is restored, the humeral head can centralize in the glenoid fossa and not be forced anteriorly. A tight posterior capsule forces the humeral head anteriorly, creating unwanted tension in the biceps-labrum complex as the phenomenon occurs. Stretching and mobilization of the posterior capsule should be emphasized because tightness of the posterior shoulder structures has been linked to a loss of IR ROM.[27] Loss of mobility potentially can limit progress; a tight posterior capsule is thought to cause anterosuperior migration of the humeral head with forward elevation of the shoulder, which can contribute to a SLAP tear.[28] If posterior shoulder tightness and a decrease in IR ROM is observed, careful assessment must be taken. The Tyler test for posterior shoulder tightness can be performed to determine if posterior shoulder tightness is present (Figure 5).[27,29] To further determine if the loss of IR is due to capsular contracture, a posterior glide must be performed (Figure 6). An effective method of stretching this area is to stabilize the patient's scapula at the inferior angle manually while the patient provides a cross-chest adduction force in the supine position (Figure 7). Farther stretch can be felt by having the patient add slight pressure into IR by pressing inferiorly on the dorsal aspect of his or her hand or wrist. Passive range of motion of ER and abduction should be limited to 65° and 70°, respectively, so stress is not put on the healing biceps-labrum complex. Initial ROM goals are to achieve within 10° of full IR and 150° to 165° of passive flexion in the plane of the scapula. The ulti-

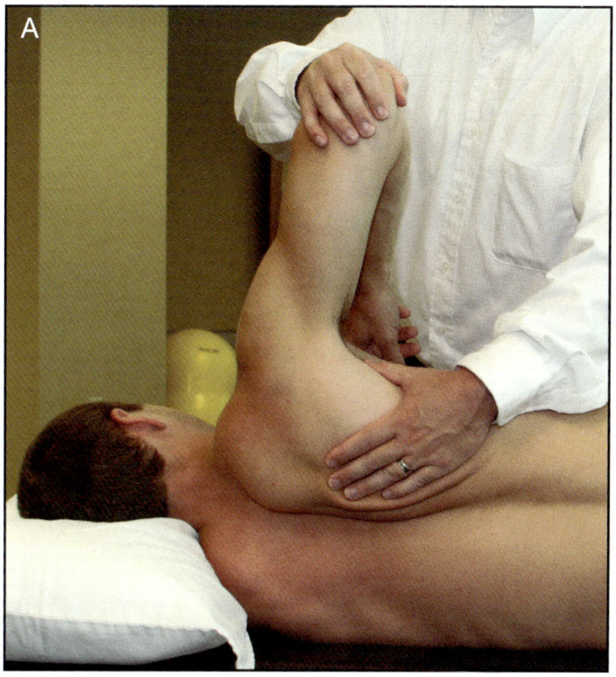

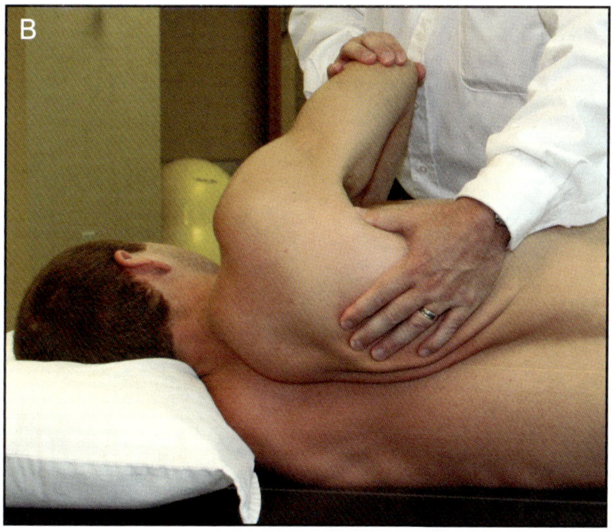

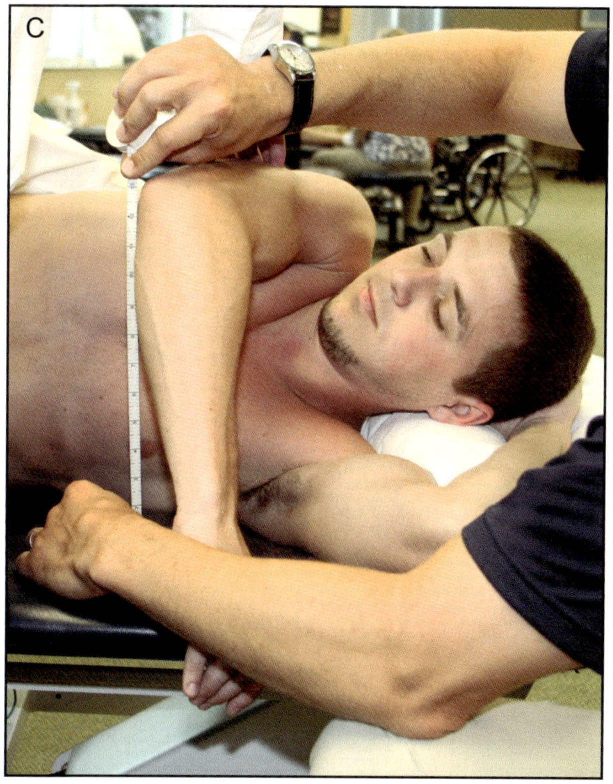

Figure. 5. The Tyler test for posterior shoulder tightness. A, Starting position. B, Middle position. C, Finished position.

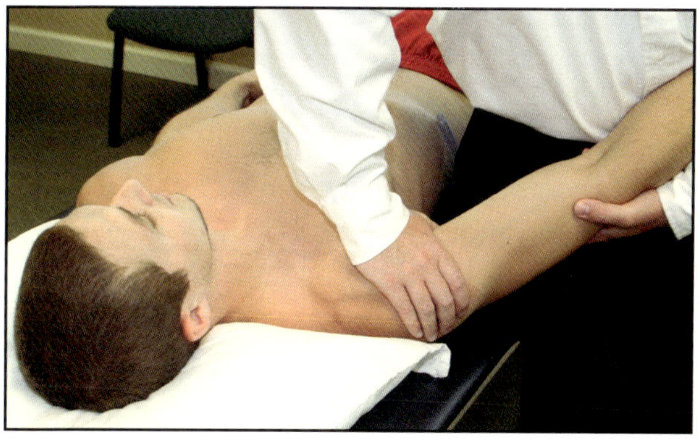

Figure 6. A posterior glide in the plane of the scapula to distinguish posterior capsule tightness.

mate goal is to maintain available mobility and prevent excessive scarring. Similar to Burkhart and Morgan[30] and Burkhart et al,[31] isotonic strengthening exercises are initiated for abduction, scaption, IR, and ER in the scapular plane.[32] In addition, rhythmic stabilization at the end ROM can be performed at this time. To have normal scapulohumeral rhythm, dynamic scapular stability of this joint needs to be restored.

Scapular exercises are encouraged in this phase of rehabilitation to counteract scapulohumeral dissociation and provide a stable base of support for active

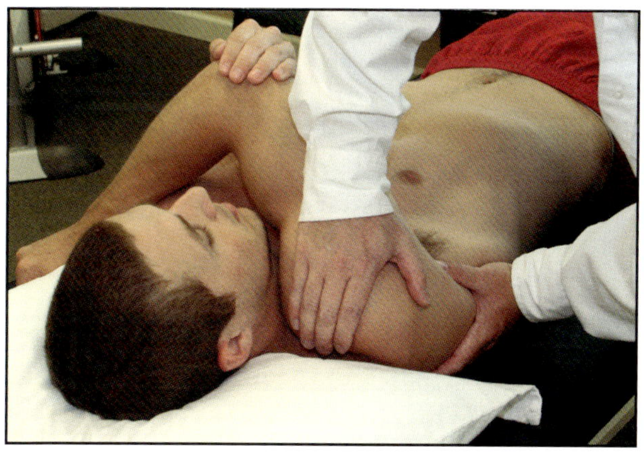

Figure 7. Supine posterior shoulder stretch with the rehabilitation provider stabilizing the scapula.

ROM (AROM) to be performed.[33] Recently, Tyler et al[34] reported on the importance of scapular stability in generating shoulder rotation torque in patients with microinstability. They found that patients with microinstability exhibited a large decrease in peak shoulder ER and IR torque after exercise-induced fatigue of the scapular stabilizer.[34] Many authors have examined the electromyographic (EMG) activity during scapular strengthening exercises; however, when choosing the appropriate exercise, the rehabilitation provider must keep the activity pain-free and must protect the repair.[35–37] Three relatively low-level exercises that we use after SLAP repair are (1) elastic-resistance rows (not to break the frontal plane with the involved elbow); (2) standing scapular retraction against elastic resistance with straight extremities just below 90° of shoulder flexion; and (3) shoulder oscillation in the plane of the scapula, keeping the wrist, elbow, and shoulder steady (Figure 8). Finally, in the later phases of rehabilitation, the patient can progress to more demanding open and closed kinetic chain scapular strengthening exercises.

Strengthening exercises should progress to resistance training with elastic bands for IR, ER, abduction, and extension. Maintaining the GH joint in the scapular plane (30°–45° anterior to the frontal plane) will minimize the tensile stress placed on the labral repair.[38] We have found that giving oral feedback to lift the chest up and pinch the shoulders back can facilitate scapular stabilization while the patient trains the external rotators. Hintermeister et al[39] found shoulder elastic-resistance training placed a low load on the shoulder and, therefore, was safe postoperatively.

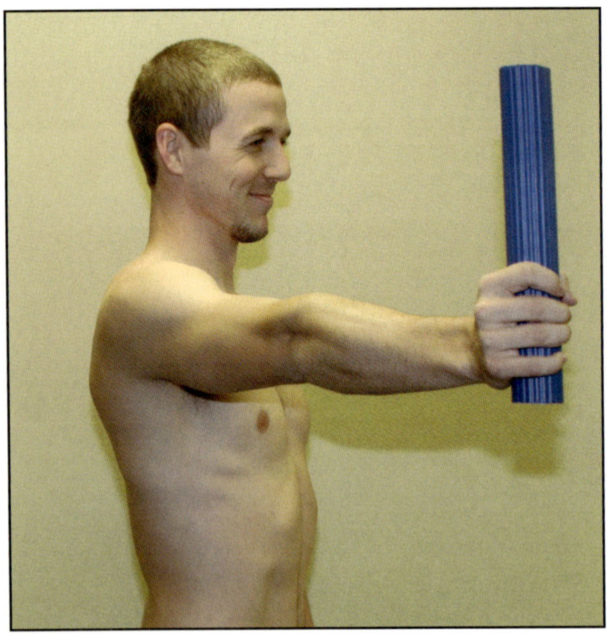

Figure 8. Shoulder oscillation in the scapular plane, keeping the wrist, elbow, and shoulder steady.

We believe that the use of free weights with the upper extremity in a dependent position should be used accordingly during this period to minimize the potential for detrimental humeral head translation. Sidelying ER typically is initiated during the later portion of this phase (Figure 9). Proper technique, weight, and ROM are important to execute this safely. Stabilizing the humerus to the thorax and not allowing the elbow to drift past the frontal plane of the body places minimal winding upon the labral repair.

At this phase, minimal weight should be used within the comfortable ROM to prevent placing stress on the biceps-labrum complex, which could damage the healing tissues. The rehabilitation provider also might recommend that the patient wait until the end of the intermediate postoperative period to initiate jogging or running for this same reason, as the humeral head might be forcibly thrust anteriorly. The rehabilitation provider must supervise the ROM progression during this period to protect the healing tissue.[32] Clinical milestones for progressing to the next phase of rehabilitation include achieving (1) 160° of flexion in the scapular plane, (2) ER to 65° in the scapular plane, (3) ER at 90° of abduction to 45°, (4) nearly full IR in the scapular plane, (5) IR at 90° of abduction to 45°, (6) 150° of abduction, (7) symmetrical posterior shoulder flexibility, and (8) improved isotonic internal and external strength in the available ROM.

Phase 3 (Strengthening Phase)

Time: Weeks 9 to 14 after surgery

Goals: Normalization of ROM, progression of strength, normalization of scapulothoracic motion and strength, and overhead activities without pain

During weeks 9 to 14 (usually 2–3 treatment sessions per week), rehabilitation continues to progress toward achieving full GH ROM and dynamic stability of the humeral head in the glenoid fossa. Gaining or maintaining full AROM within 10° of flexion in the sagittal plane and ER are to be achieved later dur-

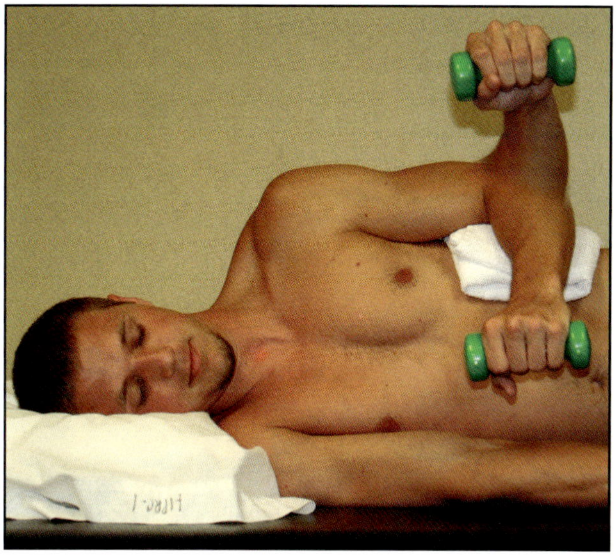

Figure 9. External rotation strengthening in the side-lying position with a free weight.

ing this phase. At this time, regaining ER, abduction, and flexion does not seem to be a limiting factor for recovery. When the patient has achieved the milestone of 70° to 80° of ER in the plane of the scapula, he or she will begin to acquire ER ROM at 90° of abduction. In the past, the patient has been expected to have full AROM 8 weeks after a SLAP repair, but most patients do not achieve this at week 8. Depending on the patient, we have found that an individual typically does not achieve full ER and IR ROM measured in the supine position with the GH joint abducted to 90° until 10 to 12 weeks or longer after a SLAP repair. This corresponds with the findings of other authors who have demonstrated a lack of full return of ROM in patients 12 weeks after a SLAP repair.[18,30,31,40] Therefore, during this phase, the patient can safely use a sleeper stretch to regain passive IR ROM (Figure 10). We believe that the key to a successful rehabilitation of these patients at this phase is finding the balance between stretching ER and letting them naturally regain their ROM.

At this time, an upper body ergometer (UBE) with light resistance can facilitate ROM and initiate active muscular control of the shoulder. The axis of rotation of the UBE should remain below the level of the shoulder joint so forward flexion is not forced above 80°. To avoid stress to the biceps-labrum complex, the patient should be positioned at a distance from the axis of rotation that does not allow the elbow to move posterior to the frontal plane when performing ergometer revolutions. This exercise is not initiated earlier because the amount of stress placed on the biceps-labrum complex during the use of a UBE is unknown.

When designing the strengthening program, matching the patients' needs with their limitations and goals is important. A properly designed strengthening program addresses their needs by attempting to gain the most benefit from each exercise prescription. In electromyography studies, researchers have set forth the shoulder exercises that activate particular muscles, and they should be considered as the clinician prescribes a program.[22–24,36,37] We have combined many of these programs to address generalized to specific weaknesses. From these studies, we have developed the "prone program plus" to address scapular stability and generalized weakness. The prone program plus can be started in this phase of the rehabilitation if the exercises can be accomplished without pain. The prone program plus includes prone GH horizontal abduction with GH IR (thumb down), prone scapular adduction with GH ER (thumb up), prone rows, prone shoulder flexion in the scapular plane, prone 90°/90° ER, push-ups with a plus (rehabilitation provider initiates exercise in quadruped), and ball press-downs. Patients can easily develop poor habits or can begin performing these exercises with improper form. We recommend that rehabilitation providers educate their patients about these exercises and allow ample time for them to develop proper form before prescribing these as part of a home program.

Proprioceptive neuromuscular facilitation (PNF) can be described as movements that combine rotational and diagonal (D) components that closely resemble the

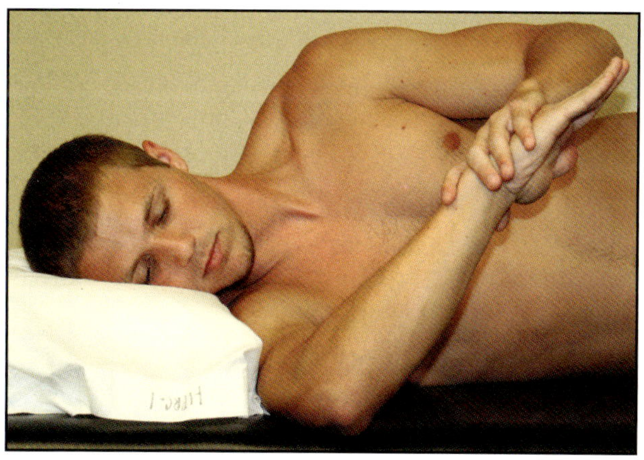

Figure 10. The sleeper stretch for gaining internal rotation.

movement patterns required for sport and work activities. Proprioceptive neuromuscular facilitation acts to enhance the proprioceptive input and neuromuscular responses while stressing motor relearning in the post-operative phases of rehabilitation. The PNF patterns are initiated with the scapula because scapular stability is essential for total function of the shoulder. Scapular patterns generally are performed in the side-lying position with the head and neck in neutral alignment. The coupled patterns of anterior elevation and posterior depression and of anterior depression and posterior elevation are used. Trunk rotation eventually should be combined with scapular and extremity PNF patterns to maximize combined muscular movement patterns. Techniques, such as hold-relax, slow reversals, and contract-relax, are used specifically to improve motion, whereas rhythmic stabilization, repeated contractions, and combination isotonics are used to enhance concentric and eccentric muscle action. Specifically, the D2-flexion pattern combines flexion, abduction, and ER, emphasizing the posterior rotator cuff and posterior deltoid. These neuromuscular control exercises are used to re-establish scapular positioning and stability of the humeral head in the glenoid.[33]

As the patient progresses through the program, periodic re-evaluation of the scapular dyskinesis is highly recommended. We stress this especially as the patient gains full ROM and may no longer be inhibited by tight soft tissue structures. Although indicating that an alteration exists, *scapular dyskinesis* is a qualitative collective term that does not differentiate between types of scapular positions or motions.[41] Therefore, scapular evaluation and categorization is challenging. The most common techniques for objective quantification include visual evaluation, the lateral scapular slide test, and 3-dimensional techniques. Kibler et al[41] introduced a visual technique that can help rehabilitation providers standardize categorizations. This dynamic technique categorizes the dyskinesis in 1 of 4 groups: type I, inferior angle prominence (horizontal-plane movement); type II, medial border prominence dorsally (frontal-plane movement); type III, shoulder shrug motion without winging (sagittal-plane movement); and type IV, bilaterally symmetrical movement (normal movement).

As with all scapular categorization techniques, the rehabilitation provider must be concerned with combined movements, a learning curve, and patient experience; however, this technique does present clinicians with a valuable tool that with practice, might enhance our clinical communication.

We also believe that exercises directed toward facilitation of functional muscular firing patterns in both the open and closed chains can provide useful input for return to function after SLAP repair. Lear and Gross[38] demonstrated that scapular muscle activity increases with a wall push-up progression. However, the strain on the biceps-labrum complex is unknown and might be too great for patients after a SLAP repair. The patient should gradually build up to and cautiously proceed with this exercise. Clinicians should reserve this exercise for the advanced strengthening phase to protect the healing tissue.

Isotonic exercises that emphasize light resistance and increased repetitions are used for isolated and combined movement patterns of the shoulder. We use a progression from 3 sets of 10 to 2 sets of 15 and to 1 set of 30 repetitions. If the patient can perform 1 set of 30 repetitions with good form and no substitution, he or she can progress to using 1- to 2-pound (0.45-kg–0.90-kg) weights for resistance and repeating the cycle, beginning with the 3 sets of 10. This rationale is based on lending objectivity to the progression and the tonic nature of the rotator cuff muscles and the scapular stabilizers. Isolated exercises are used to enhance or increase the strength of a particular muscle. Isotonic exercises are combined in functional movement patterns and are performed with PNF patterns using elastic resistance or the cable column to enhance coordinated movement. For a swimmer, the D1 pattern with elastic resistance will carry over to his or her athletic function. Initiation of isokinetic strengthening at this phase might enhance the shoulder's ability to strengthen in a pain-free ROM. Slower speeds should be used when strengthening patients with shoulder instability. Isokinetic principles suggest that faster isokinetic speeds create greater translational forces, whereas slower speeds create stronger compressive forces, which would stabilize the shoulder. Milestones that should be met before moving to the next rehabilitation phase include (1) within 10° of full AROM in flexion, abduction, IR, and ER in the plane of the scapula; (2) normalized scapulothoracic motion and strength; (3) moderate overhead activities without pain; and (4) isometric internal and external strength that is at least 50% of the uninjured side.

Phase 4 (Advanced Strengthening Phase)

Time: Weeks 15 to 24 after surgery

Goals: Pain-free full ROM, improvement of muscular endurance, and improvement of dynamic stability

After 15 weeks, the patient is in the final phase of rehabilitation. Full AROM should be attained at this time. The only restriction on ROM is that the GH joint should not be stretched in ER beyond 90°. Allowing the athlete to regain additional degrees of ER over time might be preferable to stressing the biceps-labrum complex, potentially stretching the repair. Stretching of the posterior capsule is appropriate if full IR has not been obtained yet. Performing the side-lying sleeper stretch encourages ROM for IR (Figure 10). At this phase of rehabilitation, treatment should begin to streamline toward the functional demands of the patient.[42]

At the onset of this phase, a thorough strength assessment is needed to evaluate the direction of strengthening needed for the patient. This assessment might include manual muscle testing, hand-held dynamometry, and isokinetic strengthening (or a combination of these techniques). Assessment should include the primary shoulder movers, shoulder rotators, and scapular stabilizers. Results of this assessment should be addressed with a well-rounded strengthening program to include isotonic-loading, concentric-loading, and eccentric-loading exercises. When designing these programs, consider the everyday demands of each patient. For an overhead-throwing athlete, strengthening in the throwing position is imperative (Figure 11).

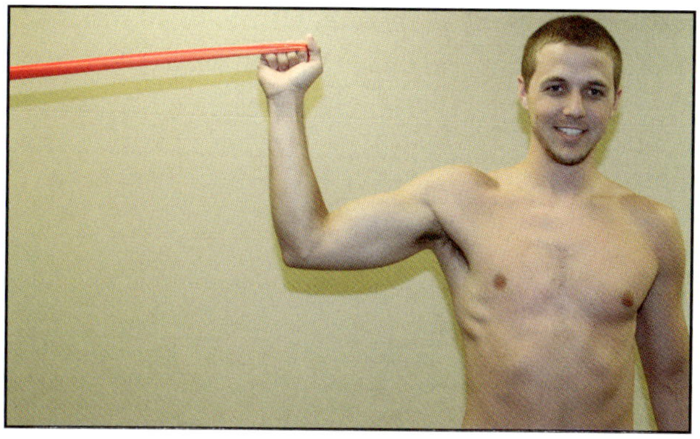

Figure 11. External rotation strengthening in the 90°/90° position with elastic resistance.

Initiation of a properly designed plyometric training program is often the missing link to discharging a high-level patient. Plyometric training for the upper extremity is used to generate rapid and powerful muscular contractions in response to a dynamic stretch-inducing load to a muscle or group of muscles. We suggest that plyometrics train the entire neuromuscular system, using the principles of stored elastic energy to use strength as quickly and forcefully as possible. The myotatic reflex develops stored elastic potential. If the exercise movement is slow, such as in weight training, the energy is dissipated and nonproductive. However, with rapid movement, this stored elastic energy can be used to generate a force greater than that of the concentric contraction of the muscle alone. Plyometrics use the principles of progressive loading with the ultimate goal of power development. Using a trampoline increases the EMG activity and elevates the level of eccentric loading of the shoulder rotators.[43] Therefore, a progression from 2-hand side-to-side throws to overhead throws and to 1-hand overhead throws is encouraged to maximize the power development of the overhead athlete. A well-rounded program addresses both the internal and external rotators of the shoulder and the core muscles of the trunk. Externally challenging the patient by permitting stability from a naturally unstable surface, such as a ball, challenges the entire kinetic chain. Advanced exercises, such as walk outs with a large exercise ball, exemplify this concept (Figure 12). As the patient walks out from the ball with his or her hands, core stabilizers and GH stabilizers are challenged. Milestones to progress to the final phase of

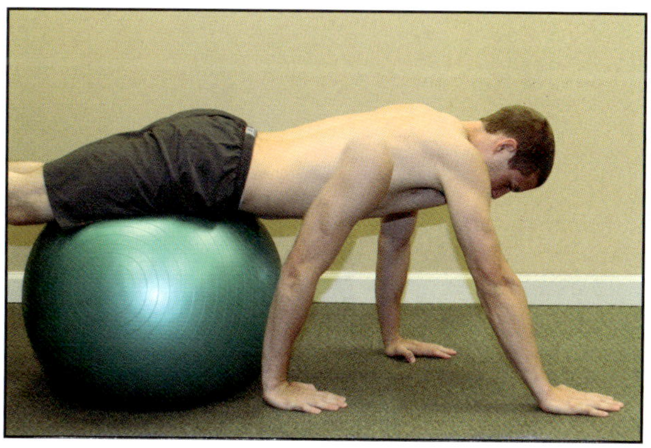

Figure 12. Exercise ball walk out.

rehabilitation include (1) pain-free full ROM, (2) less than 20% strength deficits for IR and ER at 90°/s, and (3) 20% strength deficits in all positions.

Phase 5 (Return-to-Activity and Return-to-Sport Phase)

Time: Months 4 to 6 after surgery

Goals: Pain-free full ROM, normalized strength, and return-to-sport or return-to-activity program

This is the phase of rehabilitation at which very few rehabilitation providers have the opportunity to discharge their patients. Too often patients loose interest, exhaust insurance coverage, or just neglect the importance of fine-tuning their shoulders before fully returning to their lifestyles. This stage is designed to prepare patients to return without hesitation to full participation in all activities. Milestones to successful completion of this phase include (1) total confidence in the shoulder, (2) pain-free full ROM, and (3) less than 10% deficit in all positions for isokinetic or hand-held dynamometry.[44]

Exercises in this phase continue to emphasize functional positions. During this phase, a progression of the plyometric program to PNF D2 plyometrics is initiated (Figure 13). A gradual return to sport is permitted when the patient is pain-free; has nearly full ROM in all planes; has confidence in the affected shoulder; and has 85% to 90% of the strength of the opposite side on isokinetic testing at 90°/s, 180°/s, and 300°/s for the motions of IR and ER. Confidence is achieved when the patient can perform pain-free functional movement in his or her sport. In our experience, the throwing athlete requires an additional 1 to 2 months to allow the shoulder to accommodate to the motion. Patients also report that it takes up to 1 year for their affected shoulders to feel "normal" after a SLAP repair. We currently use the American Shoulder and Elbow Surgeons shoulder evaluation form to standardize the documentation of pain, motion, strength, stability, and function. Although gathering enough data to determine a criterion score for return to sport when 6 months have passed and clinical milestones have been met remains difficult, the athlete is cleared for full throwing. This timeframe is in agreement with other authors' findings (Table).[45]

In conclusion, considerations must be given if additional procedures are performed for reattachment of the labrum, ligaments, or the biceps tendon. However, stronger fixation techniques have allowed the rehabilitation to progress more rapidly after these procedures. These guidelines are a continuum of rehabilitation phases based on the effect that the operative procedure has on the tissue and the surrounding structures. Scientific rationale is applied whenever possible; however, rehabilitation must evolve as surgical procedures

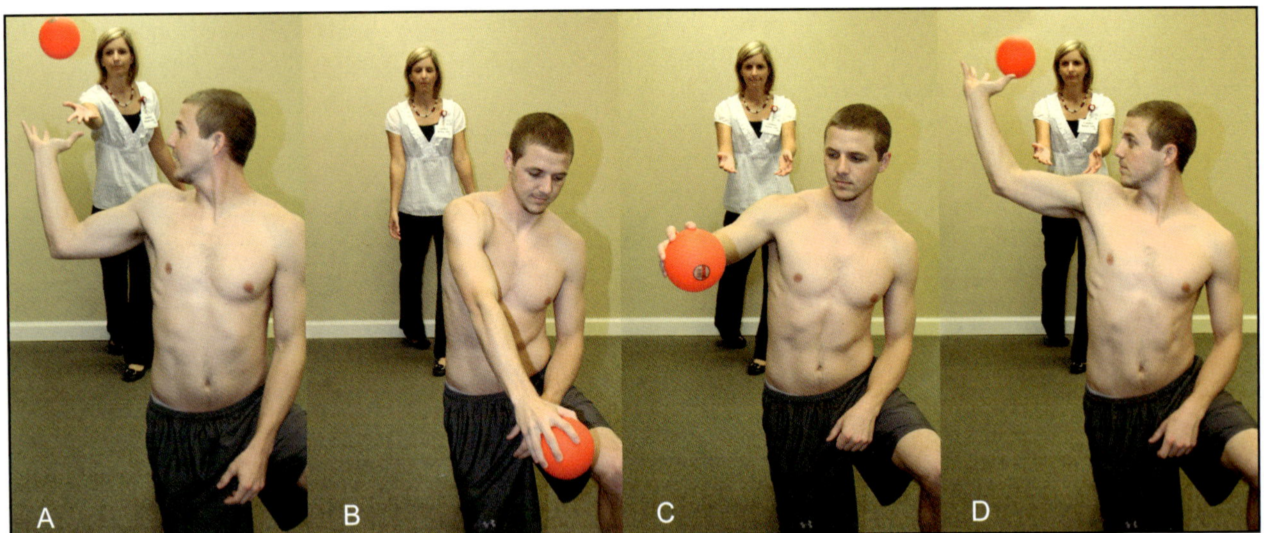

Figure 13. Plyometric proprioceptive neuromuscular facilitation diagonal 2 reverse throws. A, The rehabilitation provider throws the ball over the patient's shoulder. B, The patient catches the ball and decelerates it down to the foot. C, The patient begins to accelerate the ball and, D, throws it back over the shoulder to the rehabilitation provider.

Superior Labrum Anterior-Posterior (SLAP) Lesion Repair

Table. Time to Return to Participation in Sports After Superior Labrum Anterior-Posterior Lesion Surgery[46]

Study	Year	Procedure	Type of SLAP Lesion	Population	Return to Sports[a]	Full Throwing
Yoneda et al[17]	1991	Repair	II	Athletes	ND	ND
Resch et al[11]	1993	Repair	II	NS	6 mo	ND
Cordasco et al[18]	1993	Debridement	II	NS	ND	ND
Pagnani et al[5]	1995	Repair	II, IV	NS	4 mo	6 mo (NS)
Field and Savoie[14]	1993	Repair	II, IV	NS	ND	ND
Berg and Ciullo[47]	1997	Repair	II, IV	NS	ND	ND
Segmüller et al[48]	1997	Repair	II, IV	NS	6 mo	ND
Morgan et al[49]	1998	Repair	II	Athletes, nonathletes	4 mo	7 mo
Samani et al[50]	2001	Repair	II	Athletes, nonathletes	ND	ND
O'Brien et al[46]	2002	Partial anterolateral acromioplasty, repair	II	Athletes, nonathletes	ND	ND
Jazrawi et al[51]	2003	Repair/arthroscopic thermal capsular shift	II	Athletes	3–4 mo	11.2 mo

[a] In most studies, *time to return* refers to the initial return rather than the full return.
Abbreviations: SLAP, superior labrum anterior-posterior; NS, not specified; and ND, not documented.

evolve. These guidelines are not set in stone, and all exercises are not distinct to particular phases. The goals and exercises need to be modified based on the patient, pathologic lesion, and performance demands. Exercise prescriptions should be viewed as guidelines upon which to base the rehabilitation rather than as a protocol.

REFERENCES

1. Andrews JR, Carson WG Jr, McLeod WD. Glenoid labrum tears related to the long head of the biceps. *Am J Sports Med.* 1985;13(5):337–341.
2. Synder SJ, Karzel RP, Del Pizzo W, Ferkel RD, Friedman MJ. SLAP lesions of the shoulder. *Arthroscopy.* 1990;6(4):274–279.
3. Prodromos CC, Ferry JA, Schiller AL, Zarins B. Histological studies of the glenoid labrum from fetal life to old age. *J Bone Joint Surg Am.* 1990;72(9):1344–1348.
4. Stetson WB, Snyder SJ, Karzel RP, Banas MP, Rahal SE. Long-term clinical follow-up of isolated SLAP lesions of the shoulder. Paper presented at the 64th Annual Meeting of the American Academy of Orthopaedic Surgeons; San Francisco, CA; February 13–17, 1997.
5. Pagnani MJ, Speer KP, Altchek DW, Warren RF, Dines DM. Arthroscopic fixation of superior labral lesions using a biodegradable implant: a preliminary report. *Arthroscopy.* 1995;11(2):194–198.
6. Itoi E, Kuechle DK, Newman SR, Morrey BF, An KN. Stabilising function of the biceps in stable and unstable shoulders. *J Bone Joint Surg Br.* 1993;75(4):546–550.
7. Maffet MW, Gartsman GM, Moseley B. Superior labrum-biceps tendon complex lesions of the shoulder. *Am J Sports Med.* 1995;23(1):93–98.
8. Pal GP, Bhatt RH, Patel VS. Relationship between the tendon of the long head of the biceps brachii and the glenoidal labrum in humans. *Anat Rec.* 1991;229(2):278–280.
9. Rodosky MW, Harner CD, Fu FH. The role of the long head of the biceps muscle and superior glenoid labrum in anterior stability of the shoulder. *Am J Sports Med.* 1994;22(1):121–130.
10. Vangsness CT Jr, Jorgenson SS, Watson T, Johnson DL. The origin of the long head of the biceps from the scapula and glenoid labrum: an anatomical study of 100 shoulders. *J Bone Joint Surg Br.* 1994;76(6):951–954.
11. Resch H, Golser K, Thoeni H, Sperner G. Arthroscopic repair of the superior glenoid labral detachment (the SLAP lesion). *J Shoulder Elbow Surg.* 1993;2(3):147–155.
12. Synder SJ, Banas MP, Karzel RP. An analysis of 140 injuries to the superior glenoid labrum. *J Shoulder Elbow Surg.* 1995;4(4):243–248.
13. Cooper DE, Arnoczky SP, O'Brien SJ, Warren RF, DiCarlo E, Allen AA. Anatomy, histology, and vascularity of the glenoid labrum: an anatomical study. *J Bone Joint Surg Am.* 1992;74(1):46–52.
14. Field LD, Savoie FH III. Arthroscopic suture repair of superior labral detachment lesions of the shoulder. *Am J Sports Med.* 1993;21(6):783–790.
15. O'Brien SJ, Pagnani MJ, Fealy S, McGlynn SR, Wilson JB. The active compression test: a new and effective test for diagnosing labral tears and acromioclavicular joint abnormality. *Am J Sports Med.* 1998;26(5):610–613.
16. Kim TK, Queale WS, Cosgarea AJ, McFarland EG. Clinical features of the different types of SLAP lesions: an analysis of one hundred and thirty-nine cases. *J Bone Joint Surg Am.* 2003;85(1):66–71.

17. Yoneda M, Hirooka A, Saito S, Yamamoto T, Ochi T, Shino K. Arthroscopic stapling for detached superior glenoid labrum. *J Bone Joint Surg Br*. 1991;73(5):746–750.
18. Cordasco FA, Steinmann S, Flatow EL, Bigliani LU. Arthroscopic treatment of glenoid labral tears. *Am J Sports Med*. 1993;21(3):425–431.
19. Chandnani VP, Yeager TD, DeBerardino T, et al. Glenoid labral tears: prospective evaluation with MRI imaging, MR arthrography, and CT arthrography. *AJR Am J Roentgenol*. 1993;161(6):1229–1235.
20. Karzel RP, Synder SJ. Magnetic resonance arthrography of the shoulder: a new technique of shoulder imaging. *Clin Sports Med*. 1993;12(1):123–136.
21. Tirman PF, Applegate GR, Flannigan BD, Stauffer AE, Crues JV III. Magnetic resonance arthrography of the shoulder. *Magn Reson Imaging Clin N Am*. 1993;1(1):125–142.
22. Ellsworth AA, Mullaney MJ, Nicholas SJ, McHugh MP, Tyler TF. Electromyography of selected shoulder musculature during unweighted and weighted pendulum exercises. *J Orthop Sports Phys Ther*. 2004;34(1):A57.
23. Decker MJ, Hintermeister RA, Faber KJ, Hawkins RJ. Serratus anterior muscle activity during selected rehabilitation exercises. *Am J Sports Med*. 1999;27(6):784–791.
24. Tyler TF, Calabrese GJ, Parker RD, Nicholas SJ. Electrothermally-assisted capsulorrhaphy (ETAC): a new surgical method for glenohumeral instability and its rehabilitation considerations. *J Orthop Sports Phys Ther*. 2000;30(7):390–400.
25. Burkhart SS, Morgan CD. The peel-back mechanism: its role in producing and extending posterior type II SLAP lesions and its effect on SLAP repair rehabilitation. *Arthroscopy*. 1998; 14(6):637–640.
26. Kuhn JE, Lindholm SR, Huston LJ, Soslowsky LJ, Blasier RB. Failure of the biceps superior labral complex: a cadaveric biomechanical investigation comparing the late cocking and early deceleration positions of throwing. *Arthroscopy*. 2003;19(4):373–379.
27. Tyler TF, Roy T, Nicholas SJ, Gleim GW. Reliability and validity of a new method of measuring posterior shoulder tightness. *J Orthop Sports Phys Ther*. 1999;29(5):262–274.
28. Harryman DT II, Sidles JA, Clark JM, McQuade KJ, Gibb TD, Matsen FA III. Translation of the humeral head on the glenoid with passive glenohumeral motion. *J Bone Joint Surg Am*. 1990;72(9):1334–1343.
29. Tyler TF, Nicholas SJ, Roy T, Gleim GW. Quantification of posterior capsule tightness and motion loss in patients with shoulder impingement. *Am J Sports Med*. 2000;28(5):668–673.
30. Burkhart SS, Morgan C. SLAP lesions in the overhead athlete. *Orthop Clin North Am*. 2001;32(3):431–441.
31. Burkhart SS, Morgan CD, Kibler WB. The disabled throwing shoulder: spectrum of pathology part II. Evaluation and treatment of SLAP lesions in throwers. *Arthroscopy*. 2003;19(5):531–539.
32. Diederichs S, Harndorf M, Stempfle J. Follow-up treatment with physiotherapy after arthroscopic reconstruction in SLAP lesions [in German]. *Orthopade*. 2003;32(7):647–653.
33. Kibler WB. Shoulder rehabilitation principles and practice. *Med Sci Sports Exerc*. 1998;30(suppl 4):S40–S50.
34. Tyler TF, Cuoco A, Schachter AK, Thomas GC, McHugh MP. The effect of scapular-retractor fatigue on external and internal rotation in patients with internal impingement. *J Sport Rehabil*. 2009;18(2):229–239.
35. McCann PD, Wooten ME, Kadaba MP, Bigliani LU. A kinematic and electromyographic study of shoulder rehabilitation exercises. *Clin Orthop Relat Res*. 1993;288:179–188.
36. McMahon PJ, Jobe FW, Pink MM, Brault JR, Perry J. Comparative electromyographic analysis of shoulder muscles during planar motions: anterior glenohumeral instability versus normal. *J Shoulder Elbow Surg*. 1996;5(2 pt 1):118–123.
37. Moseley JB Jr, Jobe FW, Pink M, Perry J, Tibone J. EMG analysis of the scapular muscles during a shoulder rehabilitation program. *Am J Sports Med*. 1992;20(2):128–134.
38. Lear LJ, Gross MT. An electromyographical analysis of the scapular stabilizing synergists during a push-up progression. *J Orthop Sports Phys Ther*. 1998;28(3):146–157.
39. Hintermeister RA, Lange GW, Schultheis JM, Bey MJ, Hawkins RJ. Electromyographic activity and applied load during shoulder rehabilitation exercises using elastic resistance. *Am J Sports Med*. 1998;26(2):210–220.
40. Warner JJ, Kann S, Marks P. Arthroscopic repair of combined Bankart and superior labral detachment anterior and posterior lesions: technique and preliminary results. *Arthroscopy*. 1994;10(4):383–391.
41. Kibler WB, Uhl TL, Maddux JW, Brooks PV, Zeller B, McMullen, J. Qualitative clinical evaluation of scapular dysfunction: a reliability study. *J Shoulder Elbow Surg*. 2002;11(6):550–556.
42. Burkhart SS, Morgan CD, Kibler WB. Shoulder injuries in overhead athletes: the "dead arm" revisited. *Clin Sports Med*. 2000;19(1):125–158.
43. Cordasco FA, Wolfe IN, Wooten ME, Bigliani LU. An electromyographic analysis of the shoulder during a medicine ball rehabilitation program. *Am J Sports Med*. 1996;24(3):386–392.
44. McFarland EG, Park HB, Chronopolous E, Yokota A, Kim TK. Results of repair of SLAP lesion [in German]. *Orthopade*. 2003;32(7):637–641.
45. Park HB, Lin SK, Yokota A, McFarland EG. Return to play for rotator cuff injuries and superior labrum anterior posterior (SLAP) lesions. *Clin Sports Med*. 2004;23(3):321–334, vii.
46. O'Brien SJ, Allen AA, Coleman SH, Drakos MC. The transrotator cuff approach to SLAP lesions: technical aspects for repair and a clinical follow-up of 31 patients at a minimum of 2 years. *Arthroscopy*. 2002;18(4):372–377.
47. Berg EE, Ciullo JV. The SLAP lesion: a cause of failure after distal clavicle resection. *Arthroscopy*. 1997;13(1):85–89.
48. Segmüller HE, Hayes MG, Saies AD. Arthroscopic repair of glenolabral injuries with an absorbable fixation device. *J Shoulder Elbow Surg*. 1997;6(4):383–392.
49. Morgan CD, Burkhart SS, Palmeri M, Gillespie M. Type II SLAP lesions: three subtypes and their relationships to superior instability and rotator cuff tears. *Arthroscopy*. 1998;14(6):553–565.
50. Samani JE, Marston SB, Buss DD. Arthroscopic stabilization of type II SLAP lesions using an absorbable tack. *Arthroscopy*. 2001;17(1):19–24.
51. Jazrawi LM, McCluskey GM III, Andrews JR. Superior labral anterior and posterior lesions and internal impingement in the overhead athlete. *Instr Course Lect*. 2003;52:43–63.

REHABILITATION GUIDELINES FOR SUPERIOR LABRUM ANTERIOR-POSTERIOR (SLAP) LESION REPAIR

Nicholas Institute of Sports Medicine and Athletic Trauma

All information contained in this rehabilitation guideline is to be used as a general guideline only. Specific variations might be appropriate for each patient and might be specified by the physician. In all cases, it is acceptable to advance the program more slowly than stated. If the patient experiences excessive pain, discontinue exercise until the physician is contacted. ***Achieving and maintaining a low level of pain and inflammation and protecting the surgical repair are the guiding principles in all stages of rehabilitation, even if less passive and active range of motion are accomplished.***

SYMBOLS AND ABBREVIATIONS

AAROM, active-assistive range of motion
AC, acromioclavicular
AROM, active range of motion
ER, external rotation
GH, glenohumeral
IR, internal rotation
LT, lower trapezius
MT, middle trapezius
POM, postoperative month
POW, postoperative week
PROM, passive range of motion
RHM, rhomboid
ROM, range of motion
SC, sternoclavicular
ST, scapulothoracic
UBE, upper body ergometer

EARLY PROTECTIVE PHASE: POW 0 TO 4

Goals

°Protect the surgical procedure
°Educate the patient about the procedure and the therapeutic progression
°Regulate pain and control the inflammation
°Initiate ROM and dynamic stabilization
°Neuromuscular re-education of external rotators and ST muscles

Treatment Plan: POW 0 to 2

°Sling immobilization for 2 to 4 weeks
°Gripping exercises
°Elbow, wrist, and hand ROM
°Pendulum exercises
°Shoulder PROM forward, abduction, IR, and ER
  °**DO NOT** go beyond the position set at the time of surgery for ER (progress flexion to AAROM)

°IR and ER proprioception training (controlled range)
°Initiate gentle alternating isometrics for IR and ER in the scapular plane to 0° of abduction
°Initiate passive forward flexion to 90°
°Initiate scapular mobility

Treatment Plan: POW 2 to 4

°ROM progression
°Forward flexion to 110° to 130°
°ER in the scapular plane to 35° (position set at the time of surgery)
°IR in the scapular plane to 60°
°Progress submaximal alternating isometrics for IR and ER in the scapular plane
°Initiate scapular strengthening
°Manual scapular retraction
°Resistance-band retraction
    °Ensure no shoulder extension past the trunk
°Deltoid isometrics in all directions
°Biceps and triceps strengthening
°Initiate light elastic-resistance-band work for IR and ER

Milestones for Progression

°Forward flexion to 90°
°Abduction to 70°
°ER in the scapular plane to 30°
°IR in the scapular plane to 20°
°Tolerance of submaximal isometrics
°Knowledge of home care and contraindications
°Normalize mobility of related joints (AC, SC, ST)

INTERMEDIATE PHASE: POW 5 TO 8

Goals

°Normalize arthrokinematics
°Gains in neuromuscular control
°Normalization of posterior shoulder flexibility
°Limit PROM of ER and abduction to 65° to 70° to protect the healing biceps-labrum complex

Treatment Plan

°ROM progression
°Flexion in the scapular plane passively to 150° to 165°
°ER in the scapular plane to 65°
°IR in the scapular plane: full or to within 10°
°Initiate joint mobilizations as necessary
°Initiate posterior capsule stretching
°Progress strengthening

°IR and ER (with GH in the scapular plane) with elastic-resistance band
°Side-lying ER
°Scaption full can (no weight if substitution patterns)
°Clockwise and counterclockwise ball against wall
°Body blade at neutral or rhythmic stabilization

Milestones for Progression

°Forward flexion to 160°
°ER in the scapular plane to 65°
°Full IR in the scapular plane
°Symmetrical posterior capsular mobility
°Progressing isotonic strength with IR and ER in available range

STRENGTHENING PHASE: POW 9 TO 14

Goals

°Normalize ROM
°Progression of strength
°Normalize ST motion and strength
°Overhead activities without pain

Treatment Plan

°ROM progression: stretching ER at 90° of GH abduction
°Within 10° of full AROM in all planes
°Progression of scapular retractors and stabilizers
°Prone program: LT, MT, and RHM
°LT: scapular depression
°Progress strengthening
°Challenging rhythmic stabilization
°UBE
°Initiate isokinetic IR and ER in the scapular plane
°Initiate IR and ER at 90° of GH abduction
°Isotonic strengthening: flexion and abduction
°Closed kinetic chain exercise

Milestones for Progression

°Within 10° of full AROM in the scapular plane
°Less than 50% isometric strength deficits: IR and ER
°Less than 30% strength deficits: primary shoulder muscles and scapular stabilizers

ADVANCED STRENGTHENING PHASE: POW 15 TO 24

Goals

°Pain-free full ROM
°Improve muscular endurance

°Improve dynamic stability

Treatment Plan

°Maintain flexibility
°Progress strengthening
°Advanced closed kinetic chain exercise
°Wall push-ups: with and without ball
°Continue with overhead strengthening
°Continue with isokinetic IR and ER strengthening: 90° of GH abduction
°Advance isotonic strengthening
°Advance rhythmic stabilization training in various ranges and positions
°Initiate plyometric strengthening
°Chest passes
°Trunk twists
°Overhead passes
°90°/90° single-arm plyometrics

Milestones for Progression

°Full pain-free ROM
°Less than 20% strength deficits: IR and ER at 90° of GH abduction
°Less than 20% strength deficits throughout

RETURN-TO-ACTIVITY AND RETURN-TO-SPORT PHASE: POM 4 TO 6

Goals

°Pain-free full ROM
°Normalized strength
°Return-to-activity or return-to-sport program

Treatment Plan

°Continue isokinetic training
°Continue with stability training
°Advance plyometric training
°Continue with closed kinetic chain exercise

Milestones for Activity

°Confidence in shoulder
°Less than 10% strength deficits throughout
°Pain-free full ROM
°Completion of return-to-sport or return-to-activity program

III-6

Rehabilitation After Subacromial Decompression, Excision of the Distal Clavicle, or Acromioplasty

Brian J. Phillips, PT, DPT

CHAPTER CONTENTS

WHAT PATIENTS ARE APPROPRIATE FOR THE USE OF THIS GUIDELINE?

- Patients who have undergone isolated arthroscopic subacromial decompression, distal clavicle excision, or acromioplasty. If concomitant with surgical repair of the rotator cuff, labrum, or capsule, defer to that specific postoperative protocol.
- Patients who have undergone arthroscopic debridement of a partial rotator cuff tear or labrum tear, or both, with no formal repair.
- Patients who have undergone arthroscopic bursectomy or debridement of the glenohumeral joint.
- Patients who have undergone one of the procedures listed with concomitant biceps tenodesis or biceps tenotomy.

Clinical pearls are highlighted in yellow throughout the text.

THE MOST IMPORTANT FACTOR THAT SHOULD GUIDE CLINICAL DECISION MAKING

One of the top priorities for the rehabilitation provider treating a patient who has undergone shoulder surgery is to minimize the amount of postoperative pain and inflammation. In our clinic, this largely is achieved by my facility's philosophy of treatment that is **always gentle**. This treatment approach allows the patient to experience less pain, enabling better relaxation and tolerance to therapeutic exercises and passive range of motion (PROM) stretching and, in turn, promoting a faster return of range of motion (ROM). Obtaining smooth, comfortable ROM in a timely manner will help prevent postoperative shoulder stiffness, which can severely limit a patient from regaining full functional use of his or her shoulder. Chapter II-I provides a more detailed explanation of our always gentle philosophy. The use of an always gentle treatment approach will help the rehabilitation provider achieve the 2 most important goals of rehabilitation after subacromial decompression, excision of the distal clavicle, or acromioplasty: minimizing postoperative pain and inflammation and establishing normal or nearly normal

PROM in the first 6 postoperative weeks (POWs). Accomplishing these 2 goals as quickly as possible will dictate the speed and intensity at which the patient can be progressed through the postoperative rehabilitation protocol.

KEY PRINCIPLES IN REHABILIATION OF THIS PROBLEM

As with rehabilitation after any surgical procedure, the rehabilitation provider must consider certain key principles when treating patients who have undergone shoulder surgery. These factors include knowledge of the details of the surgical procedure; factors that can affect the healing of tissues involved during the operation; knowledge of the stresses that each therapeutic intervention places on the shoulder; and an understanding of how to progress these patients through a structured, systematic, evidence-based protocol. Close communication among the physician, rehabilitation provider, and patient is paramount to ensure that the patient is progressed through his or her postoperative rehabilitation program in a safe and effective manner.

Knowledge of the Surgical Procedure

The rehabilitation provider must know the details of the surgical procedure performed before evaluating and treating a patient who has had shoulder surgery. He or she must know and understand the specific surgical technique used, if any concomitant procedures were performed, and the severity of the affected tissues before initiating a treatment plan. Knowledge of each of these factors will help to determine contraindications of treatment, the risk of postoperative stiffness, the potential need for modalities, the amount of stress that should be applied to the involved structures during rehabilitation, and proper progression of therapeutic exercises.

The most important factor that dictates the rehabilitation guideline after subacromial decompression or excision of the distal clavicle, or both, is whether the operation involved an open or arthroscopic technique. Postoperative considerations for an open approach for either subacromial decompression or distal clavicle excision include protection of the deltoid and trapezius muscles, which are detached or split to obtain access to the surgical site.[1] Specific adaptations to the base rehabilitation guideline must be made and are detailed in the Special Considerations section.

Arthroscopic subacromial decompression typically is performed using standard anterior, midlateral, and posterior arthroscopic portals. A subtotal bursectomy is performed to give better visualization of the subacromial space. The periosteum on the undersurface of the acromion is removed using a radiofrequency ablator, exposing the anterolateral ridge and anterior aspect of the acromion. After release of the coracoacromial ligament, a motorized burr is inserted to remove the anterior lip of the acromion and to bevel the anterolateral edge, creating a smooth surface for rotator cuff articulation (Figure 1).

Arthroscopic excision of the distal clavicle can be performed using the same portals as

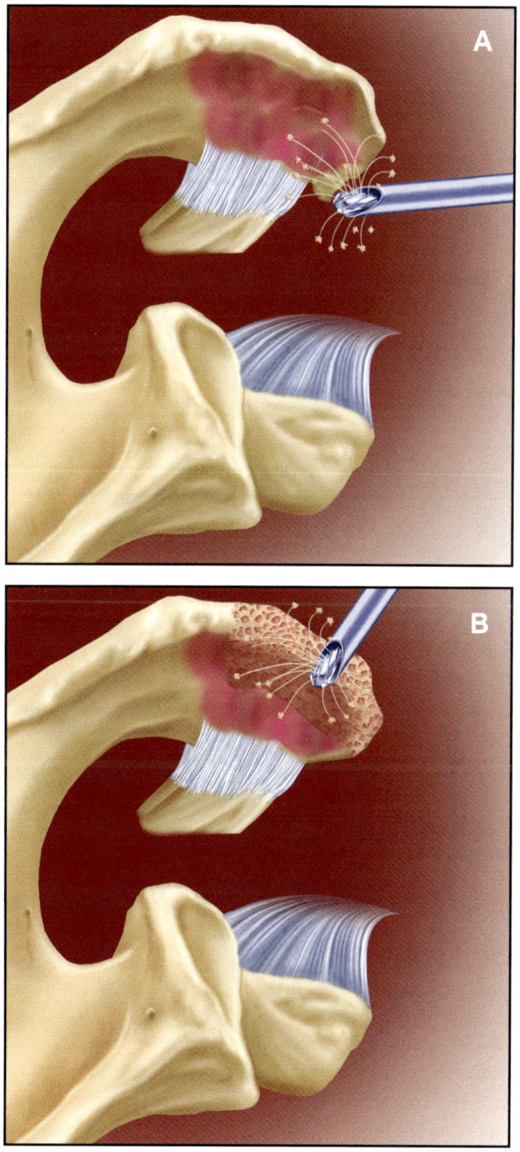

Figure 1. A, The anterior lip of the acromion and the calcific burr are removed. B, The anterolateral ridge is beveled to allow the rotator cuff to encounter a smoother surface with active elevation.

those used for the subacromial decompression, with 1 accessory portal usually added just anterior to the acromioclavicular (AC) joint. The radiofrequency ablator is used to expose the inferior aspect of the joint and remove the inferior capsule up to the superior AC joint. Care is taken to not disrupt the superior capsule of the AC joint to ensure joint stability.[1] Using the anterior accessory portal, 3 to 4 mm of the medial acromion are removed (Figure 2). Attention now is directed to the distal clavicle where 5 to 7 mm of it are removed (Figure 3). In total, approximately 10 mm of the AC joint are resected to complete the surgical procedure.

Advantages of the arthroscopic technique include a smaller surgical incision; preservation of the AC ligaments and capsule during the distal clavicle excision procedure; and reduced trauma to the deltoid and trapezius, allowing for an accelerated rehabilitation program and faster return of functional use of the upper extremity.[2] Researchers have shown that both the superior and subacromial approach for arthroscopic excision of the distal clavicle result in successful clinical outcomes, including return to participation in sporting activities in an athletic population.[3] Good to excellent short-term and long-term results also have been noted when a distal clavicle excision procedure is performed concomitantly with a subacromial decompression.[2,4]

Factors That Can Affect the Healing of Involved Tissues

Many factors can slow the healing process after arthroscopic shoulder surgery. These include, but are not limited to, certain comorbidities (diabetes, vascular compromise, immunodeficiencies), smoking, advanced age of the patient, increased inflammation, poor tolerance to or compliance with administration of pain medication, and lack of adherence to postoperative precautions. The presence of large amounts of inflammation or synovitis, which can be present before the patient undergoes shoulder surgery, is thought to be a risk factor for postoperative stiffness and can negatively affect a patient's level of pain after surgery. Another potential source of postoperative stiffness includes bleeding into the subacromial space after subacromial decompression, excision of the distal clavicle, or any other surgical procedure in which a bleeding bone bed is created. We believe that trauma from the surgical procedure creates an inflammatory response and bleeding in the subacromial space, increasing the risk of adhesion formation. Increased postoperative pain, stiffness, and inflammation can slow the postoperative progression of rehabilitation if appropriate modifications, which are detailed later in this chapter, are not made. Therefore, because postoperative stiffness is

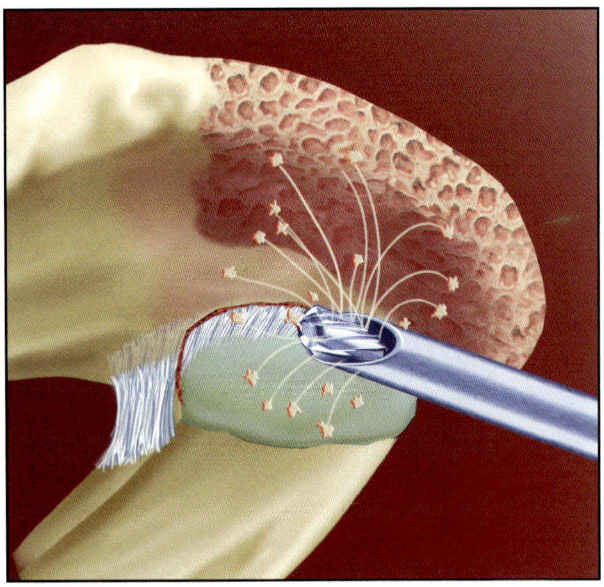

Figure 2. A burr is used to remove 3 to 4 mm of the medial acromion to allow better visualization of the acromioclavicular joint.

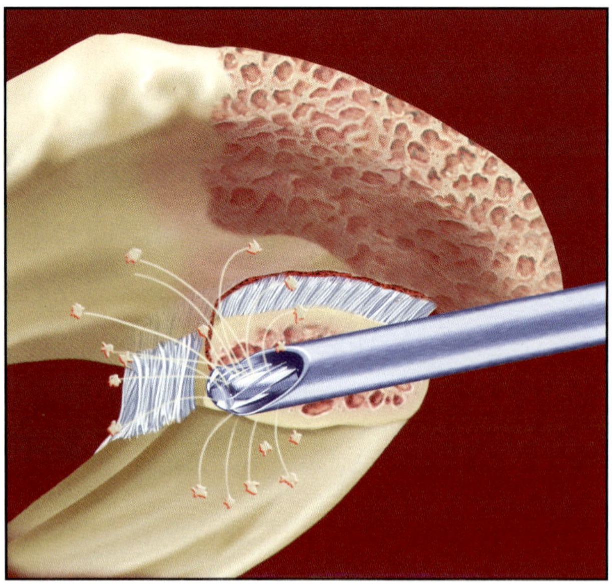

Figure 3. A burr is used to remove 5 to 7 mm of the distal clavicle.

a risk after any shoulder surgery, the rehabilitation provider must be aware of any factors or situations that are slowing or preventing the return of full ROM and rectify them as quickly as possible.

The use of modalities (eg, cryotherapy, iontophoresis, ultrasound) can help decrease the amount of inflammation and pain after surgery and allow for better tolerance to physical therapy and performance of a home exercise program. The most commonly used modality at our facility for the reduction of pain, inflammation, and swelling is ice. Patients typically are instructed to place ice on their shoulders for 10 to 20 minutes after each exercise session and when needed throughout the day to minimize pain and inflammation.

Knowledge of the Stresses Applied by Therapeutic Exercises

When beginning rehabilitation after shoulder surgery, the rehabilitation provider must ensure that any therapeutic exercise that the patient performs does not place excessive stress on the surgical site. This is extremely important after surgical repair of tissue, such as tendon, cartilage, or bone, and is also important in cases of isolated tissue debridement when no tissue repair is performed. Allowing adequate healing time for the operatively treated tissues is important to ensure that the patient can be progressed through each stage of his or her rehabilitation without causing unnecessary complications. Performing an exercise or participating in an activity that places large amounts of stress on the surgical site can lead to increased levels of inflammation and pain, which not only can slow the healing of the involved tissues, but can lead to decreased ROM and decreased use of the upper extremity for functional activities due to the increase in pain.

Although no formal tissue repair usually is performed during subacromial decompression or distal clavicle excision operations, structural changes occur (eg, bone spurs removed, inflamed tissue excised) that can contribute to increased inflammation and pain after surgery. Because of this, the initiation of certain passive and active-assistive exercises should be delayed to avoid increased stress and pain to the shoulder. Our facility's philosophy is that passive coronal-plane shoulder abduction should be limited to 90° to avoid potential impingement of the rotator cuff against the acromion. Another shoulder position that can lead to impingement symptoms is horizontal adduction of the shoulder, so we also limit ROM in that plane during the early postoperative period. Finally, we have noticed that patients typically poorly tolerate the active-assistive exercise for functional shoulder internal rotation (Figure 4), using either a towel or the contralateral hand, in the early phases of rehabilitation. A more detailed explanation of our specific postoperative rehabilitation guideline is discussed in the following section.

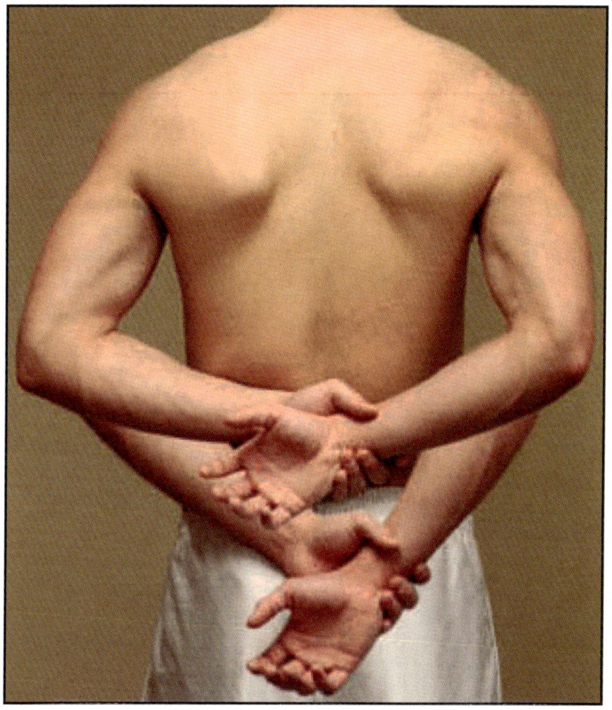

Figure 4. Functional shoulder internal rotation. This exercise is typically poorly tolerated in the early phase of rehabilitation and is best reserved for the later phases of rehabilitation.

Finally, the rehabilitation provider needs to thoroughly educate the patient in specific activities of daily living (ADLs) that are acceptable immediately after surgery and in which ADLs need to be modified or withheld during the immediate postoperative period to avoid applying unnecessary amounts of stress to the shoulder. Chapter II-1 provides a more detailed explanation about specific areas of importance in patient education. Highlights of patient education and a detailed rehabilitation protocol after subacromial decompression, distal clavicle excision, or acromioplasty can be found in the Appendix.

SPECIFIC REHABILITATION GUIDELINE

My facility has divided the postoperative rehabilitation after subacromial decompression, distal clavicle excision, or acromioplasty into 3 phases based on the timeframe since surgery. Phase 1 begins on postoperative day (POD) 1 and typically lasts until POW 6. Phase 2 begins at POW 6 and lasts until POW 12. Phase 3 begins at POW 12 and lasts until the patient has full functional use of the shoulder or is able to return to full participation in work or sporting activities. Each phase of the rehabilitation protocol addresses specific exercises and activities that can be performed safely during that specific timeframe and follows a systematic progression of increased resistance and stress applied to the shoulder as the patient gains more ROM, strength, and muscle endurance while keeping pain and inflammation minimized.

The following postoperative guideline should be tailored to each patient based on his or her level of pain and inflammation, ability to meet the staged ROM goals both comfortably and easily, and desired level of return to function after completing rehabilitation. Some patients quickly and easily regain ROM with very little exercise or need of therapist-assisted stretching. These patients do not need to perform every exercise listed in this guideline, might be advanced more rapidly through the guideline, and might require fewer visits to therapy. Other patients will have a more challenging time regaining ROM due to the continuation of preoperative pain and stiffness; increased postoperative pain and inflammation, especially if synovitis is present; or poor tolerance to the stretching exercises. These patients have a greater likelihood of developing postoperative stiffness. The rehabilitation provider should pay close attention to these patients during the early postoperative period. If excessive stiffness is present or if the patient has difficulty achieving the staged ROM goals, modifications, including increased frequency of visits to therapy and increased frequency of gentle stretching at home, should be made. Advancement from one rehabilitation phase to the next might be delayed if excessive pain or inflammation is present, if staged ROM goals are not met, or if the patient demonstrates poor tolerance to or compliance with the current exercise program.

Phase 1

Phase 1 of our postoperative program begins on POD 1 and continues until the patient returns to the surgeon for his or her follow-up examination, which typically occurs at POW 6. The primary goal of phase 1 is for the patient to comfortably regain as much PROM as possible, especially passive forward elevation (PFE) and passive external rotation (PER), while minimizing pain and inflammation. Early glenohumeral PROM traditionally has been encouraged after shoulder surgery to help minimize the negative effects of immobilization, such as the formation of scar tissue and joint contracture, muscle atrophy, and degradation of articular cartilage.

Many of the exercises prescribed for the patient during phase 1 are the same as described in the previous 5 chapters in this section, Specific Shoulder Girdle Rehabilitation Guidelines. Specific exercises that the patient performs independently include the pendulum exercise; table step-back exercise for PFE (Figure 5); PER walk-around exercise (Figure 6); shoulder shrugs and scapular retractions; and elbow, wrist, and hand exercises. The rehabilitation provider will perform assisted PFE (Figure 7) and assisted PER (Figure 8) in sitting to further progress PROM in these planes. If the patient poorly tolerates these exercises, which is demonstrated by increased muscle guarding, pain, and patterns of muscle substitution, a family member can be instructed to assist with the exercises at home to encourage increased ROM and improved relaxation by the patient during these exercises. As an adjunct,

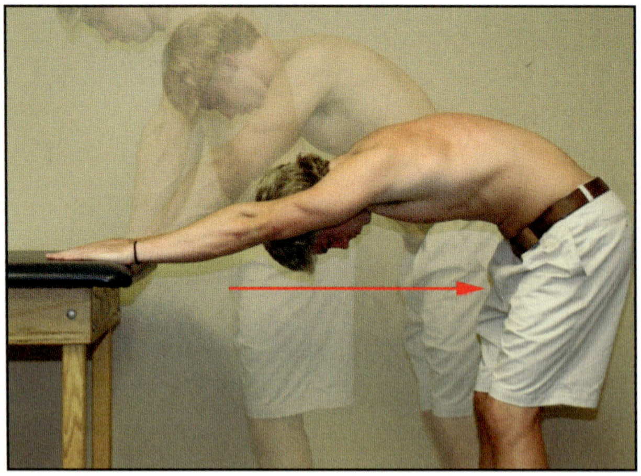

Figure 5. Table step-back exercise for passive forward elevation.

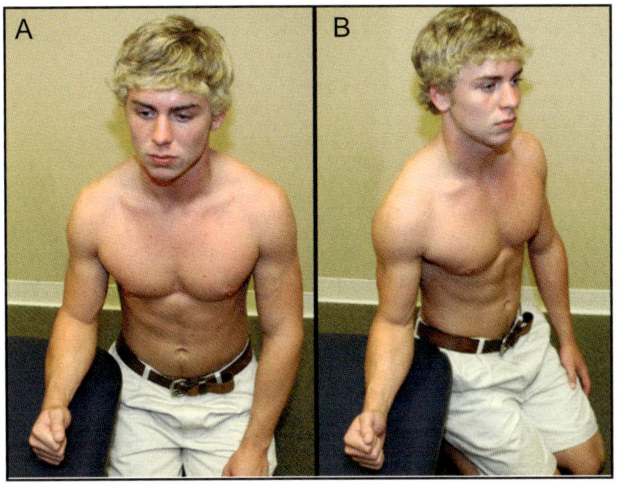

Figure 6 A and B. Passive external rotation walk-around exercise.

the rehabilitation provider can initiate the following therapist-assisted stretches in the supine position: PER at approximately 20° of abduction, PFE in the scapular plane, passive internal rotation at a variety of degrees (45°, 60°, 80°) below 90° of abduction, and passive shoulder abduction to a maximum of 90°. Care is taken not to advance the shoulder above 90° in straight-plane abduction to minimize the potential of impingement symptoms. One way that end-range abduction can be achieved without substantial risk of impingement is by positioning the extremity in approximately 90° of forward elevation and moving horizontally into abduction (Figure 9).

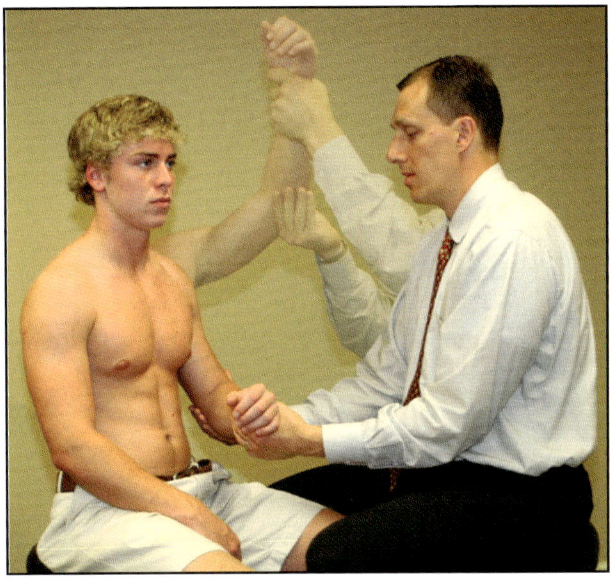

Figure 7. Assisted seated passive forward elevation.

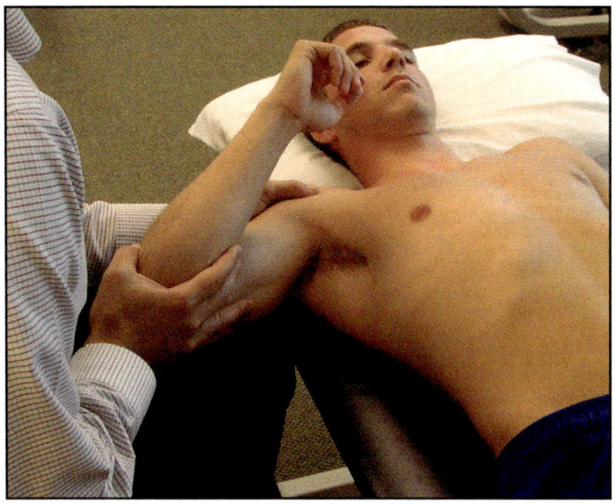

Figure 9. Alternative technique for passive shoulder abduction starting in approximately 90° of forward elevation and moving in a horizontal direction into abduction.

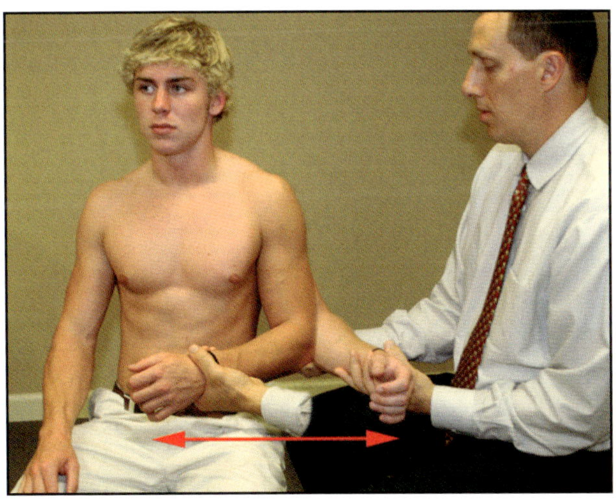

Figure 8. Assisted seated passive external rotation.

As patients achieve the staged goals for PROM in this protocol, they can be advanced to progressive stretching exercises to promote further increases in ROM. Progression from the table step-back exercise for PFE to the pulley is allowed around POW 3 after approximately 110° to 130° of forward elevation can be achieved in a comfortable manner without signs of altered scapular mechanics, including a shoulder shrug sign. Additional exercises added between POW 3 and

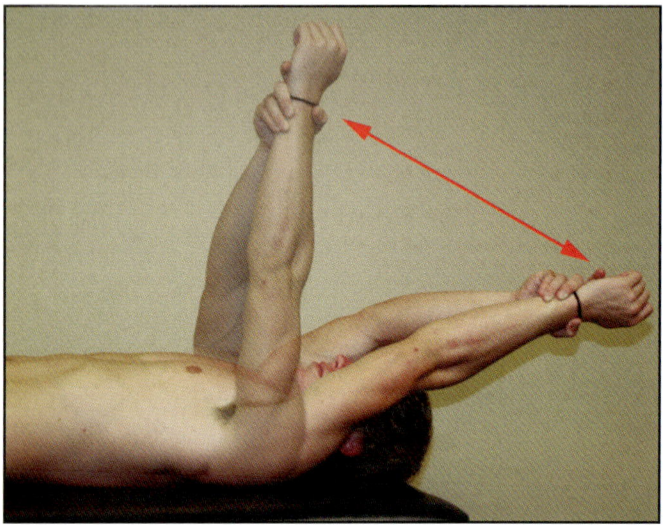

Figure 10. Self-assisted supine active-assistive forward elevation.

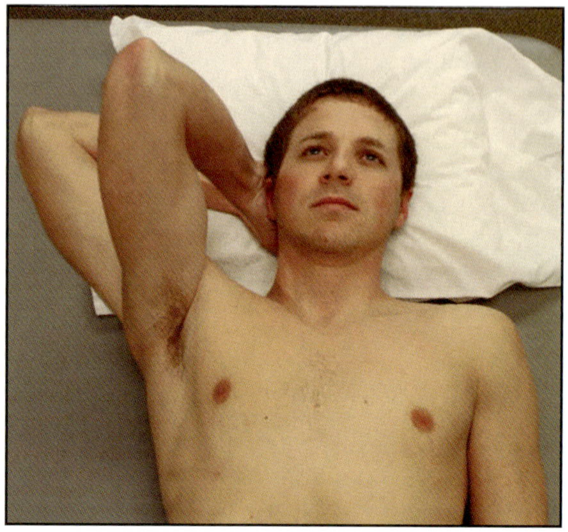

Figure 11. Supine hand-behind-head stretch.

POW 6 to progress terminal ROM include self-assisted supine active-assistive forward elevation (Figure 10); supine hand-behind-head stretch (Figure 11); horizontal adduction (Figure 12); sleeper stretch (Figure 13); and external rotation stretching at 70° to 90° of abduction (Figure 14). Adjunctive therapist-assisted stretching can be performed in all planes in the supine position with the goal of comfortably obtaining full PROM in all planes by the end of phase 1. In our experience, the amount of ease or difficulty in rehabilitating a patient after shoulder surgery usually can be predicted based on the amount of ROM achieved, how easily this ROM is obtained, and the patient's level of pain and inflammation at the end of phase 1. We believe that extra attention spent early in the rehabilitation process to address these issues can help to progress the patient through his or her postoperative rehabilitation more effectively and efficiently, with less pain and residual complications in the long term.

Although some rehabilitation protocols[5,6] do initiate active range of motion (AROM) and resistive strengthening exercises within the first 4 weeks after subacromial decompression, our philosophy is that for most patients, this immediate postoperative period is better used ensuring that the patient regains his or her PROM easily and that the levels of pain and inflammation are reduced as much as possible. In some patients, we have noticed that if we start AROM and strengthening exercises during this early period, their levels of pain and inflammation remain elevated or they emphasize the AROM and strengthening exercises to the detri-

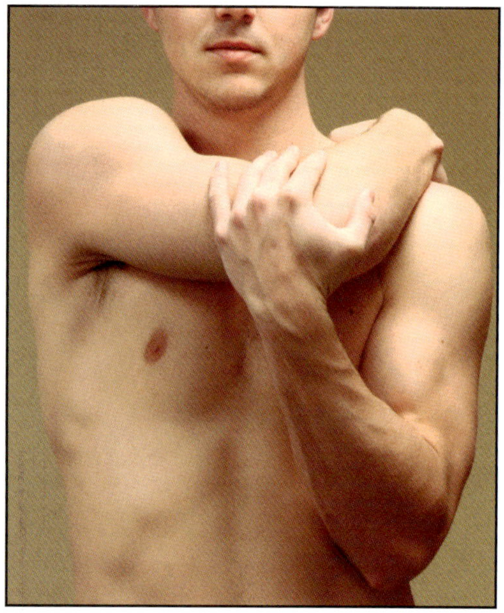

Figure 12. Horizontal adduction stretch.

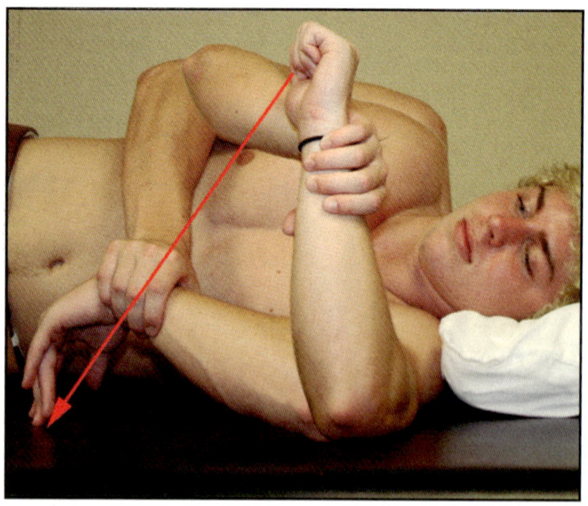

Figure 13. Sleeper stretch.

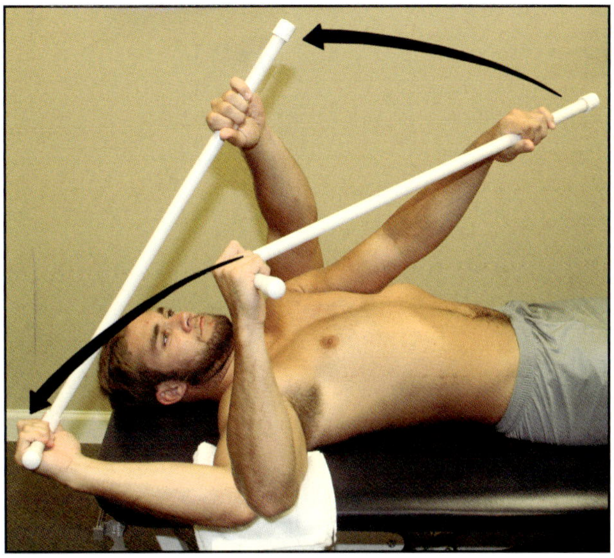

Figure 14. Supine passive external rotation with a wand in approximately 70° to 90° of abduction.

ment of their PROM. Submaximal isometrics to the muscles of the shoulder girdle, as well as table dusting, can be incorporated at this time to minimize muscle atrophy. Whereas Hultenheim Klintberg et al[6] noted that early activation of the upper extremity using a supervised physical therapy protocol can be achieved safely after subacromial decompression, we agree with Ellman[7] that strenuous overhead activities, strengthening exercises, and full ADL use with the operated upper extremity should be deferred for at least 4 to 6 weeks.

Phase 2

The focus of phase 2, which typically begins at POW 6 and continues to POW 12, is to continue to promote low levels of shoulder pain and inflammation during all activities, to ensure full PROM in all planes of motion, and to begin a structured strengthening program progressing from waist level to shoulder level and to overhead strengthening. If staged ROM goals have been met and full to nearly full ROM has been achieved, minimal stretching might be necessary. If ROM deficits persist or if increased amounts of pain and inflammation are encountered, addressing these issues takes priority over beginning a strengthening program.

A strengthening program is initiated during phase 2 to strengthen the rotator cuff, deltoids, and scapular stabilizers to allow for increased functional use of the upper extremity. We use both a base strengthening program and an elevation strengthening progression, which is termed the *assistive-to-active shoulder elevation progression* (AASEP). It begins with waist-level and gravity-minimized strengthening exercises and advances to an upright elevation strengthening program that incorporates upright active exercises and upright resistive exercises to further strengthen the shoulder girdle muscles. The goal by the end of phase 2 is for the patient to be ready to advance from upright active forward elevation with light resistance to advanced strengthening exercises that incorporate exercises that maximally activate the muscles of the shoulder girdle. These advanced strengthening exercises will prepare the shoulder for the increased demands required to perform heavy lifting; repetitive overhead activities; or high-velocity, powerful activities if the patient's normal activity level requires these demands. A more detailed explanation of this strengthening progression can be found in chapter II-4.

The base strengthening program includes resistive exercises performed below shoulder level in nonprovocative positions to strengthen the entire rotator cuff and scapular muscles. These exercises, which are performed with the resistance of an elastic band, include shoulder internal and external rotation with the upper extremity near the side, forward reaching beginning at waist level and progressing to chest level (Figure 15), and scapular retractions. All band exercises are performed with a 5- to 6-foot (1.5-m–1.8-m) elastic band and emphasize light resistance and progression to a large number (range, 30–50) of repetitions. As the pa-

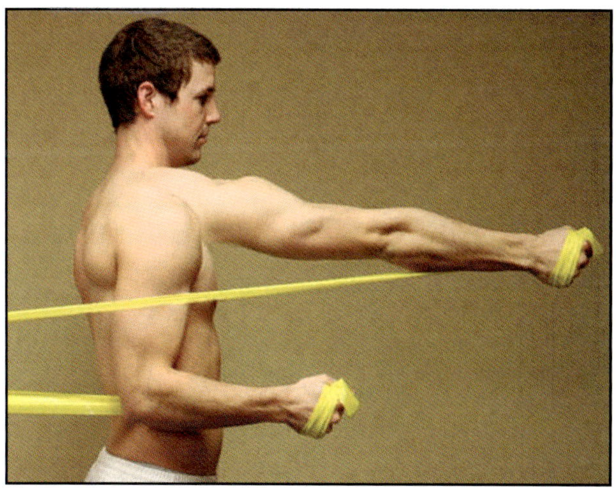

Figure 15. Forward reach with an elastic band.

tient can perform a greater number of repetitions with minimal fatigue, advancing to a more resistive elastic band can help facilitate increased shoulder girdle strength and endurance. Understanding the different physical characteristics of elastic-resistance-band exercises is essential for rehabilitation providers to ensure that the specific exercises performed are appropriate, efficient, and safe for their patients. The physical characteristics of elastic-resistance-band exercises are detailed in chapter II-5.

The AASEP program begins with gravity-minimized, active-assistive ROM (AAROM) exercises in which gravity provides assistance to complete the concentric portion of the exercise or exercises in which the primary movement is perpendicular to gravity while the weight of the upper extremity is supported.[8] These exercises include horizontal table dusting; supine forward elevation with elastic resistance; side-lying, gravity-eliminated active forward elevation (AFE); and the supine reaching progression (Figure 16). They are intended to strengthen the shoulder girdle musculature to allow for progression to upright assistive AAROM exercises.

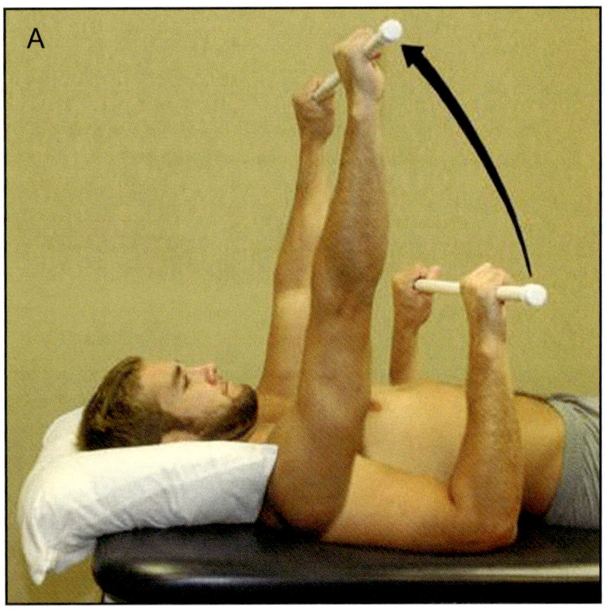

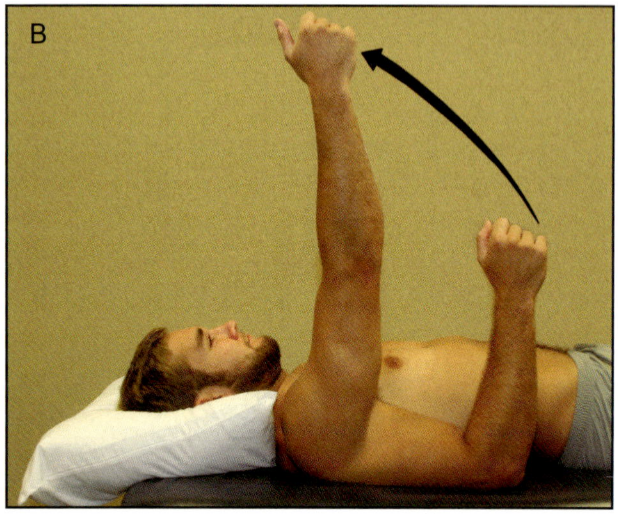

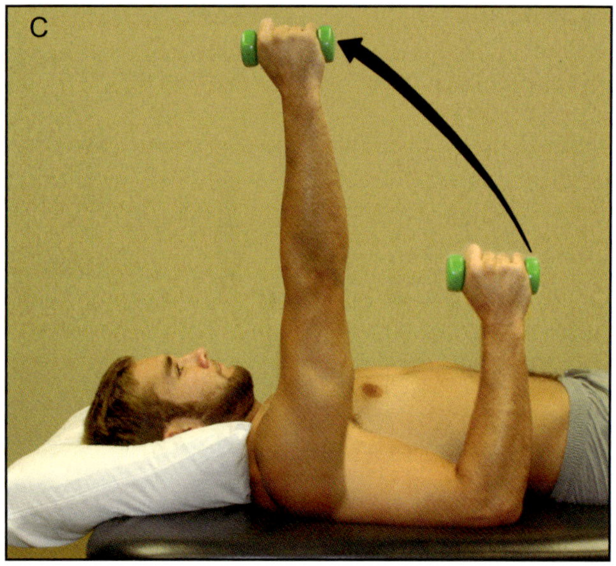

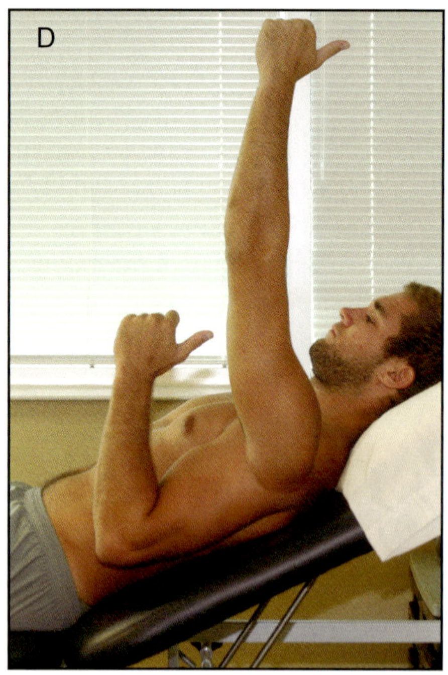

Figure 16. Supine reaching progression. In all levels of the progression, reaching begins with the elbow bent and ends with the elbow straight. All levels of the progression do not need to be used clinically. A, Step 1: assistive reaching from 0° to 90° with support via a polyvinyl chloride pipe. B, Step 2: active reaching from 0° to 90°. C, Step 3: resistive reaching from 0° to 90° with 1 to 2 lb (0.45–0.90 kg). D, Step 4: incline reaching to the ceiling with or without 1 to 2 lb (0.45–0.90 kg).

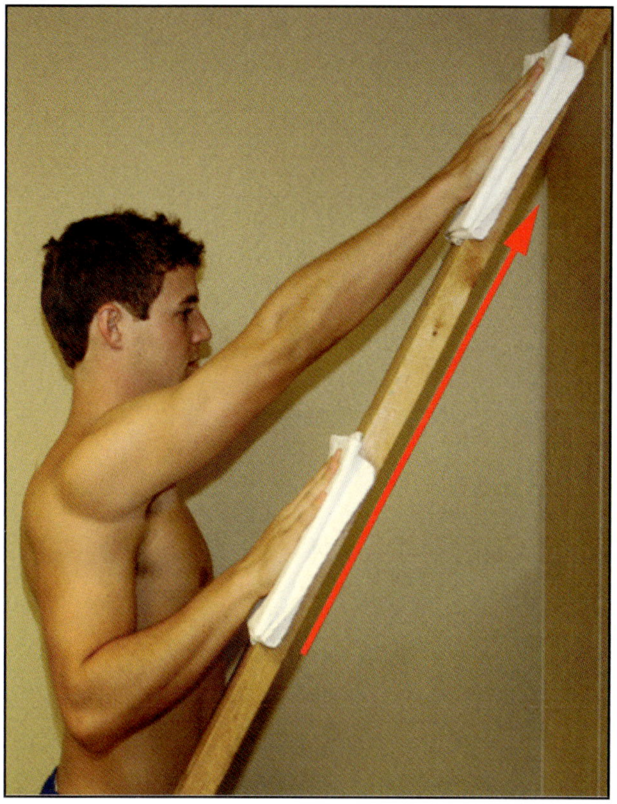

Figure 17. Incline dusting.

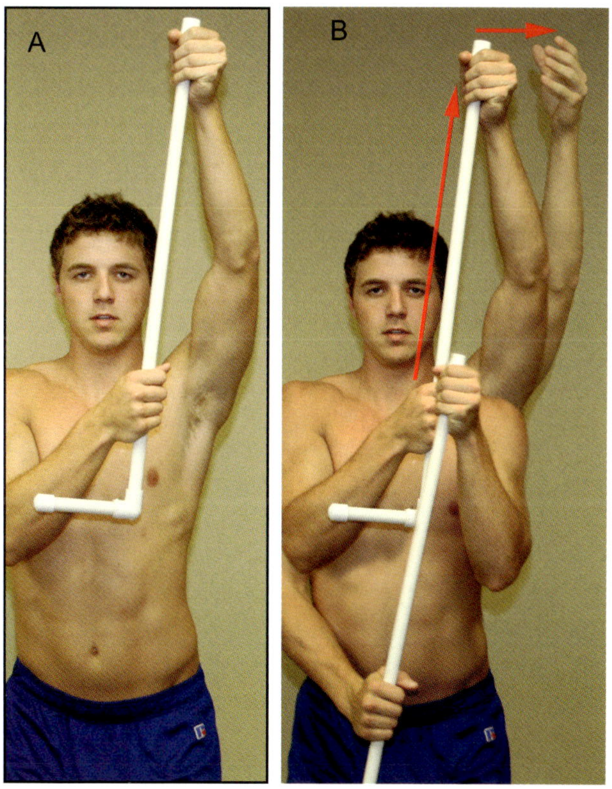

Figure 18. A, Standing active-assistive forward elevation and lowering with a wand. B, Standing active-assistive forward elevation with a wand and active lowering.

Upright assistive AAROM exercises are any exercises during which the patient is in the upright position and is elevating the upper extremity against gravity during the concentric phase of motion with assistance.[8] These exercises include the rope-and-pulley exercise, incline dusting (Figure 17), standing active-assistive forward elevation with a stick or bar (Figure 18), and the wall-walk exercise. These exercises are designed to further enhance the strength of the rotator cuff, anterior deltoid, and scapular muscles so that the patient ultimately can achieve upright AFE unsupported against gravity.

Upright AFE unsupported against gravity is the third level of the AASEP and the goal of the elevation strengthening program. This exercise should be performed only if full or nearly full AROM is possible, and the exercise should be both comfortable to the patient and free of substantial substitution patterns during its performance. No weight is used initially with this exercise, and the patient is progressed to more repetitions (up to 20–30) as the upper extremity is strengthened and the exercise becomes easy for the patient to perform. After minimal fatigue is noted with a large number of repetitions, weight is added to advance the difficulty of the exercise. The goal of phase 2 strengthening for most patients is to successfully perform the AFE exercise with correct form and minimal pain or soreness, progressing to using 1 to 3 pounds (0.45–1.35 kg) of resistance.

Not all steps or exercises of the AASEP might be necessary to perform during the strengthening progression of phase 2. Some patients naturally have good strength in their shoulders and, therefore, can be progressed more rapidly through the AASEP or might be better served by skipping certain levels of the AASEP for more appropriate strengthening exercises. The AASEP might not be necessary if painless AFE can be performed with full ROM and normal mechanics of the upper extremity and scapula. The rehabilitation provider should use sound judgment to discern which exercises are appropriate for each patient.

Certain patients, such as the elderly, those whose work demands typically are below shoulder level, or those who have lower demands of activity with their upper extremities, can be discharged at the end of phase 2 after their functional goals have been met. These functional goals typically include independence in grooming activities, independence in donning and doffing shirts and jackets, and independence in reaching into an overhead cabinet to retrieve dishes. Athletes, those with high demands in overhead use of their upper extremities, and those with high demands of heavy lifting are progressed to phase 3 for sport- and work-specific training.

Phase 3

Phase 3 of our postoperative protocol begins at POW 12 and is designed to address any ROM or strength deficits that still might exist and prevent the patient from returning to full functional use of the upper extremity. The goal of phase 3 is to normalize the strength, endurance, and power of the shoulder girdle muscles to allow the patient to return to full participation in ADLs, work responsibilities, and recreational activities. The necessity, extent, and makeup of phase 3 rehabilitation is highly individualized based on the patient's daily activities, work demands, and recreational participation. Each patient's rehabilitation program must match his or her expected functional demands. Therefore, for patients with sedentary work and limited recreational demands, phase 3 rehabilitation might be only the completion or continuation of phase 2 rehabilitation activities. For those with an increased demand for overhead or repetitive shoulder-level activities, overhead athletes, or patients wanting to return to participation in a higher level of physical fitness, a formal phase 3 rehabilitation program can be prescribed.

Exercises and activities that are addressed in phase 3 include the initiation of the overhead shoulder press, prone strengthening exercises, sport-specific strengthening exercises, and a work-conditioning or work-simulation program. The overhead shoulder press exercise has been delayed until this time in the protocol because of the increased potential of impingement symptoms if the exercise is performed before adequate glenohumeral ROM, rotator cuff or deltoid strength, or normal scapulohumeral rhythm has been achieved. Prone strengthening exercises, such as prone forward elevation, prone horizontal abduction, and prone external rotation at 90° of abduction, are used as advanced strengthening exercises for the rotator cuff, deltoid, and scapular muscles because of the increased levels of muscle activation needed to perform these exercises, as noted in electromyography studies.[9–12] These exercises also are used to functionally strengthen the shoulder because they might be provocative positions for functional impingement in this patient population.

Sport-specific training exercises include elastic-resistance-band training in a proprioceptive neuromuscular facilitation diagonal 2 pattern to simulate the throwing motion; internal and external rotation at 90° of shoulder abduction and 90° of elbow flexion (Figure 19); and simulated batting, golf, or tennis forehand and backhand movements. Finally, a modified weight-training program, plyometric strengthening, and interval sport program (eg, interval throwing program, interval tennis program, interval golf program) are initiated when approved by the physician to return the patient to full athletic participation.

SPECIAL CONSIDERATIONS

The rehabilitation provider needs to take into account a few special considerations when formulating a postoperative plan of care after subacromial decompression, excision of the distal clavicle, or acromioplasty. These special considerations include, but are not limited to, the use of an open surgical technique; concomitant procedures performed at the time of surgery; the presence of synovitis or primary shoulder stiffness, or both; and concomitant biceps tenodesis or tenotomy procedures.

Use of an Open Surgical Technique

In 1972, Neer[13] described the indications and surgical technique for open acromial decompression. Open resection of the distal clavicle initially was described in 1941 by Mumford[14] and Gurd.[15] The use of arthroscopic techniques for these procedures is now widespread because of decreased postoperative weakness, decreased restrictions in motion, a smaller scar, and the use of a single set of portals for performing both techniques.[4] Despite these advantages, the

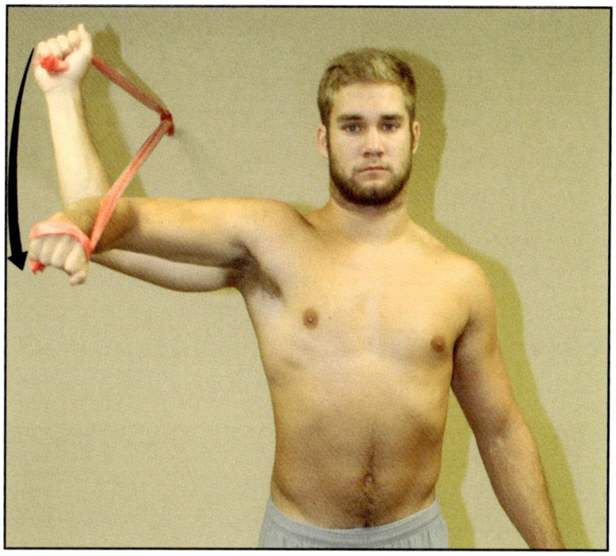

Figure 19A. Internal rotation at 90° of abduction with elastic resistance.

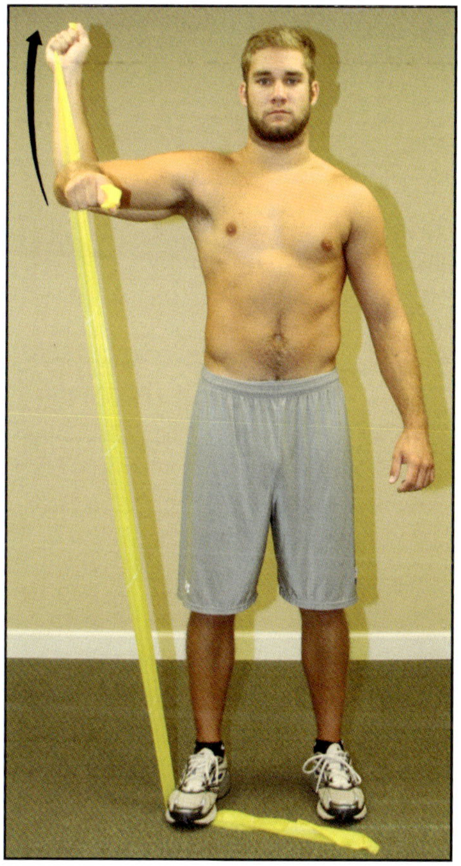

Figure 19B. External rotation at 90° of abduction with elastic resistance.

rehabilitation provider needs to be aware of how the use of an open technique for either or both of these procedures will require modification to the postoperative rehabilitation protocol.

Open subacromial decompression involves violating the origin of the deltoid to gain access to the surgical site. This is achieved by splitting and taking down the deltoid from its attachment on the acromion.[13] After the decompression is complete, the deltoid is reattached to its origin on the acromion.[13] Postoperative rehabilitation considerations after open subacromial decompression include the protection of the deltoid muscle to allow for adequate healing before high levels of stress are placed on the repaired tissue. To achieve this, AROM and strengthening of the anterior deltoid are contraindicated for 6 weeks. Protecting the deltoid in this manner is vitally important because the deltoid repair is very fragile and relatively easy to pull off from its surgical attachment, even more so than the typical rotator cuff repair. In addition, unlike a postoperative retear of a rotator cuff repair that can be relatively asymptomatic and not adversely affect function, the complication of deltoid pull-off is typically a devastating complication, resulting in pain, cosmetic deformity, and limited function above waist level because no other effective muscle compensates for the loss of this powerful shoulder flexor.[16] Repairing a deltoid pull-off also is challenging, and the results of this procedure are modest at best, with very low rates of patient satisfaction.[16,17] After enough time has passed for tissue healing to occur, submaximal isometrics can be initiated to begin strengthening the deltoid. Progression to AROM exercises and progressive resisted exercises are based on the patient's level of pain, tolerance to the exercises, and lack of substitution patterns (ie, shoulder shrug sign during forward reach) during deltoid activation. Avoidance of horizontal shoulder adduction for 6 weeks also is recommended to further minimize stress to the repair site.

The use of an open technique for excision of the distal clavicle also involves anatomic dissection that will alter postoperative rehabilitation exercises. The open technique involves detachment of the deltoid and trapezius muscles and their adjacent fascia.[1] As with the open subacromial decompression, protecting these repaired tissues is paramount during the postoperative period to avoid complications due to excessive stresses prematurely being placed on them. The use of AROM or strengthening exercises for the deltoid and upper trapezius is prohibited for 6 weeks after surgery. This includes the use of the active shoulder shrug exercise, which commonly is included in early postoperative shoulder rehabilitation protocols for scapular mobility and strengthening. Progression to AROM and progressive resisted exercises is permitted after adequate time for tissue healing has passed and again is based on the patient's level of pain, tolerance to the exercises, and lack of substitution patterns.

Complex Concomitant Procedures Performed at the Time of Surgery

When formulating a postoperative rehabilitation progression, the rehabilitation provider must consider the inclusion of more complex, concomitant surgical procedures that might be performed at the time of surgery. When not performed in isolation, subacromial decompression, excision of the distal clavicle, or other acromioplasty procedures typically are performed in conjunction with repair of the rotator cuff. When other, more complex procedures, such as a rotator cuff or labral repair, are performed concomitantly, the treatment protocol that should take precedence is the one for the more complicated surgical procedure. This will allow for better protection of all tissues involved and will reduce the risk of postoperative morbidity, complications, and operative failure.

The Presence of Synovitis or Primary Shoulder Stiffness

The presence of synovitis or primary shoulder stiffness can affect the progression of the rehabilitation protocol after subacromial decompression, excision of the distal clavicle, or acromioplasty. The presence of a large amount of synovitis or shoulder stiffness before any surgical procedure can greatly influence the patient's tolerance to and progression of ROM after surgery. These patients tend to demonstrate a high risk for excessive postoperative stiffness and increased pain after surgery. They almost always require an increased frequency and volume of stretching to regain shoulder mobility. Because of the need to ensure a steady and gentle return of ROM for these patients, the initiation of strengthening exercises or advanced stretching exercises might be delayed if high levels of pain or stiffness, or both, are present after surgery. We have found that patients with synovitis and early postoperative stiffness respond favorably with our facility's philosophy of **always gentle** PROM stretching.

Concomitant Biceps Tenodesis or Biceps Tenotomy Procedures

Finally, the rehabilitation provider must consider modifications that will need to be made to the postoperative plan of care for patients who have undergone concomitant biceps tenodesis or tenotomy procedures. Biceps tenodesis is a procedure in which the long head of the biceps tendon is detached from its origin spanning the glenohumeral joint and is reattached to the humeral head near the bicipital groove (Figure 20). It is indicated for symptomatic tears of the long head of the biceps tendon and is performed to relieve pain. The tendon is stabilized by various soft tissue or bone tenodesis methods, all of which provide secure fixation for early protected motion. Occasionally, a physician might prefer only passive elbow flexion for 3 to 6 weeks; however, generally, active-assistive elbow flexion that progresses to active elbow flexion as comfortable is tolerated well by the patient immediately after surgery. Refraining from resistive biceps activity for a minimum of 6 weeks is vitally important after biceps tenodesis surgery. Patients must receive extensive and repeated education that emphasizes the avoidance of lifting anything of consequential weight in the hand during this period. This weight depends on many factors, including the age, mass, and tendon quality of the patient, and should be determined on an individual basis. No other change to the standard rehabilitation guideline is needed.

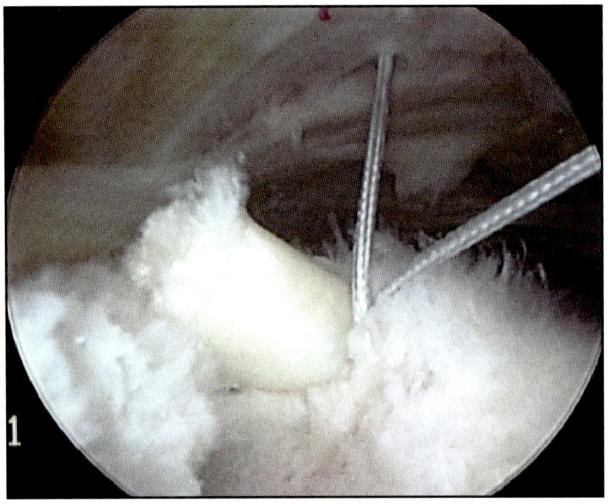

Figure 20. Biceps tenodesis.

Biceps tenotomy is a procedure in which the long head of the biceps tendon is released from its origin and is not reattached. The goal is for the released tendon to scar to an area near the bicipital grove, maintaining a relatively normal-looking biceps. It is indicated to relieve pain in patients who have symptomatic tears of the long head of the biceps tendon. Typically, it is performed instead of tenodesis in patients who are elderly, in patients whose proximal biceps tendons are diseased and of such poor quality that they might not hold a secure tenodesis repair, and in patients who do not use their biceps for regular heavy lifting. To give the released tendon the best chance to scar to the proximal humerus, elbow PROM is allowed, and resistive biceps activity is not suggested. Active flexion of the elbow should be minimized during the first 6 weeks after surgery to prevent retraction that would result in a "Popeye" deformity. Although the reported incidence of Popeye deformities after biceps tenotomy is 62% to 70%, the resultant negative consequences of the deformity are relatively benign and are more of a cosmetic issue due to the deformity rather than any noticeable loss of function.[18]

REFERENCES

1. Lesko PD. Arthroscopic Mumford procedure variation of technique. *Iowa Orthop J.* 1999;19:93–98.
2. Martin SD, Baumgarten TE, Andrews JR. Arthroscopic resection of the distal aspect of the clavicle with concomitant subacromial decompression. *J Bone Joint Surg Am.* 2001;83(3):328–335.
3. Charron KM, Schepsis AA, Voloshin I. Arthroscopic distal clavicle resection in athletes: a prospective comparison of the direct and indirect approach. *Am J Sports Med.* 2007;35(1):53–58.
4. Kay SP, Dragoo JL, Lee R. Long-term results of arthroscopic resection of the distal clavicle with concomitant subacromial decompression. *Arthroscopy.* 2003;19(8):805–809.
5. Wilk KE, Andrews JR. Rehabilitation following arthroscopic subacromial decompression. *Orthopedics.* 1993;16(3):349–358.
6. Hultenheim Klintberg I, Gunnarsson AC, Styf J, Karlsson J. Early activation or a more protective regime after arthroscopic subacromial decompression: a description of clinical changes with two different physiotherapy treatment protocols. A prospective, randomized pilot study with a two-year follow-up. *Clin Rehabil.* 2008;22(10–11):951–965.
7. Ellman H. Arthroscopic subacromial decompression: analysis of one- to three-year results. *Arthroscopy.* 1987;3(3):173–181.
8. Gaunt BW, McCluskey GM, Uhl TL. An electromyographic evaluation of subdividing active-assistive shoulder elevation exercises. *Sports Health.* 2010;2(5):424–432.
9. Reinold MM, Wilk KE, Fleisig GS, et al. Electromyographic analysis of the rotator cuff and deltoid musculature during common shoulder external rotation exercises. *J Orthop Sports Phys Ther.* 2004;34(7):385–394.
10. Reinold MM, Macrina LC, Wilk KE, et al. Electromyographic analysis of the supraspinatus and deltoid muscles during 3 common rehabilitation exercises. *J Athl Train.* 2007;42(4):464–469.
11. Blackburn TA, McLeod WD, White B, Wofford L. EMG analysis of posterior rotator cuff exercises. *Athl Train J Natl Athl Train Assoc.* 1990;25(1):41–45.
12. Townsend H, Jobe FW, Pink M, Perry J. Electromyographic analysis of the glenohumeral muscles during a baseball rehabilitation program. *Am J Sports Med.* 1991;19(3):264–272.
13. Neer CS II. Anterior acromioplasty for the chronic impingement syndrome in the shoulder: a preliminary report. *J Bone Joint Surg Am.* 1972;54(1):41–50.
14. Mumford EB. Acromioclavicular dislocation: a new operative treatment. *J Bone Joint Surg.* 1941;23(4):799–802.
15. Gurd FB. The treatment of complete dislocation of the outer end of the clavicle: an hitherto undescribed operation. *Ann Surg.* 1941;113(6):1094–1098.
16. Groh GI, Simoni M, Rolla P, Rockwood CA. Loss of the deltoid after shoulder operations: an operative disaster. *J Shoulder Elbow Surg.* 1994;3(4):243–253.
17. Gumina S, Di Giorgio G, Perugia D, Postacchini F. Deltoid detachment consequent to open surgical repair of massive rotator cuff tears. *Int Orthop.* 2008;32(1):81–84.
18. Krupp RJ, Kevern MA, Gaines MD, Kotara S, Singleton SB. Long head of the biceps tendon pain: differential diagnosis and treatment. *J Orthop Sports Phys Ther.* 2009;39(2)55–70.

ISOLATED SUBACROMIAL DECOMPRESSION, EXCISION OF THE DISTAL CLAVICLE, OR ACROMIOPLASTY REHABILITATION GUIDELINE

St. Francis Orthopaedic Institute and St. Francis Rehabilitation Center

All information contained in this protocol is to be used as a general guideline only. Specific variations might be appropriate for each patient and might be specified by the physician. In all cases, it is acceptable to advance the program more slowly than stated. If the patient experiences excessive pain, discontinue exercise until the physician is contacted. ***Achieving and maintaining a low level of pain and inflammation and protecting the surgical repair are the guiding principles in all stages of rehabilitation, even if less passive and active range of motion are accomplished.***

SYMBOLS AND ABBREVIATIONS

AAFE, active-assistive forward elevation
AAROM, active-assistive range of motion
AASEP, assistive-to-active shoulder elevation progression
ADLs, activities of daily living
AFE, active forward elevation
AROM, active range of motion
CPM, continuous passive motion
ER, external rotation
FE, forward elevation
IR, internal rotation
MMT, manual muscle testing
NA, not applicable
PER, passive external rotation
PFE, passive forward elevation
PNF, proprioceptive neuromuscular facilitation
POD, postoperative day
POM, postoperative month
POW, postoperative week
PRN, as needed
PROM, passive range of motion
ROM, range of motion
T-Band, Thera-Band
(The Hygenic Corporation, Akron, OH)
WNL, within normal limits

Forward elevation, either active or passive, is the plane of motion in which an individual naturally lifts his or her arm that is anterior to the plane of the scapula and lateral to flexion.

STAGED GOALS FOR RANGE OF MOTION

Specific limits might be specified by the physician. These are approximate targets for range of motion. These ranges can be exceeded, but care must be taken to ensure that all ROM stretching remains comfortable.

Time	PFE	PER at 20° of Abduction	PER at 90° of Abduction	AFE
POD 1	70°	0°–20°	NA	NA
POW 1	115°	20°–40°	NA	NA
POW 3	135°–150°	35°–60°	45°–75°	NA
POW 6	155°–WNL	60°–70°	80°–WNL	120°+
POW 9	WNL	WNL	WNL	145°+
POW 12	WNL	WNL	WNL	WNL

PHASE 1

Goals

°Minimize pain and inflammatory response
°Achieve staged ROM goals

- °Maximally protect the healing tissue
- °Establish a stable scapula
- °Patient education

POD 1 to POW 3

- °Elbow, wrist, and hand AROM with no weight
- °Scapular elevations and retractions (no weight) in or out of the sling
- °Pendulum exercises
  - °Lean over a table a comfortable amount
  - °Let the arm hang down relaxed
  - °Keep the body still
  - °As able, move the arm in small comfortable circles only
- °Upright PER in slight abduction until mild stretch and discomfort
  - °10 to 15 repetitions 2 times per day
  - °Preferred exercises
    - °Sit with family member or rehabilitation provider rotating the arm (Figure 8)
    - °PER walk-around (stand with the arm supported on a table and rotate the body) (Figure 6)
- °PFE in the plane of the scapula until mild stretch and discomfort
  - °10 to 15 repetitions 2 times per day
  - °Preferred exercises
    - °Sit with family member or therapist lifting the arm (Figure 7)
    - °Table step-back exercise (Figure 5)
    - °+/- Kinex (Kinex Medical Company, LLC, Waukesha, WI) shoulder CPM machine
    - °After achieving 110° to 130° of PFE, progress to self-assisted AAFE in the supine position (Figure 10) and rope-and-pulley AAFE as tolerated
- °Ice for pain reduction
- °Patient education
  - °Primary focus of phase 1: decrease pain and inflammation and achieve staged PROM
  - °Use of sling
    - °As instructed by physician; typically, full time in the community and when up for more than 5 to 10 minutes at home
- °Minimal use of the arm for light waist-level activities as comfortable
  - °Ensure the level of pain is not increasing because of excessive use of the arm for ADLs or work
- °Sleep in a recliner
  - °3 weeks (required)
  - °6 weeks (preferred)

Adjunctive Exercises

- °Therapist-assisted supine PROM within a comfortable ROM to
  - °Decrease muscle guarding
  - °Gain patient confidence
  - °Achieve staged PROM goals
- °Cervical spine AROM
- °Moist heat before exercise (after POW 1)
- °Pain-control agents PRN

°Aquatic therapy for AAROM progression to AROM (no swimming strokes) after incision has healed completely

Interventions To Avoid

°Exercises that result in moderate or severe pain
°Exercises that result in excessive guarding or splinting of muscles
°Weighted exercises
°Full-motion straight-plane abduction
°Repetitive activity with affected extremity

POW 3 to POW 6

°Achieve staged ROM goals in FE
  °Preferred exercises
    °Rope-and-pulley exercise (elbows remain straight in the plane of the scapula)
    °Patient-assisted supine AAFE exercise (use unaffected arm for assistance)
°Achieve staged ROM goals in ER at 20° using upright exercises
°Initiate the horizontal adduction (Figure 12) and/or sleeper stretch (Figure 13) PRN
°Progressive exercises to increase ER at 90° of abduction
  °Initiate supine hand-behind-head stretch (Figure 11)
  °Progress to gentle ER stretching in 70° to 90° of abduction using a wand (Figure 14)
°Therapist-assisted PROM to achieve staged ROM goals with mobilizations PRN
°Horizontal dusting
°Submaximal isometrics
°Patient education
  °Increase frequency of stretching if difficulty achieving staged goals
  °Sling use PRN
  °Use of the arm as tolerated for waist-level activities and limited use of the arm for shoulder-level and over head ADLs

PHASE 2

Goals

°Normalize PROM and AROM
°Minimize shoulder pain
°Begin to increase strength and endurance
°Increase functional activities

POW 6 to 12

°Continue PROM in all planes as described above PRN
°Initiate functional IR AAROM and stretching as tolerated (Figure 4)
°Initiate base strengthening progression
  °Includes standard rotator cuff, deltoid, and scapular strengthening program
  °2 times per day at most with light resistance and increasing repetitions
  °T-Band ER and IR strengthening with the arm near the side
    °5- to 6-foot band length and light or no pretension in a 3- to 6-inch arc of motion
    °Can use side-lying ER instead of T-Band

°T-Band forward reach (Figure 15)

°Initially, 5- to 6-foot band length and light or no pretension

°Start with the elbow bent and by the side and the band tied behind the patient

°Reach **forward** with the hand at waist level, progressing to reaching **forward** at chest level

°Do not initiate until forward reach at waist level is pain-free and can be accomplished without resistance

°If forward reach is painful or difficult, replace with a gravity-minimized exercise from the AASEP (described below) until the forward reach can be done comfortably

°Scapular strengthening emphasizing scapular retractions and scapular upward rotators

°Low-level closed chain strengthening (chapter II-4)

°No prone FE, abduction, or ER

°Initiate the AASEP as comfortable (chapter II-4)

°A stepwise progression in difficulty of strengthening exercises from PFE to active elevation of the arm (or AFE) against gravity

°Goal of the progression is to achieve pain-free full AFE

°All exercises are performed in the plane of the scapula (FE)

°If scapular or glenohumeral substitutions or pain are present, choose an easier exercise in the progression

°The order of the exercise sequence has some variability

°The goal of exercise selection is to select an exercise that is pain-free but fatiguing

°Usually not all exercises need to be performed

°Not necessary if AFE can be performed in full, pain-free ROM without substitution

°Ensure that these exercises do not increase signs and symptoms

°Exercises are divided into 3 levels of difficulty

1. Gravity-minimized exercises

°Horizontal dusting

°Perform straight ahead

°Perform at 20° angles medially and laterally if comfortable

°T-Band supine FE

°Must start the involved arm at 90° of elevation

°Pull the arm into FE

°Side-lying, gravity-eliminated AFE

°Lie on the uninvolved side

°Place the involved arm on an ironing board

°Slide the hand on the board

°Supine reaching progression

°Begin at 0° of elevation with the elbow bent and end at 90° of elevation with the elbow extended

°Start with the assistance of a cane or wand (Figure 16A)

°Progress to active (Figure 16B)

°Can progress to using 1 to 2 pounds of weight (Figure 16C)

°Can progress to inclined position, continuing to reach to ceiling (Figure 16D)

2. Assistive elevation exercises

°Rope-and-pulley AAFE

°Incline dusting (Figure 17)

°Standing AAFE (assistive elevation and descent via T-bar or unaffected arm) (Figure 18A)

°Standing AAFE and active independent eccentric lowering (Figure 18B)

°Wall-walk AAFE

°Ensure that the patient is in FE and is not in flexion

°Must be pain-free and natural when performing

3. Unsupported elevation exercises

°Overhead wall taps

°AFE

°Initiate AFE after the AASEP is complete

°Only perform if full or nearly full AROM is possible and comfortable

°Eventually progress to 1 to 3 pounds for resistance, depending on body size

°Gradually progress T-Band resistance for base strengthening

Adjunctive Exercises

°Moist heat or ice

°Aquatic exercises: AAROM, AROM, and light strengthening

°Spine therapy assessment and mobilization if

°Nonneurogenic cervical or scapular pain or

°Limitation in end-range shoulder FE

°Trunk stabilization and strengthening

°Initiate return-to-golf progression beginning with chipping and putting

°Initiate progressive replication of moderate-intensity ADLs and work at the end of this phase

Interventions To Avoid

°Initiating base strengthening program or overhead strengthening progression before overall level of pain is low

°Exercises that significantly increase signs and symptoms

°Strengthening if PROM is significantly below staged ROM

°Heavy lifting with the elbows away from the body

°Highly repetitive rehabilitation activities with the elbow at or above chest level, including the upper extremity ergometer

°Strengthening into straight-plane abduction

PHASE 3

Goals

°Normalize strength, endurance, and power

°Return to full participation in ADLs, work, and recreation

POM 3 to 4

°PROM, stretching PRN, and warm-up stretching

°Continue base strengthening program

°Continue AFE with progressive but light weight

°Discharge when functional goals are met

°Many patients, especially those who are elderly or have lower demands, do not progress to any of the rehabilitation described below

°Participate in dumbbell overhead shoulder press **PRN**

°Must meet the criteria to start the advanced strengthening progression (described below)

- °Place hands in front of the shoulder with elbows bent and naturally reach overhead
- °Sets of 15 to 20 repetitions with 3 pounds or more 3 to 7 times per week

°Initiate the advanced strengthening progression **PRN** (chapter II-4)

- **°Strict criteria to start program**
  - **°Approval of physician**
  - °MMT at least 4+/5 of shoulder girdle
  - °Pain-free with basic ADLs and all phase 2 strengthening activities
  - °Full AFE
  - °Goal of returning to participation in sports, heavy labor, or repetitive or heavy overhead work
  - °Use of the following principles to develop exercises to gradually progress the patient from the current level of functioning to desired goals
- **°Exercise principles**
  - °Decrease the amount of external stabilization provided to the shoulder girdle
  - °Integrate functional patterns
  - °Increase speed of movements
  - °Integrate kinesthetic awareness drills into strengthening activities
  - °Decrease rest time to improve endurance
  - °Initiate prone strengthening PRN
  - °Train larger upper extremity muscles wisely
- **°Sample exercises**
  - °T-Band standing PNF-type patterns
  - °T-Band IR (Figure 19A) and ER (Figure 19B) at 90° of abduction with or without arm support
  - °T-Band simulation of batting, golf, or tennis forehand and backhand
  - °Modified weight training

°Initiate progressive replication of demanding ADLs and work

°Initiate modified return-to-weight-training program

°Initiate plyometric program **(PRN and when approved by physician)**

°Can begin interval throwing program after 2 to 4 weeks of plyometrics **(PRN and when approved by physician)**

Interventions To Avoid

°Any rehabilitation activity that is significantly more demanding than daily or expected activities

°Any rehabilitation activity that is a moderate to large increase in demand compared with previous rehabilitation

°Any rehabilitation activity that results in a level of pain high enough that the patient needs to use modalities

III-7

Traditional Shoulder Arthroplasty

Bryce W. Gaunt, PT, SCS

CHAPTER CONTENTS

WHAT PATIENTS ARE APPROPRIATE FOR THE USE OF THIS GUIDELINE?

- Patients with standard total shoulder arthroplasty due to the following conditions:
  - Osteoarthritis
  - Rheumatoid arthritis
  - Avascular necrosis
  - Posttraumatic arthritis (postfracture)
  - Arthritis of dislocation
- Patients with humeral head replacement (excluding replacement due to cuff tear arthropathy)

Clinical pearls are highlighted in yellow throughout the text.

THE MOST IMPORTANT FACTOR THAT SHOULD GUIDE CLINICAL DECISION MAKING

Understanding the surgical goals of shoulder arthroplasty and protecting the subscapularis repair are of paramount importance for successful rehabilitation after traditional anatomic total shoulder arthroplasty (TSA). The primary surgical goals of shoulder arthroplasty are to relieve pain and maintain stability of the prosthesis (no subluxation and no dislocation). Whereas improved active range of motion (AROM), improved passive range of motion (PROM), and improved function are also goals of this procedure, rehabilitation providers always must remember these goals are of secondary importance. Improved range of motion (ROM) or function cannot be gained at the expense of substantial pain or a stable joint. Therefore, in some cases, a slower progression of rehabilitation is used or less aggressive interventions are chosen for the long-term benefit of the patient. Understanding the issues discussed in the next section of this chapter along with using the precise priority for clinical decision making detailed in chapter II-1 will give you the knowledge needed to make these decisions.

All traditional TSAs require surgical takedown and subsequent repair of the subscapularis. Protecting this repair is the single most important specific component of rehabilitation after TSA because this repair is fairly easy to damage, often overlooked if torn, and demonstrates relatively poor outcomes if re-repaired. This topic will be detailed in the next section of this chapter.

KEY PRINCIPLES IN REHABILITATION OF THIS PROBLEM

At the St. Francis Orthopaedic Institute and the St. Francis Rehabilitation Center, we believe 5 key principles are critically important to follow to optimally rehabilitate the patient after TSA. They are (1) understand the surgical procedure and challenge of TSA rehabilitation, (2) know the expected outcome of your patient, (3) protect the subscapularis repair, (4) maximize passive forward elevation (PFE), and (5) use a gradual strengthening progression and have patience.

Understand the Surgical Procedure and Challenge of TSA Rehabilitation

As with the rehabilitation of other shoulder conditions, optimal rehabilitation of the patient after TSA requires that the rehabilitation provider have a basic understanding of the surgical procedure and what structures must be protected during rehabilitation. To summarize the surgical procedure, the TSA typically is performed using the deltopectoral approach (Figure 1). The subscapularis is taken down for later repair either by releasing it near its insertion at the lesser tuberosity (Figure 2) or by performing an osteotomy of the lesser tuberosity. The anterior aspect of the joint capsule and glenohumeral ligaments are reflected back along with the subscapularis. The humeral head is dislocated and then is resected with the help of an alignment system (Figures 3 and 4). Osteophytes around the anatomic neck of the humerus are removed (Figure 5), and a trial humeral stem is inserted in the humerus. A series of releases are performed to the subscapularis, glenohumeral capsule, and ligaments (Figure 6), including an anterior capsulectomy to improve postoperative ROM and help balance the glenohumeral joint. The glenoid

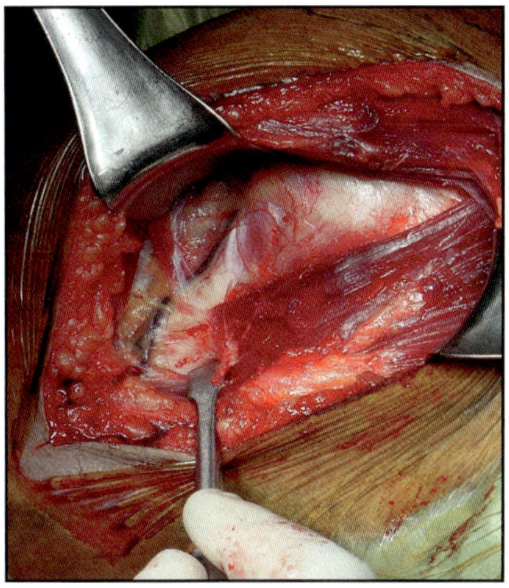

Figure 1. Anterior exposure through the deltopectoral approach. The surgeon retracts the deltoid superiorly and the pectoralis major inferiorly.

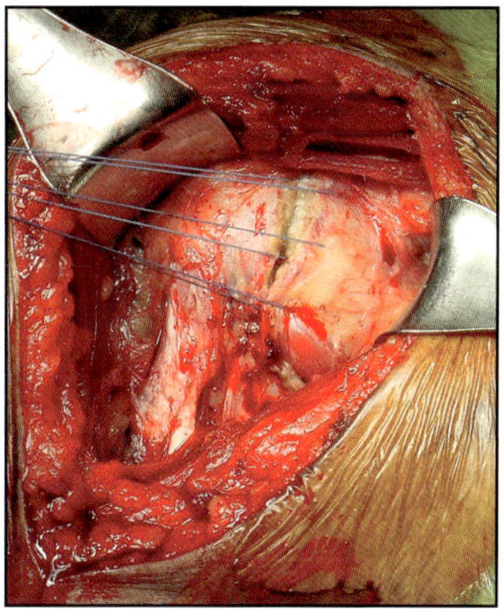

Figure 2. Takedown of the subscapularis tendon and capsule incision 1 cm medial to its insertion on the lesser tuberosity with tagging sutures placed.

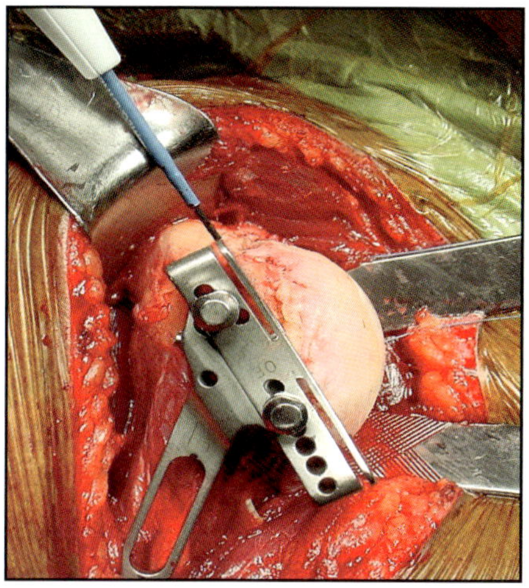

Figure 3. An alignment system is positioned on the proximal humerus to guide the cutting and removal of the humeral head while sparing the tuberosities.

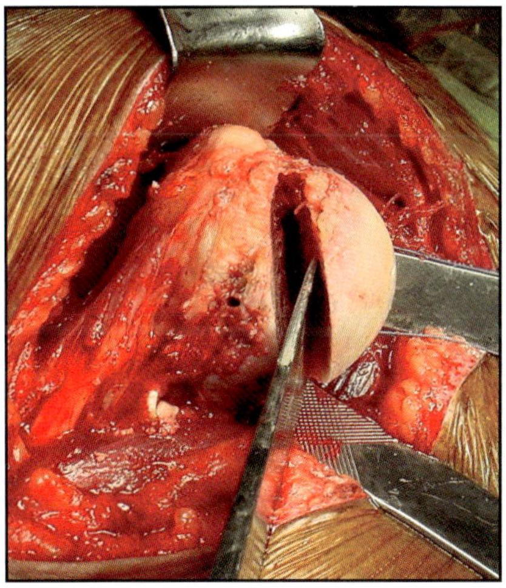

Figure 4. After using and removing the proximal cutting guide, the surgeon uses an osteotome to remove the humeral head.

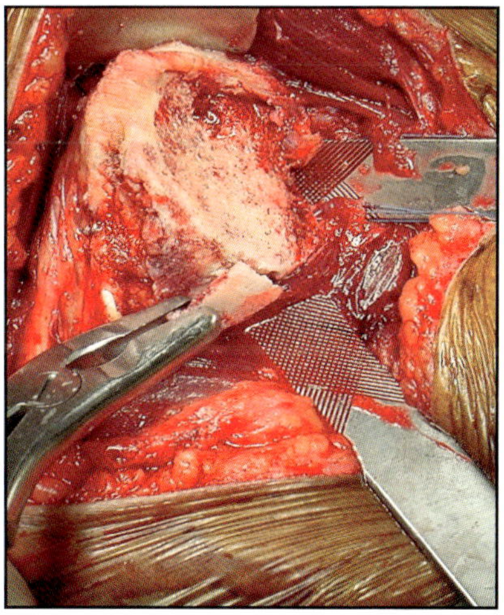

Figure 5. The humeral head has been removed. Osteophytes are removed with a rongeur and an osteotome.

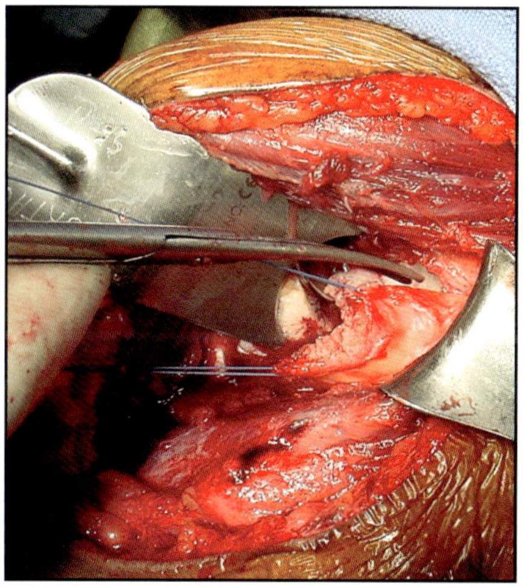

Figure 6. The superior portion of the subscapularis is released back to the base of the coracoid as part of the extra-articular and intra-articular release of the subscapularis.

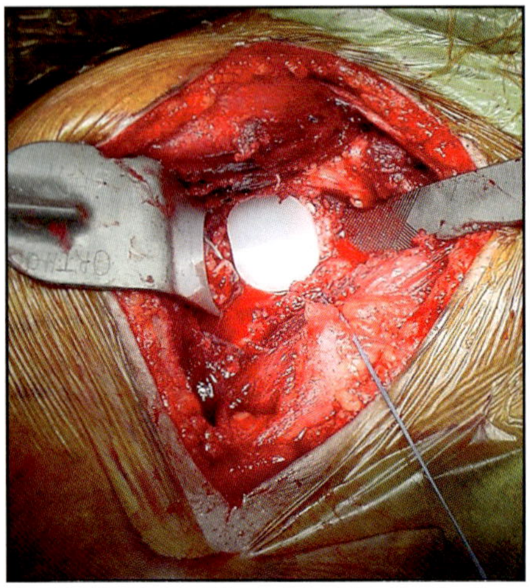

Figure 7. Completed glenoid polyethylene component (bright white).

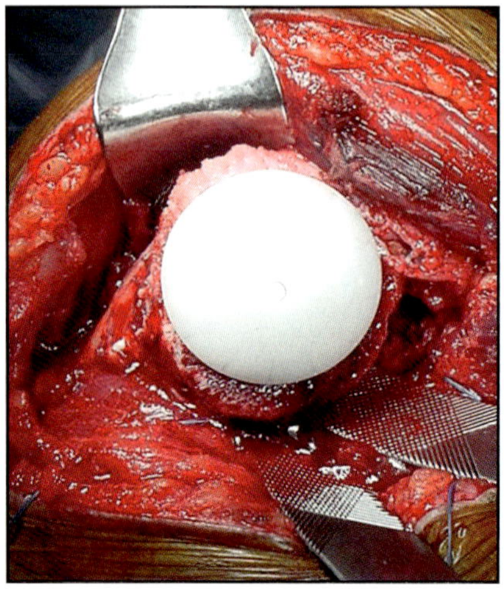

Figure 8. Trial humeral head with the humerus dislocated.

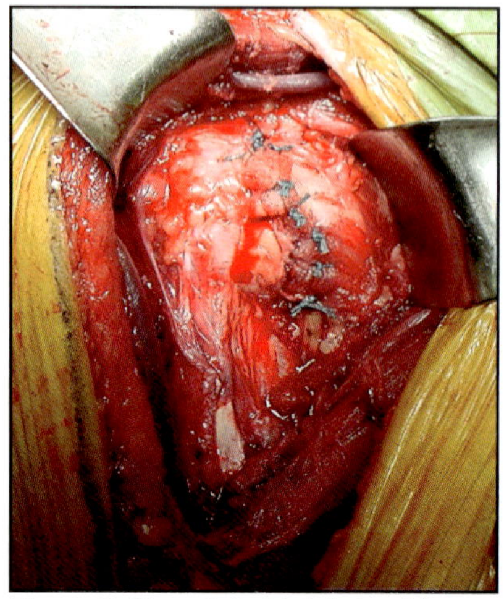

Figure 9. Completed total shoulder arthroplasty with the repaired subscapularis. Notice the sutures.

then is sequentially cleaned, aligned, prepared, and cemented in place (Figure 7), which occasionally requires bone grafting to re-establish normal alignment. Various trials of humeral head (Figure 8) are used to determine the best fit and stability of the glenohumeral joint. After the humeral component is finalized and the glenohumeral joint has been reduced, the subscapularis is repaired anatomically (Figure 9), ROM and stability are tested again, and the various tissue layers are closed. A typical early postoperative radiograph is shown in Figure 10.

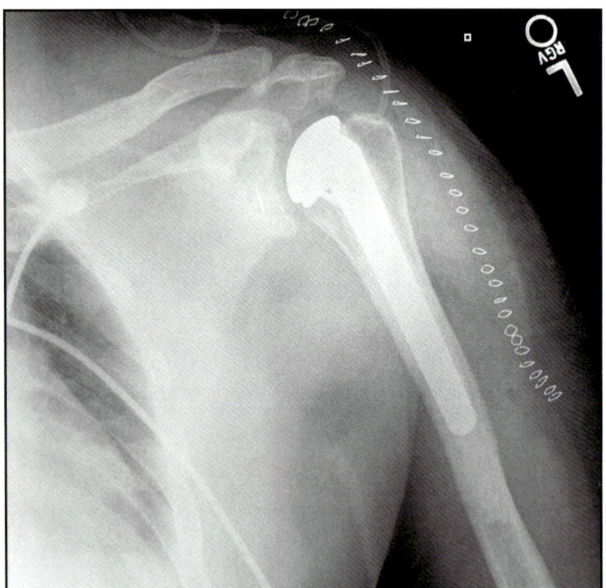

Figure 10. A typical early postoperative radiograph shows a standard total shoulder arthroplasty.

It is easy to mistakenly think that rehabilitation after TSA is very simple if you believe that the surgery is directed exclusively toward the bony structures of the humeral head and glenoid fossa. In actuality, rehabilitating a patient after TSA is an individualized, arduous task because of the complex and variable nature of the surgical procedure and the patient's pathologic condition. The often unrecognized challenge of rehabilitation after TSA is that in addition to longstanding bony abnormalities that are present with arthritis, soft tissues that have been abnormal and often of poor quality for a prolonged period are always present around the shoulder joint. Therefore, in addition to restoring the normal bony architecture of the glenohumeral joint through replacement as mentioned, the surgeon also attempts as much as possible to normalize the abnormal soft tissue through surgical releases, repair, or reconstruction, depending on the specific need. As rehabilitation providers, our challenge is to normalize the ROM, strength, and function of the patient as much as possible while respecting the limits of the soft tissues around the shoulder joint that have been released, repaired, or reconstructed after being in a weakened, abnormal state for a prolonged period. Rehabilitation of a patient after TSA means we are working with a patient who has had a rotator cuff repair (of the subscapularis), release of adhesions, and occasionally a capsular tightening during 1 procedure!

Know the Expected Outcome of Your Patient

Understanding this challenge, it is easy to appreciate that patients have quite variable outcomes after TSA, and it is quite helpful to appreciate the expected outcome of each patient with whom you are working so that the rehabilitation can match his or her expected outcome. Many factors can affect a patient's outcome and rehabilitation, some of which are listed in Table 1. The factors that are thought to have the biggest effect on rehabilitation and overall outcome are (1) the preoperative diagnosis, (2) the extent and skill of soft tissue balancing by the surgeon, and (3) the size and position of the humerus and glenoid components.[1–4]

Table 1. Factors Affecting Rehabilitation of Patients With Traditional Shoulder Arthroplasty

Patient Variables
- Preoperative diagnosis
- Preoperative range of motion
- Comorbidities
- Tissue quality
- Motivation

Surgical Variables
- Size and position of components
- Extent and skills of soft tissue balancing
- With or without rotator cuff repair of supraspinatus or infraspinatus
- With or without bone grafts

The preoperative diagnosis, or the type of arthritis that requires shoulder arthroplasty, plays a large role in the expected outcome of the patient because each form of shoulder arthritis has a relatively characteristic cluster of problems that allows surgeons to group each diagnosis into a general category of expected outcome. Table 2 lists common preoperative TSA diagnoses and the associated rehabilitation category or expected outcome associated with each diagnosis.[1,2] Patients with preoperative osteoarthritis (OA) and osteonecrosis, which is known as *avascular necrosis*, are placed in the good rehabilitation category because these disease processes typically have minimal involvement of the soft tissue of the glenohumeral joint, such as the capsule, ligaments, and rotator cuff. This means these tissues are generally more normal and stronger than that with the other disease processes, so more normal AROM, PROM, strength, and function likely are to be obtained postoperatively. However, this does not mean that tissue abnormalities are not present. Patients with moderate to severe OA often have very limited external rotation and elevation before surgery that possibly has been present for many years. Outcomes of patients in this category are expected to approach normal or to be normal for basic activities of daily living (ADLs). Passive forward elevation and active forward elevation (AFE) are often from 140° to 165°, passive external rotation (PER) with the upper extremity in about 20° of abduction is often from 45° to 60°, and functional internal rotation behind the back eventually might reach the L1-T9 spinal level.

Table 2. Common Preoperative Diagnosis of Patients With Traditional Shoulder Arthroplasty and the Associated Rehabilitation Category or Expected Patient Outcome

Preoperative Diagnosis	Rehabilitation Category
Osteoarthritis	Good
Osteonecrosis	Good
Rheumatoid arthritis	Fair
Posttraumatic arthritis	Fair
Arthritis of dislocation	Fair or limited goals
Cuff tear arthropathy	Limited-goals or reverse total shoulder arthroplasty

Patients with preoperative rheumatoid arthritis (RA) and patients with posttraumatic arthritis, which is arthritis due to trauma (eg, proximal humerus fracture), are placed in the fair rehabilitation category. Because RA is a systemic inflammatory disease, the rotator cuff, capsule, ligaments, and synovium all are affected negatively by this disease process, resulting in poorer-quality tissues, increased inflammation, inflammatory stiffness, and poorer tolerance to exercise. Patients with posttraumatic arthritis have substantial injury to the soft tissues of the shoulder that can result in rotator cuff tears and dense adhesions and in large distortions in bony anatomy due to the trauma. Patients in the fair rehabilitation category are expected to have much more modest outcomes. Passive forward elevation is often from 120° to 140°, AFE is often from 80° to 125°, PER is often from 30° to 50°, and functional internal rotation eventually might reach the L3-L1 spinal level. Functional use of the upper extremity overhead with reasonable strength to allow the patient to perform activities, such as reaching a 2- to 3-pound (0.90-kg–1.35-kg) can out of an overhead cupboard is variable.

Arthritis due to multiple dislocations or due to a longstanding fixed subluxation or dislocation is called *arthritis of dislocation*. The surgeon places these patients in either the fair rehabilitation category or limited-goals category. These patients have longstanding abnormalities of the static and dynamic stabilizers and often require repair or reconstruction of the glenohumeral ligaments and joint capsule in addition to releases in other parts of the shoulder. The rotator cuff is also typically of poor quality or damaged. Gross distortion of the humeral head or glenoid might be present. Severe glenoid bone loss or erosion might require bone grafting, which complicates recovery. Modifications to rehabilitation due to glenoid bone grafting is addressed in the Special Considerations section of this chapter. If the patient is placed in the fair rehabilitation category, expectations are as mentioned.

Limited-goals rehabilitation is reserved for patients for whom the surgeon expects only very limited long-term functional use of the upper extremity to be appropriate. The main goals of this type of rehabilitation are to achieve and maintain a stable joint with a low level of pain. Use of the upper extremity for basic waist-level activities is variable, use of the upper extremity for activities requiring shoulder-level reaching, such as combing hair, occurs only occasionally. Functional use of the upper extremity overhead is not expected. Rehabilitation for these patients is very minimal and is detailed in chapter III-18.

Patients with arthritis due to fixed superior migration of the humeral head caused by a longstanding massive rotator cuff tear have cuff tear arthropathy. With TSA, these patients are placed in the limited-goals category because whereas pain often can be relieved, function is not restored because of the irreparable rotator cuff damage. However, if these patients are managed with a reverse shoulder arthroplasty, they can have much better short-term and long-term outcomes because of the biomechanical advantages, including improved active elevation of the extremity, that the reverse arthroplasty provides. Therefore, rehabilitation of this problem and rehabilitation of patients after reverse TSA are detailed in chapter III-7.

Several technical aspects of the surgery also have a large effect on the rehabilitation and outcomes of patients with TSA.[4–6] For the patient to optimize his or her outcome, the surgeon must choose the proper-sized humeral head; orient both the humerus and glenoid correctly; and balance the soft tissues around the glenohumeral joint, such as the rotator cuff and posterior capsule, through releases or tensioning to attempt to restore normal biomechanics, length-tension relationships, and force couples to the glenohumeral joint. Doing this correctly is challenging even to the accomplished surgeon because at the time of surgery, usually both the osseous structures and soft tissues are distorted. Overstuffing the humeral head occurs when a prosthetic humerus that is too large is used. If this occurs, if the orientation of the humerus or glenoid is not correct, or if appropriate releases are not performed, then abnormal biomechanics are present in the glenohumeral joint, and available ROM is limited severely regardless of the rehabilitation employed.[6] In this situation, gentle ROM and light strengthening both done in a very comfortable way are all that is appropriate. A humerus that is too small or improper orientation of the humerus or glenoid also can result in instability of the replaced glenohumeral joint.

Protect the Subscapularis Repair

Although listed as the third key rehabilitation principle, protecting the subscapularis repair that is a part of all typical TSAs (Figure 9) is considered the single most important part of rehabilitation after TSA because this repair is fairly easy to damage,[4,7,8] often overlooked,[4] and demonstrates inconsistent results if re-repaired.[4,9] The subscapularis repair is often very delicate because at the time of repair, the tendon might be torn; is often of very poor quality even to the point of resembling toilet paper; might be retracted with adhesions that might make an anatomic repair difficult; and might be compromised due to comorbidities, such as RA or diabetes.

The tendon can be damaged easily by inappropriate rehabilitation or during daily activities, especially in the first 6 to 12 postoperative weeks (POWs).[2,4,7] Gonzalez et al[4] examined the complication rate of unconstrained TSAs with a minimum 2-year follow-up (average = 6 years; range, 2–25 years) from multiple case series in a pooled review of 4010 prostheses. Overall, the authors included 1595 complications, giving an overall incidence of 39.8%. They found 45 secondary ruptures of the subscapularis tendon, with an incidence of 1.1% (2.8% of all complications), and reoperation was performed in 33 of the 45 patients (73%). However, they believed their figure underestimated this complication because it was reported in only 10 of the 47 series reviewed. Miller et al[7] specifically studied subscapularis function after shoulder arthroplasty and found the muscle was dysfunctional in 67% of patients. Rupture or dysfunction results in variable clinical signs and symptoms, ranging from asymptomatic[10] to limited functional internal rotation,[7,11] to limited overall functional use,[12] and to anterior instability.[4,9]

The integrity of the subscapularis is vital for maintaining stability of the glenohumeral joint because it is the primary restraint to anteriorly directed forces after a TSA, during which the anterior capsule and ligaments commonly are excised. Thus, if the subscapularis is ruptured or is dysfunctional, the patient has an increased risk of anterior shoulder instability. Additionally, if the subscapularis is damaged, re-repair of it has been shown to have inconsistent results, especially for eliminating recurrent instability.[4,9] Therefore, protecting the subscapularis during all stages of rehabilitation is of the utmost importance.

Inappropriate rehabilitation can damage the subscapularis by being either too forceful or too excessive during PER or by strengthening the subscapularis too soon or too aggressively. To protect the subscapularis repair during PER, ROM limits commonly are used, careful exercise selection is needed, and regular patient education is required. Many surgeons specify PER limits during early rehabilitation, such as no PER past neutral for 3 weeks after surgery and 30° maximum until 6 weeks after surgery. The surgeons at the St. Francis Orthopaedic Institute typically do not employ strict limits but instead usually use staged ROM goals or targets (Appendix) that allow for a range of ROM to be achieved with a target of 35° to 50° of PER at POW 6.

In all situations during PER exercise, PER should never be forcefully performed, and if a patient is on target or ahead of his or her PER goals, then no stretching is performed. For patients with TSA, we believe 30° provides satisfactory ROM for typical ADLs if that is all that can be achieved by gentle stretching, whereas 45° to 60° is the maximum that is required for patients with TSA for ADLs. Therefore, when patients with TSA achieve 45° of PER easily, we discontinue all PER PROM and find that ROM gradually improves over time. Typically, the amount of PER that the patient can achieve easily after TSA depends on the size and position of the surgical components, as mentioned, and the length of the subscapularis that the physician obtained in surgery. Therefore, we believe that gentle PER stretching allows the patient to achieve appropriate ROM and that forceful stretching risks damaging the repair. In fact, we believe that having limited PER via gentle stretching is better for the patient than having a larger amount of PER obtained forcefully that might have damaged the subscapularis.

I feel very strongly that appropriate exercise selection is important to protect the subscapularis during PER exercises performed both at home and in the clinic to ensure that the patient is not guarding or actively contracting the internal rotators during PER ROM. Our facility's preferred exercises are family-

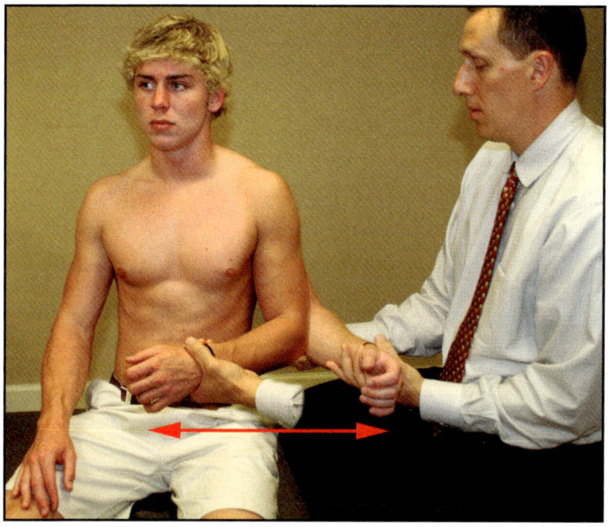

Figure 11. Assisted sitting passive external rotation.

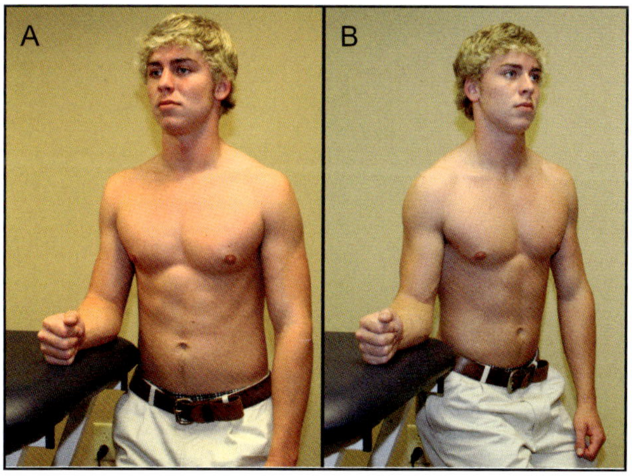

Figure 12 A and B. Passive external rotation walk-around exercise.

assisted or therapist-assisted PER in 20° of abduction while seated (Figure 11) or the PER walk-around exercise (Figure 12). With manual assistance of another person, determining if the patient is contracting the internal rotators is easy, and the motion can be stopped appropriately. To help minimize guarding, cueing the patient to lightly assist with external rotation during PER reflexively inhibits the internal rotators. The PER walk-around exercise is used because there is no counterpressure to internal rotation during the exercise. That is, if the patient guards with his or her internal rotators, the PER motion will be limited, but excessive tension on the subscapularis will not be generated because nothing restrains the forearm (Figure 12). On the other hand, PER via a wand or other apparatus provides an object against which the hand can push and might result in excessive tension being placed on the subscapularis if the subscapularis contracts excessively during the exercise. Detailed descriptions of the proper technique for the exercises we use can be found in chapter II-2. Educating patients about the importance of protecting the subscapularis repair during passive, active, and strengthening exercises is very important so they do not adopt a "harder-the-better" attitude.

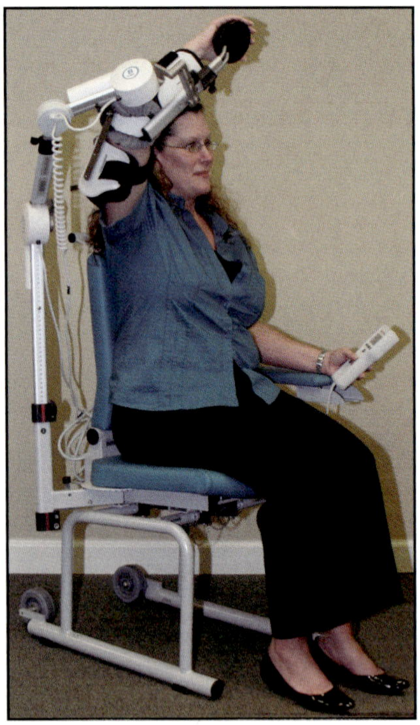

Figure 13. The Kinex KS2 (Kinex Medical Company, LLC, Waukesha, WI) shoulder continuous passive motion machine.

Maximize Passive Forward Elevation

Maximizing PFE is important in patients with TSA because this motion often is very limited preoperatively, sometimes for many years, so gaining functional ROM overhead after surgery can be a slow, difficult process. However, it is important to achieve because authors of several studies have demonstrated that compared with other planes of ROM, overhead ROM has the highest correlation with good function.[13,14] Surgeons try to facilitate good PFE during surgery by sizing and orienting the humerus and glenoid properly and through soft tissue releases. Because the benefits of these soft tissue releases might be lost if PFE is not gained quickly after surgery, the rehabilitation provider needs to emphasize and maximize PFE PROM during the first 1 to 2 postoperative months, remembering that not all patients will have the potential for full PFE. Therefore, communication with the surgeon is vital so the entire team agrees on realistic ROM goals. The exercises we prefer to use to maximize PFE in the first 2 to 3 postoperative months in patients with TSA are shown in Figures 13–16.

Use a Gradual Strengthening Progression and Have Patience

The final key principle in TSA rehabilitation is to use a gradual strengthening progression and have patience. Much like PFE, AROM and rotator cuff strength, especially in the overhead position, often have been limited for months or even years preoperatively so their return after surgery can be very gradual and slow, especially in patients in the fair to poor rehabilitation categories. Having patience and using

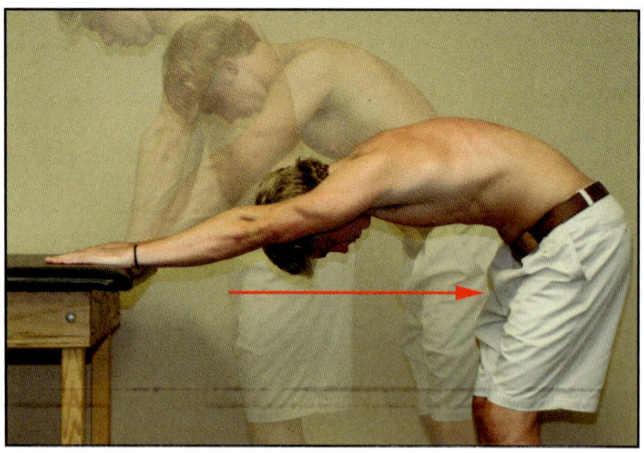

Figure 14. Table step-back exercise.

the AROM and strengthening principles of progression that are detailed in chapter II-1 are of the utmost importance. For instance, not setting a timetable for progression of exercise, having the strengthening exercises that are chosen match or be behind the patient's comfortable use of his or her upper extremity, ensuring that pain does not increase with the advancement of exercises, and exercising at a submaximal level or intensity are all critical principles that must guide the progression of strengthening exercises in patients with TSA.

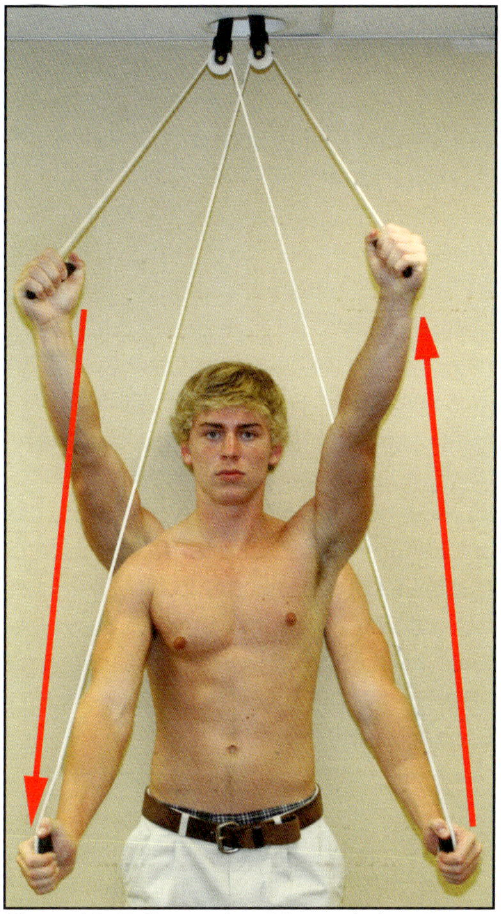

Figure 15. Pulley-assisted forward elevation. Note that the elbows are straight and the thumbs are up.

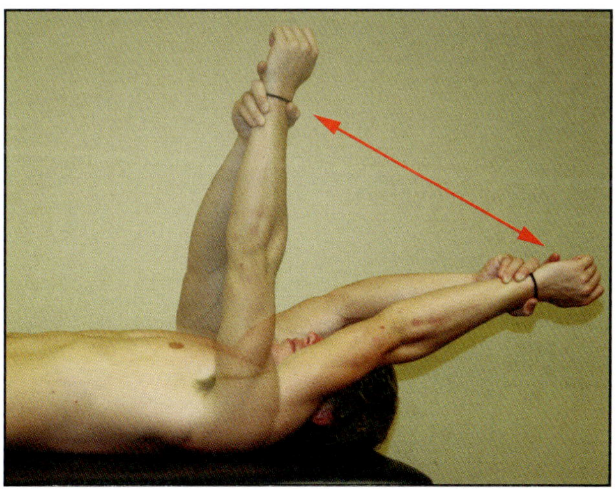

Figure 16. Self-assisted supine active-assisted forward elevation. The hand-assisted exercise is preferred.

SPECIFIC REHABILITATION GUIDELINE

The Appendix contains our complete rehabilitation guideline for standard TSA. In this section, I explain the rationale for selected components of the guideline. It is divided into 3 phases based on general timeframes of healing and staged ROM targets. To advance from one rehabilitation phase to the next, the patient must gain approval from the physician, successfully complete the core components of the previous rehabilitation activities, and meet the time criteria.

Phase 1

The primary focus of phase 1 rehabilitation, which constitutes the first 6 POWs, is to maximally protect the surgical repair, especially the subscapularis repair; ensure prosthetic or joint stability; control edema; achieve the staged ROM goals, especially in PFE; minimize pain; and educate the patient about postoperative precautions. The importance of most of these factors and how to achieve them have been detailed earlier in the chapter, but the importance of controlling edema has not been mentioned. A moderate to large amount of edema is common in the operated extremity in the early postoperative period, and the edema can lead to a wide variety of complications if it is not managed aggressively in the first POW. During the patient's hospital stay and during the first few POWs, the operated upper extremity is evaluated visually for edema. If present, an edema glove and Tubigrip (Mölnlycke Health Care US, LLC, Norcross, GA) are used to lightly compress the extremity from the fingers to the axilla (Figure 17). During the application, the tubing should be sized so only light compression is provided, and a slit should be made in the tubing near the axilla so the lymphatic system is not compressed excessively, which would result in reduced lymphatic drainage. In addition to elbow, wrist, and hand AROM that all patients begin on postoperative day 1, this edema management program typically resolves the problem in 7

Figure 17 A–C. Management of acute edema with an edema glove and Tubigrip (Mölnlycke Health Care US, LLC, Norcross, GA). Ensure only light compression is used and a slit is made in the tubing in the region of the axilla so lymphatic drainage is not impeded.

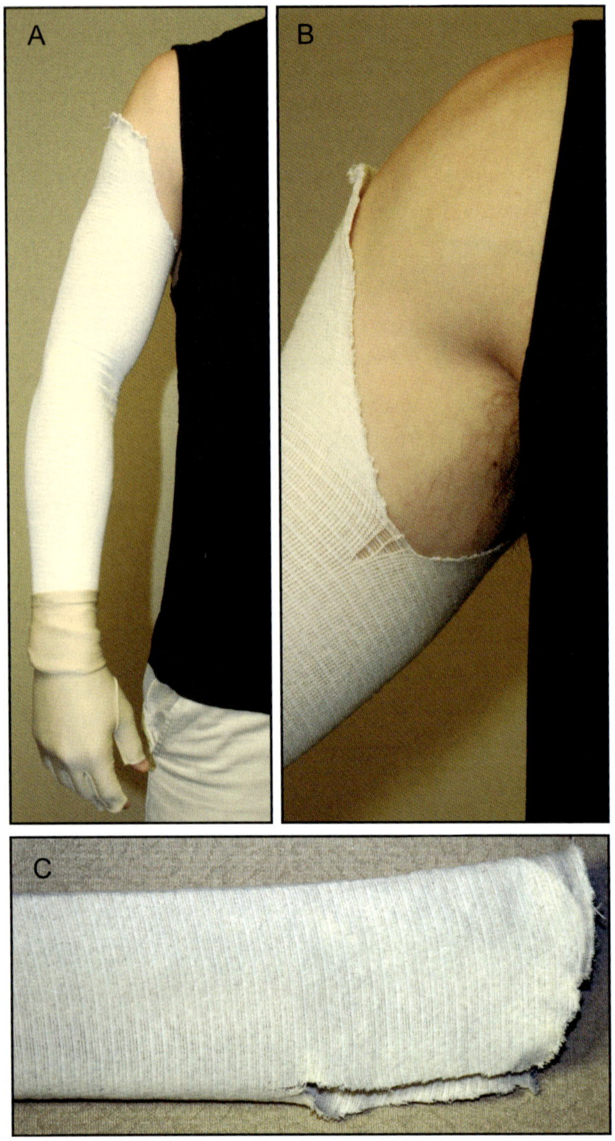

to 10 days, making more formal lymphedema therapy generally unnecessary.

The level of pain that patients have after TSA is typically very low within the first POW and is often lower than it was preoperatively. Therefore, patient education is important to emphasize that whereas some active use of the upper extremity is allowed, most ADLs still must be limited to protect the surgical repair. Patients especially are educated about not forcefully performing PER, not forcefully contracting their internal rotators during exercise or ADLs, and the importance of quickly gaining PFE in a comfortable manner based on their expected functional outcomes.

Phase 2

The focus of phase 2 rehabilitation, which typically constitutes POWs 6 through 12, is to continue to achieve staged ROM using an expanded PROM and stretching program and to begin an AROM and strengthening progression. The amount of PROM and stretching that is needed varies and depends on the patient's expected outcome (good, fair, or limited-goals rehabilitation category) and progress to his or her staged goals. Passive external rotation at 20° of abduction typically is discontinued for home and clinic exercises in late phase 1 or early phase 2 when 45° of ROM is obtained easily to protect the subscapularis. Passive forward elevation ROM continues to be emphasized both in clinic and home exercises, stressing gentle stretching performed by the rehabilitation provider and also stressing educating the patient about the importance of frequent (4 to 7 times each day), brief, gentle self-stretching to improve this ROM if it is below expected amounts. During this time, we prefer the home exercises that are shown in Figures 15 and 16 to improve PFE. Staged ROM goals for patients in the good rehabilitation category are listed in the Appendix; in the fair rehabilitation category, Table 3; and in the limited-goals rehabilitation category, chapter III-18.

During phase 2 rehabilitation, PROM in planes of motion other than PER in slight abduction and PFE can be added to the home exercise program as needed, keeping in mind the functional needs of patients with TSA and their expected outcomes that the surgeon determined. Compared with a competitive baseball player after a capsulolabral repair who needs to obtain greater than 90° of external rotation while the upper extremity is abducted at shoulder level, most patients with TSA do not have these functional demands and likely have not had this amount of PROM before surgery for many years. Therefore, working to achieve extremes of PROM in the combined position of abduction with external rotation or in other planes of PROM is likely unrealistic and might compromise the primary surgical goals of arthroplasty (pain relief and a stable joint).

Instead, achieving functional PROM that maximizes the patient's expected outcome is the goal of stretching for the patient with TSA during phases 2 and 3 rehabilitation. For abduction combined with external rotation, having enough PROM to allow the patient to easily reach the back of the head to comb his or her hair, reaching across the body to the opposite shoulder and underarm, and reaching behind the back to at least the small of the back are important. All of these ROMs are essential for basic hygiene, dressing, and self-care. To facilitate these motions, exercises, such as the hand-behind-head, or quadrant, stretch (Figure 18) and the horizontal adduction stretch (Figure 19), can begin as early as POW 6. Functional internal rotation stretching behind the back often begins about POW 8 using the opposite hand to assist (Figure 20).

The need for these stretching exercises is variable and should be considered carefully. For example, the quadrant stretch (Figure 18) stretches the subscapularis, so it should be used with care. If deemed realistic by the physician for the patient, we aim for functional PROM in abduction and external rotation and cross-body abduction at about postoperative month 3 and at about a month later for functional internal rotation. For motions that do not have specific staged goals, such as ROM in these planes, ROM of the operated side can be compared with ROM of the nonoperated side. For instance, to attain functional ROM at 12 POWs in a gradual way, about 50% of the motion of the uninvolved side would be expected at 6 POWs and about 75% of normal motion should be attained at 9 POWs with a normal end feel of the joint. A variable amount of stretching is needed to achieve these functional ROM goals in patients with TSAs based on the number of directions that are behind staged ROM goals, the size of the deficit, and the end feel of the joint that is noted during ROM assessment. Often, no structured stretching or only very selective and very gentle stretching is necessary to achieve the desired ROM. However, a comprehensive stretching program occasionally is appropriate. Therefore, phase 2 PROM exercises require a selective and individualized approach. The Appendix contains typical examples of stretches we consider using during this stage at the St. Francis Rehabilitation Center.

Structured AROM and strengthening can begin at POW 6 as long as PROM is not substantially behind staged goals. If it is, AROM and strengthening would be delayed so PROM could continue to be emphasized exclusively. As mentioned in the Key Principles in Rehabilitation of This Problem section, the AROM and strengthening progression for these patients is fairly straightforward and has predictable success as long as a gentle progression and much patience are used. To protect the subscapularis repair, only very gentle IR strengthening should be performed, especially during the first half of phase 2. Therefore, only exceptionally light resistance is used, and in patients who tend to be overexuberant, internal rotation strengthening is delayed.

Some patients with TSA, often those in the good rehabilitation category, might gain AROM and strength very quickly and only need a minimal strengthening program of basic strengthening with an elastic band

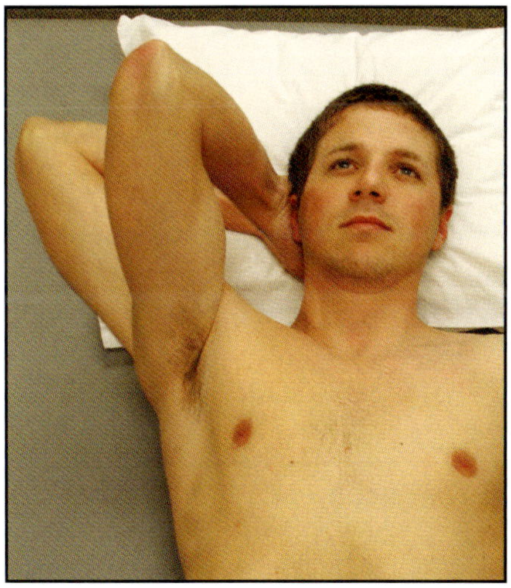

Figure 18. Supine hand-behind-head stretch.

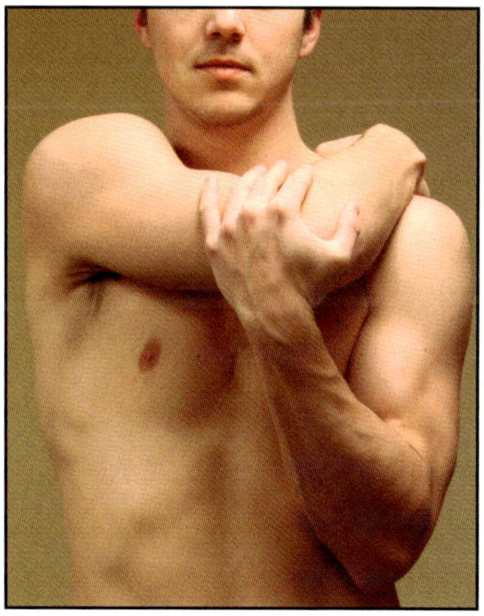

Figure 19. Horizontal adduction stretch.

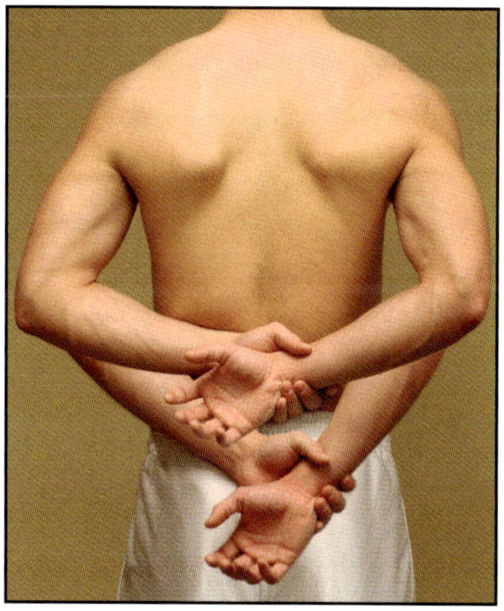

Figure 20. Functional internal rotation stretching with the assistance of the unaffected hand.

and AFE (Figure 21) without weight then progressing to 1 to 2 pounds (0.45–0.90 kg) of weight. Patients who are progressing very quickly should be cautioned about refraining from heavy lifting and forceful internal rotation during all of phase 2. Other patients with TSA, especially those in the fair or poor rehabilitation category or those who had very limited preoperative function, might gain AROM and strength slowly. In these patients, the use of elastic bands might need to be delayed for several weeks to focus on gravity-minimized strengthening. Often, these patients also require extensive use of the assistive-to-active elevation progression, including a very slow progression that might last well into phase 3 rehabilitation. The St. Francis Rehabilitation Center's AROM and strengthening progression is outlined in the Appendix and detailed in chapter II-4.

Phase 3

Phase 3 TSA rehabilitation is basically a continuation of phase 2 rehabilitation. Patients still emphasize achieving functional PROM for essential ADLs and continuing the AROM and strengthening progression outlined in phase 2 of the Appendix. Patients are discharged when functional PROM, functional AROM, and functional goals are met, considering their expected outcomes. Patients who progress slowly might require structured rehabilitation through postoperative months 5 or 6 or even longer. In these situations, especially in patients in whom PROM is functional and the main deficits are in AROM and strength, clinic visits can be very occasional, usually only 1 time every 2 to 4 weeks to advance the patient's home exercise program. In patients with moderate PROM deficits, we find that more regular structured rehabilitation visits are helpful.

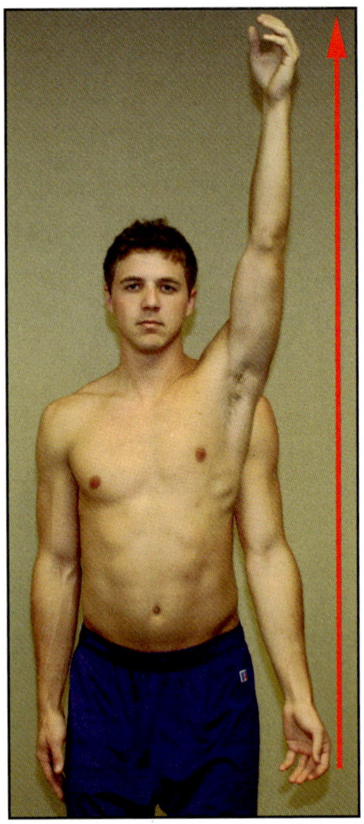

Figure 21. Active forward elevation.

Patients who are doing well begin phase 3 with functional to nearly normal PROM, AROM, and strength. These patients might be ready to be discharged to a maintenance home exercise program at the beginning of phase 3 that typically consists of our base strengthening program with appropriate resistance, AFE with light weight, and sometimes selected stretching exercises. These patients also are interested in resuming their normal leisure activities that might include hobbies, such as golfing, bowling, weight training, swimming laps, bicycling, hiking, and snow skiing. The appropriateness of returning to these activities at the beginning of phase 3 or even long term for some of the more vigorous activities is controversial, and even experienced shoulder surgeons disagree.[15] Therefore, the return to recreational activities, especially demanding recreational activities (eg, upper body weight training), and occupations that require repetitive lifting or moderate to heavy lifting, or both, is individualized and must be determined jointly by the physician and patient after extensive counseling and considering each patient's unique case. Of concern is whether the greater loading of the joint with higher-level activities or activities that carry the risk of falling will lead to more rapid wear and a higher rate of loosening of the prosthesis with time. Therefore, return to specific recreational activities should begin only with approval of the physician.

SPECIAL CONSIDERATIONS

Humeral Head Replacement

Rehabilitation does not change just because a humeral head replacement was performed instead of a TSA; the structures we directly treat during rehabilitation are the soft tissues surrounding the glenohumeral joint rather than the glenoid itself. However, rehabilitation is different for patients with humeral head replacement based on the reason the humeral head replacement was performed. In current practice, humeral head replacement most commonly is performed for arthritis due to osteonecrosis or proximal humerus fracture. As mentioned in the Know the Expected Outcome of Your Patient subsection, patients with the preoperative diagnosis of osteonecrosis are placed in the good rehabilitation category and are expected to have nearly normal ROM and basic shoulder function. Along with patients with OA, they use the rehabilitation guidelines detailed in the Appendix without modification. Patients with humeral head replacement due to a proximal humerus fracture are placed in the fair rehabilitation category and have lower expectations as discussed earlier in this chapter. Specific rehabilitation modifications are discussed in the next section.

Posttraumatic Arthritis

Patients with humeral head replacements due to the preoperative diagnosis of posttraumatic arthritis also have significant injury to the soft tissues of the shoulder that can result in rotator cuff tears and dense adhesions, as well as large distortions in bony anatomy due to the trauma that caused the injury. Patients in the fair rehabilitation category are expected to have much more modest outcomes. Passive forward elevation is often from 120° to 140°, AFE is often from 80° to 125°, PER is often from 30° to 50°, and functional internal rotation eventually might reach the L3-L1 spinal level. Functional use of the extremity overhead with reasonable strength to allow the patient to perform activities, such as reaching a 2- to 3-pound (0.90-kg–1.35-kg) can in an overhead cupboard, is variable.

Compared with the standard TSA rehabilitation detailed in the Appendix, the rehabilitation provider must be much more careful with PROM in this situation because the greater and lesser tuberosities might have been displaced during the injury, which requires mobilization and stabilization during the surgery. Because the rotator cuff tendons are attached directly to the tuberosities, extremes of PROM, forceful PROM, or overly active early ROM can cause displacement and incorrect healing of the tuberosities, resulting in long-term complications.[16] Therefore, the surgeon might specify PROM limits or delayed initiation of PROM. For the same reason, AROM and strengthening might be delayed or limited as determined by the surgeon. Given the significant trauma of the initial injury, preoperative adhesions, and rotator cuff damage, AROM and strengthening progresses very slowly and rarely progresses beyond light base strengthening and the elevation progression even if allowed to progress to tolerance. Further details on the rehabilitation of proximal humerus fractures are presented in chapter III-11.

Rheumatoid Arthritis

Patients with RA must be treated much differently from patients with TSA secondary to OA because RA is a systemic inflammatory disease. The rotator cuff, capsule, ligaments, and synovium are affected negatively by this disease process, which results in poorer-quality tissues, increased inflammation, inflammatory stiffness, and poorer tolerance to exercise. Even in the long term, less ROM and lower levels of function are expected as mentioned earlier in the chapter and as noted in the staged ROM tables (Appendix and Table 3). The standard TSA rehabilitation protocol needs to be adapted mainly by progressing rehabilitation at a slower pace; being more gentle in PROM, AROM,

Table 3. Staged Range-of-Motion Goals for Patients in the Fair Rehabilitation Category

Postoperative Time	Passive Forward Elevation	Passive External Rotation at 20° of Abduction	Passive External Rotation at 90° of Abduction	Active Forward Elevation
Week 1	70°–100°	0°–15°	Not applicable	Not applicable
Week 3	90°–115°	15°–30°	Not applicable	Not applicable
Week 6	120°–135°	30°–50°	45°	45°–100°
Week 12	120°–145°	<50°	<60°	80°–125°
Month 5	130°–150°	<50°	<60°	80°–135°

and strengthening; and often keeping the rehabilitation more simple. For example, in some patients, it might be best to delay the initiation of the AROM and strengthening progressions until POW 10 to 12 to allow a decrease in inflammation and improved ease of PROM. Similarly, expanding PROM and stretching beyond basic PFE and PER stretches even at POWs 6 to 8 sometimes is tolerated poorly. If so, then an extended time with only basic phase 1 stretching is warranted. I always progress AROM and strengthening slower and gentler in this patient population, minimizing repetitions, using active-assistive ROM more than AROM and resistive strengthening during phase 2, and emphasizing lower-level elevation progression exercises. Slower progress is expected in patients with TSA due to RA, so much patience is needed when rehabilitating them.

Arthritis of Dislocation

The surgeon places patients with arthritis of dislocation in either the fair or limited-goals rehabilitation category. These patients have long-standing abnormalities of the static and dynamic stabilizers due to recurrent dislocations and often require repair or reconstruction of the glenohumeral ligaments and joint capsule in addition to releases in other parts of the shoulder along with their TSAs. The rotator cuff is also typically of poor quality or damaged in these patients. In addition, gross distortion of the humeral head or glenoid might be present. Severe glenoid bone loss or erosion might require bone grafting, which complicates recovery. Modifications to rehabilitation due to glenoid bone grafting are addressed next in the Special Considerations section.

If placed in the fair rehabilitation category, patients need individualized PROM. Some patients require aggressive PROM to establish new ROMs that have not been available for years, whereas some patients must have PROM that is very gentle or restricted with ROM limits due to tissue damage or profound preoperative laxity in that direction. An extended period with passive stretching might be required due to preoperative stiffness in certain directions that is unique to each patient. Similarly, the AROM and strengthening progression must be individualized for each patient. Some patients use our standard progression at a normal pace of recovery; however, in some patients, only limited strengthening is appropriate, or the normal progressions might be appropriate but might be accomplished at a slower pace. Therefore, for this problem, excellent communication among the surgeon, rehabilitation provider, and the patient is required so all members of the team are in unity regarding contraindications, expected ROM, expected functional use, and specific areas of rehabilitation to emphasize.

Limited-goals rehabilitation for this patient population is reserved for patients for whom the surgeon expects only very limited long-term functional use of the upper extremity to be appropriate. The main goals of this type of rehabilitation are to achieve and maintain a stable joint with a low level of pain. Use of the upper extremity for basic waist-level activities is variable, and use of the upper extremity for shoulder activities requiring shoulder-level reaching, such as combing hair, occurs only occasionally. Functional use of the upper extremity overhead is not expected. Rehabilitation for these patients is very minimal and is detailed in chapter III-18.

Glenoid Bone Grafting

Patients who require glenoid bone grafting with their TSAs to restore proper orientation of the glenoid require modification of the base rehabilitation guideline, especially during phase 1 and the early part of phase 2, to promote incorporation of the bone graft. The surgeon often will place limits on the amount of PROM that is safe to achieve in the first 4 to 8 POWs to avoid overstressing the graft. The surgeon occasionally might delay the initiation of PROM, as well. Modifications to the later stages of rehabilitation are rare, but some patients require a slower progression because early rehabilitation was limited.

Subscapularis Takedown Versus Osteotomy of the Lesser Tuberosity

All typical TSAs require takedown of the subscapularis for later repair by either releasing it near its insertion to the lesser tuberosity (Figure 2) or by performing an osteotomy of the lesser tuberosity. Whereas each method of subscapularis takedown has proposed advantages for the surgeon[17,18] and the lesser tuberosity osteotomy might heal quicker than the tendon repair,[18,19] no differences in rehabilitation are needed based on the method of subscapularis takedown. Protecting the subscapularis repair that is a part of all typical TSAs is considered the single most important part of rehabilitation after TSA because this repair is fairly easy to damage, often overlooked, and demonstrates relatively poor outcomes if re-repaired. Why this protection is important and how to protect the subscapularis repair during rehabilitation was detailed earlier in this chapter.

TSA With Concomitant Rotator Cuff Repair of the Supraspinatus and/or Infraspinatus

Finally, in addition to the takedown and subsequent reattachment of the subscapularis, changes to the standard TSA rehabilitation guideline are required if a patient undergoes a rotator cuff repair of the supraspinatus and/or infraspinatus concomitant with his or her TSA. The subscapularis protection is the same as the standard TSA rehabilitation. Otherwise, the routine or massive rotator cuff repair rehabilitation guideline is used rather than the TSA rehabilitation guideline because the rotator cuff repair rehabilitation guideline is the factor that limits the speed of rehabilitation. These patients usually progress through the entire rehabilitation process slower than if either procedure was performed in isolation. Passive ROM usually is gained more slowly, and a longer time typically is required to achieve functional AROM and strength. Occasionally, physicians might choose to delay starting AROM strength until postoperative month 2 or 3 even if the only rotator cuff repair was to the supraspinatus.

REFERENCES

1. McCluskey GM III, Uhl T. Total shoulder replacement. In: Donatelli RA, ed. *Clinics in Physical Therapy: Physical Therapy of the Shoulder*. 3rd ed. New York, NY: Churchill Livingstone; 1997:459–476.
2. Wilcox RB, Arslanian LE, Millett P. Rehabilitation following total shoulder arthroplasty. *J Orthop Sports Phys Ther*. 2005;35(12):821–836.
3. Maybach A, Schlegel TF. Shoulder rehabilitation for the arthritic glenohumeral joint: preoperative and postoperative considerations. *Semin Arthroplasty*. 1995;6(4):297–304.
4. Gonzalez JF, Alami GB, Baque F, Walch G, Boileau P. Complications of unconstrained shoulder prostheses. *J Shoulder Elbow Surg*. 2011;20(4):666–682.
5. Hammond JW, Queale WS, Kim TK, McFarland EG. Surgeon experience and clinical and economic outcomes for shoulder arthroplasty. *J Bone Joint Surg Am*. 2003;85(12):2318–2324.
6. Figgie HE III, Inglis AE, Goldberg VM, Ranawat CS, Figgie MP, Wile JM. An analysis of factors affecting the long-term results of total shoulder arthroplasty in inflammatory arthritis. *J Arthroplasty*. 1988;3(2):123–130.
7. Miller SL, Hazrati Y, Klepps S, Chiang A, Flatow EL. Loss of subscapularis function after total shoulder replacement: a seldom recognized problem. *J Shoulder Elbow Surg*. 2003;12(1):29–34.
8. Scheibel M, Habermeyer P. Subscapularis dysfunction following anterior surgical approaches to the shoulder. *J Shoulder Elbow Surg*. 2008;17(4):671–683.
9. Moeckel BH, Altcheck DW, Warren RF, Wickiewicz TL, Dines DM. Instability of the shoulder after arthroplasty. *J Bone Joint Surg Am*. 1993;75(4):492–497.
10. Armstrong A, Lashgari C, Teefey S, Menendez J, Yamaguchi K, Galatz LM. Ultrasound evaluation and clinical correlation of subscapularis repair after total shoulder arthroplasty. *J Shoulder Elbow Surg*. 2006;15(5):541–548.
11. Ponce BA, Ahluwalia RS, Mazzocca AD, Gobezie RG, Warner JJ, Millet PJ. Biomechanical and clinical evaluation of a novel lesser tuberosity repair technique in total shoulder arthroplasty. *J Bone Joint Surg Am*. 2005;87(suppl 2):1–8.
12. Edwards TB, Boulahia A, Kempf JF, Boileau P, Nemoz C, Walch G. The influence of rotator cuff disease on the results of shoulder arthroplasty for primary osteoarthritis: results of a multicenter study. *J Bone Joint Surg Am*. 2002;84(12):2240–2248.
13. Rundquist PJ, Ludewig PM. Correlation of 3-dimensional shoulder kinematics to function in subjects with idiopathic loss of shoulder range of motion. *Phys Ther*. 2005;85(7):636–647.
14. Boström C, Harms-Ringdahl K, Nordemar R. Shoulder, elbow and wrist movement impairment: predictors of disability in female patients with rheumatoid arthritis. *Scand J Rehabil Med*. 1997;29(4):223–232.
15. Magnussen RA, Mallon WJ, Willems WJ, Moorman CT III. Long-term activity restrictions after shoulder arthroplasty: an international survey of experienced shoulder surgeons. *J Shoulder Elbow Surg*. 2011;20(2):281–289.
16. Noyes MP, Kleinhenz B, Markert RJ, Crosby LA. Functional and radiographic long-term outcomes of hemiarthroplasty for proximal humeral fractures. *J Shoulder Elbow Surg*. 2011;20(3):372–377.
17. Caplan JL, Whitfield B, Neviaser JR. Subscapularis function after primary tendon to tendon repair in patients after replacement arthroplasty of the shoulder. *J Shoulder Elbow Surg*. 2009;18(2):193–198.
18. Gerber C, Yain EH, Pfirrmann CA, Zumstein MA, Werner CM. Subscapularis muscle function and structure after total shoulder replacement with lesser tuberosity osteotomy and repair. *J Bone Joint Surg Am*. 2005;87(8):1739–1745.
19. Jandhyala S, Unnithan A, Hughes S, Hong T. Subscapularis tenotomy versus lesser tuberosity osteotomy during total shoulder replacement: a comparison of patient outcomes. *J Shoulder Elbow Surg*. 2011;20(7):1102–1107.

REHABILITATION GUIDELINE FOR TOTAL SHOULDER ARTHROPLASTY OR HUMERAL HEAD REPLACEMENT WITH THE PREOPERATIVE DIAGNOSIS OF OSTEOARTHRITIS OR AVASCULAR NECROSIS

St. Francis Orthopaedic Institute and St. Francis Rehabilitation Center

All information contained in this protocol is to be used as a general guideline only. Specific variations might be appropriate for each patient and might be specified by the physician. In all cases, it is acceptable to advance the program more slowly than stated. If the patient experiences excessive pain, discontinue exercise until the physician is contacted. ***Achieving and maintaining a low level of pain and inflammation and protecting the surgical repair are the guiding principles in all stages of rehabilitation, even if less passive and active range of motion are accomplished.***

SYMBOLS AND ABBREVIATIONS

AAFE, active-assistive forward elevation
AAROM, active-assistive range of motion
AASEP, assistive-to-active shoulder elevation progression
AFE, active forward elevation
AROM, active range of motion
CPM, continuous passive motion
EMG, electromyography
ER, external rotation
FE, forward elevation
IR, internal rotation
NA, not applicable
PER, passive external rotation
PFE, passive forward elevation
POD, postoperative day
POM, postoperative month
POW, postoperative week
PRN, as needed
PROM, passive range of motion
ROM, range of motion
T-Band, Thera-Band (The Hygenic Corporation, Akron, OH)
WNL, within normal limits

Forward elevation, either active or passive, is the plane of motion in which an individual naturally lifts his or her arm that is anterior to the plane of the scapula and lateral to flexion.

STAGED GOALS FOR RANGE OF MOTION

These are approximate targets for ROM. Specific limits might be specified by the physician. **Emphasize PFE, which can be gained at a faster rate than the staged goals if comfortable. Because of the subscapularis repair, protect PER at 20° of abduction and 90° of abduction by not being forceful with stretching and by not exceeding the staged goals.**

Time	PFE	PER at 20° of Abduction	PER at 90° of Abduction	AFE
POW 1	80°–100°	0°–15°	NA	NA
POW 3	115°–130°	20°–30°	NA	NA
POW 6	130°–145°	35°–50°	45°	90°–130°
POW 12	140°–155°	<60°	<70°	125°–155°
POM 5	WNL	<60°	<70°	145°+

PHASE 1

Goals

- °Maximally protect the repair (especially the subscapularis repair)
- °Ensure prosthetic or joint stability
- °Control edema
- °Achieve staged ROM goals, especially PFE
- °Minimize pain and inflammatory response
- °Educate the patient about postoperative precautions

POW 1 to POW 6

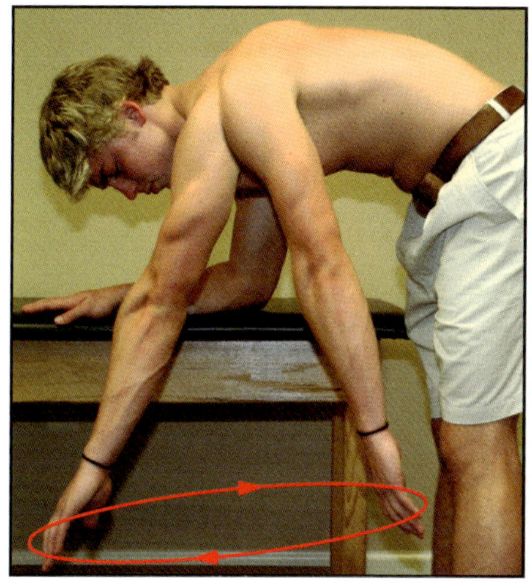

Figure 22. Pendulum exercise. Use smaller circles initially.

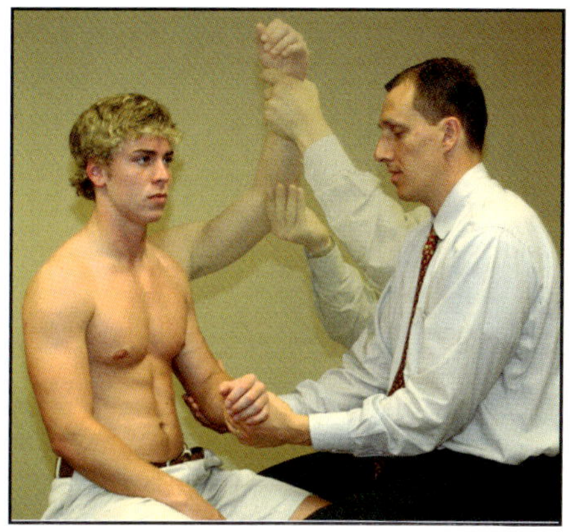

Figure 23. Assisted passive forward elevation. The assistant typically stands diagonally in front of the patient.

- °Elbow, wrist, and hand AROM with no weight starts on POD 1
- °Edema control PRN, including edema glove, Tubigrip (Mölnlycke Heath Care US, LLC, Norcross, GA), and retrograde massage starts on POD 1
- °Scapular elevations and retractions (no weight) in or out of sling
- °Pendulum exercise (Figure 22)
  - °Lean over the table a comfortable amount
  - °Let the arm hang down relaxed
  - °Keep the body still
  - °As able, move the arm in only small comfortable circles
- °PFE until mild stretch and discomfort
  - °7 to 12 repetitions starting with 2 times per day
  - °**Emphasize gaining ROM in this plane**
  - °Preferred exercises
    - °Sit with family member or therapist lifting the arm (Figure 23)
    - °Table step-back exercise (Figure 14)
    - °Kinex KS2 (Kinex Medical Company, LLC, Waukesha, WI) shoulder CPM as ordered by the physician (Figure 13)
    - °After achieving more than 110° of PFE, progress to self-assisted AAFE in the supine position as tolerated (Figure 16)
- °Upright PER at 20° of abduction until mild stretch and +/- discomfort
  - °7 to 12 repetitions starting with 2 times per day
  - °ROM limits might be specified by physician
  - °**Protect ROM in this plane; do not exceed staged goals and no forceful stretching**
  - °Preferred exercises
    - °Sit with family member or therapist rotating the arm (Figure 11)
    - °PER walk-around (Figure 12)
- °Ice for pain reduction
- °Fit the sling properly, providing a lift to the shoulder girdle
- °Patient education
  - °Use of the sling as instructed by physician
  - °Typically, full time in community and when up for more than 5 to 10 minutes at home
  - °Can use the arm for light waist-level activities as comfortable
  - °Ensure the level of pain is not increasing because of excessive use of the arm for activities of daily living or work
  - °Sleep in a recliner

Adjunctive Exercises

- °Therapist-assisted supine PROM within comfortable ROM to
  - °Decrease muscle guarding
  - °Gain patient confidence
  - °Achieve staged PROM goals (no mobilizations)
- °Cervical spine AROM

°Pain-control agents PRN
°Aquatic therapy for gentle pain-free AAROM (no swimming strokes) after incision has healed completely

Interventions to Avoid

°Glenohumeral PROM, except PFE and PER, for home exercise
°Forceful PER stretching to protect the subscapularis repair
°Exercises that result in moderate or severe pain
°Exercises that result in excessive guarding or splinting of muscles
°Weighted exercises and the upper body ergometer

PHASE 2

Goals

°Protect the subscapularis repair
°Ensure prosthetic or joint stability
°Achieve staged ROM goals, especially PFE
°Begin to increase AROM, strength, and endurance
°Increase functional activities

POW 6 to POM 3

- °Achieve staged ROM goals in FE
  - °**Continue to emphasize increasing ROM in this plane**
  - °Preferred exercises
    - °Rope-and-pulley in FE (elbows straight) (Figure 15)
    - °Patient-assisted supine AAFE exercise (use unaffected arm for assistance) (Figure 16)
- °**Discontinue ROM exercises for PER** at 20° of abduction unless ROM is less than 35° to 40°
- °Initiate horizontal adduction (Figure 19) or sleeper stretch, or both, **PRN**
- °Goals of obtaining functional flexibility at POM 3
- °Initiate supine hand-behind-head stretch **PRN** (Figure 18)
  - °To facilitate the PROM necessary to comb hair by POM 3
- °Functional IR AAROM stretching **PRN** using opposite hand to assist (Figure 20)
  - °Typically, do not start before POW 8 and only then to help the patient reach the small of the back during phase 2
- °Therapist-assisted PROM to achieve staged ROM goals with mobilizations PRN
- °Initiate base strengthening progression
  - °Includes standard rotator cuff, deltoid, and scapular strengthening program
  - °2 times per day at most with light resistance and increasing repetitions (generally 25–40)
  - °Yellow T-Band for ER and IR
    - °5- to 6-foot band length and light or no pretension in a 3- to 6-inch arc of motion
    - °**Be especially careful and gentle with IR because of subscapularis repair.** Wait to begin if painful.

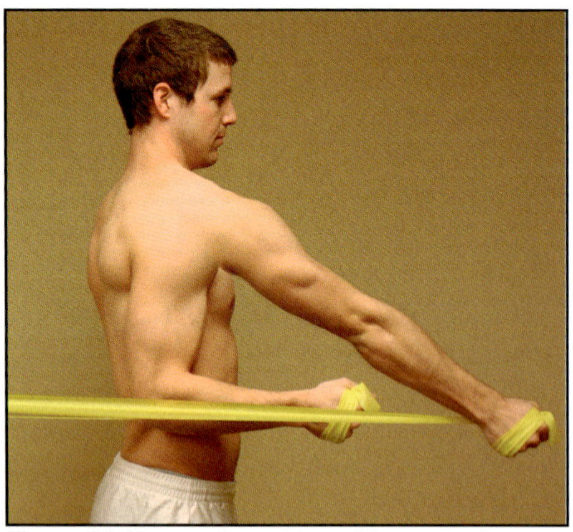

Figure 24. Forward reaching with an elastic band at waist level.

- °Can use side-lying ER instead of T-Band
- °Yellow T-Band forward reach (Figure 24)
  - °Initially, 5- to 6-foot band length and light or no pretension with progressive tension as tolerated
  - °Reach forward with the hand at waist level, progressing to reaching forward at chest level
  - °**Do not initiate until active forward reach at waist level is pain-free**
  - °If forward reach is painful or difficult, replace with a "gravity-minimized" exercise from the AASEP (described below) until the forward reach can be done comfortably
- °Scapular strengthening emphasizing scapular retractions and scapular upward rotators
- °**No prone FE, abduction, or ER**

°Initiate the AASEP as comfortable (chapter II-4)

- °A stepwise progression in difficulty of strengthening exercises from PFE to AFE against gravity
- °Goal of the progression is to achieve pain-free full AFE
- °EMG demonstrates progressive activation of cuff, deltoid, and scapular upward rotators during the progression
- °If scapular or glenohumeral substitutions or pain are present, choose an easier exercise in the progression
- °The order of the exercise sequence has some variability
- °Usually not all exercises need to be performed. **Choose an exercise that is comfortable and can be performed without deviations but that is fatiguing.**
- °**Ensure that these exercises do not increase pain**
- °Exercises are divided into 3 levels of difficulty
  1. **Gravity-minimized exercises**
     - °Horizontal dusting (Figure 25)
       - °Perform straight ahead
       - °Perform at 20° angles medially and laterally if comfortable
     - °T-Band supine FE (Figure 26)
       - °Must start involved arm at 90° of elevation
       - °Pull the arm into FE
     - °Side-lying, gravity-eliminated AFE (Figure 27)
       - °Lie on uninvolved side
       - °Place involved arm on an ironing board
       - °Slide hand on the board
     - °Supine reaching progression
       - °Begin at 0° with the elbow bent and end at 90° of elevation with the elbow extended
     - °Start with the assistance of a cane or wand
       - °Progress to active motion (Figure 28)

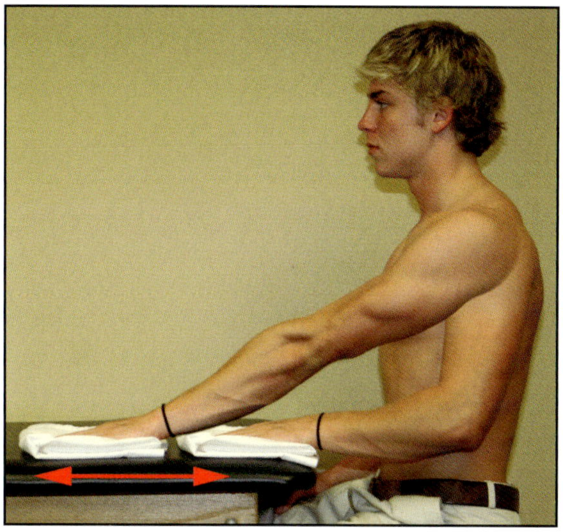
Figure 25. Horizontal dusting.

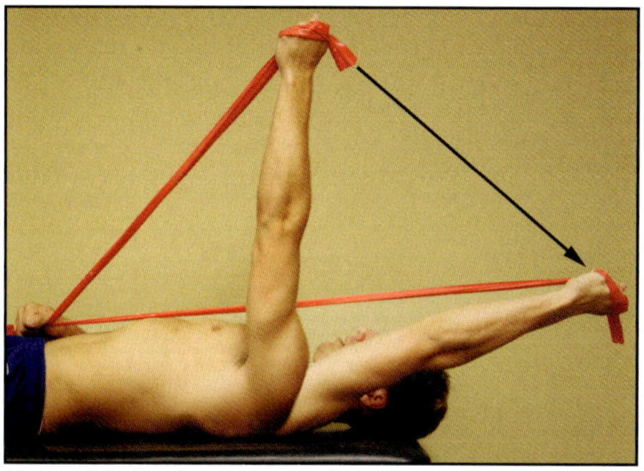
Figure 26. Supine forward elevation with an elastic band.

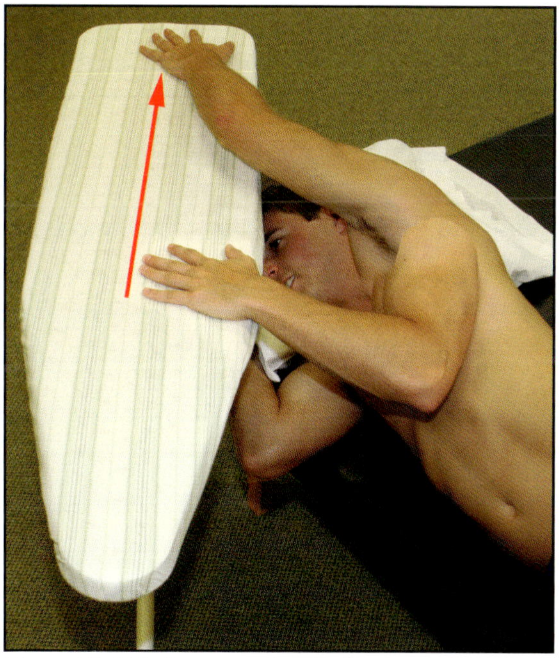
Figure 27. Side-lying, gravity-eliminated active forward elevation.

°Can progress to using 1 to 2 pounds of weight

°Can progress to inclined position, continuing to reach to ceiling

2. Assistive elevation exercises

°Rope-and-pulley AAFE

°Incline dusting (Figure 29)

°Standing AAFE (assistive elevation and descent via T-bar or unaffected arm)

°Standing assistive elevation and active independent eccentric lowering

°Wall-slide AAFE

°Ensure that patient is in FE and is not in flexion

°Must be pain-free and natural when performing

3. Unsupported elevation exercises

°Overhead wall taps

°AFE (Figure 21)

°Initiate AFE when the AASEP is complete

°Only perform if full or nearly full AROM is possible and comfortable

°Eventually progress to 1 to 3 pounds for resistance depending on body size

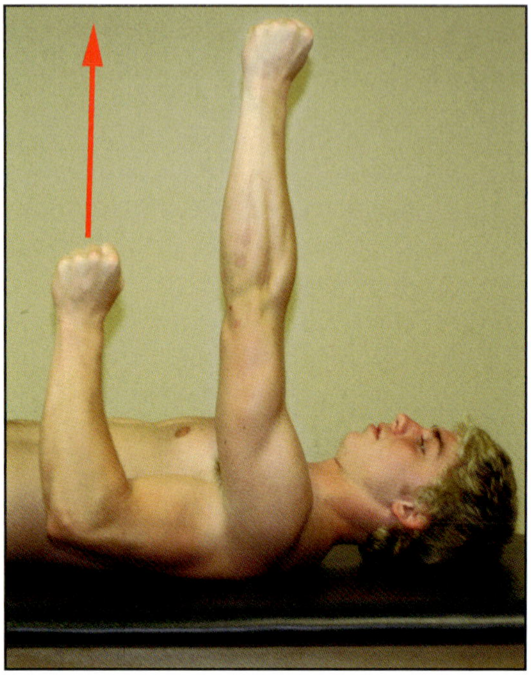

Figure 28. Supine active reaching from 0° to 90°.

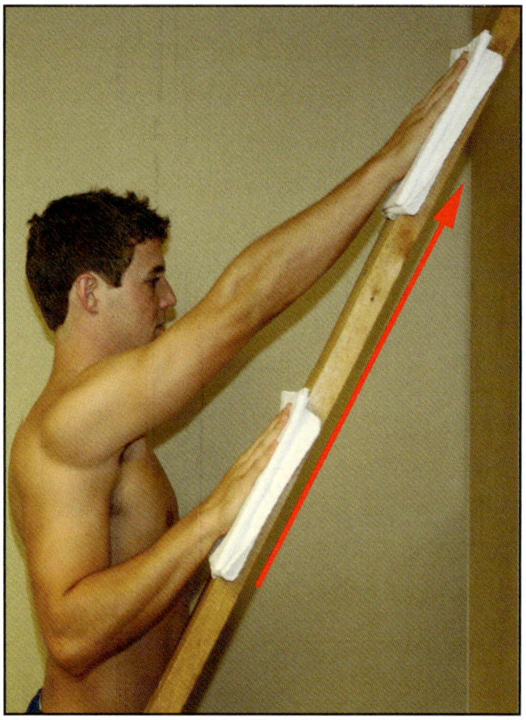

Figure 29. Incline dusting.

Adjunctive Exercises

°Cryotherapy

°Modalities as needed

°Aquatic exercises

°AAROM, AROM, and light strengthening

°Spine therapy assessment and mobilization if

°Nonneurogenic cervical or scapular pain or

°Limitation in end-range shoulder FE

°Golf chipping and putting when physician allows

Interventions to Avoid

°**Initiating strengthening exercises if PROM is behind staged goals**

°Initiating base strengthening program or overhead strengthening progression before overall level of pain is low

°Exercises that greatly increase signs and symptoms

°Heavy lifting with elbows away from body

°The upper extremity ergometer

°Strengthening into straight-plane abduction

°Prone FE, abduction, or ER

PHASE 3

Goals

°Functional AROM and PROM
°Normalize strength and endurance
°Return to activities of daily living, work, and recreation

POM 3 to 5+

°PROM, stretching as needed, and warm-up stretching to achieve **functional** PROM and staged goals. Functional IR to bra line is allowed for female patients.
 °Some patients will need an extensive amount of phase 2 stretching that will be the primary thrust of phase 3 rehabilitation
 °Some patients will need almost no PROM or stretching because functional PROM already will be achieved
°Continue base and elevation strengthening program
 °Progress T-Band color very gradually
 °Continue progressive AFE as previously described
°**Discharge when functional goals are met**
°Individualized return to recreational activities and demanding work activities as determined **by physician** to protect the longevity of the prosthesis
 °Return-to-golf program and recreational swimming generally are allowed at this time but still require physician approval
 °Tennis when physician allows
 °**Return to demanding recreational activities, including throwing sports; upper body weight training; and occupations requiring repetitive lifting or moderate to heavy lifting, or both, is extremely individualized and must be determined by the physician after counseling the patient. Begin only with specific approval by physician.**

Adjunctive Exercises

°Therapist-assisted stretching and mobilizations PRN

Interventions to Avoid

°Any rehabilitation activity that is much more demanding than daily or expected activities
°Any rehabilitation activity that is a moderate to large increase in demand compared with previous rehabilitation
°Any rehabilitation activity that results in a level of pain high enough that the patient needs to use modalities
°Strengthening in straight-plane abduction
°The upper extremity ergometer

III-8

Reverse Shoulder Arthroplasty

Brian G. Leggin, PT, DPT, OCS

CHAPTER CONTENTS

- What patients are appropriate for the use of this guideline?
- Overview of rotator cuff tear arthropathy
- Shoulder arthroplasty with rotator cuff deficiency
- Reverse total shoulder arthroplasty
- Rehabilitation after reverse shoulder arthroplasty

WHAT PATIENTS ARE APPROPRIATE FOR THE USE OF THIS GUIDELINE?

- Patients who have received a reverse shoulder arthroplasty due to shoulder arthritis associated with irreparable rotator cuff tear arthropathy
- Patients who have received a reverse shoulder arthroplasty due to a severe shoulder fracture with associated rotator cuff deficiency
- Patients who have received a reverse shoulder arthroplasty for revision of a conventional total shoulder arthroplasty with a loss of rotator cuff function

Clinical pearls are highlighted in yellow throughout the text.

In the earliest description of the pathoanatomic features of rotator cuff tear arthropathy (CTA), Adams[1] characterized chronic rotator cuff tears leading to localized destructive arthritis.[1] Codman[2] later expanded the description when he reported recurrent swelling of the shoulder, absence of the rotator cuff, cartilaginous bodies attached to the synovial tissue, and severe destructive glenohumeral arthritis in a 51-year-old woman. In 1983, Neer et al[3] coined the term *cuff tear arthropathy* to explain a recognized clinical entity of the shoulder consisting of severe disorganization of the glenohumeral joint with collapse of the humeral head that occurs after some massive tears of the rotator cuff. In association with chronic full-thickness rotator cuff tears, they noted erosion of the osseous structures, humeral osteopenia, and restricted shoulder motion.[3,4] Subsequently, the massive rotator cuff tear allows superior migration of the humerus into the subacromial space, eventually resulting in "femoralization" of the humeral head, which describes erosion of the greater tuberosity, and "acetabularization" of the coracoacromial arch, which results in reshaping of the arch so it creates a socket for the proximal aspect of the humerus (Figure 1).[3,4]

Several theories about the development of CTA have been postulated, but the exact cause is unknown.[4] Associations between CTA and the presence of basic calcium phosphate crystals in synovial fluid and tissue have been identified and termed *Milwaukee Shoulder*.[5–7] Reports on the Milwaukee Shoulder have included clinical aspects and studies of synovial fluid, as well as morphologic and biochemical studies of excised synovial tissue.[8] Visotsky et al[4] proposed that

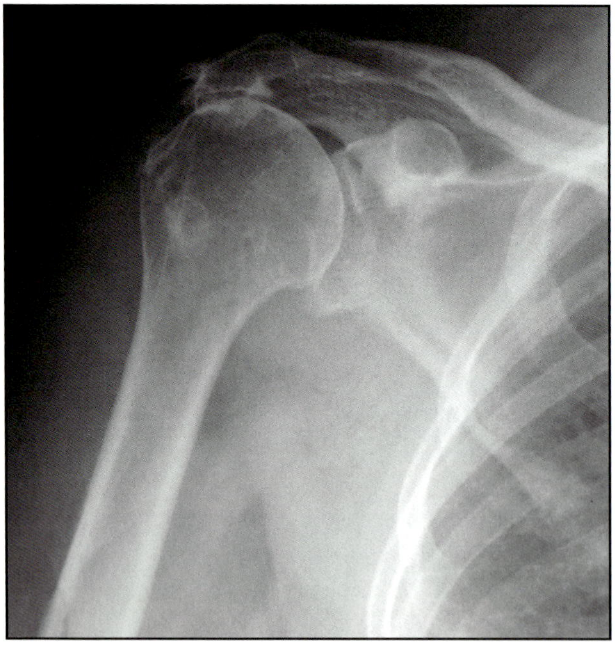

Figure 1. Radiographic anteroposterior view of a shoulder with rotator cuff tear arthropathy.

calcium phosphate crystals induce an immunologic cascade and release of collagenase. These activated enzymes destroy periarticular and articular structures.[4]

Neer et al[3] believed that both nutritional and mechanical factors are involved in the development of CTA. Nutritional factors imposed by the massive tear include loss of a closed joint space and impaired movement of the glenohumeral joint.[3] The loss of a "water-tight" joint space with leaking synovial fluid under reduced pressure deters the perfusion of nutrients into the articular cartilage.[3] Impaired joint movement or inactivity can lead to structural changes in the articular cartilage and to biochemical changes in the water and glycosaminoglycan content of the cartilage and capsule.[3]

Mechanical factors that Neer et al[3] proposed include unbalanced muscle forces, which lead to gross instability of the humeral head on the glenoid and to upward migration of the head against the acromion and acromioclavicular joint. The superior migration of the humeral head imposes destructive forces on the anterior soft tissue structures and the osseous constraints, leading to an accelerated process of further rotator cuff destruction and arthropathy.[4]

Three radiographic classifications have been developed to define the bony changes that occur in CTA. Although overlapping characteristics are considered with each of these classifications, each focuses on a different set of findings associated with these disorders.[9] The Seebauer classification targets superior migration of the humeral head and its containment within the coracoacromial arch.[4] The Hamada classification system characterizes the associated structural changes within the coracoacromial arch.[10] The Favard classification focuses on bone loss of the glenoid.[11] Iannotti et al[9] found that the Seebauer classification and clinical examination for active elevation and superior instability of the humeral head were the most important factors in recommending surgical options for the treatment of CTA.

SHOULDER ARTHROPLASTY WITH ROTATOR CUFF DEFICIENCY

Surgical treatment of shoulders with an arthritic or damaged glenohumeral joint associated with a deficient or nonfunctional rotator cuff has had limited success.[12,13] Surgeons must face this challenging combination in at least 3 situations: (1) arthritis associated with a massive and irreparable rotator cuff tear; (2) fracture sequelae in which distortion of the proximal humeral anatomy around the insertion of the cuff results in a functionally useless rotator cuff; and (3) revision after failure of a previous arthroplasty in which the rotator cuff is deficient, scarred, or retracted or has undergone fatty infiltration.[12,14–16] Neer et al[3] performed total shoulder arthroplasty (TSA) for 26 patients with CTA and reported 25 of 26 patients improved. Although TSA provides good pain relief in patients with rotator cuff deficiency, loosening of the glenoid component is a recognized long-term complication.[17–19] In patients with superior migration of the humerus, a "rocking horse" phenomenon might develop and contribute to glenoid loosening.[17] Therefore, given that fewer patients developed these complications with hemiarthroplasty, it became the surgical treatment of choice for patients with rotator cuff arthropathy.[8] This option has resulted in only modest improvements in pain and function.[16,20–24] Furthermore, with superior humeral migration, the humerus might become "locked" under the acromion.[25]

Recognizing the poorer outcomes of arthroplasty when the rotator cuff was not functional, Neer explored constrained arthroplasty designs to obviate the need for rotator cuff reconstruction.[26] He designed 3 variations of constrained TSAs, each having a reversed glenohumeral articulation.[26] However, each prosthesis resulted in various complications, convincing Neer that rotator cuff repair rather than constraint was essential for improved shoulder function.[26] Therefore, he abandoned his pursuit of constrained shoulder arthroplasty.

Several surgeons continued to pursue fixed-fulcrum designs that maintained the standard ball-and-socket glenohumeral articulation with increased constraint.[26–32] However, complication rates were high and improvement was "inconsistent and disappointing."[26,30] The most notable complication requiring revision was loosening of the glenoid component.[26,33] Kessel and Bayley[29] recognized that one factor limiting a satisfactory shoulder prosthesis was the unsuitability of the scapula for holding a prosthesis with acrylic cement. As more researchers reported loosening of the glenoid, shoulder arthroplasty designs included glenoid component fixation without cement, relying on flanges, pegs, and screws.[26] Given a concern for scapular fractures, constrained prostheses were designed to dislocate at lower forces than required for scapular fracture.[26,32] Despite these changes, failures continued, and researchers reported high rates of revision.[34,35]

REVERSE TOTAL SHOULDER ARTHROPLASTY

Given the challenges of constrained shoulder arthroplasty, many investigators began to explore reversing the normal anatomy by placing the socket in the proximal humerus and the prosthetic ball on the glenoid.[26] In the 1970s, several researchers designed reverse arthroplasty systems with various forms of scapular fixation.[36–44] These prostheses tended to fail because their designs resulted in excessive torque and shear forces at the glenoid component-bone interface.[45] The clinical results of these prostheses were unsatisfactory because of poor motion and prosthetic instability, and most are no longer available.[45]

In the early 1980s, Grammont and 2 engineers concluded that when the cuff is absent, the solution is to intrinsically balance the middle deltoid to strengthen its abduction component and decrease the elevation component responsible for loosening stress on the glenoid.[46] Grammont's system focused on 4 key features: (1) the prosthesis must be inherently stable; (2) the weight-bearing part must be convex; (3) the center of the sphere must be at or within the glenoid neck; and (4) the center of rotation must be medialized and distalized. Grammont noted the deltoid function could be increased by moving the center of rotation distally and medially compared with the native glenohumeral articulation.[26,41] His new concept was that the glenoid component should be fixed with a central peg and some screws of divergent direction to counteract the initial shearing forces.[25,45] The glenoid component (glenosphere) is a half sphere to place the center of rotation directly in contact with the glenoid surface, decreasing lateral offset at the glenohumeral articulation and thus decreasing shearing forces (Figure 2).[45] The humeral component has a small cup, oriented with a nonanatomic inclination of 155° that covers less than half the glenosphere (Figure 3). This system developed by Grammont has the advantage of lowering the

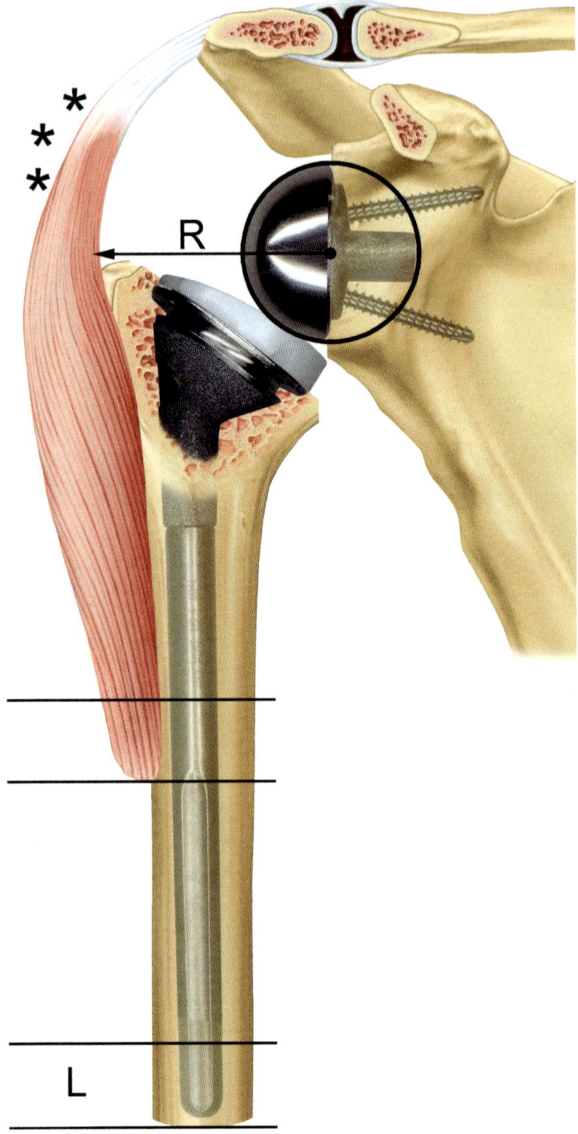

Figure 2. Illustration of the arthroplasty demonstrating key design concepts.

humerus, resulting in overtensioning of the deltoid.[45] Reverse shoulder arthroplasty prostheses that are currently available vary in some design details, but their intrinsic design remains based on Grammont's principles.[26] However, the degree of medialization differs among implants, and the optimal amount is not known.

The reverse shoulder arthroplasty has been available in the United States since 2004 but has been used in Europe for 2 decades.[47] The collective experience suggests that the reverse shoulder arthroplasty is best used for the patient who has end-stage, severe CTA; is elderly; and places low demand on the shoulder, with active elevation to less than 120°. In addition, the del-

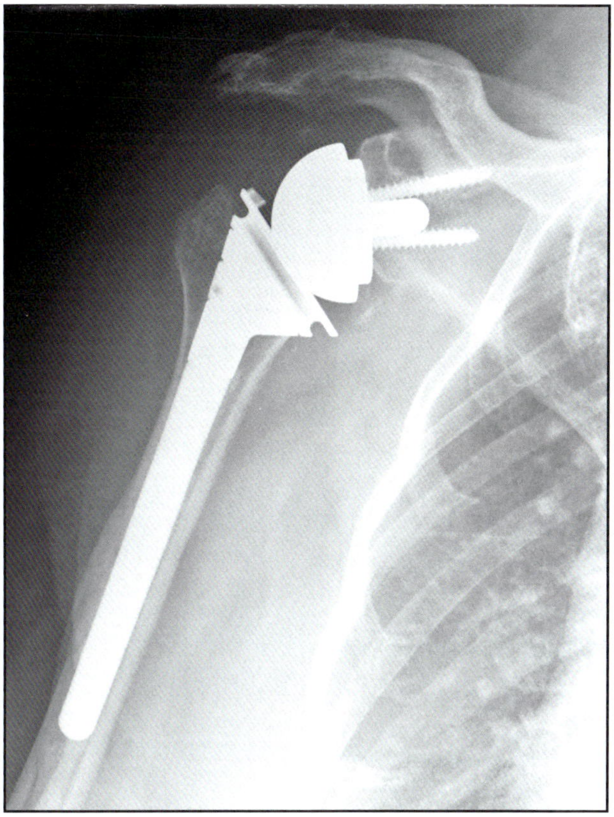

Figure 3. Radiographic anteroposterior view of a shoulder after reverse total shoulder arthroplasty.

toid must be functional, and bone on the glenoid side needs to be sufficient to allow for secure screw fixation of the component.

REHABILITATION AFTER REVERSE SHOULDER ARTHROPLASTY

Rehabilitation after reverse shoulder arthoplasty is not standardized. Early motion depends on the preference of the surgeon and the quality of the glenoid fixation. Some authors have reported initiating no postoperative rehabilitation and allowing patients to use their upper extremities freely for functional activities. Researchers also have advocated immobilization up to 4 to 6 weeks after surgery.[48] Others have initiated passive range of motion (PROM) on the first postoperative day with limits of 90° of passive elevation and 0° of external rotation for the first 6 weeks and have allowed active movement after 6 weeks.[49]

The rehabilitation provider and the patient need to understand the risks of positioning and functional activity after reverse TSA. The risk of shoulder dislocation is higher after reverse TSA than conventional TSA. The most dangerous position for the reverse TSA is internal rotation and adduction in conjunction with extension. Therefore, exercises in this position should be limited. In addition, functional activities, such as tucking in a shirt or reaching the back pocket, should be avoided especially in the first 12 postoperative weeks.

Patients also need to understand that the primary goal of this procedure is to allow pain-free elevation of the shoulder. Activities or positions involving external rotation also are limited because little if any rotator cuff musculature remains and external rotation provided by the deltoid is decreased due to medialization of the center of rotation.

Our approach to rehabilitation depends on the patient's preoperative deltoid function and postoperative stiffness. Patients with good deltoid function are allowed to use their upper extremities for waist-level activities for the first 6 postoperative weeks. Thereafter, they are allowed unrestricted use of their extremities. Patients with postoperative stiffness in forward elevation begin early PROM exercises within the first 7 to 10 days after surgery. Patients with poor deltoid function begin strengthening and functional training at 6 weeks.

Phase 1: Postoperative Weeks 0 to 6

The rehabilitation process begins with patient education. Patients should expect swelling and discoloration of the affected extremity and occasionally of the chest wall due to surgery. They typically are immobilized in a sling that positions the extremity in slight abduction to keep it in the plane of the scapula. Patients also are instructed in the use of ice to help control pain and inflammation. They can use the extremity for waist-level activities and can bring their hands to their mouths with their elbows held at their sides. Patients should not sleep on or make sudden movements with the operated side. In addition, they should avoid lifting, carrying, pushing, pulling, and leaning on the affected side. Evaluation should include documentation of distal neurovascular status and passive arc of forward elevation. The shoulder can be externally rotated passively to neutral.

The rehabilitation provider should emphasize that all exercises are to be performed 4 to 6 times per day. To maintain strength and decrease swelling in the distal aspect of the upper extremity, patients are instructed in hand-squeezing exercises and elbow active range of motion (AROM). They also are instructed in pendulum exercises, which are to be performed 25 times in each direction. Supine passive forward elevation with the opposite hand (Figure 4) and external rotation with a stick or the opposite hand to neutral rotation can be added at this time. Ten repetitions of the exercises are performed with a 10-second hold for each repetition.

Patients with bilateral shoulder disease or polyarticular arthritis might require modification of the exercise program that includes the assistance of a family member or arrangement of home or outpatient therapy. The exercise can be modified with the patient seated next to a table and the operated extremity placed on the table. He or she slides the extremity into elevation by leaning forward until a slight stretch is achieved (Figure 5). Patients in this category and patients with large or heavy upper extremities also might perform a chair stretch exercise to help with forward elevation range of motion (ROM).

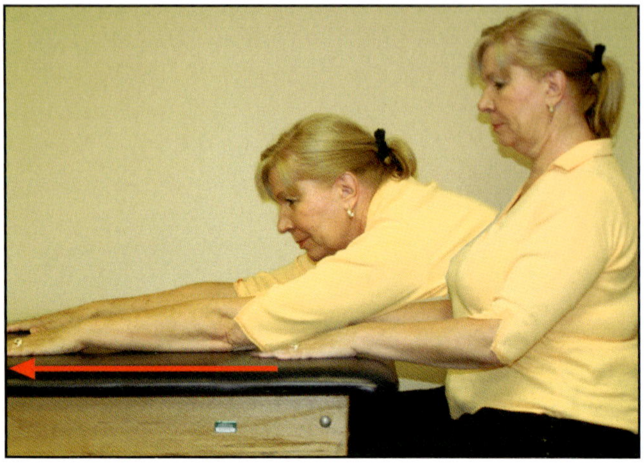
Figure 5. Table elevation stretch.

Phase 2: Postoperative Weeks 6 to 12

Soft tissue healing at 6 weeks after surgery allows for a progression to full PROM and the addition of active-assistive ROM and AROM exercises. Patients also can perform a pulley exercise to help improve passive and active forward elevation (Figure 6). They are encouraged to "unweight" the operated extremity to tolerance by using the nonoperated extremity. Deltoid strengthening is emphasized with a supine elevation progression. Gravity virtually is eliminated, and the patient can practice raising the extremity past 90° while strengthening the deltoid. The patient begins with the elbow bent to 90° to decrease the lever arm and weight of the extremity. When he or she can

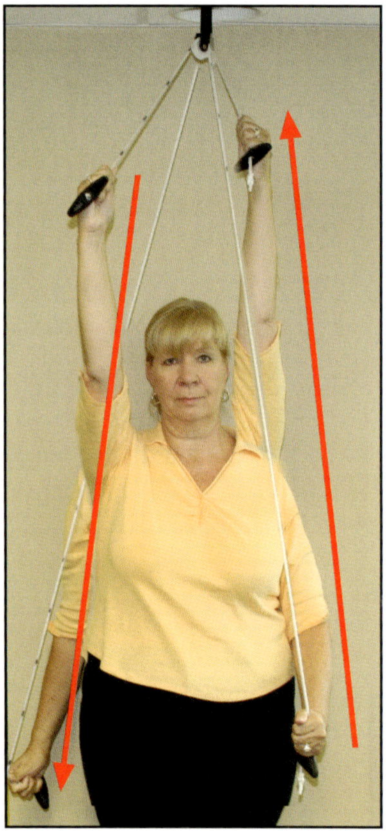
Figure 6. Rope-and-pulley exercise.

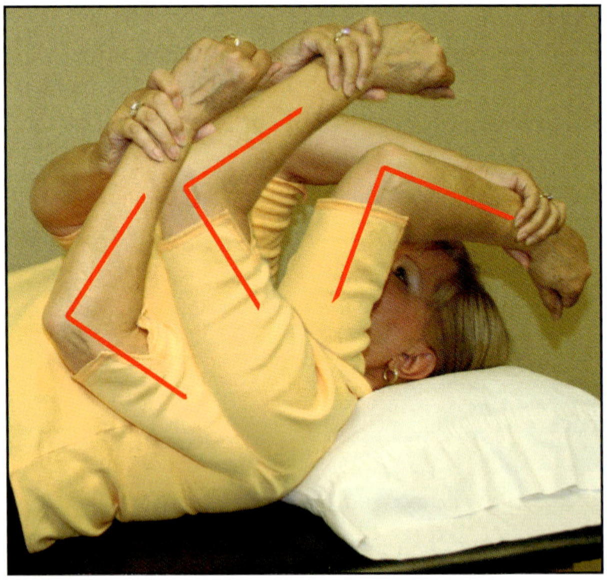
Figure 4. Supine passive forward elevation with the opposite hand.

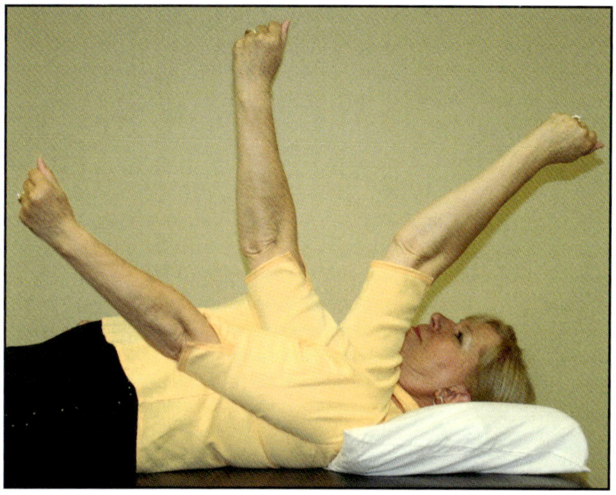

Figure 7. Supine active elevation with the elbow fully extended.

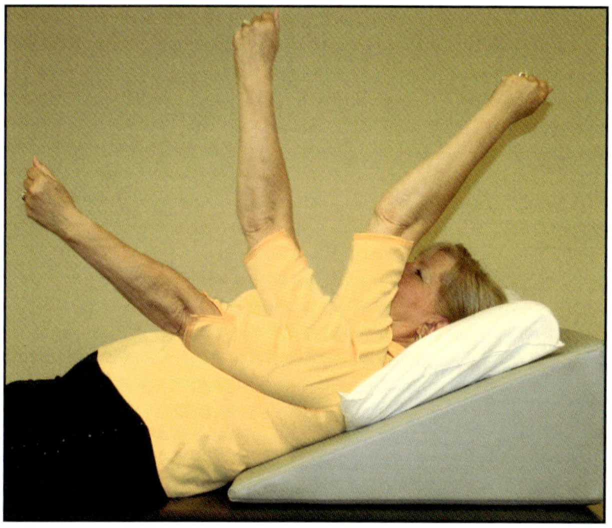

Figure 8. Supine active elevation with the torso elevated to 30°.

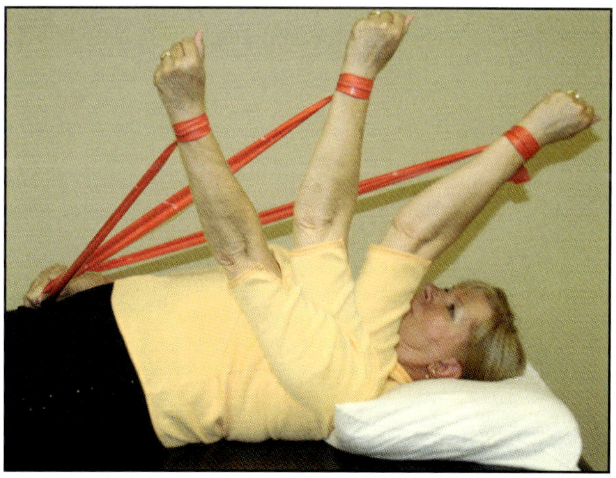

Figure 9. Supine elevation with elastic resistance.

comfortably perform 30 repetitions in this position, the patient gradually extends the elbow to increase the weight of the extremity until he or she can perform 30 repetitions with the elbow fully extended (Figure 7). Next, the patient's head is elevated slightly with pillows, a wedge, or an elevated table to gradually add the weight of gravity to the exercise (Figure 8). This sequence continues until the patient can raise the extremity while standing upright. In addition to deltoid strengthening, patients perform periscapular strengthening exercises, including scapular retraction with and without resistance. Manual resistance to elevation with the extremity supported is helpful to gain contraction of the deltoid in a safe position.

Phase 3: Postoperative Week 12+

Phase 3 begins when the patient has nearly full PROM and can actively elevate the extremity in supine with the elbow fully extended. The supine elevation progression is enhanced with the use of weighted balls, dumbbells, or elastic resistance (Figure 9). The UE Ranger (Rehab Innovations, Inc, Omaha, NE) is a useful device to help gain functional ROM of the shoulder (Figure 10). Manual resistance in unsupported positions can be progressed using alternating isometrics and proprioceptive neuromuscular facilita-

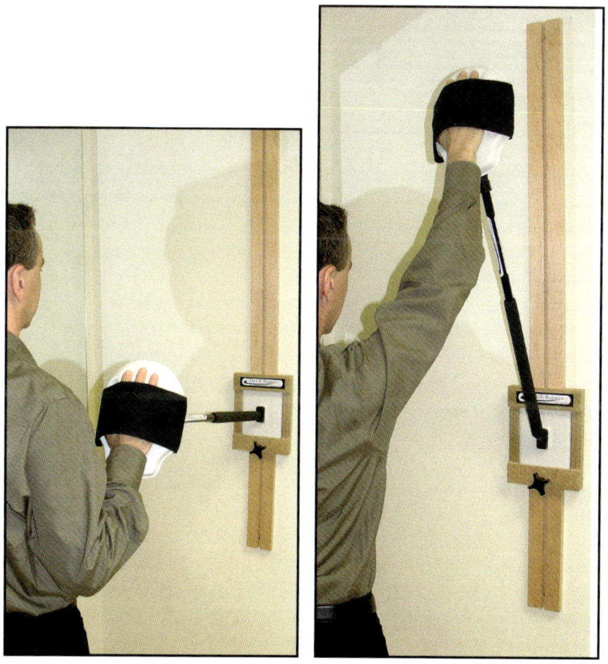

Figure 10. The UE Ranger (Rehab Innovations, Inc, Omaha, NE).

tion diagonals. In addition, manual resistance to the short-arc ranges of shoulder elevation in supine can be instituted.

Phase 4: Postoperative Week 16+

This phase begins when the patient is ready to be discharged to a home exercise program. He or she should demonstrate full and functional AROM and should be independent with the home exercise program. Expected AROM for a patient with good deltoid function is at least 120°. Patients can return to light household work and leisure activities. They should be reminded that this procedure is designed to allow only functional use of the shoulder and excessive use or strenuous activities should be avoided. In addition to the typical complications after reverse TSA, we have seen patients who have developed an overuse syndrome of their shoulders and have had to undergo secondary rehabilitation to return to pain-free functional use.

In conclusion, the reverse TSA should be considered a salvage procedure for patients with a rotator cuff deficiency and associated damage to the glenohumeral joint. Successful outcome of this procedure depends on good ROM and a good-functioning deltoid. The rehabilitation after reverse TSA is not standardized. However, the principles of postoperative rehabilitation are similar and include protection of the joint by avoidance of stressful positions, gradual return of PROM, and progression to AROM and strengthening. The goal of this procedure is to allow pain-free functional use of the shoulder in the plane of elevation with little to no rotation.

REFERENCES

1. Adams R. *Illustrations of the Effects of Rheumatic Gout or Chronic Rheumatic Arthritis on All the Articulations: With Descriptive and Explanatory Statements*. London, UK: John Churchill and Sons; 1857.
2. Codman EA. *The Shoulder: Rupture of the Supraspinatus Tendon and Other Lesions in or About the Subacromial Bursa*. Boston, MA: T. Todd; 1934:478–480.
3. Neer CS II, Craig EV, Fukuda H. Cuff-tear arthropathy. *J Bone Joint Surg Am*.1983;65(9):1232–1244.
4. Visotsky JL, Basamania C, Seebauer L, Rockwood CA, Jensen KL. Cuff tear arthropathy: pathogenesis, classification, and algorithm for treatment. *J Bone Joint Surg Am*. 2004;86(suppl 2):35–40.
5. McCarty DJ, Halverson PB, Carrera GF, Brewer BJ, Kozin F. "Milwaukee shoulder": association of microspheroids containing hydroxyapatite crystals, active collagenase, and neutral protease with rotator cuff defects. I. Clinical aspects. *Arthritis Rheum*. 1981;24(3):464–473.
6. Halverson PB, Cheung HS, McCarty DJ, Garancis J, Mandel N. "Milwaukee shoulder": association of microspheroids containing hydroxyapatite crystals, active collagenase, and neutral protease with rotator cuff defects. II. Synovial fluid studies. *Arthritis Rheum*. 1981;24(3):474–483.
7. Garancis JC, Cheung HS, Halverson PB, McCarty DJ. "Milwaukee shoulder": association of microspheroids containing hydroxyapatite crystals, active collagenase, and neutral protease with rotator cuff defects. III. Morphologic and biochemical studies of an excised synovium showing chondromatosis. *Arthritis Rheum*. 1981;24(3):484–491.
8. Jensen KL, Williams GR Jr, Russell IJ, Rockwood CA Jr. Rotator cuff tear arthropathy. *J Bone Joint Surg Am*. 1999;81(9):1312–1324.
9. Iannotti JP, McCarron J, Raymond CJ, et al. Agreement study of radiographic classification of rotator cuff tear arthropathy. *J Shoulder Elbow Surg*. 2010;19(8):1243–1249.
10. Hamada K, Fukuda H, Mikasa M, Kobayashi Y. Roentgenographic findings in massive rotator cuff tears: a long-term observation. *Clin Orthop Relat Res*. 1990;254:92–96.
11. Sirveaux F, Favard L, Oudet D, Huquet D, Walch G, Molé D. Grammont inverted total shoulder arthroplasty in the treatment of glenohumeral osteoarthritis with massive rupture of the cuff: results of a multicentre study of 80 shoulders. *J Bone Joint Surg Br*. 2004;86(3):388–395.
12. Boileau P, Watkinson D, Hatzidakis AM, Hovorka I. Neer Award 2005: The Grammont reverse shoulder prosthesis. Results in cuff tear arthritis, fracture sequelae, and revision arthroplasty. *J Shoulder Elbow Surg*. 2006;15(5):527–540.
13. Edwards TB, Boulahia A, Kempf JF, Boileau P, Nemoz C, Walch G. The influence of rotator cuff disease on the results of shoulder arthroplasty for primary osteoarthritis: results of a multicenter study. *J Bone Joint Surg Am*. 2002;84(12):2240–2248.
14. Barrett WP, Franklin JL, Jackins SE, Wyss CR, Matsen FA III. Total shoulder arthroplasty. *J Bone Joint Surg Am*. 1987;69(6):865–872.
15. Boileau P, Trojani C, Walch G, Krishnan SG, Romeo A, Sinnerton R. Shoulder arthroplasty for the treatment of the sequelae of fractures of the proximal humerus. *J Shoulder Elbow Surg*. 2001;10(4):299–308.
16. Williams GR Jr, Rockwood CA Jr. Hemiarthroplasty in rotator cuff-deficient shoulders. *J Shoulder Elbow Surg*. 1996;5(5):362–367.
17. Franklin JL, Barrett WP, Jackins SE, Matsen FA III. Glenoid loosening in total shoulder arthroplasty: association with rotator cuff deficiency. *J Arthroplasty*. 1988;3(1):39–46.
18. Torchia ME, Cofield RH, Settergren CR. Total shoulder arthroplasty with the Neer prosthesis: long-term results. *J Shoulder Elbow Surg*. 1997;6(6):495–505.
19. Sneppen O, Fruensgaard S, Johannsen HV, Olsen BS, Sojbjerg JO, Andersen NH. Total shoulder replacement in rheumatoid arthritis: proximal migration and loosening. *J Shoulder Elbow Surg*. 1996;5(1):47–52.

Reverse Shoulder Arthroplasty

20. Sanchez-Sotelo J, Cofield RH, Rowland CM. Shoulder hemiarthroplasty for glenohumeral arthritis associated with severe rotator cuff deficiency. *J Bone Joint Surg Am.* 2001;83(12):1814–1822.
21. Field LD, Dines DM, Zabinski SJ, Warren RF. Hemiarthroplasty of the shoulder for rotator cuff arthropathy. *J Shoulder Elbow Surg.* 1997;6(1):18–23.
22. Arntz CT, Jackins SE, Matsen FA III. Prosthetic replacement of the shoulder for the treatment of defects in the rotator cuff and the surface of the glenohumeral joint [erratum in *J Bone Joint Surg Am.* 1993;75(7):1112]. *J Bone Joint Surg Am.* 1993;75(4):485–491.
23. Boyd AD Jr, Thomas WH, Scott RD, Sledge CB, Thornhill TS. Total shoulder arthroplasty versus hemiarthroplasty: indications for glenoid resurfacing. *J Arthroplasty.* 1990;5(4):329–336.
24. Zuckerman JD, Scott AJ, Gallagher MA. Hemiarthroplasty for cuff tear arthropathy. *J Shoulder Elbow Surg.* 2000;(3):169–172.
25. Grammont PM, Baulot E. Delta shoulder prosthesis for rotator cuff rupture. *Orthopedics.* 1993;16(1):65–68.
26. Flatow EL, Harrison AK. A history of reverse total shoulder arthroplasty. *Clin Orthop Relat Res.* 2011;469:2432–2439.
27. Linscheid RL, Cofield RH. Total shoulder arthroplasty: experimental but promising. *Geriatrics.* 1976;31(4):64–69.
28. Coughlin MJ, Morris JM, West WF. The semiconstrained total shoulder arthroplasty. *J Bone Joint Surg Am.* 1979;61(4):574–581.
29. Kessel L, Bayley I. Prosthetic replacement of shoulder joint: preliminary communication. *J R Soc Med.* 1979;72(10):748–752.
30. Lettin AW, Copeland SA, Scales JT. The Stanmore total shoulder replacement. *J Bone Joint Surg Br.* 1982;64(1):49–51.
31. Lettin AW, Scales JT. Total replacement of the shoulder joint (two cases). *Proc R Soc Med.* 1972;65(4):373–374.
32. Post M, Jablon M, Miller H, Singh M. Constrained total shoulder joint replacement: a critical review. *Clin Orthop Relat Res.* 1979;144:135–150.
33. Cofield RH. Status of total shoulder arthroplasty. *Arch Surg.* 1977;112(9):1088–1091.
34. Post M. Constrained arthroplasty of the shoulder. *Orthop Clin North Am.* 1987;18(3):455–462.
35. Post M, Haskell SS, Jablon M. Total shoulder replacement with a constrained prosthesis. *J Bone Joint Surg Am.* 1980;62(3):327–335.
36. Ahir SP, Walker PS, Squire-Taylor CJ, Blunn GW, Bayley JI. Analysis of glenoid fixation for a reversed anatomy fixed-fulcrum shoulder replacement. *J Biomech.* 2004;37(11):1699–1708.
37. Bodey WN, Yeoman PM. Prosthetic arthroplasty of the shoulder. *Acta Orthop Scand.* 1983;54(6):900–903.
38. Broström LA, Wallensten R, Olsson E, Anderson D. The Kessel prosthesis in total shoulder arthroplasty: a five-year experience. *Clin Orthop Relat Res.* 1992;277:155–160.
39. Buechel FF, Pappas MJ, DePalma AF. "Floating-socket" total shoulder replacement: anatomical, biomechanical, and surgical rationale. *J Biomed Mater Res.* 1978;12(1):89–114.
40. Fenlin JM Jr. Total glenohumeral joint replacement. *Orthop Clin North Am.* 1975;6(2):565–583.
41. Grammont PM, Trouilloud P, Laffay J, Deries X. Concept study and realization of a new total shoulder prosthesis. *Rhumatologie.* 1987;39:407–418.
42. Gristina AG, Webb LX. The Trispherical total shoulder replacement. In: Bayley JI, Kessel L, eds. *Shoulder Surgery.* New York, NY: Springer-Verlag; 1982:153–157.
43. Reeves B, Jobbins B, Dowson D, Wright V. A total shoulder endoprosthesis. *Eng Med.* 1974;1:64–67.
44. Reeves B, Jobbins B, Flowers F, Dowson D, Wright V. Some problems in the development of a total shoulder endoprosthesis. *Ann Rheum Dis.* 1972;31(5):425–426.
45. Boileau P, Watkinson DJ, Hatzidakis AM, Balg F. Grammont reverse prosthesis: design, rationale, and biomechanics. *J Shoulder Elbow Surg.* 2005;14(1 suppl S):147S–161S.
46. Baulot E, Sirveaux F, Boileau P. Grammont's idea: the story of Paul Grammont's functional surgery concept and the development of the reverse principle. *Clin Orthop Relat Res.* 2011;469:2425–2431.
47. Seebauer L. Total reverse shoulder arthroplasty: European lessons and future trends. *Am J Orthop (Belle Mead NJ).* 2007;36(12 suppl 1):22–28.
48. Frankle M, Levy JC, Pupello D, et al. The reverse shoulder prosthesis for glenohumeral arthritis associated with severe rotator cuff deficiency: a minimum two-year follow-up study of sixty patients. Surgical technique. *J Bone Joint Surg Am.* 2006;88(suppl 1 pt 2):178–190.
49. Rittmeister M, Kerschbaumer F. Grammont reverse total shoulder arthroplasty in patients with rheumatoid arthritis and nonreconstructible rotator cuff lesions. *J Shoulder Elbow Surg.* 2001;10(1):17–22.

REVERSE SHOULDER ARTHROPLASTY REHABILITATION GUIDELINE

Good Shepherd Penn Partners, Penn Therapy and Fitness, and Penn Presbyterian Medical Center

All information contained in this protocol is to be used as a general guideline only. Specific variations might be appropriate for each patient and might be specified by the physician. In all cases, it is acceptable to advance the program more slowly than stated. If the patient experiences excessive pain, discontinue exercise until the physician is contacted. ***Achieving and maintaining a low level of pain and inflammation and protecting the surgical repair are the guiding principles in all stages of rehabilitation, even if less passive and active range of motion are accomplished.***

SYMBOLS AND ABBREVIATIONS

AAROM, active-assistive range of motion
ADLs, activities of daily living
AFE, active forward elevation
AROM, active range of motion
FE, forward elevation
NA, not applicable
PER, passive external rotation
PFE, passive forward elevation
PIR, passive internal rotation
PNF, proprioceptive neuromuscular facilitation
POD, postoperative day
POM, postoperative month
POS, plane of the scapula
POW, postoperative week
PROM, passive range of motion
ROM, range of motion

STAGED GOALS FOR RANGE OF MOTION

Time	PFE	PER at 20° of Abduction	PER at 90° Abduction	PIR Behind the Back	AFE
POD 1	60°	0°	NA	NA	NA
POW 1	70°–120°	0°	NA	NA	NA
POW 3	90°–120°	0°–20°	NA	NA	NA
POW 6	120°–135°	10°–30°	NA	NA	80°–120°
POW 12	120°–150°	20°–45°	30°–45°	Hip	90°–135°
POM 6	120°–150°	20°–45°	45°–75°	Buttock	110°–150°

PHASE 1: WEEKS 0 TO 6

Goals

°Patient education on goals of rehabilitation and precautions
°Protect the surgical incision
°Achieve staged ROM goals

POD 1 to POW 6

°Elbow, wrist, and hand AROM with no weight
°Pendulum exercises
  °Lean over a table or chair
  °Let the arm hand down relaxed
  °Keep the body still
  °Move the arm in small arcs forward and back, side to side, clockwise, and counterclockwise
  °Perform 25 repetitions in each direction 4 to 6 times per day

- °PFE in the POS to a tolerable stretch or discomfort
    - °Preferred exercises
        - °Supine PFE with the opposite hand, family member, or therapist and with the elbow flexed to 90° throughout (Figure 4)
        - °Table or chair step-back exercise
        - °Table slide (Figure 5)
    - °Hold each exercise for 10 to 20 seconds and perform 10 repetitions 4 to 6 times per day
- °PER in slight abduction to staged ROM goals
    - °Preferred exercises
        - °Supine with the elbow on a pillow in the POS and flexed to 90°
        - °Apply a slight force with a cane, stick, or dowel
    - °Hold each exercise for 10 to 20 seconds and perform 10 repetitions 4 to 6 times per day
- °Ice for pain reduction
- °Position the arm in a sling in the POS
- °Patient education
    - °Primary focus of phase 1: encourage healing and protection of the incision
    - °Use of a sling and support of the arm in the POS
    - °Minimal use of the arm for light, waist-level ADLs
    - °Be cautious of excessive use of the arm for ADLs or work
    - °Sleep in a recliner with the arm supported in the POS

Adjunctive Exercises

- °Therapist-assisted supine PROM within comfortable ROM to
    - °Decrease muscle guarding
    - °Gain the patient's confidence
    - °Achieve staged ROM goals
- °Cervical spine ROM
- °Moist heat before exercises (after POW 1)
- °Pain-control agents and modalities as needed

Interventions to Avoid

- °Aggressive PROM, especially in patients who are muscle guarding
- °Exercises that result in moderate to severe pain
- °Reaching behind the back, cross-body adduction, extension, rope and pulley
- °Weighted exercises
- °Upper body ergometer

PHASE 2: WEEKS 6 TO 12

Goals

- °Achieve staged ROM goals
- °Minimize shoulder pain
- °Work toward AFE above shoulder level

POW 6 to 12

- °Achieve staged ROM goals in PFE
  - °Preferred exercises
    - °Supine AAROM FE with a cane or stick
    - °Table or chair step-back exercise
    - °Table slide
    - °Rope-and-pulley exercise (Figure 6)
- °Achieve staged ROM goals in PER
  - °Continue supine PER with a cane or stick
- °Achieve staged ROM goals for AFE
  - °Preferred exercises
    - °Supine elevation progression (Figure 7), gradually introducing gravity by elevating the head (Figure 8)
    - °UE Ranger (Rehab Innovations, Inc, Omaha, NE) (Figure 10)
    - °Ball roll on a table

Adjunctive Exercises

- °Therapist-assisted PROM and light stretching
- °Manual resistance to elevation by the therapist with alternating isometrics
- °Scapular retraction and elevation with and without elastic resistance
- °Gentle stretching into shoulder extension
- °Moist heat or ice, or both
- °Modalities as needed

Interventions to Avoid

- °Exercises that significantly increase pain or reactivity
- °Excessive use of the arm for ADLs or work

PHASE 3: WEEKS 12+

Goals

- °Achieve staged ROM goals
- °Minimize shoulder pain
- °Increase deltoid strength
- °Increase functional activities

POW 12+

- °Continue PROM, AAROM, and AROM exercises
- °Increase intensity of elevation progression exercises
  - °Supine elevation with dumbbell or weighted ball
  - °Supine elevation with elastic resistance (Figure 9)
  - °Ball roll up a wall

HPRC at St. Francis Rehabilitation Center

- °Manual resistance in unsupported positions
  - °Alternating isometrics
  - °PNF diagonals
  - °Short-arc ranges
- °Total body flexibility and strengthening
  - °Trunk and lower extremity flexibility exercises
  - °Total arm strengthening
  - °Trunk and lower extremity strengthening
- °Gradual return to light leisure activities
- °Remind the patient that this procedure is designed to return some functional use of the shoulder and excessive use or strenuous activities should be avoided

III-9

Manipulation Under Anesthesia, Lysis of Adhesions, and Capsular Release

Joseph H. Kostuch, PT, SCS

CHAPTER CONTENTS

- What patients are appropriate for the use of this guideline?
- The most important factor that should guide clinical decision making
- Key principles in rehabilitation of this problem
- Specific rehabilitation guideline
- Special considerations
  - Concomitant diabetes
  - Postoperative captured shoulder
  - Partial-thickness rotator cuff tear
  - Concomitant synovitis

WHAT PATIENTS ARE APPROPRIATE FOR THE USE OF THIS GUIDELINE?

- Patients with arthroscopic lysis of adhesions due to
  - Adhesive capsulitis
  - Postoperative captured shoulder
- Patients with manipulation under anesthesia for adhesive capsulitis
- Patients without concomitant synovial debridement or soft tissue repair

Clinical pearls are highlighted in yellow throughout the text.

THE MOST IMPORTANT FACTOR THAT SHOULD GUIDE CLINICAL DECISION MAKING

The factor that most substantially affects the patient's full recovery after manipulation under anesthesia (MUA) or lysis of adhesions (LOA) is the performance of passive range-of-motion (PROM) stretching by the rehabilitation provider with every attempt to achieve full PROM measures into each plane of motion each day. The physician restores range of motion (ROM) into all glenohumeral directions with the procedure. Failure to achieve these maximum measures each day thereafter reinforces the body's tendency to return to its previous level of capsular restriction.

KEY PRINCIPLES IN REHABILITATION OF THIS PROBLEM

When possible, the rehabilitation provider initially should perform PROM while the nerve block still is intact. This provides the patient with visual encouragement of initial gains and moves the upper extremity beyond the previous point of capsular restriction. The patient must perform regular home stretching to a terminal range. Encouragement from the rehabilitation provider and appropriate patient counseling is especially important for success.

Failure to conservatively manage shoulder stiffness, whether from adhesive capsulitis or from postoperative stiffness, can result in a recommendation for surgery from the physician. The decision to recommend a closed manipulation or an arthroscopic procedure will be specific to the clinical presentation and the cause of stiffness. Closed manipulation most commonly is performed for patients who have adhesive capsulitis (Figure 1) and have not improved with at least 6 months of conservative treatment. Reported results are excellent, with follow-ups documented up to 15 years.[1–4] Arthroscopic release procedures have become

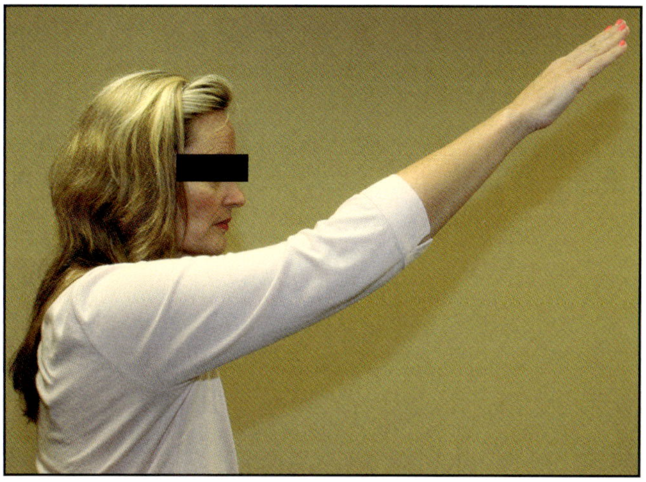

Figure 1. Patient with adhesive capsulitis.

increasingly commonplace for treating both adhesive capsulitis and refractory postoperative stiffness. Although timeframes for recommending this procedure for postoperative stiffness vary based on multiple factors and facilities, the range can be as short as 3 to 4 months, but the average is closer to 8 months, from primary surgery.[5] Documented results for arthroscopically releasing adhesive capsulitis have revealed good results at up to 5 years after surgery, with significant improvement noted in functional outcome scores and PROM measures.[6–8] Similarly good results have been shown after release of postoperative stiffness, with good results up to 3 years after the procedure.[5,7]

SPECIFIC REHABILITATION GUIDELINE

The Appendix specifies our complete Manipulation Under Anesthesia, Lysis of Adhesions, and Capsular Release Rehabilitation Guideline. In this section, I explain the rationale for selected components of the guideline. It is divided into 3 phases based on general timeframes of healing and normalized PROM. To advance from one rehabilitation phase to the next, the patient must gain approval from his or her physician, successfully complete the core components of the previous rehabilitation activities, and meet the time criteria.

Phase 1

The sole focus of our phase 1 program is to maintain the PROM that the surgeon gained during the procedure. The stretching exercises performed during these first few weeks remain entirely passive, that is, without muscle contraction about the shoulder. The home exercises and the stretching by the rehabilitation provider are soley intended to normalize PROM. No attempt is made in phase 1 to perform any active ROM (AROM), muscle strengthening, or functional training. As mentioned, a short window of time exists to regain PROM, whereas the muscle strengthening and functional recovery can be achieved later without detrimental effect. Attempts to strengthen during the first phase also may keep the inflammatory response high in the shoulder, slowing the pain relief that patients are seeking.

During the first several weeks after the MUA or LOA, the rehabilitation provider performs manual stretching in all planes of motion about the shoulder. These planes encompass both phase 1 and phase 2 PROM described in chapter II-3. With the surgeon having released the tissue and achieved normal ROM under anesthesia during the procedure, the rehabilitation provider strives to achieve these same measures each session with the patient (Figures 2 and 3). Often during this stretching, the shoulder is sore and painful not only due to the surgical procedure, but also due to the musculotendon contraction that has occurred about the joint from the pathologic condition. The rehabilitation provider must work through this soreness with the patient because these maximum measures must be achieved at each session to allow for the

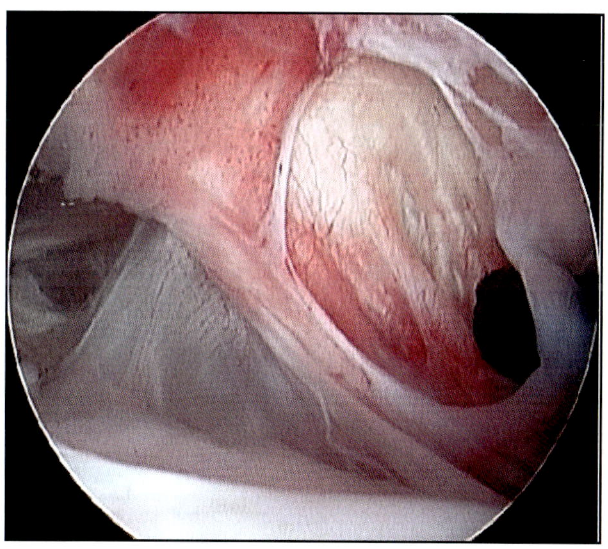

Figure 2. Arthroscopic image depicts postoperative subacromial adhesions.

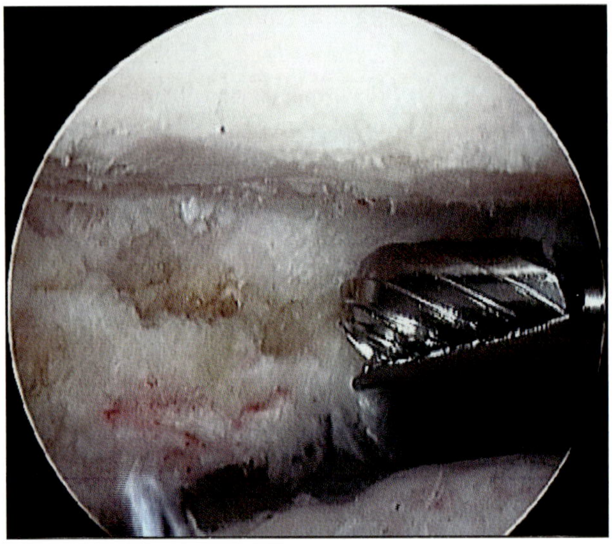

Figure 3. Arthroscopic image depicts the same patient as Figure 2 after subacromial lysis of adhesions and subacromial decompression.

tissue to remain stretched while it heals and matures in this lengthened position. Therefore, the patient also must work very hard at home to consistently (up to 4 times a day) perform the home stretching program to maintain his or her ROM. Understanding that pain and soreness are involved with this process, the surgeon prescribes pain medication, which the patient should take at regular intervals. In addition, the rehabilitation provider educates the patient about reduced functional use, icing, and positioning to help reduce the soreness (Figure 4).

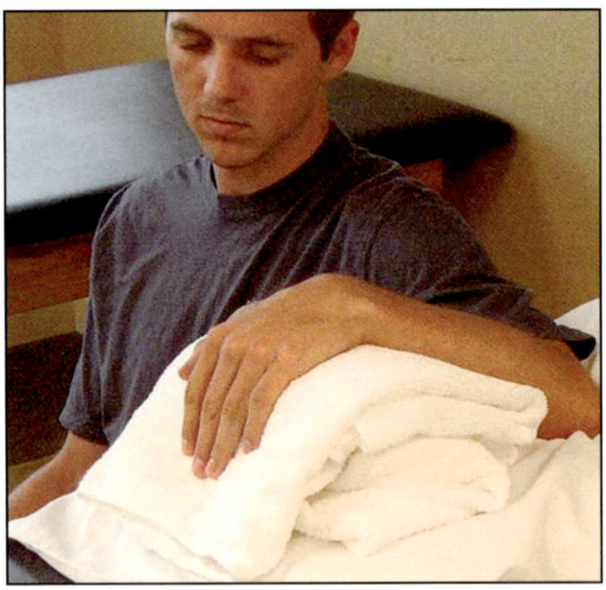

Figure 4. Positioning for icing in a comfortable amount of abduction and external rotation to aid in maintaining passive range of motion.

When the procedure is performed, the patient is reintroduced quickly to physical therapy. Generally, within just a few hours, the patient is discharged from the outpatient facility and taken directly to the therapy clinic before going home. Because the nerve block that the surgeon placed remains intact between 8 and 12 hours after the procedure, the patient presents to the rehabilitation provider without any sensation or motor control of his or her upper extremity. During this initial visit, the rehabilitation provider moves the shoulder into passive external rotation (PER) at the side, PER with the upper extremity in abduction, passive forward elevation (PFE), and functional internal rotation with the patient sitting or standing (Figures 5–8).

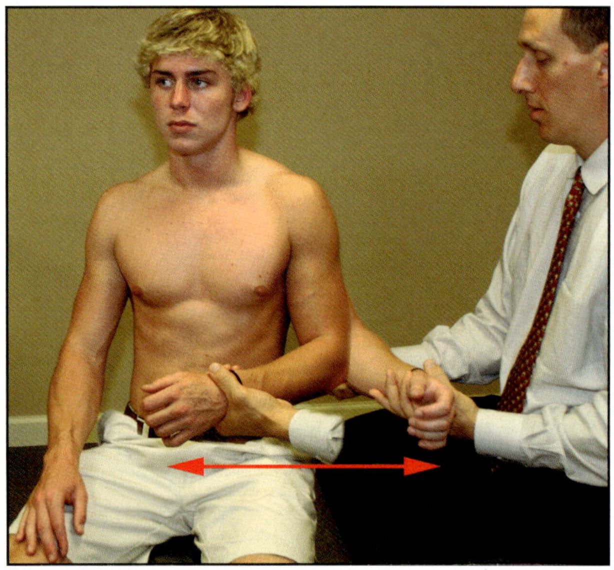

Figure 5. Passive external rotation at the side.

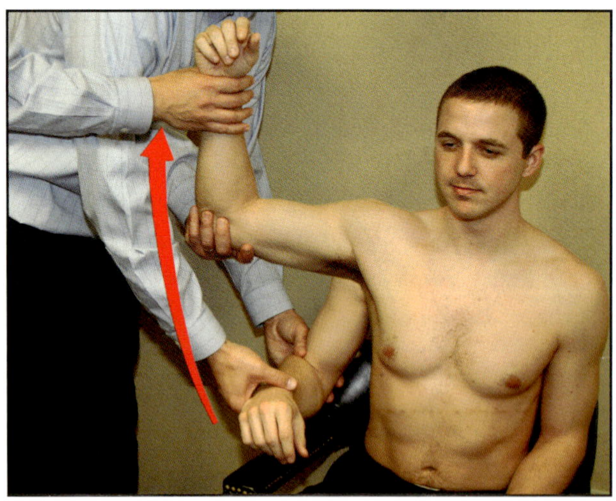

Figure 6. Passive external rotation in abduction.

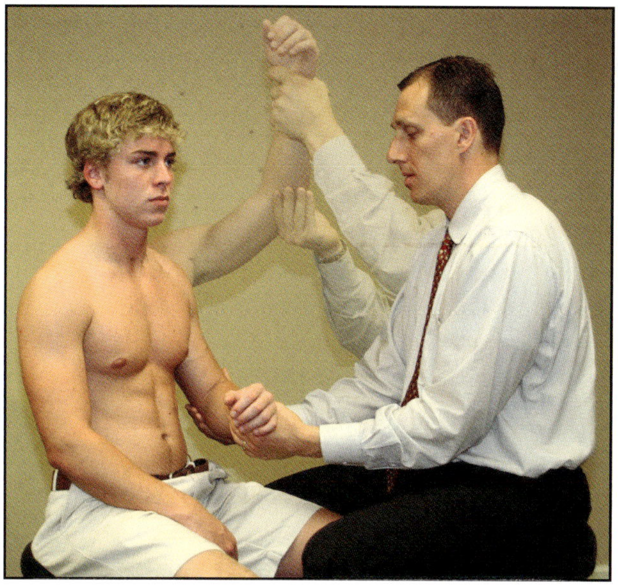

Figure 7. Passive forward elevation.

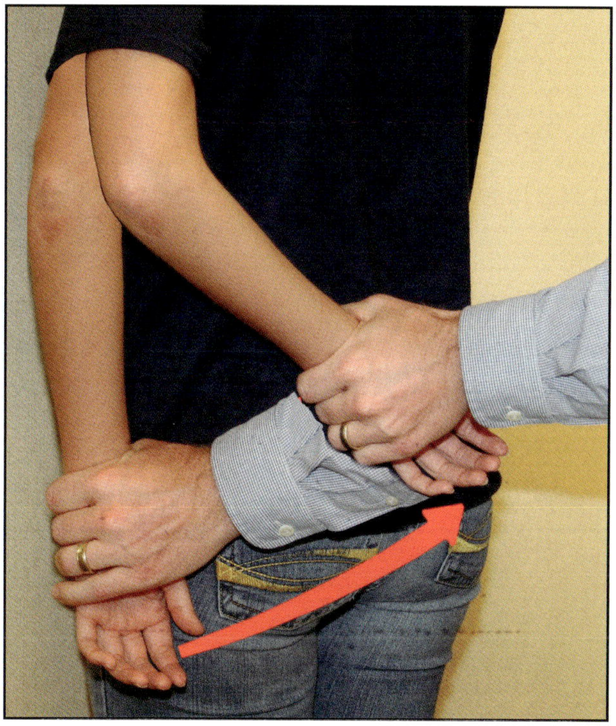

Figure 8. Active-assistive internal rotation.

This initial PROM, which is achieved by the rehabilitation provider when the scalene nerve block is intact, is important for several reasons. Conscious or unconscious muscle guarding seems to be one factor that can limit shoulder PROM either before or after MUA or LOA. We anecdotally have noticed that when the upper extremity is moved through a complete ROM while the nerve block is intact, this muscle guarding is much less or eliminated even after the patient regains active control of the extremity. We have noticed that after the patient regains active control of the extremity, muscle guarding is much greater if the extremity has not moved through a complete ROM while the scalene nerve block is intact. For maximum success, I have found that the rehabilitation provider must move the extremity past the preoperative point of restriction for several repetitions to reduce or eliminate this muscle guarding. In addition at my clinic, we believe that when the patient sees that his or her upper extremity can move through a full ROM while flaccid, his or her confidence increases and anxiety about ROM after the nerve block has worn off decreases.[7]

This urgency of reintroducing therapy is necessary because of the bleeding that occurs inside the shoulder with either the breaking up or surgical release of the adhesions (Figures 3 and 9).[7] If the shoulder were manipulated and then simply left by the side, it would begin to readhere down after only a short period. During the initial therapy visit on the day of the procedure, the rehabilitation provider moves the extremity through the range as described, then the patient and

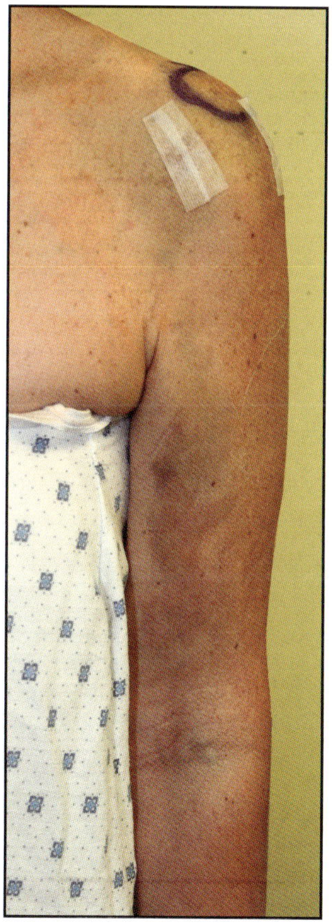

Figure 9. Bruising and swelling after lysis of adhesions.

family member are instructed how to perform sitting PFE, sitting PER at the side, and PER in abduction at home until the nerve block resolves. After the block has resolved, patients add scapular AROM and Codman exercises to their home programs. These patients are seen 5 days per week for the first 2 weeks after an MUA or LOA. The frequency of outpatient visits then is reduced to 3 visits per week between postoperative weeks 3 and 6. This occurs when the patient can achieve normal PROM measures with his or her self-stretches that are equal to the measures achieved by the rehabilitation provider.

At St. Francis Rehabilitation Center, these patients also receive a Kinex K2 (Kinex Medical Company, LLC, Waukesha, WI) shoulder continuous passive motion (CPM) machine for home PFE stretching (Figure 10). This unit is custom fit to the patient preoperatively to ensure a smooth arc of motion and full PFE. Because the nerve block is intact, PFE is not performed with the CPM machine at the first therapy visit but is instructed and begun at the second therapy visit when sensory and motor control have returned. The CPM machine is instructed for home use up to 4 times per day for 20-minute sessions. Successful use of the CPM machine for PFE above the patient's previous point of restriction is an excellent indicator of desired recovery.

Because the shoulder has so many planes of motion, the home stretching program encompasses all 3 planes of motion (coronal, sagittal, transverse). Within the first week after the procedure, the patient performs at least 1 stretch into each plane. These home stretches are described specifically in Figures 1 and 12 of chapter II-3. Each stretch is held for 10 to 15 seconds, and sets of 5 to 8 repetitions are performed 4 to 5 times per day. Because up to 8 stretches are used, this program takes a time commitment from the patient to perform appropriately. Most patients are encouraged by their immediate motion, so they willingly commit the time necessary to perform them.

The patient should begin to comfortably achieve full PROM with self stretches between postoperative weeks 3 and 6. As the pain decreases and ease of PROM increases, the patient enters phase 2 of recovery.

Phase 2

During phase 2, the rehabilitation provider sees the patient less often because he or she now is achieving nearly normal PROM independently, so intense stretching by the rehabilitation provider is not needed as frequently. The intensity and duration of the patient's home program also decreases. He or she is instructed to perform light warm-up stretches and then advanced stretches (as described in Figures 12 and 13 of chapter II-3) only in the planes of motion that might have some lingering stiffness. These motions might include functional internal rotation, horizontal adduction, or external rotation and abduction. This shorter stretching program still is prescribed multiple times per day, but stretches are performed with a comfortable intensity and fewer repetitions.

The patient now can begin a strengthening program. The program, which is detailed in chapter II-4, is initiated at waist level and progresses to shoulder level as the patient can tolerate. The rotator cuff and scapular stabilizers are isolated and strengthened to allow increased functional use of the upper extremity. The patient must achieve comfortable forward reaching

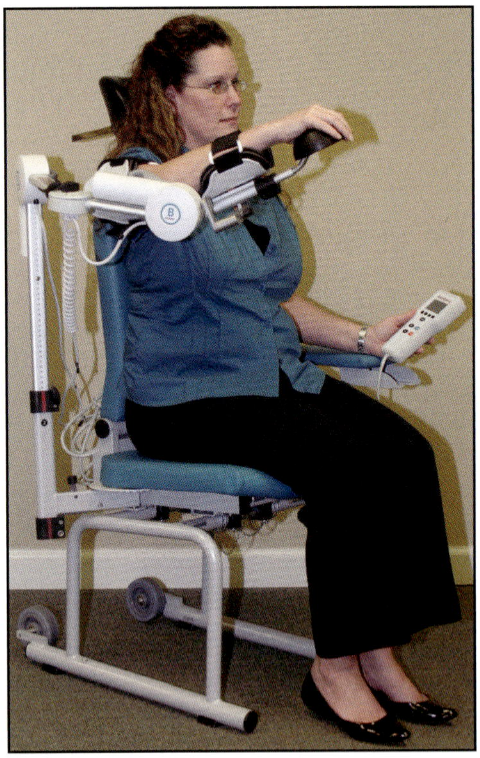

Figure 10. Passive forward elevation with the continuous passive motion machine.

before initiating a Thera-Band (The Hygenic Corporation, Akron, OH) program for strength. If the patient remains too weak or has too much pain with the forward reach, we initiate our movement strengthening program with gravity eliminated and then against gravity before advancing to external Thera-Band resistance. Unlike the stretching program that is performed multiple times per day, the strengthening program is performed only up to 2 times per day. This base Thera-Band program is advanced with repetitions then with resistance over several weeks. After the patient's endurance of these important muscles has improved, functional use of the extremity has returned to chest level, and the level of pain remains low, we advance to our elevation progression.

Depending on the severity and duration of the preoperative condition, the patient might not have actively raised the extremity above shoulder level for several months. Now that joint flexibility has been restored, the muscles must be retrained and strengthened to actively lift the extremity. We use our assistive-to-active elevation progression, which is a series of strengthening exercises shown to systematically and progressively recruit the appropriate muscles for lifting the upper extremity overhead (Figure 11) (chapter II-4).[9] Each patient tolerates and progresses through this stage to full active forward elevation at various speeds. The rehabilitation provider must keep in mind that the shoulder girdle muscles have not been engaged at these length-tension positions for a long time, so the patient's tolerance to this progression might be slow and require frequent adjustment in both exercise selection and intensity. When the body can elevate the extremity overhead without substitution, the muscles are strengthened to allow normal return to overhead use of the extremity.

Phase 3

Progression of overhead strength and full return to normal functional use of the upper extremity is achieved in phase 3. Scaption is progressed in repetition, and weight is progressed in proportion to the patient's overall size and strength and in consideration of his or her functional, occupational, or recreational demands. During this phase, progressing strength specific to a recreational fitness program, light tennis, or golf along with group exercise programs can be achieved. If appropriate, diagonal and abduction-external rotation strength can be initiated if required for recreational or occupational demands.

The patient's speed of progression through this recovery largely depends on his or her preopera-

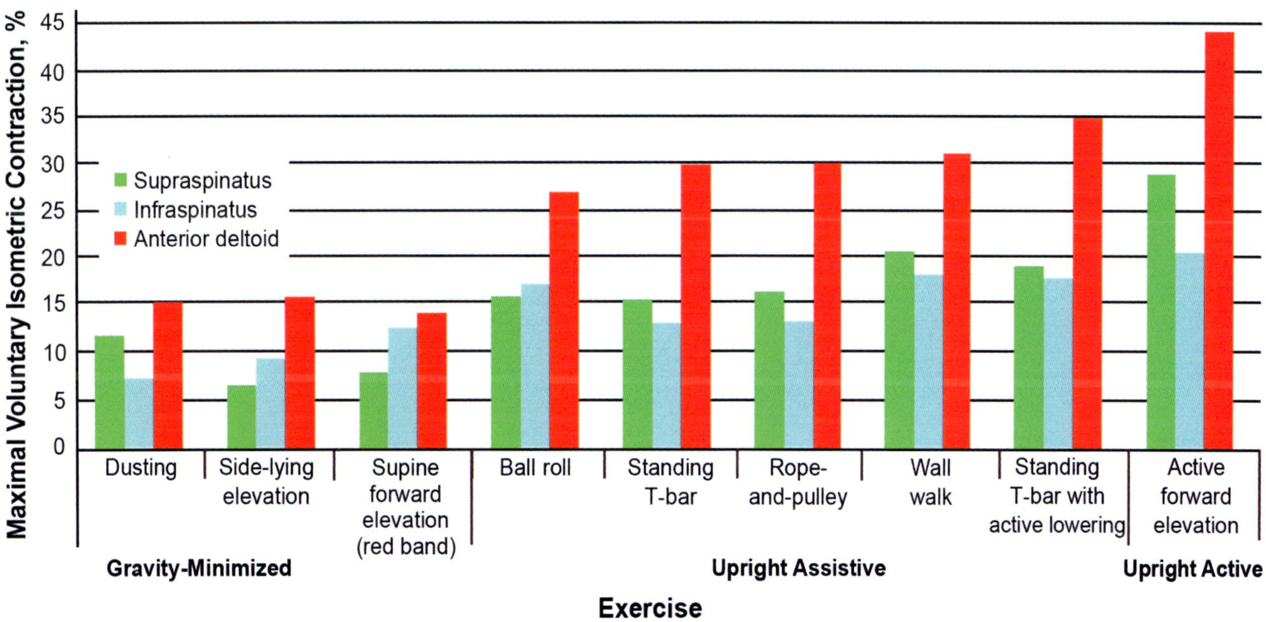

Figure 11. Maximum electromyographic activity of the supraspinatus, infraspinatus, and anterior deltoid during gravity-minimized exercises, upright assistive exercises, and active forward elevation evaluated by Gaunt et al.[9]

tive condition. The MUA or LOA provides a reliable means of regaining PROM, but the speed at which the patient regains his or her strength and functional use of the extremity is more variable. A 3-month onset of symptoms is much different from a 6-month preoperative duration of symptoms; the body requires longer to regain its strength and function when the symptoms have been present longer. Generally, patients should expect to return to normal household and light work demands within 2 to 3 months. Recreational sports or physically demanding jobs require a longer recovery of 3 to 5 months.

SPECIAL CONSIDERATIONS

Concomitant Diabetes

Because of the relatively poor healing tendencies and the high probability of recurrent stiffness specific to people with diabetes, these patients must be managed aggressively with their PROM and pain control.[5] In addition, their introduction to strengthening might be delayed slightly, and more time might be spent with their terminal stretching well into phase 3.

Postoperative Captured Shoulder

Because postoperative stiffness is a potential complication after repair or reconstructive surgery, LOA might become appropriate if the patient develops substantial stiffness while the repair heals (Figure 12). At the St. Francis Orthopaedic Institute, we recommend that this procedure always is performed arthroscopically and is never manipulated without visualization and specific structures released. In addition, the surgeon must inspect and verify that the previous repair has healed adequately so that our normal LOA rehabilitation guideline can be followed safely.

Partial-Thickness Rotator Cuff Tear

When adhesive capsulitis does not resolve with a typical intervention of stretching by the rehabilitation provider, an MUA might be the physician's choice of management. Some patients also might have a partial-thickness rotator cuff tear underlying their more prominent stiffness. This condition likely will become evident during the second phase of recovery when these patients have difficulty managing their pain with strength and functional advances. Maintaining full PROM remains critical while managing their rotator cuff symptoms with appropriate exercise modification.

Concomitant Synovitis

Patients with concomitant synovitis require a much more guarded and symptom-directed recovery. The different rehabilitation program is detailed in chapter III-10.

In conclusion, MUA or LOA is a quicker and more reliable means of regaining PROM for patients who do not improve with nonoperative intervention from the rehabilitation provider. These procedures are very specific for the patients for whom they are intended to help. In addition, the patient's general health and any contraindications need to be addressed thoroughly.

REFERENCES

1. Dodenhoff RM, Levy O, Wilson A, Copeland SA. Manipulation under anesthesia for primary frozen shoulder: effect on early recovery and return to activity. *J Shoulder Elbow Surg*. 2000;9(1):23–26.
2. Farrell CM, Sperling JW, Cofield RH. Manipulation for frozen shoulder: long-term results. *J Shoulder Elbow Surg*. 2005;14(5):480–484.
3. Pollock RG, Duralde XA, Flatow EL, Bigliani LU. The use of arthroscopy in the treatment of resistant frozen shoulder. *Clin Orthop Relat Res*. 1994;304:30–36.

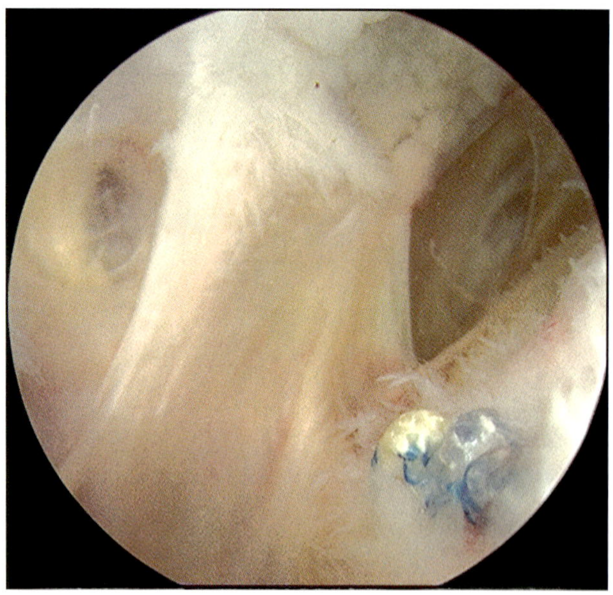

Figure 12. Postoperative captured shoulder after rotator cuff repair.

4. Warner JJ, Allen A, Marks PH, Wong P. Arthroscopic release for chronic, refractory adhesive capsulitis of the shoulder. *J Bone Joint Surg Am*. 1996;78(12):1808–1816.
5. Huberty DP, Schoolfield JD, Brady PC, Vadala AP, Arrigoni P, Burkhart SS. Incidence and treatment of postoperative stiffness following arthroscopic rotator cuff repair. *Arthroscopy*. 2009;25(8):880–890.
6. Cinar M, Akpinar S, Derincek A, Circi E, Uysal M. Comparison of arthroscopic capsular release in diabetic and idiopathic frozen shoulder patients. *Arch Orthop Trauma Surg*. 2010;130(3):401–406.
7. Elhassan B, Ozbaydar O, Massimini D, Higgins L, Warner JJ. Arthroscopic capsular release for refractory shoulder stiffness: a critical analysis of effectiveness in specific etiologies. *J Shoulder Elbow Surg*. 2010;19(4):580–587.
8. Musil D, Sadovský P, Stehlík J, Filip L, Vodicka Z. Arthroscopic capsular release in frozen shoulder syndrome [in Czech]. *Acta Chir Orthop Traumatol Cech*. 2009;76(2):98–103.
9. Gaunt BW, McCluskey GM, Uhl TL. Electromyographic evaluation of subdividing active-assistive shoulder exercises. *Sports Health*. 2010;2(5):424–432.

MANIPULATION UNDER ANESTHESIA, LYSIS OF ADHESIONS, AND CAPSULAR RELEASE REHABILITATION GUIDELINE

St. Francis Orthopaedic Institute and St. Francis Rehabilitation Center

All information contained in this protocol is to be used as a general guideline only. Specific variations might be appropriate for each patient and might be specified by the physician. In all cases, it is acceptable to advance the program more slowly than stated. If the patient experiences excessive pain, discontinue exercise until the physician is contacted. ***Achieving and maintaining a low level of pain and inflammation while achieving maximum range-of-motion measures are the guiding principles in all stages of rehabilitation.***

SYMBOLS AND ABBREVIATIONS

AAFE, active-assistive forward elevation
AAROM, active-assistive range of motion
AASEP, assistive-to-active shoulder elevation progression
AFE, active forward elevation
AROM, active range of motion
ER, external rotation
FE, forward elevation
IR, internal rotation
PER, passive external rotation
PFE, passive forward elevation
POD, postoperative day
POM, postoperative month
POW, postoperative week
PRN, as needed
PROM, passive range of motion
ROM, range of motion
T-Band, Thera-Band (The Hygenic Corporation, Akron, OH)
WNL, within normal limits

Forward elevation, either active or passive, is the plane of motion in which an individual naturally lifts his or her arm that is anterior to the plane of the scapula and lateral to flexion.

PHASE 1: POD 0 TO POW 6

Goals

- °Establish a tolerance to a comprehensive stretching program that achieves normal PROM measures into FE and ER and progressively stretches into all planes of motion
- °Control reactivity by minimizing pain and the inflammatory response
- °Educate the patient about modified activity, controlling the inflammatory response, and cryotherapy

Exercises

- °***Note: If the patient is seen on the day of the procedure with his or her nerve block intact, we recommend following this initial evaluation and treatment.***
- °Therapist PROM with the patient seated into ER near the side, ER at 90° of abduction, and FE (Figures 13–15)
    - °3 to 5 repetitions
    - °Diligent attempt should be made to achieve normal ranges while the patient is awake and the arm is flaccid
    - °Patient and family members are instructed to perform these 3 assisted motions every 4 waking hours until the nerve block has resolved
    - °**Begin performing home exercises as listed below after all sensory and motor control have returned to the arm**
- °Pendulum exercises
    - °Perform for 30 to 60 seconds 8 to 12 times per day
    - °Lean over a table a comfortable amount with the arm hanging down relaxed

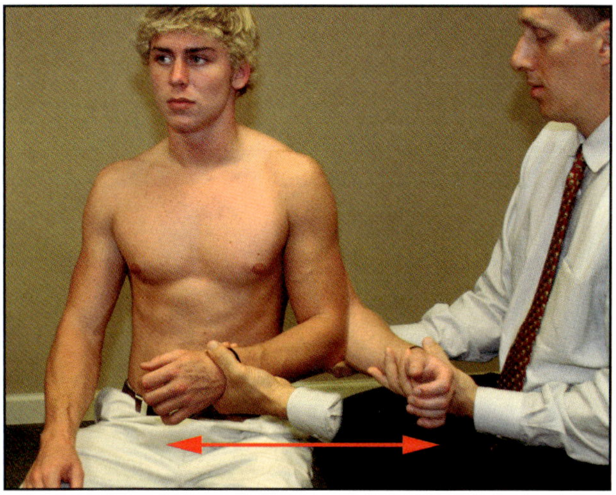

Figure 13. Passive external rotation at the side.

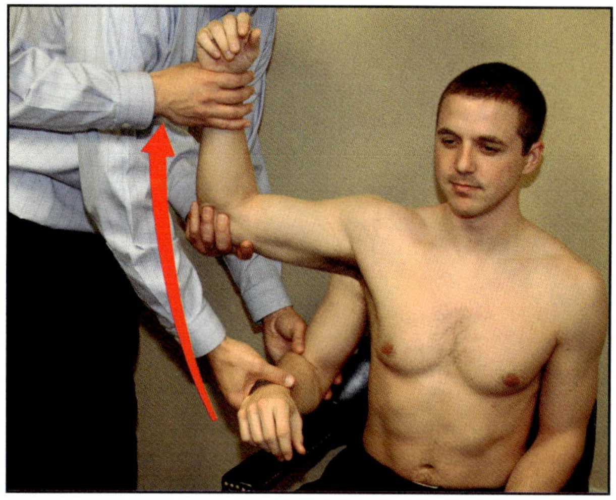

Figure 14. Passive external rotation in abduction.

- °Keep the body still and move the arm in small comfortable circles only
- °Upright PER in slight abduction until moderate stretch and discomfort
  - °7 to 12 repetitions 3 to 4 times per day
  - °Preferred exercises
    - °Sit with family member or therapist rotating the arm
    - °PER walk-around (stand with the arm supported on a table and rotate the body)
- °PFE until moderate stretch and discomfort
  - °7 to 12 repetitions 3 to 4 times per day
  - °Preferred exercises
    - °Sit with family member or therapist lifting the arm
    - °Table step-back exercise
    - °Continuous passive motion machine for PFE
    - °After achieving more than 120° of PFE, progress to self-assisted AAFE in the supine position or pulley PFE as comfortable

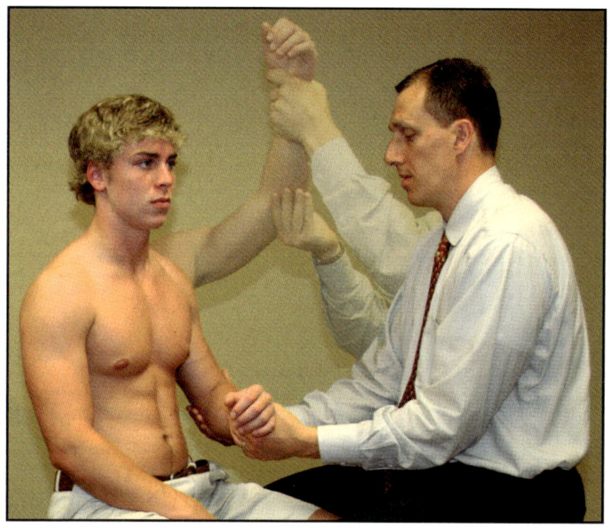

Figure 15. Passive forward elevation.

- °Therapist-assisted seated PROM into PER, PER to 90°, and PFE
- °Therapist-assisted supine PROM into PER, PER to 90°, and PFE with the goal of achieving nearly normal ROM into FE and ER planes (chapter II- 3)
  - °Performed 5 days per week for the first 2 weeks after the procedure then decreased to 3 days per week only after the patient can more easily achieve normal ranges with his or her self-stretching
    - °Decrease pain and muscle guarding
    - °Achieve and maintain ROM gained during the procedure
    - °Additional planes of therapist stretching should be added into a comfort tolerance only
      - °ER at 20°, 45°, and 90° of abduction
      - °IR in progressive abduction up to 90°
      - °Horizontal adduction
      - °Diagonal elevation from 90° of FE to 140° of abduction

°Forward elevation progressing to flexion
°Coracohumeral ligament stretch (Figure 16)
°Patient education
°Education of the pathogenesis and recovery process
°Importance of frequent use of ice and prescribed medicine for pain reduction
°Minimal use of the arm for light waist-level activities as comfortable
°Ensure that the level of pain is not increasing because of excessive use of the arm for activities of daily living or work

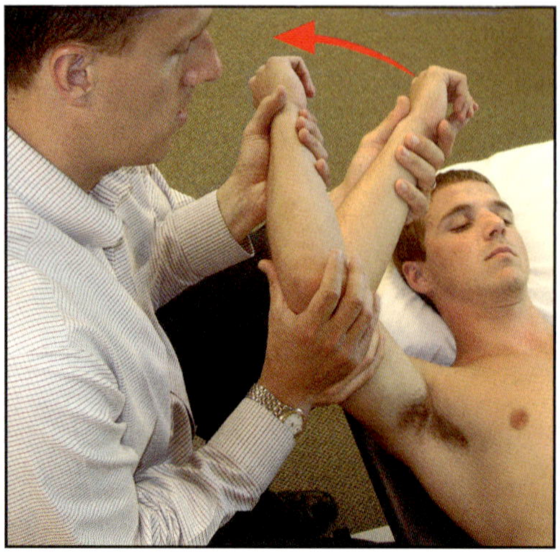

Figure 16. Coracohumeral ligament stretch.

Adjunctive Exercises

Progressively can add to the home program if the patient responds favorably to these planes of manual therapist stretching
°Horizontal adduction
°Sitting with the uninvolved hand assisting the elbow across the body
°Sleeper stretch
°Performed in the side-lying position on the involved side with the arm elevated to 70°
°The uninvolved hand rotates the involved hand down to a mat table
°Supine hand-behind-head stretch
°With a pillow under the head
°Progress to gentle ER stretching
°70° to 90° of abduction supine with a T-stick (Figure 17)
°Functional IR AAROM
°The uninvolved hand assists the involved arm directly
°Horizontal thigh dusting
°10 to 20 repetitions 3 to 5 times per day
°Perform straight ahead on an outstretched leg while seated
°Aquatic therapy for gentle pain-free AAROM (no swimming strokes)

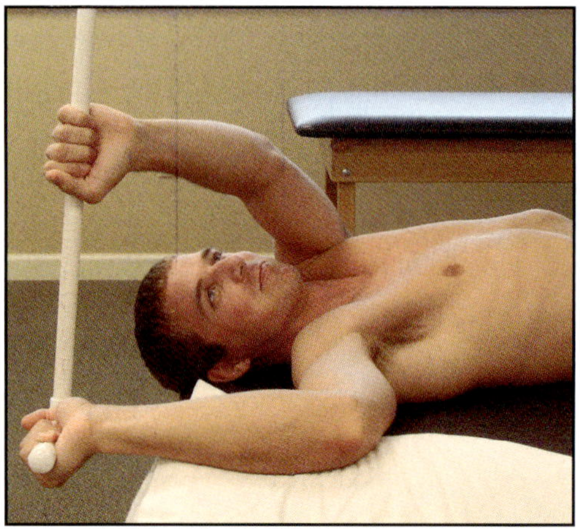

Figure 17. Supine T-stick PER to 90°.

Interventions to Avoid

°Exercises that result in severe immediate or delayed pain
°Exercises that result in excessive guarding or splinting of muscles
°Home exercises into straight-plane abduction
°Strengthening exercises
°Repetitive daily activity with the affected arm above waist level

PHASE 2: POW 6 TO POW 12

Criteria to Begin

°Successful tolerance to PFE and PER stretching
°Low reactivity (stretch sensation before pain and no delayed pain)

- °Improving ease and amount of ROM
- °Low pain at rest and with active forward reaching at waist level
- °Low reactivity when assessing tolerance to PROM in different planes
- °Physician approval

Goals

- °Further reduce shoulder pain
- °Continue a comprehensive PROM and stretching program for the clinic
- °Fully implement a comprehensive terminal stretching program for the home program
- °Achieve normal PROM into FE and ER at the side and nearly normal PROM in all planes
- °Improve AROM
- °Increase functional activities

Exercises

Comprehensive home stretching program: Assess each of the motions below to determine if stretching is needed. Stretching should be performed if (1) motion is limited more than 10° to 15° and (2) the level of pain is less than or equal to the sensation of stretch. If a particular ROM is limited due to only pain, then inflammation rather than stiffness is limiting the ROM; therefore, home stretching is NOT appropriate in this particular plane of motion at this time **BUT** should be performed by the therapist in the clinic.

- °PFE stretching
  - °Preferred exercises
    - °Rope-and-pulley exercise (elbows remain straight)
    - °Patient-assisted supine AAFE exercise (use the unaffected arm for assistance)
    - °Wall terminal-elevation stretch (Figure 18)
- °PER stretching
  - °Preferred exercises
    - °PER sitting with the wand upright and the hand in neutral
    - °PER walk-around (stand with the arm supported on a table and rotate the body)
    - °PER corner walk-around (stand with the hand propped on a doorway)
- °Horizontal adduction or sleeper stretch, or both
- °Supine hand-behind-head stretch
  - °ER stretching at 70° to 90° of abduction
  - °ER stretching at 90° of abduction against a wall
- °Functional IR AAROM
  - °The uninvolved hand assists the involved arm directly
  - °Towel or pulley active-assistive IR
- °Therapist-assisted supine PROM into all planes targeting a stretch greater than pain-limited end feel and progressively including all of the following:
  - °ER at 20°, 45°, and 90° of abduction
  - °IR in progressive abduction up to 90°
  - °Horizontal adduction
  - °Diagonal elevation from 90° of FE to 140° of abduction

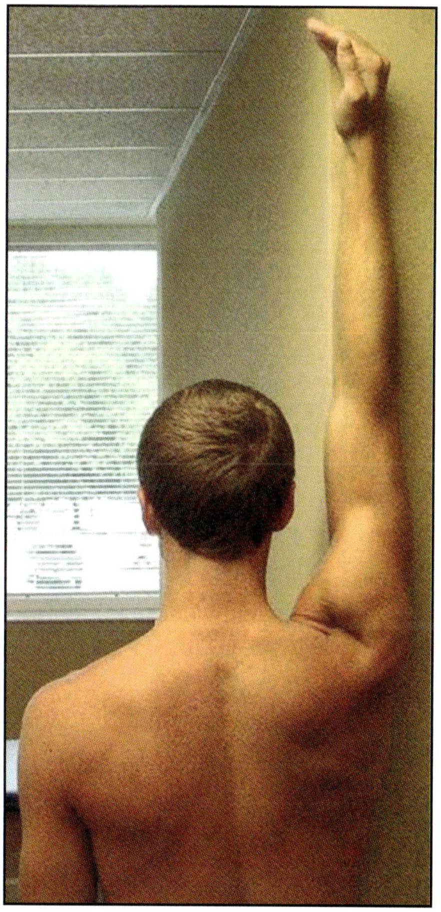

Figure 18. Wall terminal-elevation stretch.

- °Forward elevation progressing to flexion
- °Coracohumeral ligament stretch (Figure 16)

°Initiate base strengthening program if PROM is steadily advancing and if pain and inflammation are well controlled

- °Includes standard rotator cuff, deltoid, and scapular strengthening program
- °2 times per day at most with light resistance and increasing repetitions
- °Yellow T-Band for ER and IR
  - °Initially, 4- to 6-foot band length and light pretension in a 3- to 6-inch arc of motion
  - °Can use side-lying ER instead of T-Band to begin
- °Yellow T-Band forward reach
  - °Initially, 4- to 6-foot band length and light pretension
  - °Start with the elbow bent and by the side and the band tied behind the patient
  - °Reach forward with the hand at waist level, progressing to reaching **forward** at chest level
- °Scapular strengthening emphasizing scapular retractions and scapular upward rotators (chapter IV-2)
- °**No prone FE, abduction, or ER strenghthening**

°Initiate the AASEP as comfortable (chapter II-4)

- °A stepwise progression in difficulty of strengthening exercises from PFE to AFE against gravity
- °Goal of the progression is to achieve pain-free full AFE
- °Start with a level of exercise that is challenging but not painful
- °If scapular or glenohumeral substitution or pain is present, choose an exercise that is a step easier in the progression
- °Usually not all exercises need to be performed
- °Exercises are divided into 3 levels of difficulty
  1. Gravity-minimized exercises
     - °T-Band supine FE
       - °Must start the involved arm at 90° of elevation
       - °Pull the arm into FE
     - °Side-lying, gravity-eliminated AFE
       - °Lie on the uninvolved side
     - °Jackins supine reaching progression
       - °Begin at 0° with the elbow bent and end at 90° of elevation with the elbow extended
         - °Start with the assistance of a cane or wand
         - °Progress to active motion
         - °Can progress to using 1 to 2 pounds of weight
       - °Can progress to the inclined position, continuing to reach to the ceiling
  2. Assistive elevation exercises
     - °Rope-and-pulley AAFE
     - °Incline dusting
     - °Standing AAFE (assistive elevation and descent via a T-bar or the unaffected arm)
     - °Standing assistive elevation and active independent eccentric lowering
     - °Wall-slide AAFE
       - °Ensure that the patient is in FE and is not in flexion
       - °Must be pain-free and natural when performing
  3. Unsupported elevation exercises
     - °AFE

°Initiate progressive replication of moderate-intensity activities of daily living and work

°AFE without weight progressing to a maximum of 1 to 3 pounds

Adjunctive Exercises

If the patient has convenient access to a pool or is having difficulty managing a comfortable strength progression on land or seeking additional means of strengthening beyond the T-Band program, use aquatic strengthening exercises (chapter IV-9)

Interventions to Avoid

°Advanced strengthening except as described above
°Exercises that greatly increase signs and symptoms
°Highly repetitive rehabilitation activities with the elbow at or above chest level, including upper extremity ergometer
°Stretching into straight-plane abduction during home exercise

PHASE 3: POW 12 TO POM 6

Criteria to Begin

°Low reactivity: low pain with passive stretching and no delayed pain after stretching
°Nearly normal PROM in all planes of motion
°Physician approval

Goals

°Discharge when functional goals are met. Full AROM and PROM are goals, but if not all planes are WNL while the patient is in therapy, this does not preclude discharge.
°Transition to maintenance home exercise program
°Normal PROM
°Normal to nearly normal strength and endurance
°Return to full activities of daily living, work, and recreation

Exercises

°PROM and stretching
- °Continue home-based PROM and stretching as detailed in phase 2 for all planes of motion that are limited due to stiffness
- °Continue terminal stretches, such as those listed below PRN
  These should be used only if residual stiffness remains and symptoms are not exacerbated.
  - °Wall terminal-elevation stretch (Figure 18)
  - °PER stretching with the arm near the side using a wall
  - °PER stretching at 90° of abduction
  - °Functional IR stretching using towel or pulley

°Continue base strengthening progression
- °Includes standard rotator cuff, deltoid, and scapular strengthening program
- °2 times per day at most with progressive resistance and repetitions
- **°No prone FE, abduction, or ER strengthening**

°Initiate or continue the AASEP as needed (chapter II-4)

°Initiate advanced strengthening progression as needed and ensure comfort (chapter III-4)

°Only participate in advanced strengthening exercises, including heavier dumbbell strengthening, higher speed exercises, and powerful activities **in very rare circumstances where these functional demands are regularly required**

Adjunctive Exercises

°Initiate if the patient demonstrates substantial capsular limitation precluding full PROM

°Therapist-assisted stretching and mobilizations PRN

Interventions to Avoid

°Any rehabilitation activity that is substantially more demanding than daily or expected activities

°Any exercise that substantially increases signs and symptoms

°Typically no prone FE, abduction, or ER

°No strengthening in straight-plane abduction

III-10

Synovectomy

Joseph H. Kostuch, PT, SCS

CHAPTER CONTENTS

WHAT PATIENTS ARE APPROPRIATE FOR THE USE OF THIS GUIDELINE?

- Patients with arthroscopic synovectomy
- Patients without concomitant rotator cuff or labral repair

Clinical pearls are highlighted in yellow throughout the text.

THE MOST IMPORTANT FACTOR THAT SHOULD GUIDE CLINICAL DECISION MAKING

Whereas the goal after synovectomy is achieving normal passive (PROM) and active range of motion (AROM) as quickly as possible, the primary issue remains the rehabilitation provider's ability to monitor and control the patient's pain and inflammation. Our ability to successfully control the reactivity of his or her shoulder will dictate both the speed and aggressiveness of our exercise progression.

KEY PRINCIPLES IN REHABILITATION OF THIS PROBLEM

Synovitis about the shoulder is an extremely painful and functionally limiting diagnosis (Figures 1 and 2). Specifically termed *hypervascular synovial hyperpla-*

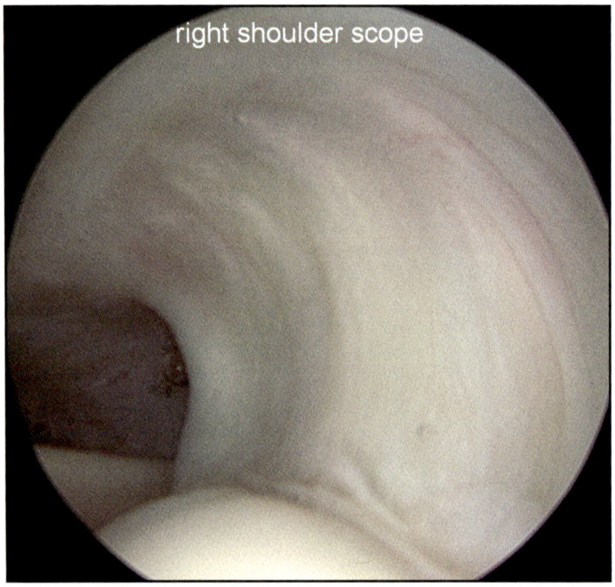

Figure 1. Normal synovial tissue.

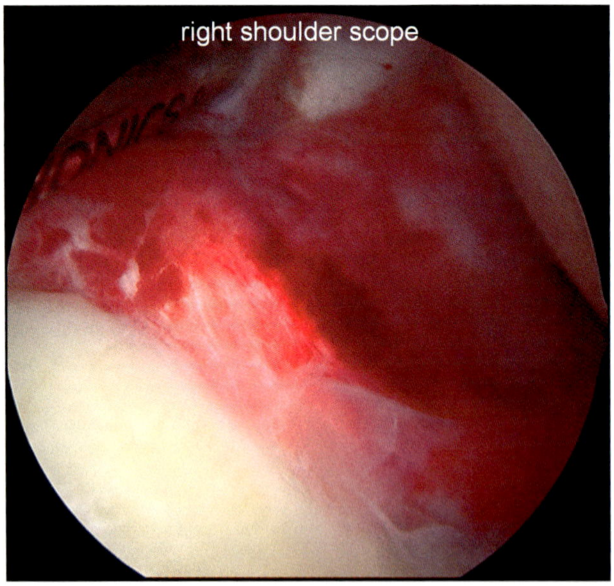

Figure 2. Active synovitis.

sia, the inflamed synovium creates a loss of inferior capsular redundancy, a thickened fibrosis of the capsule and ligament complex, and decreased volume of synovial fluid. This process is thought to be most active during the initial "freezing" stage of adhesive capsulitis. It is during this phase that fibroblasts and myofibroblasts lay down a dense matrix of type I and type III collagen within the capsule, creating the contraction.[1–6]

The physician's decision to proceed with surgical intervention for synovitis must be paired with a comprehensive postoperative plan of care along with extensive preoperative patient counseling. Given the strong tendency to lose range of motion (ROM) and function with overly aggressive rehabilitation,[7] strict attention must be paid to the patient's response to treatment. Monitoring and adjusting the exercise variables, such as the frequency and intensity of stretching, to achieve optimal patient comfort is crucial for success. When managed appropriately, results have been positive in these patients when compared with patients who have traumatic or postoperative captured shoulders.[8,9] In addition, active synovitis that is present during a surgical repair, such as a rotator cuff repair, places this population at additional risk for developing postoperative stiffness[10] if it is not properly identified and managed with an altered postoperative plan of care.

SPECIFIC REHABILITATION GUIDELINE

The Appendix specifies our complete Synovectomy Rehabilitation Guideline. In this section, I explain the rationale for selected components of the guideline. It is divided into 3 phases based on general timeframes of healing and expected reduction of inflammation. To advance from one rehabilitation phase to the next, the patient must gain approval from the physician to advance, successfully complete the core components of the previous rehabilitation activities, and meet the time criteria.

Phase 1

The sole focus of our phase 1 program is to maintain a comfortable PROM program that steadily improves to achieve the same ROM that the surgeon gained during the procedure. The stretching exercises performed during phase 1 remain entirely passive: that is, without muscle contraction about the shoulder. The home exercises and stretching by the rehabilitation provider are solely intended to address the patient's PROM. No attempt is made in phase 1 to perform any AROM, muscle strengthening, or functional training. Any attempt to strengthen during phase 1 usually keeps the inflammatory response high in the shoulder, slowing the ROM progression and pain relief that patients are seeking.

Because active synovitis about the glenohumeral joint is highly painful, the rehabilitation provider must adjust both the clinic PROM stretching and the patient's home program accordingly based on his or her response to pain both during and after treatment. During the first several weeks after synovectomy, the rehabilitation provider performs manual stretching primarily into passive external rotation (PER) and passive forward elevation (PFE) planes of motion about the shoulder. These planes encompass phase 1 PROM described in chapter II-3. With the surgeon having improved ROM and removed the inflamed synovial tissue during the procedure (Figures 3), the rehabilitation provider strives to steadily progress the PROM measures over the course of phase 1 recovery. Differing from the program for manipulation under anesthesia (MUA) or arthroscopic lysis of adhesions (LOA), the PROM program after synovectomy is not forced or

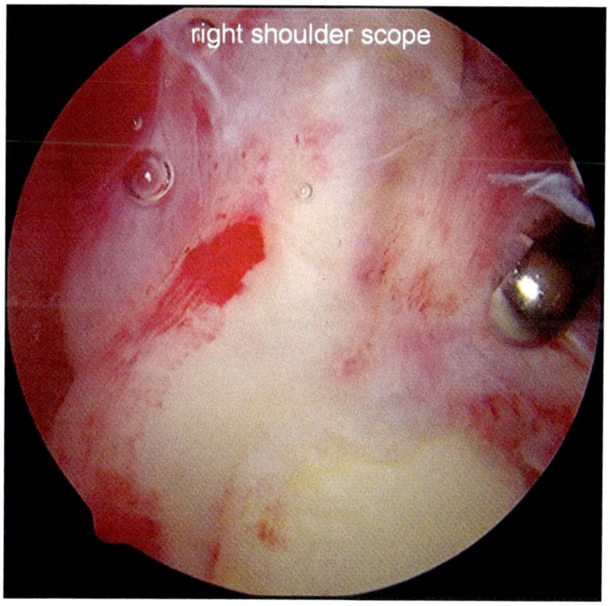

Figure 3. Rotator interval after synovectomy.

aggressively stretched into painful end ranges. Figure 4 compares the expected course of PROM progression relative to recovery after LOA and synovectomy. Note the highlighted area where steady and comfortable ROM progress is desired compared with a forced maintenance found with MUA or after LOA.

The patient must work very diligently at home to consistently (up to 4 times a day) perform his or her home stretching program to maintain and advance ROM. Educating the patient about performing comfortable and not forced home stretching is crucial. Patients must be aware that gains will be slow to recognize but that comfort and overall pain control are of primary importance for their home exercise programs. A certain amount of soreness remains from the surgical procedure and from the musculotendon contraction that has occurred about the joint from the condition. The rehabilitation provider must teach the patient to respect a painful end point and avoid stretching into this soreness. Appreciating that pain and soreness are involved from the procedure, the surgeon provides prescription pain medication and possibly nonsteroidal anti-inflammatory drugs, which should be taken at regular, prescribed intervals. When educating the patient, the rehabilitation provider needs to emphasize reduced functional use, icing, and positioning to help reduce soreness.

The patient typically is reintroduced to physical therapy within the first 3 days after surgery; however, there are situations in which the physician might want to begin PROM immediately and send patients to physical therapy directly from surgery with their nerve blocks intact. With either situation, the initial visit will consist of the rehabilitation provider moving the shoulder into PER and PFE with the patient sitting (Figures 5 and 6).

This urgency of reintroducing therapy is necessary because of the bleeding that occurs inside the shoulder with the removal of synovitis. If the shoulder were simply left by the side after surgery, it would begin to readhere down after only a short period. During the initial therapy visit after the procedure, the rehabilitation provider moves the extremity as described. Sometimes, the patient is seen after synovectomy while his or her nerve block is still intact, and a family member is instructed how to perform sitting PER and PFE at home. After the block has resolved, patients add scapular AROM and Codman exercises to their home programs. The home exercises are performed only within a pain-free range. These patients then are seen 3 to 4 times per week for the first 2 weeks after their synovectomies. The frequency of outpatient visits might be reduced to 3 times per week for stretching by the rehabilitation provider between postoperative

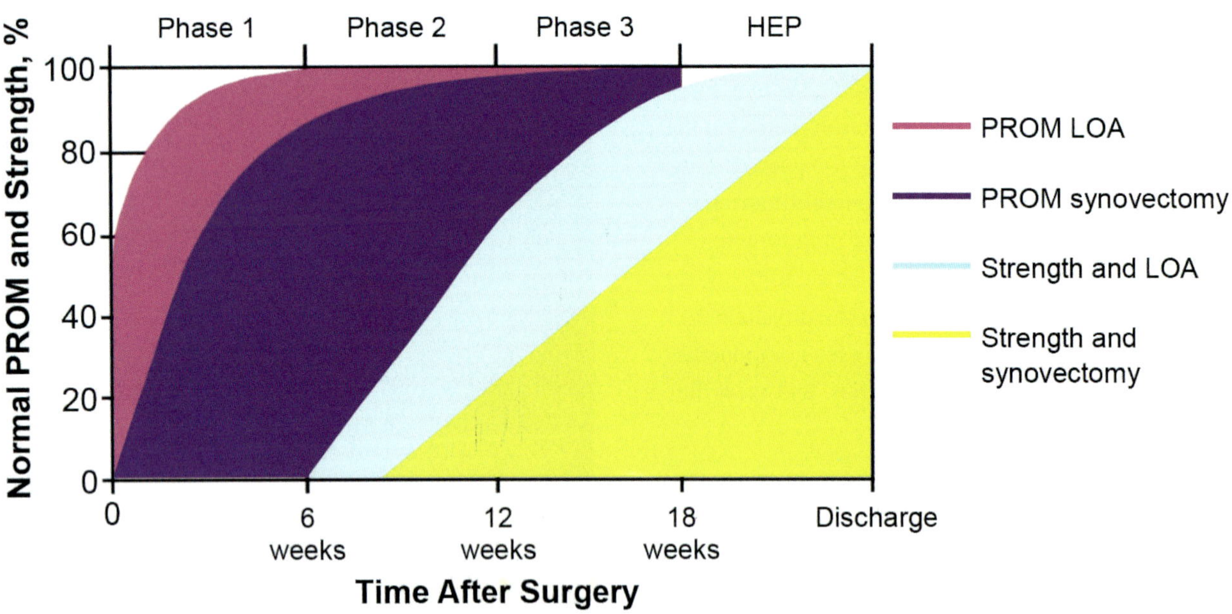

Figure 4. Expected course of passive range of motion (PROM) progression for recovery after lysis of adhesions (LOA) and synovectomy. Abbreviation: HEP, home exercise program.

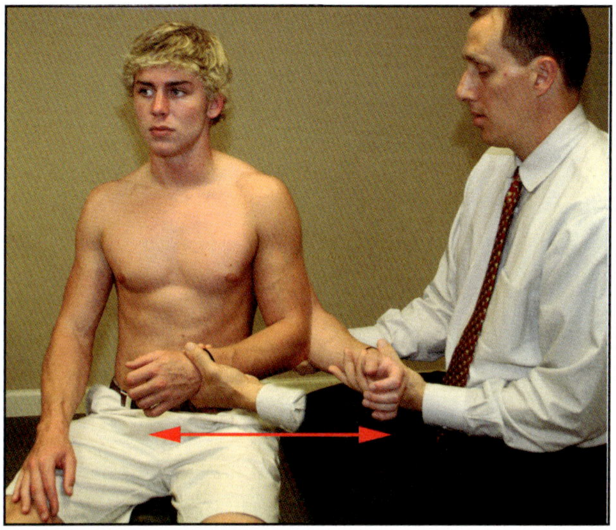

Figure 5. Therapist-assisted passive external rotation.

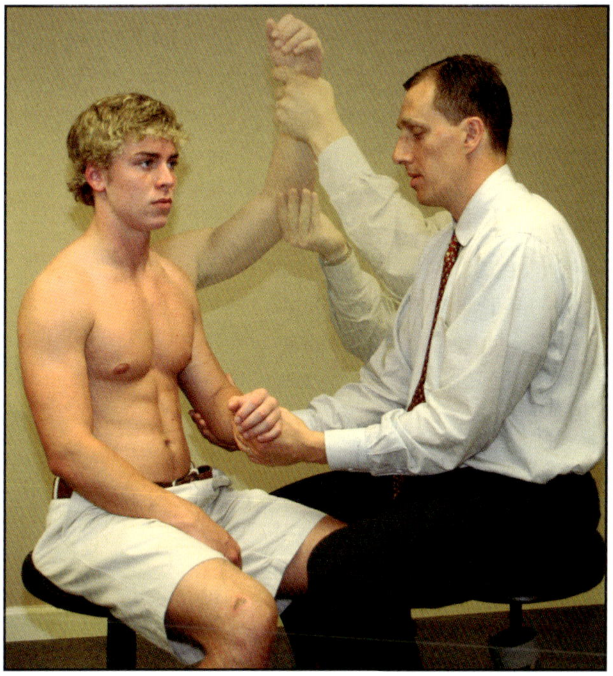

Figure 6. Therapist-assisted passive forward elevation.

weeks 3 and 6. When the patient can more comfortably perform PROM self stretches that are close to equal to the measures achieved by the rehabilitation provider, his or her frequency of visits can decrease.

At St. Francis Rehabilitation Center, these patients also receive a Kinex K2 (Kinex Medical Company, LLC, Waukesha, WI) shoulder continuous passive motion (CPM) machine for home PFE stretching. This unit is custom fit to the patient preoperatively to ensure a smooth arc of PFE. If the patient is seen the day of surgery and the nerve block is still intact, PFE is not performed with the CPM machine at the first therapy visit but is instructed and begun at the second therapy visit when sensory and motor control have returned. The CPM machine is instructed for home use up to 3 times per day for 15-minute sessions. Successful use of the CPM machine for PFE to the patient's point of comfort is an excellent means of achieving our desired goal of steady PFE progression.

Because increased emphasis is placed on maintaining patient comfort, the home stretching program remains straightforward and encompasses only exercises for PER and PFE, progressing toward active-assistive forward elevation. Initially, the rehabilitation provider also adheres to these primary planes but then slowly and progressively works into all 3 planes of motion (coronal, sagittal, transverse) with his or her hands-on stretching. Within the first few weeks after the procedure, the rehabilitation provider begins clinic-only movement into passive abduction, 90° of PER, horizontal adduction stretch, and 90° of passive internal rotation. These rehabilitation-provider-only stretches are described specifically in Figure 12 (Manual Therapist Technique) of chapter II-3. They are light intensity, each stretch is held for 10 seconds, and sets of 5 repetitions are performed. While keeping the intensity low and communicating with the patient about appropriate recovery time, the rehabilitation provider successfully and slowly introduces these additional planes of clinic stretching. The patient is taught specifically that although the PROM stretching by the rehabilitation provider might result in some increased soreness during and shortly after the session, the home stretching should be kept mild and below his or her perceived intensity of soreness with clinic stretching.

The patient should be comfortably achieving increased PFE and PER with his or her self stretches by postoperative week 6. As the pain decreases and ease of PROM increases, the patient enters phase 2 of recovery.

Phase 2

During phase 2 of recovery, the rehabilitation provider directs the patient into an expanded home stretching program. This program gradually encompasses all the planes that the rehabilitation provider has been stretching in the clinic but are now added for the home. These stretches are described specifically in Figure 12 (Home Patient Technique) of chapter II-3. The additional planes of stretching must be added individually, and comfort must be emphasized. The rehabilitation provider should be able to best identify the patient's easiest planes of motion from his or her hands-on stretching and add those to the home stretches first. As the patient's tolerance to the new home stretches improves, he or she is seen less often by the rehabilitation provider. Remember that just as in phase 1 of recovery, the additional planes of stretching advance in a steady, progressive manner. The duration of the patient's home program steadily increases. He or she is instructed to perform this expanded stretching 3 to 4 times per day and work up to performing 10 repetitions of each stretch.

Although most patients who have had synovectomy will continue with active-assistive ROM stretching only during phase 2, a select group of patients with synovectomy is appropriate to begin a strengthening program during the later stages of phase 2. Our strengthening program is detailed in chapter II-4. This program is initiated at waist level, and comfort above all else is emphasized. The rotator cuff and scapular stabilizers are isolated and strengthened to allow increased functional use of the upper extremity below shoulder level. The patient must achieve comfortable forward reaching before initiating a Thera-Band (The Hygenic Corporation, Akron, OH) program for strength. If the patient remains too weak or has too much pain with his or her forward reach, we initiate our movement strengthening program first with gravity eliminated and then against gravity before advancing to Thera-Band resistance. Unlike the stretching program that was performed multiple times per day, performance of the strengthening program is recommended only 1 time per day. When the patient reaches a tolerance to strength training, a second daily session is added. This base Thera-Band program is advanced with repetitions then with resistance over the course of the next several weeks.

Phase 3

For most patients who have had synovectomy, strengthening begins during phase 3 of recovery. This base strengthening program that we have detailed emphasizes muscle activation and recruitment rather than targeting muscle hypertrophy and growth. When the patient's endurance of these important muscles is improved, functional use of the upper extremity returns to chest level, and the level of pain remains low, we advance to our assistive-to-active elevation progression. This strengthening phase of recovery often takes several months and likely produces frustration in patients because their functional use and strength remain limited. Patient counseling and education to appropriately set expectations for functional use of the upper extremity are very important.

Depending on the severity and duration of the preoperative condition, the patient might not have actively raised the extremity above shoulder level for several months. Now that joint flexibility has been restored, the muscles must be retrained and strengthened to actively lift the extremity. We use our elevation strengthening progression, which is a series of strengthening exercises demonstrated to systematically and progressively recruit the appropriate muscles for lifting the upper extremity overhead (chapter II-4).[11] Each patient tolerates and progresses through this stage to full active forward elevation (AFE) at various speeds. The rehabilitation provider must keep in mind that the shoulder girdle muscles have not been engaged at these length-tension positions for a long time, so the patient's tolerance to this progression might be slow and require frequent adjustment in both exercise selection and intensity. When the body can elevate the upper extremity overhead without substitution, the muscles are strengthened to allow normal return to overhead use of the extremity.

As strength is progressed above shoulder level, terminal stretching often is still required from both the rehabilitation provider in the clinic and with the regular home program. The patient needs to be taught that although full, normalized ROM is close, the intensity of stretching must not increase. The intensity of the program is accounted for in the advancement of the home stretching technique or position rather than the patient forcing the terminal range.

Rehabilitation providers and patients often confuse lack of terminal AROM with a strength deficit when in fact a small amount of capsular tightness remains and requires continued stretching. Often, full AFE is trained specifically by ordering the program to include terminal forward elevation stretching then working actively into these recently stretched ranges in the appropriate elevation strengthening progression that is best tolerated by the patient. In addition, achieving normalized flexibility of the posterior capsule is often necessary to gain terminal PFE or AFE.

This progression of overhead strength and full return to normal functional use of the upper extremity is achieved in the later stages of phase 3. Full AFE might take longer than expected because of mild residual capsular tightness as described earlier. Active forward elevation is progressed in repetition, and weight is progressed in proportion to the patient's overall size and strength and in consideration of his or her functional, occupational, or recreational demands. During this phase, progressing strength specific to a recreational fitness program, light tennis, or golf along with group exercise programs can be achieved as directed by the surgeon.

SPECIAL CONSIDERATIONS

Concomitant Diabetes

Because of the relatively poor healing tendencies and high risk for recurrent stiffness specific to people with diabetes, these patients must be managed delicately, balancing their PROM and pain control. In addition, their introduction to strengthening might be delayed slightly, and more time might be spent with their terminal stretching well into phase 3.

Postoperative Captured Shoulder

Because postoperative stiffness is a potential complication after repair or reconstructive surgery, an LOA might become appropriate if the patient develops substantial stiffness while the repair heals. At St. Francis Orthopaedic Institute, we recommend that this procedure always is performed arthroscopically and is never manipulated without visualization and specific structures released. Specific situations exist in which active synovitis is present during this arthroscopy. These patients must be treated more delicately than patients with typical LOA, balancing their reactivity and PROM. The surgeon also must inspect and verify that the previous repair has healed adequately so that our normal synovectomy protocol can be followed safely.

Combined Rotator Cuff Repair and Synovectomy

Patients who have had a rotator cuff repair combined with a synovectomy present a great rehabilitation challenge (Figure 7). We have observed that overly aggressive PROM appears to exacerbate the inflammatory response and results in a large increase in long-term stiffness and pain.[7,10] This observation is supported by work from Diercks and Stevens.[7] Overly aggressive early PROM also might be detrimental to the healing of the rotator cuff repair, which remains the first priority in this situation. Our preferred management is to start PROM on postoperative day 1, striving for the same ROM targets as the typical rotator cuff repair but realizing that ROM likely will be more painful and limited. Because of their increased pain both at rest and with PROM exercises, patients are encouraged to take appropriate pain medications, especially in conjunction with their exercises, and to ice their shoulders more often. With the higher level of pain, patients often have difficulty managing their home stretching programs; therefore, we prefer an increased frequency of clinic treatments, especially the first month after surgery. This increased exposure to manual PROM by the rehabilitation provider will increase the patient's chances of achieving the desired staged PROM goals as concisely as possible in the early weeks.

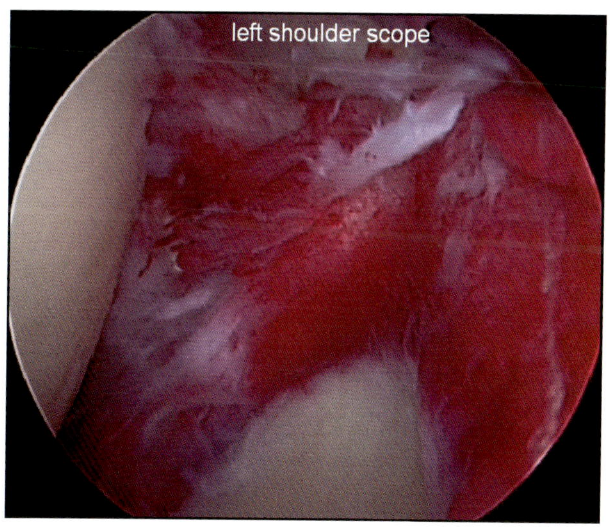

Figure 7. Rotator cuff tear with synovitis.

During the later phases of rehabilitation, we recommend continued gentle stretching only to a point of minimal discomfort because we have found that an exacerbation in inflammation and subsequent stiffness can result if terminal PROM is aggressively attempted. This preference often means settling for functional ROM rather than ROM that is normalized to the contralateral side, but it empirically appears to achieve joint homeostasis quicker. Because the joint remains sensitive to rapid changes, the initiation of AROM and strengthening also is delayed until the overall level of inflammation is low and a functional amount of PROM is well established. A 1- to 2-month delay in AROM and strengthening is common.

Partial-Thickness Rotator Cuff Tear

When stiffness and pain do not resolve with a typical intervention of stretching by the rehabilitation provider, an arthroscopic synovectomy might be the surgeon's choice of management. Some patients also might have a small partial-thickness rotator cuff tear that is managed by debridement underlying their more prominent stiffness and pain. These patients participate in a longer phase 2 and 3 program to address the unrepaired partial-thickness rotator cuff injury. An extended base strengthening program might be necessary if they have difficulty managing their pain while attempting to increase strength and functional advances. Maintaining full PROM remains critical while managing their rotator cuff symptoms with appropriate exercise modification and advancement.

In conclusion, the patient's speed of progression through this recovery largely depends on his or her preoperative condition. The synovectomy provides a reliable means of regaining PROM and releasing the inflamed tissue, but the speed at which the patient regains his or her strength and functional use of the extremity is more variable. Generally, patients should expect to return to normal household and light work demands within 3 to 4 months. To return to participation in recreational sports or physically demanding jobs, patients require a longer recovery of 4 to 6 months.

REFERENCES

1. Bunker TD, Reilly J, Baird KS, Hamblen Dl. Expression of growth factors, cytokines and matrix metalloproteinases in frozen shoulder. *J Bone Joint Surg Br*. 2000;82(5):768–773.
2. Neviaser JS. Adhesive capsulitis of the shoulder: a study of the pathological findings in periarthritis of the shoulder. *J Bone Joint Surg Am*. 1945;27(2):211–222.
3. Omari A, Bunker TD. Open surgical release for frozen shoulder: surgical findings and results of the release. *J Shoulder Elbow Surg*. 2001;10(4):353–357.
4. Reeves B. The natural history of the frozen shoulder syndrome. *Scand J Rheumatol*. 1975;4(4):193–196.
5. Uitvlugt G, Detrisac DA, Johnson LL, Austin MD, Johnson C. Arthroscopic observations before and after manipulation of frozen shoulder. *Arthroscopy*. 1993;9(2):181–185.
6. Wiley AM. Arthroscopic appearance of frozen shoulder. *Arthroscopy*. 1991;7(2):138–143.
7. Diercks RL, Stevens M. Gentle thawing of the frozen shoulder: a prospective study of supervised neglect versus intensive physical therapy in seventy-seven patients with frozen shoulder syndrome followed up for two years. *J Shoulder Elbow Surg*. 2004;13(5):499–502.
8. Warner JJ, Allen A, Marks PH, Wong P. Arthroscopic release for chronic, refractory adhesive capsulitis of the shoulder. *J Bone Joint Surg Am*. 1996;78(12):1808–1816.
9. Elhassan B, Ozbaydar O, Massimini D, Higgins L, Warner JJ. Arthroscopic capsular release for refractory shoulder stiffness: a critical analysis of effectiveness in specific etiologies. *J Shoulder Elbow Surg*. 2010;19(4):580–587.
10. Huberty DP, Schoolfield JD, Brady PC, Vadala AP, Arrigoni P, Burkhart SS. Incidence and treatment of postoperative stiffness following arthroscopic rotator cuff repair. *Arthroscopy*. 2009;25(8):880–890.
11. Gaunt BW, McCluskey GM, Uhl TL. Electromyographic evaluation of subdividing active-assistive shoulder exercises. *Sports Health*. 2010;2(5):424–432.

SYNOVECTOMY REHABILITATION GUIDELINE

St. Francis Orthopaedic Institute and St. Francis Rehabilitation Center

All information contained in this protocol is to be used as a general guideline only. Specific variations might be appropriate for each patient and might be specified by the physician. In all cases, it is acceptable to advance the program more slowly than stated. If the patient experiences excessive pain, discontinue exercise until the physician is contacted. ***Achieving and maintaining a low level of pain and inflammation are the guiding principles in all stages of rehabilitation, even if less passive and active range of motion are accomplished.***

SYMBOLS AND ABBREVIATIONS

AAFE, active-assistive forward elevation
AAROM, active-assistive range of motion
ADL, activity of daily living
AFE, active forward elevation
AROM, active range of motion
ER, external rotation
FE, forward elevation
IR, internal rotation
PER, passive external rotation
PFE, passive forward elevation
POD, postoperative day
POM, postoperative month
POW, postoperative week
PRN, as needed
PROM, passive range of motion
ROM, range of motion
T-Band, Thera-Band (The Hygenic Corporation, Akron, OH)
WNL, within normal limits

Forward elevation, either active or passive, is the plane of motion in which an individual naturally lifts his or her arm that is anterior to the plane of the scapula and lateral to flexion.

PHASE 1: POD 1 TO POW 6

Goals

- °Control reactivity by minimizing pain and the inflammatory response
- °Educate the patient about modified activity, controlling the inflammatory response, and cryotherapy
- °Establish a tolerance to a stretching program that progressively increases PROM measures into FE and ER
- °Progressively stretch into selected additional planes of motion with the assistance of the rehabilitation provider

Exercises

Note: If the patient is seen on the day of the procedure with his or her nerve block intact, we recommend following this initial evaluation and treatment.

- °Therapist PROM with the patient seated into FE and ER near the side
  - °3 to 5 repetitions
  - °Comfortable attempt should be made to achieve normal ranges while the patient is awake and the arm is flaccid
  - °Patient and family members are instructed to perform these 3 assisted motions for 1 to 2 sessions at home until the nerve block has resolved
  - °**Begin performing home exercises as listed below after all sensory and motor control have returned to the arm**
- °Pendulum exercises
  - °Perform for 30 to 60 seconds 8 to 12 times per day
  - °Lean over a table a comfortable amount with the arm hanging down relaxed

°Keep the body still and move the arm in small comfortable circles only

°Upright PER in slight abduction until mild stretch and discomfort

°7 to 12 repetitions 3 to 4 times per day

°Preferred exercises

°Sit with family member or therapist rotating the arm

°PER walk-around (stand with the arm supported on a table and rotate the body)

°PFE until mild stretch and discomfort

°7 to 12 repetitions 3 to 4 times per day

°Preferred exercises

°Sit with family member or therapist lifting the arm

°Table step-back exercise

°Continuous passive motion machine for PFE (Figure 8)

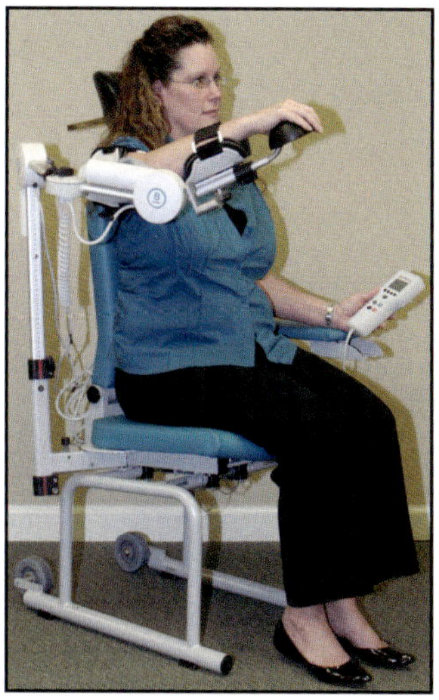

Figure 8. Continuous passive motion machine for PFE.

°Therapist-assisted seated PER and PFE, emphasizing comfortable range only

°Therapist-assisted supine PROM, specifically emphasizing comfortable PER and PFE

°Pending tolerance to FE and ER stretching, the therapist might selectively add the following to clinic stretching only:

°PER to 45° and 90°

°Passive IR to 45° and 90°

°Cross-body adduction (Figure 9)

°Performed 3 to 5 days per week for the first 2 weeks after the procedure then decreased to 3 days per week only after the patient more easily can maintain the PROM achieved in the clinic during the home exercise program with

°Decreased pain and muscle guarding

°Steadily increased ROM gained during the procedure

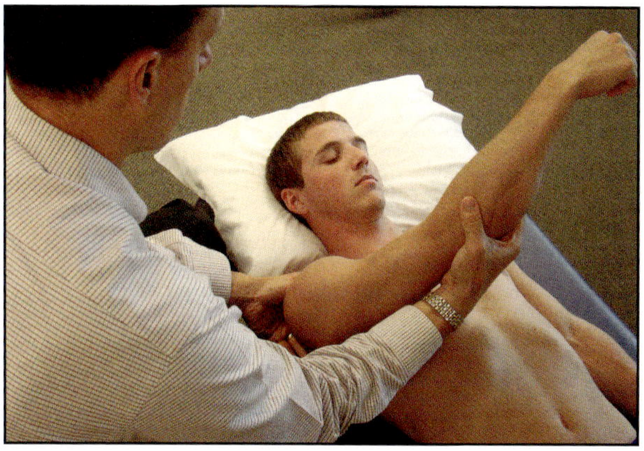

Figure 9. Cross-body adduction.

°Patient education

°Education about the pathogenesis and recovery process

°Importance of frequent use of ice and prescribed medicine for pain reduction

°Minimal use of the arm for light waist-level activities as comfortable

°Ensure pain level is not increasing because of excessive use of the arm for ADLs or work

Adjunctive Exercises

°Progressively can add to the home program if the patient responds favorably to manual therapist stretching and issued only if pain-free and relieves stiffness

°Horizontal table or thigh dusting (Figure 10)

°10 to 20 repetitions 3 to 5 times per day

°Perform straight ahead on an outstretched leg while seated

°Aquatic therapy for gentle pain-free PROM and AAROM (no swimming strokes)

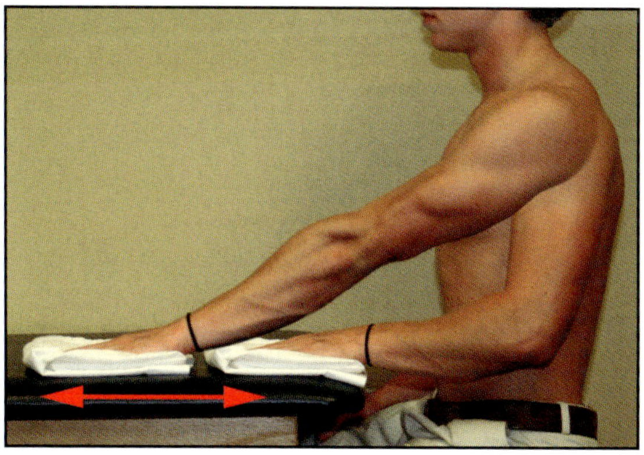

Figure 10. Horizontal dusting.

Interventions to Avoid

°Exercises that result in moderate immediate or delayed pain
°Exercises that result in guarding or splinting of muscles
°Aggressive home or clinic stretching
°Home exercises into straight-plane abduction
°Strengthening exercises
°Repetitive daily activity with the affected arm above waist level

PHASE 2: POW 6 TO POW 12

Criteria to Begin

°Successful tolerance to PFE and PER PROM stretching
  °Low reactivity (stretch sensation before pain and no delayed pain)
  °Improved ease and amount of PROM with therapist stretching
°Low pain at rest and reactivity is controlled and predictable
°Physician approval

Goals

°Establish a tolerance to a comprehensive therapist and home stretching program that includes all planes of motion
°Targeting nearly normal PFE and PER ROM
°Control reactivity by minimizing pain and the inflammatory response
°Educate the patient about modified activity, controlling inflammatory response, and cryotherapy

Exercises

Comprehensive home stretching program: Assess each motion below to determine if stretching is needed. Stretching should only be performed if (1) motion is limited more than 10° to 15° and (2) the level of pain is less than or equal to the sensation of stretch. If a particular ROM is limited due to only pain, then inflammation rather than stiffness is limiting the ROM; therefore, home stretching is NOT appropriate in this particular plane of motion at this time **BUT** should be performed by the therapist in the clinic.
°PFE stretching
  °Preferred exercises
    °Rope-and-pulley exercise (elbows remain straight and thumbs are up)
    °Patient-assisted supine AAFE exercise (use the unaffected arm for assistance)
°PER stretching
  °Preferred exercises
    °PER sitting with the wand upright and the hand in neutral
    °PER walk-around (stand with the arm supported on a table and rotate the body)
°Supine hand-behind-head stretch
  °Progressing to ER stretching with the wand in 70° to 90° of abduction
°Horizontal adduction
  °Sitting with the uninvolved hand assisting the elbow across the body
°Functional IR AAROM
  °Uninvolved hand assists involved arm directly
°Horizontal thigh dusting

    - °10 to 20 repetitions 3 to 5 times per day
    - °Perform seated on the outstretched leg and straight ahead
- °Therapist-assisted supine PROM in all planes with the goal of achieving normal ROM into FE and ER planes and increased tolerance to all rotational planes of motion
    - °Performed 2 to 3 times per week
    - °Decrease pain and muscle guarding
- °Progressively add additional planes of therapist stretching to comfortable tolerance only
    - °ER at 20°, 45°, and 90° of abduction
    - °IR in progressive abduction up to 90°
    - °Horizontal adduction
    - °Diagonal elevation from 90° of FE to 140° of abduction
    - °Forward elevation progressing to flexion
- °Patient education
    - °Education of the specific stage of the recovery process
    - °Importance of the continued use of ice and prescribed medicine for pain PRN
    - °Minimal use of the arm for light waist- to chest-level activities as comfortable
        - °Ensure the level of pain is not increasing because of excessive use of the arm for ADLs or work

Adjunctive Exercises

- °Progressively can add to the home program if the patient responds favorably to these planes of manual therapist stretching
- °Sleeper stretch
    - °Performed in the side-lying position on the involved side with the arm elevated to 70°
    - °Uninvolved hand rotates the involved hand down to the mat table
- °Functional IR PROM
    - °Uninvolved hand or towel assists the involved arm directly
- °Aquatic therapy
    - °PROM and AAROM
    - °AROM
    - °Light waist-level strengthening
- °Base strengthening progression only if PROM is steadily improving in both ease and measurement and if the level of pain and inflammation is well controlled (details in phase 3)

Interventions to Avoid

- °Exercises that result in severe immediate or delayed pain
- °Exercises that result in excessive guarding or splinting of muscles
- °Home exercises into straight-plane abduction
- °Strengthening exercises
- °Repetitive daily activity with the affected arm above waist level

PHASE 3: POW 12 TO POM 6

Criteria to Begin

- °Successful tolerance to all planes of PROM stretching
    - °Low reactivity (stretch sensation before pain and no delayed pain)
    - °Improved ease and amount of PROM

°No pain at rest and with active forward reaching at waist level
°Low reactivity for waist- to chest-level ADLs
°Physician approval

Goals

°Resolve shoulder pain
°Continue comprehensive PROM and stretching program for the clinic
°Implement and advance the comprehensive terminal stretching program for the home program
°Achieve normal PROM into all planes
°Improve AROM to nearly normal
°Achieve nearly normal strength and endurance
°Increase functional activities, including work, home, and recreational ADLs
°Discharge when functional goals are met. Full AROM and PROM are goals, but if not all planes are WNL while the patient is in therapy, this does not preclude discharge
°Transition to a maintenance home exercise program

Exercises

Comprehensive home stretching program using criteria specifically described in phase 2
°PFE stretching
  °Preferred exercises
    °Rope-and-pulley exercise (elbows remain straight)
    °Patient-assisted supine AAFE exercise (use the unaffected arm for assistance)
    °Wall terminal-elevation stretch
°PER stretching
  °Preferred exercises
    °PER sitting with the wand upright and the hand in neutral
    °PER walk-around (stand with the arm supported on a table and rotate the body)
    °PER corner walk-around (stand with the hand propped on a doorway)
°Horizontal adduction or sleeper stretch, or both
°ER stretching in abduction
  °ER stretching at 70° to 90° of abduction
  °ER stretching at 90° of abduction against a wall
°Functional IR AAROM
  °Uninvolved hand assists the involved arm directly
  °Towel or pulley active-assistive IR
°Therapist-assisted supine PROM into all planes of restricted motion (use the same criteria as listed above for the comprehensive home stretching program)
°Initiate base strengthening progression if PROM is steadily improving in both ease and measurement and if pain and inflammation are well controlled
  °Includes standard rotator cuff, deltoid, and scapular strengthening program
  °2 times per day at most with light resistance and increasing repetitions
  °Yellow T-Band for ER and IR
    °Initially, 4- to 6-foot band length and light pretension in a 3- to 6-inch arc of motion
    °Can use side-lying ER instead of T-Band

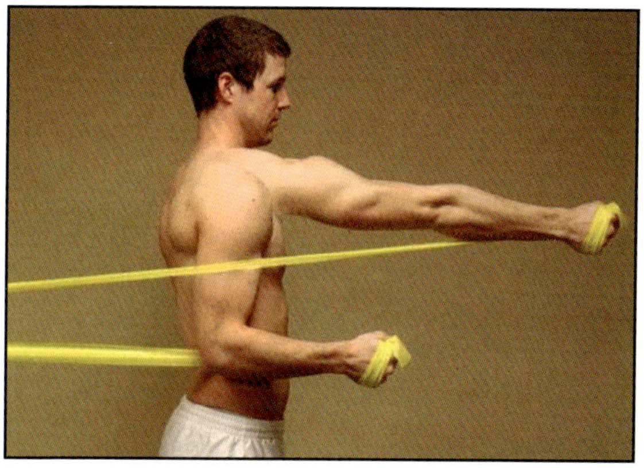

Figure 11. Forward reaching with an elastic band at chest level.

°Yellow T-Band forward reach (Figure 11)
°Initially, 4- to 6-foot band length and light pretension
°Start with the elbow bent and by the side and the band tied behind the patient
°Reach **forward** with the hand at waist level, progressing to reaching **forward** at chest level
°Scapular strengthening emphasizing scapular retractions and scapular upward rotators (chapter IV-2)
°No prone FE, abduction, or ER strengthening
°Initiate the AASEP as comfortable (chapter II-4)
°A stepwise progression in difficulty of strengthening exercises from PFE to AFE against gravity
°Goal of the progression is to achieve pain-free full AFE
°Start with whatever level of exercise is challenging but not painful
°If scapular or glenohumeral substitution or pain are present, choose an easier exercise in the progression
°Usually not all exercises need to be performed
°Exercises are divided into 3 levels of difficulty
1. Gravity-minimized exercises
°T-Band supine FE
°Must start the involved arm at 90° of elevation
°Pull the arm into FE
°Side-lying, gravity-eliminated AFE
°Lie on the uninvolved side
°Jackins supine reaching progression
°Begin at 0° with the elbow bent and end at 90° of elevation with the elbow extended
°Start with the assistance of a cane or wand
°Progress to active motion
°Can progress to using 1 to 2 pounds of weight
°Can progress to the inclined position, continuing to reach to the ceiling
2. Assistive elevation exercises
°Rope-and-pulley AAFE
°Incline dusting
°Standing AAFE (assistive elevation and descent via a T-bar or the unaffected arm)
°Standing assistive elevation and active independent eccentric lowering
°Wall-slide AAFE (Figure 12)
°Ensure that the patient is in FE and is not in flexion
°Must be pain-free and natural when performing
3. Unsupported elevation exercises
°AFE
°AFE without weight progressing to a maximum of 1 to 3 pounds

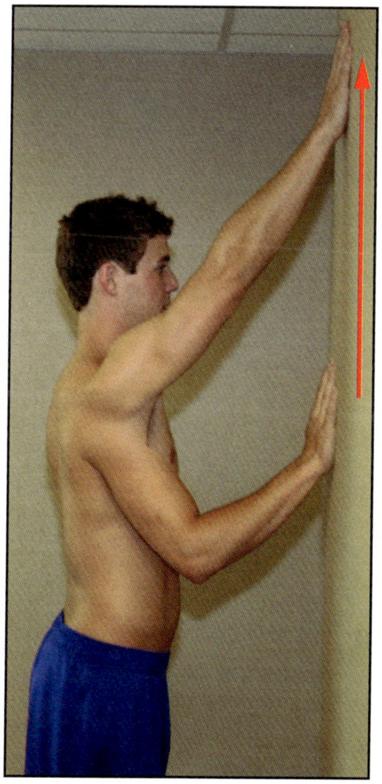

Figure 12. Wall-slide AAFE.

- °Participate in advanced strengthening exercises, including heavier dumbbell strengthening, higher speed, and powerful activities **ONLY in very rare circumstances where functional demands are regularly required**

Adjunctive Exercises

- °Therapist-assisted stretching and mobilizations PRN

Interventions to Avoid

- °Any rehabilitation activity that is much more demanding than daily or expected activities
- °Any exercise that substantially increases signs and symptoms
- °Typically no prone FE, abduction, or ER
- °No strengthening in straight-plane abduction

III-11

Postoperative and Nonoperative Rehabilitation of Proximal Humerus Fractures

John J. Basti, PT

CHAPTER CONTENTS

- What patients are appropriate for the use of this guideline?
- The most important factor that should guide clinical decision making
- Key principles in rehabilitation of this problem
- Specific rehabilitation guidelines
- Special considerations

WHAT PATIENTS ARE APPROPRIATE FOR THE USE OF THIS GUIDELINE?

- Patients with closed reduction; open reduction and internal (ORIF) for 2-part fractures; ORIF or humeral head replacement for some 3-part, 4-part, articular, or head-splitting fractures; and fracture dislocations. The decision for surgery is based on an array of clinical factors, which primarily are the number of bony fragments, the amount of displacement, and angulations of the segments. In 3-part fractures with poor-quality bone and comminution, humeral head replacement might be indicated and preferred by the surgeon. In patients who have 3-part or 4-part fractures and rotator cuff deficiency, reverse total shoulder arthroplasty might be indicated and the surgeon's treatment of choice.
- Older patients who have osteoporosis and poor-quality soft tissue and who have had a minor fall on an outstretched hand. They have a high incidence of proximal humerus fractures.
- Younger patients who have good-quality bone and soft tissue and incur substantial high-velocity bone and soft tissue trauma.
- Patients who have undergone ORIF after undiagnosed posterior fracture-dislocation, incomplete closed reduction, tuberosity pull-off, nonunion, malunion, and avascular necrosis.
- Patients with concomitant rotator cuff tears, neurovascular injury, and degenerative arthritis.

Clinical pearls are highlighted in yellow throughout the text.

THE MOST IMPORTANT FACTOR THAT SHOULD GUIDE CLINICAL DECISION MAKING

Multiple factors direct our clinical decision making when rehabilitating patients with these complex fractures. The primary concern after the initial trauma managed by closed reduction or ensuing surgery for reduction is maintaining stability of the fracture segments and integrity of the soft tissue repair. Limited motion in designated anatomic planes and intensity of exercise appropriate to preserving fixation strength address this concern. Attention to these variables ensures safe early mobilization that will not put the repair at risk while avoiding early stiffness and contracture. Motion and intensity of exercise increase as healing progresses and as postinjury pain diminishes.

KEY PRINCIPLES IN REHABILITATION OF THIS PROBLEM

The substance of a well-defined rehabilitation program lies in the principles of treatment. The complexity of the fracture, the type of reduction and soft tissue repair, and the patient and his or her presentation will determine the treatment progression.

Team Approach

Through the entire process of recovery, the team approach is advocated. Close communication among the surgeon, patient, rehabilitation provider, and care givers will optimize clinical decision making, avoid unanticipated complications, and maximize functional outcome.

Early Passive Motion

Many consider the concept of early, controlled, passive motion tailored to the surgical repair to be the keystone of successful management of proximal humerus fractures, providing the fracture is stable and adequate control of pain is achieved.[1–4] The principles of early passive motion are to establish motion before maturation of scar tissue and development of adhesions while protecting the repair.

Scapular Plane

The *scapular plane* has been defined as the plane of maximum elevation (Figure 1).[1] This position allows the humeral head to remain centered on the glenoid, enabling the capsule to be relaxed and the ligaments and muscles to be balanced. Positioning in this plane allows for more comfort after surgery. Comfortable motion in this plane helps attain maximum functional elevation.

Proximal and Distal Joints

Proximal and distal joints always should be incorporated in the exercise program. Many times, these patients have substantial swelling and ecchymosis of the extremity. Elbow and hand range-of-motion exercises facilitate improved circulation, reduced edema, and reduced stiffness.

Gradual Introduction of Exercise

Gradually introduce exercise. The shoulders of some patients might be too reactive, or the patient might not have the ability to comprehend more than 1 or 2 exercises at a time. They also might have difficulty understanding the exercise. Gradual introduction tailored to the patient's ability to comprehend and execute the prescribed exercise avoids confusion, potential for harm, increased reactivity, and delayed progress.

Stiffness and Weakness

In cases of excessive stiffness, focus your treatment program on increasing flexibility and range of motion. If you are at a point in the rehabilitation progression where resistive exercise can be initiated, your focus should continue to be on stretching with limited strengthening if excessive stiffness and reactivity are present. Strength with excessive stiffness can contribute to poor function, impingement, chronic pain, and a poor outcome. The reverse is also true; in cases of excessive weakness, focus on strengthening when active motion and resistive exercise are appropriate for the healing bone and soft tissue.

Strengthening

When strengthening, ensure the patient avoids substitution, such as leaning back with the trunk, excessive elevation of the shoulder girdle (shrug sign), and anterosuperior translation of the humeral head. These substitutions might be due to weakness or stiffness, or

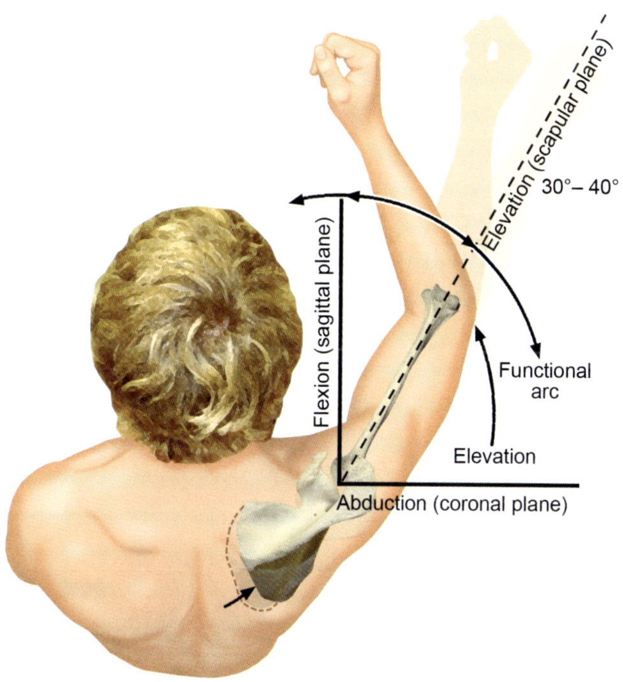

Figure 1. The scapular plane is the plane of maximum elevation and is the preferred plane for overhead motion of the shoulder for all levels of rehabilitation. The humeral head is centered on the glenoid in the scapular plane rather than the coronal plane (abduction) or the sagittal plane (flexion). The scapular plane enhances balanced, relaxed soft tissue and joint capsule, allowing the greatest amount of comfortable motion. It is considered the plane of functional motion.[1]

both. More attention to strengthening exercises in the supine position with presentations of this kind might be more prudent. When excessive stiffness is present, more attention to stretching might be indicated. The rehabilitation provider must monitor the biomechanics of the shoulder during exercise and loading. Overloading creates aberrant movement patterns that create abnormal stress on some structures and might injure the healing tissue. In my experience, the most common result of overloading has been impingement. Overloading of the rotator cuff during forward flexion results in a shrug sign. The humeral head rides up and becomes impinged under the coracoacromial arch. Repeated exercise with this poor biomechanical construct might result in bursal-tendon inflammation, causing substantial reactivity, slowing recovery, and creating unnecessary pain and distress for the patient.

Locked Elbow

At my institution, we advocate exercising the upper extremity in functional patterns that avoid a locked elbow. Straight-arm strengthening increases the lever-arm effect and might be too aggressive for most patients, putting them at risk of injury. With the younger and more athletic population and in specific cases, this is modified but only under the direction and supervision of the clinician.

Pain Medication

Appropriate analgesics and pain medication should be incorporated and administered before exercise to help reduce pain and muscle spasm. Educating patients about the importance of controlling pain helps accomplish early goals and helps with the compliance and willingness of the patient to do the exercise.

Home Program

A home program consists of instruction for coordination of medication, application of heat or ice, and positioning for comfort to help manage pain. Instruction to family and friends and a precise exercise program with diagrams and written instructions will make what is expected clear to all.

Severity of the Injury

Patients who present for postoperative rehabilitation of these injuries demonstrate symptoms of pain, swelling, substantial tenderness about the shoulder and upper quarter, stiffness, and loss of function due to the acute trauma or the ensuing surgical repair. The tissue can be indurated with ecchymosis present in the arm, forearm, chest wall, and sometimes as far down as the flank. The patient should be assured that this is not unusual and will resolve gradually.

Because we see these patients days or weeks after surgery, we must understand the progression of their injuries, how they occurred, the type of fracture, and how the fracture was reduced. A thorough neurovascular examination should be performed because the brachial plexus and axillary nerve are in close proximity and injury to these structures is not uncommon (Figure 2).[3] On further observation, one might see a transient deltoid atony and inferior subluxation (sulcus sign), which can be due to deltoid muscle fatigue rather than axillary nerve palsy (Figure 3). If the condition persists for more than 4 weeks. it should be differentiated as

Figure 2. The proximity of the brachial plexus as it traverses medial to the glenohumeral joint.

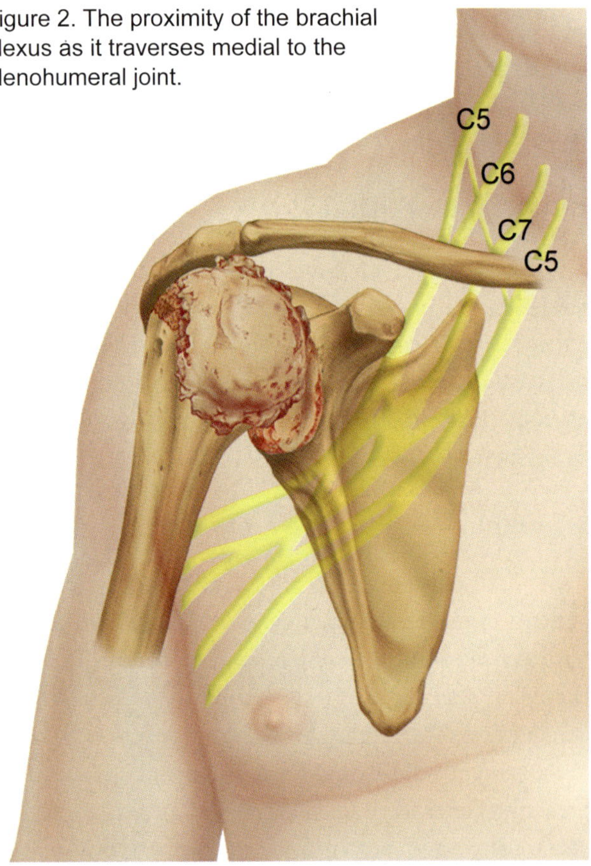

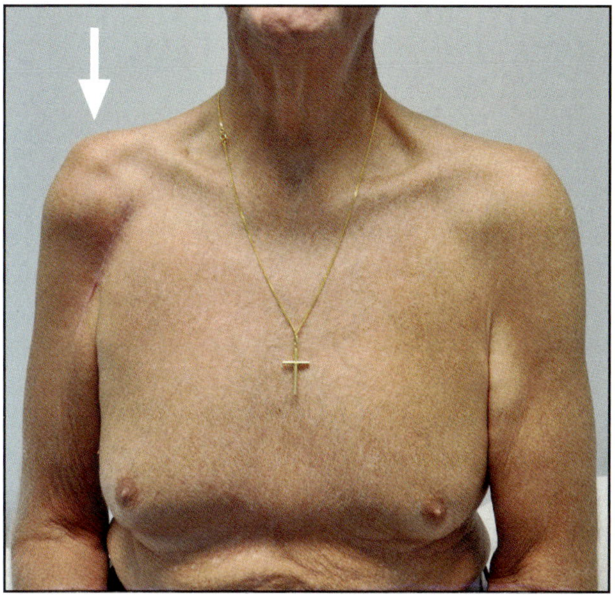

Figure 3. This patient had open reduction and internal fixation of a 4-part fracture. Atrophy of the deltoid and a sulcus sign are apparent. Given the weakness of the rotator cuff and deltoid, the humeral head is subluxed inferiorly and sucks in the tissue in the subacromial space, creating the sulcus sign. The sulcus sign sometimes disappears with initiation of active movement then reappears in the relaxed state.

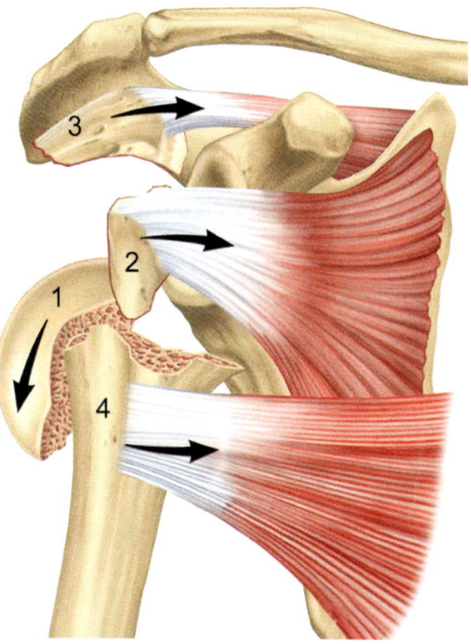

Figure 4A. Fracture segments and the influence of muscle traction on each segment. These patterns are considered when diagnosing and planning the management of these complex fractures.

true axillary nerve palsy. Loss of sensation over the lateral deltoid at the C5 dermatome usually is compromised if an axillary nerve injury is present. This should be well documented.

The amount of trauma and the resulting fracture patterns can be quite complex; therefore, management can be difficult in some cases and can have a less predictable outcome (Figure 4). Knowing the type of fracture classification and how the segments are displaced and reduced will enhance your understanding of why excessive loading and overaggressive treatment in the early and sometimes late stage of recovery can have devastating consequences. In addition, the rotator cuff can be torn in older patients, in whom most proximal humerus fractures occur, or a tear that existed before the fracture can extend.[2] In surgical-neck and anterior fracture-dislocation, one would suspect possible vascular and axillary nerve injury. The clinician always should be watchful because this can become more apparent as rehabilitation progresses. Posterior fracture-dislocation is misdiagnosed frequently because the injury is difficult to evaluate with plain radiographs. Patients usually present with unrelenting pain and have locked external rotation if it is not reduced. They

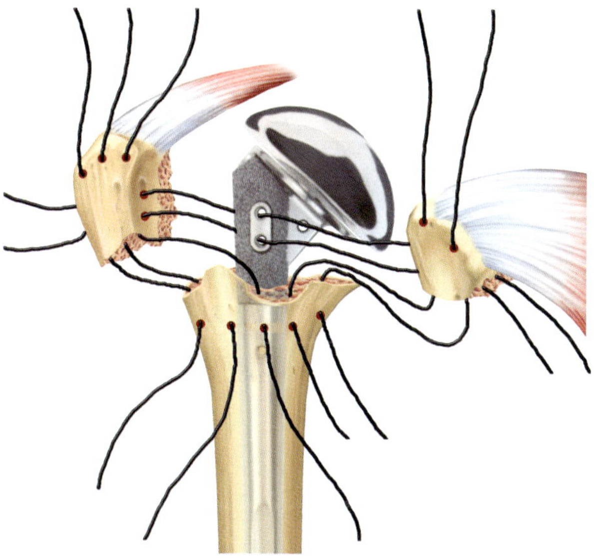

Figure 4B. Four-part fracture with humeral head replacement. The "flying tuberosities" are reduced by suturing them to the humeral head and shaft. Early motion and progression in the rehabilitation program depend on the surgeon's confidence in the repair and tuberosity fixation. In shoulder hemiarthroplasty, the subscapularis repair also must be protected. Motion is limited usually to 30° of external rotation and 130° of elevation in the early rehabilitation phase. Extension and internal rotation are deferred for 6 weeks, and external rotation is limited because these motions put traction across the greater tuberosity repair and subscapularis repair.

usually develop avascular necrosis of the humeral head and subsequently have an ORIF with hemiarthroplasty or a total shoulder arthroplasty, depending on the extent of the glenoid injury.

It is important to understand the forces that we are required to exert at the shoulder and the effect they have on the repaired structures. The goals of closed and surgical management of fractures are to realign and reconstruct bony and soft tissue anatomy. Rehabilitation should be adjusted to the type of fracture (open or closed), the stability of the reduction or fixation, the quality of the bone and soft tissue, the surgical approach, and soft tissue repair.

SPECIFIC REHABILITATION GUIDELINES

An appropriate rehabilitation program after closed reduction and ORIF of proximal humerus fractures ensures a level of maximum recovery that optimizes range of motion, strength, and function but that does not put the patient and repaired structures at risk of failure. This guideline is a working document that when applied appropriately, will help ensure a safe and optimal recovery. The program consists of application of heat or ice; appropriate use of electrical stimulation; gentle mobilization; therapeutic massage; early passive motion (EPM); active-assistive, isometric, stretching, and active exercises; special stretching and resistive exercises; and a home program. These multiple levels of exercise increase in intensity and are applied over

Table 1. Closed Reduction of a Nondisplaced or Minimally Displaced Fracture of the Surgical Neck and the Anatomic Neck and Tuberosity Fracture Displaced Less Than 1 cm

Time After Fracture to Initiate Interventions	Type of Exercise	Specific Exercises
7–10 d[a]	Early passive motion	Pendulum Passive forward elevation Passive external rotation
10 d to 3 wk[a] (when pain has diminished and the patient is less apprehensive)	Active-assistive	Pendulum Active-assistive forward elevation with the opposite hand Active-assistive external rotation to 30° with a stick
4–6 wk[a]	Isometrics (submaximal)	Internal rotation External rotation (at 6 wk) Forward flexion (anterior deltoid) Extension (posterior deltoid) Abduction (middle deltoid)
6–8 wk[b]	Active exercise	Supine active forward elevation with a stick Supine active forward elevation Supine active forward elevation with weights Erect forward elevation with a stick Active extension with a stick Internal rotation up the back Concentric pulleys Eccentric pulleys
8–12 wk[b]	Resistive exercise	Resistive exercises Stretching Advanced stretching

[a] Indicates the goals are to control pain and swelling; protect the fracture site and tuberosity fixation or repair; prevent adhesion formation; increase range of motion in the scapular plane; educate the patient about the importance of medication, ice and heat application, compliance with the program, frequent gentle exercise, rest, and positioning for comfort at home; instruct family or friend; and establish a well-understood home program with a gradual introduction of exercises.
[b] Indicates the goals are to control pain and swelling, increase active range of motion, increase strength, develop neuromuscular control of the shoulder complex, improve proprioception, and normalize response to dynamic challenges.

Table 2. Open Reduction and Internal Fixation for Displaced 2-Part and 3-Part Fractures and Fracture-Dislocations

Time After Fracture to Initiate Interventions	Type of Exercise	Specific Exercises
3–5 d[a]	Early passive motion	Supine external rotation to 30° Supine forward elevation to 130°
7–10 d[a]	Active-assistive	Pendulum External rotation with a stick to 30° Forward elevation with the opposite hand to 140°
4–9 wk[a]	Isometrics (submaximal)	Forward flexion (anterior deltoid) Extension (posterior deltoid) Abduction (lateral deltoid) Internal and external rotation begin at 6–9 wk with a tuberosity fracture
6 wk[b]	Active exercise	Supine active forward elevation with a stick Supine active forward elevation with weights Erect forward elevation with a stick Concentric pulleys Eccentric pulleys Extension Side-lying internal and external rotation
12 wk[b]	Resistive exercise	Resistive exercises Stretching Special stretching

[a] Indicates the goals are to control pain and swelling; protect the fracture site and tuberosity fixation or repair; prevent adhesion formation, increase range of motion in the scapular plane; educate the patient about the importance of medication, ice and heat application, compliance with the program, frequent gentle exercise, rest, and positioning for comfort at home; instruct family or friend; and establish a well-understood home program with a gradual introduction of exercises.
[b] Indicates the goals are to control pain and swelling, increase active range of motion, increase strength, develop neuromuscular control of the shoulder complex, improve proprioception, and normalize response to dynamic challenges.

time as healing and the patient's response dictate. The management and level of recovery depend on several factors. Primary considerations include the complexity of the fracture, the type of reduction, the extent of soft tissue involvement, the patient's age and compliance, degenerative joint disease, concomitant rotator cuff tear, and dislocation. The patients are protected in a sling for 6 weeks. They are encouraged to remove the sling for frequent elbow, wrist, and hand motion performed for 2 to 3 minutes frequently throughout the day. The progression and intensity of treatment then are individualized and based on the configuration of the fracture, the apparent and tested stability of the fracture, signs of fracture healing and callus formation determined by radiography, and the patient's response and tolerance to the exercises.

Pendulum exercises and EPM are initiated with closed reduction after approval of the surgeon, which is usually 7 to 10 days after closed reduction (Table 1). With ORIF, pendulum exercises and EPM can be started sooner (usually the second or third postoperative day) because of the more stable surgical fixation (Table 2). Patients with hemiarthroplasty are managed in a similar manner with some modified requirements and precautions (Table 3). Patients are encouraged to perform the pendulum exercises 4 to 5 times per day. In our program, we use a modified pendulum exercise that is less demanding but accomplishes the expected goals. We consider the pendulum exercise to be a relaxation and warm-up exercise and a precursor to increasing range of motion rather than an exercise to increase range of motion. The patient is instructed to bend forward slowly at the waist and allow the upper extremity to relax and hang in the dependent position. The patient should support the upper body on a stable surface, such as a countertop or tabletop, to protect and take stress off of the low back. The weight of the extremity initiates a gentle traction across the joint, facilitating relaxation of the periscapular, rotator cuff, and deltoid muscles. The patient gently rocks his or her

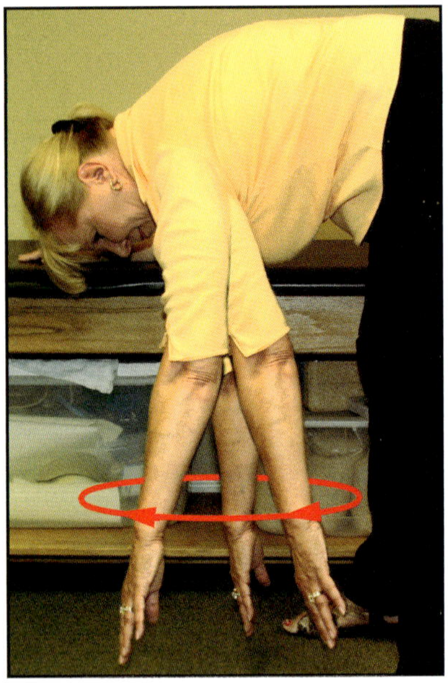

Figure 5. Pendulum exercise. The patient bends at the waist supported by a countertop and gently rocks her body to create momentum and small clockwise and counter-clockwise circles, performing 10 clockwise then 10 counterclockwise circles.

body to create a momentum that in turn allows stress-free, small circular motion to occur at the shoulder. The rotational motion at the glenohumeral joint and scapulothoracic articulation further enhance relaxation and easy motion (Figure 5).

Early Passive Motion

Early passive motion is considered the cornerstone of a successful result if bony and soft tissues are not overstressed and adequate pain control is achieved.[1–4] McCann et al[5] found that in the supine position, passive external rotation and elevation in the scapular plane demonstrated the least electromyographic (EMG) activity of the rotator cuff and deltoid muscles. They reported that providing oral cues to the patient to allow his or her extremity to become like a rag doll

Table 3. Postoperative Rehabilitation Guidelines for Hemiarthroplasty for 4-Part Fractures, Some 3-Part Fractures, Fracture-Dislocations, Head-Splitting Fractures, and Impression Fractures Involving More Than 40% of the Articular Surface

Time After Fracture to Initiate Interventions	Type of Exercise	Specific Exercises
3–5 d[a]	Early passive motion	Supine external rotation to 30° Supine forward flexion to 130° Elbow, wrist, and hand range of motion
7–10 d[a]	Active-assistive	Pendulum External rotation with a stick Forward flexion Internal rotation and extension with a stick begin at 6 wk
4–9 wk[a]	Isometrics (submaximal)	Anterior, posterior, and middle deltoid Multiangle Internal or external rotation begin at 6–9 wk
6 wk[b]	Active exercise	Pulley Supine forward flexion with a stick Supine forward flexion with a stick and weight (1–2 lb) Supine forward flexion Eccentric pulleys Side-lying active external rotation Eccentric pulleys Standing press with a stick Eccentric standing press with a stick Active forward flexion Prone extension and abduction
12 wk[b]	Advanced stretching Resistive exercise	Follow exercise figures Progress as tolerated

[a] Indicates the goals are to control pain and swelling; protect the fracture site and tuberosity fixation or repair; prevent adhesion formation; increase range of motion in the scapular plane; educate the patient about the importance of medication, ice and heat application, compliance with the program, frequent gentle exercise, rest, and positioning for comfort at home; instruct family or friend; and establish a well-understood home program with a gradual introduction of exercises.
[b] Indicates the goals are to control pain and swelling, increase active range of motion, increase strength, develop neuromuscular control of the shoulder complex, improve proprioception, and normalize response to dynamic challenges.

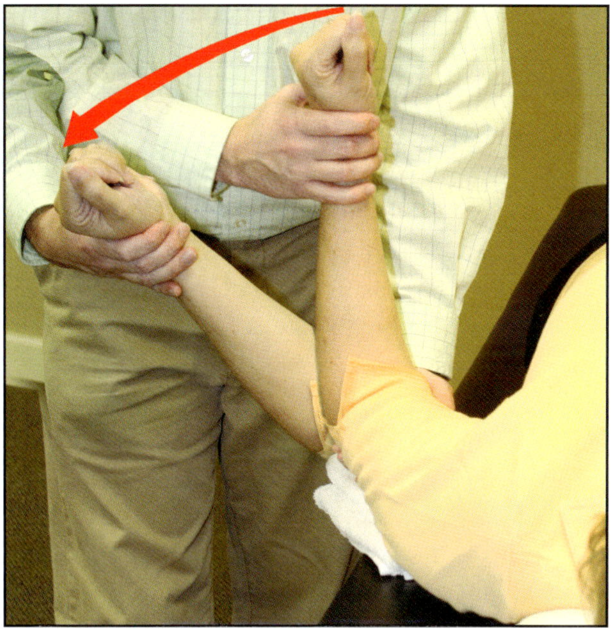

Figure 6A. Supine passive external rotation. The rehabilitation provider supports the elbow and holds the wrist. Giving oral cues for the patient to relax, the rehabilitation provider externally rotates the upper extremity to a point of stiffness and then repeats the activity.

is an important factor in facilitating relaxed passive motion. Elevation with a bent rather than extended elbow also generated significantly less activity of the supraspinatus and middle deltoid. They demonstrated that early safe motion and protection of the repaired bone and soft tissue can be accomplished. Our program initiates with instruction in the pendulum exercise followed by passive external rotation with the upper extremity placed comfortably on a pillow at the side in the supine (Figure 6A) or sitting (Figure 6B) position based on comfort or preference and supine passive forward flexion in the scapular plane (Figure 7). The upper extremity is placed on a pillow to avoid extension by keeping it in the neutral position. With the extremity supported at the elbow and held at the wrist, gentle oscillations are started for muscle relaxation before gentle external rotation. Depending on the type of fracture, limits of motion sometimes are not imposed in closed reduction. During the procedure, the surgeon determines the amount of motion after ORIF through trial motion, assessing the bone and soft tissue stability; it usually is 30° of external rotation and 130° of forward flexion. Slow gentle motion with the elbow in slight flexion is undertaken initially. Constant communication with the patient and feedback during

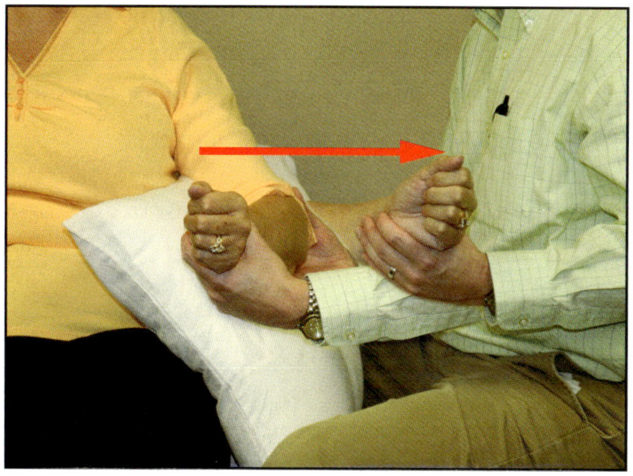

Figure 6B. Sitting external rotation. The extremity is supported with a pillow in the plane of the scapula. The rehabilitation provider supports the elbow; holds the wrist; and after giving oral cues to relax, externally rotates the extremity.

the exercise guide the amount of motion for each treatment session. Forward elevation is accomplished in a similar manner, with the arc of motion going no higher than 130° in the scapular plane. To ensure true passive motion, the rehabilitation provider must give oral cues to relax the extremity throughout the activity. In some instances, the sitting position (Figure 6B) might be more comfortable. One should proceed cautiously in this position when performing elevation. After elevating the extremity to 130°, bringing the extremity back

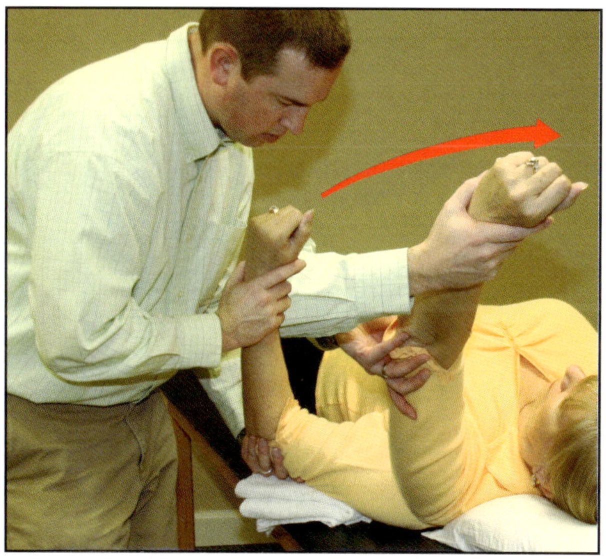

Figure 7. Supine passive forward flexion. The patient lies supine with a towel under the elbow. The rehabilitation provider holds the wrist, supports the elbow, and performs forward flexion in the plane of the scapula. Oral cues from the rehabilitation provider to relax the shoulder and upper extremity accompany the motion.

down might be difficult because some people begin to actively guard if they feel discomfort. Support and oral cues to let the extremity go can help avoid any undue discomfort. In this situation, the exercise becomes eccentric if relaxation is not accomplished, thus putting stress on the bone and soft tissue repair. If this occurs, revert to the supine position. The development of trust between the rehabilitation provider and patient is initiated on the first meeting. Fostering this relationship cannot be overemphasized as you proceed through the recovery process. Educating the patient about the intended goals of treatment and being responsive to his or her feedback will ensure a positive working relationship throughout this sometimes lengthy process.

Active-Assistive Exercise

Limited external rotation with a stick (Figure 8) and supine forward flexion using the opposite extremity (Figure 9) are initiated usually at 10 days to 3 weeks after closed reduction or at 7 to 10 days after ORIF. Limits of motion can vary in closed reduction according to the surgeon. With ORIF, motion usually is limited to 30° of external rotation and 130° of forward flexion in the plane of the scapula. The patient is instructed to move to the point of stiffness, proceed into the tightness, and hold for a count of 5. This is repeated 10 times 4 to 5 times per day. Exercise should

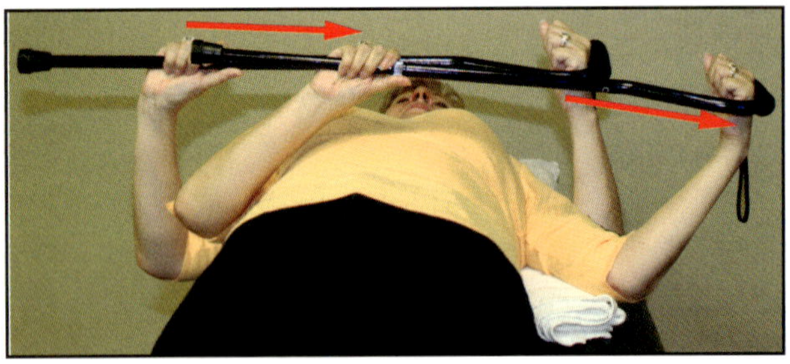

Figure 8. Active-assistive external rotation. The patient lies supine with a small pillow underneath the affected elbow as illustrated, maintaining the arm in the plane of the scapula instead of extension. The end of the stick is placed in the affected hand, and the opposite hand pushes the affected hand gently outward on a slight angle, keeping the elbow flexed to 90°. The position is held for the count of 5 to 10. The patient then returns to the starting position.

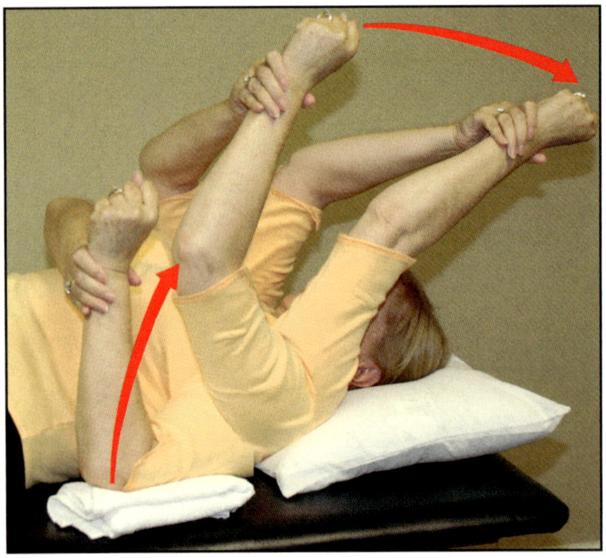

Figure 9. Supine active-assistive forward flexion. The patient lies supine with a pillow under the affected extremity. The hand on the unaffected side reaches across the body; grasps the wrist of the affected extremity; lifts the extremity above the head to a target, such as a headboard or a wall; and returns it back to the starting position. As end range of motion becomes easier, the patient moves slightly away from the wall or headboard to increase elevation.

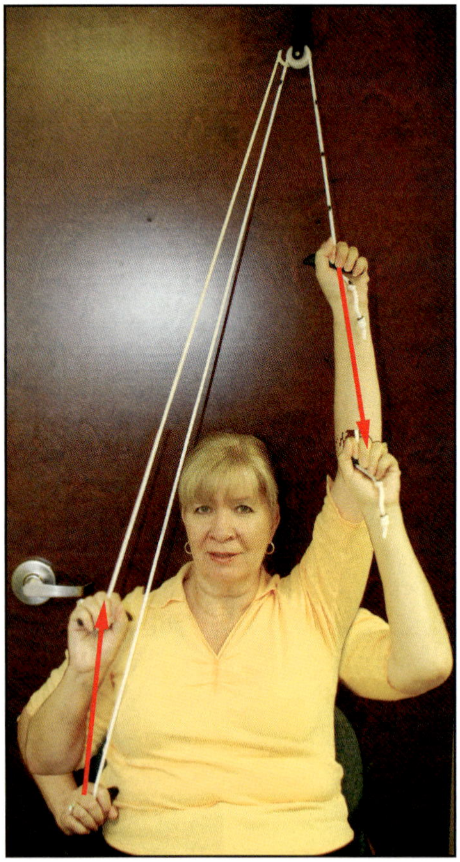

Figure 10. Active-assistive pulleys. The patient is instructed to sit in a chair and hold the handles of the pulley system. Next, she is instructed to relax the involved extremity and use the unaffected extremity to pull the involved extremity gently above the head. The patient is continually instructed to relax the involved extremity. Note the pulley block is located over the involved extremity, which ensures elevation in the plane of the scapula.

be coordinated with medication, preceded by heat or ice, and followed by ice as needed. These exercises continue for 6 weeks with the limits of 30° of external rotation and 130° of elevation in the case of ORIF.

At 6 weeks, adequate healing has occurred to initiate the pulley exercise, extension with the stick, and internal rotation up the back. The pulley exercise develops a substantial increase in EMG activity of the spinati and deltoid muscles (Figure 10). With large and massive rotator cuff tears and tuberosity fixation in fractures, the activity can put undue stress across the repaired rotator cuff and tuberosity. By the nature of motion, extension (Figure 11) and internal rotation (Figure 12) put stress across the rotator cuff and tuberosity fixation. Therefore, these exercises are delayed until 6 weeks when adequate healing has occurred. Gentle motion is encouraged with internal rotation, especially with tuberosity and rotator cuff conditions.

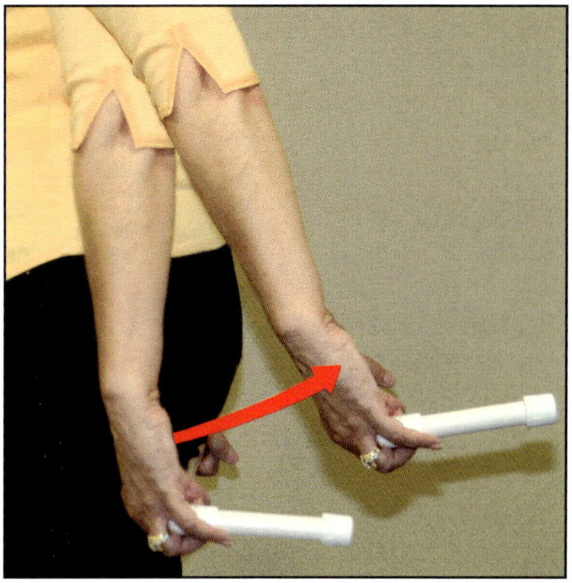

Figure 11. Standing active-assistive extension. The patient grasps the stick behind the back and lifts it away from the body with the unaffected extremity helping the affected extremity. She maintains an erect posture and avoids bending forward. Standing in front of a wall or a door might assist in this exercise.

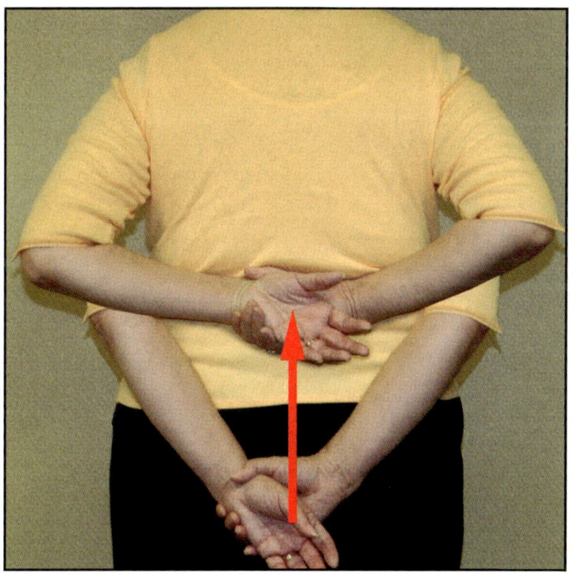

Figure 12. Active-assistive internal rotation. The patient is instructed to grasp the affected extremity at the wrist or the thumb. Using the unaffected extremity, she supplies power to bend the elbow and slide the hand up the middle of the back to the point of stiffness. She holds the position for the count of 5 then returns to the starting position.

Isometric Exercise

The introduction of submaximal isometric exercise can vary depending on the type of fracture and the surgeon's preferred application. More conservative variables of management defer isometrics until 9 weeks after injury with fractures involving the tuberosities. Earlier, more aggressive management initiates submaximal isometrics at 4 to 6 weeks after closed reduction and ORIF (eg, nondisplaced fractures, impaction fractures, surgical-neck and head-splitting fractures). As with all exercise application, specific instruction from the surgeon must be followed on a patient-by-patient basis. Submaximal isometric exercises, including anterior deltoid (Figure 13A), middle deltoid (Figure

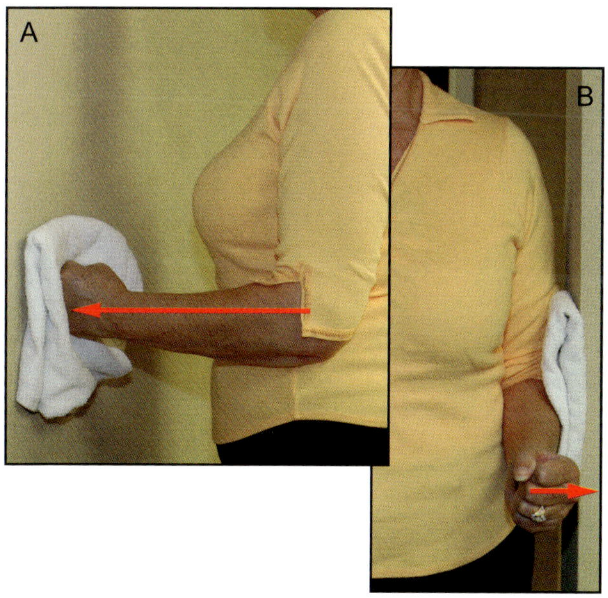

Figure 13. Isometric exercises to the anterior deltoid, A, and middle deltoid, B. The patient uses a towel and presses into the wall for the count of 10 then relaxes. These exercises are repeated 5 to 10 times.

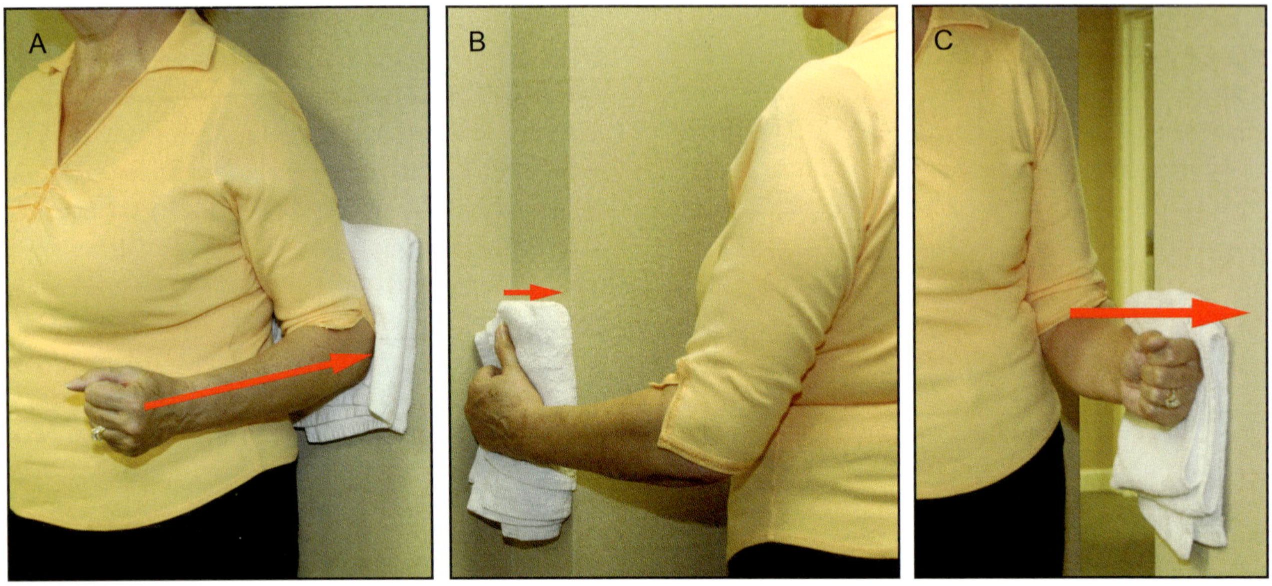

Figure 14. Isometric exercises to the posterior deltoid, A, internal rotators, B, and external rotators, C. The patient uses a towel and presses into the wall for the count of 10 then relaxes. Exercises are repeated 5 to 10 times.

13B), posterior deltoid (Figure 14A), and internal and external rotation (Figure 14 B and C), can be initiated with the upper extremity at the side. Exercise should be pain-free and gentle. Five repetitions held to a count of 5 are adequate initially and can increase to 10 repetitions as the exercise becomes more familiar and comfortable. Isolating selected muscles helps the patient identify and initiate a comfortable muscle contraction that might have been difficult to perform previously. Given that isometric exercise can demonstrate a marked increase in EMG activity if performed to maximum contraction, internal and external rotation are deferred for 6 to 9 weeks in greater tuberosity fractures and fractures managed with shoulder replacement. This prevents direct pull across the subscapularis and tuberosity repairs, avoiding the risk of avulsion or displacement.[5]

Isometrics are an important step in neuromuscular re-education. The patient should not feel pain during this exercise progression. Younger patients usually progress quickly through this phase, whereas older patients might require more attention and instruction to perform the exercises properly. In cases of excessive weakness with external rotation, patients might benefit from performing multiangle supine external rotation isometrics (Figure 15).

Active Exercise (Early Strengthening)

Active exercise is considered early strengthening. Patients are out of the sling and are encouraged to use their affected extremities in a functional manner below the horizontal plane. Patients are discouraged from lifting weighted objects at this time. Exercise in the supine position is the initial step for undertaking progressive strengthening of the shoulder muscles. The upper extremity weighs approximately 5% of body mass.[6] In the erect position, the effects of gravity and subacromial contact increase when approaching the critical

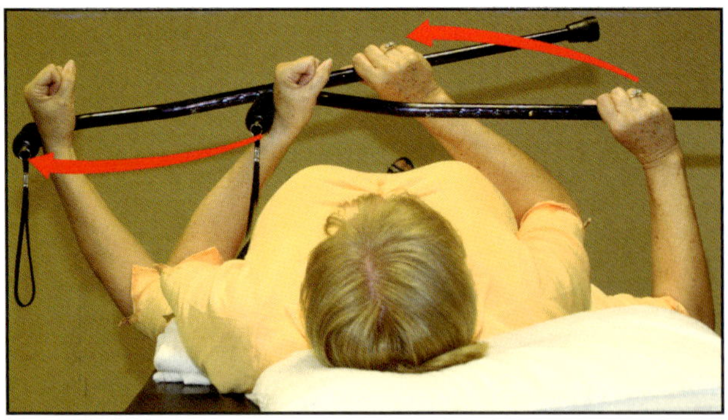

Figure 15. Multiangle external rotation isometric. The patient lies supine with a folded towel under the affected extremity. The cane is held in the unaffected hand, and the hook of the cane is put over the wrist of the involved extremity. The patient pushes out at different points in the range of motion, holds for the count of 10, relaxes, moves out slightly, holds for the count of 10, and progresses through the full range.

point of 60° to 120° of forward flexion. This arc of motion is considered the arc of maximum subacromial contact.[7] One can ascertain that the rotator cuff must have adequate compressive and depressive force to maintain the head centered in the glenoid, avoiding excessive riding up under the coracoacromial arch during the elevation phase. After the substantial trauma, these patients probably do not have adequate rotator cuff and surrounding muscle strength to perform this activity without pain and substitution. One of our goals during rehabilitation is to maintain good mechanics during comfortable exercise. Exercise in the supine position lends itself to accomplishing this goal. The trunk is supported and relaxed in this position with a pillow placed under the elbow to maintain good alignment in neutral. The relaxed supine position allows the patient to focus on shoulder motion. He or she holds a stick in both hands (Figure 16) and initiates flexion, moving toward the ceiling then overhead. This closed loop activity provides support from the opposite extremity as the patient moves through the motion. Patients tend to be more comfortable with this exercise because it allows them to control discomfort and weakness during forward flexion if it presents. As motion approaches 60° of elevation, the effects of gravity and the weight of the extremity begin to diminish. As 90° of elevation is approached, gravity has no essential effect on the weight of the extremity. As the patient approaches 120° of elevation, gravity facilitates flexion. In this position, motion is more comfortable while maintaining good mechanics under the coracoacromial arch, facilitating neuromuscular re-education and strengthening of the rotator cuff and deltoid. Normal posterior and downward accessory motion of the humeral head also is enhanced by this position. Gradual loading to a 2-pound (0.90-kg) weight and conditioning in this position can progress (Figure 17). Single-extremity elevation follows (Figure 18). At 12 weeks, the extremity can be gradually loaded with 1 to 2 pounds (0.45–0.90 kg) of weight to initiate resistive exercise in this supine position if the patient has weakness in the erect position. Active external rotation in the

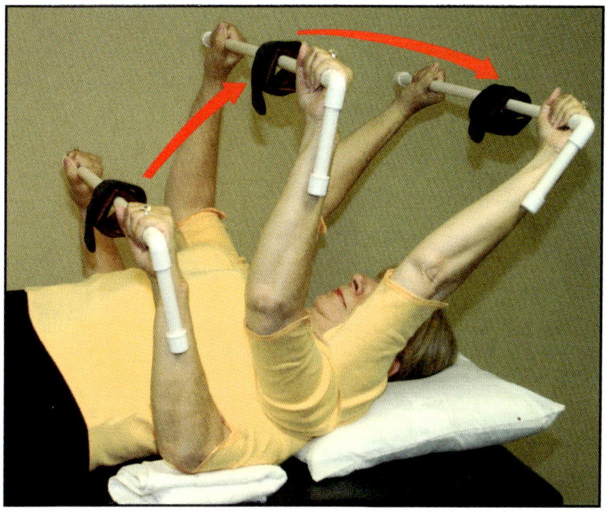

Figure 17. Active forward flexion with a weighted stick. Attach a light weight (1–2 lb [0.45–0.90 kg]) to the stick and repeat the motions of the forward-flexion-with-a-stick exercise.

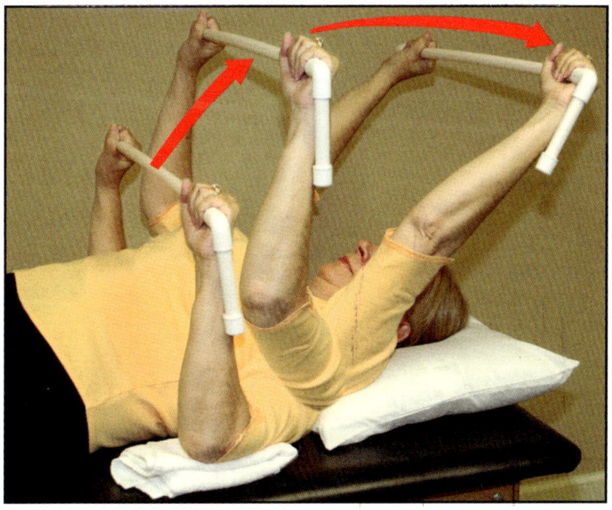

Figure 16. Active forward flexion with a stick. The patient is instructed to lie supine holding a stick, slowly raise the stick across her face and over her head to the point of stiffness, then return to the starting position.

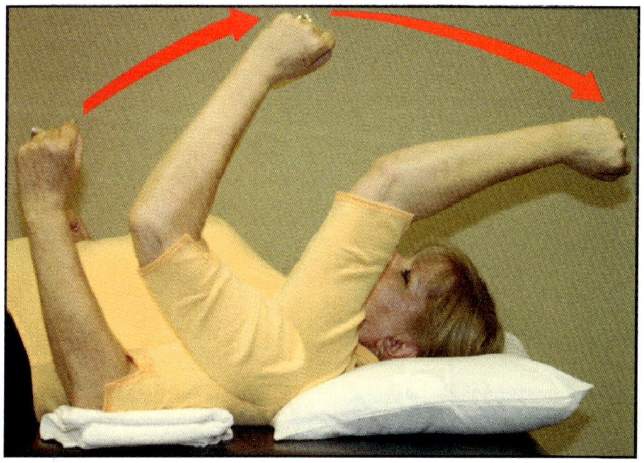

Figure 18. Active forward flexion. The extremity is supported on a pillow. The patient is instructed to slowly raise her hand over her head with a bent elbow. As she proceeds with the hand moving over the head, the elbow begins to straighten. The extremity is lowered in the same manner.

side-lying position also is initiated (Figure 19). This position can be used at 12 weeks with light weight for isolated supraspinatus, infraspinatus, and teres minor exercise. Active forward flexion with a stick (closed loop) in the erect position facilitates the controlled loading and support for the involved extremity (Figure 20). Watching for proper mechanics at this transition is important. Prone exercise isolates the posterior cuff and periscapular muscles. The patient lies in the prone position with the extremity over the side of the plinth and performs prone abduction with the palm down (Figure 21) followed by the more demanding prone abduction with the thumb pointing up (Figure 22). All exercises are performed to a limit below the horizontal and ensure protection of the anterior structures. These exercises are useful for strengthening the cuff while avoiding irritation of a sometimes reactive subacromial space. Manual resistive exercise and a weight of 1 to 2 pounds (0.45–0.90 kg) can be added at 12 weeks when resistive exercise is appropriate. The patient is advanced as he or she responds to the exercise and develops comfort, strength, control, and confidence.

Eccentric loading is initiated using the pulley system (Figure 23) and the standing press with a stick (Figure 24). The pulley block must be positioned over the involved shoulder. This position maintains the upper extremity in the plane of the scapula during exercise. The patient pulls up the involved extremity to the limits of motion. He or she then lowers the involved extremity under his or her own power, following the handle down. Following the handle is a safety precaution in case of pain, weakness, or loss of control and protects the involved shoulder. A critical point for which to watch during this exercise is at 120° of flexion because the presence of pain or weakness will become apparent at this position. Substitution, shrug sign, or giving way due to the pain will present if this exercise is too

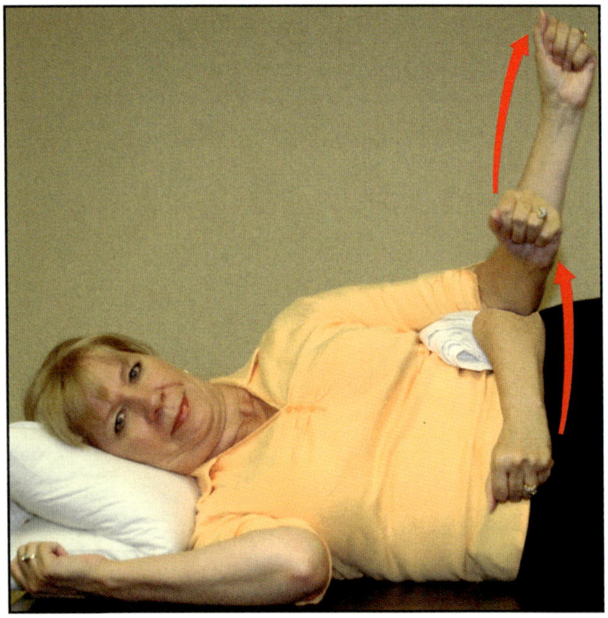

Figure 19. Side-lying active external rotation. The patient lies on her side with a pillow under the affected extremity and her elbow flexed to 90°. She slowly rotates the forearm away from the center of the body to a comfortable end range.

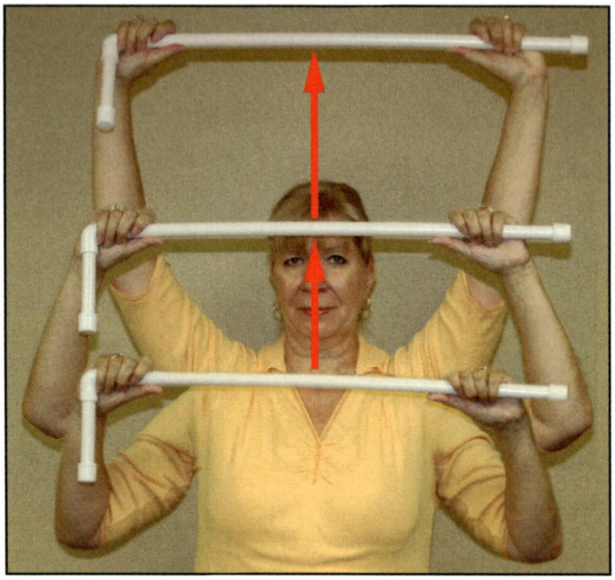

Figure 20. Standing active press. The patient holds the stick, performs a standing press over the head, then lowers it to the starting position.

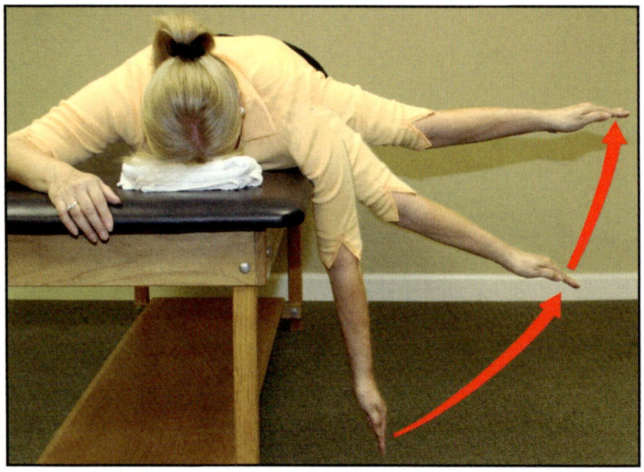

Figure 21. Prone active modified abduction with the palm down. The patient lies prone with the extremity hanging over the table and the palm facing down. She raises the extremity in an abduction motion to three-fourths the distance to the horizontal then lowers to the starting position.

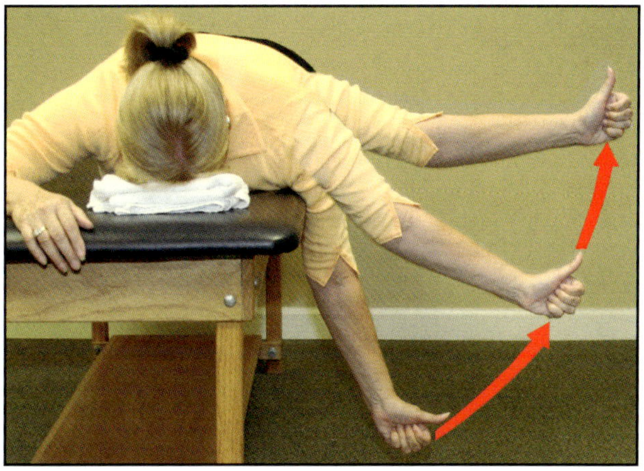

Figure 22. Prone active modified abduction with the thumb pointing up. The patient hangs the extremity over the side of the table and rotates the palm so the thumb is facing up. She is instructed to slowly raise the extremity to three-fourths the distance to the horizontal then to lower to the starting position.

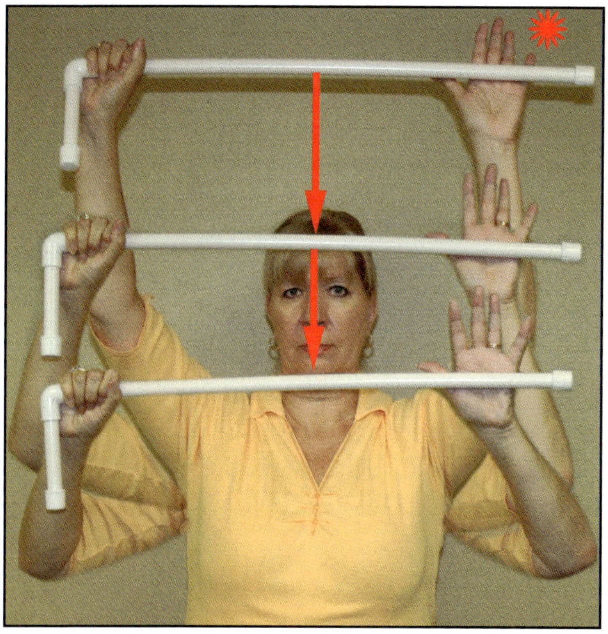

Figure 24. Standing active eccentric press. The patient performs the activity as the standing press; however, when the patient gets to maximum elevation, she lifts the hand off the bar and follows the bar down using her own power to lower the extremity to the starting position.

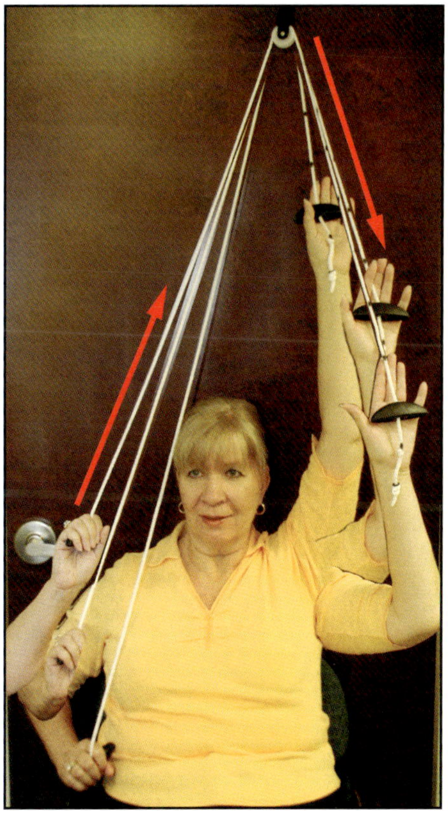

Figure 23. Active eccentric pulleys. The patient stretches the affected extremity as high as it can go. Next, she opens the hand; lifts off the pulley handle; and under her own power, lowers the hand as it follows the pulley down to the starting position. The exercise is repeated 10 times.

aggressive. The substitution suggests that the shoulder is not strong enough to maintain stability, the head rides up, and impingement occurs. More support of the opposite extremity is helpful. If the patient cannot adjust, then the exercise should be performed at a later time because substantial irritation usually will develop.

Advanced Stretching Exercise

The fracture is sufficiently healed at 12 weeks to tolerate more forceful stretching. Advanced stretching is one of the most important exercise progressions because it addresses the combination and melding of the planar motions to optimize global movement, most specifically at the glenohumeral joint. Active sliding of the hand up the wall to gain range of motion with the assistance of the uninvolved extremity and initiation of periscapular upward rotation in the erect position is one of the first advanced stretching exercises. The patient then attempts to press the axilla into the wall as he or she stretches upward (Figure 25). Patients can be quite stiff and sore with this exercise because it stretches the anteroinferior structures and can increase compression in the subacromial space. A slow, gentle progression of intensity of stretching is encouraged. As the patient progresses to 140° of forward elevation comfortably, a combined flexion, external rotation, and abduction stretch is initiated and performed in the supine position (Figure 26). At the end position, the patient presses the extremities into the table. This combined stretch tends to open up and stretch the anteroinferior structures of the glenohumeral joint and axilla. The over-the-door-hang is more aggressive and applies more force to the overhead stretch (Figure 27). Patients are reminded that this is not a pull-up but a hang-down exercise. They are instructed to reach the top of the door or chin-up bar by only tightening with their finger tips and relaxing the rest of the upper extremity. Next, they can apply stretch by bending their knees, allowing the weight of their bodies to increase the force applied to the soft tissues of the shoulder. This stretch should be gradual because of the potential for substantial force. The standing 90°/90° stretch continues to address the anteroinferior soft tissues of the glenohumeral joint (Figure 28). When patients are instructed to assume this position of combined planar motion, limitations are noted. The opposite side can approach the normal external rotation in the abducted position while the involved side appears adducted and internally rotated due to the shortened soft tissues in the area of the anterior and inferior glenohumeral joint. Patients are instructed to assume the corner position and lean into the corner with

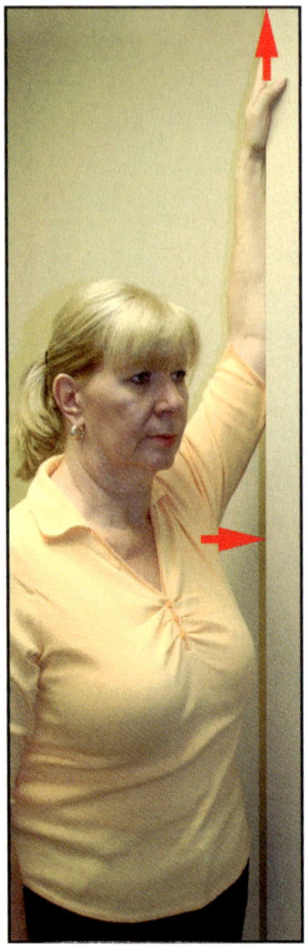

Figure 25. Advanced stretching with 1 extremity. The patient places her hand on the wall and slides her hand up the wall, reaching and stretching in an attempt to press the axilla into the flat surface.

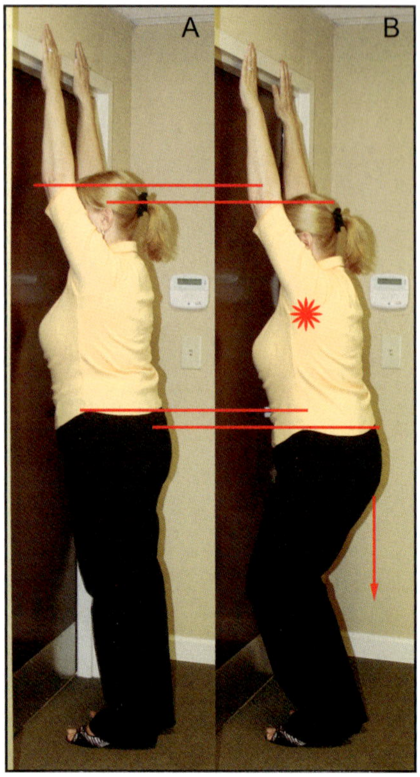

Figure 27. Over-the-door hang. A, The patient slides both hands to the top of the door and grasps the top of the door with her fingertips. B, She gently applies the stretch by slowly bending her knees. She increases the weight and stretches as tolerated by taking more weight off the lower extremities and by bending the knees.

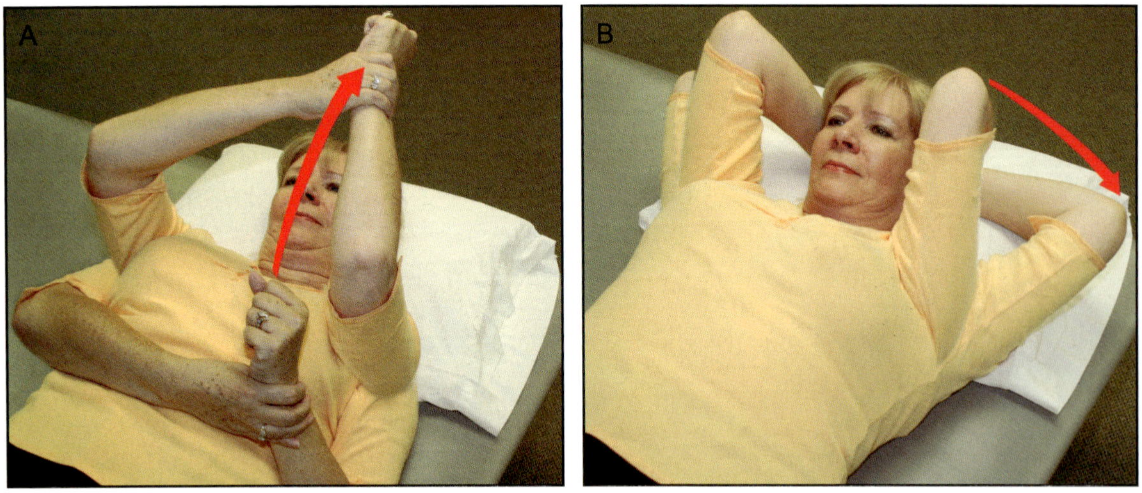

Figure 26. Hands clasped behind the head with the elbows abducted. A, In 1 motion, the patient brings her hands above her head. B, Reaching behind her head, she clasps her hands and brings her elbows back into the mat, then she reverses the action, bringing the elbows together.

their upper bodies (Figure 28). The advanced version of internal rotation involves the use of a towel or a countertop (Figures 29A and 29B). Finally, a posterior capsular stretch is accomplished by horizontally adducting the upper extremity with force applied from the opposite extremity (Figure 30). The presence of posterior capsular tightness can add to anterosuperior humeral head translation, contributing to impingement and development of anterior shoulder pain. If the scapula is very mobile, the supine position is used to stabilize it against the thoracic wall.

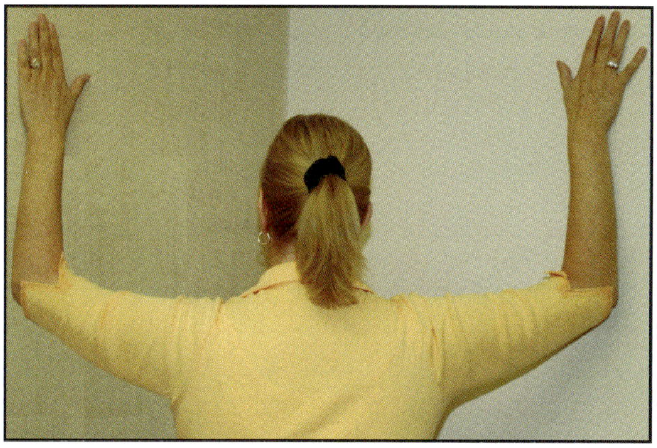

Figure 28. Standing 90°/90° of external rotation corner stretch. The patient is instructed to put her extremities out to the side with the shoulders at 90° of abduction and the elbows bent to 90° in the 90°/90° position. She is instructed to slowly lean into the corner to stretch. She holds the position for the count of 5 or 10 then repeats the stretch.

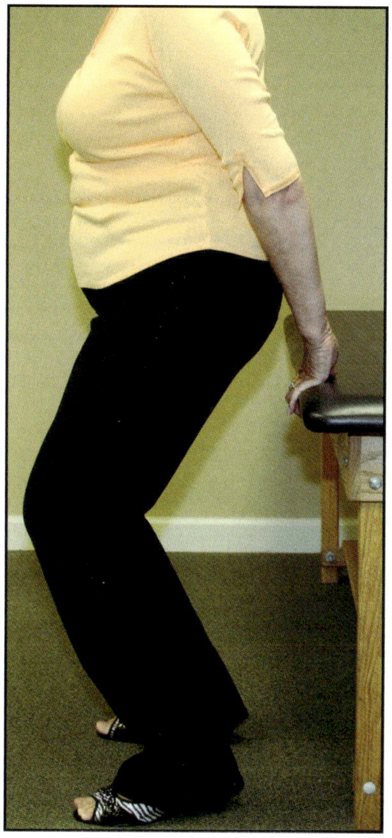

Figure 29B. The patient stands in front of a countertop and places her hand behind her back, holding onto the counter with the affected extremity. Next, she is instructed to bend her knees so the hand slides up the back.

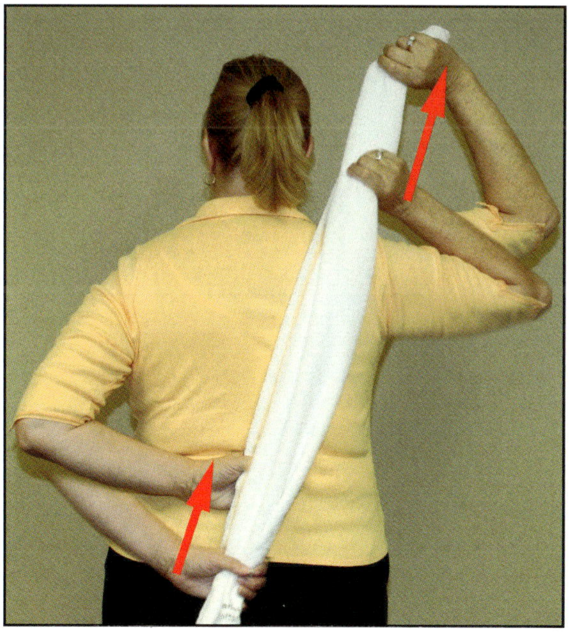

Figure 29A. Advanced internal rotation stretch. With a towel, the patient pulls the affected extremity up the center of the back using the opposite extremity overhead.

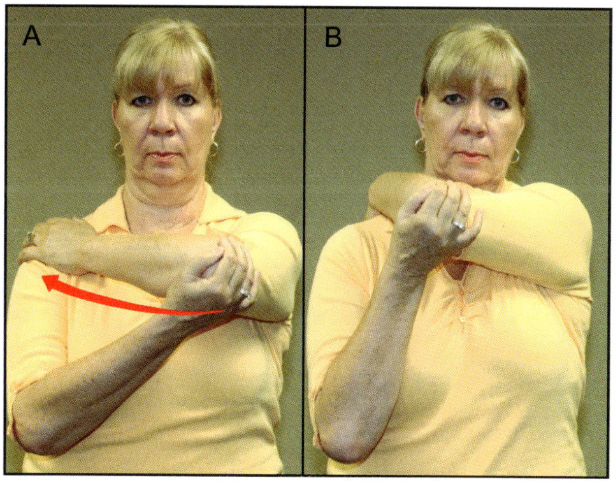

Figure 30 A and B. Posterior capsule stretch. The patient is instructed to raise her extremity to the horizontal position and, with the other hand, to press the extremity toward the opposite shoulder. The position is held for the count of 5 to 10 then repeated.

Resistive Exercise

At 12 weeks after surgery, the fractures and repaired soft tissues are healed. Pain-free strengthening begins with a 1- to 3-pound (0.45-kg–1.35-kg) weight and elastic bands or tubes. The focus of strengthening is on the rotator cuff, deltoid, and periscapular muscles. In younger patients who have higher functional demands, a program of plyometrics, timing exercises, and conditioning might be undertaken after the standard resistive exercise program. Poppen and Walker[6] and Inman et al[8] found that joint reaction force at the glenohumeral joint while raising the upper extremity in abduction approximates body mass. A considerable amount of force occurs at the glenohumeral joint with elevation and should be considered during resistive exercise. Attention must be paid to the arthrokinematics when resistance is applied. In all cases during rehabilitation, be mindful that exercises that are too strenuous and cause aberrant movement and poor mechanics can result in irritation of the soft tissues and development of pain, so they should be avoided. The strengthening exercises should be pain-free as a progressive system of increasing resistance is applied with light weight, elastic bands, and elastic tubing. Resisted external rotation strengthens the posterior rotator cuff muscles. Attention should be paid to the excursion and the position of the scapula (Figure 31). If retraction of the scapula and riding back of the shoulder girdle are noted, the patient can perform this exercise in the supine position to stabilize the scapula so more excursion occurs at the glenohumeral joint (Figure 32). External rotation while abducting the elbows is a complex exercise that requires a coordinated activation of multiple muscles (Figure 33). This exercise simultaneously activates the infraspinatus and teres minor for external rotation and the supraspinatus and deltoid to accomplish abduction while the periscapular muscles also stabilize. The hands must lead and continue through an arc of motion to approximately 45° of abduction. Internal rotation is performed by bringing the hand to the stomach (Figure 34). Some patients bring the hand across the trunk, which alters the focus of the exercise and should be corrected. Observation of this exercise for good form and correction for substitution and poor technique are important to ensure the exercise is effective. Extension is performed to the midline of the trunk from a flexed position (Figure 35). Resisted forward flexion starts with the extremity at the side (Figure 36). The patient is instructed to perform an upper cut to approximately 90° of elevation. Scapular mechanics should be observed with this exercise. Anterior shoulder pain or the shrug sign, or both, is an indication of overloading,

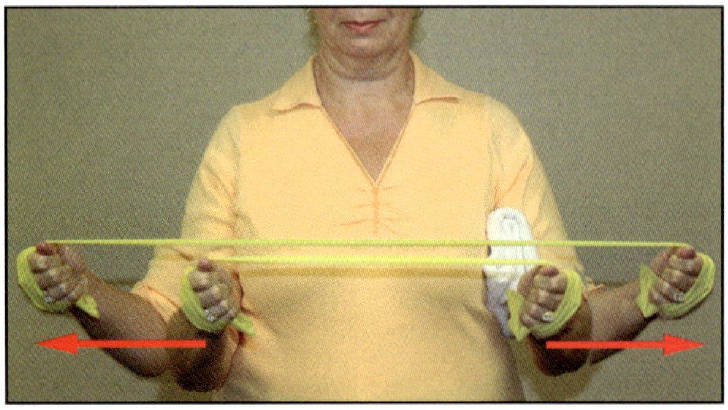

Figure 31. Erect resisted external rotation. The patient places a folded towel between the waist and arm. Keeping the elbow close to the waist, she pulls the elastic-resistance band outward.

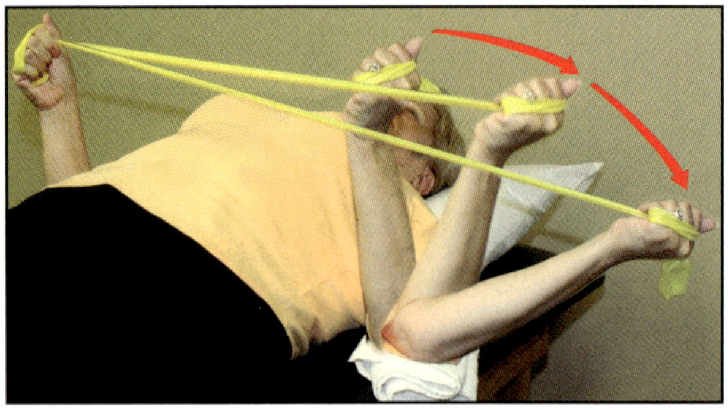

Figure 32. Supine resisted external rotation. With a pillow under the elbow and the extremity bent to 90°, the patient externally rotates the involved extremity against the resistance of the elastic band.

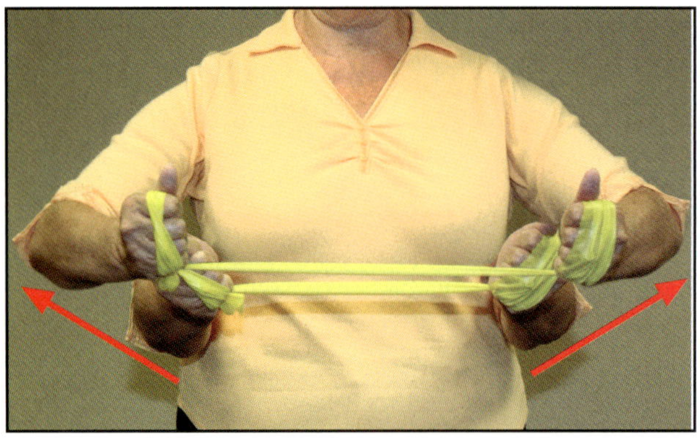

Figure 33. Resisted abduction. The patient holds the elastic-resistance band. With the elbows held at 90°, she brings her hands and elbows away from the sides of her body to approximately 45° of abduction, keeping the elbow and hand in the same plane.

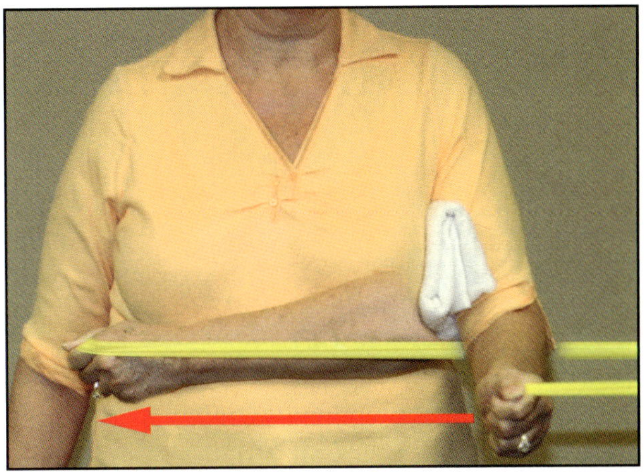

Figure 34. Resisted internal rotation. Attach 1 end of the elastic-resistance band to a stationary object. Instruct the patient to place a folded towel under the affected extremity. She stands at a right angle to the attachment and with the extremity pressed to the towel, internally rotates, bringing the hand to the stomach.

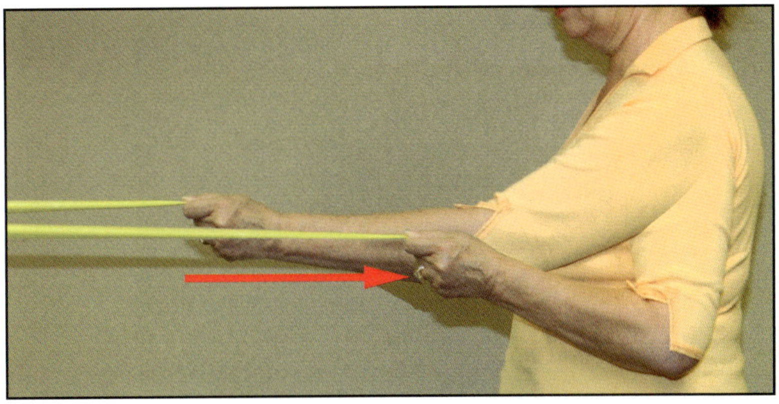

Figure 35. Resisted extension. The patient attaches the elastic-resistance band to a stationary object or doorknob and with the extremity positioned as illustrated, brings the elbow back to the plane of the trunk.

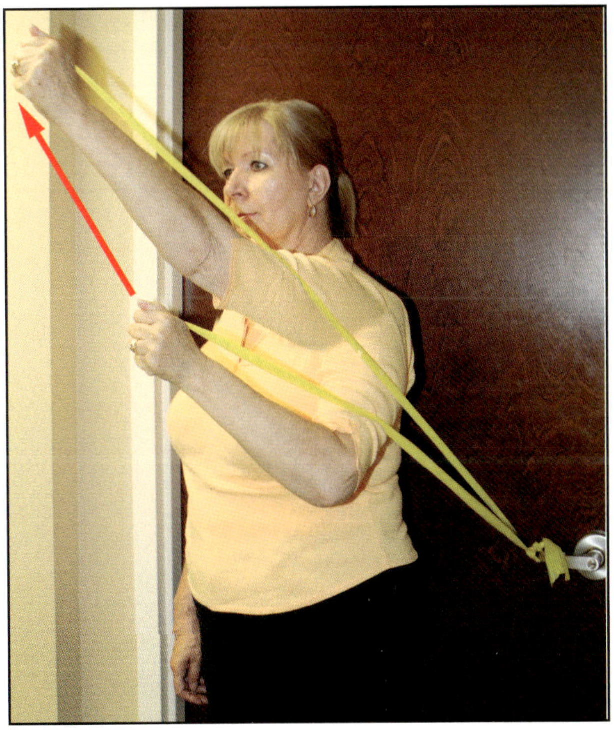

Figure 36. Resisted flexion. The patient attaches the elastic-resistance band to a doorknob and stands at a right angle to the door so the doorknob is by the elbow. Next, she performs an upper cut.

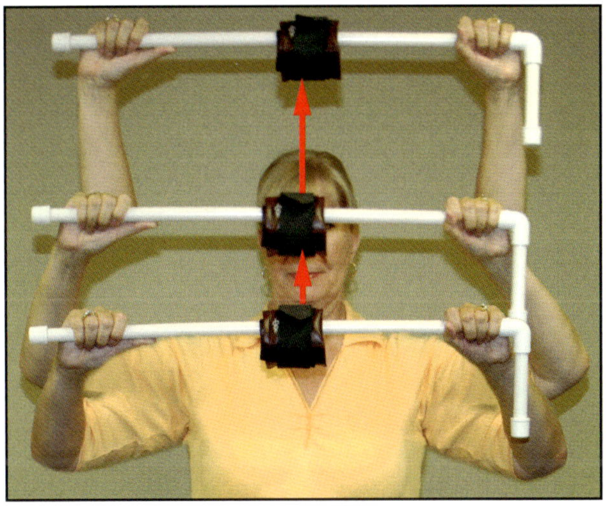

Figure 37. Standing press with a stick and a 1 or 2 lb (0.45-kg or 0.90-kg) weight.

thus resistance should be reduced. The standing press initiates strengthening through a full arc of flexion with the stick and a 1- to 2-pound (0.45-kg–0.90-kg) weight (Figure 37). This closed loop activity supports the involved extremity as it elevates with resistance. The 1-arm standing press is the next progression in overhead resistive exercise (Figure 38). It is not uncommon to observe a transient shrug sign during elevation initially. If it persists, the resistance should be reduced. The scapula also should be observed because it might not be providing a stable base from which the upper extremity can work. Supine scapular protraction with resistance (Figure 39), chair push-ups for scapular depression (Figure 40), and wall push-ups with and without a ball address scapular stabilization (Figure 41).

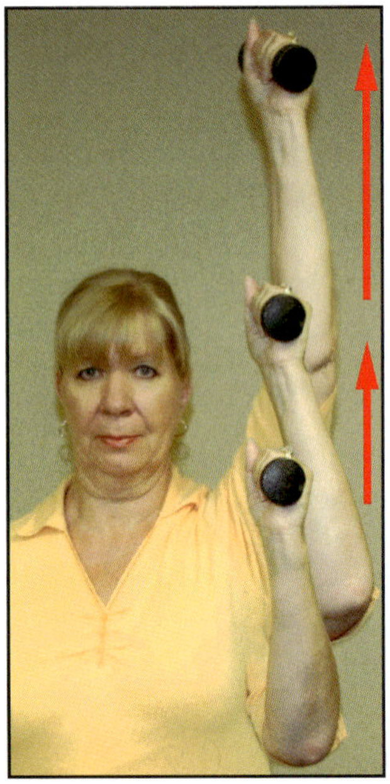

Figure 38. Standing 1-arm press. Using a weight that is appropriate to a maximum of 5 lb (2.25 kg), the patient performs a press-up through maximum range.

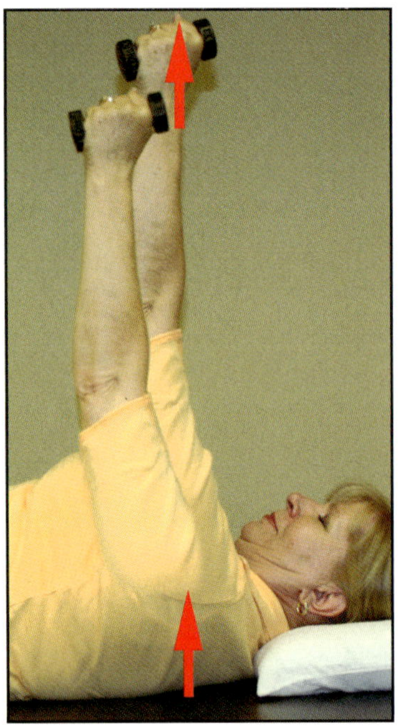

Figure 39. Scapular protraction with a weight. Lying supine, the patient reaches toward the ceiling, moving the shoulder girdle forward.

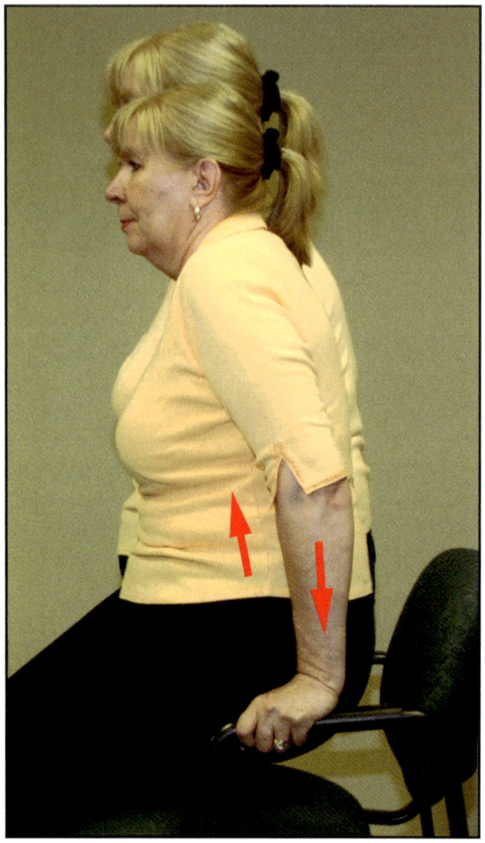

Figure 40. Scapular depression-sheer press-up plus. The patient lifts her body from the sitting position using her lower and upper extremities. Next, instruct the patient to push down on her upper extremities, lifting the body to enhance scapular depression.

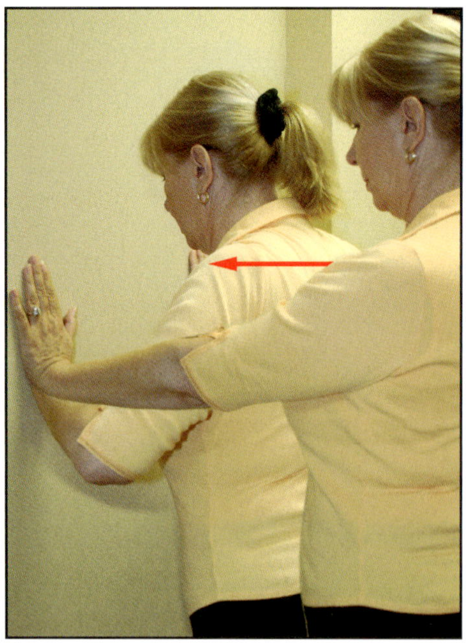

Figure 41. Wall push-up plus. The patient places both hands on the wall and rounds out her back by pushing away from the wall. This also can be performed on an exercise ball.

As resistance increases, exercise sessions can be reduced to 1 time per day and eventually every other day. Patients are encouraged to continue stretching daily if they continue to have residual stiffness.

SPECIAL CONSIDERATIONS

We need to understand the forces that we are required to exert at the shoulder and the effect they have on the repaired structures during rehabilitation.

Tuberosity Fractures

Avoid placing stress across the fracture site on the tuberosity whether treated with closed or open reduction. Overly aggressive rehabilitation has been identified as one of the contributing factors in tuberosity pull-off. Tuberosity pull-off and tuberosity nonunion or malunion can be attributed to premature, overly aggressive stretching or loading, especially with passive internal rotation, extension, and active and resistive external rotation in cases of greater tuberosity fracture that includes some 2-part, 3-part, and 4-part fractures. Judicious application of exercise is imperative to avoid this most significant complication.

Shoulder Arthroplasty

Protecting the repairs of the tuberosity and subscapularis muscle while starting early gentle motion is imperative for an uncomplicated recovery. If avulsion of the subscapularis muscle occurs with the disruption of the repair, instability and loss of function are devastating consequences and more than likely require additional surgery and rerepair.

Reverse Shoulder Arthroplasty

No consensus exists on rehabilitation guidelines for reverse shoulder arthroplasty. Postoperative management can vary from surgeon to surgeon. The design of the prosthetic components also differs slightly depending on what named prosthesis is used. The rudimentory difference from a conventional anatomically designed prosthesis is the reversal of the ball and socket. The reverse shoulder prosthesis has a large hemispherical glenoid component with no neck, which brings the center of shoulder rotation to a more medial position than the anatomic center of rotation. This in turn reduces stress from the fixed fulcrum on the bone-prosthesis interface and increases the movement arm of the deltoid.[9] The humeral side is a cup. In addition, tension of the deltoid muscle is accomplished by tilting the glenoid component in a caudal direction, elongating the deltoid. This increases muscle tension, strength, and joint compression, increasing stability and function. The deltoid and design properties of the prosthesis implement and direct motion in a shoulder with rotator cuff deficiency. The major amount of inherent stability of the shoulder now is shifted to the prosthesis, which maintains a fulcrum for elevation. This is unlike a conventional prosthesis, which is more anatomically designed and relies much more heavily on the soft tissues (capsule, ligaments, rotator cuff, and deltoid) for stability and function.

Dislocation and infection are 2 major early concerns in the immediate and ensuing postoperative periods. The patient can put the prosthesis at risk of dislocation through internal rotation and reaching behind himself or herself. These motions are avoided for 6 weeks. A late complication can be a spontaneous fracture of the acromion. The main factors that are considered to attribute to this are the increased tensioning of the deltoid and a thin acromion that might be inherent to the patient or might be due to intentionally reduced acromial thickness with a previous acromioplasty.

During the course of rehabilitation, the patient will present with the onset of pain and palpable tenderness at the top of the shoulder over the acromion. These patients usually heal with rest and modified activity. Patients also are cautioned about applying force when the extremity is in extension with an internal rotation component, such as reaching behind and forcefully pushing oneself up from a chair.

Goals for rehabilitation are to maintain stability and improve function above and below the horizontal plane. Functional motion within 30° of external rotation and 130° of forward elevation in the scapular plane is acceptable; however, active motion and function can be much better and can vary from patient to patient. The hornblower's sign usually is present due to a deficient rotator cuff and lack of active external rotation. Difficulty reaching behind is inherent to this procedure.

Postoperative management can vary from immobilization in a sling for 6 weeks to a home program of exercise directed by the surgeon. Patients then are encouraged to use their affected upper extremity functionally during activities of daily living on an independent basis without a formal rehabilitation program. Other approaches include early limited motion and a formal rehabilitation program, which the surgeon directs. The pendulum exercise and passive external rotation to 0° to 15° and 0° to 90° progressing to 120° of forward flexion as the patient tolerates is initiated at 2 to 3 weeks after surgery if the surgeon believes he or she has achieved good tuberosity fixation. At 6 weeks as healing continues, patients are moved through a modified gentle progression of pulley exercises, stretching, strengthening, and a home exercise program depending on whether they present with stiffness or weakness, or both. Therefore, you must have close communication with the surgeon and must prudently apply exercises as the patient moves through the rehabilitation progressions.

Understanding the complexities of proximal humerus fractures and their management is crucial to attain the best possible outcome. The concept of early controlled passive range of motion and a progression of exercise intensity applied to fracture stability lends itself to a safe, efficient approach in the rehabilitation of these patients. The pitfalls and complications related to rehabilitation have been defined and always should be a consideration in the recovery process. The model of the team approach enhances individualized care and maximizes the goals and abilities of each patient. The understanding of this program, its exercises, and its levels of intensity gives you a platform to effectively treat and customize the rehabilitation program with respect to the patient's condition, response to treatment, and progress during the recovery process.

REFERENCES

1. Neer CS II. Glenohumeral arthroplasty. In: Neer CS II, ed. *Shoulder Reconstruction*. Philadelphia, PA: WB Saunders; 1990:143–271.
2. Basti J. Rehabilitation of shoulder arthroplasty. In: Bigliani LU, Flatow EL, eds. *Shoulder Arthroplasty*. New York, NY: Springer; 2005:167–207.
3. Cofield RH. Degenerative and arthritic problems of the glenohumeral joint. In: Rockwood CA, Matsen FA II, eds. *The Shoulder*. Philadelphia, PA: WB Saunders; 1990:678–749.
4. Norris RT. Fractures of proximal humerus and dislocation of the shoulder. In: Browner BD, Jupiter JB, Levine AM, Trafton PG, eds. *Skeletal Trauma: Fractures, Dislocations, Ligamentous Injuries*. Vol 2. Philadelphia, PA: WB Saunders; 1992:1201–1290.
5. McCann PD, Wootten ME, Kadaba MP, Bigliani LU. A kinematic and electromyographic study of shoulder rehabilitation exercises. *Clin Orthop Relat Res*. 1993;288:179–188.
6. Poppen NK, Walker PS. Forces at the glenohumeral joint in abduction. *Clin Orthop Relat Res*. 1978;135:165–170.
7. Soslowsky LJ, Flatow EL, Pawluk RJ, et al. Subacromial contact (impingement) on the rotator cuff in the shoulder. Paper presented at: 38th Annual Meeting of the Orthopaedic Research Society; February 17–20, 1992; Washington, DC.
8. Inman VT, Saunders JBDM, Abbott LC. Observations on the function of the shoulder joint. *J Bone Joint Surg Am*. 1944,26(1):1–30.
9. Grassi FA, Murena L, Valli F, Alberio R. Six-year experience with the Delta III reverse shoulder prosthesis. *J Orthop Surg (Hong Kong)*. 2009;17(2):151–156.

RECOMMENDED READING

Bigliani LU, Kelkar R, Flatow EL, Pollock RG, Mow VC. Glenohumeral stability: biomechanical properties of passive and active stabilizers. *Clin Orthop Relat Res*. 1996;330:13–30.

Bigliani LU, Flatow EL, McCluskey GM, Fisher RA. Failed prosthetic replacement for displaced proximal humerus fractures. *Orthop Trans*. 1991;15:747–748.

Boileau P, Trojani C, Walch G, Krishnan SG, Romeo A, Sinnerton R. Shoulder arthroplasty for the treatment of the sequelae of fractures of the proximal humerus. *J Shoulder Elbow Surg*. 2001;10(4):299–308.

Prakash U, McGurty DW, Dent JA. Hemiarthroplasty for severe fractures of the proximal humerus. *J Shoulder Elbow Surg*. 2002;11(5):428–430.

Marx RG, McCarty EC, Montemurno TD, Altchek DW, Craig EV, Warren RF. Development of arthrosis following dislocation of the shoulder: a case-control study. *J Shoulder Elbow Surg*. 2002;11(1):1–5.

Neer CS II, McCann PD, Macfarlane EA, Padilla N. Early passive motion following shoulder arthroplasty and rotator cuff repair: a prospective study. *Orthop Trans*. 1987;11:231.

Hughes M, Neer CS II. Glenohumeral joint replacement and postoperative rehabilitation. *Phys Ther*. 1975;55(8):850–858.

Post M, Bigliani LU, Flatow EL, Pollack RG. *The Shoulder: Operative Technique*. Philadelphia, PA: Lippincott Williams & Wilkins; 1998.

III-12

Conservative Rehabilitation of Subacromial Impingement and Internal Impingement

Joseph H. Kostuch, PT, SCS, and Amee L. Seitz, PT, PhD, DPT, OCS

CHAPTER CONTENTS

WHAT PATIENTS ARE APPROPRIATE FOR THE USE OF THIS GUIDELINE?

- Patients with primary or secondary subacromial impingement
- Patients with internal impingement
- Patients without substantial global capsular tightness or active synovitis
- Patients without frank instability
- Patients without full-thickness rotator cuff tears

Clinical pearls are highlighted in yellow throughout the text.

THE MOST IMPORTANT FACTOR THAT SHOULD GUIDE CLINICAL DECISION MAKING

Shoulder impingement presents with multiple biomechanical and anatomic variables that must be considered when prescribing an appropriate rehabilitation program. Treatment should focus on addressing modifiable contributing factors, such as muscle strength, imbalance, flexibility, and coordination. Whereas the objective evaluation helps the clinician select the appropriate evidence-based treatment interventions, assessing the overall level of reactivity of the patient's shoulder dictates the intensity of the prescribed program. Patients who have highly reactive shoulders and are experiencing almost constant pain and difficulty sleeping must be managed very differently from patients who only have pain with specific positions or activities. A thorough evaluation of the patient to determine the individualized approach to rehabilitation is the key to a successful outcome.

KEY PRINCIPLES IN REHABILITATION OF THIS PROBLEM

Given that shoulder impingement can be caused by multiple factors, thorough subjective and objective evaluations must be performed to identify all the contributing, modifiable biomechanical impairments in each patient. Failure to thoroughly evaluate the entire shoulder girdle often results in only partial resolution of symptoms and continued functional limitations. A comprehensive rehabilitation program for shoulder impingement includes a combination of flexibility and strength training, recruitment and timing exercises, and endurance of the muscles at the glenohumeral and scapulothoracic joints. In addition, mobility of the cervical and thoracic spine should be considered. Thoroughly evaluating and training all implicated structures unique to each patient allows for an optimal recovery of function and resolution of symptoms.

CONTRIBUTING FACTORS

Subacromial impingement syndrome classically has been defined as compression of the rotator cuff tendons and associated tissues under the anterior aspect of the acromion or surrounding structures[1,2] that results in pain and disability (Figure 1). Narrowing of the subacromial space, the interval between the coracoacromial arch/anterior acromion and the humeral head[3] can result from both anatomic and biomechanical factors. Anatomic factors include variations in the shape of the acromion,[4–7] orientation of the slope and angle of the acromion,[8–10] and prominent subacromial spurs (Figure 2).[7,11,12] Biomechanical factors of impingement contribute to narrowing of the subacromial space during movement. These impairments typically are modifiable with rehabilitation, such as dynamic strength and control of the rotator cuff muscles and scapular stabilizers. All potential contributing biomechanical factors must be evaluated, and the clinician must address each impairment to maximize the clinical outcome of rehabilitation.

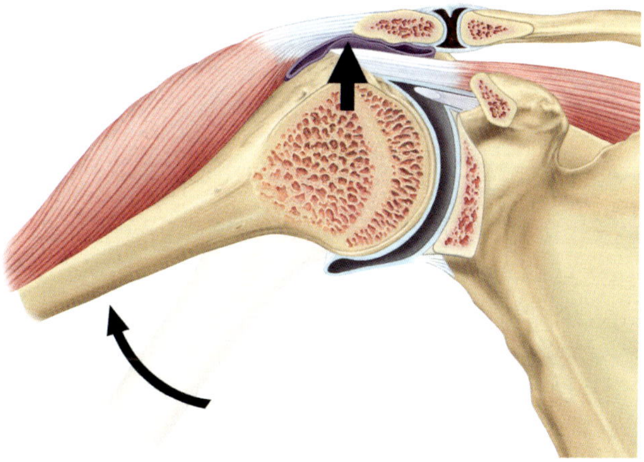

Figure 1. Subacromial impingement with an intact rotator cuff but pinched bursa.

Deficits in dynamic control of the rotator cuff muscles can lead to proximal migration of the humeral head on the glenoid and result in compression of the subacromial tissues.[13–15] Therefore, a complete evaluation of rotator cuff strength, peak force, endurance, and dynamic control during elevation is necessary. In addition, the posteroinferior aspect of the glenohumeral joint capsule and posterior aspect of the shoulder must have adequate flexibility in both horizontal adduction and internal rotation to prevent excessive obligate anterosuperior translation of the humeral head during elevation (Figure 3).

Because the scapula plays a critical role in controlling the position of the glenoid,[16] acromion process, and coracoacromial arch in relation to the humerus, relatively small alterations in scapular movement, in theory, can greatly affect the dimensions of the subacromial space. The scapula normally upwardly rotates, externally rotates, and posteriorly tilts during humeral elevation. Alterations in scapular motion during humeral motion, which is termed *scapular dyskinesis*, can be related to decreased flexibility of the pectoralis minor muscle,[17–19] poor strength or timing of the scapular muscles,[19] or an increase in flexion or kyphosis of the thoracic spine.[19–21] Scapular motion

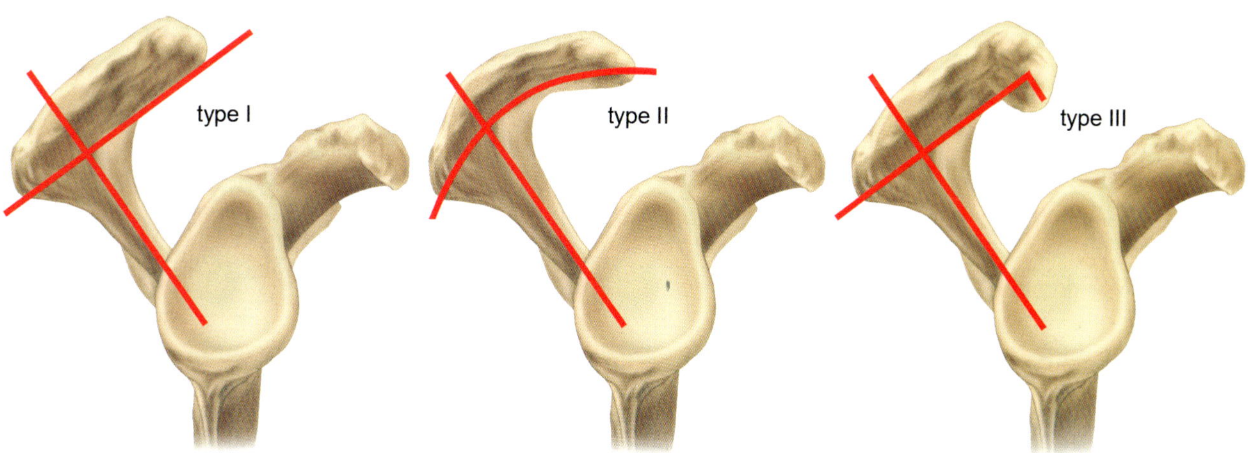

Figure 2. The 3 types of acromions: type I (flat), type II (curved), and type III (hooked).

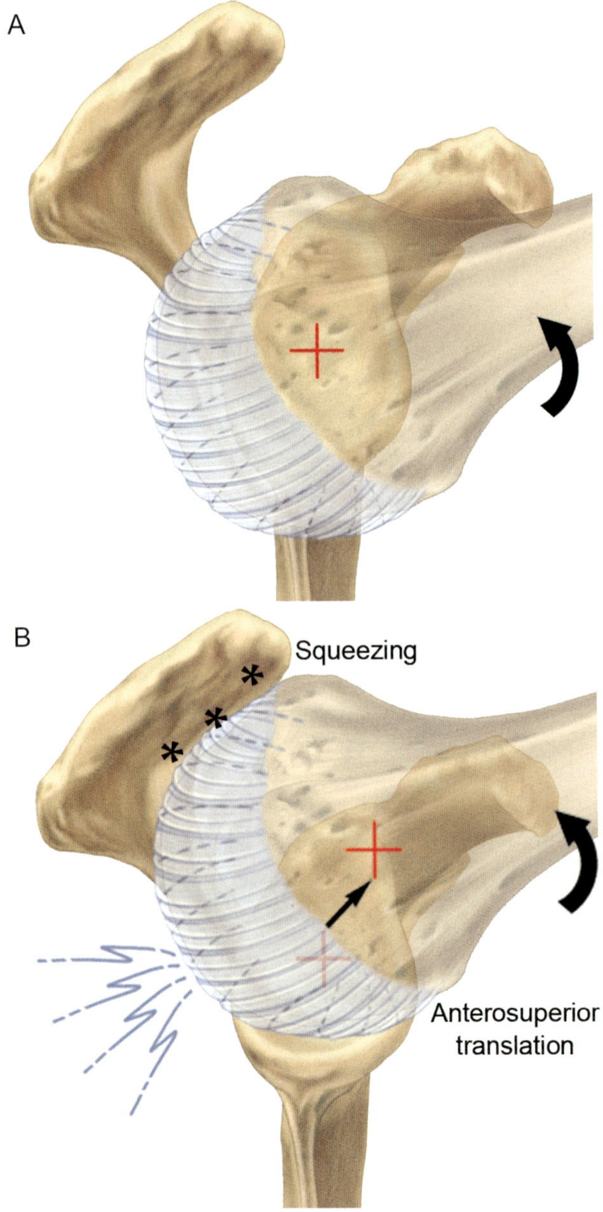

Figure 3. A, Normal biomechanics. B, Excessive anterosuperior translation causing subacromial impingement due to posterior capsule tightness.

should be evaluated during humeral elevation with light weights (3 or 5 pounds [1.35 kg or 2.25 kg]) for at least 5 repetitions in flexion (Figure 4) and abduction along with positioning against resistance in a closed chain position to determine whether dyskinesis is present. Correcting deficits in muscle performance of the upper and lower serratus anterior muscles and trapezius muscles that stabilize the scapula and induce normal scapular motion[22–24] to allow the humeral head to clear the acromion with elevation[25] is critical to the successful rehabilitation of patients with impingement. In addition, adequate flexibility of the pectoralis minor (Figure 5) and thoracic spine is necessary for normal scapular motion to occur.[17,20,26]

SPECIFIC REHABILITATION GUIDELINE

The Appendix specifies our complete Conservative Rehabilitation Guideline for Subacromial Impingement and Internal Impingement. In this section, we explain the rationale for selected components of the

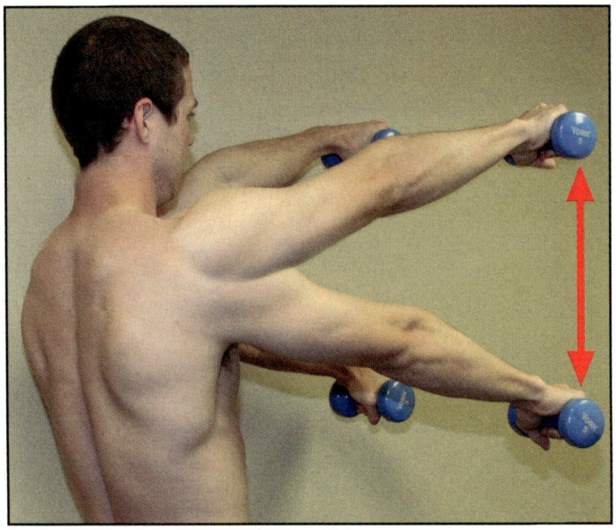

Figure 4. Evaluation of dynamic scapular mechanics during weighted shoulder flexion.

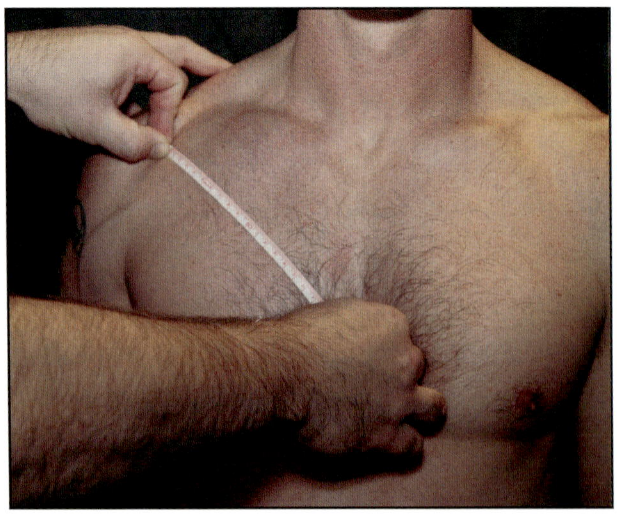

Figure 5. Borstad's[17] pectoralis minor muscle length assessment. The pectoralis minor muscle length is assessed as the distance between the coracoid process and fourth rib. The measurement is taken at the inferomedial edge of the coracoid to the anteroinferior edge of the fourth rib 1 finger-width lateral to the sternum.

guideline. It is divided into 3 phases based on general timeframes of inflammatory response along with the time necessary to gain physiologic strength. Advancement from one rehabilitation phase to the next is not directed specifically by time but rather by constant re-evaluation of the patient's symptoms and ability to meet the specified treatment goals established in the current phase in conjunction with re-evaluation by the physician. Patients also enter into this guideline at various phases depending on their specific impingement classifications and the reactivity of their shoulders.

Primary Impingement

Primary impingement can create substantial bursal irritation and injury to the bursal surface of the rotator cuff tendons and has been described as a progressive disorder that results initially in acute tendinitis, progresses to rotator cuff tendonosis with degeneration and partial-thickness tears, and eventually can result in full-thickness rotator cuff tendon rupture.[2] The progression of rotator cuff disease is specifically described in chapter III-13. Impingement might be due to an acute episode, such as a specific lifting or reaching incident or repetitive overuse. Typically, patients describe symptoms with movement of the upper extremities against resistance and elevation at or above shoulder height and behind the back. A painful arc with reproduction of symptoms between 60° and 120° of elevation is characteristic of this disorder (Figure 6). The combination of a painful arc, pain with external rotation or elevation, and a positive Hawkins impingement sign yields a 10.6 times greater likelihood of subacromial impingement.[27] Suspicion for the presence of a full-thickness rotator cuff tear during a clinical examination warrants referral to an orthopaedist for further evaluation.

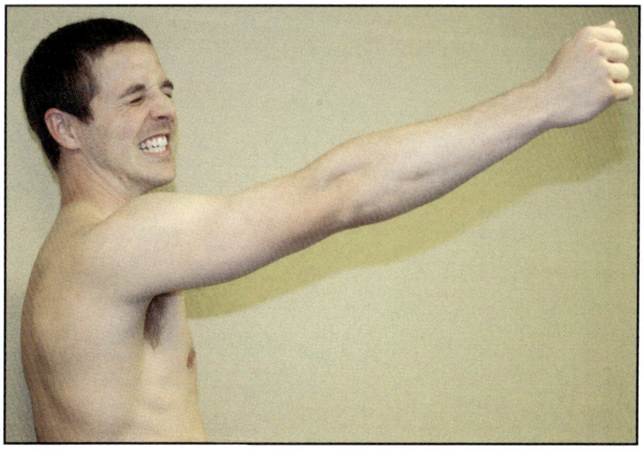

Figure 6. Painful arc that is characteristic with subacromial impingement.

If accurately diagnosed early, **acute** primary subacromial impingement should respond fairly quickly and predictably to a subacromial injection followed by a generalized course of rotator cuff scapular strengthening and activity modification. If warranted by the physician, the injection calms the inflammation, allowing pain-free recruitment and strengthening of the weakened rotator cuff muscles. If good pain relief is noted with the bursal injection, simple active-assistive range of motion is often helpful for 7 to 14 days. In addition, our base rotator cuff strengthening program often is initiated and should be prescribed in a manner that would have been appropriate for the patient's level of preinjection symptoms. We have found that being extra gentle is important with any rotator cuff strengthening immediately after a subacromial injection for 7 to 14 days to help maximize the benefits of the injection. After this time, patients typically can advance their strengthening programs rapidly because their weakness most likely is due to reflexive pain inhibition than true muscle weakness. Full resolution of symptoms can occur quickly, often within 4 to 6 weeks. Advancing to phase 2 to 3 strengthening for fitness or occupational demands can be initiated after 6 weeks, pending adequate relief of symptoms for all household activities of daily living (ADLs) and tolerance to the full base strengthening program. Maintenance of this home strengthening program also should yield good long-term results.

However, in many cases, the problem has become chronic and might have progressed through multiple episodes of inflammation and calming based on functional use of the upper extremity. In these situations, treatment more commonly is initiated after several months or even years of repetitive aggravation of the subacromial tissue. In these chronic situations, simple bursal irritation has progressed into rotator cuff irritation (tendinitis or tendonosis) or partial-thickness tearing of the rotator cuff. Given the chronicity of the injury, the scapula and potentially the cervical spine likely have adapted substitution patterns with associated muscle weakness and terminal capsular tightness.

In addition, the posterior aspect of the capsule has tightened adaptively, and this creates an anterosuperior translation of the humerus, gliding the humerus farther into the offending spur (Figure 3).

These combined factors make the evaluation and treatment of chronic impingement more specific and detailed. The patient often requires a substantially longer and more detailed rehabilitation. Substantial modification of activities also might be required for several weeks or months to allow for reduction of tissue irritation. His or her progression through phase 1 and phase 2 will be much longer, and most of these patients might not experience great improvement in their shoulders for closer to 6 to 12 weeks due to the changes that must occur about the scapula, cervical spine, posterior capsule, and rotator cuff. The additional recovery time specific to this patient population is related to multiple factors, including the time needed for the body to gain strength and hypertrophy of these muscles. Muscles hypertrophy, and growth typically requires 3 to 6 weeks,[28] which might be necessary to appropriately center and rotate the humeral head to allow pain-free elevation. In addition, passive range-of-motion (PROM) stretching into terminal planes of motion might need to be integrated and allowed several weeks to normalize (see Figures 12 and 13 in chapter II-3). After rotator cuff strength is improved and elevation strengthening is initiated successfully, the patient can progress to a full phase 2 then to a phase 3 program, allowing return to normal ADLs.

Secondary Impingement

Secondary impingement also involves mechanical compression of the subacromial tissues, but it is due to underlying glenohumeral pathologic conditions, such as anterior or multidirectional capsular instability of the glenohumeral joint or underlying labral lesions creating altered glenohumeral arthrokinematics and thus a microinstability. A poorly stabilized humerus migrates superiorly on the glenoid particularly in positions that stress the glenohumeral ligaments, such as combined humeral abduction and external rotation. Treatment of a secondary impingement might not differ greatly from a primary impingement, but the ultimate outcome of treatment might be compromised if the underlying instability is not addressed.

Given a lack of a frank instability of the glenohumeral joint with dislocation, the instability associated with secondary impingement often is termed *microinstability*. This instability typically occurs with moderate- to high-level ADLs, occupational activities, or athletic activities in which the shoulder is placed in a high-demand position when the rotator cuff and scapula must work near maximum recruitment to stabilize the glenohumeral joint. If underlying microinstability exists and the cuff and scapula cannot dynamically stabilize the humerus, impingement likely will occur. Therefore, the strengthening program for these patients initially must be basic but should quickly progress to more challenging positions because of the need for maximum recruitment specific to the positions of impingement. These patients rarely require active-assistive range-of-motion exercises unless their shoulders are highly reactive and should begin with a phase 1 or phase 2 strengthening program, again being specific to address the scapular component. After a comprehensive strengthening program is well tolerated, the rehabilitation program may advance into phase 3, now focusing on strengthening the positions where symptoms occur for full return to recreational and occupational activities (Figure 7). Depending on the reactivity

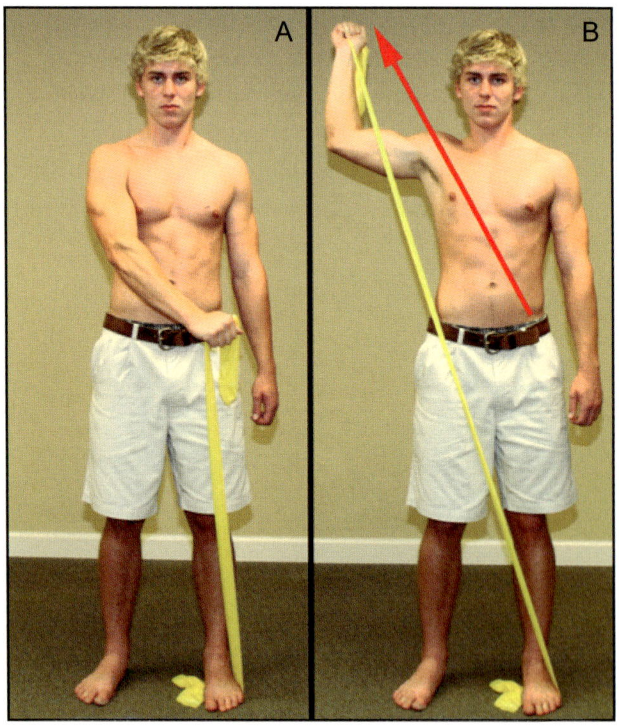

Figure 7 A and B. Diagonal resisting elevation and external rotation with an elastic band.

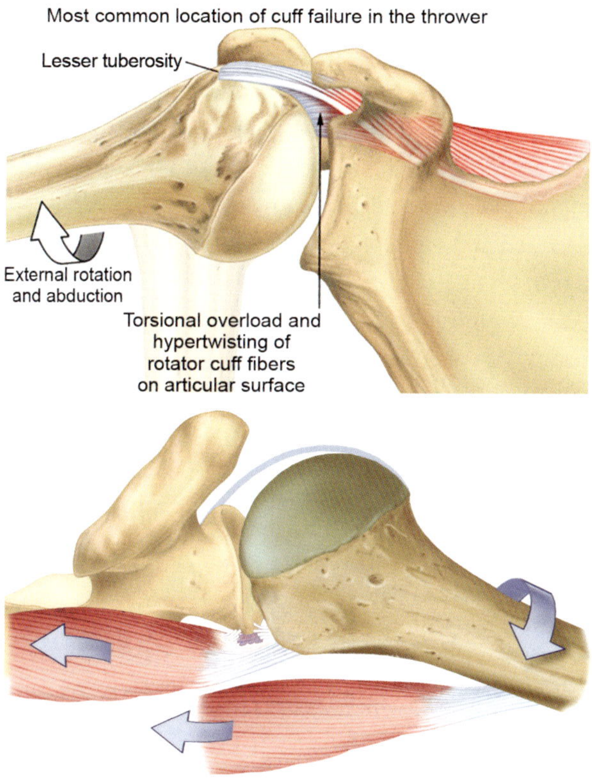

Figure 8. Internal impingement during external rotation.

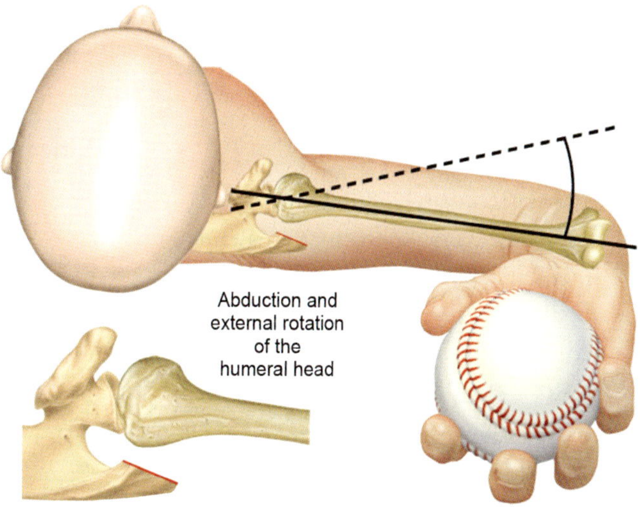

Figure 9. Hyperangulation of the humerus.

of their shoulders and concominent need for maintaining their current levels of activity, most patients should expect to see improvement with this diagnosis from 6 to 10 weeks after initiating a strengthening program.

Internal Impingement

Internal impingement is very specific to overhead athletes or laborers who repeatedly overuse their shoulders above their heads most commonly in a throwing-type abducted and externally rotated (ABDER) position.[29–32] Internal impingement is described as pinching of the articular side of the rotator cuff tendons between the posterosuperior glenoid rim and humerus when the upper extremity is in full external rotation, abduction, and extension (Figure 8).[33,34] This is accentuated with further hyperangulation of the humerus to the glenoid with anterior glenohumeral joint instability[33] or, in theory, with a reduction in scapular retraction[29,31] and posterior tilt (Figure 9).[35] Patients with internal impingement tend to present with pain located in the posterior and superior aspects of the shoulder typically while in a humeral position similar to the late-cocking phase of the throwing motion.[30,32] Because this mechanism of impingement is not due to narrowing of the subacromial space and compression between the acromion and humerus, it can be considered a unique subgroup of impingement. Treatment should address underlying impairments that contribute to articular-sided compression of the rotator cuff in the posterior portion of the shoulder, including evaluation of all potentially contributing biomechanical factors related to primary impingement.

The approach for treatment of internal impingement should include stretching of the posterior aspect of the capsule, basic progressing to advanced strengthening of the rotator cuff, and comprehensive rehabilitation of the scapula. Researchers have theorized that stretching the posterior aspect of the capsule (Figure 10) helps reduce the anterior translation forces about the humerus

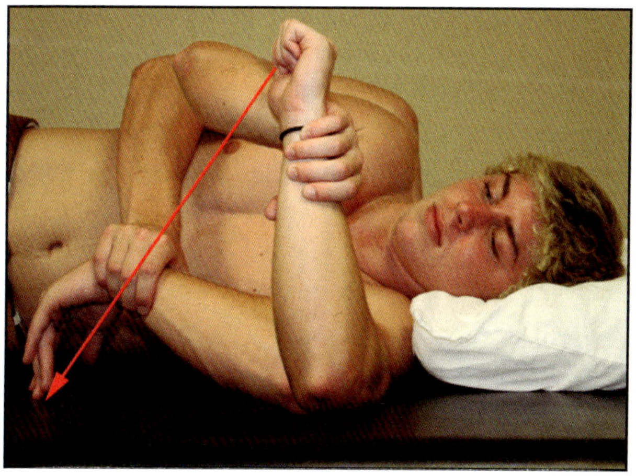

Figure 10. The sleeper stretch.

when placed into ABDER, allowing the humerus to centrally rotate about the glenoid and eliminating impingement of the posterior portion of the rotator cuff.[36] Because this type of impingement is very specific to the ABDER position of the extremity, certain exceptions apply to this rehabilitation program. As comfortable, progressively strengthening the rotator cuff and scapula in the ABDER position is critical for success as detailed in phase 3 of the Appendix. In addition, activity technique (eg, throwing, swimming) must be evaluated critically for correct biomechanical form. A core and lower extremity functional strength screening also might reveal the genesis of poor technique leading to increased stress being placed through a weakened shoulder and creating this compensatory internal impingement.

SPECIAL CONSIDERATIONS: ADHESIVE CAPSULITIS OR SYNOVITIS WITH IMPINGEMENT

Frequently, patients present to the physician's or rehabilitation provider's office with impingement symptoms on clinical or radiologic examination but display an unusually high level of stiffness or reactivity, or both. This subgroup of patients requires an altered treatment approach to their diagnoses that includes increased use of modalities and PROM stretching. Cryotherapy most often is recommended for this population because of its anti-inflamatory properties and the ease with which patients can use it at home. For patients who display capsular stiffness that is greater than the stiffness that patients with impingement normally display, a more comprehensive stretching program should be implemented and emphasized before addressing any deficits or imbalances in strength. Depending on the level of reactivity in the shoulder, this program might need to start with the phase 1 or phase 2 stretching program only (see Figures 1 and 12 in chapter II-3). These patients might require additional therapy visits initially to help normalize their PROM deficits. This additional time in therapy should be spent primarily performing PROM stretching and appropriate joint mobilizations specific to their capsular limitations. After patients have progressed to terminal planes of stretching, they are appropriate to begin addressing their imbalances in rotator cuff and scapular strength to improve their symptoms of impingement. If little progress is realized, this population of patients should be transitioned into the adhesive capsulitis rehabilitation program (see chapter III-15) and should not attempt to strengthen. In addition, a referral to the physician for re-evaluation might be appropriate. When his or her pain is well managed and more predictable, the patient can engage in progressive strengthening. This subgroup of patients likely requires an additional 4 to 6 weeks of supervised therapy beyond the "typical" impingement program to help normalize their flexibility.

REFERENCES

1. Neer CS II. Anterior acromioplasty for the chronic impingement syndrome in the shoulder: a preliminary report. *J Bone Joint Surg Am*. 1972;54(1):41–50.
2. Neer CS II. Impingement lesions. *Clin Orthop Relat Res*. 1983;173:70–77.
3. Neer CS, Poppen NK. Supraspinatus outlet. *Orthop Trans*. 1987;11:234.
4. Bigliani LU, Ticker JB, Flatow EL, Soslowsky LJ, Mow VC. The relationship of acromial architecture to rotator cuff disease. *Clin Sports Med*. 1991;10(4):823–838.
5. Epstein RE, Schweitzer ME, Frieman BG, Fenlin JM Jr, Mitchell DG. Hooked acromion: prevalence on MR images of painful shoulders. *Radiology*. 1993;187(2):479–481.
6. Gill TJ, McIrvin E, Kocher MS, Homa K, Mair SD, Hawkins RJ. The relative importance of acromial morphology and age with respect to rotator cuff pathology. *J Shoulder Elbow Surg*. 2002;11(4):327–330.
7. Ogawa K, Yoshida A, Inokuchi W, Naniwa T. Acromial spur: relationship to aging and morphologic changes in the rotator cuff. *J Shoulder Elbow Surg*. 2005;14(6):591–598.
8. Toivonen DA, Tuite MJ, Orwin JF. Acromial structure and tears of the rotator cuff. *J Shoulder Elbow Surg*. 1995;4(5):376–383.
9. Edelson JG. The "hooked" acromion revisited. *J Bone Joint Surg Br*. 1995;77(2):284–287.
10. Vaz S, Soyer J, Pries P, Clarac JP. Subacromial impingement: influence of coracoacromial arch geometry on shoulder function. *Joint Bone Spine*. 2000;67(4):305–309.
11. Nicholson GP, Goodman DA, Flatow EL, Bigliani LU. The acromion: morphologic condition and age-related changes. A study of 420 scapulas. *J Shoulder Elbow Surg*. 1996;5(1):1–11.
12. Farley TE, Neumann CH, Steinbach LS, Petersen SA. The coracoacromial arch: MR evaluation and correlation with rotator cuff pathology. *Skeletal Radiol*. 1994;23(8):641–645.
13. Chen SK, Simonian PT, Wickiewicz TL, Otis JC, Warren RF. Radiographic evaluation of glenohumeral kinematics: a muscle fatigue model. *J Shoulder Elbow Surg*. 1999;8(1):49–52.
14. Royer PJ, Kane EJ, Parks KE, et al. Fluoroscopic assessment of rotator cuff fatigue on glenohumeral arthrokinematics in shoulder impingement syndrome. *J Shoulder Elbow Surg*. 2009;18(6):968–975.
15. Deutsch A, Altchek DW, Schwartz E, Otis JC, Warren RF. Radiologic measurement of superior displacement of the humeral head in the impingement syndrome. *J Shoulder Elbow Surg*. 1996;5(3):186–193.

16. Cools AM, Declercq GA, Cambier DC, Mahieu NN, Witvrouw EE. Trapezius activity and intramuscular balance during isokinetic exercise in overhead athletes with impingement symptoms. *Scand J Med Sci Sports*. 2007;17(1):25–33.
17. Borstad JD. Resting position variables at the shoulder: evidence to support a posture-impairment association. *Phys Ther*. 2006;86(4):549–557.
18. Hébert LJ, Moffet H, McFadyen BJ, Dionne CE. Scapular behavior in shoulder impingement syndrome. *Arch Phys Med Rehabil*. 2002;83(1):60–69.
19. Ludewig PM, Cook TM. Alterations in shoulder kinematics and associated muscle activity in people with symptoms of shoulder impingement. *Phys Ther*. 2000;80(3):276–291.
20. Kebaetse M, McClure P, Pratt NA. Thoracic position effect on shoulder range of motion, strength, and three-dimensional scapular kinematics. *Arch Phys Med Rehabil*. 1999;80(8):945–950.
21. Wang CH, McClure P, Pratt NE, Nobilini R. Stretching and strengthening exercises: their effect on three-dimensional scapular kinematics. *Arch Phys Med Rehabil*. 1999;80(8):923–929.
22. Johnson GR, Pandyan AD. The activity in the three regions of the trapezius under controlled loading conditions: an experimental and modelling study. *Clin Biomech (Bristol, Avon)*. 2005;20(2):155–161.
23. Kronberg M, Németh G, Broström LA. Muscle activity and coordination in the normal shoulder: an electromyographic study. *Clin Orthop Relat Res*. 1990;257:76–85.
24. Bagg SD, Forrest WJ. A biomechanical analysis of scapular rotation during arm abduction in the scapular plane. *Am J Phys Med Rehabil*. 1988;67(6):238–245.
25. McQuade KJ, Dawson J, Smidt GL. Scapulothoracic muscle fatigue associated with alterations in scapulohumeral rhythm kinematics during maximum resistive shoulder elevation. *J Orthop Sports Phys Ther*. 1998;28(2):74–80.
26. Borstad JD, Ludewig PM. The effect of long versus short pectoralis minor resting length on scapular kinematics in healthy individuals. *J Orthop Sports Phys Ther*. 2005;35(4):227–238.
27. Park HB, Yokota A, Gill HS, El Rassi G, McFarland EG. Diagnostic accuracy of clinical tests for the different degrees of subacromial impingement syndrome. *J Bone Joint Surg Am*. 2005;87(7):1446-1455.
28. Bosco C, Rusko H, Hirvonen J. The effect of extra-load conditioning on muscle performance in athletes. *Med Sci Sports Exerc*. 1984;18(4):415–419.
29. Burkhart SS, Morgan CD, Kibler WB. The disabled throwing shoulder: spectrum of pathology part III. The SICK scapula, scapular dyskinesis, the kinetic chain, and rehabilitation. *Arthroscopy*. 2003;19(6):641–661.
30. Jobe CM. Posterior superior glenoid impingement: expanded spectrum. *Arthroscopy*. 1995;11(5):530–536.
31. Kibler WB. The role of the scapula in athletic shoulder function. *Am J Sports Med*. 1998;26(2):325–337.
32. Kvitne RS, Jobe FW. The diagnosis and treatment of anterior instability in the throwing athlete. *Clin Orthop Relat Res*. 1993;291:107–123.
33. Davidson PA, Elattrache NS, Jobe CM, Jobe FW. Rotator cuff and posterior-superior glenoid labrum injury associated with increased glenohumeral motion: a new site of impingement. *J Shoulder Elbow Surg*. 1995;4(5):384–390.
34. Edelson G, Teitz C. Internal impingement in the shoulder. *J Shoulder Elbow Surg*. 2000;9(4):308–315.
35. Laudner KG, Myers JB, Pasquale MR, Bradley JP, Lephart SM. Scapular dysfunction in throwers with pathologic internal impingement. *J Orthop Sports Phys Ther*. 2006;36(7):485–494.
36. Tyler TF, Nicholas SJ, Lee SJ, Mullaney M, McHugh MP. Correction of posterior shoulder tightness is associated with symptom resolution in patients with internal impingement. *Am J Sports Med*. 2010;38(1):114–119.

CONSERVATIVE REHABILITATION GUIDELINE FOR SUBACROMIAL IMPINGEMENT AND INTERNAL IMPINGEMENT

St. Francis Orthopaedic Institute and St. Francis Rehabilitation Center

All information contained in this protocol is to be used as a general guideline only. Specific variations might be appropriate for each patient and might be specified by the physician. ***Patients do not have to begin with phase 1 rehabilitation****. They can begin at whatever level of rehabilitation matches their current signs and symptoms, but most patients begin with phase 1 rehabilitation.* ***Achieving and maintaining a low level of pain and inflammation are the guiding principles in all stages of rehabilitation****.*

SYMBOLS AND ABBREVIATIONS

AAFE, active-assistive forward elevation
AAROM, active-assistive range of motion
AASEP, assistive-to-active shoulder elevation progression
AFE, active forward elevation
ADL, activity of daily living
ER, external rotation
FE, forward elevation
IR, internal rotation
MMT, manual muscle testing
PFE, passive forward elevation
PNF, proprioceptive neuromuscular facilitation
PRN, as needed
PROM, passive range of motion
ROM, range of motion
T-Band, Thera-Band (The Hygenic Corporation, Akron, OH)

Forward elevation, either active or passive, is the plane of motion in which an individual naturally lifts his or her arm that is anterior to the plane of the scapula and lateral to flexion.

PHASE 1

Goals

- °Initiate a therapeutic level of rotator cuff, deltoid, and scapular strengthening that does not increase inflammation or the reactivity level of the shoulder
- °Educate the patient about modifying activity, controlling the inflammatory response, and using cryotherapy
- °Identify and address secondary factors contributing to current symptoms as long as they do not place the shoulder in impingement positions or exacerbate impingement symptoms
- °Decrease reactivity of the shoulder PRN through gentle AAROM
- °Use of the shoulder for pain-free ADLs below end ranges of motion

Exercises

Note: Patients might receive a cortical steroid injection in the subacromial bursa from their physicians to decrease their pain and inflammation and thus allow greater participation in their prescribed therapy programs. If patients present to therapy within 7 to 10 days of this injection, great care should be taken to prescribe exercises that are not beyond their described preinjection level of function.

- °Comfortable AAROM exercises to relieve pain and to improve confidence are used if the level of reactivity of the shoulder is high
    - °Preferred exercises
        - °Codman
        - °Rope and pulley (elbows remain straight with the thumb up) (Figure 11)
        - °Table step-back
- **°Initiate base strengthening program as soon as the patient can perform it comfortably**

°Includes rotator cuff, deltoid, and scapular strengthening performed at or below chest level (chapter II-4)
°2 times per day at most with light resistance and increasing repetitions
°Yellow T-Band (initially) for ER and IR
°Initially, 4- to 6-foot band length and light pretension in a small arc of motion
°Can use side-lying ER instead of T-Band ER to begin
°Yellow T-Band forward reach
°Initially, 4- to 6-foot band length and light pretension
°Start with the elbow bent and by the side and the band tied behind the patient
°Reach **forward** with the hand at waist level, progressing to reaching **forward** at chest level (Figure 12)
°Scapular strengthening emphasizing scapular retractions and scapular upward rotators (chapter IV-2)
°No prone FE, abduction, or ER strengthening
°Initiate progressive overhead strengthening to improve AFE via the AASEP (chapter II-4) ***ONLY when a tolerance to base strengthening is established and when the AASEP is comfortable***
°It is a stepwise progression in difficulty of strengthening exercises from PFE to AFE against gravity
°The goal of the progression is to achieve pain-free full AFE
°Start with whatever level of exercise is challenging but not painful
°If scapular or glenohumeral substitutions or pain are present, choose an easier exercise in the progression
°Only the exercises that are most often used for these patients are listed below
°Full motion AFE without weight is the goal of phase 1 for the AASEP
°See chapter II-4 for a comprehensive discussion of this program
°Exercises are divided into 3 levels of difficulty
1. Gravity-minimized exercises
°T-Band supine FE
°Must start the involved arm at 90° of elevation
°Pull the arm into FE
2. Assistive elevation exercises
°Rope-and-pulley AAFE (Figure 11)
°Incline dusting (Figure 13)
°Wall-slide AAFE
3. Unsupported elevation exercises
°AFE
°Patient education
°Pathogenesis and rehabilitation process
°Importance of frequent use of ice
°Minimal use of the arm for provocative positions or recreational activities

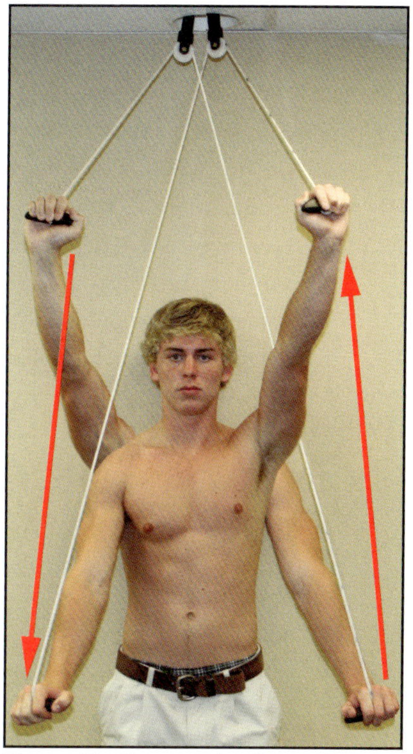
Figure 11. Rope-and-pulley active-assistive forward elevation.

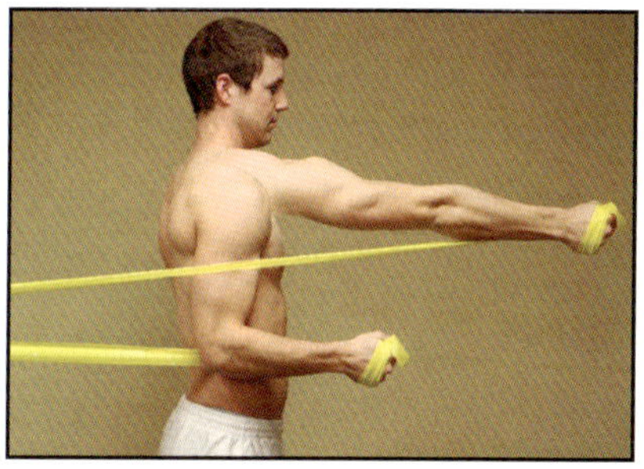
Figure 12. Forward reaching with an elastic band at chest level.

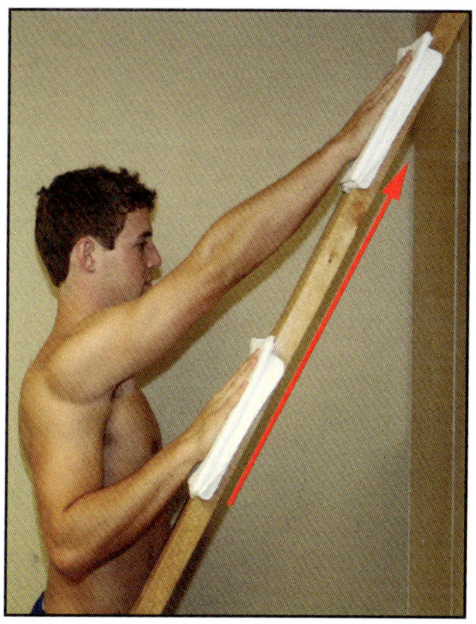
Figure 13. Incline dusting.

- °Ensure the level of pain is not increasing because of excessive use of the arm for ADLs, work, or recreation

°Identify and address secondary factors contributing to current symptoms as long as they do not place the shoulder in impingement positions or exacerbate impingement symptoms. These might include, but are not limited to, assessing for and treating

- °Pectoralis minor tightness (chapters IV-1 and IV-2)
- °Scapular dyskinesia (chapters IV-1 and IV-2)
- °Spinal facet dysfunction or other cervical spine disorders (chapter IV-3)
- °Thoracic outlet syndrome
- °Myofascial syndrome or other soft tissue disorders

Adjunctive Exercises

°Modalities as needed to reduce resting or constant pain

- °Cryotherapy and ice massage
- °Electrical stimulation only in patients who are not responding well to standard phase 1 rehabilitation (chapter IV-12)

°Aquatic therapy acutely for pain-free AAROM and comfort (no swimming strokes) (chapter IV-9)

°Aquatic therapy subacutely for progressive base rotator cuff, scapular, and deltoid strengthening (chapter IV-9)

Interventions to Avoid

°Exercises that result in severe immediate or delayed pain

°Exercises that result in excessive guarding or splinting of muscles

°Home or clinic exercises into straight-plane abduction or other exercises that place the shoulder in positions of impingement, such as horizontal adduction

°Repetitive daily activity with affected extremity that provokes symptoms

PHASE 2

Criteria to Begin

°No pain with the arm at rest and symptoms limited to specific and predictable activities with or without pain at night

°Pain-free tolerance to base strengthening program and the AASEP with only reported fatigue

Goals

°Progressively advance rotator cuff and scapular strength and endurance with a comprehensive strengthening program specific to the patient's evaluated deficits

°Progressively normalize PROM and flexibility deficits, specifically deficits of the posterior capsule and pectoralis minor, that are limited due to stiffness into all planes of motion

°Address core and lower extremity deficits because they might contribute to functional limitation

°Allow pain-free return to normal household and low-demand occupational ADLs along with recreational sports that do not require repetitive or powerful overhead use of the arm

Exercises

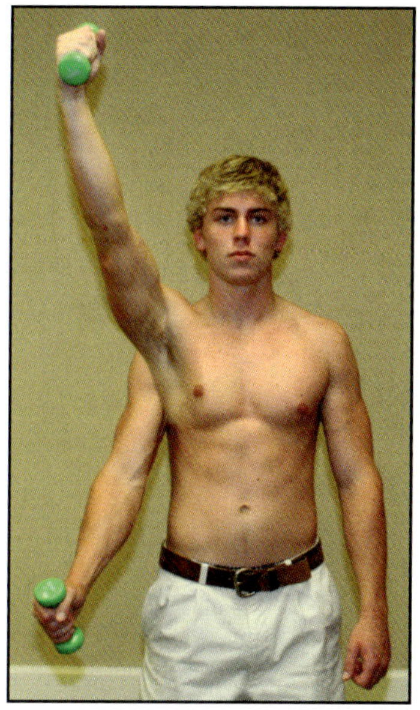

Figure 14. Active forward elevation with light weight.

- °Progress the base strengthening program established in phase 1
  - °Increase strength and endurance by increasing repetitions and resistance while still using the philosophy of relatively low resistance during rotator cuff strengthening and allowing no visible mechanical deviations (chapter II-1)
  - °Increase the size of ROM
  - °Perform 2 times per day to perceived level of fatigue
- °Progress the AASEP established in phase 1
  - °Achieve full-motion AFE without weight if that has not been achieved in phase 1
  - °Progress to AFE with very light resistance (typically 1 to 3 pounds) (Figure 14)
- °Implement a home-based stretching program to normalize PROM and flexibility deficits that are limited due to stiffness into all planes of motion as long as impingement symptoms are not exacerbated
  - °Assess each plane of the motions to determine if stretching is needed. Stretching should be performed if (1) motion is limited more than the contralateral side and (2) the level of pain is minimal or none. If a particular ROM is limited only due to pain, then mechanical pinching or inflammation rather than stiffness is limiting the ROM. Home stretching would NOT be appropriate at this time.
  - °Especially evaluate the posterior capsule, forward elevation, and pectoralis minor
  - °Preferred posterior capsule stretches include
    - °Horizontal adduction or cross-body stretching
    - °Sleeper stretch (Figure 10)

Adjunctive Exercises

- °Aquatic therapy for progressive base rotator cuff, scapular, and deltoid strengthening (chapter IV-9)
- °Closed kinetic chain exercises for shoulder girdle and core stabilization
- °Kinethetic awareness drills
- °Lower extremity and core training if deficits are present and thought to contribute to the patient's signs and symptoms

Interventions to Avoid

- °Advanced strengthening or unrestricted return to overhead sports or weight training
- °Exercises that greatly increase signs and symptoms
- °Home or clinic exercises into straight-plane abduction
- °Highly repetitive rehabilitation activities with the arm positioned overhead

Note: Most patients will be discharged at the completion of phase 2 into an independent home exercise program. This program will focus on progressive or maintenance shoulder girdle strengthening. ***Only patients who require return to vigorous sports or moderate to heavy occupational demands should progress to phase 3.***

PHASE 3

Criteria to Begin

- °Goals of returning to sports, heavy labor, or repetitive or heavy overhead work
- °No pain with the arm at rest and symptoms limited to specific and predictable high-level activities, such as competitive sports or high-demand occupations
- °Successfully normalize all PROM and capsular deficits
- °Pain-free tolerance to progressive base and overhead strengthening program with 5/5 MMT of the rotator cuff and scapular muscles
- °Physician approval

Goals

- °Normalize dynamic strength and endurance of the rotator cuff and scapula
- °Full return to recreational or high-demand occupational ADLs
- °Discharge when functional goals are met
- °Transition to maintenance home exercise program

Exercises

- °Advance base strengthening progression and AFE
  - °Increase elastic resistance and repetitions to 50
  - °Larger, more functional full arc of motion
  - °Increase speed to replicated functional activity without losing eccentric control
  - °AFE up to to 5 pounds depending on body size and functional demands
- °Initiate the advanced strengthening progression **PRN** (chapter II-4)
  - °**Strict criteria to start the program listed above**
  - °**Exercise principles**
    - °Decrease the amount of external stabilization provided to the shoulder girdle
    - °Integrate functional patterns, including abduction and ER
    - °Increase speed of movements
    - °Integrate kinesthetic awareness drills into strengthening activities
    - °Include the entire kinetic chain
    - °Decrease rest time to improve endurance
    - °Initiate prone strengthening PRN
    - °Train larger upper extremity muscles wisely
  - °**Sample exercises**
    - °Prone rotator cuff strengthening: light weight with emphasis on the scapula
      - °Hang to abduction with external rotation (Figure 15)
      - °Extension
      - °Abduction
      - °Scaption

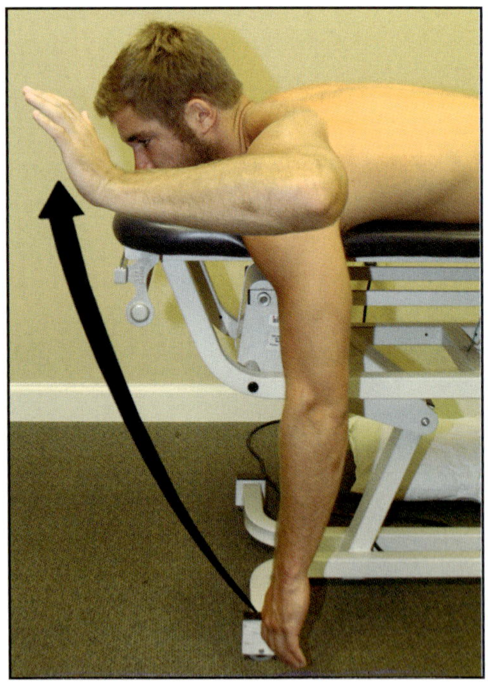

Figure 15. Prone hang to external rotation near 90° of abduction without support.

- °T-Band standing PNF-type patterns (Figure 7 A and B)
- °T-Band 90°/90° ER and IR with or without arm support (Figures 16)
- °T-Band simulation of batting, golf, or tennis forehand and backhand
- °Weighted shoulder shrugs
- °Dumbbell overhead shoulder press **PRN** (Figure 17)
    - °Place hands in front of the shoulder with the elbows bent and naturally reach overhead
    - °Sets of 15 to 20 repetitions with 3 pounds or more 3 to 7 times per week
- °Initiate progressive replication of demanding ADLs and work
- °Can begin interval throwing program or return to tennis program (**when approved by physician**) (chapter IV-6 and chapter IV-8)
- °Initiate modified return to weight-training program (**when approved by physician**) (chapter IV-4)

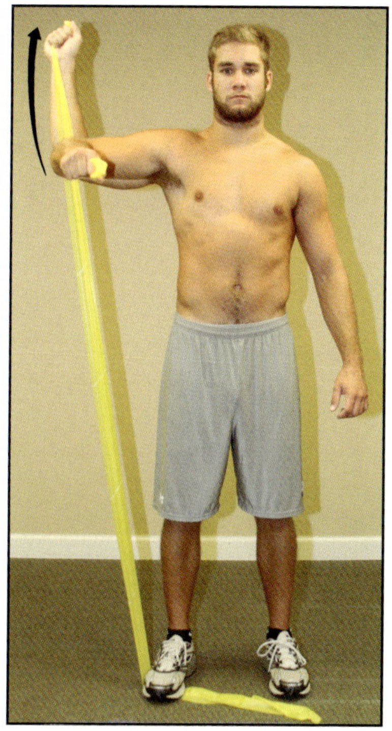

Figure 16. External rotation at 90° of abduction with an elastic band.

Adjunctive Exercises

- °Initiate plyometric program (**PRN for overhead athletes and if approved by physician**)
    - °Can begin after 2 to 3 weeks of advanced strengthening program
    - °Do not begin until 5/5 MMT for the rotator cuff and scapula
    - °Use only 2 to 3 times per week
    - °Begin with a beach ball or tennis ball and progress to weighted balls
- °Progressions
    - °2-handed tosses
        - °Waist level
        - °Overhead
        - °Diagonally
    - °1-handed drop-and-catch drills
    - °1-handed tosses, varying the amount of
        - °Abduction
        - °Arm support

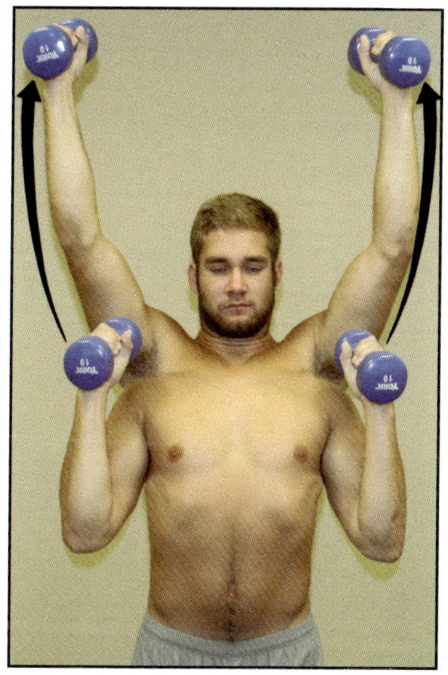

Figure 17. Dumbbell overhead press with hands starting in front of the shoulders.

Interventions to Avoid

- °Any rehabilitation activity that is significantly more demanding than daily or expected recreational activities
- °Any exercise that significantly increases signs and symptoms

III-13

Conservative Rehabilitation of Rotator Cuff Disorders

Joseph H. Kostuch, PT, SCS, and Amee L. Seitz, PT, PhD, DPT, OCS

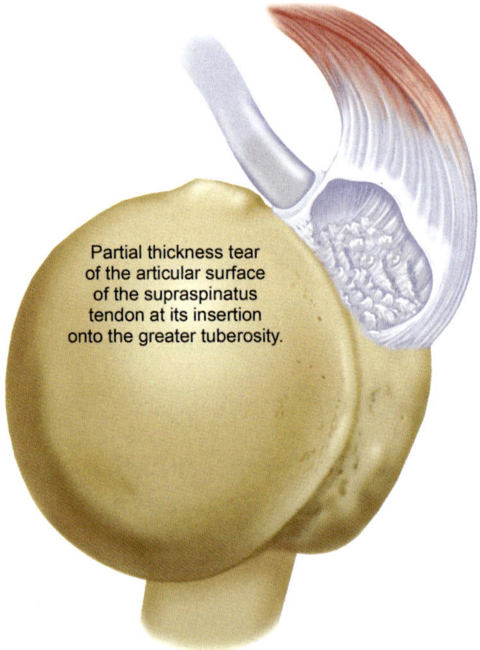

CHAPTER CONTENTS

WHAT PATIENTS ARE APPROPRIATE FOR THE USE OF THIS GUIDELINE?

- Patients with chronic age-related or activity-related rotator cuff disease
- Patients with a documented rotator cuff tendon tear that is being managed nonoperatively by choice or because it is inoperable
- Patients with rotator cuff overuse or strain injuries
- Patients without concomitant synovitis or adhesive capsulitis
- Patients with chronic complete rotator cuff tears of multiple tendons occasionally might use this guideline but are often more appropriate to use the Partial Repair of the Massive Rotator Cuff Tear guideline (chapter III-3) even if nonoperative treatment is chosen

Clinical pearls are highlighted in yellow throughout the text.

THE MOST IMPORTANT FACTOR THAT SHOULD GUIDE CLINICAL DECISION MAKING

The stage of rotator cuff disease as indictated by the underlying pathologic condition likely dictates the recommended treatment. For individuals with symptomatic full-thickness rotator cuff tears, surgical treatment is recommended.[1] However, nonoperative rehabilitation might be indicated to help restore range of motion (ROM) preoperatively and to treat individuals for whom surgery is not an option. Most partial-thickness and some full-thickness tears can be managed successfully with rehabilitation that progresses slowly. Exercise prescription is based on the level of irritation, an individualized assessment of the patient's impairments, and the patient's overall physical health. The rehabilitation provider should address all of the impairments that exist to maximize the likelihood of success with nonoperative treatment, with the focus placed on strengthening the rotator cuff and deltoid, educating the patient about modification of activities, and resolving passive ROM limitations.

KEY PRINCIPLES IN REHABILITATION OF THIS PROBLEM

The outcome of rehabilitation can vary based on the size and location of the tear and on the individual's overall functional demands. Treatment should be based on improving the individual's specific impairments and should include increasing ROM, strengthening both the damaged and remaining intact rotator cuff and the surrounding deltoid and scapular muscles, and educating the patient about modification of activities. Pain should guide the intensity of treatment. When treating large rotator cuff tears, the goal is to maximize overall function and to progressively strengthen the rotator cuff and deltoid. With smaller or partial-thickness rotator cuff tears, the response to treatment will be slower in older individuals with chronic symptoms, and they might use a home program for up to 1 year after discharge from formal physical therapy.[2]

SPECTRUM OF ROTATOR CUFF TENDON DISEASE

Rotator cuff disease has been classically described as a continuum of pathologic conditions of the rotator cuff tendons characterized by 3 age-dependent stages.[3] Acute tendinitis with edema and hemorrhage, which is common in individuals less than 25 years, defines *Stage 1*, and the onset probably is due to overuse or a particular traumatic event. *Stage 2* is common in individuals from age 25 to 40 years, is characterized by fibrosis and tendonosis with or without partial-thickness tears, and can become a chronic condition. *Stage 3* is defined as a full-thickness tendon tear that is attributed to attrition of the rotator cuff tendons and characteristically is found in individuals 40 years of age or older, but it can occur in younger individuals due to trauma (Figure 1). The relevance of age in rotator cuff disease and tears is indisputable.

The natural history of rotator cuff tendon tears in both symptomatic and asymptomatic shoulders has been investigated using magnetic resonance imaging and ultrasonography. The prevalence of tendon degeneration, including partial- and full-thickness tears has been found to increase linearly each decade starting at age 40 years[4–7] and reaching more than 50% of individuals between 60 and 70 years of age[5,6] and more than 80% of individuals more than 80 years of age (Figure 2).[8] In ad-

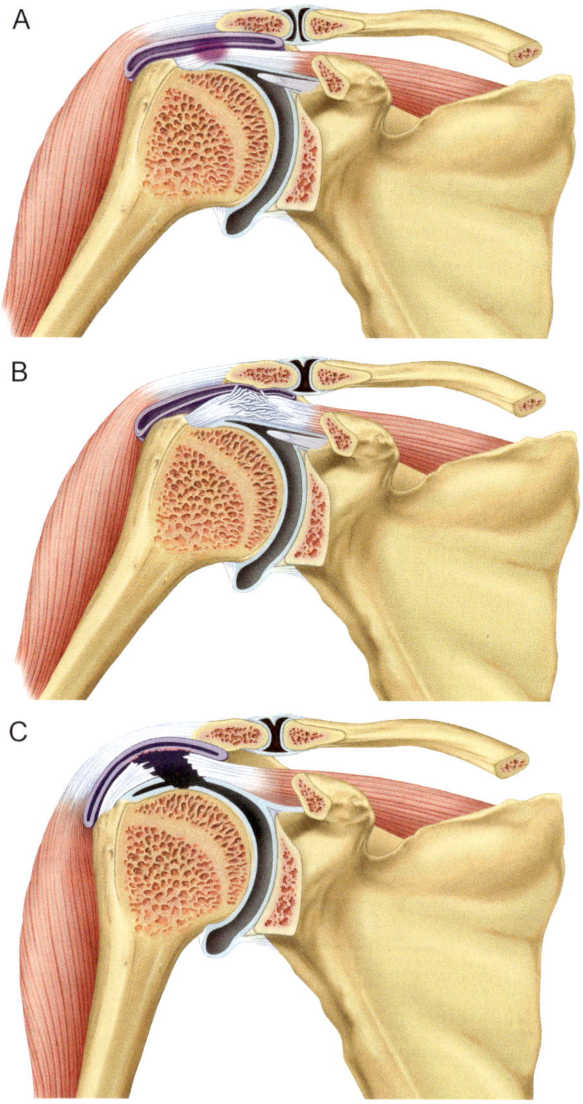

Figure 1. Neer's[3] 3 stages of rotator cuff disease. A, Stage 1, edema and hemorrhage. B, Stage 2, fibrosis and tendonosis. C, Stage 3, full-thickness rotator cuff tear.

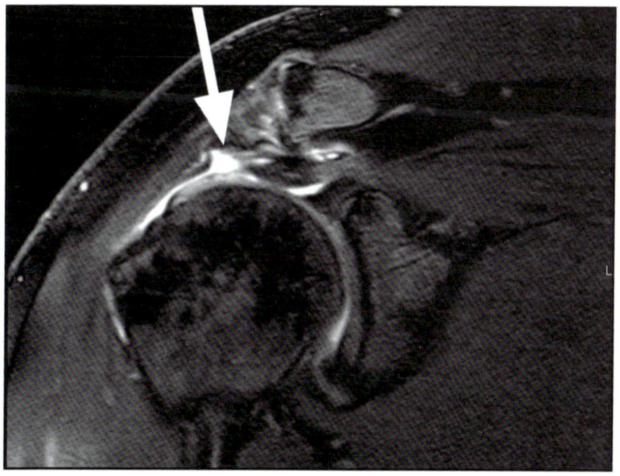

Figure 2. Magnetic resonance imaging scan of a partial-thickness rotator cuff injury.

dition, investigators have shown that asymptomatic rotator cuff tears are progressive and result in pain and disability in more than 50% of previously asymptomatic individuals in less than 4 years after diagnosis.[9]

Neer[3,10] originally proposed an extrinsic mechanism for rotator cuff disease involving compression of the rotator cuff tendons and associated tissues under the anterior aspect of the acromion or surrounding structures[10] and called it *subacromial impingement syndrome*[3] (see chapter III-12). However, Codman and Akerson[11] postulated that the origin of rotator cuff disease was intrinsic due to degeneration within the tendon, which has been attributed to the natural process of aging,[4–7] poor vascularity,[12–17] altered biology,[18–20] and inferior mechanical properties or excessive tensile or shear strain.[21–24] Despite the debate over the pathogenesis, evidence suggests that rotator cuff disease has many causes and perhaps both intrinsic and extrinsic mechanisms play a role.

The structure of the rotator cuff tendons has been shown to interdigitate to form 5 axial-plane layers from the bursal to articular side,[25] which coincides with the region where tendon pathologic conditions are most prevalent (Figure 3).[26] Partial-thickness rotator cuff tears can extend through several layers and commonly are described as bursal-sided, midsubstance, or articular-sided tears (Figure 4 A–D). The size of a full-thickness tear is determined by the number of tendons affected or by the overall size in centimeters of the tear. From a rehabilitation perspective, treatment should focus on maximizing the function of the remaining intact and damaged rotator cuff tendons and surrounding muscles. Rotator cuff tendon tears have not been shown to heal spontaneously.[7,9,27]

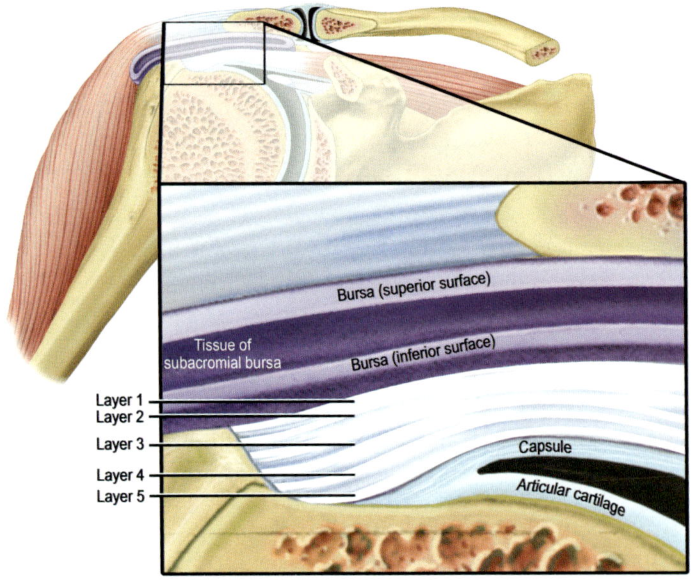

Figure 3. Five axial-plane layers where rotator cuff tears occur.

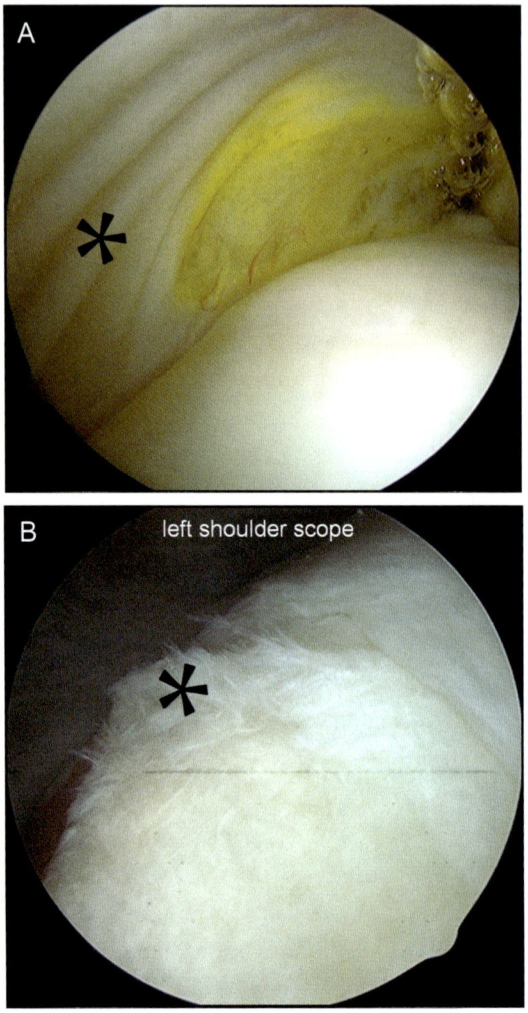

Figure 4 A and B. Arthroscopic view shows a partial-thickness rotator cuff tear involving the bursal side. Note the intact articular fibers, A, and the fraying of the bursal surface, B.

FACTORS INFLUENCING THE OUTCOMES OF REHABILITATION

The success rate for nonoperative treatment of rotator cuff tears has been shown to vary widely.[1,2,28] Little information is available to help guide our expectations about the ultimate outcome for nonoperative treatment. Limited evidence suggests a few factors might be related to a successful outcome of rehabilitation,[29] including preserved ROM in external rotation, little to no atrophy of the supraspinatus muscle, and characteristics of the remaining supraspinatus muscle (presence of the central tendon). These factors suggest smaller tears, including partial-thickness tears, might

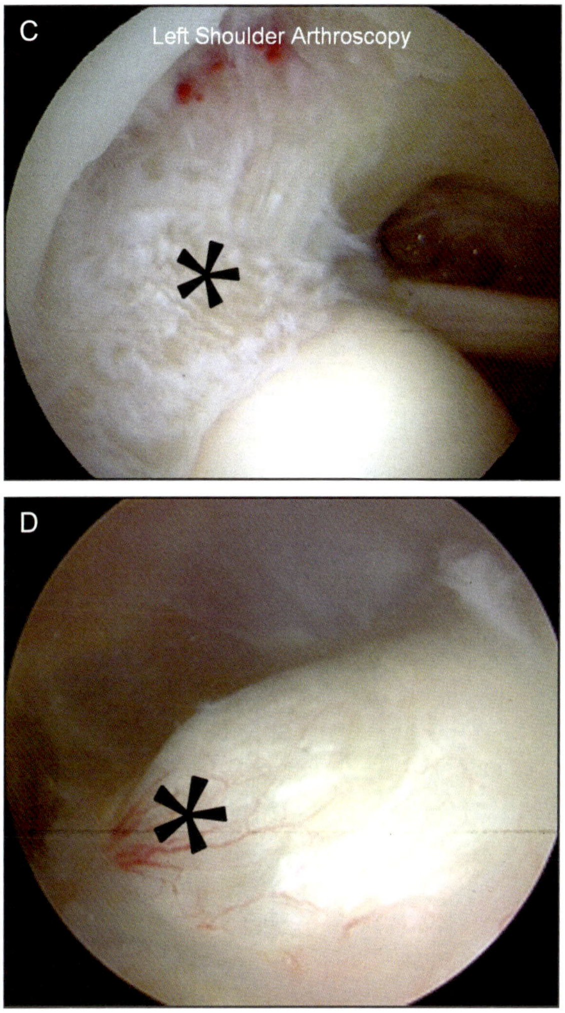

Figure 4 C and D. Arthroscopic view of an articular-sided, partial-thickness rotator cuff tear. C, Disruption of the articular fibers. D, Intact bursal surface of the cuff.

respond to nonoperative rehabilitation. However, comparison of surgery and rehabilitation for individuals with small- to medium-sized rotator cuff tears has shown more favorable results at 1 year after surgery than with rehabilitation alone.[1]

In addition, the shape of the acromion can be an underlying extrinsic mechanism of rotator cuff tears that is associated with a negative outcome of rehabilitation. The shape of the acromion, which is described as type I (flat), type II (curved), or type III (hooked),[30] has been associated with the severity of the rotator cuff tendon condition,[31–34] with a greater prevalence of type III, or hooked, acromion in patients with impingement[32] and full-thickness rotator cuff tears (Figure 5).[31–33,35] In addition, the success of nonoperative treatment for patients with rotator cuff tears has been related to the shape or type of acromion. Wang et al[28] reported that patients with type I acromions responded in 89% of cases of nonoperative treatment; patients with type II, in 73%; and patients with type III, in 58.3%.

SPECIFIC REHABILITATION GUIDELINE

The Appendix specifies our complete 3-phase Conservative Rehabilitation Guideline for Rotator Cuff Disorders. In this section, I explain the rationale for selected components of the guideline. The patient's advancement from one rehabilitation phase to the next phase is not directed specifically by time but rather by the patient's level of symptoms, tolerance to exercise, specific functional goals, and re-evaluation by the phy-

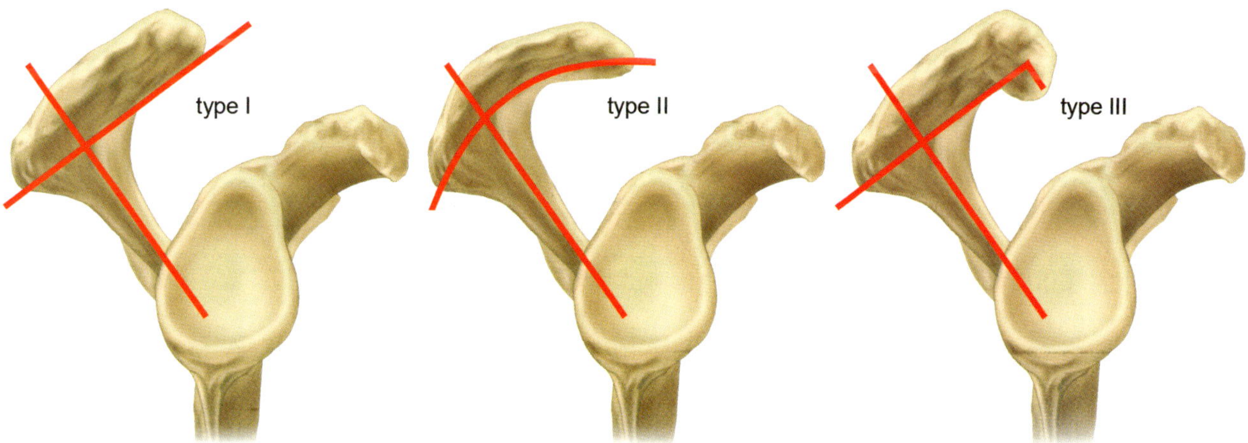

Figure 5. The 3 types of acromions: type I (flat), type II (curved), and type III (hooked).

sician. Patients will enter into this guideline at varying phases depending on their specific impairments and reactivity of their shoulders. In addition, not every patient will complete all phases of rehabilitation because their specific impairment might not respond appropriately to the more advanced rehabilitation activities that are included in the later phases of rehabilitation. The recovery of many patients is most efficient when a prolonged period is spent in phase 1 rehabilitation before a very small advancement in rehabilitation is made. Rapidly progressing rehabilitation in either exercise choice or intensity of the current exercise through increased resistance or repetitions often can result in exacerbation of the patient's symptoms.

Therapeutic Interventions for Rotator Cuff Disease

As described, accurate diagnosis and staging of rotator cuff disease are of primary importance when discussing physical therapy management of this problem with the patient. A thorough clinical examination and imaging studies as described in chapter I-3 will provide the information necessary for the physician to recommend a treatment plan best suited for this patient. The physician's recommendation can vary from an immediate surgical repair to conservative rehabilitation depending on the findings of the clinical examination. This orthopaedic evaluation and consultation with the patient are important so he or she presents to therapy with appropriate expectations for recovery.

Stage 1: Edema and Hemorrhage. Typically, a young patient who presents with stage 1 rotator cuff disease has a short onset of symptoms and a relatively unimpressive magnetic resonance imaging (MRI) report, which usually is prescribed only if the patient experienced a large trauma. Although variable, the therapy examination usually reveals some degree of rotator cuff weakness or pain with strength testing or active ROM (AROM). In addition, the patient will experience varying levels of pain during functional activities, when sitting, and at night depending on his or her level of inflammation and whether he or she received a subacromial steroid injection from the physician. Minimal secondary or compensatory impairments or capsular limitations are generally present, and most patients can expect a fairly short recovery.

Phase 1 management with therapy includes specific education about and modifications to activities of daily living (ADLs) to reduce or eliminate any offending activities that are sustaining or increasing inflammation. Researchers have not shown that modalities beyond cryotherapy are beneficial for patients with rotator cuff tears; however, some researchers have shown that ultrasound is beneficial for patients with calcific tendinitis, subdeltoid bursitis, and subacromial bursitis (see chapter IV-12 for specific details). Anecdotally, we have found that cryotherapy is almost universally well received by patients and provides excellent pain control. We also use comfortable active-assistive ROM, especially rope-and-pulley forward elevation and pendulum, to help reduce inflammation and pain. The base strengthening program and the assistive-to-active elevation progression that are detailed in chapter II-4 and that are light rotator cuff and scapular strengthening should be initiated as soon as comfortable. They are the most important parts of our conservative rehabilitation program for rotator cuff disease and the interventions we find to be most helpful in improving pain with AROM, at night, and with basic functional activities. They often can be started with the initial treatment or very soon after that time.

After the base strengthening program and active forward elevation (Figure 6) are well tolerated (generally

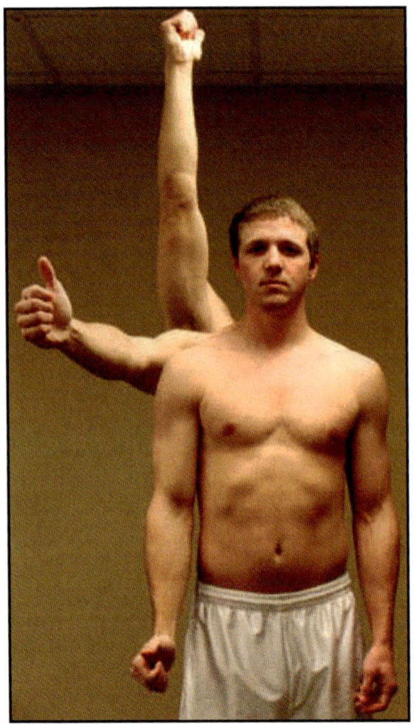

Figure 6. Active forward elevation.

within the first several weeks), the patient's strengthening program is advanced to phase 2, in which weight and repetition are progressed to his or her tolerance while emphasizing high repetitions that can improve the strength of the tendon. During this phase, most patients are released to full ADLs without restriction and will progress to participation in light recreational activities. Most patients are discharged in this level of rehabilitation when their symptoms have resolved or have become minimal. After discharge, patients are expected to continue their rotator cuff strengthening programs for the next 4 to 6 weeks. Patients with significantly higher demands in their occupations or sports are progressed to phase 3, in which the rotator cuff is strengthened in activity-specific positions and the specific technique for the given activity or gymnasium exercise is evaluated. This higher-demand population also is educated that although a full, normal return to participation in all preinjury activities is anticipated, continuing to use the maintenance program for the long term is recommended.

Stage 2: Fibrosis and Tendonosis. A more chronic and more difficult problem to manage about the shoulder is stage 2 rotator cuff tendonosis or partial-thickness rotator cuff tear in which the tendon is degenerating. The overall quality and mechanical properties of the tendon and musculotendon juncture decline,[12–14,16–20] which leads to a longer and potentially more limited recovery. These patients generally are referred to therapy, but if the partial tearing involves more than half of the tendon and/or they have had multiple episodes that have now greatly reduced their quality of life, the orthopaedist might discuss surgery as a treatment option.

When beginning therapy, these patients probably have not received a steroid injection but might have received oral nonsteroidal anti-inflammatory drugs to reduce their symptoms. Phase 1 management might be longer and requires a greater commitment from the patient to reduce occupational activities or ADLs that are causing symptoms. With evaluation, rotator cuff weakness and pain, scapular dyskinesia, cervical dysfunction, or deficits in glenohumeral passive ROM commonly are identified. These impairments in joints other than the glenohumeral joint must be addressed during phase 1 treatment through a combination of strengthening, manual stretching, and mobilization by the rehabilitation provider in addition to appropriate home exercises. Introduction of rotator cuff strengthening might be minimal during the first several weeks of recovery or might begin at the first treatment depending on the level of inflammation, ROM, and basic pain-free use for ADLs.

The phases of rehabilitation and progression of exercise are the same with these types of patients in stage 2 as with patients in stage 1. As with patients in stage 1, rotator cuff strengthening is a crucial component of the treatment plan but requires more diligent monitoring by the rehabilitation provider to adjust the intensity, frequency, and duration of the strength program. Rotator cuff strengthening must be progressed much slower than described for patients in stage 1, with the overall goal being submaximal work that results in minimal fatigue or postworkout soreness (see chapter II-1 for details). Repetitions are valued more than weight, and transition to pain-free forward elevation likely requires the rehabilitation provider to implement the assistive-to-active arm elevation progression described in detail in chapter II-4. During this progression, continued patient compliance with reduced ADLs and recreational activities is required to optimize results. Because the importance of structured rehabilitation is to select and gradually progress the patient's home exercise program, these patients normally can be managed with only occasional clinic visits. The rehabilitation provider needs to spend specific time educating these patients about long-term changes that they need to make to their current occupational or recreational activities. Given the chronic nature of their rotator cuff disease, they will continue to be susceptible to additional episodes of inflammation and potentially can extend their rotator cuff tears if permanent lifestyle changes are not implemented. Advanced or aggressive rotator cuff strengthening, such as outlined in phase 3 of the Appendix, is almost never recommended for this patient population unless they have unavoidable occupational or very specific competitive sport demands and unless the physician specifically approves this level of rehabilitation. In this situation, the physician usually counsels the patient about the likelihood of progressive injury if these functional activities are performed frequently.

Stage 3: Full-Thickness Rotator Cuff Tears. Patients with stage 3 rotator cuff disease have a suspected

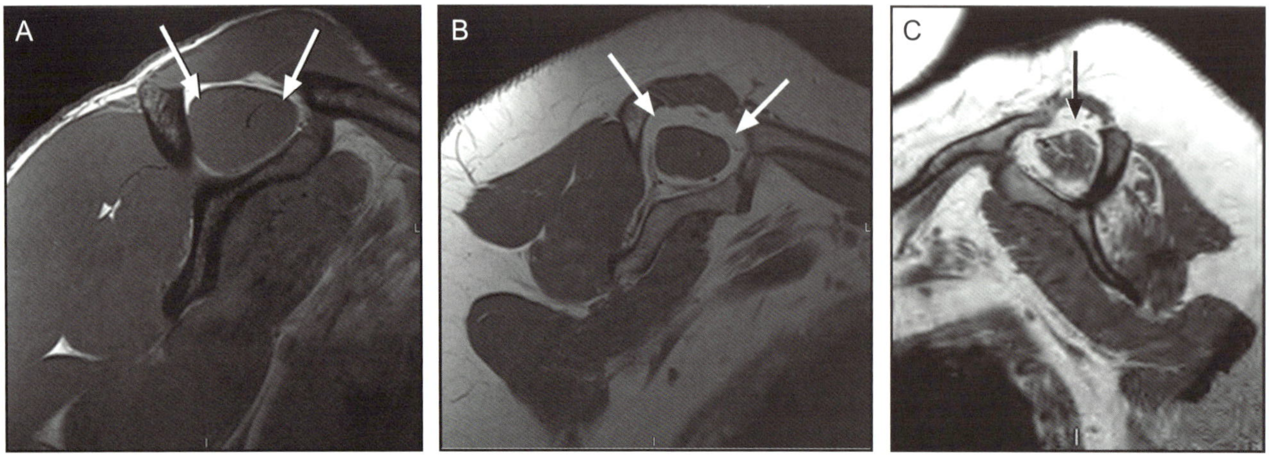

Figure 7. Sagittal-oblique images of the rotator cuff tendons and musculature. A, Normal. B, Muscle atrophy. C, Muscle atrophy and fatty infiltration indicating a large or massive rotator cuff tear.

or confirmed full-thickness tear that is more likely treated surgically than the other stages of rotator cuff disease depending on the patient's level of symptoms, overall health, desired quality of life, and current pain and functional limitations. Whereas some patients with full-thickness rotator cuff tears have a large amount of pain, very limited AROM, and very poor function, some patients with even very large rotator cuff tears that are longstanding primarily might report moderate to severe pain at night with very good AROM and minimal functional limitations. Researchers have shown that even these patients tend to improve with conservative rehabilitation but not typically as much as patients with stage 1 or stage 2 rotator cuff disease.[1,2,28]

Some patients may present with complete tears of multiple rotator cuff tendons or large tears with significant atrophy and fatty infiltration (Figure 7). If a referral to conservative rehabilitation is made in this situation, the rehabilitation provider must realize that because the normal stabilizing force couples of the rotator cuff are damaged (Figure 8), the "standard" rehabilitation guideline is not appropriate. After inflammation has decreased, the remaining dynamic stabilizers of the glenohumeral joint must be trained to attempt to compensate for the torn rotator cuff tendons. Often, the rehabilitation guideline that is used for patients after partial repair of the massive rotator cuff tear (chapter III-3) is the most appropriate guideline to use for nonoperative rehabilitation of the patient with a complete tear of multiple rotator cuff tendons.

The treatment plan for patients with full-thickness rotator cuff tears varies greatly depending on the severity of the cuff tear, clinical presentation of the patient's shoulder, and overall physical health of the patient. Therapy for many older individuals with poor health or inoperable tears often will not move beyond a phase 1 program. The patient's goals must be discussed early and candidly to help the patient understand that his or her final outcomes cannot be accurately well predicted. Preserving and maximizing their AROM and passive ROM through primarily a home exercise program while balancing pain control throughout treatment is important. Often, the goal is to accomplish functional and pain-free ROM rather than to proceed with painful terminal stretching, understanding that their active use of the upper extremity likely is limited due to their rotator cuff damage. Developing a functional strengthening program focused on the damaged and

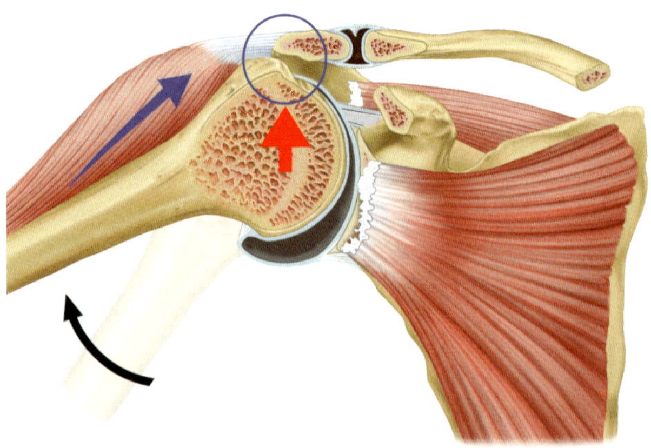

Figure 8. Excessive superior migration of the humeral head, which is shown by the red arrow and blue circle, occurs due to some multitendon rotator cuff tears where the rotator cuff does not adequately stabilize the superior pull of the deltoid.

remaining rotator cuff, deltoid and scapular muscles is emphasized when it can be performed comfortably. Strengthening still can be introduced early in treatment as long as gentle interventions are selected, proper instruction and technique are used, and interventions are progressed very slowly, often waiting several weeks before small advancements are made (see the Appendix and chapters II-1, II-4, II-5, and III-3). In patients with larger rotator cuff tears, selecting interventions that focus on improving the force couples of the rotator cuff and deltoid as detailed in chapter III-2 is especially important (Figure 9). This population also might benefit from regular aquatic therapy exercise for both ROM and strengthening as described in chapter IV-9.

Patients who are in good physical health and have small- to moderate-sized supraspinatus tears and who are referred for conservative rehabilitation require a thorough evaluation to formulate a treatment plan that addresses any ROM or capsular deficits present in addition to a comprehensive rotator cuff, deltoid, and scapular strengthening program described in the Appendix and chapter II-4. The progression of their strengthening programs, similar to that of patients with stage 2 rotator cuff disease, will need to be submaximal to ensure that pain and inflammation are not increased and to ensure that the humeral head remains centered in the glenoid. Overhead active elevation for basic function and rehabilitation usually is achieved with this group, but their ultimate strength and symptoms rarely allow for consistent return to overhead ADLs that are repetitive or that require large amounts of strength. If the patient wants to return to participation in a fitness program, he or she can use a modified weight-training program that withholds exercises that place a large load on the rotator cuff in provocative positions, such as dips, behind-the-head shoulder press, and heavy full-range dumbbell chest presses. Chapter IV-4 details modifications that are important to make in weight-training programs in many clinical situations.

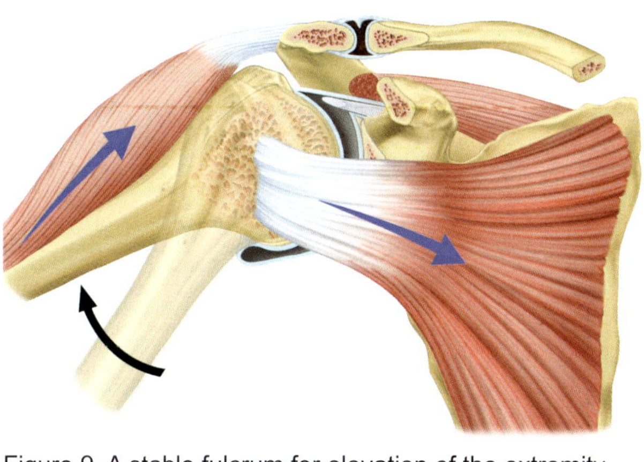

Figure 9. A stable fulcrum for elevation of the extremity can be achieved with a complete supraspinatus tear with stabilization from the subscapularis, infraspinatus, and teres minor.

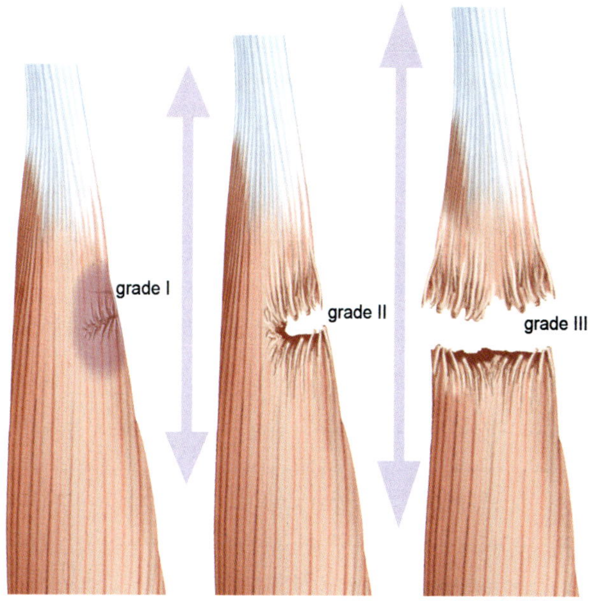

Figure 10. Diagram of muscle strain grades.

SPECIAL CONSIDERATIONS

Acute Strain

As with the lower extremities, the rotator cuff is susceptible to a musculotendon strain injury. These injuries vary greatly in mechanism, and they do not always require substantial force overload but often are more position specific. By definition, a *muscle strain* is an overstretching of the muscle tissue and tendon. Strains are classified by severity as grade I (*overstretched and inflamed*), grade II (*partially torn but competent*), and grade III (*complete rupture and incompetent*) (Figure 10). Initial diagnosis and treatment of this injury might include MRI or ultrasound to rule out a full-thickness rotator cuff injury that might necessitate a recommendation for surgery. Patients presenting to therapy with grade I or II strains should progress in speed and nature as patients with stage 1 rotator cuff disease.

Altering their recreation and daily upper extremity activities is required for 2 to 3 weeks, but they should expect a fairly fast and full recovery.

Athletic "Thrower's Shoulder" or Occupational Overuse Injury

Whether through recreational or occupational demands, repetitive overuse can lead to progressive shoulder pain, weakness, and decreased performance. Often, no specific injury has occurred, but rather a sudden or gradual increase in upper quarter activity has created this injury. Unlike patients with acute tendinitis, this population, when seen shortly after symptom onset, only demonstrates symptoms during their offending activities but may progress into a more severely inflamed state if overuse continues. Imaging may reveal no rotator cuff condition with an acute onset; instead, repetitive overuse of the shoulder creates a constant state of rotator cuff fatigue that the body cannot overcome without intervention.

This is commonly seen in occupational settings in which an employee transitions to a new position with increased upper extremity demands or in an athlete who is just beginning a new sports season. In either case, the shoulder, and more specifically the rotator cuff, has not had a specific and progressive build-up of strength and endurance to successfully perform these increased tasks without fatigue and subsequent breakdown. Most patients will begin to experience symptoms within 3 to 6 weeks of beginning this new activity. Their symptoms will begin with their specific activity, and if not addressed, they progressively will increase to include symptoms with basic ADLs and often will interfere with sleeping. It is not uncommon for these patients rather quickly to develop periscapular pain and often cervical stiffness and soreness to compensate for their rotator cuff weakness.

Treatment received from the rehabilitation provider should proceed similar to the plan described for stage 1 rotator cuff disease. Activity modification or more often stopping the offending activity is required for 3 to 6 weeks. During phase 1, active-assistive ROM stretching and cryotherapy for comfort can be progressed into base strengthening as symptoms decrease. Advancement to phase 2 can occur seamlessly as strength and endurance improve and allow a limited return to activity with advancement to phase 3 activity-specific rotator cuff training, which is very important for this patient population. A gradual reintroduction to the offending activity yields optimal results. The physician often manages this reintroduction by reducing work exposure in the occupational setting and progressing the overhead athlete through an interval throwing program before allowing competitive throwing or pitching in a game.

REFERENCES

1. Moosmayer S, Lund G, Seljom U, et al. Comparison between surgery and physiotherapy in the treatment of small and medium-sized tears of the rotator cuff: a randomised controlled study of 103 patients with one-year follow-up. *J Bone Joint Surg Br*. 2010;92(1):83–91.
2. Bennell K, Wee E, Coburn S, et al. Efficacy of standardised manual therapy and home exercise programme for chronic rotator cuff disease: randomised placebo controlled trial. *BMJ*. 2010;340:c2756.
3. Neer CS II. Impingement lesions. *Clin Orthop Relat Res*. 1983;173:70–77.
4. Iannotti JP, Zlatkin MB, Esterhai JL, Kressel HY, Dalinka MK, Spindler KP. Magnetic resonance imaging of the shoulder: sensitivity, specificity, and predictive value. *J Bone Joint Surg Am*. 1991;73(1):17–29.
5. Milgrom C, Schaffler M, Gilbert S, van Holsbeeck M. Rotator-cuff changes in asymptomatic adults: the effect of age, hand dominance and gender. *J Bone Joint Surg Br*. 1995;77(2):296–298.
6. Sher JS, Uribe JW, Posada A, Murphy BJ, Zlatkin MB. Abnormal findings on magnetic resonance images of asymptomatic shoulders. *J Bone Joint Surg Am*. 1995;77(1):10–15.
7. Tempelhof S, Rupp S, Seil R. Age-related prevalence of rotator cuff tears in asymptomatic shoulders. *J Shoulder Elbow Surg*. 1999;8(4):296–299.
8. Milgrom C, Mann G, Finestone A. A prevalence study of recurrent shoulder dislocations in young adults. *J Shoulder Elbow Surg*. 1998;7(6):621–624.
9. Yamaguchi K, Tetro AM, Blam O, Evanoff BA, Teefey SA, Middleton WD. Natural history of asymptomatic rotator cuff tears: a longitudinal analysis of asymptomatic tears detected sonographically. *J Shoulder Elbow Surg*. 2001;10(3):199–203.
10. Neer CS II. Anterior acromioplasty for the chronic impingement syndrome in the shoulder: a preliminary report. *J Bone Joint Surg Am*. 1972;54(1):41–50.
11. Codman EA, Akerson IB. The pathology associated with rupture of the supraspinatus tendon. *Ann Surg*. 1931;93(1):348–359.
12. Biberthaler P, Wiedemann E, Nerlich A, et al. Microcirculation associated with degenerative rotator cuff lesions: in vivo assessment with orthogonal polarization spectral imaging during arthroscopy of the shoulder. *J Bone Joint Surg Am*. 2003;85(3):475–480.
13. Brooks CH, Revell WJ, Heatley FW. A quantitative histological study of the vascularity of the rotator cuff tendon. *J Bone Joint Surg Br*. 1992;74(1):151–153.

14. Fukuda H, Hamada K, Yamanaka K. Pathology and pathogenesis of bursal-side rotator cuff tears viewed from en bloc histologic sections. *Clin Orthop Relat Res*. 1990;254:75–80.
15. Goodmurphy CW, Osborn J, Akesson EJ, Johnson S, Stanescu V, Regan WD. An immunocytochemical analysis of torn rotator cuff tendon taken at the time of repair. *J Shoulder Elbow Surg*. 2003;12(4):368–374.
16. Rathbun JB, Macnab I. The microvascular pattern of the rotator cuff. *J Bone Joint Surg Br*. 1970;52(3):540–553.
17. Rudzki JR, Adler RS, Warren RF, et al. Contrast-enhanced ultrasound characterization of the vascularity of the rotator cuff tendon: age- and activity-related changes in the intact asymptomatic rotator cuff. *J Shoulder Elbow Surg*. 2008;17(1 suppl):96S–100S.
18. Kumagai J, Sarkar K, Uhthoff HK. The collagen types in the attachment zone of rotator cuff tendons in the elderly: an immunohistochemical study. *J Rheumatol*. 1994;21(11):2096–2100.
19. Riley GP, Harrall RL, Constant CR, Chard MD, Cawston TE, Hazleman BL. Glycosaminoglycans of human rotator cuff tendons: changes with age and in chronic rotator cuff tendinitis. *Ann Rheum Dis*. 1994;53(6):367–376.
20. Riley GP, Harrall RL, Constant CR, Chard MD, Cawston TE, Hazleman BL. Tendon degeneration and chronic shoulder pain: changes in the collagen composition of the human rotator cuff tendons in rotator cuff tendinitis. *Ann Rheum Dis*. 1994;53(6):359–366.
21. Huang CY, Wang VM, Pawluk RJ, et al. Inhomogeneous mechanical behavior of the human supraspinatus tendon under uniaxial loading. *J Orthop Res*. 2005;23(4):924–930.
22. Reilly P, Amis AA, Wallace AL, Emery RJ. Mechanical factors in the initiation and propagation of tears of the rotator cuff: quantification of strains of the supraspinatus tendon in vitro. *J Bone Joint Surg Br*. 2003;85(4):594–599.
23. Lake SP, Miller KS, Elliott DM, Soslowsky LJ. Effect of fiber distribution and realignment on the nonlinear and inhomogeneous mechanical properties of human supraspinatus tendon under longitudinal tensile loading. *J Orthop Res*. 2009;27(12):1596–1602.
24. Bey MJ, Song HK, Wehrli FW, Soslowsky LJ. Intratendinous strain fields of the intact supraspinatus tendon: the effect of glenohumeral joint position and tendon region. *J Orthop Res*. 2002;20(4):869–874.
25. Clark JM, Harryman DT II. Tendons, ligaments, and capsule of the rotator cuff: gross and microscopic anatomy. *J Bone Joint Surg Am*. 1992;74(5):713–725.
26. Codman EA. *The Shoulder: Rupture of the Supraspinatus Tendon and Other Lesions in or About the Subacromial Bursa*. Boston, MA: T Todd; 1934.
27. Mazzocca AD, Rincon LM, O'Connor RW, et al. Intra-articular partial-thickness rotator cuff tears: analysis of injured and repaired strain behavior. *Am J Sports Med*. 2008;36(1):110–116.
28. Wang JC, Horner G, Brown ED, Shapiro MS. The relationship between acromial morphology and conservative treatment of patients with impingement syndrome. *Orthopedics*. 2000;23(6):557–559.
29. Tanaka M, Itoi E, Sato K, et al. Factors related to successful outcome of conservative treatment for rotator cuff tears. *Ups J Med Sci*. 2010;115(3):193–200.
30. Bigliani LU, Morrison DS, April EW. The morphology of the acromion and its relationship to rotator cuff tears. *Orthop Trans*. 1986;10:228.
31. Bigliani LU, Ticker JB, Flatow EL, Soslowsky LJ, Mow VC. The relationship of acromial architecture to rotator cuff disease. *Clin Sports Med*. 1991;10(4):823–838.
32. Epstein RE, Schweitzer ME, Frieman BG, Fenlin JM Jr, Mitchell DG. Hooked acromion: prevalence on MR images of painful shoulders. *Radiology*. 1993;187(2):479–481.
33. Gill TJ, McIrvin E, Kocher MS, Homa K, Mair SD, Hawkins RJ. The relative importance of acromial morphology and age with respect to rotator cuff pathology. *J Shoulder Elbow Surg*. 2002;11(4):327–330.
34. Ogawa K, Yoshida A, Inokuchi W, Naniwa T. Acromial spur: relationship to aging and morphologic changes in the rotator cuff. *J Shoulder Elbow Surg*. 2005;14(6):591–598.
35. Toivonen DA, Tuite MJ, Orwin JF. Acromial structure and tears of the rotator cuff. *J Shoulder Elbow Surg*. 1995;4(5):376–383.

CONSERVATIVE REHABILITATION GUIDELINE FOR ROTATOR CUFF DISORDERS

St. Francis Orthopaedic Institute and St. Francis Rehabilitation Center

All information contained in this protocol is to be used as a general guideline only. Specific variations might be appropriate for each patient and might be specified by the physician. Patients do not have to begin with phase 1 rehabilitation. They can begin at whatever level of rehabilitation matches their current signs and symptoms, but most patients begin with phase 1 rehabilitation. ***Achieving and maintaining a low level of pain and inflammation are the guiding principles in all stages of rehabilitation****.*

SYMBOLS AND ABBREVIATIONS

AAFE, active-assistive forward elevation
AAROM, active-assistive range of motion
AASEP, assistive-to-active shoulder elevation progression
AFE, active forward elevation
ADL, activity of daily living
ER, external rotation
FE, forward elevation
IR, internal rotation
MMT, manual muscle testing
PFE, passive forward elevation
PNF, proprioceptive neuromuscular facilitation
PRN, as needed
PROM, passive range of motion
ROM, range of motion
T-Band, Thera-Band (The Hygenic Corporation, Akron, OH)

Forward elevation, either active or passive, is the plane of motion in which an individual naturally lifts his or her arm that is anterior to the plane of the scapula and lateral to flexion.

PHASE 1

Goals

°Initiate a therapeutic level of rotator cuff, deltoid, and scapular strengthening that does not increase inflammation or the level of reactivity of the shoulder
°Educate the patient about modifying activity, controlling the inflammatory response, and using cryotherapy
°Identify and address secondary factors contributing to current symptoms as long as they do not place the shoulder in impingement positions or exacerbate impingement symptoms
°Decrease reactivity of the shoulder PRN through gentle AAROM
°Use of the shoulder for pain-free ADLs below end ranges of motion

Exercises

Note: Patients might receive a cortical steroid injection in the subacromial bursa from their physicians to decrease their pain and inflammation and thus allow greater participation in their prescribed therapy programs. If patients present to therapy within 7 to 10 days of this injection, great care should be taken to prescribe exercises that are not beyond their described preinjection level of function.

Progression of the current level of exercise resistance and volume or advancement to challenging exercises should be done very slowly and cautiously. Often, several weeks of the same program is prudent before small advancements are made.

°Comfortable AAROM exercises to relieve pain and to improve confidence are used if the level of reactivity of the shoulder is high
  °Preferred exercises

°Codman
°Rope and pulley (elbows remain straight with the thumb up)
°Table step-back

°**Initiate base strengthening program as soon as the patient can perform it comfortably**
- °Includes rotator cuff, deltoid, and scapular strengthening performed at or below chest level (chapter II-4)
- °2 times per day at most with light resistance and increasing repetitions
- °Yellow T-Band (initially) for ER (Figure 11) and IR
  - °Initially, 4- to 6-foot band length and light pretension in a small arc of motion
  - °Can use side-lying ER instead of T-Band ER to begin
- °Yellow T-Band forward reach
  - °Initially, 4- to 6-foot band length and light pretension
  - °Start with the elbow bent and by the side and the band tied behind the patient
  - °Reach **forward** with the hand at waist level, progressing to reaching **forward** at chest level (Figure 12)
- °Scapular strengthening emphasizing scapular retractions and scapular upward rotators (chapter IV-2)
- °**No prone FE, abduction, or ER strengthening**

°Initiate progressive overhead strengthening to improve AFE via the AASEP (chapter II-4) ***ONLY when a tolerance to base strengthening is established and when the AASEP is comfortable***
- °It is a stepwise progression in difficulty of strengthening exercises from PFE to AFE against gravity
- °The goal of the progression is to achieve pain-free full AFE
- °Start with whatever level of exercise is challenging but not painful
- °If scapular or glenohumeral substitutions or pain are present, choose an easier exercise in the progression
- °Only the exercises that are most often used for these patients are listed below
- °**Full motion AFE without weight is the goal of phase 1 for the AASEP**
- °See chapter II-4 for a comprehensive discussion of this program
- °Exercises are divided into 3 levels of difficulty
  1. Gravity-minimized exercises
     - °T-Band supine FE
       - °Must start the involved arm at 90° of elevation
       - °Pull the arm into FE

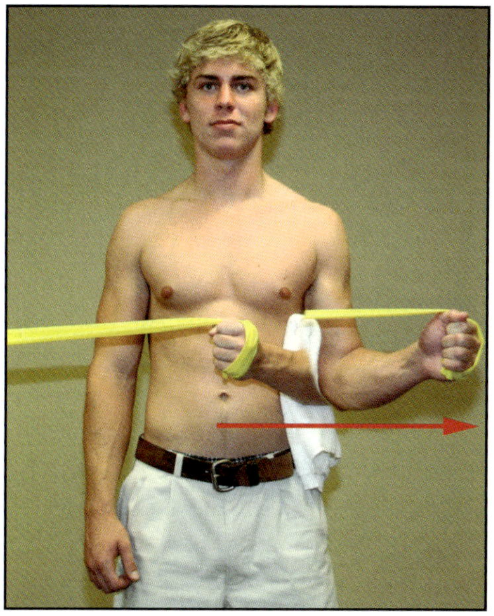

Figure 11. External rotation with an elastic band.

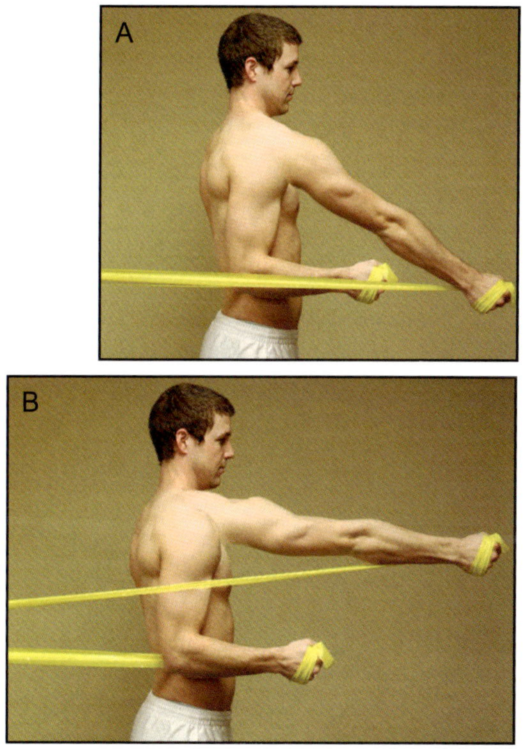

Figure 12. Forward reaching with an elastic band at waist level, A, and at chest level, B, which is more difficult.

- °Jackins supine reaching progression
  - °Begin at 0° with the elbow bent and end at 90° of elevation with the elbow extended
    - °Start with the assistance of a cane or wand
    - °Progress to active motion (Figure 13)
    - °Can progress to using 1 to 2 pounds of weight
  - °Can progress to the inclined position, continuing to reach to the ceiling

2. Assistive elevation exercises
   - °Rope-and-pulley AAFE (Figure 14)
   - °Incline dusting
   - °Wall-slide AAFE
3. Unsupported elevation exercises
   - °AFE

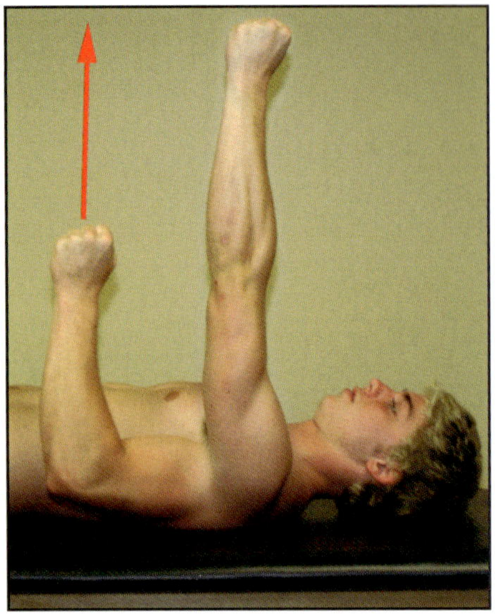

Figure 13. Supine active reaching from 0° to 90°.

- °Patient education
  - °Pathogenesis and rehabilitation process
  - °Importance of frequent use of ice
  - °Minimal use of the arm for provocative positions or recreational activities
    - °Ensure the level of pain is not increasing because of excessive use of the arm for ADLs, work, or recreation
- °Identify and address secondary factors contributing to current symptoms as long as they do not place the shoulder in impingement positions or exacerbate impingement symptoms. These might include, but are not limited to, assessing for and treating
  - °Pectoralis minor tightness (chapters IV-1 and IV-2)
  - °Scapular dyskinesia (chapters IV-1 and IV-2)
  - °Spinal facet dysfunction or other cervical spine disorders (chapter IV-3)
  - °Thoracic outlet syndrome
  - °Myofascial syndrome or other soft tissue disorders

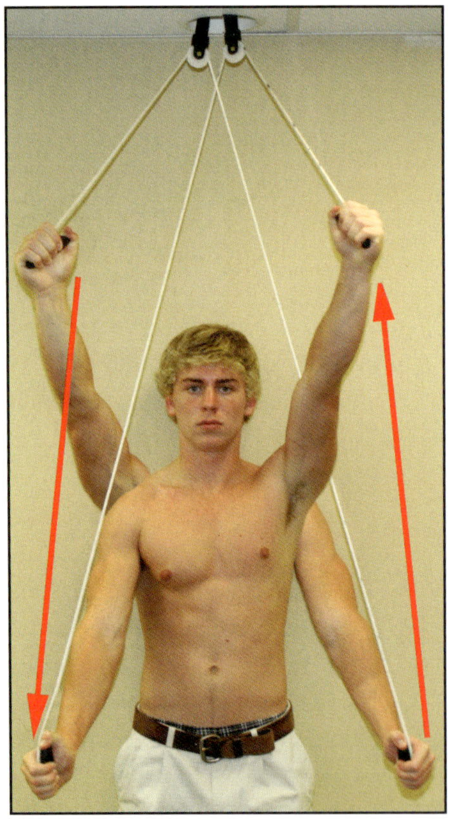

Figure 14. Rope-and-pulley AAFE.

Adjunctive Exercises

- °Modalities as needed to reduce resting or constant pain
  - °Cryotherapy and ice massage
  - °Electrical stimulation only in patients who are not responding well to standard phase 1 rehabilitation (chapter IV-12)
- °Aquatic therapy acutely for pain-free AAROM and comfort (no swimming strokes) (chapter IV-9)
- °Aquatic therapy subacutely for progressive base rotator cuff, scapular, and deltoid strengthening (chapter IV-9)

Interventions to Avoid

- °Exercises that result in severe immediate or delayed pain
- °Exercises that result in excessive guarding or splinting of muscles

°Home or clinic exercises into straight-plane abduction or other exercises that place the shoulder in positions of impingement, such as horizontal adduction
°Repetitive daily activity with affected extremity that provokes symptoms

PHASE 2

Criteria to Begin

°No pain with the arm at rest and symptoms limited to specific and predictable activities with or without pain at night
°Pain-free tolerance to base strengthening program and the AASEP with only reported fatigue
°Note: Many patients, especially elderly patients or those with larger full-thickness tears may never progress to phase 2 rehabilitation or they may stay in phase 1 rehabilitation for at least 4 to 6 weeks.

Goals

°Progressively advance rotator cuff and scapular strength and endurance with a comprehensive strengthening program specific to the patient's evaluated deficits
°Progressively normalize PROM and flexibility deficits, specifically deficits of the posterior capsule and pectoralis minor, that are **limited due to stiffness** into all planes of motion
°Address core and lower extremity deficits because they might contribute to functional limitation
°Allow pain-free return to normal household and low-demand occupational ADLs along with recreational sports that do not require repetitive or powerful overhead use of the arm

Exercises

°Progress the base strengthening program established in phase 1
  °Increase strength and endurance by increasing repetitions and resistance while still using the philosophy of relatively low resistance during rotator cuff strengthening and allowing no visible mechanical deviations (chapter II-1)
  °Increase the size of ROM
  °Perform 2 times per day to perceived level of fatigue
°Progress the AASEP established in phase 1
  °Achieve full-motion AFE without weight if that has not been achieved in phase 1
  °Progress to AFE with very light resistance (typically 1 to 3 pounds) (Figure 15)
°Implement a home-based stretching program to normalize PROM and flexibility deficits that are limited due to stiffness into all planes of motion as long as impingement symptoms are not exacerbated
  °Assess each plane of the motions to determine if stretching is needed. Stretching should be performed if (1) motion is limited more than the contralateral side and (2) the level of pain is minimal or none.

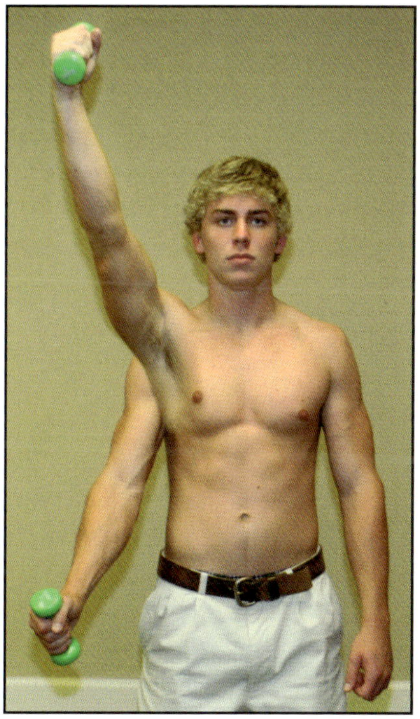

Figure 15. Active forward elevation with light weight.

- °If a particular ROM is limited only due to pain, then mechanical pinching or inflammation rather than stiffness is limiting the ROM. Home stretching would NOT be appropriate at this time
- °Especially evaluate the posterior capsule, forward elevation, and pectoralis minor
- °Preferred posterior capsule stretches include
  - °Horizontal adduction or cross-body stretching
  - °Sleeper stretch

Adjunctive Exercises

- °Aquatic therapy for progressive base rotator cuff, scapular, and deltoid strengthening (chapter IV-9)
- °Closed kinetic chain exercises for shoulder girdle and core stabilization
- °Kinethetic awareness drills
- °Lower extremity and core training if deficits are present and thought to contribute to the patient's signs and symptoms
- °Modified weight-training program PRN (when approved by physician) (chapter IV-4)
  - °Use high repetitions (15–25 repetitions) for at least 1 month and relatively light weight
  - °Initially no chest training or deltoid training beyond rehabilitation exercises
  - °Depending on the size of the tear and the level of symptoms, can progress to chest and shoulder training exercises that do not place a large load on the rotator cuff in provocative positions; for example, do not perform dips, behind-the-head-shoulder press, and heavy full-range dumbbell chest presses

Interventions to Avoid

- °Advanced strengthening or unrestricted return to overhead sports or weight training
- °Exercises that greatly increase signs and symptoms
- °Home or clinic exercises into straight-plane abduction
- °Highly repetitive rehabilitation activities with the arm positioned overhead

Note: Most patients will be discharged at the completion of phase 2 into an independent home exercise program. This program will focus on progressive or maintenance shoulder girdle strengthening. ***Only patients who require return to frequent participation in vigorous sports or moderate to heavy occupational demands and who have stage 1 and occasionally stage 2 rotator cuff disease should progress to phase 3. This level of exercise is not used for most patients with rotator cuff disease.***

PHASE 3

Criteria to Begin

- °Goals of returning to sports, heavy labor, or repetitive or heavy overhead work
- °No pain with the arm at rest and symptoms limited to specific and predictable high-level activities, such as competitive sports or high-demand occupations
- °Successfully normalize all PROM and capsular deficits
- °Pain-free tolerance to progressive base and overhead strengthening program with 5/5 MMT of the rotator cuff and scapular muscles
- °Physician approval

Goals

- °Normalize dynamic strength and endurance of the rotator cuff and scapula
- °Full return to recreational or high-demand occupational ADLs
- °Discharge when functional goals are met
- °Transition to maintenance home exercise program

Exercises

- °Advance base strengthening progression and AFE
  - °Increase elastic resistance and repetitions to 50
  - °Larger, more functional full arc of motion
  - °Increase speed to replicated functional activity without losing eccentric control
  - °AFE up to 5 pounds depending on body size and functional demands
- °Initiate the advanced strengthening progression **PRN** (chapter II-4)
  - °**Strict criteria to start the program listed above**
  - °**Exercise principles**
    - °Decrease the amount of external stabilization provided to the shoulder girdle
    - °Integrate functional patterns, including abduction and ER
    - °Increase speed of movements
    - °Integrate kinesthetic awareness drills into strengthening activities
    - °Include the entire kinetic chain
    - °Decrease rest time to improve endurance
    - °Initiate prone strengthening PRN
    - °Train larger upper extremity muscles wisely
  - °**Sample exercises**
    - °Prone rotator cuff strengthening: light weight with emphasis on the scapula
    - °Hang to abduction with external rotation (Figure 16)
    - °Extension
    - °Abduction
    - °Scaption
- °T-Band standing PNF-type patterns (Figure 17)
- °T-Band 90°/90° ER and IR with or without arm support
- °T-Band simulation of batting, golf, or tennis forehand and backhand
- °Weighted shoulder shrugs
- °Dumbbell overhead shoulder press **PRN**
  - °Place hands in front of the shoulder with the elbows bent and naturally reach overhead
  - °Sets of 15 to 20 repetitions with 3 pounds or more 3 to 7 times a week
- °Initiate progressive replication of demanding ADLs and work

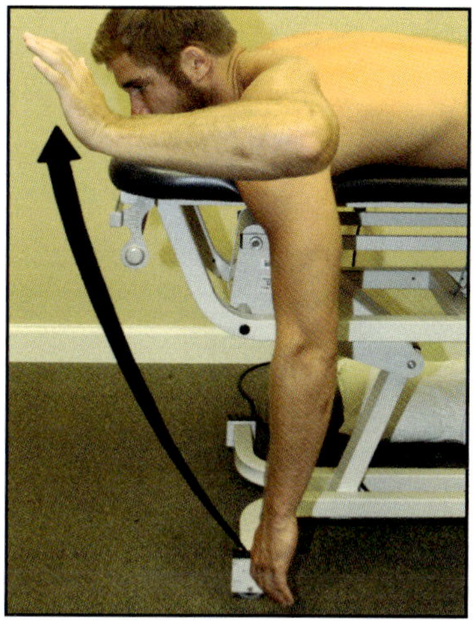

Figure 16. Prone hang to external rotation near 90° of abduction without support.

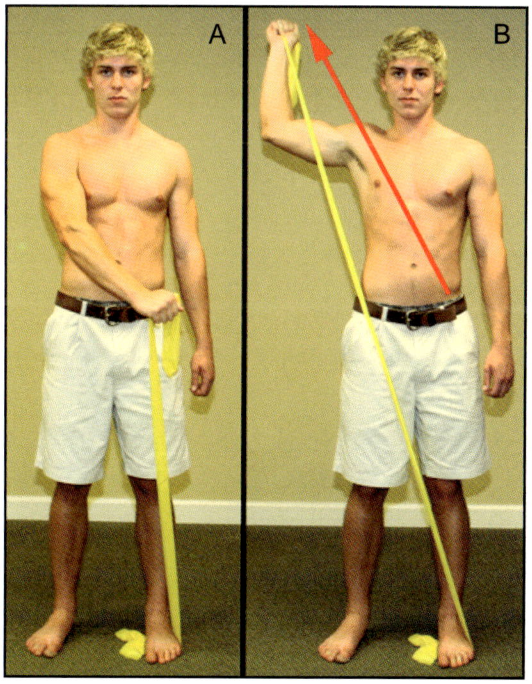

Figure 17 A and B. T-Band standing PNF-type patterns.

- °Can begin interval throwing program or return to tennis program (**when approved by physician**) (chapter IV-6 and chapter IV-8)
- °Initiate modified return to weight-training program (**when approved by physician**) (chapter IV-4)

Adjunctive Exercises

- °Initiate plyometric program (**PRN for overhead athletes and if approved by physician**)
    - °Can begin after 2 to 3 weeks of advanced strengthening program
    - °Do not begin until 5/5 MMT for the rotator cuff and scapula
    - °Use only 2 to 3 times per week
    - °Begin with a beach ball or tennis ball and progress to weighted balls
- °Progressions
    - °2-handed tosses
        - °Waist level
        - °Overhead
        - °Diagonally
    - °1-handed drop-and-catch drills
    - °1-handed tosses, varying the amount of
        - °Abduction
        - °Arm support

Interventions to Avoid

- °**Any rehabilitation activity that is significantly more demanding than daily or expected recreational activities**
- °Any exercise that significantly increases signs and symptoms

III-14

Conservative Rehabilitation of Glenohumeral Instability

Turner A. "Tab" Blackburn, Jr, MEd, PT, ATC

CHAPTER CONTENTS

Clinical pearls are highlighted in yellow throughout the text.

To understand and develop appropriate principles for rehabilitation of the unstable glenohumeral joint, it is important to explore the mechanisms of stability found in the body's most mobile joint and the influences rehabilitation programs have on those mechanisms. The rehabilitation provider also must understand how injury (trauma, congenital conditions, or overuse mechanisms), healing tissue rates, and biomechanical issues affect treatment paradigms.

The ability to translate the glenohumeral joint in multiple directions with the application of nonphysiologic stresses depends on the tissue stiffness about the joint. Stiffness of soft tissue varies in humans; one person can have "tight" joints, and another person can have "loose" joints. During physiologic movement in normal joint mobility, the humeral head can translate upward slightly on the glenoid in scaption from 30° to 60° and then return more to the geometric center as the upper extremity continues to be elevated; nevertheless, it remains close to its geometric center. The main goal of rehabilitation for the unstable glenohumeral joint is to enable the patient to unconsciously maintain joint congruency during all activities.

STABILIZATION MECHANISMS

Stabilization of the humeral head occurs through several mechanisms. Matsen et al[1] pointed out that simply because the joint surfaces are moist, they adhere to each other as 2 glass slides stick together when wet. Building on this minor stability factor, the glenohumeral joint is a concave-convex joint that although not deep, provides resistance to translation. The humeral head must move away from the joint (distraction) to slide off the glenoid and dislocate. The glenoid labrum provides more stability because it deepens the socket, requiring more joint distraction for subluxation or dislocation of the humeral head. The glenohumeral joint is compressed with any movement of the upper extremity, and the capsule is watertight and airtight, creating a vacuum to assist in stabilizing the joint.

The coracohumeral ligament is the only extra-articular ligament of the glenohumeral joint. The remaining ligamentous support comes through the joint capsule. The capsule can vary in its tightness, and a "loose-jointed" person needs more muscular involvement to stabilize the joints. The capsule appears to play most of its role in stabilization at the extremes of range of motion. When the extremity is in the neutral plane-of-the-scapula (POS) position between 80° and 120° of elevation, little stress is placed on the capsule. When the extremity is in full external rotation for example, the anterior capsule tightens, influencing the position of the humeral head.

The tone of all the muscles that affect the glenohumeral joint provides most of the shoulder stability when a person sits relaxed in a chair, sleeps, or moves the upper extremity through various ranges. Muscle tone increases stiffness about the joint and compresses the joint, which in turn allows the mechanisms of stability that I have described to be used. In a patient without muscle tone about the shoulder, any stability probably comes entirely from the capsule.

The dynamic stabilizers, which are the stability components the rehabilitation provider can affect, surround the scapula and the glenohumeral joint. The primary stabilizers are the supraspinatus, infraspinatus, teres minor, subscapularis, biceps brachii, and deltoid muscles. The teres major, latissimus dorsi, and pectoralis major provide secondary stability. At the scapula, the serratus anterior and the trapezius control position for optimal rotator cuff function. As indicated in chapter II-1, electromyography studies have shown the best positions to activate these muscles. The important elements of rehabilitating the unstable shoulder are the biomechanical properties discussed here. Balancing these muscle forces is the art of shoulder rehabilitation.

As mentioned, muscular contraction provides compressive forces and helps stiffen the capsule. The neuromuscular control of these muscles involves efferent and afferent activities of the central nervous system with input from the proprioceptors about the shoulder. The patient must know consciously and unconsciously where the extremity is in space. Lephart et al[2] reported that patients with instability had less ability to reposition the joint even with training before surgery than after surgery, showing that too much instability is difficult to overcome even with the best rehabilitation program.

ARTHROKINEMATICS

The position of the joint and the translational forces also affect glenohumeral joint stability. With the upper extremity at the side, the superior glenohumeral ligament provides anterior stability, and the posterior capsule provides posterior stability. The coracohumeral ligament and the superior capsule provide inferior stability.

As the extremity is elevated overhead, the superior glenohumeral ligament slides up and away, the middle glenohumeral ligament provides anterior stability, the posterior capsule protects the posterior side, and the upper and middle capsules provide inferior support. This continues as the extremity is elevated to 90° except that the inferior glenohumeral ligament supplies the anterior support. Because this is the most commonly damaged ligament in acute anterior dislocations, care should be taken in early rehabilitation to protect the glenohumeral joint from extreme external rotation in the frontal plane with the upper extremity at 90° of elevation.

When the extremity is positioned completely overhead, the anterior glenohumeral ligaments are not stressed; the inferior capsule is taut, supporting inferior stability; and the anterior and posterior bands protect anterior and posterior stability. Depending on the mechanism of injury and the tissue damage, care should be taken to protect these positions. This principle shows that exercising in the POS is necessary for the unstable shoulder.

If a portion of the capsuloligamentous complex is stretched out, the humeral head translates abnormally.[3] In the stable shoulder, external rotation of the humerus at 90° actually causes the humeral head to move posteriorly from the geometric center. When the extremity is internally rotated, the humeral head moves anteriorly. Care must be taken in rehabilitation to position the extremity appropriately to control translation.

Another concept of shoulder stability that can affect rehabilitation programs is the circle concept that Warren et al[4] described. Basically, if a dislocation has occurred, both sides of the capsule lose integrity and, therefore, should be protected in early rehabilitation.

SHOULDER INSTABILITY AND MANAGEMENT

Matsen et al[5] described 2 scenarios that might simply explain shoulder instability and its management: (1) atraumatic, multidirectional, bilateral, responds to rehabilitation and inferior capsular shift (AMBRI) and (2) traumatic event that is unidirectional associated with Bankart lesion requiring surgery (TUBS). With AMBRI, the shoulder has sustained no injury, has laxity in all directions in both shoulders but is symptomatic with pain and dysfunction in the involved shoulder, and most likely will respond to rehabilitation. If not, a more extensive capsular procedure is required to restore stability. With TUBS, the shoulder has a Bankart lesion that more than likely needs operative treatment if the patient wants to return to the activity in which the injury occurred.

Of course, any variation can occur between these 2 situations, but the exercises for both groups are based on the same core exercises. The exercise application can be modified to protect healing tissue.

Three basic types of acute dislocation can lead to shoulder instability that can be treated nonoperatively: acute dislocation with capsular stretch, with capsular tear, and with capsular tear and labral tear (Bankart lesion). Congenital or atraumatic instability and acquired instability also can be treated nonoperatively. Each situation might require some adjustment of upper extremity positioning and limitation of certain movements. Healing restraints can vary in each of these situations.

Acute Dislocation

Initial management of acute dislocation includes reduction, support of the affected extremity, and gradual return to activity. Rowe et al[6] indicated that up to 86% of patients aged less than 20 years who have an acute dislocation will redislocate the shoulder upon return to the activity in which the dislocation occurred (As people age, more type I collagen is produced in the shoulders, so the dislocation and redislocation rates decrease). The rate of redislocation does not seem to change regardless of the postinjury treatment. Although immobilization has been recommended, Hovelius[7] demonstrated that immobilization in internal rotation and adduction for any time did not reduce redislocation in his patients. Itoi et al[8] found that the best way to promote healing in the shoulder after an acute anterior dislocation was to position the extremity in a more externally rotated position and in adduction, which allowed better approximation of the damaged tissue. Other investigators have disputed this finding.

At this point, immobilization or support of the acutely anteriorly or posteriorly dislocated shoulder appears to revolve around symptomatic immobilization. During rehabilitation exercises, protecting the tissues in the first 6 weeks of healing is important. For the anteriorly dislocated shoulder, this means avoiding excessive external rotation and abduction; for the posteriorly dislocated shoulder, this means avoiding excessive internal rotation and across-midline activities. This is another reason to exercise in the POS.

Unfortunately, most investigators using immobilization and exercise have not had consistently successful outcomes (range, 7–75%).[9] Many variables affect the outcomes in these studies. It might boil down to the fact that, if the capsule and labrum are damaged, nonoperative treatment cannot restore stability to enable the patient to return to the activity in which the injury occurred.

First-time traumatic dislocations can result in many acute symptoms. Baker et al[10] indicated that 3 injury scenarios exist. First, patients who have loose joints can have a stretched capsule with intact glenoid labrum after anterior dislocation. Second, patients can have an anteroinferior capsular tear. Third, patients can have a torn anteroinferior capsule and Bankart lesion. In their study, almost all patients with the third type of injury did not improve with rehabilitation and needed operative treatment to return to their active military duties.[10] The first group responded well to rehabilitation, and the second group had mixed results. Consider this information when counseling patients about their treatment choices.

When shoulder dislocation becomes a recurrent problem, the patient has fewer symptoms of trauma, and the shoulder might not require immobilization. Some patients can reduce the joint themselves or with the help of the treating clinician, and they can return to play immediately.

Bracing is most likely to be used to treat the patient with an acute or recurrent shoulder dislocation. Most braces are constructed to prevent extreme external rotation and abduction. How much can they control this extreme of motion? Using 2 commercial braces, Weise et al[11] demonstrated and supported the results of previous investigators, showing that these braces do not limit the shoulder at their preset motions but do prevent hyperabduction and external rotation (Figure 1).

Chu et al[12] demonstrated that with a Neoprene (DuPont Performance Elastomers, Wilmington, DE) shoulder brace, active repositioning was improved in external rotation and abduction in unstable shoulders. The appliance did not limit range of motion.[12] If increase in active repositioning indicates an improved ability to control translation of the humeral head dur-

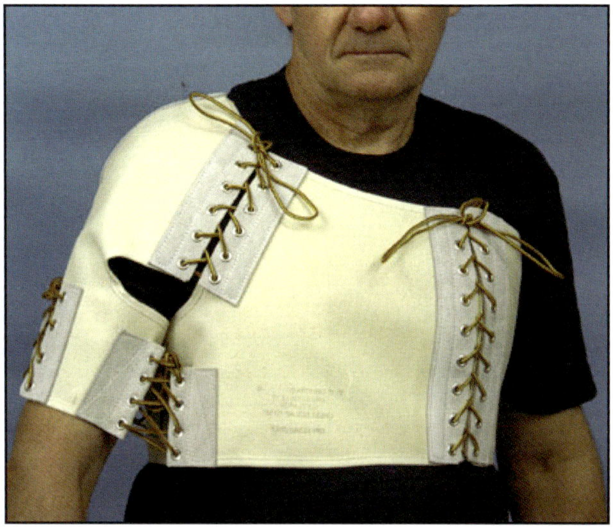

Figure 1. Denison and Duke Wyre harness.

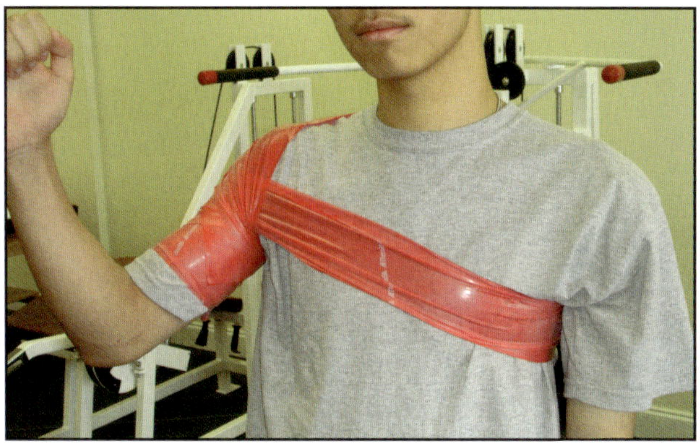

Figure 2. Figure-of-8 strap.

ing activity, then proprioceptive appliances can give patients with unstable shoulders another protective device (Figure 2). To date, no researchers have demonstrated the performance of restrictive or proprioceptive devices on the field, but they are an option.

Initial treatment consists of cryotherapy and electrical stimulation to reduce pain and inflammation. Because initial treatment should be based on the patient's symptoms, avoid extremes of range of motion. In addition, relatively pain-free, early activities include pendulum; shoulder shrug and scapular retraction; and elbow, wrist, and hand active range-of-motion exercises.

As symptoms diminish, core rotator cuff and scapular exercises (chapter II-4) are started (Figures 3 and 4). They should be done in the POS. If the patient has soreness that causes poor exercise technique, the reha-

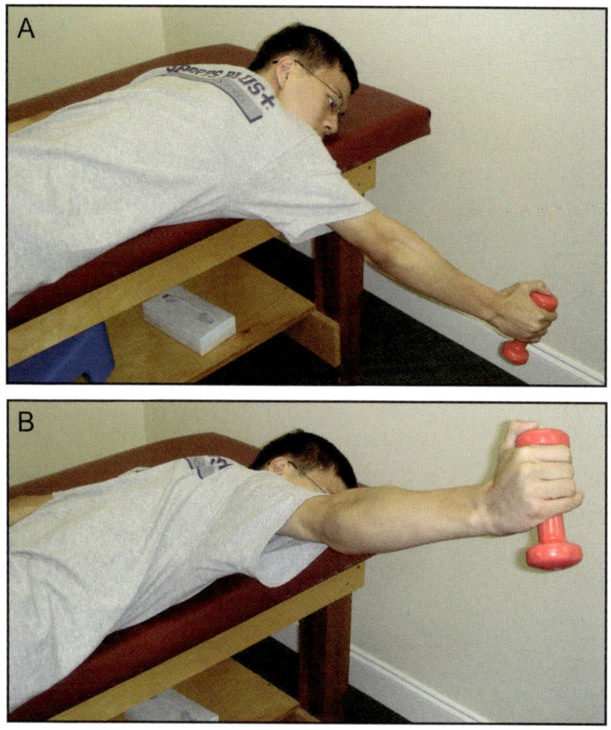

Figure 3. Modification of prone horizontal abduction. A, Correct positioning. B, Incorrect positioning.

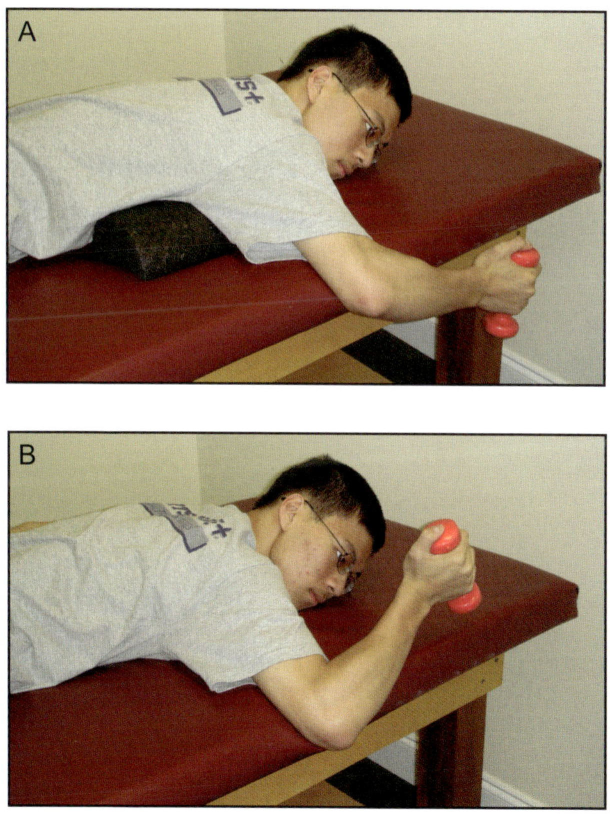

Figure 4. Modification of prone external rotation. A, Correct positioning. B, Incorrect positioning.

bilitation provider initially should use exercises with gravity reduced. Range of motion is usually not an issue. Proprioceptive exercises as described in chapter IV-2 should also be started as soon as comfortable and should be performed in the POS.

If the patient is returning to an activity that will stress the shoulder in the position of dislocation, proprioceptive and strengthening activities should be performed into the more stressful area after at least 3 weeks of healing and aggressively after 6 weeks. If the patient is still apprehensive and his or her shoulder in not stable in that position, return to activity will be slowed.

When the patient returns to more normal weight-training activities, care should be taken to stay in the POS with all activities. Exercises, such as push-ups, bar dips, and bench presses should be done with limited motion so the glenohumeral joint does not go past the frontal plane. A narrow grip on the bench press or narrow hand placement with push-ups puts less stress on the anterior capsule. A wide grip protects the posterior capsule (Figures 5 and 6).

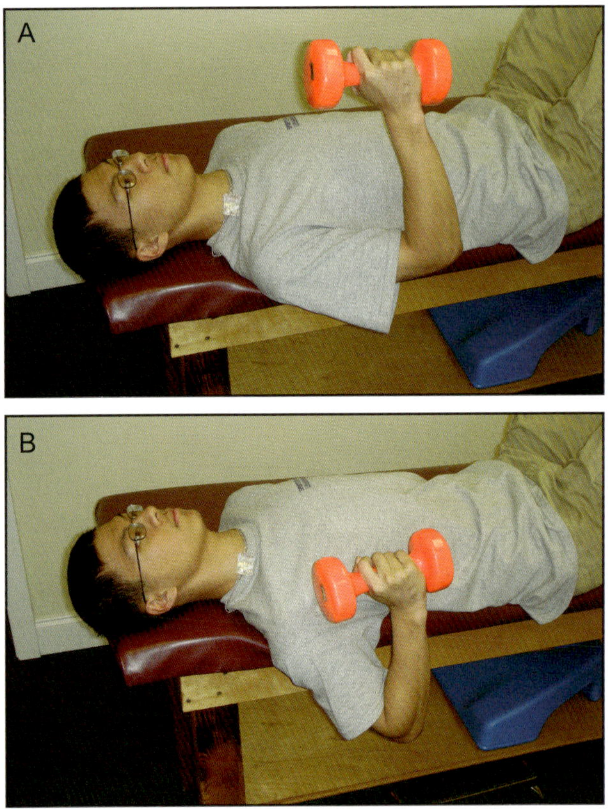

Figure 5. Protective bench press. A, Correct positioning. B, Incorrect positioning.

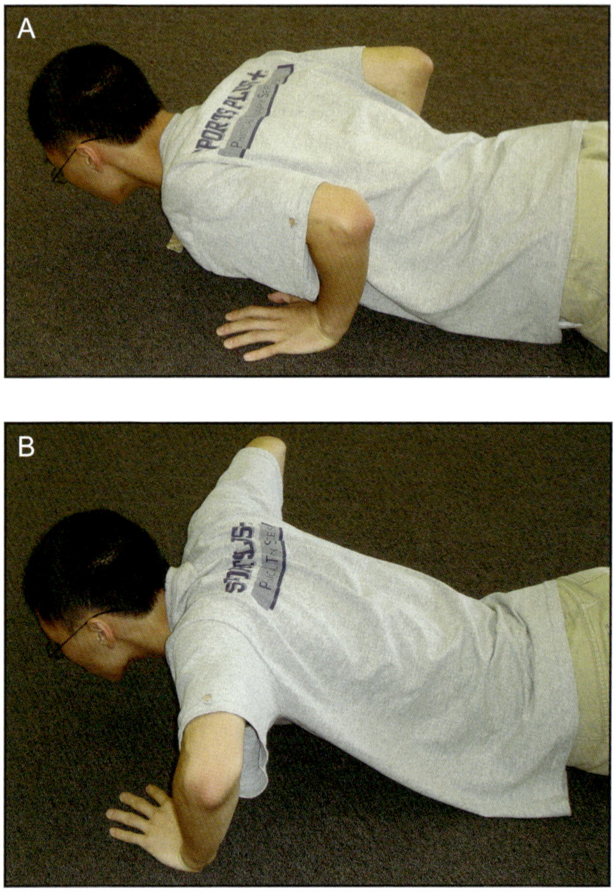

Figure 6. Protective push-up. A, Correct form. B, Incorrect form.

Congenital or Atraumatic Instability

In some patients, the shoulder partially or completely dislocates with very little force. These patients usually have generalized ligament laxity. Many times, their instability is termed *multidirectional instability*. It usually is not related to a torn labrum or capsule. This condition might be related to a connective tissue disorder, poor motor coordination, or deficiency in the rotator cuff interval. However, Burkhead and Rockwood[13] showed that with appropriate rotator cuff and scapular strengthening and with proprioceptive training, almost 80% of these patients improved. Modification of activity also is needed. These patients can have an episode of dislocation or subluxation but usually do not have many acute symptoms. The challenge is when certain upper extremity positions cause the subluxation. Because subluxation occurs easily in these patients, finding positions to perform the appropriate exercises is difficult. They also might have pain from impingement, requiring modalities and a more gradual approach to exercise. These patients generally need little flexibility training.

I start atraumatic patients on core rotator cuff and scapular exercises. It is important to start proprioceptive exercises gently but immediately in the program, paying attention to the POS. Avoid impingement pain with any of the exercises.

Acquired Instability

The overhead athlete is most likely to have acquired instability. Through repetitive overhead activity in external rotation and abduction, baseball, volleyball, water polo, and various racquet-sport athletes seem to be the most commonly affected. High forces developed across the anterior aspect of the shoulder in the cocking phase and dramatic forces developed during deceleration stress the entire capsule. These patients seem to have increased laxity in all directions.

Other theories point to tightening of the posterior aspect of the capsule with the deceleration; this trauma forces the humeral head superiorly, stressing and injuring the superior labrum and thus increasing overall shoulder laxity. Many times these patients have symptoms of impingement that cause them to seek treatment.

Treatment focuses on reducing pain due to impingement and carefully progressing into the core rotator cuff and scapular program. If the patient has posterior capsule tightness, then the rehabilitation provider stretches the posterior capsule. When symptoms are reduced, these patients likely progress through a return-to-overhead-activity program that must balance rest and activity for safe return.

In conclusion, giving attention to the arthrokinematics, healing rates of damaged tissues, and the stresses that various exercises apply to the glenohumeral joint is important in successful nonoperative treatment of the unstable shoulder. Although most stretching activities are limited in this shoulder condition, a tight posterior capsule might need stretching. Appropriate strengthening and proprioceptive exercises are the keys to a satisfactory outcome.

REFERENCES

1. Matsen FA III, Harryman DT II, Sidles JA. Mechanics of glenohumeral instability. *Clin Sports Med*. 1991;10(4):783–788.
2. Lephart SM, Warner JJP, Borsa PA, FH. Proprioception of the shoulder joint in healthy, unstable, and surgically repaired shoulders. *J Shoulder Elbow Surg*. 1994;3(6):371–380.
3. Howell SM, Galinat BJ, Renzi AJ, Marone PJ. Normal and abnormal mechanics of the glenohumeral joint in the horizontal plane. *J Bone Joint Surg Am*. 1988;70(2):227–232.
4. Warren RF, Kornblatt IS, Morehand R. Static factors affecting posterior shoulder stability. *Orthop Trans*. 1984;8:89.
5. Matsen FA III, Thomas SC, Lippitt SB, Rockwood CA Jr, Wirth MA. Glenohumeral instability. In: Rockwood CA Jr, Matson FA III, Wirth MA, Lippitt SB, eds. *The Shoulder*. 3rd ed. Philadelphia, PA: Saunders; 2004:633–639.
6. Rowe CR, Patel D, Southmayd WW. The Bankart procedure: a long-term end-result study. *J Bone Joint Surg Am*. 1978;60(1):1–16.
7. Hovelius L. Anterior dislocation of the shoulder in teen-agers and young adults: five-year prognosis. *J Bone Joint Surg Am*. 1987;69(3):393–399.
8. Itoi E, Hatakeyama Y, Sato T, et al. Immobilization in external rotation after shoulder dislocation reduces the risk of recurrence: a randomized controlled trial. *J Bone Joint Surg Am*. 2007;89(10):2124–2131.
9. Walton J, Paxinos A, Tzannes A, Callanan M, Hayes K, Murrell GA. The unstable shoulder in the adolescent athlete. *Am J Sports Med*. 2002;30(5):758–767.
10. Baker CL, Uribe JW, Whitman C. Arthroscopic evaluation of acute initial anterior shoulder dislocations. *Am J Sports Med*. 1990;18(1):25–28.
11. Weise K, Sitler MR, Tierney R, Swanik KA. Effectiveness of glenohumeral-joint stability braces in limiting active and passive shoulder range of motion in collegiate football players. *J Athl Train*. 2004;39(2):151–155.
12. Chu JC, Kane EJ, Arnold BL, Gansneder BM. The effect of a Neoprene shoulder stabilizer on active joint-reposition sense in subjects with stable and unstable shoulders. *J Athl Train*. 2002;37(2):141–145.
13. Burkhead WZ Jr, Rockwood CA Jr. Treatment of instability of the shoulder with an exercise program. *J Bone Joint Surg Am*. 1992;74(6):890–896.

CONSERVATIVE REHABILITATION GUIDELINE FOR GLENOHUMERAL INSTABILITY

Sports Plus Physical Therapy

All information contained in this protocol is to be used as a general guideline only. Specific variations might be appropriate for each patient and might be specified by the physician. In all cases, it is acceptable to advance the program more slowly than stated. If the patient experiences excessive pain, discontinue exercise until the physician is contacted. ***Achieving and maintaining a low level of pain and inflammation are the most important goals in all stages of rehabilitation, even if less passive and active range of motion are accomplished.***

SYMBOLS AND ABBREVIATIONS

AROM, active range of motion
POS, plane of the scapula

FIRST-TIME ACUTE DISLOCATION

Acute: Initial Care

°Protection with sling
°Relative rest
°Ice and pain modalities
°Nonsteroidal anti-inflammatory drugs and pain medication as needed

Weeks 1 to 3: Progress as Symptoms Subside and out of Sling as Tolerated and Perform in the POS or Forward

°Pendulum
°Elbow, wrist, and hand AROM and light resistance
°Shoulder shrug
°Scapular retraction
°Limited weight bearing with weight shifts

Weeks 4 to 6: Perform in the POS or Forward

°Progress forward elevation activities
°Progress scapular activities
°Progress rotator cuff activities
°Progress proprioceptive activities

Weeks 7 to 12: Progress Toward Abduction and External Rotation as Tolerated

°When rotator cuff and scapular exercises are performed well, can progress to weight training, monitoring arm positions and symptoms
°Continued emphasis on proprioception

Weeks 13 to 16: Return to Participation in Sport Activity

°Use protective harness
°Return when symptoms are controlled

CONGENITAL OR ATRAUMATIC INSTABILITY

Weeks 1 to 6: Avoid Impingement Pain Positions

°Use modalities as needed
°Progress scapular activities
°Progress rotator cuff activities
°Progress proprioceptive activities

Week 7 to 12: Return to Sport Activity

°Maintain core program for maintenance

III-15

Conservative Rehabilitation of Adhesive Capsulitis

Sachiko T. Garner, PT, MS

CHAPTER CONTENTS

- What patients are appropriate for the use of this guideline?
- The most important factor that should guide clinical decision making
- Key principles in rehabilitation of this problem
- St. Francis Rehabilitation Center's staged rehabilitation program
- Special considerations
- Clinical pearls

WHAT PATIENTS ARE APPROPRIATE FOR THE USE OF THIS GUIDELINE?

- Patients with primary adhesive capsulitis
- Patients with secondary adhesive capsulitis
- Patients with long-term stiffness secondary to shoulder surgery
- Patients with long-term stiffness secondary to healed proximal humerus fracture
- Patients with synovitis

Clinical pearls are highlighted in yellow throughout the text.

Adhesive capsulitis was first described by Duplay[1,2] in 1872 as *scapula-humeral periarthritis* and named *frozen shoulder* by Codman in 1934.[1,3] Neviaser[1,4] defined the pathologic anatomy and coined the term *adhesive capsulitis* in 1945. He described the condition as characterized by inflammation of the synovial lining and capsule that causes dense formation of adhesions globally within the joint.[1,4] The condition results in pain and restriction of both passive range of motion (PROM) and active range of motion (AROM) in conjunction with a normal radiograph and affects from 2% to 5% of the population, with a higher incidence in those with diabetes and thyroid disease (10–38%). If affects women more often than men and usually appears between the ages of 40 and 65 years. *Primary adhesive capsulitis* is defined as an entity of unknown cause, resulting in painful and limited active and passive shoulder motion with a characteristic history, presentation, and recovery.[5] This characteristic presentation can be shown through the continuum of 3 phases.[5] The disease begins in a painful, freezing phase with progressive, involuntary stiffness in most cases. Less often, the stiffness precedes the pain and generally lasts from 10 to 36 weeks. The second phase is considered the frozen stage during which pain typically decreases but motion restriction continues to be limited and can last from 4 to 12 months. The final phase in the continuum is the thawing phase that can last from 5 to 20 months with gradual improvement in motion and pain. The total course of the disease has a mean duration of 30 months, with symptoms ranging from 1 to 3.5 years. *Secondary adhesive capsultis* results from other known systemic, extrinsic, or intrinsic diseases, such as alcoholism, thyroid disease, diabetes, cancer, cardiac disease, low estrogen, and strain or sprain.[5] Refer to chapter I-6 for detailed phases of adhesive capsulitis.

THE MOST IMPORTANT FACTOR THAT SHOULD GUIDE CLINICAL DECISION MAKING

Controlling the level of irritability through gentle interventions and modification of activities should always dictate clinical decision making. This is the key principle in the rehabilitation process of adhesive capsulitis. Inflammation is required for the appropriate healing of all injured and operatively repaired tissues; however, researchers have shown that excessive inflammation can increase the chance of developing shoulder stiffness and also results in increased pain.[6,7] Diercks and Stevens[6] examined 77 patients with idiopathic adhesive capsulitis in a prospective, randomized study of supervised neglect versus intense physical therapy. The supervised neglect (gentle) group performed pendulum exercises and range of motion (ROM) within a painless range. The intense physical therapy (aggressive) group performed ROM up to and beyond the threshold of pain and maximum stretching. All patients were re-examined every 3 months for 24 months. Outcomes were measured by the Constant shoulder score. For the gentle group, 64% had a Constant score greater than 80 by 12 months, and 89% had a Constant score greater than 80 at 24 months. For the aggressive group, 0% of patients had a Constant score greater than 80 at 12 months, and only 63% had a Constant score greater than 80 at 24 months. Therefore, the gentle group had vastly superior outcomes in both the short and longer term and even long after rehabilitation had finished. The authors in part concluded, ". . . we believe that the effect of intensive passive stretching, as was done in our physical therapy group, probably had an adverse effect on the natural course of the disease process in the active phase."[6] Several researchers have demonstrated that very gentle stretching is highly effective in restoring ROM and reducing pain over time[8–10] in patients with adhesive capsulitis compared with the decreased effectiveness with other methods of exercise.[11–13]

KEY PRINCIPLES IN REHABILITATION OF THIS PROBLEM

Interventions of Primary Importance

The purpose of formal physical therapy is for education about the pathophysiology of adhesive capsulitis and to establish a home exercise program (HEP) in which gentle stretching, exercise instruction, exercise progression, and use of cryotherapy are emphasized. Rehabilitation progression should be guided by each patient's response to treatment. The typical visit frequency for treatment is an evaluation then a visit at 10 days, 3 to 4 weeks, 6 weeks, and every 4 to 6 weeks as needed thereafter.

The ultimate goal is to decrease levels of pain and inflammation and subsequently increase ROM using patient-specific, short-duration, nearly pain-free stretching to allow the individual to resume his or her desired activities without limitation. However, when inflammation is present, some pain is also present. Slight discomfort is reasonable when stretching with the assistance of a rehabilitation provider and self-stretching at home, but the stretch should never go beyond the threshold of pain. If the pain is too substantial for even minimal stretching, then the goal initially needs to be directed at minimizing the pain with rest; ice; modification of activities; and on occasion, use of modalities, which is discussed later in this chapter. The low-intensity, short-duration stretches alter the input of the joint receptors, resulting in reduced pain, decreased muscle guarding, and increased motion over time.[14] Again, the goal is to increase motion without increasing the patient's overall level of pain. Progression should take place by increasing the frequency and duration but not the intensity of the stretch. It is also important to avoid scapular compensation to minimize abnormal movement patterns and to allow for expansion of the planes of motion that are stretched.

Interventions of Secondary Importance and Adjunct Rehabilitation Options

Manual therapy and modalities can be included in the rehabilitation program as an adjunct as needed. Joint mobilizations can be used in the first phase of rehabilitation and should be low-grade mobilizations for patients with high levels of irritability and higher grades of mobilizations for patients with low levels of irritability. The key to successful joint mobilization is reinforcement in the HEP of the newly gained ROM. Posterior joint mobilizations, especially to increase external rotation, are encouraged. Gerber et al[15] demonstrated that selective tensioning of the posterior capsule decreased ROM in multiple planes of motion. Johnson et al[16] showed a great improvement in external rotation if posterior joint mobilizations at the end range of abduction and external rotation were performed compared with only very small gains in ROM after anterior mobilizations in a group of patients with adhesive capsulitis (Figure 1).[15,16]

Modalities, especially cryotherapy, might be beneficial in the rehabilitation process, but little data exist to support their use. The general consensus is that the best results come when the patient adheres to a combination of physical therapy and an HEP. Ice substantially reduces pain and inflammation, and heat

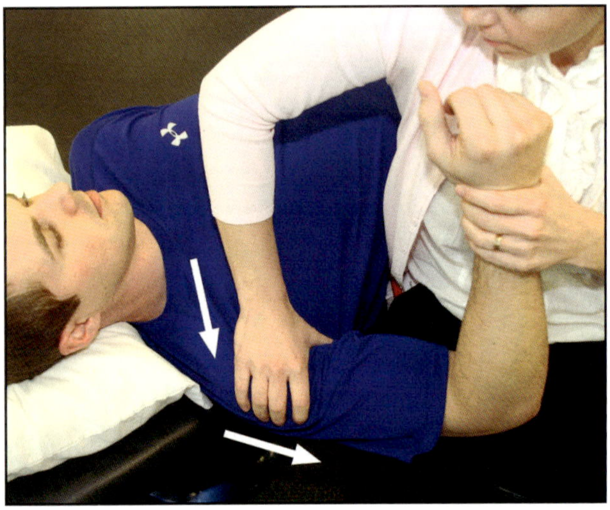

Figure 1. Posterior joint mobilizations performed by the rehabilitation provider.

increases muscle extensibility. Jewell et al[17] found no significant benefit of ultrasound over sham ultrasound. Electrical stimulation uses the gate control theory and can be used as an adjunct to physical therapy for acute pain relief. Many investigators have shown that steroid injections help decrease pain and improve ROM.[18–22] This can allow a patient, who otherwise has too much pain, to better participate in a rehabilitation program. Oral corticosteroids also are used but might not be as effective as an intra-articular steroid injection.[23]

Strengthening only should be initiated in the later stages of rehabilitation when the patient achieves nearly normal PROM in all planes. If these exercises are issued too early in the rehabilitation process, they will hinder control of inflammation, hinder gains in ROM, and increase the overall length of recovery from insidious adhesive capsulitis.

ST. FRANCIS REHABILITATION CENTER'S STAGED REHABILITATION PROGRAM

The reactivity and the subjective history of the patient were the basis for developing this guideline, and they determine the progression through it. It is a 3-stage program that is criteria-based on the patient's presentation and level of irritability in the shoulder. Usually, patients begin in phase 1, but in some cases, a patient initially can begin in phase 2. For example, a patient who has completed the freezing phase of adhesive capsulitis before beginning therapy or who is beginning therapy early enough that he or she has not obtained a severely inflamed and irritated shoulder and has motion that has not become substantially limited initially could begin in phase 2. Progressing from one phase to the next also is determined by the reactivity of the patient and the subjective history. The shoulder needs to have a progressive decrease in pain and inflammation, and ROM needs to improve gradually. Pushing to the next level without improvement will be detrimental and increase inflammation, thus slowing overall recovery.

Phase 1

Phase 1 includes almost everyone, especially those with inflamed, painful shoulders. These patients might present with moderate to high levels of pain, limitations in all planes of AROM and PROM, an empty end feel, and relentless aching or pain at rest. The goal is to educate patients about the pathogenesis and recovery process, the levels of irritability, and the importance of using ice and modifying activity levels; to minimize pain; and to establish tolerance to a gentle stretching program as defined in this chapter. These patients might have a limited therapeutic exercise program due to their levels of pain. Exercises might include Codman circles (Figure 2), passive forward elevation (PFE) using a table (Figure 3) or pulley (Figure 4), passive external rotation (PER) walk-around exercise (Figure 5), lap dusting, and scapular AROM. Adjunct exercises to phase 1 might include rehabilitation-provider-assisted stretching and aquatic therapy. The patient should avoid all exercises that result in immediate or delayed pain that is moderate or severe, exercises that result in excessive muscle guarding, straight-plane abduction activity, strengthening activity, and repetitive activity with the affected extremity. The patient is ready to begin phase 2 after he or she achieves a low level of pain at rest; can reach forward at chest level without pain; is successful with PFE and PER exercises; and has a low level of reactivity when testing ROM in expanded directions, such as passive external rotation and internal rotation at 90° of abduction. Pain still might be present with AROM and activity above shoulder level. The patient typically needs 4 to 6 weeks of phase 1 rehabilitation to meet these goals and then is appropriate to begin phase 2 rehabilitation.

Phase 2

Phase 2 rehabilitation includes a comprehensive PROM program with a low level of pain, with or without joint mobilizations, and addressing associated impairments. The goal of this phase is to expand on phase 1 stretching, further reduce pain, increase the patient's pain-free ROM up to 80% or greater of normal PROM, and increase functional use. The comprehensive stretching program should focus on planes in which the motion is limited more than 10° to 15° and planes in which the level of pain is equal to or less than that of a stretch. Decision making should include understanding that the patient's shoulder should not be stretched into a direction that is not stiff and avoiding stretches that are too painful or reactive. If the patient stretches into a painful plane without a sensation of stretch, then inflammation is limiting the motion, and stretching is not appropriate in that plane. A stretching progression might include the rope and pulley (Figure 4), PER walk-around (Figure 5), patient-assisted

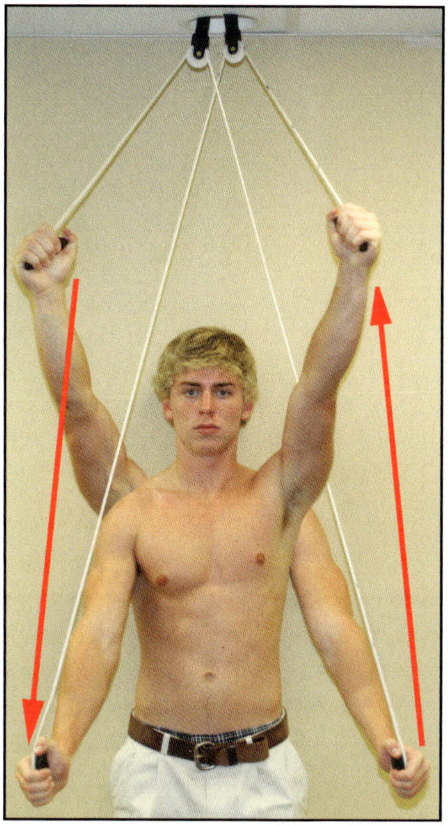

Figure 4. Passive forward elevation using a pulley.

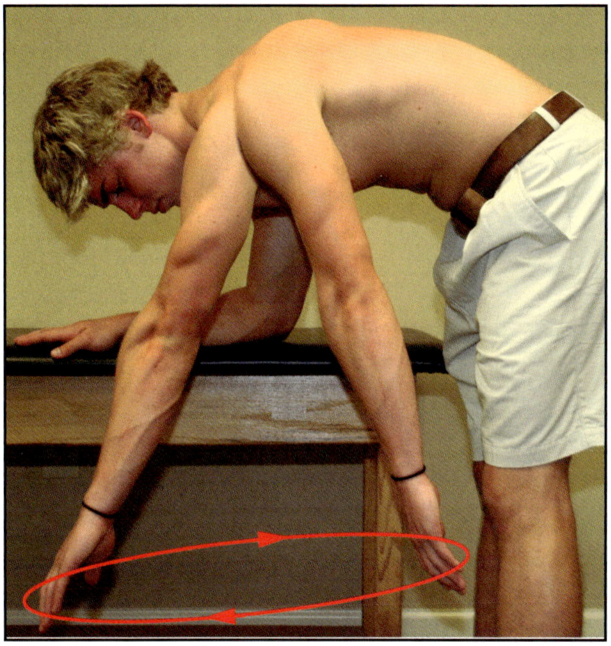

Figure 2. Codman exercise.

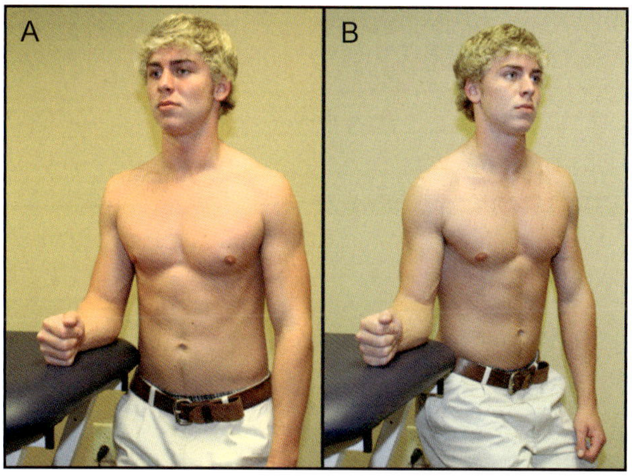

Figure 5 A and B. Passive external rotation stretch using a table.

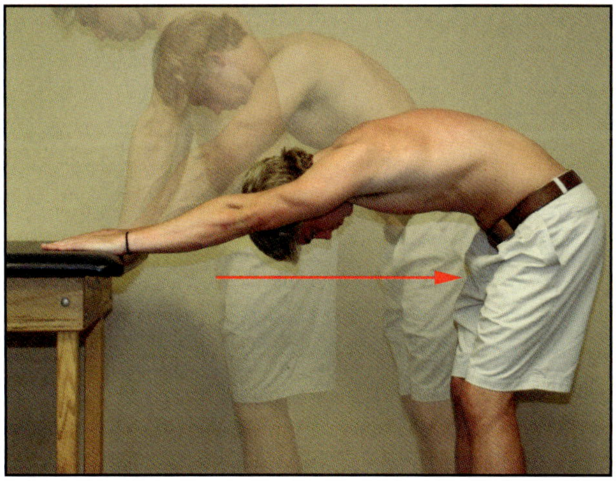

Figure 3. Passive forward elevation stretch using a table.

active-assistive forward elevation (Figure 6), PER with a wand (Figure 7), horizontal adduction stretch (Figure 8), sleeper stretch (Figure 9), functional internal rotation stretch (Figure 10), and supine hand-behind-head stretch (Figure 11). Refer to the comprehensive PROM program in chapter II-3 for further details. In addition to limitations in glenohumeral ROM, other associated impairments that can cause pain and limit ROM and function might be present. Therefore, looking for and fixing associated problems that might be contributing to the patient's clinical signs and symptoms are important. Impairments that commonly can occur with adhesive capsulitis include spine dysfunction, scapular dyskinesia, thoracic outlet syndrome, postural abnormalities, soft tissue problems, and acromioclavicular or sternoclavicular joint hypomobility. Progression to phase 3 rehabilitation should take place when the patient achieves up to or greater than 80% of normal PROM and has substantial decrease in pain.

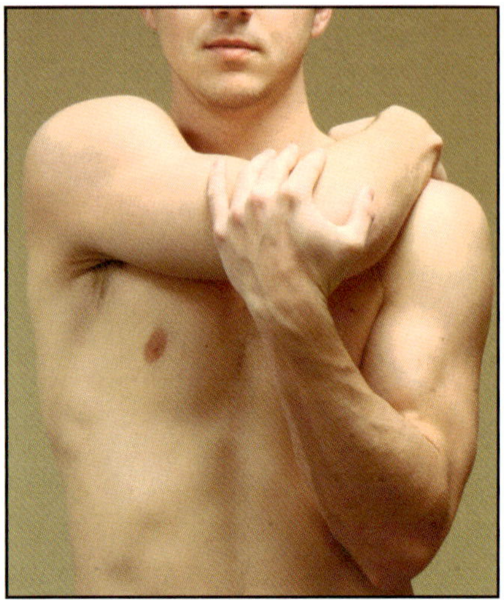

Figure 8. Horizontal adduction stretch.

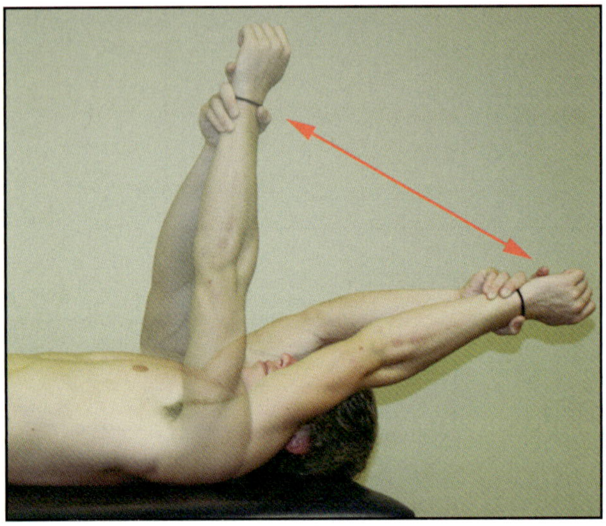

Figure 6. Supine active-assistive forward elevation stretch.

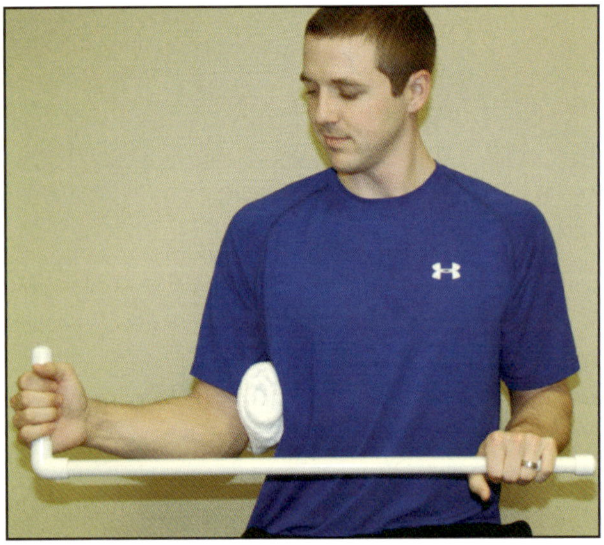

Figure 7. Seated passive external rotation using a wand.

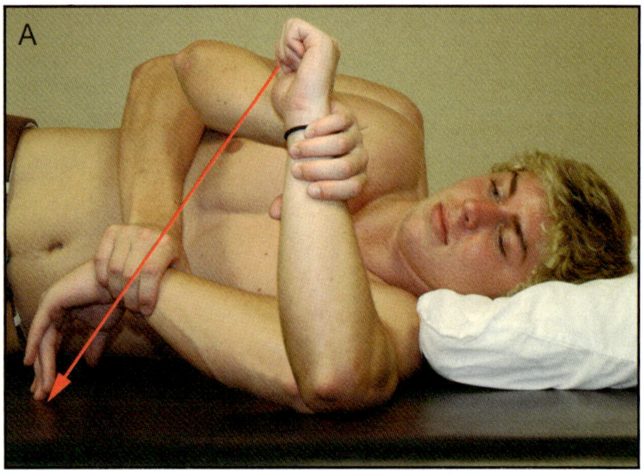

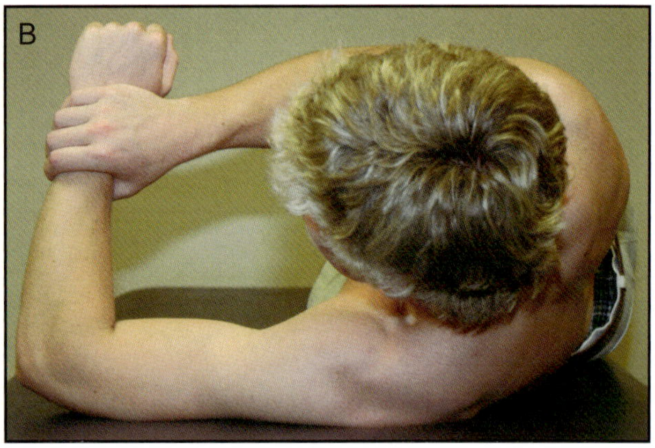

Figure 9. Sleeper stretch. A, Anteroposterior view. B, Aerial view.

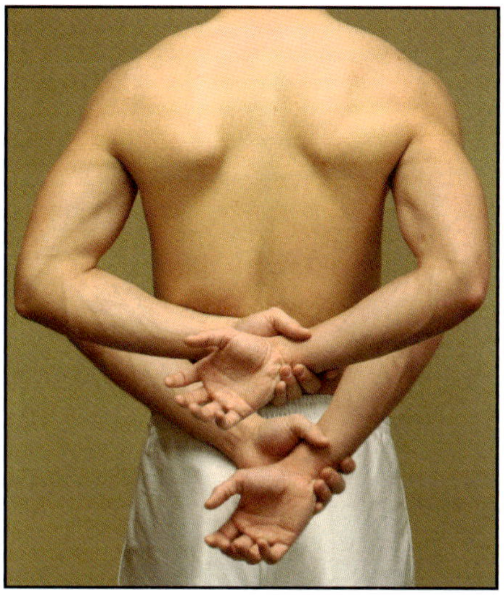

Figure 10. Functional internal rotation stretch.

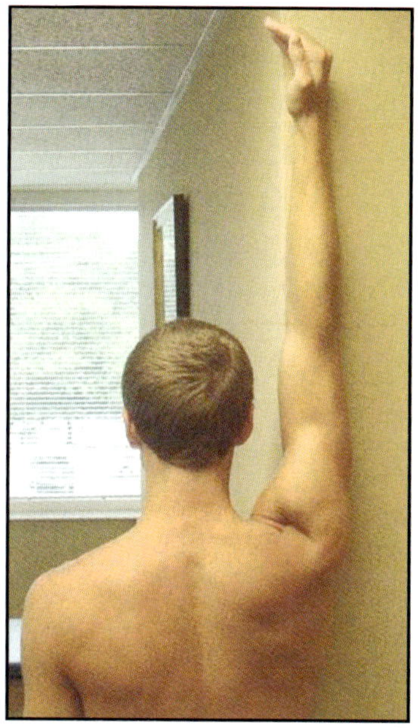

Figure 12. Wall terminal forward elevation stretch.

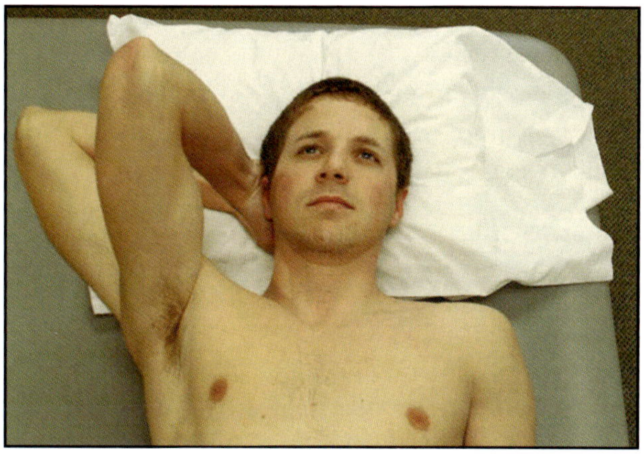

Figure 11. Supine hand-behind-head stretch.

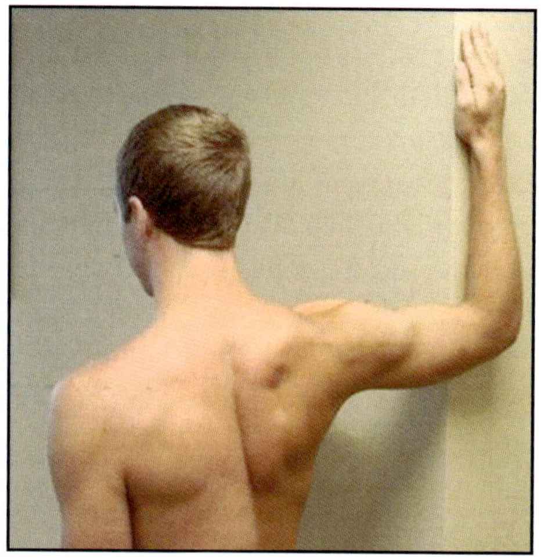

Figure 13. Wall abduction external rotation stretch at 90°/90°.

Phase 3

Phase 3 rehabilitation consists of terminal PROM stretching and progressive strengthening and continues to address associated impairments when the patient has nearly normal PROM. Low reactivity in the shoulder continues to be the focus: low pain with passive stretching and no delayed pain after stretching. Some patients do not require phase 3 rehabilitation to meet their functional goals, so they are discharged after phase 2 rehabilitation. Terminal stretching is advanced in phase 3 when the patient achieves greater than 80% of normal motion in most planes of motion. A patient might perform phase 3 terminal stretches in one or more planes while still using phase 2 stretches in other planes. Care must be taken to continue monitoring reactivity with these stretches. If the reactivity of the patient's shoulder increases with the terminal stretches, then he or she should resume phase 2 stretches until the reactivity decreases. Phase 3 terminal stretching can include wall PFE (Figure 12), wall PER at 90° of abduction (Figure 13) or supine 90°/90° stretch (Figure 14), and supine

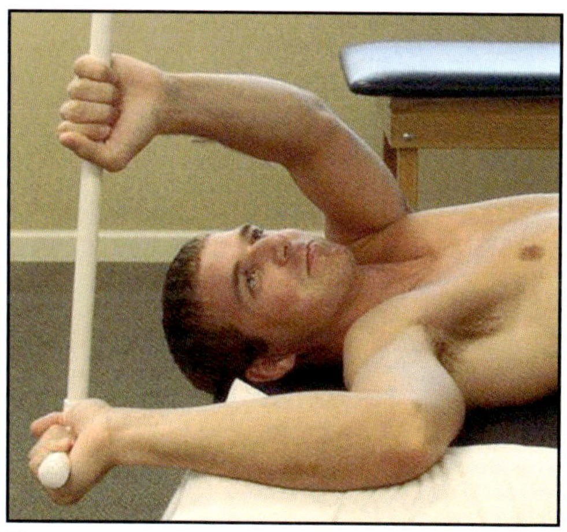

Figure 14. Supine abduction external rotation stretch at 90°/90°.

active-assistive forward elevation with a stick (Figure 15) and can progress functional internal rotation with a towel or pulley (Figure 10). Although strengthening is not the primary focus of treatment, it can be addressed in phase 3 to progress the patient to independence with all activities. A comprehensive strengthening progression is provided in chapter II-4. The strengthening progression also should follow the same progression criteria as the stretching progression. If the reactivity, irritability, or inflammation of the shoulder increases upon advancing with strength, then he or she is not ready and needs to resume only comfortable stretching. The goal of phase 3 is to get the patient to nearly normal function.

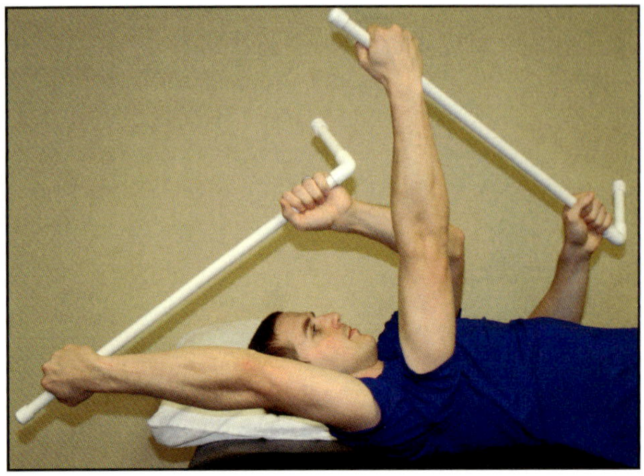

Figure 15. Supine active-assistive forward elevation with a stick.

Discharge Criteria

A successful outcome includes improved pain, ROM gains, improved function, and patient satisfaction. Occasionally, mild signs and symptoms upon discharge are normal for some patients. The discharge goal is a low level of pain; functional ROM; and independence with the HEP, including the comprehensive stretching program and prescribed strengthening to allow for continued improvements independently. Other discharge criteria might include plateaued ROM or a quality of life that is compromised and the patient is considering a manipulation or lysis of adhesions. Discharge can take place during any of the 3 phases of rehabilitation.

SPECIAL CONSIDERATIONS

Primary Adhesive Capsulitis

Patients with primary adhesive capsulitis as defined earlier generally respond predictably and relatively quickly to the standard rehabilitation guideline as outlined in this chapter.

Secondary Adhesive Capsulitis

Secondary adhesive capsulitis is due to systematic pathologic conditions, such as diabetes and thyroid disease. Adhesive capsulitis is more common in patients with type 1 or 2 diabetes (10–23%) than those without the comorbidity (2–5%).[1] Extrinsic predispositions include cervical disc problems, cardiopulmonary disease, humerus fractures, and Parkinson disease. Intrinsic factors include rotator cuff conditions, biceps tendinitis, acromioclavicular joint arthritis, and calcific tendinitis. Patients in this group usually present with increased levels of pain and reactivity. Their signs and symptoms are much easier to exacerbate during rehabilitation interventions and activities of daily living. Standard rehabilitation typically is modified to include increased use of cryotherapy, decreased level of intensity of PROM exercises, and a longer duration with phase 1 stretching exercises. These patients tend to tolerate a comprehensive stretching program poorly until their levels of reactivity are very low. They also tend to have a poor tolerance to strengthening interventions unless their levels of reactivity are exceptionally low. Thus, because of these factors, we have found at the St. Francis Rehabilitation Center that their overall recovery is slower, less predictable, and more frustrating for all parties involved in their care.

Long-Term Stiffness Secondary to Shoulder Surgery

Long-term postoperative stiffness is thought to be a type of stiffness that is much different from primary or secondary adhesive capsulitis. As mentioned, primary and secondary adhesive capsulitis have insidious onsets or result from other systemic diseases. On the other hand, ROM limitations due to postoperative stiffness typically result from dense adhesions that are located in the subacromial space, within the glenohumeral joint, in the rotator interval, or within the fascial planes of the shoulder girdle. If mature, these adhesions result in a type of stiffness that is much more resistant to rehabilitation. Inflammation and the level of reactivity can be low, moderate, or severe. Patients with high levels of reactivity need an extended period of phase 1 stretching, whereas those with low levels of reactivity seem to do best with a comprehensive home program that consists of gentle stretching exercises performed 4 to 6 times each day. This group of patients might not respond well even to prolonged rehabilitation efforts and might require further surgical intervention for full restoration of ROM.

Long-Term Stiffness Secondary to Healed Proximal Humerus Fracture

The stiffness in this group of patients and subsequent management is very similar to that in patients with long-term postoperative stiffness because dense adhesions in many parts of the shoulder often limit glenohumeral motion. In addition, the patient might have bony callus or altered bony anatomy that can limit ROM. For this reason, rehabilitation of patients with long-term stiffness after healed proximal humerus fractures is individualized and depends on what the physician estimates as their ultimate potential. Some patients have the potential for limited ROM or functional use of the extremity above shoulder level and are placed in a limited-goals rehabilitation program, which is detailed in chapter III-18. Typically, patients with long-term stiffness after fracture are appropriate for phase 1 and phase 2 rehabilitation that is gentle. In addition, some of these patients might be appropriate for strengthening as directed by the physician. Terminal phase 3 stretching is almost NEVER appropriate in this patient group. Further details on rehabilitation of patient after acute proximal humerus fracture can be found in chapter III-11.

Synovitis

The natural history of painful synovitis as it progresses to fibroplasia should play a role in determining the treatment plan for patients with synovitis. An extended recovery with substantial improvement after 1 year is expected. These patients typically have limited ROM due to reactivity and pain more than stiffness. Resolution of synovitis is longer than resolution of primary or secondary adhesive capsulitis. Patients need to be gentle with stretching during this recovery period. They typically begin in phase 1 rehabilitation with a strong emphasis on education and understanding the inflamed shoulder. Progressing beyond phase 1 with advanced terminal stretching or strengthening too soon will exaccerbate the synovitis and slow the overall progression. If pain subsides and the level of reactivity in the shoulder is low, then progression to phases 2 and 3 with terminal stretching can take place in a comfortable range only. Rehabilitation is very simple and includes limited, gentle ROM in the early and middle stages of rehabilitation. As time passes without exacerbating activity and gentle ROM is performed, the pain, reactivity, and function will improve. This group of patients is also less likely to respond well even to prolonged rehabilitation efforts than those patients with primary and secondary adhesive capsulitis. They are more likely to require further surgical intervention to achieve a comfortable functional shoulder.

CLINICAL PEARLS

Formal therapy versus HEP only should be dictated by the patient, physician, and rehabilitation provider as a team to determine best results. Patients can respond dramatically to a therapist-instructed HEP with infrequent supervised visits for progression of home-based exercises. No evidence is available to support rigorous physical therapy sessions as more beneficial than a therapist-guided home exercise progression.[6]

Therapist-assisted and self-stretching should be guided by the patient's pain and reactivity to the stretch and should include capsule and muscle stretching. Activities of daily living must be modified to minimize the inflammatory response. Finally, patient education is the key, and the patient must have a vested commitment to home exercises even upon discharge.

REFERENCES

1. Levine WN, Kashyap CP, Bak SF, Ahmad CS, Blaine TA, Bigliani LU. Nonoperative management of idiopathic adhesive capsulitis. *J Shoulder Elbow Surg*. 2007;16(5):569–573.
2. Duplay S. De la peri-arthrite scapula-humerale et des raideurs de l'epaule qui en sont la consequence. *Arch Gen Med.* 1872;20:513–542.
3. Codman EA. *The Shoulder: Rupture of the Supraspinatus Tendon and Other Lesions in or About the Subacromial Bursa.* Boston, MA: T Todd; 1934:216–224.

4. Neviaser JS. Adhesive capsulitis of the shoulder: a study of pathological findings in periarthritis of the shoulder. *J Bone Joint Surg Am.* 1945;27(2):211–222.
5. Hsu JE, Anakwenze OA, Warrender WJ, Abboud JA. Current review of adhesive capsulitis. *J Shoulder Elbow Surg.* 2011;20(3):502–514.
6. Diercks RL, Stevens M. Gentle thawing of the frozen shoulder: a prospective study of supervised neglect versus intensive physical therapy in seventy-seven patients with frozen shoulder syndrome followed up for two years. *J Shoulder Elbow Surg.* 2004;13(5):499–502.
7. Lundberg BJ. The frozen shoulder: clinical and radiographical observations. The effect of manipulation under general anesthesia. Structure and glycosaminoglycan content of the joint capsule. Local bone metabolism. *Acta Orthop Scand.* 1969;119(suppl):1–59.
8. Parsons JL, Shepard WL, Fosdick WM. DMSO an adjutant to physical therapy in the chronic frozen shoulder. *Ann N Y Acad Sci.* 1967;141(1):569–571.
9. Watson-Jones R. Simple treatment of the stiff shoulder. *J Bone Joint Surg Br.* 1963;45(1):207.
10. Nicholson GG. The effects of passive joint mobilization on pain and hypomobility associated with adhesive capsulitis of the shoulder. *J Orthop Sports Phys Ther.* 1985;6(4):238–246.
11. Rizk TE, Christopher RP, Pinal RS, Higgins AC, Frix R. Adhesive capsulitis (frozen shoulder): a new approach to its management. *Arch Phys Med Rehabil.* 1983;64(1):29–33.
12. Hazleman BL. The painful stiff shoulder. *Rheumatol Phys Med.* 1972;11(8):413–421.
13. Harryman DT II, Lazarus MD, Rozencwaig R. The stiff shoulder. In: Rockwood CA, Matsen FA III, eds. *The Shoulder.* Philadelphia, PA: WB Saunders; 1998:1064–1112.
14. Kelley MJ, McClure PW, Leggin BG. Frozen shoulder: evidence and a proposed model guiding rehabilitation. *J Orthop Sports Phys Ther.* 2009;39(2):135–148.
15. Gerber C, Werner CM, Macy JC, Jacob HA, Nyffeler RW. Effect of selective capsulorrhaphy on the passive range of motion of the glenohumeral joint. *J Bone Joint Surg Am.* 2003;85(1):48–55.
16. Johnson AJ, Godges JJ, Zimmerman GJ, Ounanian LL. The effect of anterior versus posterior glide joint mobilization on external rotation range of motion in patients with shoulder adhesive capsulitis. *J Orthop Sports Phys Ther.* 2007;37(3):88–99.
17. Jewell DV, Riddle DL, Thacker LR. Interventions associated with an increased or decreased likelihood of pain reduction and improved function in patients with adhesive capsulitis: a retrospective cohort study. *Phys Ther.* 2009;89(5):419–429.
18. Izumi T, Aoki M, Muraki T, Hidaka E, Miyamoto S. Stretching positions for the posterior capsule of the glenohumeral joint: strain measurement using cadaver specimens. *Am J Sports Med.* 2008;36(10):2014–2022.
19. Zuckerman JD. Rokito A. Frozen shoulder: a consensus definition. *J Shoulder Elbow Surg.* 2011;20(2):322–325.
20. Arslan S, Çeliker R. Comparison of the efficacy of local corticosteroid injection and physical therapy for the treatment of adhesive capsulitis. *Rheumatol Int.* 2001;21(1):20–23.
21. Bulgen DY, Binder AI, Hazleman BL, Dutton J, Roberts S. Frozen shoulder: prospective clinical study with an evaluation of three treatment regimens. *Ann Rheum Dis.* 1984;43(3):353–360.
22. van der Windt DA, Koes BW, Devillé W, Boeke AJ, de Jong BA, Bouter LM. Effectiveness of corticosteroid injections versus physiotherapy for treatment of painful stiff shoulder in primary care: randomised trial. *BMJ.* 1998;317(7168):1292–1296.
23. Lorbach O, Anagnostakos K, Scherf C, Seil R, Kohn D, Pape D. Nonoperative management of adhesive capsulitis of the shoulder: oral cortisone application versus intra-articular cortisone injections. *J Shoulder Elbow Surg.* 2010;19(2):172–179.

CONSERVATIVE REHABILITATION GUIDELINE FOR ADHESIVE CAPSULITIS

St. Francis Orthopaedic Institute and St. Francis Rehabilitation Center

All information contained in this protocol is to be used as a general guideline only. Specific variations might be appropriate for each patient and might be specified by the physician. In all cases, it is acceptable to advance the program more slowly than stated. If the patient experiences excessive pain, discontinue exercise until the physician is contacted. ***Achieving and maintaining a low level of pain and inflammation are the guiding principles in all stages of rehabilitation, even if less passive and active range of motion are accomplished.***

SYMBOLS AND ABBREVIATIONS

AAFE, active-assistive forward elevation
AAROM, active-assistive range of motion
AASEP, assistive-to-active shoulder elevation progression
AFE, active forward elevation
AROM, active range of motion
ER, external rotation
FE, forward elevation
IR, internal rotation
PER, passive external rotation
PFE, passive forward elevation
PRN, as needed
PROM, passive range of motion
ROM, range of motion
T-Band, Thera-Band (The Hygenic Corporation, Akron, OH)

Forward elevation, either active or passive, is the plane of motion in which an individual naturally lifts his or her arm that is anterior to the plane of the scapula and lateral to flexion.

PHASE 1

Goals

- °Control reactivity by minimizing pain and inflammatory response
- °Educate the patient about modified activity, inflammatory response, and use of ice
- °Establish a tolerance to a limited gentle stretching program

Exercises

- °Pendulum exercises
  - °Lean over the table a comfortable amount
  - °Let the arm hang down relaxed
  - °Keep the body still
  - °As able, move the arm in small comfortable circles only
- °Upright PER in slight abduction until mild stretch and discomfort
  - °7 to 12 repetitions 4 to 5 times per day (Figure 16)
    - °Preferred exercises
    - °Sit with family member or therapist rotating the arm
    - °PER walk-around (stand with the arm supported on a table and rotate the body) (Figure 5)
- °PFE until mild stretch and discomfort
  - °7 to 12 repetitions 4 to 5 times per day (Figure 17)
  - °Preferred exercises
    - °Sit with family member or therapist lifting the arm

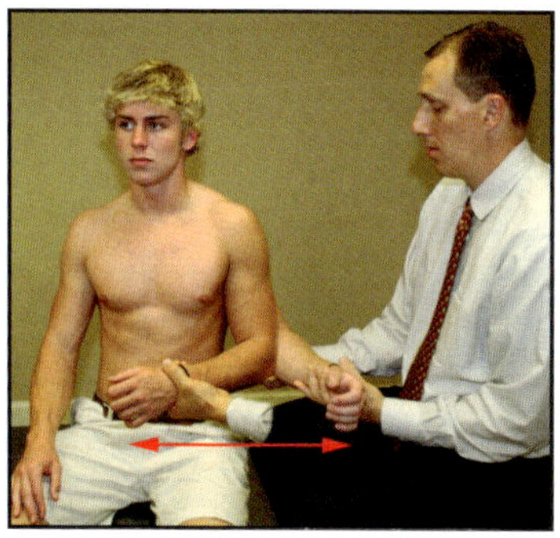
Figure 16. Seated PER.

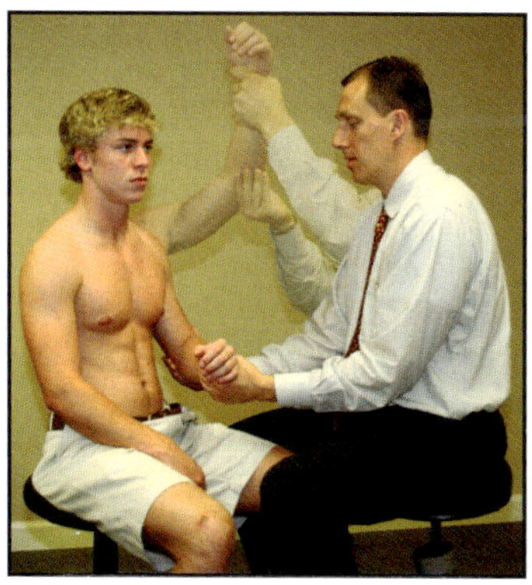
Figure 17. Seated PFE.

°Table step-back exercise (Figure 3)

°After achieving more than 120° of PFE, progress to self-assisted AAFE in the supine position (Figure 6) or rope-and-pulley PFE (Figure 4) as comfortable

°Horizontal dusting

°Perform straight ahead

°Perform at 20° angles medially and laterally if comfortable

°Patient education

°Education of pathogenesis and recovery process

°Importance of frequent use of ice for pain reduction

°Minimal use of the arm for light waist-level activities as comfortable

°Ensure the level of pain is not increasing because of excessive use of the arm for activities of daily living or work

Adjunctive Exercises

°Therapist-assisted supine PROM in all planes as tolerated within comfortable ROM to

°Decrease pain and guarding of muscles

°Achieve gentle ROM gains

°Aquatic therapy for gentle pain-free AAROM (no swimming strokes)

Interventions to Avoid

°Exercises that result in moderate or severe immediate or delayed pain

°Exercises that result in excessive guarding or splinting of muscles

°Home exercises into straight-plane abduction

°Strengthening exercises

°Repetitive activity with the affected extremity

PHASE 2

Criteria to Begin

°Successful tolerance to PFE and PER stretching

°Low reactivity (stretch sensation before pain, no delayed pain)

°Improved ROM

°Low level of pain at rest and with active forward reaching at waist level

°Moderate to low reactivity when assess tolerance to PROM in different planes

Goals

°Further reduce shoulder pain

°Implement comprehensive PROM and stretching program

°Achieve more than 80% of normal PROM

°Improve AROM

°Increase functional activities

Exercises

Comprehensive home stretching program: Assess each of the motions below to determine if stretching is needed. Stretching should only be performed if (1) motion is limited more than 10° to 15° and (2) the level of pain is equal to or less than the sensation of stretch. If a particular ROM is limited due to only pain, then inflammation and not stiffness is limiting the ROM, so stretching is NOT appropriate in this particular plane of motion at this time.

- °PFE stretching
  - °Preferred exercises
    - °Rope-and-pulley exercise (elbows remain straight) (Figure 4)
    - °Patient-assisted supine AAFE exercise (use the unaffected arm for assistance) (Figure 6)
- °Upright PER stretching
  - °Preferred exercises
    - °PER with wand upright and hand in neutral (Figure 7)
    - °PER walk-around (stand with the arm supported on a table and rotate the body) (Figure 5)
- °Horizontal adduction (Figure 8) or sleeper stretch, or both, PRN (Figure 9)
- °Supine hand-behind-head stretch (Figure 11)
  - °Progress to gentle ER stretching in 70° to 90° of abduction
- °Functional IR AAROM (Figure 10)
  - °Preferred exercise: the uninvolved hand assists the involved arm directly
- °Address associated impairments if present. Evaluate for problems, such as
  - °Spine dysfunction
  - °Scapular dyskinesia
  - °Thoracic outlet syndrome
  - °Postural abnormalities
  - °Soft tissue problems
  - °Acromioclavicular or sternoclavicular joint hypomobility
- °Cryotherapy to reduce pain and inflammation

Adjunctive Exercises

- °Therapist-assisted supine PROM in all planes as tolerated (use same criteria as listed above in comprehensive home stretching program)
  - °Consider
    - °ER at 20°, 45°, and 90° of abduction
    - °IR in progressive abduction up to 90°
    - °Horizontal adduction
    - °Diagonal elevation from 90° of FE to 140° of abduction
    - °FE progressing to flexion
- °Aquatic exercises (chapter IV-9)
  - °AAROM
  - °AROM
  - °Light strengthening
- °Consider initiating AASEP (described in phase 3) if a large discrepancy exists between PFE and AFE and if exercises are comfortable

Interventions to Avoid

- °Strengthening except as described above
- °Exercises that greatly increase signs and symptoms
- °Highly repetitive rehabilitation activities with the elbow at or above chest level, including upper extremity ergometer
- °Stretching into straight-plane abduction during home exercise

PHASE 3

Criteria to Begin

- °Low reactivity: low level of pain with passive stretching and no delayed pain after stretching
- °More than 80° of normal PROM in most planes of motion

Goals

- °Discharge when functional goals are met. Whereas full AROM and PROM are goals, they might not be attainable while the patient is in therapy, but this does not preclude discharge
- °Transition to maintenance home exercise program
- °Normal to nearly normal PROM
- °Normal to nearly normal strength and endurance
- °Return to full activities of daily living, work, and recreation

Exercises

- °PROM and stretching
  - °Continue home-based PROM and stretching as detailed in phase 2 for planes of motion that are limited due to stiffness
  - °Consider adding terminal stretches, such as those listed below PRN; **these are not needed and are not appropriate for many patients**
    - °FE stretching supine using a wand (Figure 15)
    - °PFE stretching using a wall (Figure 12)
    - °PER stretching with the arm near the side using a wall
    - °PER stretching at 90° of abduction (Figures 13 and 14)
    - °Functional IR stretching using a towel or pulley
  - **°Initiate base strengthening progression if strength deficits are present**
  - °Includes standard rotator cuff, deltoid, and scapular strengthening program
    - °2 times per day, at most, with light resistance and increasing repetitions
  - °Yellow T-Band for ER and IR
    - °Initially, 4- to 6-foot band length and light pretension in a 3- to 6-inch arc of motion
    - °Can use side-lying ER instead of T-Band
  - °Yellow T-Band forward reach
    - °Initially, 4- to 6-foot band length and light pretension
    - °Start with the elbow bent and by the side and the band tied behind the patient
    - °Reach forward with the hand at waist level, progressing to reaching forward at chest level
  - °Scapular strengthening emphasizing scapular retractions and scapular upward rotators (chapter IV-2)
  - °No prone FE, abduction, or ER strenghtening

- °Initiate the AASEP as comfortable **(chapter II-4)**
  - °A stepwise progression in difficulty of strengthening exercises from PFE to AFE against gravity
  - °Goal of the progression is to achieve pain-free full AFE
  - °Start with whatever level of exercise is challenging but not painful
  - °If scapular or glenohumeral substitutions or pain are present, choose an easier exercise in the progression
  - °Usually not all exercises need to be performed
  - °Exercises are divided into 3 levels of difficulty
    1. Gravity-minimized exercises
       - °T-Band supine FE
         - °Must start the involved arm at 90° of elevation
         - °Pull the arm into FE
       - °Side-lying, gravity-eliminated AFE
         - °Lie on the uninvolved side
       - °Jackins supine reaching progression
         - °Begin at 0° with the elbow bent and end at 90° of elevation with the elbow extended
           - °Start with the assistance of a cane or wand
           - °Progress to active motion
           - °Can progress to using 1 to 2 pounds of weight
         - °Can progress to the inclined position, continuing to reach to ceiling
    2. Assistive elevation exercises
       - °Rope-and-pulley AAFE
       - °Incline dusting
       - °Standing AAFE (assistive elevation and descent via a T-bar or the unaffected arm)
       - °Standing assistive elevation and active independent eccentric lowering
       - °Wall-slide AAFE
         - °Ensure that the patient is in FE and is not in flexion
         - °Must be pain-free and natural when performing
    3. Unsupported elevation exercises
       - °AFE without weight, progressing to a maximum of 1 to 3 pounds
- °Initiate progressive replication of moderate-intensity activities of daily living and work
- °Participate in advanced strengthening exercises, including heavier dumbbell strengthening, higher speed, and powerful activities, ONLY in very rare circumstances where functional demands are regularly required

Adjunctive Exercises

- °Therapist-assisted stretching and mobilizations PRN

Interventions to Avoid

- °Any rehabilitation activity that is much more demanding than daily or expected activities
- °Any exercise that significantly increases signs and symptoms
- °Typically no prone FE, abduction, or ER
- °No strengthening in straight-plane abduction

III-16

Conservative Rehabilitation of Glenohumeral Arthritis

Bryce W. Gaunt, PT, SCS, and Howard D. Routman, DO, FAOAO

CHAPTER CONTENTS

- What patients are appropriate for the use of this guideline?
- The most important factor that should guide clinical decision making
- Key principles in rehabilitation of this problem
  - Understanding glenohumeral arthritis
  - Effects of glenohumeral arthritis on rehabilitation
  - Principles that guide clinical decision making
- Specific rehabilitation guideline
- Special considerations
  - Mild arthritis
  - Rotator cuff tear arthropathy

WHAT PATIENTS ARE APPROPRIATE FOR THE USE OF THIS GUIDELINE?

- Patients with symptomatic moderate to severe glenohumeral arthritis due to any cause other than cuff tear arthropathy can use this guideline.
- Patients with cuff tear arthropathy are usually more appropriate to use the limited-goals program but occasionally might use this guideline.
- Patients with a minimal amount of glenohumeral arthritis typically have another pathologic condition that generates greater symptoms, and the rehabilitation guideline for that condition should be used. Examples include adhesive capsulitis, rotator cuff tear, and impingement.

Clinical pearls are highlighted in yellow throughout the text.

THE MOST IMPORTANT FACTOR THAT SHOULD GUIDE CLINICAL DECISION MAKING

The most important factor that should guide clinical decision making in rehabilitation of the patient with moderate to severe glenohumeral arthritis is to appreciate that only limited rehabilitation interventions typically are productive if the condition is advanced enough to cause moderate pain and functional limitations because the joint surfaces are abnormal, eroded, and distorted.

KEY PRINCIPLES IN REHABILITATION OF THIS PROBLEM

Understanding Glenohumeral Arthritis

The humeral head and glenoid normally articulate with smooth, congruent, and well-lubricated joint

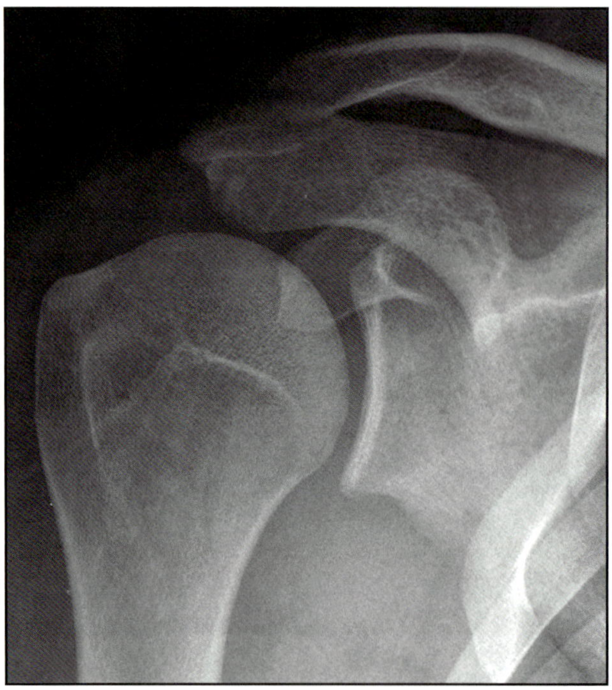

Figure 1. Normal anteroposterior view of the glenohumeral joint.

surfaces. Glenohumeral arthritis results when these joint surfaces are damaged by various factors. Loss of articular cartilage on the humeral head or glenoid, or both, can lead to shoulder pain, eventual joint-space narrowing, and deformity of the glenohumeral joint. Primary osteoarthritis (OA); rheumatoid arthritis (RA); capsulorrhaphy arthropathy; traumatic arthropathy; cuff tear arthropathy; avascular necrosis; and arthropathy due to miscellaneous causes, such as infection or gout, are different types of shoulder arthritis. Each type has a specific cause, pathologic lesions, characteristic radiographic findings, and typical findings on physical examination. Chapter I-5 provides an overview of each of these types of arthritis.

Evidence of arthritis is best found using standard radiography. To discuss the abnormal findings of the arthritic shoulder, the rehabilitation provider must understand the radiographic appearance of a glenohumeral joint without arthritis. In the nonarthritic joint, adequate space exists between the humeral head and the glenoid and between the humeral head and the acromion (Figure 1). The humeral head is round and smooth. Radiographs show a smooth contour where the proximal medial metaphysis of the humerus transitions to the articular surfaces of the humeral head and show centering of the humeral head on the glenoid. An imaginary line without large breaks can be drawn along the lateral border of the scapula to the glenoid neck, to the glenoid face, along the medial border of the humerus, and down the humeral shaft (Figure 1).

Osteoarthritis and RA are the most common types of arthritis. In contrast to a radiograph of a nonarthritic shoulder, the radiographs of the shoulder with OA usually demonstrate joint-space narrowing between the humeral head and glenoid, irregular joint surfaces, bone spurs that can be very large at times and are typically along the inferior one-half of the humeral head, sclerosis, posterior glenoid erosion, and an absence

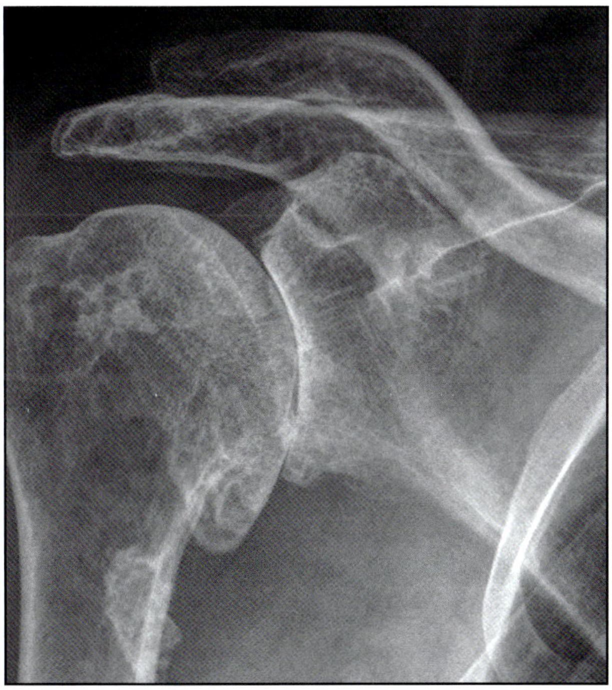

Figure 2. Anteroposterior view of 1° of osteoarthritis.

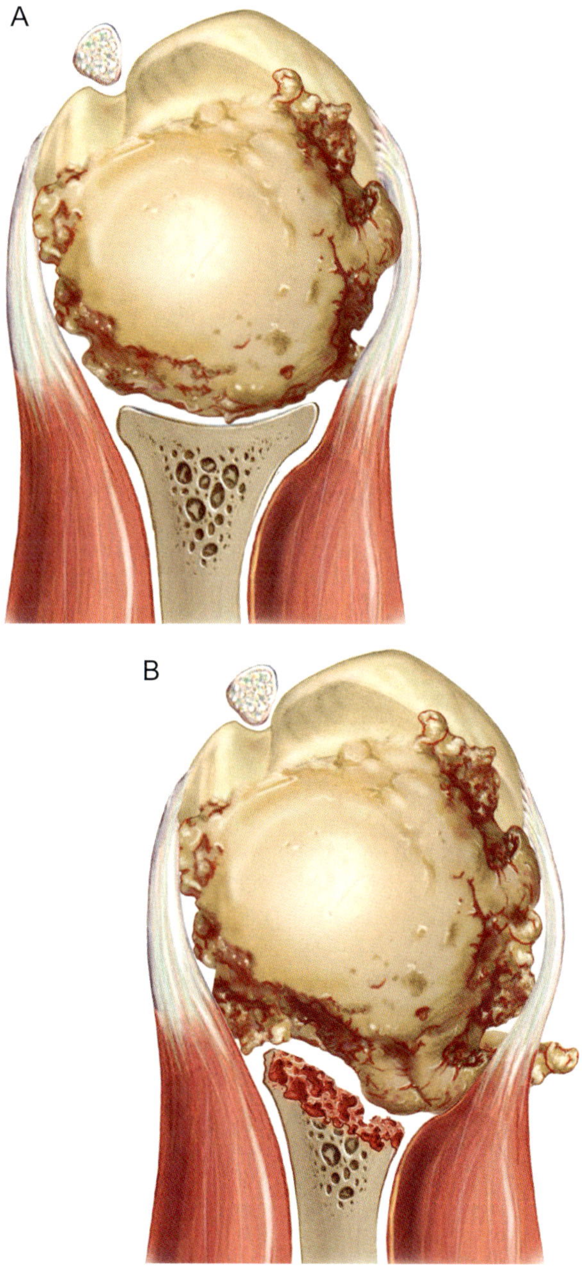

Figure 3. A, Osteoarthritis of the humeral head. B, Progressed osteoarthritis with posterior glenoid bone loss.

of other pathologic lesions (Figures 2 and 3). For example, the space between the humeral head and the acromion usually is preserved, and substantial rotator cuff tears rarely are found in patients with isolated OA. On physical examination, the patient typically presents with limited motion and function. Because the rotator cuff in most patients is intact, strength testing of the shoulder is usually good. Passive range of motion (PROM) and active range of motion (AROM) are usually similar, whereas overall range of motion (ROM) is limited. The end feel of PROM in general and especially in external rotation in the patient with OA is typically bony due to osteophyte (bone spur) contact inside the joint. This is unlike the rubbery and frequently very painful end feel of external rotation ROM in the patient with adhesive capsulitis. Pain and end feel differ among patients based on the degree of inflammation that is present. Some patients with OA have no pain at the end range of external rotation and have a solid osseous end point on palpation. Other patients have some discomfort toward the end range of rotation and pain at terminal motion, and they have crepitus from the glenohumeral joint, ranging from a palpable sensation of grinding fine sandpaper to audible popping and clunking that can be loud and painful in all available ROMs.

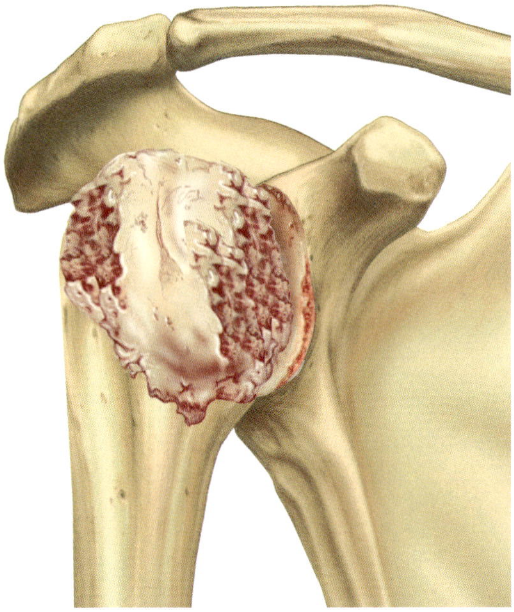

Figure 4. Rheumatoid arthritis.

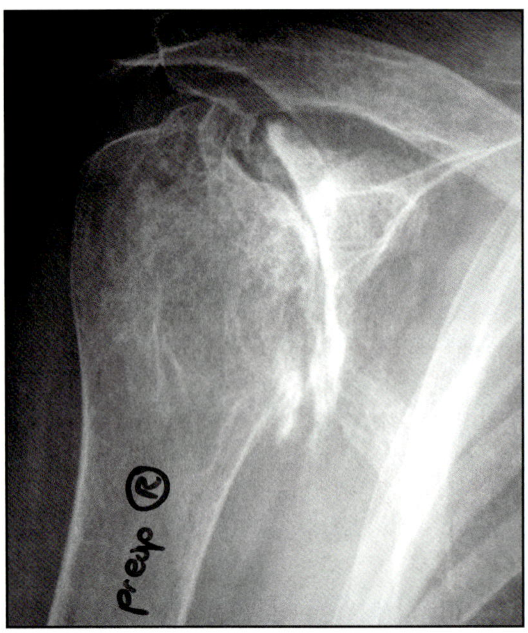

Figure 5. Rheumatoid arthritis.

Formation of pannus causes erosive changes and pain in the shoulder joint with RA. As this systemic soft tissue disease progresses, the pannus can erode into the soft tissues and bone around the joint and eventually through the rotator cuff, resulting in enzymatic degradation of the articular surfaces (Figures 4 and 5). Patients describe stiffness in the morning, periarticular soft tissue swelling around 3 or more joints, and swelling of the fingers and wrists that is typically symmetric. The patterns of arthritic change visible on radiographs (Figure 5) and the clinical presentations of RA and OA of the shoulder differ greatly. With RA, osteophyte formation and sclerosis are uncommon, glenoid erosion usually demonstrates a central rather than posterior pattern, and the bone quality usually is poor. In addition to periarticular erosions, osteopenia and large cysts can form within the humeral head and glenoid. These eventually can lead to progressive collapse of the humeral head and glenoid erosion. The rotator cuff is more likely to be torn in patients with RA, which can result in superior migration of the humeral head. Even if the rotator cuff is intact, muscle atrophy and weakness are usually present.

Effects of Glenohumeral Arthritis on Rehabilitation

Although each type of glenohumeral arthritis has a different radiographic and clinical presentation and different management by the physician, conservative rehabilitation is similar with all types. If the patient with glenohumeral arthritis presents with moderate to

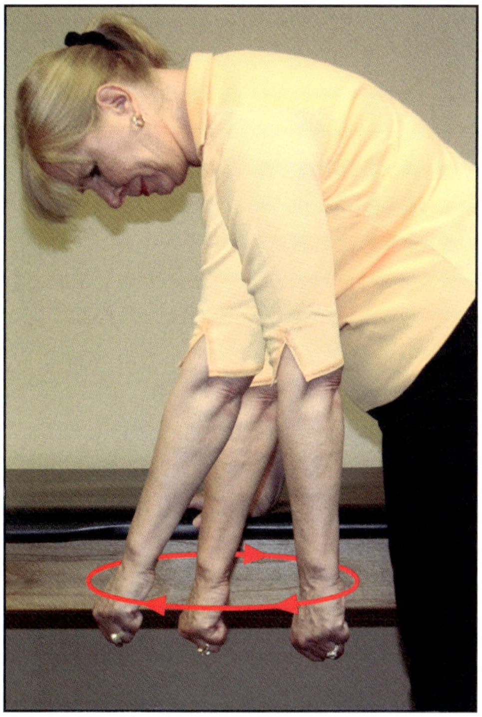

Figure 6. The pendulum exercise initially uses smaller circles.

advanced bony deformity or joint-space narrowing, or both, a simple, limited, and gentle rehabilitation program is used. The program will vary based on involvement of the rotator cuff, amount of crepitus, restriction in ROM, and the level of inflammation and pain.

Principles That Guide Clinical Decision Making

We use 5 principles to guide our clinical decision making for patients with moderate to severe symptomatic arthritis of the shoulder: (1) respect bony deformities, crepitus, and ROM restrictions; (2) minimize inflammation and pain; (3) optimize rotator cuff function; (4) implement a long-term maintenance home exercise program; and (5) help the patient prepare for the potential of shoulder arthroplasty.

Respect Bony Deformities, Crepitus, and ROM Restrictions. The rehabilitation provider needs to respect bony deformities, crepitus, and ROM restrictions that are evident during the physical examination and on radiographs during all stages of rehabilitation, including those with ROM and strengthening interventions. Not respecting these limitations is analogous to trying to fit a square peg in a round hole; you should not force the shoulder in a direction that it will no longer move due to a bony restriction. Therefore, for all ROM activities, we perform only gentle stretching sometimes to increase ROM, sometimes to prevent a decline in ROM, and sometimes to relieve pain. The pendulum (Figure 6), passive forward elevation most often performed using the rope-and-pulley (Figure 7) or table step-back (Figure 8) exercise, and passive external rotation stretching with the elbow near the side are the exercises we use most commonly, especially during phase 1 rehabilitation. Sometimes, during phase 2 rehabilitation, we use functional internal rotation stretching (Figure 9) or the hand-behind-head stretch (Figure 10).

To respect bony deformities, crepitus, and ROM restrictions during strengthening interventions, we use exercises that are performed in or near the loose pack position of the shoulder and not in near-end ranges of motion. We also do not needlessly constrain the glenohumeral joint motion during these activities. For example, during external and internal rotation strengthening with an elastic band we have found that **not** using

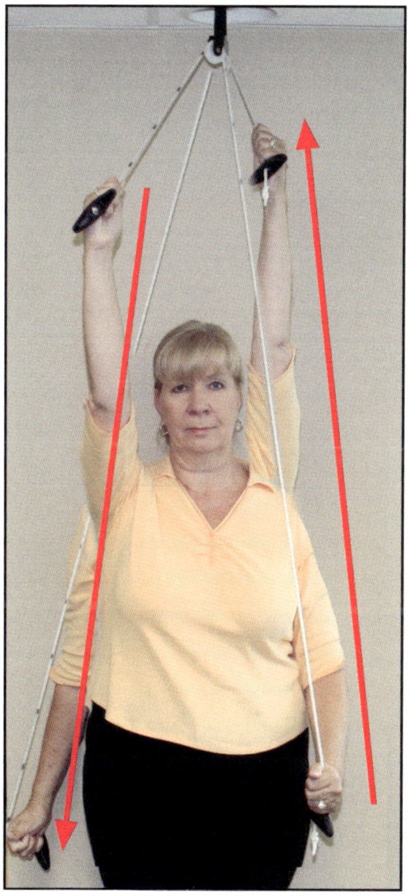

Figure 7. Rope-and-pulley active-assistive forward elevation exercise.

a towel to keep the elbow near the side minimizes joint crepitus and pain better than using a towel. For these patients, overhead rehabilitation activities must be performed in shoulder elevation or the scapular plane and should not be performed in flexion or coronal-plane abduction. If moderate or substantial crepitus, which is typically painful, is present during either PROM and strengthening interventions, the rehabilitation provider needs to modify or discontinue the intervention to prevent exacerbating the patient's symptoms.

Minimize Inflammation and Pain. Minimizing inflammation and pain is important during the rehabilitation of patients with arthritis because our rehabilitation is largely based on their symptoms. As mentioned, we cannot change the arthritic process, bony deformities, and/or osteophytes that are present; we have to work around them to decrease the patient's symptoms. We have found that a combination of gentle ROM, especially the pendulum exercise (Figure 6); comfortable forward elevation stretching (Figures 7 and 8); modification of activities of daily living (ADLs); and withholding advanced rehabilitation interventions are effective ways to meet this goal. Modalities beyond home-based application of heat and cold packs are not used in our practice to treat these patients.

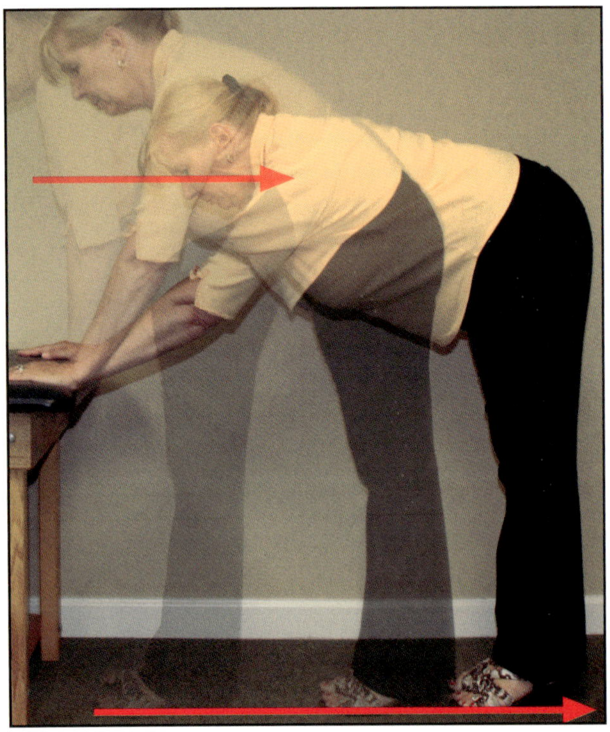

Figure 8. The table step-back exercise for passive forward elevation.

Optimize Rotator Cuff Function. Rotator cuff function needs to be optimized in patients with arthritis, especially when the rotator cuff is involved, which is more likely in patients with RA and traumatic arthropathy. However, even in patients with OA and avascular necrosis who usually do not have substantial involvement of the rotator cuff, optimizing rotator cuff function can be beneficial because the rotator cuff can be inhibited due to pain. Basic interventions performed in nonprovocative positions that follow the other hallmarks of rehabilitation are used.

Implement a Long-Term Maintenance Home Exercise Program. Implementing a long-term maintenance home exercise program is important because arthritis is a progressive disease process, and as mentioned, our treatment for this problem is based on symptoms. We have found a tendency for symptoms to return if patients stop their home exercises for a long time. A maintenance program also can help prevent or minimize further loss of ROM that can occur due to the arthritic process. We typically include a program that involves some PROM exercises along with low-level rotator cuff strengthening.

Help the Patient Prepare for the Potential of Shoulder Arthroplasty. Helping the patient prepare for the potential of shoulder arthroplasty is important physically and psychologically. Physically, comfortable PROM needs to be maximized and rotator cuff function needs to be maintained. Psychological preparation might be even more important because many patients have a negative attitude toward joint replacement, and this attitude might dissuade them from undergoing a surgical procedure that can greatly improve their pain and quality of life. Our experience is that unlike patients who have total knee replacement that is usually very painful initially and normally requires intense and painful rehabilitation, patients who undergo total shoulder arthroplasty by a surgeon who performs high volumes of the procedure usually have a very pleasant early postoperative experience, with predictable, rapid pain relief often within 2 days to 2 weeks. Compared with the preoperative level, function might be improved in as soon as 1 to 3 months after surgery. Helping a patient overcome the fear of shoulder arthroplasty, if his or her surgeon has recommended it, and understand how large and quick the benefits can be is one of the most valuable components of conservative rehabilitation.

SPECIFIC REHABILITATION GUIDELINE

The Appendix specifies our complete Conservative Rehabilitation Guideline for Glenohumeral Arthritis. The guideline is divided into 2 phases based on the reactivity of the shoulder and tolerance for exercise. To advance from one rehabilitation phase to the next, the patient must gain approval from the physician and successfully complete the core components of the previous rehabilitation activities. Patients usually spend 4 to 8 weeks in phase 1 before moving to phase 2 rehabilitation.

Phase 1

The primary focus of phase 1 rehabilitation is to establish a tolerance to a gentle exercise program, decrease inflammation and pain, seek to improve PROM in forward elevation and external rotation with the upper extremity near the side, and improve rotator cuff function. In the Appendix and Key Principles in Rehabilitation of This Problem section, we discuss the interventions we prefer to use to meet these goals along with the rationale for these choices.

Counseling the patient on appropriate modifications of ADLs is an often overlooked, but very important, component of rehabilitation of this problem. It is a large part of helping the patient's symptoms to begin to improve by ensuring that the patient appropriately minimizes his or her pain and inflammation and respects bony deformities, crepitus, and restrictions in ROM. Patients are instructed to temporarily minimize or eliminate ADLs that require use of the involved extremity in positions that cause painful crepitus, cause great pain, or require end-range ROM. For example, we discuss not reaching into the back seat of the car and not putting on a jacket with the involved shoulder first. We also discuss minimizing or eliminating activities that require a large amount of weight bearing through the shoulder, such as bench press, other weight-training activities, or vigorous cleaning. In addition, we discuss temporarily minimizing or eliminating overhead activities that are painful, especially ones that are repetitive. Patients might resist implementing these modifications, so extra education is needed to teach them that this is as important as or more important than the other components of rehabilitation for helping the shoulder to initially begin to feel better.

Phase 2

The primary focus of phase 2 rehabilitation is to expand the patient's comfortable PROM, continue to minimize inflammation and pain, and establish a long-term maintenance exercise plan that includes the components of ROM, strengthening, and modification of activities. In the Appendix and Key Principles in Rehabilitation of This Problem section, we discuss the interventions we prefer to use to meet these goals along with the rationale for these choices.

Passive ROM is important to include in phase 2 rehabilitation to minimize inflammation and pain and to minimize or prevent a decline in PROM that can occur over months and years in multiple planes of motion due to progression of the disease. For some patients, PROM exercises are expanded to include stretches for functional internal rotation behind the back (Figure 9) and the supine hand-behind-head, or quadrant, stretch (Figure 10) because both of these motions are

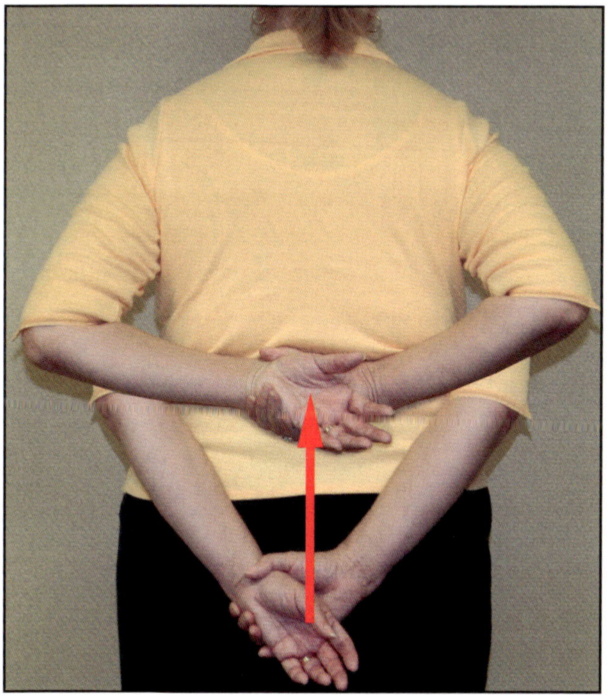

Figure 9. Functional internal rotation active-assistive range of motion.

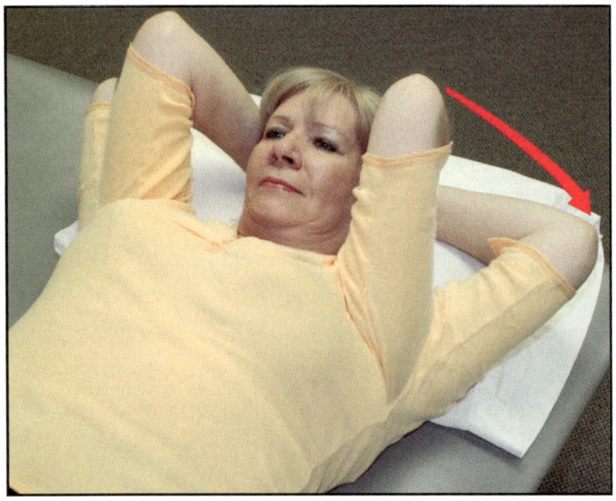

Figure 10. Supine hand-behind-head stretch to increase abduction with external rotation.

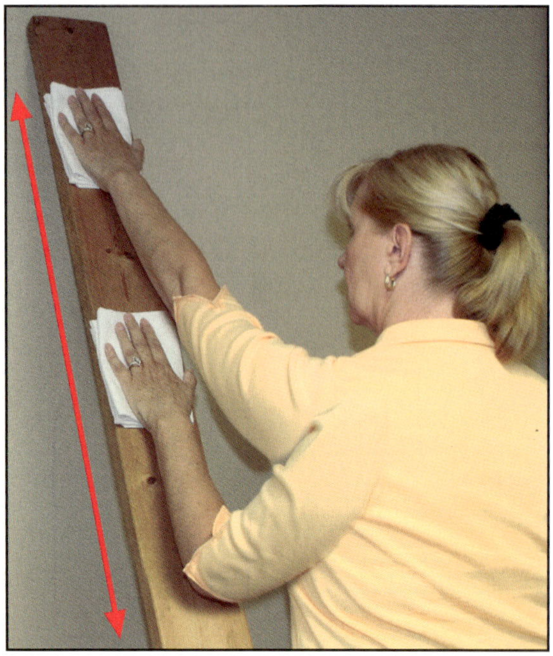

Figure 11. Incline dusting.

important for dressing and grooming. At least half of the time, only basic motions, such as passive forward elevation and passive external rotation, are well tolerated by the patient. When patients are transitioned to a maintenance program, they are encouraged to continue stretching exercises once daily.

If they are well tolerated by the patient, strengthening exercises are included in phase 2 rehabilitation to maintain or improve rotator cuff health and minimize signs and symptoms. The arthritis is so advanced in some patients that almost all strengthening interventions cause crepitus and pain. In these patients, submaximal isometrics performed with the elbow flexed to shorten the lever arm are comfortable. In patients who tolerate phase 1 strengthening well, selected elevation exercises can be considered, realizing patients are often symptomatic so these exercises are seldom used. Rope-and-pulley active-assistive ROM (Figure 7) and incline dusting (Figure 11) are the exercises we find most helpful for these patients.

An essential part of the long-term maintenance program for patients with shoulder arthritis is discussing long-term modifications of ADLs with them. Often, selected ADLs that were not performed in phase 1 so symptoms would be minimized can be performed comfortably in the long term. Overhead reaching activities and regular household cleaning are examples of activities to which patients normally can return without consistent exacerbation of symptoms. However, for some patients, minimizing or eliminating activities with large weight-bearing forces, especially in the extremes of ROM, and any activities that are especially painful can improve their quality of life over time. To help patients understand why modifications might be needed, we instruct them to think of their shoulders like old cars with rebuilt engines and worn tires. This type of vehicle can run a long time if it is regularly maintained and driven in a gentle manner. On the other hand, if regular maintenance is ignored and if the driver regularly "red lines" the engine, slams on the breaks to stop the car, and spins the wheels when accelerating, then the vehicle likely will break down much sooner.

SPECIAL CONSIDERATIONS

Mild Arthritis

Patients with a minimal amount of glenohumeral arthritis but a moderate amount of shoulder pain and functional limitations might be referred to therapy with a diagnosis of shoulder arthritis. Often, these patients have another pathologic condition, such as adhesive capsulitis, rotator cuff tear, or impingement, that is more likely the cause of their symptoms than their arthritis. A thorough examination should be performed

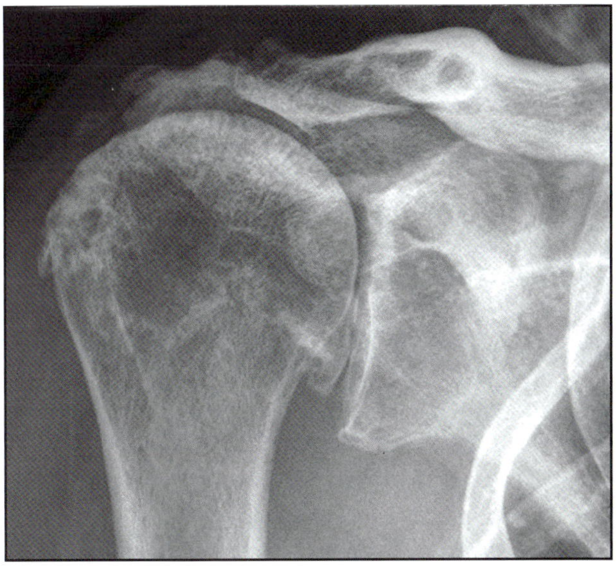

Figure 12. Anteroposterior view of rotator cuff tear arthropathy.

to help localize the cause of the symptoms. If multiple diagnoses are present and only mild arthritis is observed radiographically, the rehabilitation guideline for the other condition should be used, and modifications, such as not strengthening in extremes of ROM and incorporation of gentle stretching into the rehabilitation program, should be made as needed for the arthritis.

Rotator Cuff Tear Arthropathy

Rotator cuff tear arthropathy occurs when a chronic, massive rotator cuff defect subjects the uncovered humeral articular cartilage to abrasion by the undersurface of the coracoacromial arch. Over time, the humeral head becomes "femoralized," and the coracoacromial arch becomes "acetabularized" (Figure 12).[1] The arthritic wearing begins superiorly rather than centrally as in other forms of glenohumeral arthritis. Patients with this problem might present with pain ranging from minimal to severe and function that is almost always very limited. Currently, reverse shoulder arthroplasty is typically the surgical intervention that is most appropriate for these patients.

For many reasons, not all patients with this problem are surgical candidates, so they might receive a referral for nonoperative rehabilitation. Given longstanding multitendon rotator cuff tears and severe arthritic changes that often are associated with this problem, many patients present with active elevation and active abduction of the extremity to less than 60° and very poor rotator cuff function of the remaining cuff. Limited-goals rehabilitation, which is detailed in chapter III-18, is the best rehabilitation guideline to use for these patients.

Patients who have cuff tear arthropathy and have less severe arthritic changes and better AROM and rotator cuff function can use the shoulder arthritis guideline. If the arthritis guideline is used, PROM and stretching should use only phase 1 interventions. Strengthening with an elastic band often is not used because the infraspinatus and subscapularis commonly are completely torn. Instead, the assistive-to-active elevation progression (chapter II-4) is used more often with these patients to improve the active use of the extremity so they can perform activities, such as combing their hair and reaching into a low shelf of an overhead cupboard.

REFERENCE

1. Matsen FA III, Rockwood CA Jr, Wirth MA, Lippitt SB. Glenohumeral arthritis and its management. In: Rockwood CA Jr, Matsen FA III, Wirth MA, Harryman DT II, eds. *The Shoulder*. Vol 2. 2nd ed. Philadelphia, PA: WB Saunders; 1998:840–964.

CONSERVATIVE REHABILITATION GUIDELINE FOR GLENOHUMERAL ARTHRITIS

St. Francis Orthopaedic Institute and St. Francis Rehabilitation Center

All information contained in this protocol is to be used as a general guideline only. Specific variations might be appropriate for each patient and might be specified by the physician. In all cases, it is acceptable to advance the program more slowly than stated. If the patient experiences excessive pain, discontinue exercise until the physician is contacted. ***Achieving and maintaining a low level of pain and inflammation are the guiding principles in all stages of rehabilitation, even if less passive and active range of motion are accomplished.***

SYMBOLS AND ABBREVIATIONS

AAFE, active-assistive forward elevation
AAROM, active-assistive range of motion
AASEP, assistive-to-active shoulder elevation progression
ADLs, activities of daily living
AFE, active forward elevation
AROM, active range of motion
ER, external rotation
FE, forward elevation
IR, internal rotation
PER, passive external rotation
PFE, passive forward elevation
PRN, as needed
PROM, passive range of motion
ROM, range of motion
T-Band, Thera-Band (The Hygenic Corporation, Akron, OH)

Forward elevation, either active or passive, is the plane of motion in which an individual naturally lifts his or her arm that is anterior to the plane of the scapula and lateral to flexion.

PHASE 1

Goals

°Minimize pain and inflammatory response
°Improve or maintain PROM while respecting bony deformities and crepitus
°Consider light rotator cuff and scapular strengthening that respects bony deformities and crepitus
°Educate the patient about modifications to ADLs to avoid symptomatic positions

Exercises

°Pendulum exercises (Figure 6)
  °Lean over the table a comfortable amount
  °Let the arm hang down relaxed
  °Keep the body still
  °Move the arm in small comfortable circles only
°Comfortable PFE ROM
  °Preferred exercises
    °Rope-and-pulley AAFE (elbow straight, thumb up) (Figure 7)
    °Sit with family member or therapist lifting the arm
    °Table step-back exercise (Figure 8)

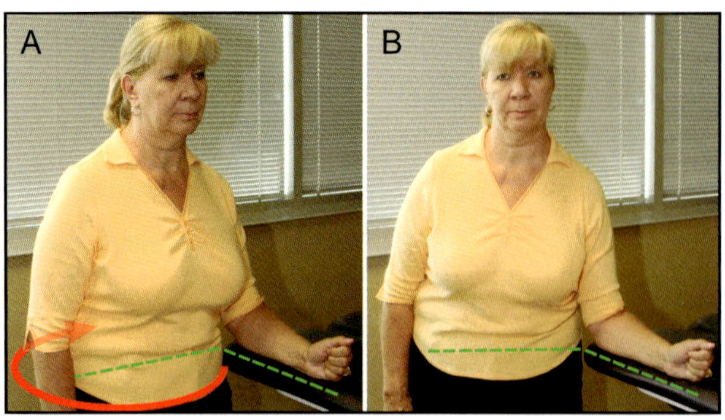

Figure 13 A and B. Passive external rotation walk-around exercise.

°Upright PER in slight abduction if ROM is restricted and comfortable to perform
  °Preferred exercises

- °PER walk-around (stand with the arm supported on a table and rotate the body) (Figure 13)
- °Sit with family member or therapist rotating the arm

°Initiate base strengthening progression only if comfortable and well tolerated

- °Includes beginning rotator cuff, deltoid, and scapular strengthening program
- °2 times per day at most with light resistance and increasing repetitions
- °Yellow T-Band for ER and IR
  - °5- to 6-foot band length and light or no pretension in a 3- to 6-inch arc of motion
  - °Modify technique and arc of motion so the patient has no substantial crepitus and pain. Usually NOT using a towel to keep the elbow by the side is helpful to this end
- °Yellow T-Band forward reach (Figure 14)
  - °Initially, 5- to 6-foot band length and light or no pretension
  - °Start with the elbow bent and by the side and the band tied behind the patient
  - °Reach forward with the hand at waist level to chest level
  - °Modify the arc of motion so the patient has no substantial crepitus and pain
- °Scapular strengthening emphasizing scapular retractions (chapter IV-2)

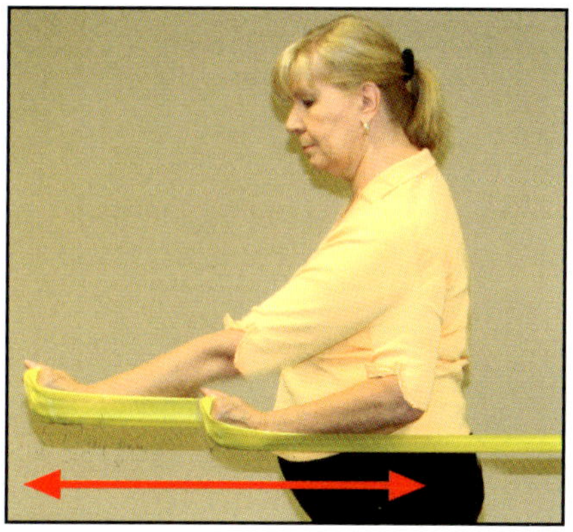

Figure 14. Forward reaching with an elastic band.

°Patient education

- °Minimize or eliminate ADLs that require use of the arm in provocative positions that cause painful crepitus or moderate to severe pain or those performed at end range
- °Minimize or eliminate activities that require a large amount of weight-bearing through the shoulder, including most upper body weight-training activities and vigorous cleaning

Adjunctive Exercises

°Aquatic therapy for gentle, comfortable AAROM, AROM, or light strengthening (no swimming strokes)

°Submaximal pain-free isometrics (consider if dynamic strengthening is not well tolerated)

- °Perform with the elbow flexed and instruct the patient to press with 1 to 2 pounds of force only
- °Flexion, ER, IR, and abduction are considered

°Instruction in ice or heat PRN for home use

°Spine therapy assessment and mobilization PRN

Interventions to Avoid

°PROM, AROM, or strengthening in coronal-plane abduction

°Exercises that result in moderate or severe pain or painful crepitus
°Prone strengthening exercises

PHASE 2

Goals

°Consider expanding PROM exercises to address functional limitations
°Optimize rotator cuff and scapular function while respecting bony deformities and crepitus
°Educate the patient about appropriate long-term modifications to ADLs
°Implement a long-term maintenance home exercise program

Interventions

°Continue comfortable ROM in FE (most often rope-and-pulley AAFE) (Figure 7)
°Can continue PER stretching depending on the amount of PROM, tolerance to the exercise, and amount functional limitations—usually discontinue this exercise
°Judiciously consider home exercise PROM into expanded directions typically only if functional limitations are present in a particular plane with a capsular end feel. If expanded stretches are included, the most common ones are
  °Supine hand-behind-head stretch PRN (Figure 10)
  °Functional IR AAROM and stretching PRN (Figure 9)
°Continue comfortable base strengthening progression that was begun in phase 1
°Consider beginning the AASEP in select patients (chapter II-4)
  °Many patients with moderate to advanced arthritis do not tolerate many of these exercises, so this progression is not used with many patients
  °Only the exercises that are most often used for these patients are listed below
  °See chapter II-4 for a comprehensive discussion of this program
  °Exercises are divided into 3 levels of difficulty
    1. Gravity-minimized exercises
      °T-Band supine FE
        °Must start the involved arm at 90° of elevation
        °Pull arm into FE
    2. Assistive elevation exercises
      °Rope-and-pulley AAFE (Figure 7)
      °Incline dusting (Figure 11)
    3. Unsupported elevation exercises
      °AFE (Figure 15)
      °Consider progressing to very light resistance (typically 1 to 2 pounds)
°Patient education
  °Educate the patient about appropriate long-term modifications to ADLs to minimize symptoms
    °Avoid activities with large weight-bearing forces through the shoulder, such as heavy bench pressing
    °Avoid repetitive activities in the extremes of ROM

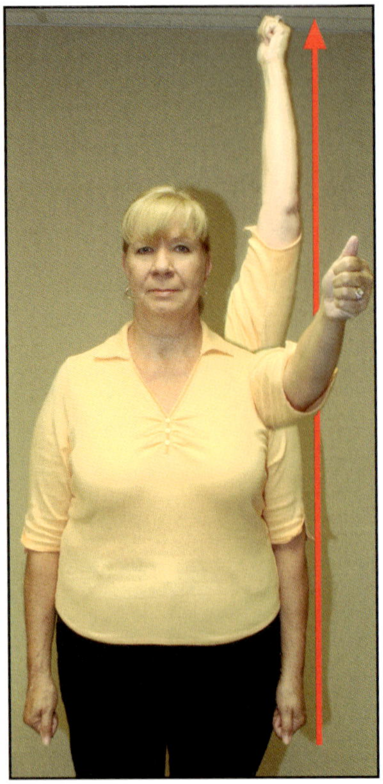

Figure 15. Active forward elevation.

HPRC at St. Francis Rehabilitation Center

- °Implement a long-term maintenance home exercise program
  - °Most often consists of the pendulum PRN, rope-and-pulley AAFE, and light elastic-band strengthening

Adjunctive Exercises

- °Aquatic exercises (chapter IV-9)

Interventions to Avoid

- °PROM, AROM, or strengthening in coronal-plane abduction
- °Prone strengthening exercises
- °Weight room activities involving chest training and shoulder presses with heavy weight
- °Exercises that greatly increase signs and symptoms

III-17

Rehabilitation of Scapular Nerve Palsies

Martin J. Kelley, PT, DPT, OCS

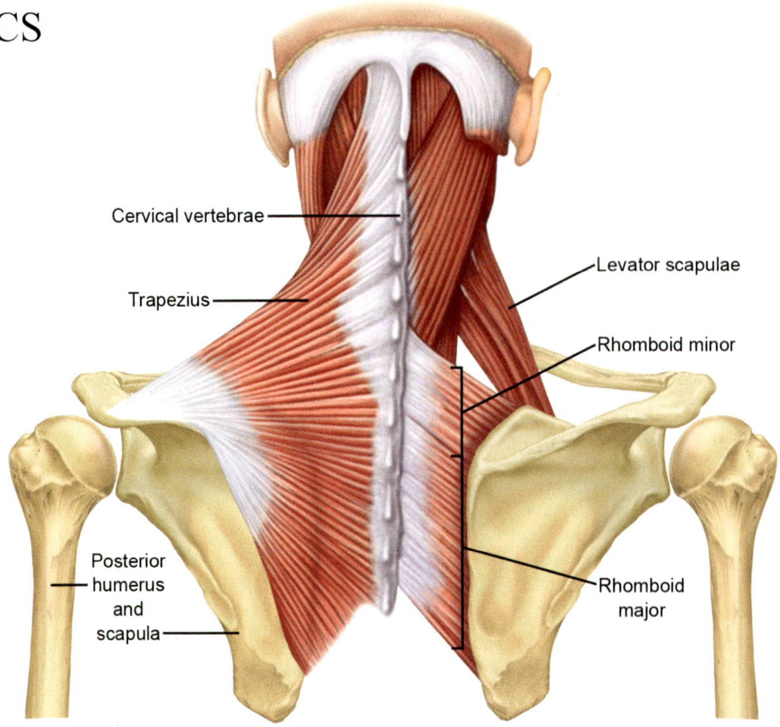

CHAPTER CONTENTS

- What patients are appropriate for the use of this guideline
- The most important factor that should guide clinical decision making
- Key principles in rehabilitation of this problem
  - Examination of long thoracic nerve palsy
  - Examination of spinal accessory nerve palsy
- Specific rehabilitation guideline
  - Education, posture, and orthosis
  - Stretching
  - Range of motion
  - Scapular muscle compensatory and primary activity training

WHAT PATIENTS ARE APPROPRIATE FOR THE USE OF THIS GUIDELINE?

- Patients with complete or incomplete long thoracic nerve palsy suspected or confirmed by clinical examination or electromyography
- Patients with complete or incomplete spinal accessory nerve palsy suspected or confirmed by clinical examination or electromyography

Clinical pearls are highlighted in yellow throughout the text.

Rehabilitation of patients with scapular nerve palsies can be a challenge, especially if regeneration is delayed, is incomplete, or does not occur. The long thoracic nerve (LTN) and spinal accessory nerve (SAN) innervate the serratus anterior and the trapezius, respectively. The serratus anterior and trapezius are large axioscapular muscles that provide a stable yet mobile scapular base for the glenohumeral joint and associated muscles. These muscles work in a force couple along with the rhomboid and levator scapulae to coordinate smooth scapular movement. The loss of serratus anterior levator trapezius function, in isolation or in combination, results in substantial scapular winging or dyskinesis, substantial impairments, functional deficits, and disability. The mechanism of injury causing nerve palsy can be blunt or penetrating trauma, iatrogenic, viral infection (ie, neuritis), stretch (separation of head and neck), exertion, or sustained compression.[1–3] Often, recovery occurs through neural regeneration, but neurolysis or nerve grafting might be required. Patients who have chronic nerve palsies for more than 1 year might require a muscle transfer stabilization procedure.

THE MOST IMPORTANT FACTOR THAT SHOULD GUIDE CLINICAL DECISION MAKING

When nerve palsy is a result of a neuraparaxia or axonotemesis, the rehabilitation provider must wait for "Mother Nature" to begin the nerve-regeneration process because therapy cannot facilitate nerve regeneration. Forcing a patient with a complete palsy to perform activities requiring recruitment from the affected muscle results in patient frustration, potential stress on the affected nerve, and possibly irritation of other tissue. After muscle activation is noted, specific exercises can be initiated to maximize neuromotor control. Usually, reinnervation begins within 3 months, and the patient requires little supervised therapy in nonoperative cases. However, if reinnervation has not started by 3 months, greater emphasis should be placed on scapular muscle compensatory and eventually on primary activation.

KEY PRINCIPLES IN REHABILITATION OF THIS PROBLEM

First, the rehabilitation provider must understand the static and dynamic scapular muscle anatomechanics. Second, the evaluation process must determine if a complete or partial palsy is present rather than some other pathologic condition or reason for dyskinesis. The same tests used to determine whether muscle activation is present often are used for intervention exercises. Third, compensatory muscle activation and patterns from unaffected muscles are used to gain scapular stabilization followed by isolation of the affected muscles when reinnervation begins. Fourth, rehabilitation providers must recognize that we have little effect on nerve regeneration, but we can educate the patient regarding the pathologic condition and encourage a friendly environment for neural recovery. If the patient has a complete palsy, demonstrates good motion, and is educated about the condition, he or she initially is treated several times then followed at 3- to 6-week intervals until muscle activation is noticed. More frequent supervised therapy is required in patients who have had surgery and in patients who have brachial plexopathies because of restricted shoulder range-of-motion concerns and other upper extremity involvement.

Examination

Scapular dyskinesis describes an alteration in the normal position or motion of the scapula during coupled scapulohumeral movements.[4] Scapular winging might be considered a type of scapular dyskinesis characterized by substantial displacement of the medial border of the scapula during shoulder elevation. A complete palsy causes dramatic winging or dyskinesis and is easy to detect (Figure 1). A patient with incomplete paralysis possibly due to partial neural regeneration might present with subdued dyskinesis, and clinical signs might vary.

Scapular winging can result from nonneurologic causes, such as scapular osteochondromas, clavicle malunions or scoliosis, scapular muscle ruptures, and congenital absence.[2,5] Glenohumeral instability, especially primary posterior instability, can result in significant scapular dyskinesis. Some patients present with motor-control dyskinesia that is related to instability, abnormal muscle-activation patterning, or voluntary effort. Kelley[6] and Leggin and Kelley[7] described an examination algorithm for scapular muscle assessment to determine if winging is due to neurologic reasons or other pathologic conditions. I discuss this algorithm and describe specific tests and findings in patients with LTN and SAN palsies.

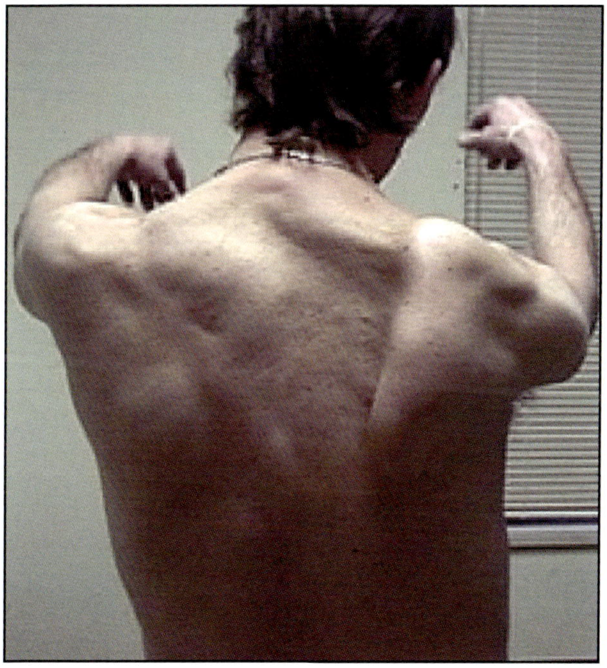

Figure 1. A patient with complete palsy of both the long thoracic and spinal accessory nerves.

Long Thoracic Nerve Palsy

Vastamäki and Kauppila[3] found that 60% of the individuals with LTN palsies affecting the serratus anterior described some traumatic or exertion event preceding the onset of symptoms. Typically, the individual is relatively young (mean age = 31 years), and his or her dominant side is affected most often. Usually, the patient presents with painless weakness.

The patient first is observed in the standing position for resting winging and obvious atrophy. Often, drooping of the affected shoulder is present. If resting winging is noted, the patient is checked for a scoliosis demonstrated by a thoracic rib hump during trunk flexion. The presence of bilateral resting medial winging rarely indicates true scapular nerve palsy. Active range of motion of both shoulders is assessed by having the patient elevate the upper extremity in the sagittal plane. Substantial scapular winging that normalizes beyond 90° during sagittal-plane flexion elevation typically is related to motor-control dyskinesia (usually, the serratus anterior). If medial winging persists beyond 90°, an LTN palsy or posterior glenohumeral instability should be suspected. A patient with primary posterior instability with or without a diagnosis of multidirectional instability almost always describes a history of instability events and demonstrates signs of instability on examination. A common finding in patients with serratus anterior palsy is attempted compensation of the lower trapezius during active shoulder elevation to stabilize the medial border of the scapula (Figure 2).

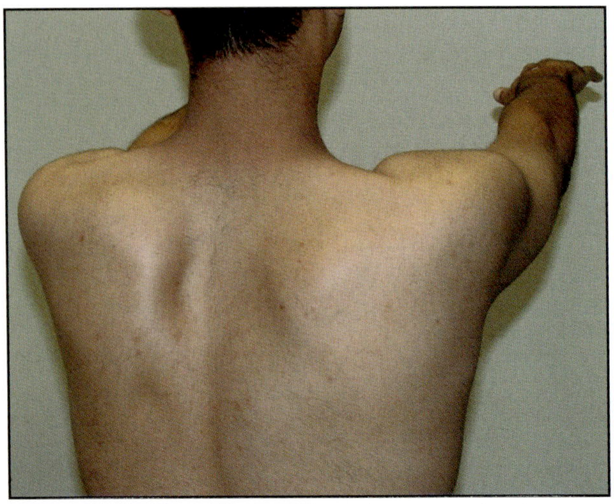

Figure 2. A patient with long thoracic nerve palsy demonstrates increased left lower trapezius activation to stabilize the medial border of the scapula.

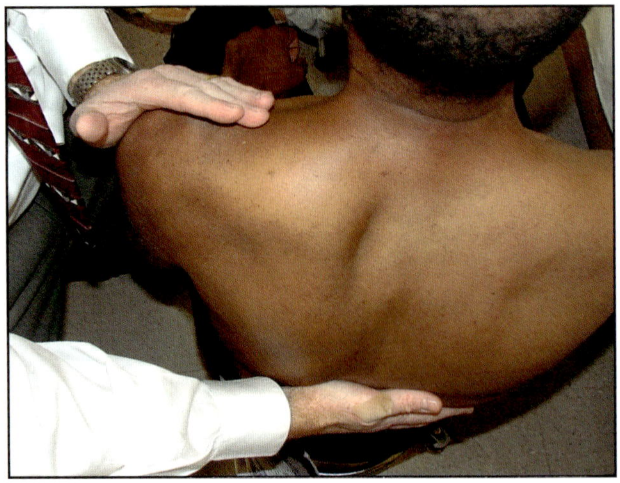

Figure 3. Serratus anterior isolation test with resistance. The medial border of the scapula is easily moved posteriorly with resistance.

Often, the patient's upper extremity will drift from the sagittal plane toward the coronal plane as the middle and lower trapezius retract the scapula. Medial winging is most notable at approximately 90°, especially upon the descent of the extremity from elevation.

The serratus anterior isolation test is performed with the extremities at the side and in external rotation. The patient actively protracts and slightly elevates the scapula. A positive test is the inability to fully displace the scapula equal to the uninvolved side. Resistance can be applied to the anterior aspect of the shoulder, attempting to displace the medial border of the scapula posteriorly. Easy posterior displacement of the scapula causing the medial border to become visible is a sign of abnormal serratus anterior weakness (Figure 3).

The plus sign is performed next. The patient lifts the extremity to 90° in the sagittal plane and reaches forward, or performs a "plus." A positive plus sign occurs when the patient is unable to protract the scapula on the thoracic wall or when scapular medial winging increases. This motion requires high levels of serratus anterior activation and concurrently inhibits the lower trapezius (Figure 4).[8] If the movement is incomplete, partial serratus anterior activity is suspected because of a recovering palsy. If the patient protracts and the scapula fully moves forward on the thoracic wall, the sign is negative, but a recovering LTN palsy cannot be ruled out because enough serratus anterior fibers might be innervated to complete the task. Next, the patient is instructed to place the extremity at 135° of sagittal-plane elevation, and the examiner resists, pushing the shoulder into extension while palpating the inferior border of the scapula.[9] Easy posterior displacement of the inferior border with minimal resistance is a sign of substantial serratus anterior weakness and likely is due to a resolving neurologic insult. Patients who have very dramatic scapular dyskinesis and who do not have glenohumeral instability but an intact neurologic system can easily maintain the scapula fixed on the thoracic wall during resisted shoulder flexion at 135°.

Spinal Accessory Nerve Palsy

A history of lymph-node excision or neck-dissection procedures should immediately cause the clinician to suspect an SAN palsy. Identification of an SAN injury is assisted by the presence of trapezius atrophy and a depressed and protracted shoulder girdle. Active shoulder range of motion is assessed in the sagittal and coronal planes, and scapular movement is noted. If good sagittal-plane elevation is present but the patient cannot lift the upper extremity above 90° in the true coronal plane without pain, an SAN palsy is suspected.[10] To further examine the trapezius, the rehabilitation provider performs the flip sign by standing to the patient's side and resisting shoulder external rotation.[10,11] The scapula is examined visually. A positive flip sign occurs when the medial border of the scapula substantially displaces, or "flips," off the thoracic wall (Figure 5). The mechanism for this sign is unopposed pull of the infraspinatus and posterior deltoid by the middle and lower trapezius. Interestingly, the rhomboid or serratus anterior muscles do not spontaneously

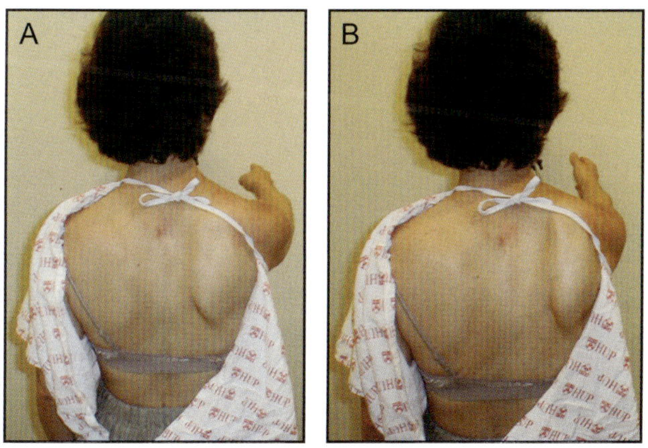

Figure 4. The plus sign. A, The patient demonstrates obvious scapular winging. B, Winging increases with attempted protraction.

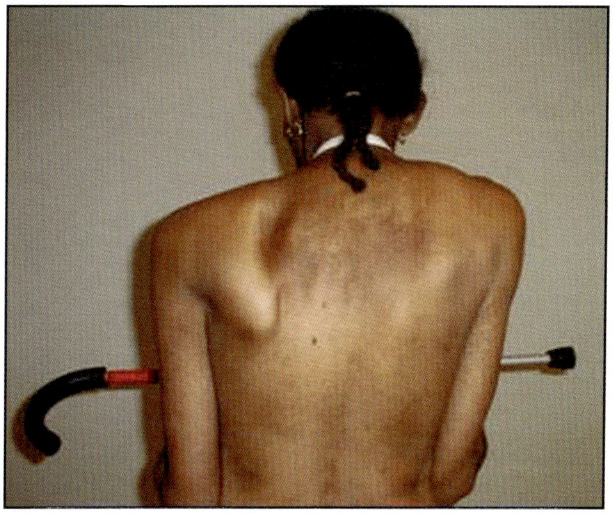

Figure 5. The flip sign. The medial border of the scapula "flips" off the thoracic wall with resisted external rotation.

activate to stabilize the scapula in this position. Further isolation of the trapezius to determine manual muscle-testing strength grade of the middle and lower trapezius can be performed with the patient lying prone, as described by Kendall and McCreary.[9]

Electrodiagnostic studies should be performed to further confirm the presence of the palsy and determine a baseline for future comparison. However, caution is required when the electrodiagnostic tests contrast with findings on physical examination because these tests are interpretive, nerve conduction velocity test rarely is done on the serratus anterior or trapezius, and the middle and lower trapezius heads rarely are tested.

SPECIFIC REHABILITATION GUIDELINE

Intervention begins after the palsy is confirmed, but the intervention will vary based on the presentation. Often, patients, especially those with an LTN palsy, already demonstrate reinnervation by the time they are referred to therapy. These patients require less intervention because the natural recovery process does the brunt of the work.

Education, Posture, and Orthosis

Rehabilitation of the individual with either an LTN or SAN palsy begins with understanding the pathologic condition and both static and dynamic scapular mechanics. In the presence of a complete palsy, the

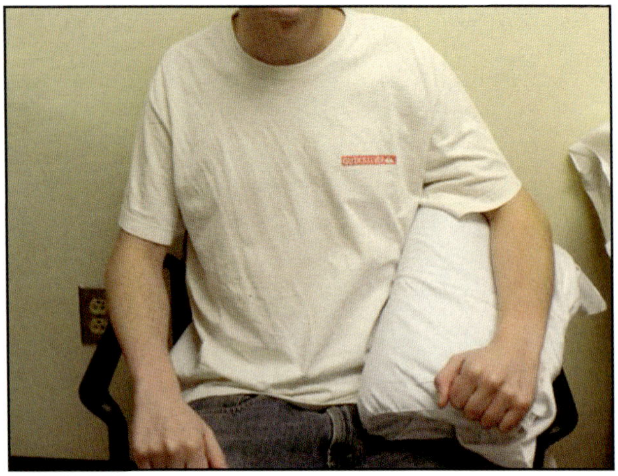

Figure 6. Placing a support under the affected upper extremity can relieve symptoms related to the upper extremity static load.

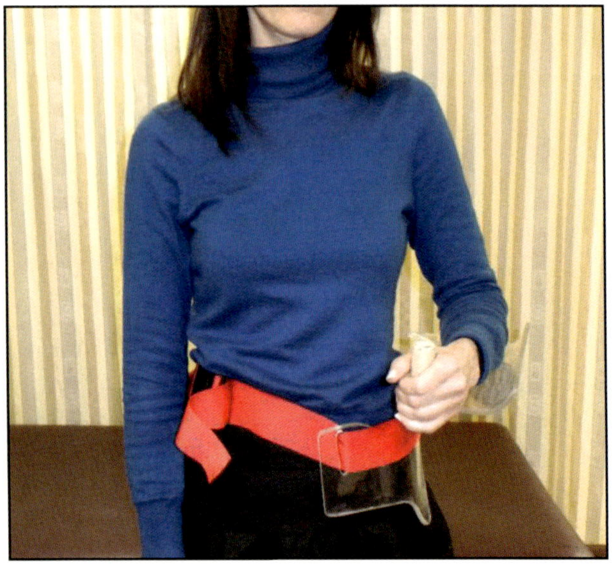

Figure 7. An orthosis that supports the upper extremity when standing is used in patients with chronic spinal accessory nerve palsy.

rehabilitation provider can do nothing to facilitate reinnervation except create a friendly environment for nerve regeneration. Patients need to understand that patience is required until the nerve recovers and the muscle or muscles activate. They need to understand that both the serratus anterior and trapezius provide static stabilization of the shoulder girdle. The loss of these muscles, particularly the trapezius, places great load upon other postural muscles that maintain appropriate thoracic, scapular, and shoulder girdle position. Therefore, postural education and upper extremity support when sitting and sometimes when standing are important. A simple, yet very effective, technique of reducing upper extremity weight is placing a pillow underneath the forearm when sitting (Figure 6). In some patients, typically those with a chronic SAN palsy, an orthosis can be fabricated to provide upper extremity support while standing and walking (Figure 7). This orthosis can be somewhat cumbersome; however, it allows support of the upper extremity yet the freedom to move it when required. Postural education that emphasizes the use of a lumbar roll when sitting in a firm chair is essential.

Another type of orthosis can be fabricated for patients with an LTN palsy when resting the upper extremity is not an option. This orthosis provides a solid posterior surface to minimize scapular winging while providing a fulcrum for the elevating upper extremity. I have only used this orthosis in combined cases of scapular nerve palsy (ie, brachial plexus injury involving more than one scapular muscle) (Figure 8).

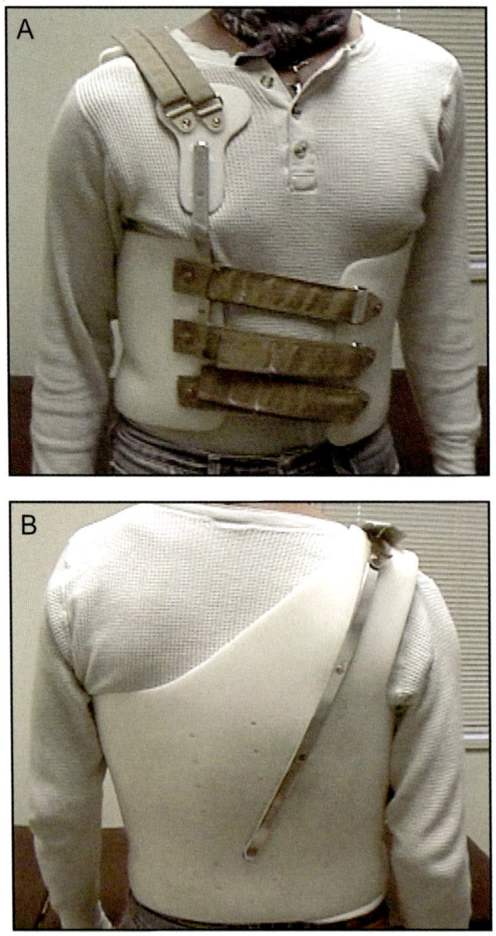

Figure 8. Orthosis used in patients who have long thoracic nerve palsy, have substantial scapular winging, and must use the upper extremity for work or activities. A, Front view. B, Back view.

Stretching

Myofascial pain might arise from unaffected scapular muscles due to increased static and dynamic load placed upon them during upper extremity use. Symptoms commonly develop in the levator scapulae and can be treated with thermal modalities, soft tissue techniques, and stretching. Care must be taken with stretching the levator scapulae because separation of the head and neck can negatively affect regeneration of the SAN or LTN.

Teaching the patient thoracic extension and pectoralis muscle stretching with a towel roll while lying supine can be very important, particularly in the case of SAN palsy. Commonly, I find that after neck dissection, patients have excessive forward head, dramatic scapular protraction, shoulder girdle depression, and substantial increase in thoracic kyphosis. These patients require stretching exercises and might need manual techniques for the cervical and thoracic spine and pectoralis muscles (Figures 9 and 10).

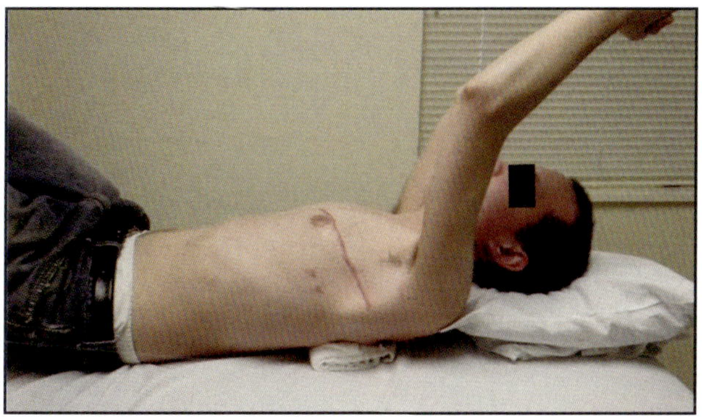

Figure 9. Thoracic extension stretch with towel roll placed at the apex of the thoracic spine.

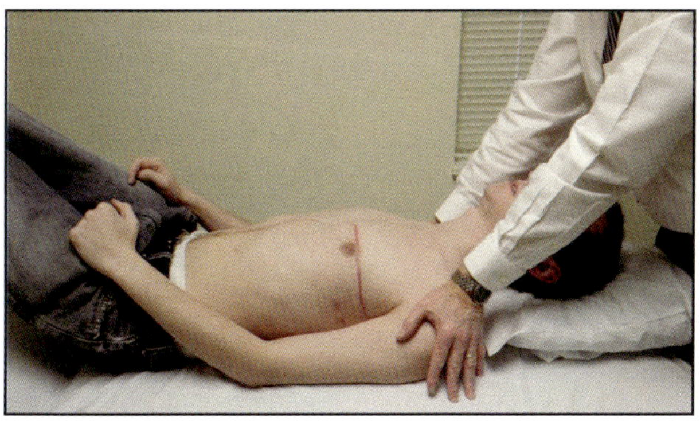

Figure 10. Pectoral stretch with towel roll placed in line with the spine. Shoulder girdles are moved into slight elevation and retraction as the patient breathes out.

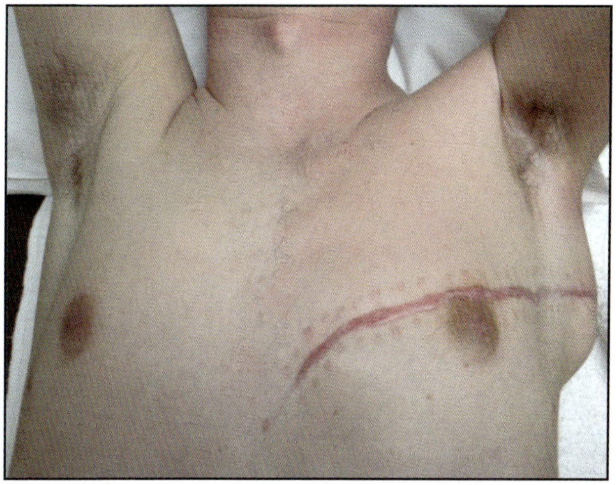

Figure 11. Patient with a crush injury to the thorax resulting in fractured ribs, long thoracic nerve palsy, and limited passive shoulder elevation. Note the excessive left scapular lateral rotation with passive elevation.

Range of Motion

Maintaining or improving shoulder range of motion might be a challenge in patients who develop scapular nerve palsy from multijoint trauma, brachial plexus injuries, or surgical procedures. Between 47% and 91% of patients who present with SAN palsies have an iatrogenic cause because of lymph-node excision or neck-dissection procedures.[1,12,13] Early shoulder range-of-motion exercises are required in this patient population. Depending on the procedure, tissue-flap transfers might be required, resulting in upper extremity immobilization. Passive and active-assistive range-of-motion exercises should be used in addition to glenohumeral and scapulothoracic joint mobilization (Figure 11). Care should be taken if performing inferior glides so that the shoulder girdle is not depressed. This can result in separation of the head and neck, causing pain and possibly aggravating nerve stretch.

Scapular Muscle Compensatory and Primary Activity Training

Improving compensatory and primary scapular muscle activity is an important aspect of rehabilitation for complete paralysis or substantial weakness of isolated scapular muscles. In other words, the rehabilitation provider should improve the patient's ability to recruit the unaffected (compensatory) scapular muscles then target the primary affected muscle when activity is noted. Therefore, we can consider 2 stages

Table 1. Staged Rehabilitation Exercises for Long Thoracic Nerve Palsy

Stage	Rehabilitation Exercise
Stage 1	Scapular retraction
	Scapular retraction with curls and triceps
	Scapular retraction with external rotation using an elastic band
	Scapular retraction with row using an elastic band
	Scapular retraction with backhand using an elastic band
	Scapular retraction and elevation (toward the scapular plane)
	Scapular retraction with forehand using an elastic band
Stage 2	Serratus anterior isolation
	Supine plus
	Side-lying plus and supported upper extremity lift with palm up
	Standing plus with palm up on ball
	Prone closed chain plus into ball
	Serratus anterior isolation and plus with upper extremity lift, palm up, and elbow bent
	Serratus anterior isolation and plus with upper extremity lift, palm up, and elbow straight
	Serratus anterior exercise with elastic an band
	Quadruped plus

Table 2. Staged Rehabilitation Exercises for Spinal Accessory Nerve Palsy

Stage	Rehabilitation Exercise
Stage 1	Rhomboid isolation
	Serratus anterior isolation
	Scapular elevation
	Rhomboid isolation and retraction with curls and triceps
	Rhomboid isolation and retraction with row using an elastic band
	Rhomboid isolation and retraction with external rotation using an elastic band
	Standing plus with palm up on ball
	Serratus anterior isolation and plus with upper extremity lift, palm up, and elbow bent
	Serratus anterior isolation and plus with upper extremity lift, palm up, and elbow straight
	Serratus anterior exercise with an elastic band
Stage 2	Retraction
	Supine middle trapezius isometric
	Supine lower trapezius isometric
	Scapular retraction with external rotation using an elastic band
	Scapular retraction with row using an elastic band
	Scapular retraction and elevation (toward the scapular plane)
	Scapular retraction with backhand using an elastic band

of muscle activity training: one related to compensatory (unaffected) muscle activation and the other related to primary (affected) muscle activation (Tables 1 and 2). The exercises might be the same or similar when targeting compensatory and primary muscles, depending on the degree of reinnervation and overlap of the muscle focus (compensatory or primary).

Consider an individual with a serratus anterior paralysis. Stage 1 rehabilitation would emphasize rhomboid and trapezius activation or "control" to gain greater stabilization and upper extremity power. Manual resistive techniques might be used to help the patient identify and strengthen the targeted unaffected scapular muscles (Figure 12). After the compensatory muscles are easily controlled by the patient, they are integrated into movement patterns. These exercises can be performed using manual resistance, elastic bands, or weights (Figure 13). Distal loading of the extremity (arms curls) by integrating compensatory scapular muscles can prepare a patient for a functional activity, such as lifting a gallon of milk out of the refrigerator. By first retracting the scapula and lifting the milk, proximal stabilization results in greater distal power. Compensatory scapular muscle integration is performed with other distal loading exercises, such as elbow extension and common rotator cuff strengthening exercises (external rotation, internal rotation, and

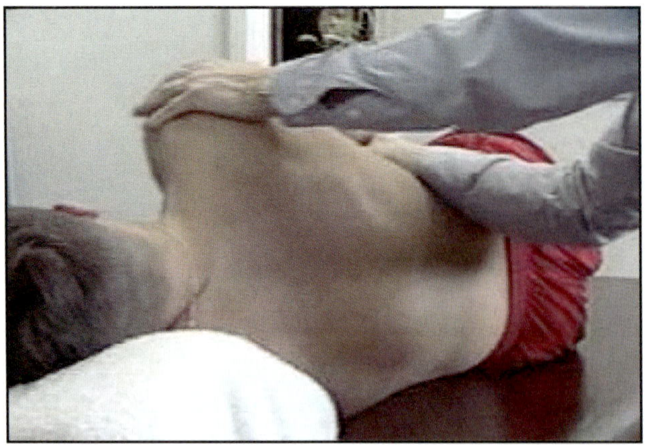

Figure 12. Manual resistance to facilitate control of the middle trapezius and rhomboid.

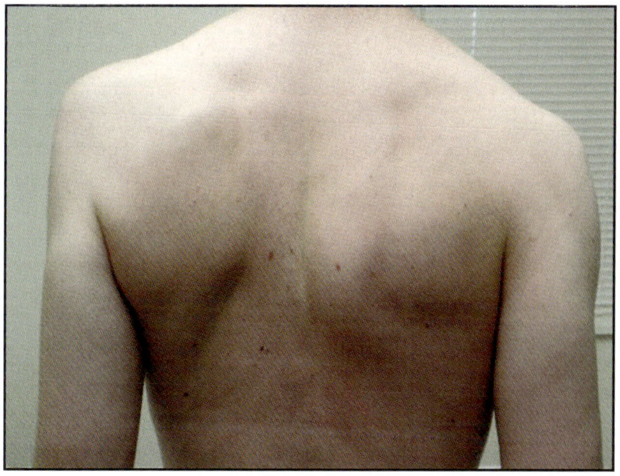

Figure 13. Scapular retraction to isolate either the middle or rhomboid muscles.

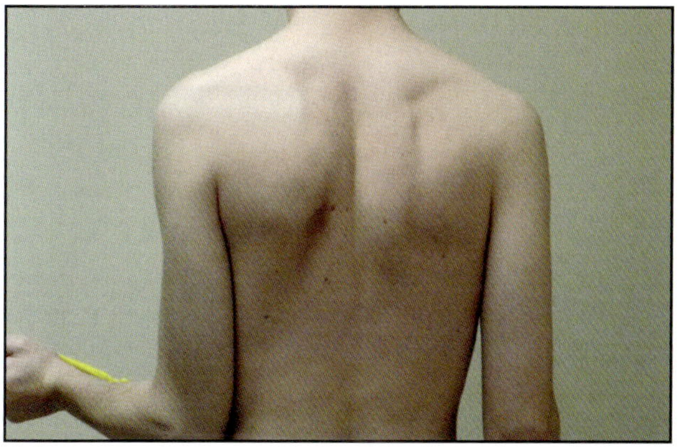

Figure 14. Scapular retraction integrated in the shoulder external rotation exercise.

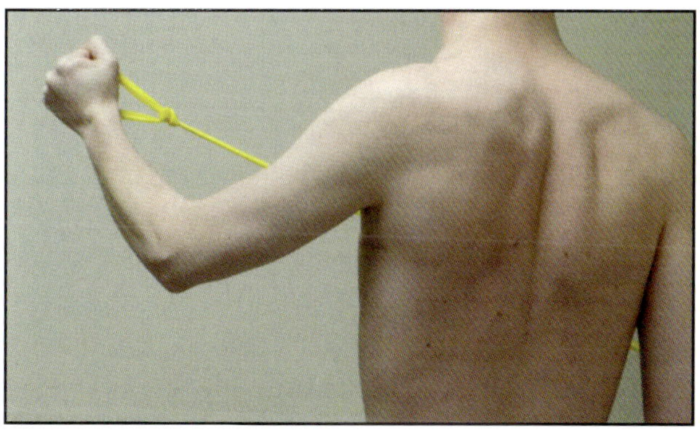

Figure 15. Scapular retraction integrated into the backhand exercise.

extension) (Figure 14). Diagonal patterns simulating a backhand are performed and emphasize scapular retraction (Figure 15).

As the patient demonstrates serratus anterior return, stage 2 activation begins with serratus anterior isolation exercises, which are performed by protracting and slightly elevating the scapula (Figure 16). The patient also might lie supine and perform a plus maneuver with the upper extremity at 90° (Figure 17). When able, activation is begun with side-lying elevation with a plus and progresses to standing ball roll plus and eventually to moving the upper extremity against gravity (Figure 18). Serratus anterior isolation and plus

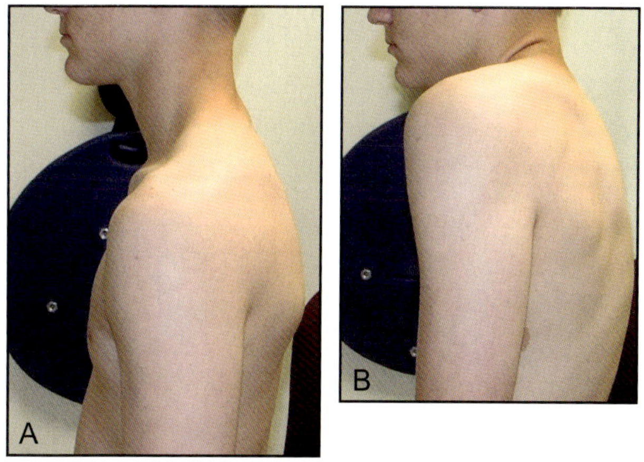

Figure 16. Serratus anterior isolation. A, At rest. B, Moving into slight elevation and protraction.

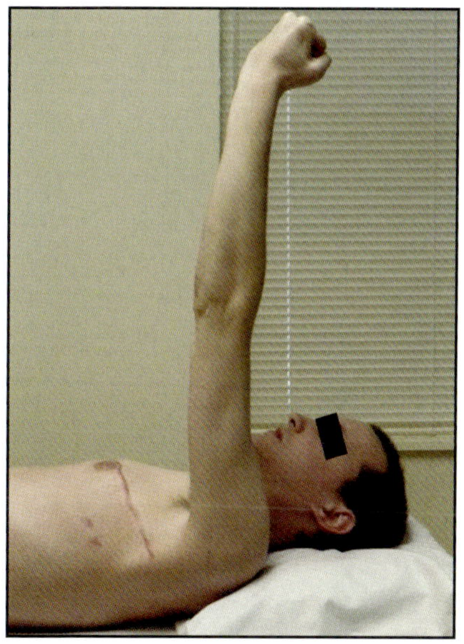

Figure 17. Supine plus at 90°.

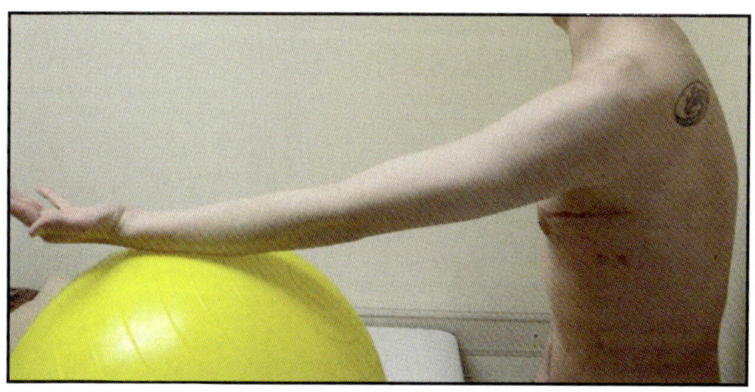

Figure 18. Standing plus on a ball with the upper extremity in external rotation (palm up).

with upper extremity lift can be performed with assistance and with the elbow either bent or straight (Figure 19). Resistance can be used to maximally recruit the serratus by reaching forward slightly medial to the sagittal plane and externally rotating the shoulder (Figure 20).[8] Progression to weight-bearing exercise is attempted in a graduated manner.

In the patient who presents with an SAN palsy, stage 1 begins with rhomboid and serratus anterior isolation. Manual resistance in the side-lying position often is required to assist the patient in proper rhomboid isolation. When achieved, distal loading can be started with

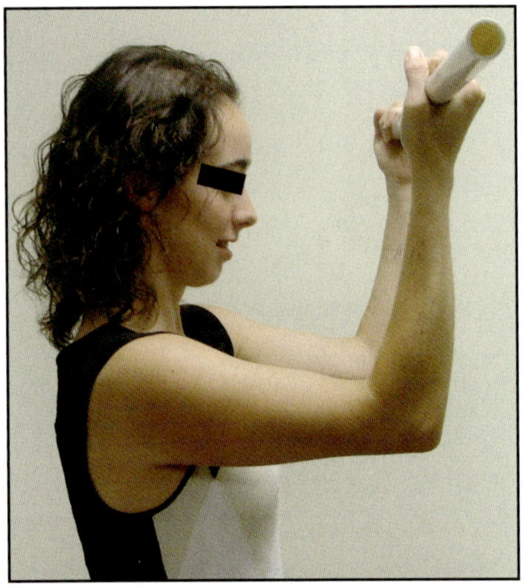

Figure 19. Serratus anterior isolation and plus with upper extremity lift, palms up, and elbows bent.

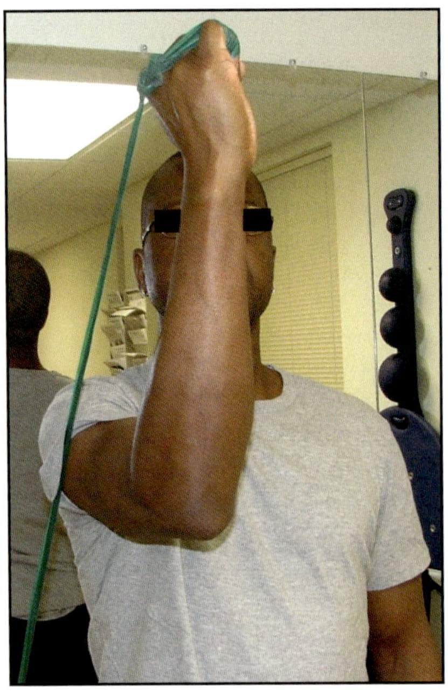

Figure 20. Serratus anterior exercise with an elastic band.

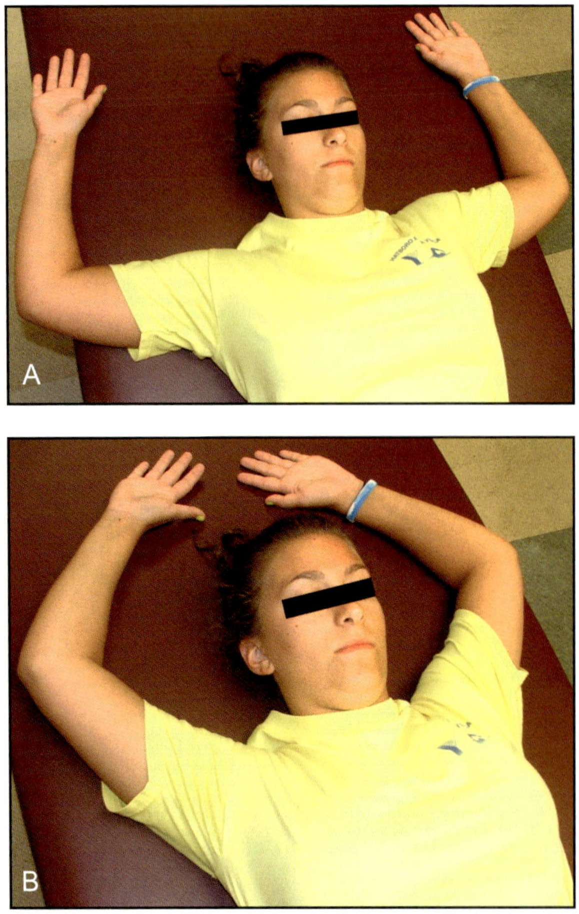

Figure 21. Middle, A, and lower, B, trapezius isometric exercises.

curls, triceps, rows, and external rotation. Many of the same exercises discussed in stage 1 for LTN treatment are performed with emphasis on recruiting the rhomboids. In addition, forward flexion with a plus is performed in stage 2. The progression includes diagonal patterns, gravity-minimized, and antigravity positions. As reinnervation of the trapezius begins, the primary focus is on activation of the trapezius using stage 1 and 2 exercises. If the patient is able, isometric activation for the middle and lower trapezius is used (Figure 21).

Supervised therapy is required initially, then usually intermittent visits are encouraged unless pain and passive motion impairments are present. Reassessment using the examination techniques is required at each session to determine if the palsy is resolving. Patience and a consistent home exercise program are important because recovery is time dependent.

Rehabilitation of patients with scapular nerve palsy requires an algorithmic examination approach to identify the pathologic condition and the appropriate intervention. A home exercise program, including postural training and possible use of orthoses, is beneficial. Specific stretching might be needed when passive range-of-motion impairments are found. Aggressive strengthening before motor control is established leads to production or perpetuation of symptoms and to frustration. Staging scapular muscle isolation and eventual integration into functional movement patterns will improve outcomes.

REFERENCES

1. Kim DH, Cho YJ, Tiel RL, Kline DG. Surgical outcomes of 111 spinal accessory nerve injuries. *Neurosurgery*. 2003;53(5):1102–1103,1106–1112.
2. Kuhn JE, Plancher KD, Hawkins RJ. Scapular winging. *J Am Acad Orthop Surg*. 1995;3(6):319–325.
3. Vastamäki M, Kauppila LI. Etiologic factors in isolated paralysis of the serratus anterior muscle: a report of 197 cases. *J Shoulder Elbow Surg*. 1993;2(5):240–243.
4. Kibler WB. Role of the scapula in the overhead throwing motion. *Contemp Orthop*. 1991;22(5):525–532.
5. Kuhn JE. The scapulothoracic articulation: anatomy, biomechanics, pathophysiology, and management. In: Iannotti JP, Williams GR, eds. *Disorders of the Shoulder: Diagnosis & Management*. Philadelphia, PA: Lippincott Williams & Wilkins; 1999:817–846.
6. Kelley MJ. An examination algorithm for examination of scapular muscle dysfunction. Paper presented at: International Congress of Shoulder Therapists; 2004; Washington, DC.
7. Leggin BG, Kelley MJ. Disease-specific methods of rehabilitation. In: Iannotti JP, Williams GR, eds. *Disorders of the Shoulder: Diagnosis and Management*. 2nd ed. Philadelphia, PA: Lippincott Williams & Wilkins; 2007:1265–1293.
8. Ekstrom RA, Donatelli RA, Soderberg GL. Surface electromyographic analysis of exercises for the trapezius and serratus anterior muscles. *J Orthop Sports Phys Ther*. 2003;33(5):247–258.
9. Kendall F, McCreary EK. *Muscles: Testing and Function*. 3rd ed. Baltimore, MD: Lippincott Williams & Wilkins; 1983.
10. Kelley MJ, Kane TE, Leggin BG. Spinal accessory nerve palsy: associated signs and symptoms. *J Orthop Sports Phys Ther*. 2008;38(2):78–86.
11. Kelley MJ, Brenneman S. The scapular flip sign: an examination sign to identify the presence of a spinal accessory nerve palsy. Paper presented at: APTA Combined Sections Meeting; 2000; New Orleans, LA.
12. Berry H, MacDonald EA, Mrazek AC. Accessory nerve palsy: a review of 23 cases. *Can J Neurol Sci*. 1991;18(3):337–341.
13. Donner TR, Kline DG. Extracranial spinal accessory nerve injury. *Neurosurgery*. 1993;32(6):907–911.

III-18

Limited-Goals Rehabilitation

Bryce W. Gaunt, PT, SCS

CHAPTER CONTENTS

WHAT PATIENTS ARE APPROPRIATE FOR THE USE OF THIS GUIDELINE?

- Any patient whom the physician believes will have a moderate to large limitation in normal shoulder function because of gross anatomic deficiencies or abnormalities in the musculotendinous, ligamentous, or bony structures. I list the most frequently used diagnoses.
- Some patients with reconstruction of their glenohumeral ligaments via allografts, such as an Achilles tendon allograft for deficiency of the anterior aspect of the capsule, glenohumeral ligaments, and labrum. Subscapularis deficiency also might be present in these patients.
- Some patients with revision repairs to treat instability.
- Some patients with rotator cuff tear arthropathy.
- Some patients with multitendon rotator cuff tears in which all tendons are irreparable or were only debrided.
- Some patients with partial repairs of massive rotator cuff tears.
- Some patients who have had revision rotator cuff repairs and who have extensive fatty degeneration.
- Some patients with revision reverse shoulder arthroplasties.
- Some patients with revision standard shoulder arthroplasties.
- Some nonoperatively treated patients with advanced end-stage arthritis and gross bony abnormalities, such as traumatic arthritis.

Clinical pearls are highlighted in yellow throughout the text.

THE MOST IMPORTANT FACTOR THAT SHOULD GUIDE CLINICAL DECISION MAKING

The most important factor that should guide clinical decision making in limited-goals rehabilitation is to appreciate that only minimal rehabilitation interventions are appropriate due to the marked anatomic deficits and abnormalities that patients in this rehabilitation category possess. Neer et al[1] originally established this rehabilitation category and an associated outcome rating classification so a patient with nonfunctioning deltoid and rotator cuff muscles could be rated as having a successful result if he or she had good pain relief and "useful" shoulder function. He defined *limited-goals rehabilitation* as an exercise program aimed at achieving a lesser range of motion (ROM), which usually was limited to 20° of external rotation and 90° of elevation, to retain more stability and allow the patient to reach his or her head and scapula for all activities of daily living.[1]

At our facility, we have expanded limited-goals rehabilitation to include any patient whom the physician believes will have a moderate to large limitation in normal shoulder function because of gross anatomic deficiencies or abnormalities in the musculotendinous, ligamentous, and/or bony structures. This can include patients with a variety of nonoperative or postoperative instability, rotator cuff conditions, or arthritis disorders. The diagnoses and surgical procedures for which limited-goals rehabilitation most commonly are prescribed are listed in the What Patients are Appropriate for the Use of This Guideline section. Our primary rehabilitation goals for these patients are to minimize pain, ensure glenohumeral stability, and achieve reasonable waist-level function. A secondary goal for most patients is to attempt to achieve shoulder-level function to allow the hand of the affected extremity to reach the top of the head for combing hair and other basic grooming activities. In all patients with limited goals, the use of the shoulder for overhead tasks is not realistic, and rehabilitation activities aimed at achieving this level of function should not be prescribed.

KEY PRINCIPLES IN REHABILITATION OF THIS PROBLEM

Physician Determines the Appropriate Level of Rehabilitation

Patients who might be considered for limited-goals rehabilitation have very complex problems with their shoulder girdles that are best evaluated and managed by an orthopaedic surgeon, preferably one who specializes in shoulder girdle disorders. Appropriate decision making regarding the best course of treatment and type of rehabilitation for these patients requires basic and often advanced imaging studies, advanced evaluation and clinical decision-making skills, and forward thinking to consider how decisions made about the patient's care today will affect the patient 10 and 20 years in the future. For patients who have had surgery, the information that the surgeon views firsthand regarding pathologic lesions, tissue quality, and the strength of any surgical repair is required to make the best rehabilitation decisions for each patient. For these reasons, an orthopaedic surgeon is the best person to determine if a patient is appropriate for limited-goals or standard rehabilitation and to determine the specific limits of limited-goals rehabilitation.

Know and Respect Anatomic Deficits

Patients are placed in limited-goals rehabilitation only if they have substantial anatomic deficits or abnormalities. To structure an appropriate rehabilitation program and understand the physician's limits on rehabilitation, the rehabilitation provider must understand, work around, and respect each patient's unique deficits. For example, no passive external rotation exercises and only limited external rotation strengthening likely would be prescribed for a patient who had a revision standard total shoulder arthroplasty due to multiple anterior dislocations before revision and a deficient anterior capsule and poor-quality glenohumeral ligaments at the time of reoperation. Similarly, no elevation strengthening exercises other than horizontal dusting likely would be prescribed for a patient who has an irreparable complete supraspinatus tear, complete infraspinatus tear, and poor deltoid function.

If anatomic deficits are not respected and too vigorous rehabilitation is used, then the primary goals of limited-goals rehabilitation (pain relief, glenohumeral stability, and waist-level function) often are jeopardized. In addition, further injury might be caused to the structures that remain. Therefore, close communication among the physician, rehabilitation provider, patient, and family is needed so everyone understands the pathologic condition that is present and the appropriate type of rehabilitation activities that should be prescribed.

Individualized Rehabilitation

Individualized rehabilitation is important for all patients, including those in standard rehabilitation programs, but it is especially important in patients in the limited-goals rehabilitation category due to the diversity and severity of the pathologic conditions that we are rehabilitating. Anatomic deficits in the shoulder girdle requiring the use of the limited-goals program can occur in musculotendinous structures, capsuloligamentous structures, and/or the bony structures. Each has its own considerations and subtleties with limited-goals rehabilitation. Some patients also have deficits in more than one anatomic area.

Anatomic deficits to the bony structures often are not considered by rehabilitation providers but might have a profound effect on limited-goals rehabilitation. Large abnormalities to the glenoid can be present in some patients with instability or arthritis. In some patients with traumatic instability, especially those with many dislocations, up to 25% to 40% of the glenoid can be missing (Figure 1). When 25% or greater of the glenoid is deficient, bone grafting to reconstruct the glenoid is recommended as part of the surgical reconstruction (Figure 2).[2-4] In these situations, ROM in directions that load the bone graft is usually limited for several months to allow healing of the graft. In patients with advanced arthritis, the glenoid can be worn abnormally or occasionally can be worn away altogether, requiring ROM limits to prevent instability.

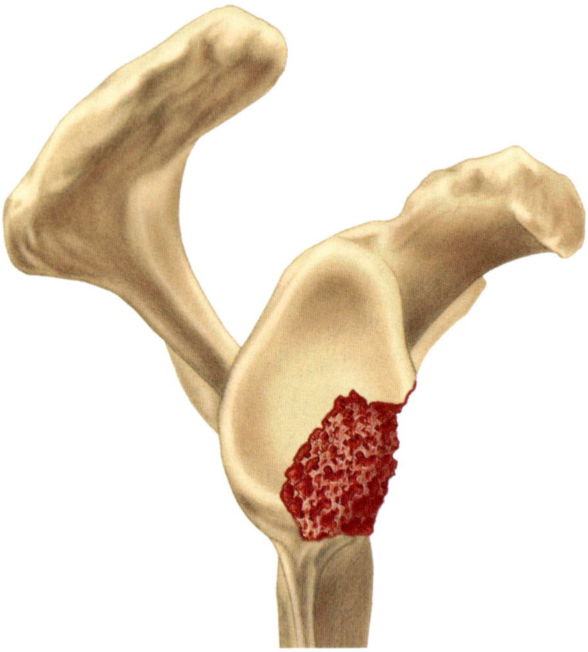

Figure 1. Glenoid bone loss of 25% to 40%.

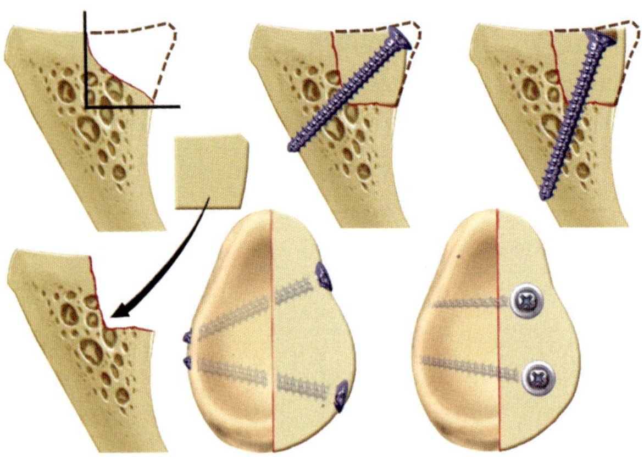

Figure 2. Structural bone grafting of the glenoid.

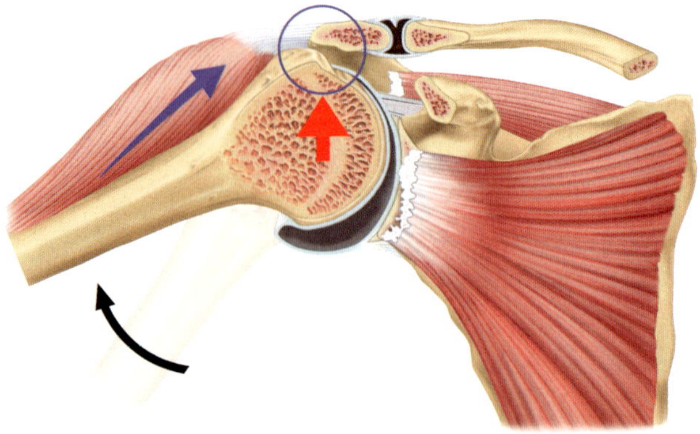

Figure 3. Excessive superior migration of the humeral head, which is shown by the red arrow and blue circle, occurs due to some multitendon rotator cuff tears where the rotator cuff does not adequately stabilize the humeral head against the superior pull of the deltoid.

Deficits to musculotendinous structures require modifications to AROM and strengthening interventions. Occasionally, training complementary muscles to make up for the job performed by the deficient or damaged muscle is possible and can result in nearly normal function. Examples and details of this type of rehabilitation are provided in chapter III-3. Limited-goals rehabilitation generally is prescribed when accessory muscles cannot perform the function of the damaged muscle or muscles due to the size of the anatomic deficit or limited capacity of the remaining muscles. For example, a patient with complete irreparable tears to the subscapularis, supraspinatus, and infraspinatus usually does not have enough remaining structures to provide a fulcrum to stabilize the humeral head against the superior pull of the deltoid during attempted elevation of the shoulder (Figure 3).[5,6] If this patient is managed nonoperatively, elevation strengthening (see chapter II-4) generally would be inappropriate because it would hasten the arthritic changes associated with rotator cuff tear arthropathy. Generally, for these patients, passive ROM (PROM) during rehabilitation also is limited to maximize pain relief and ensure joint stability because overhead active ROM (AROM) is not a realistic outcome for these patients.

For patients in limited-goals rehabilitation due to anatomic capsuloligamentous deficits, ROM must be limited during both AROM and PROM interventions to ensure joint stability. Depending on the musculotendinous structures that remain, AROM and strengthening is emphasized using low-level exercises in nonprovocative positions. Sometimes PROM and light stretching are needed in the direction that is opposite to the instability to help balance the forces acting on the glenohumeral joint. Sometimes PROM and light stretching are needed in a protected ROM as specified by the surgeon after a surgical reconstruction to restore stability, such as light external rotation stretching after an Achilles tendon allograft to reconstruct a deficient anterior capsuloligamentous complex (Figure 4).

Limited Interventions and Know What is Not Appropriate

Given the extensive anatomic deficits that are required for a person to be prescribed limited-goals rehabilitation and the low-level goals of this program, the rehabilitation provider must understand that only limited-rehabilitation activities are appropriate for these patients. Many rehabilitation activities that are common in the rehabilitation of other shoulder conditions are not appropriate in limited-goals rehabilitation. Following these guidelines helps ensure that the primary goals of a low level of pain, joint stability, and waist-level functioning have the best chance of being met and that additional structural damage is not caused by overloading the remaining structures during rehabilitation. For most patients, only very limited PROM and little to no strengthening is appropriate. During limited-goals rehabilitation, extra-gentle activities that often are more gentle than you think is necessary work best. After a patient tolerates this program well, very little exercise modification is often needed. Therefore, patients with limited goals commonly require very few in-clinic visits unless establishing a good tolerance to the exercise program is difficult, exercise technique is poor, or PROM is greatly below expectations.

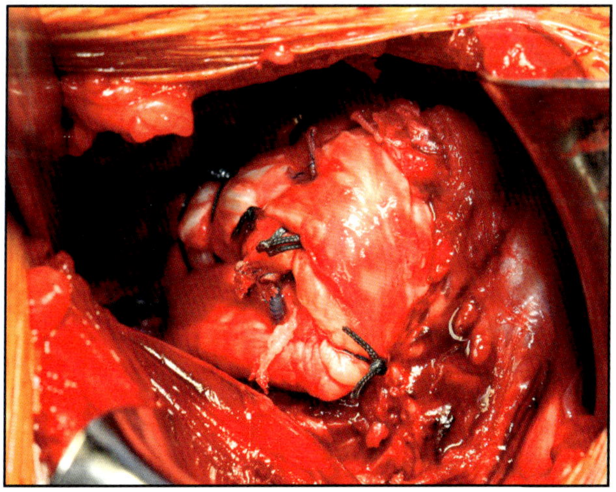

Figure 4. A completed Achilles tendon allograft for deficiency of the anteroinferior glenohumeral ligament complex.

Patient Education

Educating the patient about appropriate modifications of activities of daily living (ADLs) is an often overlooked, but very important, component of rehabilitation of this problem. It is a large part of helping the patient's symptoms to begin to improve by ensuring that the patient appropriately minimizes his or her pain and inflammation by matching ADL use with the level of the anatomic deficit. Patients are instructed to temporarily minimize or eliminate ADLs that require use of the involved extremity in positions that cause great pain, symptoms of instability, or crepitus. This typically involves minimizing the use of the upper extremity in extremes of motion, such as not putting on a jacket with the involved shoulder first and minimizing the use of the extremity for attempted overhead reaching with activities that can be performed with the other extremity. Patients might resist implementing these modifications, so extra education is needed to teach them that this is as important as or more important than the other components of rehabilitation for helping the shoulder feel better for the short and long term.

SPECIFIC REHABILITATION GUIDELINE

The Appendix specifies our complete Limited-Goals Rehabilitation Guideline. It is divided into 2 phases based on the recommendation of the physician, specific anatomic deficits, reactivity of the shoulder, and tolerance for exercise. To advance from one rehabilitation phase to the next, the patient must gain approval from the physician and successfully complete the core components of the previous rehabilitation activities. Some patients might never be appropriate to advance to phase 2 rehabilitation. The entire rehabilitation guideline is almost exclusively a home-based exercise program. Because of the limited rehabilitation goals, the use of accessory equipment and weight-training machines is not necessary and likely would exacerbate the patient's symptoms. The usefulness of clinic visits is to improve PROM by hands-on stretching if PROM is greatly below expectations, to establish and ensure correct exercise selection and performance, and occasionally to advance the program as I will discuss. Modalities beyond home-based applications of superficial heat and cold rarely are needed.

Phase 1

The primary focus of phase 1 rehabilitation is to establish a tolerance to a gentle exercise program, decrease inflammation and pain, improve or maintain PROM in forward elevation and external rotation with the upper extremity near the side, and sometimes initiate isometric exercise. In the Appendix and the Key Principles in Rehabilitation of This Problem, I discuss the interventions we prefer to use to meet these goals along with the rationale for these choices.

Of particular importance during phase 1 rehabilitation is to stay within the PROM limits that the physician specified and to ensure that the patient tolerates the exercise program comfortably. Doing both of these things keeps the priority of rehabilitation on pain relief and comfortable exercise and ensures that the damaged and remaining tissues do not receive excessive stress.

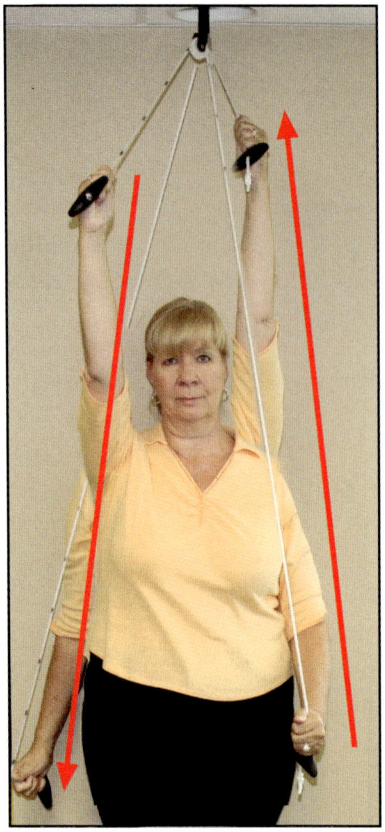

Figure 5. Rope-and-pulley active-assistive forward elevation.

Phase 2

The goals of phase 2 interventions are the same as the goals of phase 1 except that limited, gentle, dynamic strengthening is included and a long-term maintenance program is established. In the Appendix and the Key Principles in Rehabilitation of This Problem section, I discuss the interventions we prefer to use to meet these goals along with the rationale for these choices.

Phase 2 allows expanded treatment options for PROM, especially elevation ROM. However, care must be taken if rope-and-pulley active-assistive forward elevation (AAFE) (Figure 5) or supine AAFE (Figure 6) are used to ensure these exercises are comfortable and well tolerated during the initial weeks of implementation. Patients in the limited-goals category due to arthritis, rotator cuff disease, or instability might not tolerate either of these exercises, especially supine AAFE, very well. Patients also must be instructed that these exercises should not be done using "the farther, the better" mentality but instead they only

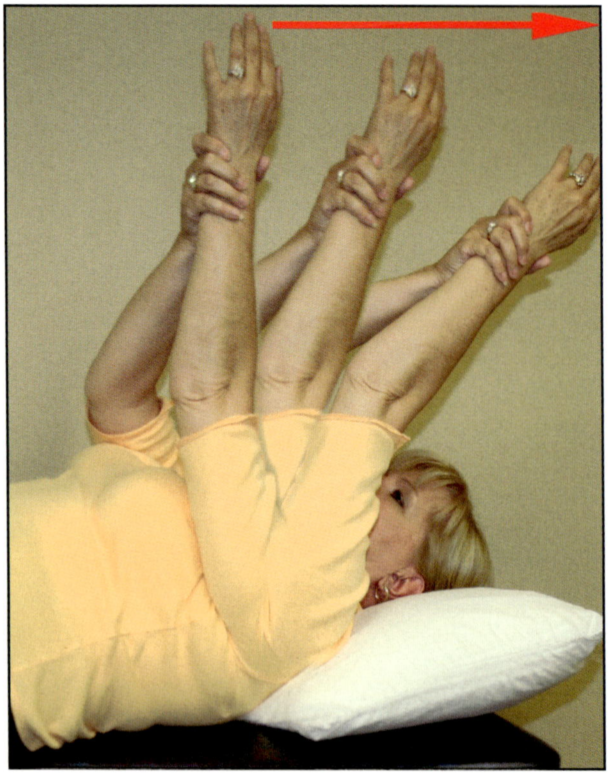

Figure 6. Self-assisted supine active-assistive forward elevation. The hand-assisted exercise is preferred.

should perform the exercises within their comfortable ROMs. In phase 2, passive external rotation exercises often are discontinued unless less than about 30° to 40° of motion is present with a capsular end feel that tends to decline without passive stretching. The hand-behind-head, or quadrant, stretch (Figure 7) is helpful if the patient has a passive limitation in abduction with external rotation that prevents him or her from reaching the back of the head and the rehabilitation provider has a reasonable expectation that the patient would be able to achieve this motion actively if the needed PROM were available. This situation applies most often for patients in the limited-goals program due to arthritis and sometimes due to rotator cuff deficiency. For most patients with limited goals, this intervention is not appropriate to use.

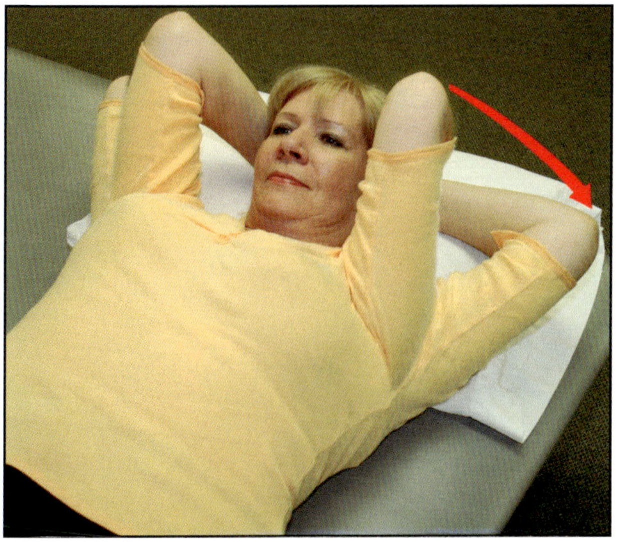

Figure 7. The hand-behind-head stretch is appropriate to use only in very specific circumstances for the patient with limited goals.

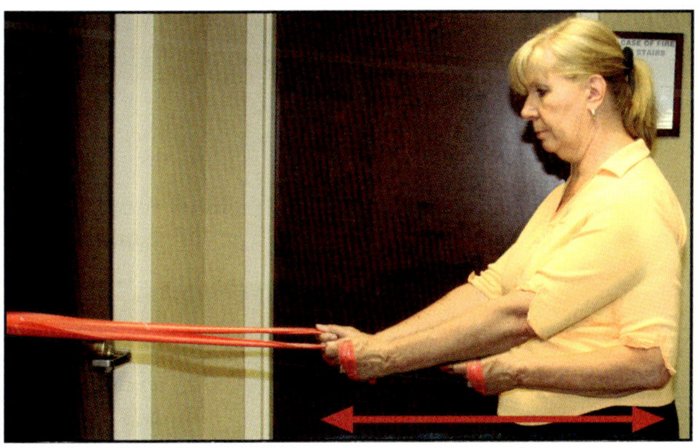

Figure 8. Scapular retraction with shoulder extension to neutral with elastic resistance.

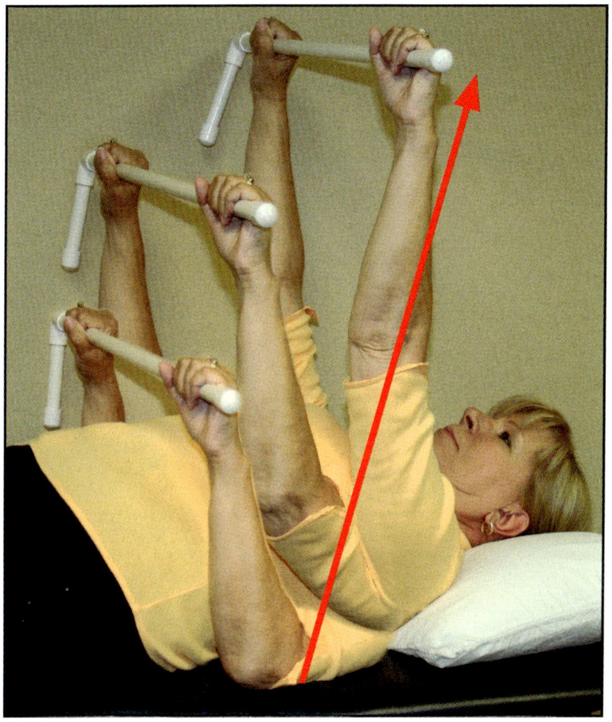

Figure 9. Supine active-assistive reaching to 90°.

Phase 2 allows for the initiation of selected dynamic strengthening activities if permitted by the physician. The physician also should specify if strengthening certain muscles or planes of motion is not appropriate due to instability, multitendon rotator cuff tears, arthritis, or bony erosion. Usually, only a very few exercises are deemed appropriate and well tolerated by each patient, and typically very little exercise progression is used for strengthening interventions. For example, internal rotation with an elastic band, scapular retraction with shoulder extension to neutral with an elastic band (Figure 8), and supine reaching progression beginning with active-assistive ROM (Figure 9) might be a good short- and long-term program for a patient with an irreparable rotator cuff tear of the supraspinatus and infraspinatus in the limited-goals program. External rotation with an elastic band performed in a protected ROM, internal rotation with an elastic band performed in a protected ROM, forward reaching with an elastic band (Figure 10), and incline dusting (Figure 11) might be a good short- and long-term strengthening program for a patient after an Achilles tendon allograft and pectoralis major transfer for multiple failed anterior instability procedures and subscapularis deficiency. Pendulum (Figure 12), rope-and-pulley AAFE (Figure 5), and side-lying external rotation (Figure 13) might be an appropriate short- and long-term program for a patient who has end-stage traumatic arthritis and is in limited-goals rehabilitation.

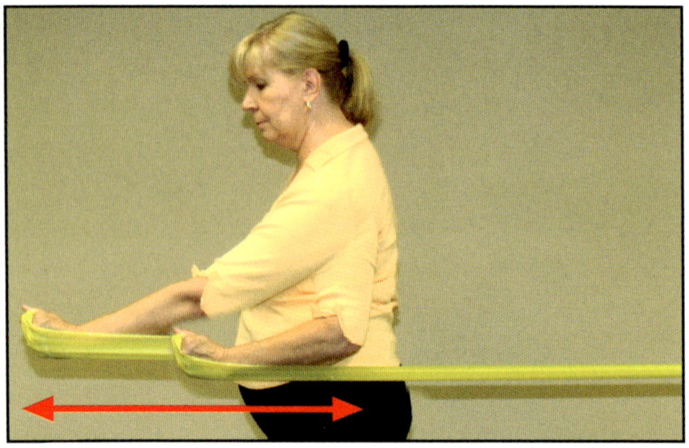

Figure 10. Forward reaching with an elastic band is used very sparingly for the patient with limited goals.

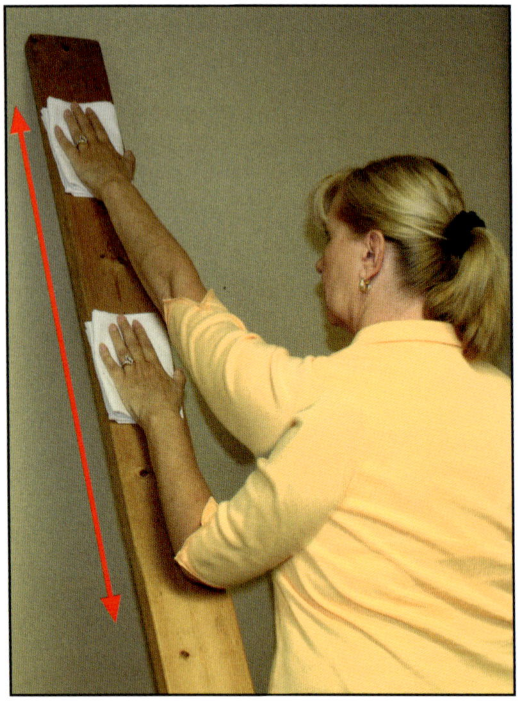

Figure 11. Incline dusting.

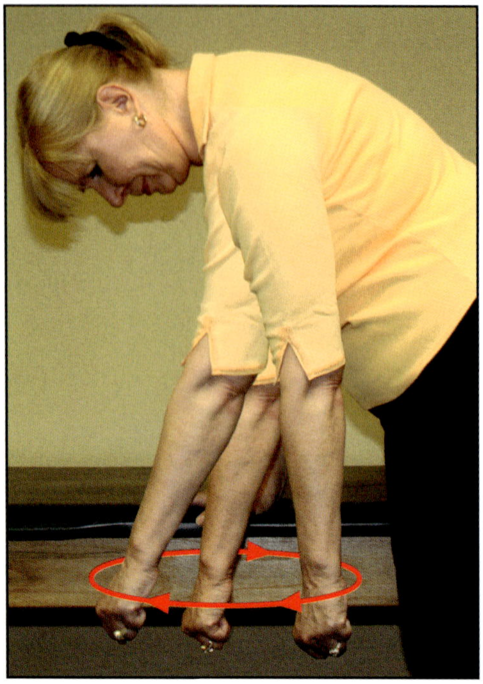

Figure 12. Pendulum exercise.

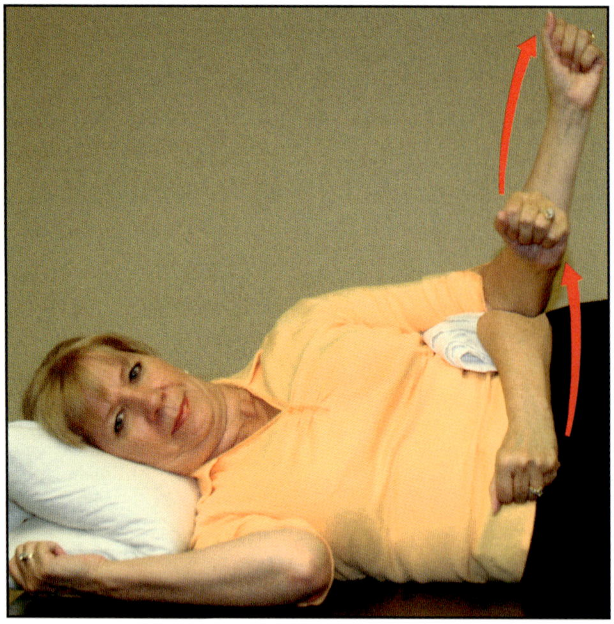

Figure 13. Side-lying external rotation.

The rehabilitation provider also needs to establish a long-term maintenance home exercise program that is well tolerated and that does not overload the damaged or remaining tissue both in the short and long term to maintain the limited function that these patients have. Implementing a long-term maintenance home exercise program is important because the pathologic condition that a patient with limited goals has generally progresses over time. A maintenance program can help maximize the structural integrity and function of the remaining structures and can help prevent a decline in ROM or function. I typically instruct the patient to continue his or her current home exercise program, which is limited, 4 to 7 times per week.

REFERENCES

1. Neer CS II, Watson KC, Stanton FJ. Recent experience in total shoulder replacement. *J Bone Joint Surg Am.* 1982;64(3):319–337.
2. Beran MC, Donaldson CT, Bishop JY. Treatment of chronic glenoid defects in the setting of recurrent anterior shoulder instability: a systematic review. *J Shoulder Elbow Surg.* 2010;19(3):769–780.
3. Lynch JR, Clinton JM, Dewing CB, Warme WJ, Matsen FA III. Treatment of osseous defects associated with anterior shoulder instability. *J Shoulder Elbow Surg.* 2009;18(2):317–328.
4. Provencher MT, Bhatia S, Ghodadra NS, et al. Recurrent shoulder instability: current concepts for evaluation and management of glenoid bone loss. *J Bone Joint Surg Am.* 2010;92(suppl 2):133–151.
5. Sharkey NA, Marder RA. The rotator cuff opposes superior translation of the humeral head. *Am J Sports Med.* 1995;23(3):270–275.
6. Thompson WO, Debski RE, Boardman ND III, et al. A biomechanical analysis of rotator cuff deficiency in a cadaveric model. *Am J Sports Med.* 1996;24(3):286–292.

LIMITED-GOALS REHABILITATION GUIDELINE

St. Francis Orthopaedic Institute and St. Francis Rehabilitation Center

All information contained in this protocol is to be used as a general guideline only. Specific variations might be appropriate for each patient and might be specified by the physician. In all cases, it is acceptable to advance the program more slowly than stated. If the patient experiences excessive pain, discontinue exercise until the physician is contacted. ***Achieving and maintaining a low level of pain and inflammation is the most important goal in all stages of rehabilitation, even if less passive and active range of motion are accomplished.***

SYMBOLS AND ABBREVIATIONS

AAFE, active-assistive forward elevation
AAROM, active-assistive range of motion
ADLs, activities of daily living
AROM, active range of motion
ER, external rotation
IR, internal rotation
PER, passive external rotation
PFE, passive forward elevation
PRN, as needed
PROM, passive range of motion
ROM, range of motion

Forward elevation, either active or passive, is the plane of motion in which an individual naturally lifts his or her arm that is anterior to the plane of the scapula and lateral to flexion.

PHASE 1

Goals

°Minimize pain and inflammatory response
°Improve or maintain PROM in basic planes while respecting the abnormal anatomy that is present
°Initiate isometric strengthening if approved by the physician and well tolerated by the patient
°Educate the patient about modifications to ADLs to avoid positions that result in symptoms

Exercises (Individualized to the Patient's Particular Situation)

°Pendulum exercises (Figure 12)
  °Lean over the table a comfortable amount
  °Keep the body still
  °Move the arm in small comfortable circles only
°Comfortable PFE ROM (specific ROM limits might be specified by the physician)
  °Preferred exercises
    °Sit with family member or therapist lifting the arm (Figure 14)
    °Table step-back exercise (Figure 15)
°Upright PER in slight abduction to 45° to 50° maximum unless a more restrictive limit is given by the physician
  °Preferred exercises

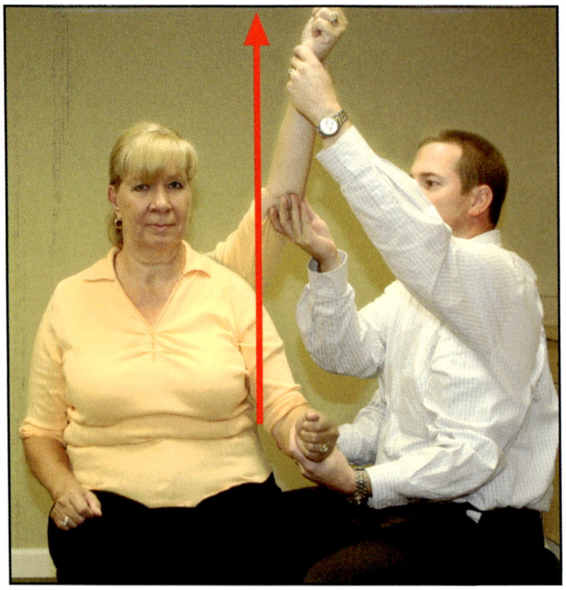

Figure 14. Assisted passive forward elevation. The assistant typically stands diagonally in front of the patient.

- °PER walk-around (stand with the arm supported on a table and rotate the body) (Figure 16)
- °Sit with family member or therapist rotating the arm (Figure 17)

°Submaximal pain-free isometrics (if approved by the physician)

- °Perform with the elbow flexed and instruct the patient to press with 1 to 2 pounds of force only
- °Flexion, ER, IR, and abduction are considered, keeping in mind anatomic deficits

°Patient education

- °Minimize or eliminate ADLs that require use of the arm in positions that cause great pain, cause crepitus, or require large amounts of abnormal movement

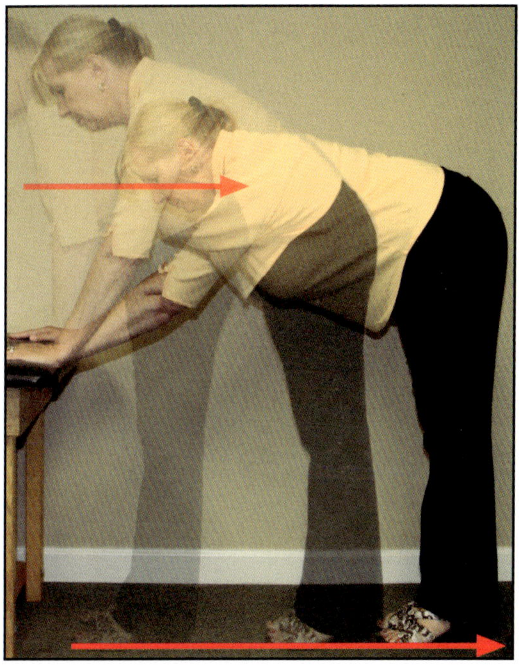

Figure 15. Table step-back exercise for passive forward elevation

Adjunctive Exercises

°Aquatic therapy for gentle, comfortable AAROM, AROM, or light strengthening (no swimming strokes)
°Instruction about ice or heat PRN for home use
°Spine therapy assessment and mobilization PRN

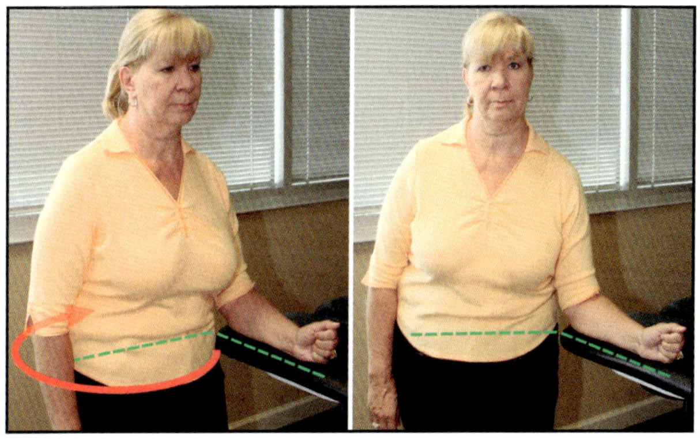

Figure 16. Passive external rotation walk-around exercise.

Interventions to Avoid

°PROM, AROM, or strengthening in coronal-plane abduction
°Advanced stretching exercises
°Moderate-level or high-level rotator cuff or deltoid strengthening activities
°Exercises that result in moderate or severe pain or painful crepitus

PHASE 2

Goals

°Minimize pain and inflammatory response
°Improve or maintain PROM in basic planes while respecting the abnormal anatomy that is present
°Consider light dynamic rotator cuff and scapular strengthening that respects anatomic abnormalities
°Educate the patient about appropriate long-term modifications to ADLs
°Implement a long-term maintenance home exercise program

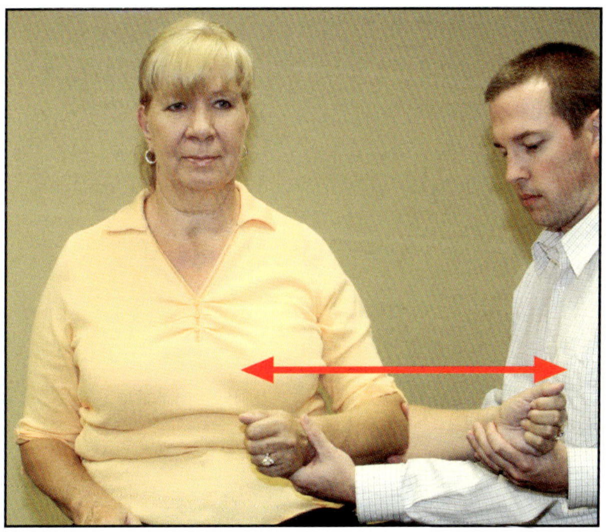

Figure 17. Assisted sitting passive external rotation.

Exercises (Individualized to the Patient's Particular Situation)

- °Continue pendulum exercise
- °Continue comfortable ROM in forward elevation
  - °Consider rope-and-pulley AAFE (Figure 5)
  - °Consider supine AAFE (Figure 6)
  - °Can continue phase 1 interventions
- °Can continue PER stretching depending on the amount of PROM, tolerance to the exercise, and amount of functional limitations
- °Consider supine hands-behind-head stretch (Figure 7) if functional limitations are present, if anterior static stability of the glenohumeral joint is adequate, and if enough shoulder girdle strength is present so reaching the top of the head with the hand of the involved arm is a realistic goal. This exercise typically is seldom used.
- °Consider limited dynamic strengthening based on the patient's anatomic deficits (if approved by the physician)
  - °All exercises should be comfortable, well tolerated, and performed with minimal or no deviation
  - °Exercises usually are performed 1 to 2 times per day with light to no resistance and limited ROM
  - °The most common exercises considered are
    - °Elastic-resistance band IR with a 5- to 6-foot band length and light or no pretension
    - °Side-lying ER (Figure 13)
    - °Scapular retraction with shoulder extension to neutral (Figure 8)
    - °Rope-and-pulley AAFE (Figure 5)
    - °Horizontal dusting (Figure 18)
    - °Supine reaching progression
      - °Begin at 0° with the elbow bent and end at 90° of elevation with the elbow extended
      - °Start with the assistance of a cane or wand (Figure 9)
      - °Can progress to active motion
      - °Occasionally can progress to using a 0.5- to 1-pound weight
  - °Incline dusting (Figure 11)
- °Patient education
  - °Educate the patient about appropriate long-term modifications to ADLs to minimize symptoms (often the same instructions as given in phase 1)
  - °Implement a long-term maintenance home exercise program
    - °Most often consists of the pendulum PRN, rope-and-pulley AAFE, and selected light strengthening

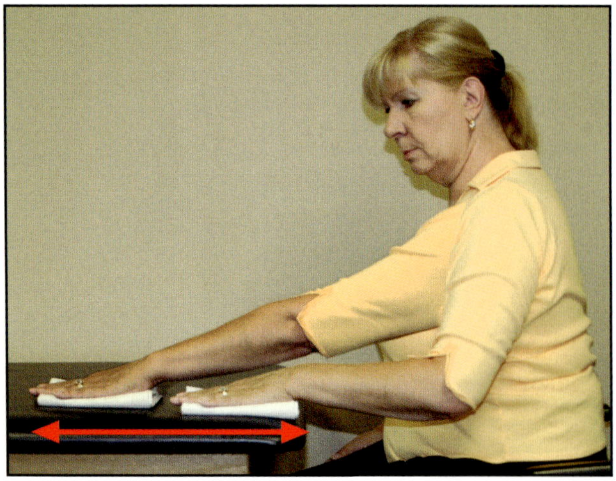

Figure 18. Horizontal dusting.

Adjunctive Exercises

- °Aquatic exercises (chapter IV-9)
- °Consider isometric strengthening if dynamic strengthening is not well tolerated or not prescribed by the physician

Interventions to Avoid

- °PROM, AROM, or strengthening in coronal-plane abduction
- °Advanced stretching exercises
- °Moderate-level or high-level rotator cuff or deltoid strengthening activities
- °Exercises that result in moderate or severe pain or painful crepitus

Miscellaneous Rehabilitation Topics and Return-To-Sports Programs

Section IV

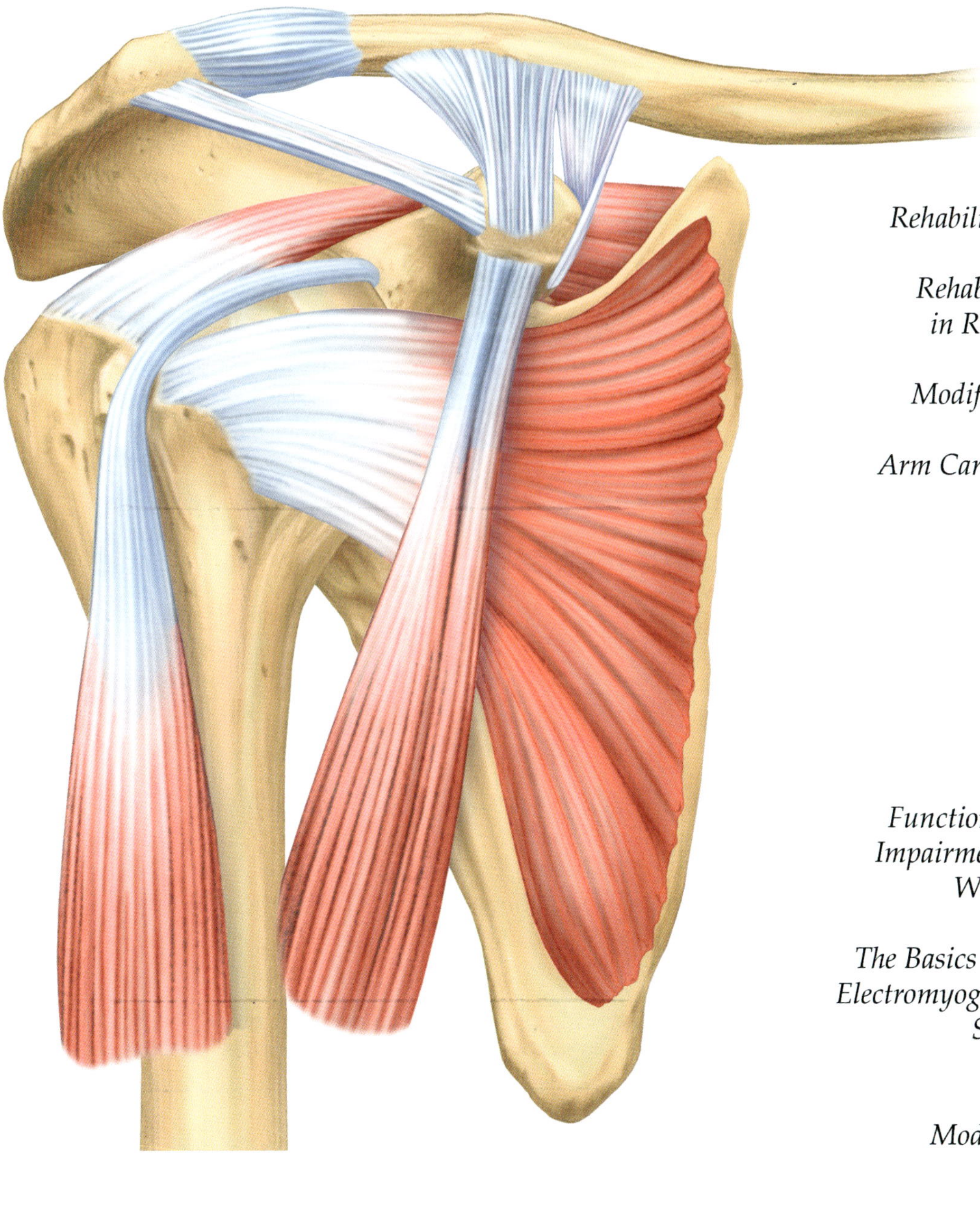

IV-1

Clinical Evaluation of Scapular Mechanics

Chuck Thigpen, PhD, PT, ATC, and Lane Bailey PT, DPT, CSCS

CHAPTER CONTENTS

- Assessment of scapular posture
  - Resting posture
  - Observation of scapular girdle height
  - Observation of scapular tilting
  - Observation of scapular upward-downward rotation
  - Observation of scapular protraction and retraction
  - Objective assessment options of resting and static scapular posture
- Scapular dyskinesis
  - Altered kinematics in athletes
  - Options for clinical assessment
- Scapular muscle performance
  - Scapular position and muscle performance
  - Alterations in muscle performance
  - Specific clinical assessment tests

Clinical pearls are highlighted in yellow throughout the text.

Scapular function is critical in the normal function of the shoulder girdle, providing a stable base for the rotator cuff and maintaining optimal alignment of the glenoid and coracoacromial arch with the humeral head. Alterations in scapular position and motion have been associated with most shoulder pathologic conditions, including impingement, rotator cuff tears, frozen shoulder, and traumatic and multidirectional instability.[1–3] Interestingly, whereas specific scapular positions have not consistently been associated with acromiohumeral distance, clinical techniques, such as the scapular assistance test (SAT), have been shown to increase acromiohumeral distance and decrease symptoms in patients with impingement.[4–7] However, McClure et al[2] reported that patients whose impingement improved with 6 weeks of rehabilitation did not display concurrent improvements in scapular kinematics. Clinically, these conflicting research reports make it difficult to fully understand the implications of scapular assessment and interventions aimed at improving scapular function. Evidence exists that intervention programs can alter scapular position, resolve dyskinesis, and prevent injury by improving scapular posture.[8–12] In this chapter, we outline a systematic assessment of scapular function based on the best available evidence combined with clinical experience for patients presenting with shoulder dysfunction.

Assessment of scapular function can easily be divided into 3 distinct parts: scapular position or posture, scapular motion or kinematics, and scapular muscle function. The assessment of scapular position or posture is the clinical assessment of how or where the scapula rests on the thoracic wall.[9,13–15] This is critical because the resting scapular position consistently has been shown to be a major determinant of scapular motion throughout shoulder elevation. In addition, researchers have suggested that altering thoracic posture strongly influences scapular position and acromiohumeral distance. After the assessment of scapular position, scapular motion should be assessed to document the range of scapular motion, as well as the ability to control the scapula during elevation and descent.[16–18] Finally, global and isolated scapular muscle performance should be assessed to differentiate deficits in individual scapular muscle function from alterations in force couple activation because both of these deficits have been demonstrated in the literature.[19–21]

ASSESSMENT OF SCAPULAR POSTURE

The assessment of scapular position is thought to be an important component of the physical examination in patients with shoulder pain.[22–30] Failure to assess the role of scapular position can lead to misinterpretation of muscle function and can decrease the effectiveness of therapeutic interventions. The clinical examination should include the observation and palpation of both shoulders, noting asymmetries, such as excessive scapular winging, inferior angle prominence, and shoulder girdle depression. Researchers have shown that overhead athletes with pathologic lesions frequently exhibit scapular malpositioning, suggesting that these asymmetries should be normalized during rehabilitation.[29–31] These asymmetries are most apparent in unilateral overhead athletes who repetitively use their dominant shoulders in a forceful manner.[22–30]

Resting Posture

After obtaining a thorough patient history, the first portion of the physical examination of the patient should be a resting assessment of the scapula. The rehabilitation provider should observe the patient and note gross positional abnormalities or asymmetries, or both, in relation to the thoracic cage and opposite shoulder girdle. He or she should carefully inspect the 3 joints, including the sternoclavicular, acromioclavicular (AC), and glenohumeral, and 1 articulation (scapulothoracic) that compose the shoulder girdle.[22] Giving emphasis to these particular sites might guide examiners to the origin of pathologic condition.

In overhead athletes, the dominant shoulder is commonly positioned lower, more anteriorly tipped, and more internally rotated than the nondominant shoulder.[32] Among the first to report this phenomenon in overhead athletes was Burkhart et al,[32] who coined the acronym *SICK* (**S**capular malposition, **I**nferior medial border prominence, **C**oracoid pain and malposition, and dys**K**inesis of scapular movement) to define the common cluster signs and symptoms in these patients. The SICK scapula syndrome is described as a muscular overuse disorder with associated ligamentous and capsular deficiencies.[29] Note that this might not be the case in every overhead athlete with a pathologic condition. Rather, a thorough examination should be completed to identify specific abnormalities before drawing diagnostic conclusions. To accurately assess the position of the scapula, clinicians must have an understanding of the scapula's bony anatomy, rotational axes, and degrees of freedom. The scapula has 2 translations (superoinferior and mediolateral), and all 3 axes of rotation.[18,33,34] (Figure 1). Effective use of observational examination and objective measurement is necessary to assess the position of the scapula.

Observation of Scapular Girdle Height

Discrepancies in the shoulder girdle height of the overhead athlete is well documented.[29,30,32] The term *infera* has been used to describe the relatively lower appearance of the affected shoulder, which is typically the dominant side, and is thought to result from increased scapular protraction, anterior tilting, and internal rotation.[32] Anatomic landmarks of reference for comparison include the superomedial border of the scapula, clavicle, spine of the scapula, AC joint, and

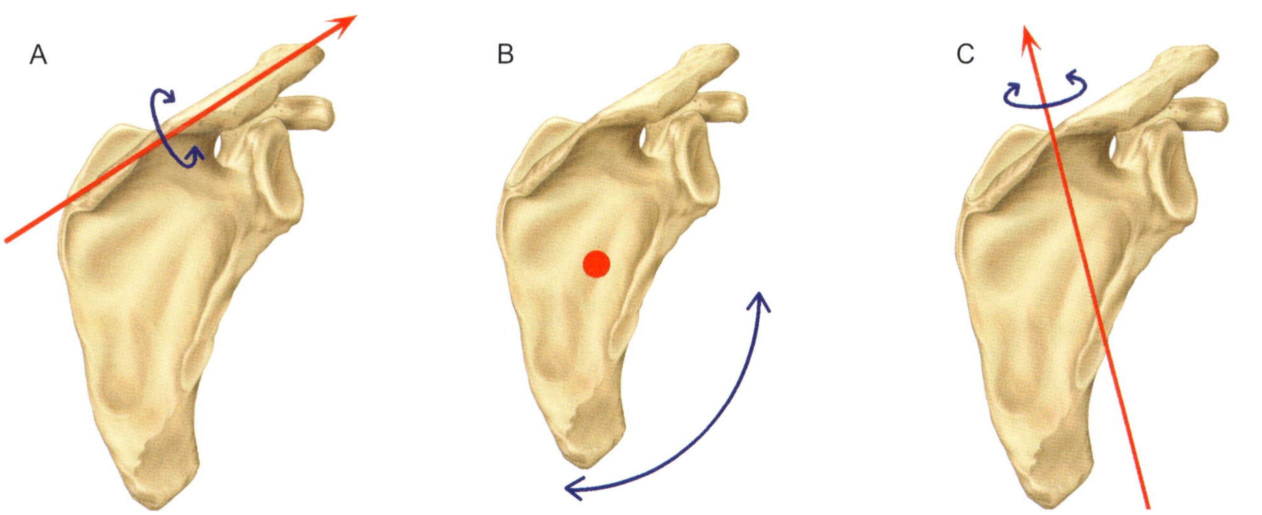

Figure 1. Scapular rotations. A, Anteroposterior tilting. B, Upward-downward rotation. C, Internal-external rotation.

inferomedial angle of the scapula (Figure 2). Specific consideration to the vertical difference between the superomedial scapular angles is used to detect the presence of this shoulder asymmetry.[35] Infera, which is a common presentation in the dominant shoulder of healthy individuals, is more severe and anecdotally attributed to the stretching of the ligaments, joint capsules, and muscles from frequent use in overhead athletes.[29]

Observation of Scapular Tilting

Marked anterior tilting of the scapula can present as a prominent inferomedial scapular angle during overhead elevation of the shoulder (Figure 3A), with the acromion resting anterior to the lumbar spine. This malposition is related to muscular imbalances of the scapula[32] and posterior capsular tightness.[35,36] These muscle imbalances include reduced pectoralis minor muscle length, which has been significantly associated with an anteriorly tilted position.The assessment of the pectoralis minor is provided in the analysis of dynamic scapular posture presented later in this chapter.

Observation of Scapular Upward-Downward Rotation

Scapular movement perpendicular to the scapular plane is known as *scapular upward-downward rotation*. Assessment of scapular upward-downward rotation in the resting position is shown in Figure 3B. Upward rotation occurs about the AC joint as the inferior angle of the scapula moves superolaterally with humeral elevation. This concomitant movement, which is known as *scapulohumeral rhythm*, is an approximate 2:1 ratio of humeral elevation to scapular upward rotation in healthy individuals.[37] Varying evidence exists regarding the specific changes that occur in scapular upward rotation in the presence of pathologic conditions.[17] Some investigators have reported increases in upward rotation,[38] whereas others have concluded decreases occur.[39,40] The rehabilitation provider should evaluate the serratus anterior (SA) muscle if deficiencies in scapular upward rotation are detected because it is the primary upward rotator of the scapula (refer to the Scapular Muscle Performance section).

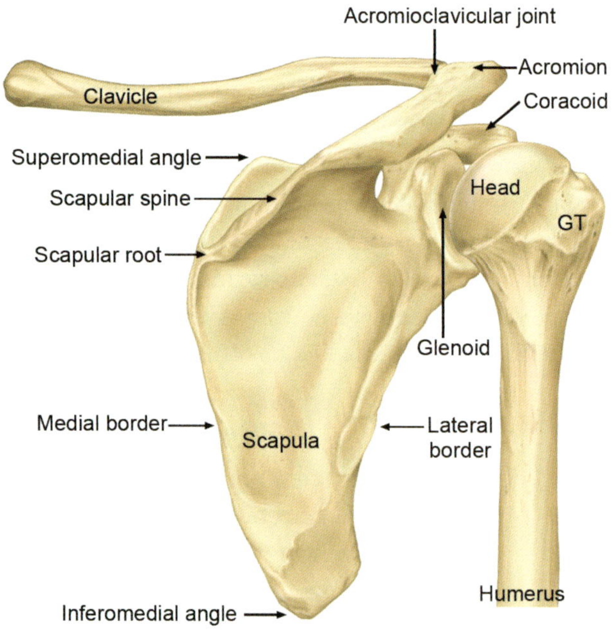

Figure 2. Scapular anatomic landmarks.
Abbreviation: GT, greater tuberosity.

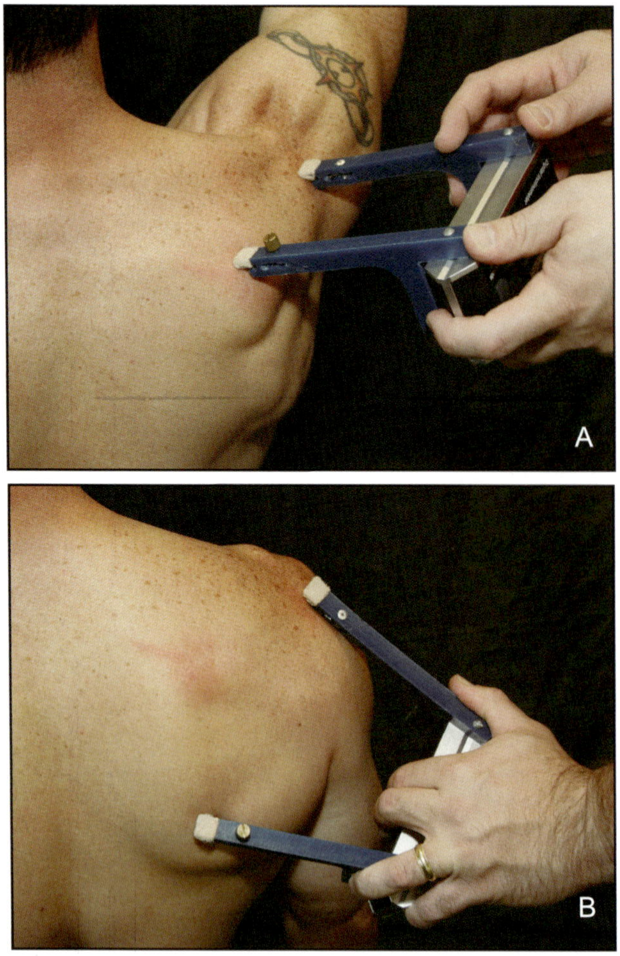

Figure 3. Clinical assessment of the scapula. A, Anteroposterior tilting. B, Upward-downward rotation.

Observation of Scapular Protraction and Retraction

Excessive forward shoulder and scapular protraction has been recognized as a factor that can contribute to head, shoulder, and neck pain.[41–43] Scapular protraction is observed posteriorly as the displacement of the medial scapular border compared with the corresponding spinous processes of the thoracic vertebrae within the transverse plane. Forward head and forward shoulder posture are thought to be associated with chronic muscle-shortening adaptations, which should be addressed with postural re-education and selective stretching and strengthening.[9]

Note that these malpositions rarely, if ever, occur independently, and classification of the asymmetry into a single scapular plane of motion is likely too restrictive.[18] Rather, these positions are thought to be interdependent because of the scapula's intimate relation and articulation with the ellipsoid thoracic cage. However, if specific positional irregularities are more pronounced, this might guide clinicians to the diagnosis and treatment of the underlying mechanism.

Objective Assessment Options of Resting and Static Scapular Posture

Several objective examination tools have been developed to help clinicians better detect resting and static scapular abnormalities. Of these clinical examination tools, the Lateral Scapular Slide Test (LSST),[27] the Greenfield method,[26] Baylor square test,[42] and Palpation Meter (PALM)[44] are among the most commonly used.

Lateral Scapular Slide Test. Developed by Kibler,[27] the LSST assesses scapular position at 0°, 45°, and 90° of humeral elevation. Specifically, this test is intended to be a measure of scapular stability in 3 static positions of humeral elevation. The LSST begins with the upper extremity resting at the patient's side. The rehabilitation provider palpates and marks the inferomedial angles of both scapulae then makes displacement comparisons from the inferomedial angles of each scapula to the nearest spinous process (approximately T7). Next, the patient rests his or her hands on the hips at approximately 45° of humeral elevation. The rehabilitation provider identifies and measures the new placement of inferomedial angles to the nearest adjacent spinous process. The procedure is repeated with the extremity positioned in 90° of humeral abduction. The presence of substantial scapular asymmetries is considered to be a positive finding.

The reported clinical value of the LSST as developed by Kibler[27] has been inconsistent and questioned by investigators. Gibson et al[45] and Odom et al[46] reported poor interrater reliability and sensitivity and specificity values, whereas McKenna et al[47] found good interrater reliability using this clinical test. Shadmehr et al[48] tried to clarify the varying evidence by using calipers instead of the previous string method. The results were varied, with variable interrater reliability from low to high (range, 0.63–0.86) and likelihood ratios that were consistently poor (positive to negative ratio range, 0.94:0.21–1.22:2.25).[48] Considering the unpredictable nature of this examination, we urge caution when reporting the findings of LSST outcomes and suggest the use of additional clinical examinations to aid in the assessment of scapular position.

Greenfield Method. Greenfield et al[26] used plain radiographs to validate a method for assessing forward scapular posture. Using geometric calculation, scapular protraction and rotation are estimated by measuring the distances between anatomic landmarks of the thorax and scapula.

To perform this method using a tape measure, palpate and mark the root of the scapular spine (A), its corresponding thoracic spine level (B), the inferior angle of the scapula (C) with its corresponding thoracic spine level (D), and the posterolateral edge of the acromion (E). A mark on the thoracic spine (B) is made to the corresponding level of the root of the scapular spine (A). Using a tape measure or 12-inch (30.48-cm) flexible ruler, take measurements between the landmarks to include in the following formulae for scapular protraction and rotation:

$$\text{Scapular protraction} = \frac{\text{line BAE}}{\text{line AE}}$$

$$\text{Scapular rotation} = \tan = \Theta \ \frac{\text{line CD}}{\text{line BC}}$$

The *BAE* is the aggregate linear distance from the mark on the corresponding thoracic spine level (B) adjacent to the root of the scapula (A) and to the tip of the acromion (E) (Figure 4).

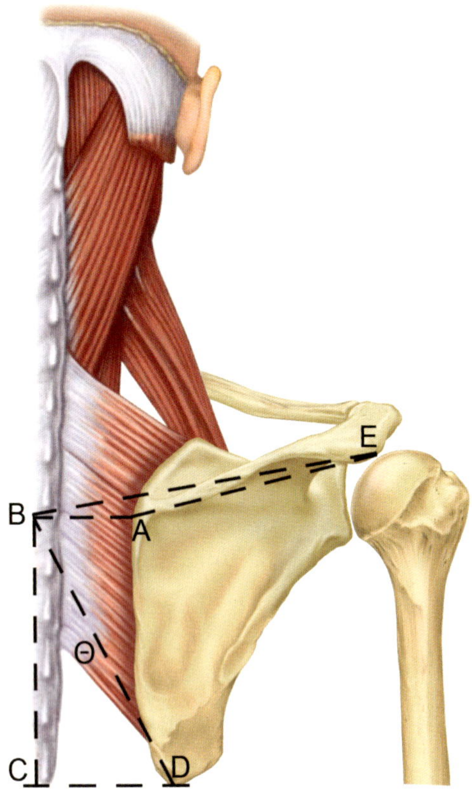

Figure 4. Greenfield method.

Baylor Square/Double-Square Test. The Baylor square test[42] uses a modified carpenter's square to measure *forward shoulder posture*, which is defined as a combination of scapular protraction and anterior tilt (Figure 5).[35] A modified version of this test, the double-square test,[42] uses 2 modified carpenter's squares affixed to each other to measure the same construct. The double-square method was recently validated,[35] with a reported intraclass correlation coefficient (ICC) of 0.84 and a standard error of measurement (SEM) of 4.6 mm. Given the increase of empirical evidence, we will discuss the double-square method.

Beginning with the participant standing with his or her back against the wall, the first square is placed above the shoulder and flush with the wall. The second square is extended along a 12-inch (30.48-cm) ruler to the anterior portion of the corresponding acromion process (Figure 5). The corresponding distance is measured, and the protocol is repeated on the opposite shoulder for comparison. Large differences in bilateral forward shoulder posture are believed to indicate the presence of scapulothoracic and posterior muscle tightness.[35] Using this method, throwing athletes have demonstrated consistent forward shoulder asymmetry in the dominant extremity when compared with the nondominant extremity.[36]

Palpation Meter Method. da Costa et al[44] recently developed the PALM method with the intent of improving on the limitations of previous measurement tools. Equipped with an inclinometer, the calipermetric device is designed to measure scapular mediolateral displacement, upward-downward rotation, and acromial height. The instrument has shown fair to good intrarater (ICC range, 0.81–0.89; SEM range, 0.56–1.17 cm) and interrater (ICC range, 0.67–0.89; SEM range, 0.59–0.98 cm) reliability; however, these methods have not been validated.[44] The measurement landmarks are similar to those used by the Greenfield method,[26] with measurements at rest, 90°, and full humeral elevation in the scapular plane (40° anterior to the frontal plane).

The participant assumes a relaxed standing posture on a reference grip with shoes removed to allow standardization of foot position for follow-up measures. Male patients are shirtless, and female patients should wear a sports bra to expose the shoulder girdle. The following landmarks are identified and marked for position measurement: the root of the spine of the scapula (A) and corresponding thoracic spine level (B), the inferomedial angle of the scapula (C) and its correspond-

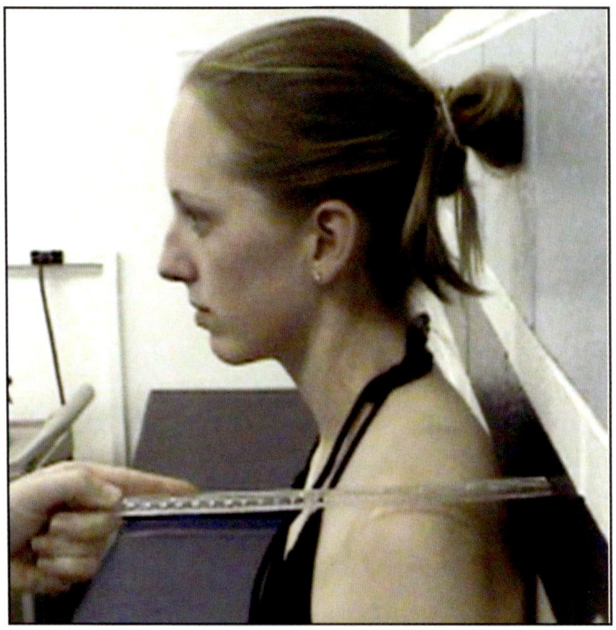

Figure 5. Assessment of forward shoulder posture using the Baylor square method.

ing thoracic spine level (D), the posteroinferior edge of the acromion (E), and the spinous process of C7 (F). To ensure that the appropriate thoracic spine level is identified within the horizontal plane, the PALM is positioned and adjusted until the inclinometer reads 0° within the transverse plane. Two measures (line A-B and line D-C) determine horizontal distance of the scapula. Vertical distance measures are determined by using the distance from the posteroinferior acromion to the spinous process of C7 (line E-F). To normalize for the differences in scapular size, the distance from the acromion to the root of the spine (line B-E) is divided by the distance of the inferior angle to the corresponding spinal level (line C-D). All procedures are repeated for the 2 static elevated positions (90° and full elevation in the scapular plane) with the exception of identifying the acromion and C7. To position the participant in elevation, reference poles and a goniometer are recommended to ensure that the movements are consistently performed with the same plane.

SCAPULAR DYSKINESIS

Altered Kinematics in Athletes

Scapular dyskinesis is a term often used to describe the visible abnormalities in scapular position and motion patterns and has been strongly associated with shoulder injury.[27] Because asymmetries might not be apparent at rest in overhead athletes, static examination of the scapula alone is not sufficient. Linear methods also do not capture the 3-dimesional motion characteristics during dynamic upper extremity movement.[16] Scapular winging, excessive scapular elevation, and excessive internal rotation are just a few commonalities seen in the dynamic assessment of these individuals. Considering the repetitive nature and extreme ranges of shoulder motion that overhead athletes use, high rates of injury are not surprising, suggesting that the dynamic stability of the scapula is vital to the health of the athlete. Scapular examination should include a functional dynamic shoulder assessment designed to elicit any irregularities to reveal the underlying cause.

Scapular dyskinesis is thought to result from abnormal muscle properties or intrinsic tightness in the posterior aspect of the shoulder, which is prevalent in overhead athletes.[35] These muscle abnormalities can include peripheral nerve damage,[16] reduced resting muscle length (ie, pectoralis minor),[49] or muscular imbalances. Muscular insufficiencies can further exacerbate scapular dyskinesis by altering normal scapulohumeral rhythm and thus the length-tension relationships of other muscles acting on the scapula and humeral head.[50–53]

Options for Clinical Assessment

Whereas 3-dimensional motion analysis of the scapula is considered the criterion standard for assessing dynamic scapular posture, this method is neither practical nor cost-effective in the clinical setting. However, clinical methods have been developed to identify which athletes potentially have abnormal dynamic scapular posture. Among these clinical methods, tools, such as inclinometers and observational classification systems, have emerged as some of the most useful.

Pectoralis Minor Muscle Length. Reduced pectoralis minor muscle length has been suggested as a possible source of scapular dyskinesis.[16,49] Considering its bony attachments, a short or overactive pectoralis minor muscle can maintain the scapula in an excessively protracted or downwardly rotated position, creating prominence of the inferomedial angle, which is a frequently observed type of abnormal scapular positioning.[54] Borstad[55] found high reliability and validity when measuring the distance between the muscular insertions of the pectoralis minor muscle. This clinical examination potentially could serve as a useful tool for the scapular evaluation of the throwing athlete, in whom asymmetry in pectoralis minor muscle length is thought to be prevelant.[32]

With the patient standing, the distance between the fourth rib and the coracoid process is measured with a tape measure to the nearest centimeter (Figure 6). The *fourth rib landmark* is defined as the anteroinferior edge of the rib 1 finger-width lateral to the sternum. This rib is located by counting down consecutively from the first rib. The coracoid process landmark is identified at its medioinferior aspect and is located by palpating below the lateral concavity of the clavicle in the deltopectoral groove.[55] Asymmetric findings between shoulders are an indication for reduced pectoralis minor muscle length.

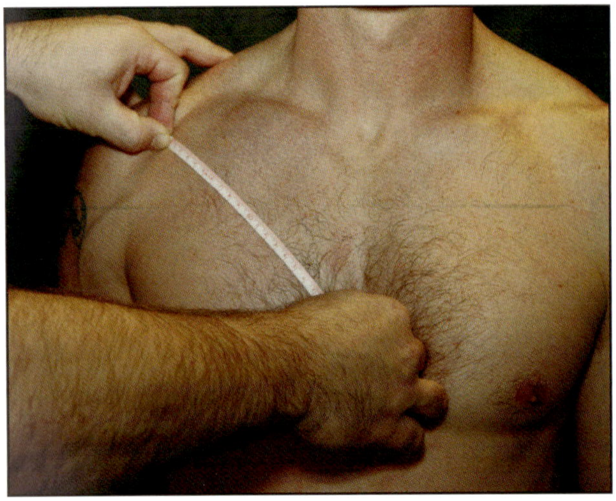

Figure 6. Pectoralis minor muscle length landmarks. The pectoralis minor muscle length is assessed as the distance between the coracoid process and fourth rib. The measurement is taken at the inferomedial edge of the coracoid to the anteroinferior edge of the fourth rib 1 finger-width lateral to the sternum.

Assessment of Scapular Upward Rotation. Johnson et al[52] found reliable and valid measurement of 4 phases of static scapular upward rotation using a modified digital inclinometer. Using locator rods that are approximately 10 cm long and are attached to the bottom of a digital inclinometer, the instrument is placed on the spine of the scapula. Each rod has square- and Y-shaped ends. When connected to the inclinometer, the square end permits adjustment (rotation) of the distal end to different widths of the patient's scapulae (Figure 3A). Before testing with the inclinometer, the locator rods are adjusted to the length of the scapular spine by moving the 2 Y-shaped ends over the root of the scapular spine and posterolateral acromion. A bubble level is attached to the left side of the inclinometer to determine anteroposterior rotation of the device about an axis parallel to the scapular spine. Scapular rotation then is assessed in 4 upper extremity positions: at rest, 60°, 90°, and 120° of static humeral elevation in the scapular plane.

Visual Classification Systems of Scapular Dyskinesis. The visual presentation of scapular dyskinesis often is reported as winging or asymmetry.[16,56] Several attempts have been made to reliably categorize the specific characteristics of scapular dyskinesis; however, few investigators have been able to effectively achieve this goal.[24,27,57] Kibler and McMullen[23] were among the first to categorize scapular dyskinesis using a 4-part visual classification system; however, reliability measures were fairly low.[16] To refine this classification system, McClure et al[16] and Tate et al[17] recently developed a modified scoring system for the scapular dyskinesis test to improve reliability of measurement.

To allow for an unobstructed view of the posterior thorax, male patients are shirtless, and female patients don a sports bra. The patient is positioned in standing with his or her upper extremities at the side. The examiner stands 2 to 3 m away and observes the patient from behind. He or she then instructs the patient to simultaneously elevate both extremities with thumbs pointed up completely overhead to a 3-second count then to lower them to a 3-second count for 5 repetitions. Depending on the participant's body mass, specific dumbbells are used to load the upper extremity: 3 lb (1.4 kg) for those weighing less than 150 lb (68.1 kg) and 5 lb (2.3 kg) for those weighing equal to or more than 150 lb (68.1 kg). The test is performed for flexion and abduction. Classifications of the observed scapular posture are as follows:

1. Normal motion: no evidence of abnormality.
2. Subtle abnormality: mild or questionable evidence of abnormality that is not consistently present.
3. Obvious abnormality: striking, clearly apparent abnormality evident on at least 3 of 5 trials (dysrhythmias or winging of 1 inch [2.54 cm] or greater displacement of scapula from the thorax).

With this method, Tate et al[17] and McClure et al[16] demonstrated acceptable validity and clinical reliability, respectively. Therefore, we suggest using the 3-part classification system rather than the 4-part design of Kibler and McMullen[23] to ensure consistency of measurement.

Scapula Reposition Test. An impairment-based classification approach to shoulder pathologic conditions also might be useful in the presence of scapular dyskinesis. The scapula reposition test (SRT) is designed to evaluate the change in strength and pain with upper extremity elevation by repositioning the scapula in a more externally rotated and posteriorly tilted position with humeral elevation.[58,59]

The SRT is performed by grasping the scapula with the fingers contacting the AC joint anteriorly and the palm and thenar eminence contacting the spine of the scapula posteriorly, with the forearm obliquely angled toward the inferior angle of the scapula for additional

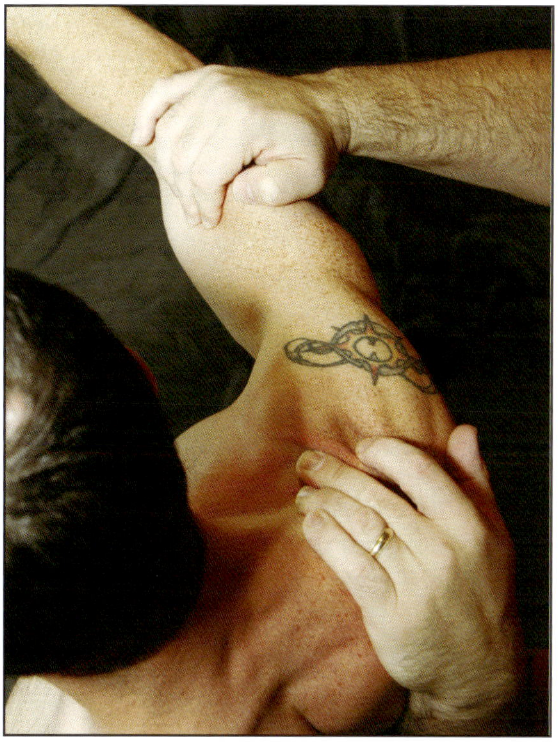

Figure 7. Scapula reposition test. The examiner grasps the scapula at the acromioclavicular joint and scapular spine with the forearm resting against the medial scapular border. Force is applied to assist in scapular posterior tilting and external rotation while the patient performs resisted shoulder elevation.

contact and support on the medial border (Figure 7). The forearm applies force to encourage scapular posterior tilting and external rotation that approximates the inferior angle and medial border to the thoracic cage, carefully avoiding end-range retraction. The test is considered positive if pain is reduced or strength is increased compared with unassisted humeral elevation.

SCAPULAR MUSCLE PERFORMANCE

Scapular Position and Muscle Performance

Muscle performance is closely related to scapular position and often is thought to be the driving factor in pathologic conditions. Excessive fatigue of the scapular stabilizers can alter scapulohumeral rhythm and potentially can lead to a decrease in rotator cuff strength.[60] Researchers have shown that individuals with pathologic shoulder conditions consistently demonstrate abnormalities in scapular rotator muscle activity.[39] To develop a successful treatment plan, clinicians must be able to identify these alterations in muscle performance. Rehabilitation interventions aimed at the correction of scapular muscle impairments might improve dysfunctional scapular movement patterns.[61] Treatment plans also should include the proper battery of tests that assess the athletes' ability to return safely to participation in their respective sports.

Alterations in Muscle Performance

Deficits in muscle performance encompass a range of impairments, including asymmetric force coupling, temporal recruitment variability,[21] and specific muscle weakness.[62] For overhead athletes who often perform forceful and repetitive movements in positions of elevation, muscular alterations include excessive activation of the upper trapezius (UT) with concomitant decreases in the middle to lower portions of the SA and the lower trapezius (LT).[19,20,21,39,63–67] Considering these consistent findings in overhead athletes, exercises promoting LT, middle trapezius (MT), and SA activation with minimal activity in the UT have been recommended.[20]

The SA is considered the primary mover of the scapula.[62,68] It is unique because it is the only scapulothoracic muscle with the ability to assist in all 3 planes of movement required for "normal" scapular movement patterns during overhead elevation of the shoulder.[62,69] Observations of scapular mechanics in healthy individuals have shown consistent patterns of upward rotation, posterior tipping, and external rotation, which often are altered in the population with injured shoulders.[1,70] The SA also is thought to prevent scapular winging by stabilizing the medial border and inferior angle of the scapula to the thorax.[62] Considering the role of the SA in scapular function, it is not surprising that overhead athletes with shoulder conditions have exhibited specific decreases in activation of this muscle, suggesting the clinical importance of improving SA strength deficits in these injured athletes.[62]

Specific Clinical Assessment Tests

The Scapular Assistance Test. The SAT[27] is a clinical evaluation tool intended to assess the integrity of dynamic scapular function. Specifically, the SAT is a muscle performance assessment designed to simulate the SA and LT force couple with upper extremity elevation.

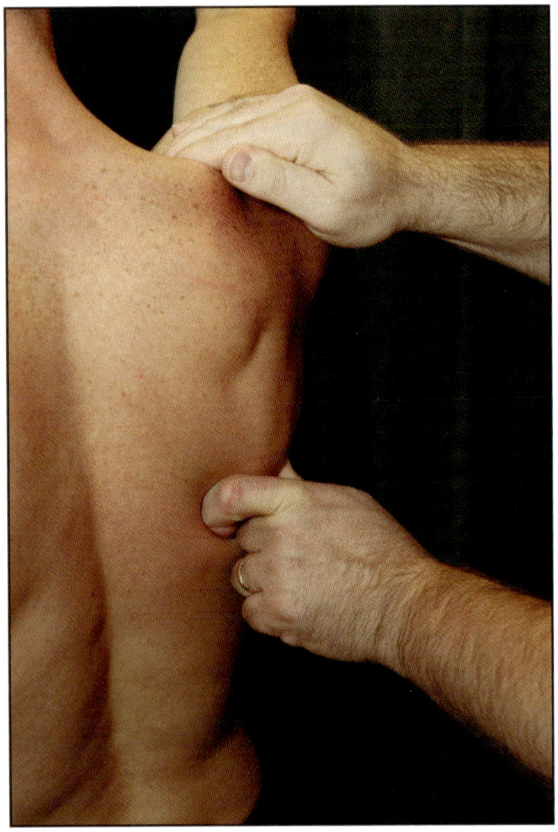

Figure 8. Scapular assistance test. The rehabilitation provider places one hand on the inferomedial scapular border and the other on the superior scapular border, providing a superolateral force in the direction of scapular protraction while the patient performs active shoulder elevation.

To perform this test, the examiner applies pressure at the inferomedial border of the scapula that is directed in a superolateral direction while the patient performs humeral elevation (Figure 8). It is considered positive if symptoms are diminished or eliminated with an examiner's assistance compared with active humeral elevation.[70] The clinical importance of a positive finding indicates deficits in motor control or muscle strength, or both, of the SA and LT. Therapeutic interventions targeted at addressing these functional deficits should be included in the athlete's plan of care. Exercises should be tailored to emphasize the lower and middle portions of the SA muscle because these areas are thought to aid most in normal scapular function.[37,62,68]

Abnormal scapular mechanics are believed to be apparent when deficits in scapular strength are present.[61] The rehabilitation provider needs to be able to reliably perform muscle testing procedures to detect potential impairments. Michener et al[61] and Ekstrom et al[71] have reported on the reliability of common manual muscle testing (MMT) procedures for the scapulothoracic muscles. Clinicians are encouraged to develop these skill sets to improve their overall ability to detect deficits in strength.

Manual Muscle Testing of Trapezius Muscles. Using surface electromyography (sEMG) and hand-held dynamometry, Michener et al[61] showed reliability in measuring the isometric strength of the UT, MT, and LT muscles first described by Hislop et al.[72] All MMT of the scapula is performed in midrange scapular position to ensure proper cross-bridge (length-tension) alignment to allow for maximum isometric contraction.

To assess the isometric strength of the LT muscle, the participant is positioned prone with the affected upper extremity placed in 140° of humeral elevation. The examiner stands on the opposite side of the table with the resistance hand placed on the spine of the scapula midway between the acromion and root of the spine. Force is applied in the direction of the long axis of the humerus (140°) and parallel to the muscle fibers of the LT (Figure 9A).

The UT muscle is assessed with the patient sitting and the examiner standing posterolateral to the patient's target shoulder. The examiner places the resistance hand over the superior border of the scapula and applies a force directed downward in the inferior direction (Figure 9B).

Manual Muscle Testing of the Serratus Anterior. Based on sEMG study, the upper portion of the SA is more active with scapular protraction and abduction,

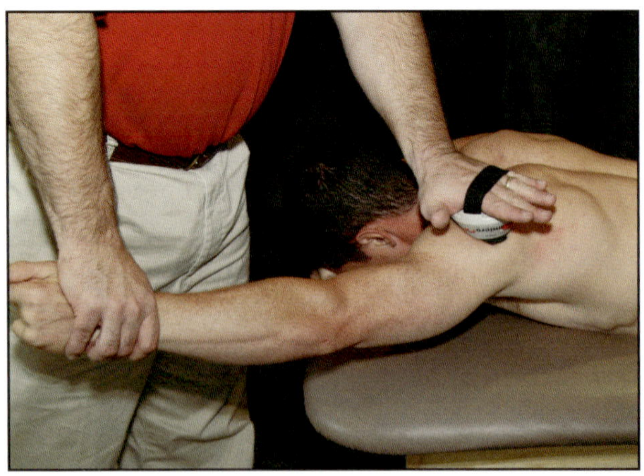

Figure 9A. Lower trapezius manual muscle test with the patient positioned prone and the examiner providing resistance at the scapula parallel to the long fiber of the muscle.

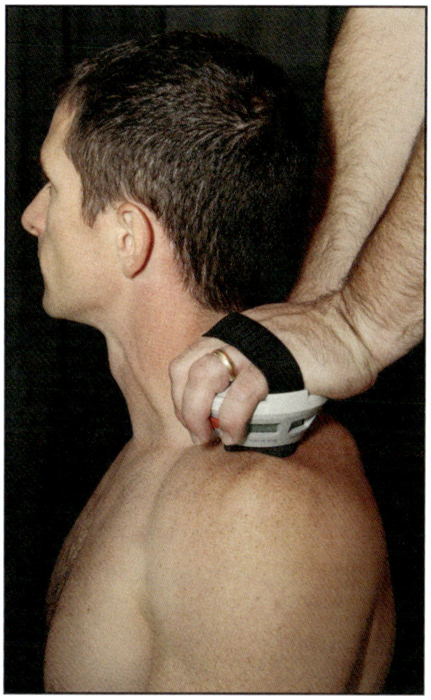

Figure 9B. Upper trapezius muscle test with the examiner providing a downwardly directed force.

whereas the lower portions are more contracted during scapular upward rotation.[71] This suggests that the role of the lower SA is critical in maintaining normal scapulohumeral rhythm by providing scapular upward rotation during humeral elevation. Therefore, clinicians must have a clinical method that specifically evaluates the strength of the lower SA muscle.

Ekstrom et al[71] reported greater sEMG activity of the lower portion of the SA muscle when the participant was seated with the upper extremity abducted to 120° in the plane of the scapula (Figure 10), providing a force directed posteroinferiorly. This increased sEMG activity indicated greater activation of the targeted lower SA muscle.

Scapular position is thought to substantially affect the strength of the rotator cuff muscles, which serve a vital role in overhead sports. The alteration of scapular position changes the length-tension relationship within the muscle, directly influencing strength. Riemann et al[73] successfully established normative muscle data for the humeral internal and external rotators, including unilateral external to internal rotation ratios, to allow clinicians to establish objective goals, address both physical and functional limitations, and guide a rehabilitation program for return to function. They suggested that the optimal position for MMT and strengthening of the rotator cuff is 30° of scaption, 30° of abduction, and 30° of internal rotation of the humerus.

Kinetic Chain. In overhead athletes, the upper extremity serves as the final piece of a very complex and powerful chain that usually begins with the lower extremities, pelvis, torso, and scapula. These individual body components function in concert through muscle activity to generate, summate, and transfer force to the upper extremity. This relation is termed the *kinetic chain*,[27] and the scapula is thought to play an integral role in this transfer of energy. When determining readiness for return to play, the evaluating clinician needs to assess not only scapular stability, but also all segments within the kinetic chain. This stands to reason because of the vital function that the scapula must play in transferring stored energy from the lower extremities and trunk to the upper extremity. The Upper Extremity Closed Kinetic Chain Test (UE CKC)[74] was developed as an objective clinical measure to aid clinicians in the assessment of scapular stability in addition to the other components that compose the kinetic chain. Goldbeck

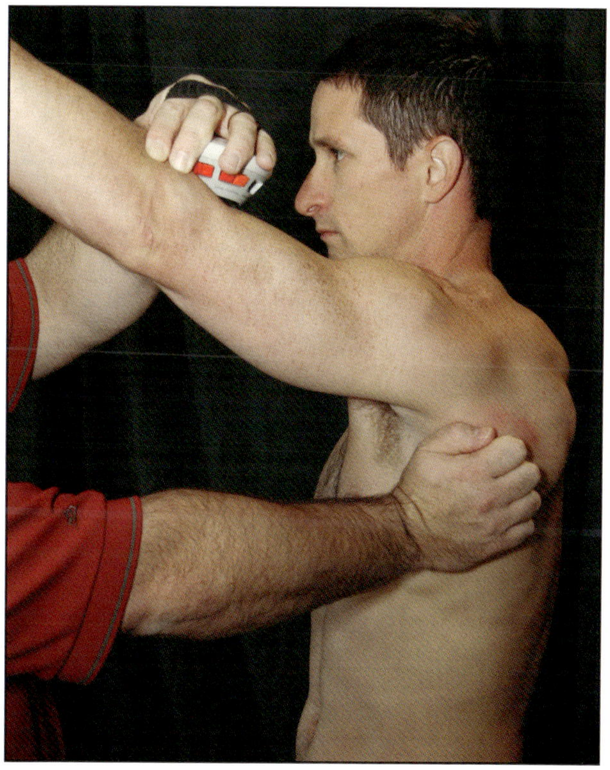

Figure 10. Serratus anterior manual muscle testing. With the patient seated, the examiner resists elevation through the forearm at 120° of shoulder elevation.

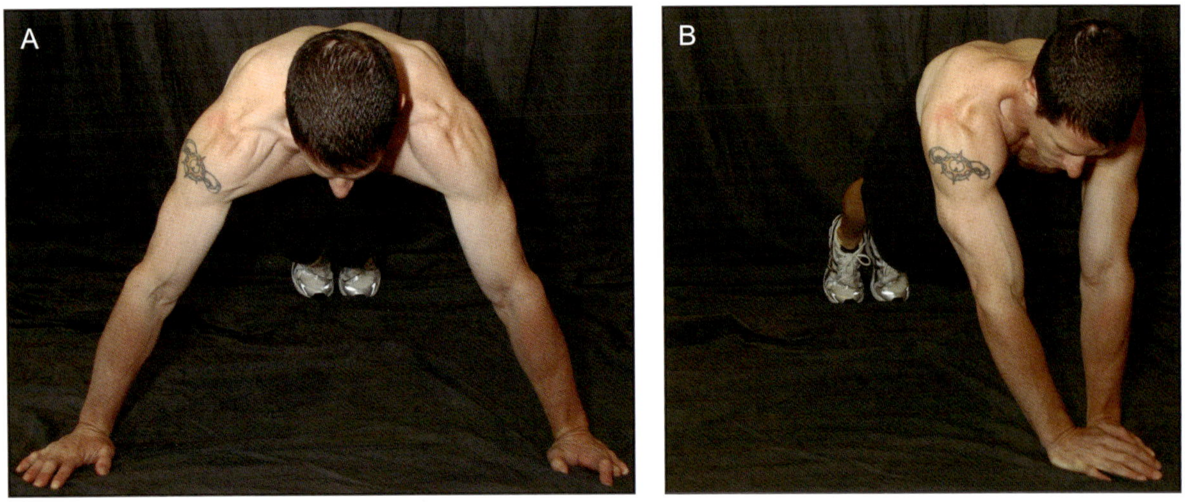

Figure 11. Upper Extremity Closed Kinetic Chain Test. A, Starting position with the hands positioned 36 inches (91.44 cm) apart. B, Second position as the patient is instructed to touch the opposite hand.

and Davies[74] used the UE CKC as a clinically efficient field test that required little time or resources to administer.

The evaluator places 2 pieces of athletic tape parallel to each other and 36 inches (91.44 cm) apart. The participant assumes a prone plank (push-up) position beginning with each hand placed on the corresponding piece of tape (Figure 11A). When the clinician gives the command, "Go," to start the test, the participant uses an alternating hand pattern to move quickly from the starting position to touch the contralateral line (Figure 11B) then to return the hand to the starting position. Using a stop watch, the examiner times each test for 15 seconds. The participant is given 3 maximum efforts in a 1:3 work to rest ratio, with each rest period totaling 45 seconds. The clinician should examine the participant for signs of muscle fatigue or weakness, including scapular winging, scapular dyskinesis, or pain, in addition to those associated with other body segments (eg, sagging of the lumbar spine, excessive elbow flexion) throughout testing. If the participant cannot successfully complete the test without signs of deteriorating mechanics, treatment should continue until these deficiencies are resolved.

REFERENCES

1. Ludewig PM, Reynolds JF. The association of scapular kinematics and glenohumeral joint pathologies. *J Orthop Sports Phys Ther*. 2009;39(2):90–104.

2. McClure PW, Bialker J, Neff N, Williams G, Karduna A. Shoulder function and 3-dimensional kinematics in people with shoulder impingement syndrome before and after a 6-week exercise program. *Phys Ther*. 2004;84(9):832–848.

3. Michener LA, McClure PW, Karduna AR. Anatomical and biomechanical mechanisms of subacromial impingement syndrome. *Clin Biomech (Bristol, Avon)*. 2003;18(5):369–379.

4. Hébert LJ, Moffet H, Dufour M, Mosian C. Acromiohumeral distance in a seated postion in persons with impingement syndrome. *J Magn Reson Imaging*. 2003;18(1):72–79.

5. Hébert LJ, Moffet H, McFadyen BJ, St-Vincent G. A method of measuring three-dimensional scapular attitudes using the Optotrak probing system. *Clin Biomech (Bristol, Avon)*. 2000;15(1):1–8.

6. Seitz AL, McClure PW, Lynch SS, Ketchum JM, Michener LA. Effects of scapular dyskinesis and scapular assistance test on subacromial space during static arm elevation. *J Shoulder Elbow Surg*. 2012;21(5):631-640.

7. Seitz AL, Reinold M, Schneider RA, Gill TJ, Thigpen C. Altered 3-dimensional scapular resting posture does not alter scapular motion in the throwing shoulder of healthy professional baseball pitchers [published online ahead of print November 16, 2011]. *J Sport Rehabil*.

8. Lynch SS, Thigpen CA, Mihalik JP, Prentice WE, Padua D. The effects of an exercise intervention on forward head and rounded shoulder postures in elite swimmers. *Br J Sports Med*. 2010;44(5):376–381.

9. Thigpen CA, Padua DA, Michener LA, et al. Head and shoulder posture affect scapular mechanics and muscle activity in overhead tasks. *J Electromyogr Kinesiol*. 2010;20(4):701–709.

10. Thigpen CA, Padua DA, Morgan N, Kreps C, Karas SG. Scapular kinematics during supraspinatus rehabilitation exercise: a comparison of full-can versus empty-can techniques. *Am J Sports Med*. 2006;34(4):644–652.

11. Thigpen CA, Padua DA, Xu N, Karas SG. Comparison of serratus anterior and upper trapezius muscle activation between subjects with and without multidirectional shoulder instability. *J Orthop Sports Phys Ther*. 2005;35(1):A80–PL22.

12. Wang HK, Cochrane T. Mobility impairment, muscle imbalance, muscle weakness, scapular asymmetry, and shoulder injury in elite volleyball athletes. *J Sports Med Phys Fitness*. 2001;41(3):403–410.

13. Thigpen CA, Padua DA, Michener LA, et al. Head and shoulder posture affect scapular mechanics and muscle activity in overhead tasks. *J Electromyogr Kinesiol.* 2010;20(4):701–709.
14. Finley MA, Lee RY. Effect of sitting posture on 3-dimensional scapular kinematics measured by skin-mounted electromagnetic tracking sensors. *Arch Phys Med Rehabil.* 2003;84(4):563–568.
15. Kebaetse M, McClure P, Pratt NA. Thoracic position effect on shoulder range of motion, strength, and three-dimensional scapular kinematics. *Arch Phys Med Rehabil.* 1999;80(8):945–950.
16. McClure P, Tate AR, Kareha S, Irwin D, Zlupko E. A clinical method for identifying scapular dyskinesis: part 1. Reliability. *J Athl Train.* 2009;44(2):160–164.
17. Tate AR, McClure P, Kareha S, Irwin D, Barbe MF. A clinical method for identifying scapular dyskinesis: part 2. Validity. *J Athl Train.* 2009;44(2):165–173.
18. Uhl TL, Kibler WB, Gecewich B, Tripp BL. Evaluation of clinical assessment methods for scapular dyskinesis. *Arthroscopy.* 2009;25(11):1240–1248.
19. Cools AM, Witvrouw EE, Declercq GA, Vanderstraeten GG, Cambier DC. Evaluation of isokinetic force production and associated muscle activity in the scapular rotators during a protraction-retraction movement in overhead athletes with impingement symptoms. *Br J Sports Med.* 2004;38(1):64–68.
20. Cools AM, Declercq GA, Cambier DC, Mahieu NN, Witvrouw EE. Trapezius activity and intramuscular balance during isokinetic exercise in overhead athletes with impingement symptoms. *Scand J Med Sci Sports.* 2007;17(1):25–33.
21. Cools AM, Witvrouw EE, Declercq GA, Danneels LA, Cambier DC. Scapular muscle recruitment patterns: trapezius muscle latency with and without impingement symptoms. *Am J Sports Med.* 2003;31(4):542–549.
22. Hoppenfeld S. *Physical Examination of the Spine & Extremities.* East Norwalk, CT: Appleton-Century-Crofts; 1976.
23. Kibler BW, McMullen J. Scapular dyskinesis and its relation to shoulder pain. *J Am Acad Orthop Surg.* 2003;11(2):142–151.
24. Kibler WB, Uhl TL, Maddux JWQ, Brooks PV, Zeller B, McMullen J. Qualitative clinical evaluation of scapular dysfunction: a reliabililty study. *J Shoulder Elbow Surg.* 2002;11(6):550–556.
25. Meister K. Injuries to the shoulder in the throwing athlete: part two. Evaluation/treatment. *Am J Sports Med.* 2000;28(4):587–601.
26. Greenfield B, Catlin PA, Coats PW, Green E, McDonald JJ, North C. Posture in patients with shoulder overuse injuries and healthy individuals. *J Orthop Sports Phys Ther.* 1995;21(5):287–295.
27. Kibler WB. The role of the scapula in athletic shoulder function. *Am J Sports Med.* 1998;26(2):325–337.
28. Burkhart SS, Morgan CD, Kibler WB. The disabled throwing shoulder: spectrum of pathology. Part II. Evaluation and treatment of SLAP lesions in throwers. *Arthroscopy.* 2003;19(5):531–539.
29. Oyama S, Myers JB, Wassinger CA, Daniel Ricci R, Lephart SM. Asymmetric resting scapular posture in healthy overhead athletes. *J Athl Train.* 2008;43(6):565–570.
30. Kendall FP, McCreary EK. *Muscles: Testing and Function.* 3rd ed. Baltimore, MD: Williams & Wilkins; 1983.
31. Magee DJ. *Orthopaedic Physical Assessment.* 2nd ed. Philadelphia, PA: WB Saunders; 1987.
32. Burkhart SS, Morgan CD, Kibler WB. The disabled throwing shoulder: spectrum of pathology part III. The SICK scapula, scapular dyskinesis, the kinetic chain, and rehabilitation. *Arthroscopy.* 2003;19(6):641–661.
33. Karduna AR, McClure PW, Michener LA, Sennett B. Dynamic measurements of three-dimensional scapular kinematics: a validation study. *J Biomed Eng.* 2001;123(2):184–190.
34. McClure PW, Michener LA, Sennett BJ, Karduna AR. Direct 3-dimensional measurement of scapular kinematics during dynamic movements in vivo. *J Shoulder Elbow Surg.* 2001;10(3):269–277.
35. Laudner KG, Moline MT, Meister K. The relationship between forward scapular posture and posterior shoulder tightness among baseball players. *Am J Sports Med.* 2010;38(10):2106–2112.
36. Borsa PA, Laudner KG, Sauers EL. Mobility and stability adaptations in the shoulder of the overhead athlete: a theoretical and evidence-based perspective. *Sports Med.* 2008;38(1):17–36.
37. Inman VT, Saunders JB, Abbott LC. Observations of the function of the shoulder joint. *J Bone Joint Surg Am.* 1944;26(1):1–30.
38. McClure PW, Michener LA, Karduna AR. Shoulder function and 3-dimensional scapular kinematics in people with and without shoulder impingement syndrome. *Phys Ther.* 2006;86(8):1075–1090.
39. Ludewig PM, Cook TM. Alterations in shoulder kinematics and associated muscle activity in people with symptoms of shoulder impingement. *Phys Ther.* 2000;80(3):276–291.
40. Graichen H, Stammberger T, Bonel H, et al. Magnetic resonance-based motion analysis of the shoulder during elevation. *Clin Orthop Relat Res.* 2000;370:154–163.
41. Sahrmann S. *Diagnosis and Treatment of Muscle Imbalances Associated With Regional Pain Syndromes.* St. Louis, MO: Washington University School of Medicine, Washington University Medical Center; 1990.
42. Peterson DE, Blankenship KR, Robb JB, et al. Investigation of the validity and reliability of four objective techniques for measuring forward shoulder posture. *J Orthop Sports Phys Ther.* 1997;25(1):34–42.
43. Griegel-Morris P, Larson K, Mueller-Klaus K, Oatis CA. Incidence of common postural abnormalities in the cervical, shoulder, and thoracic regions and their association with pain in two age groups of healthy subjects. *Phys Ther.* 1992;72(6):425–431.
44. da Costa BR, Armijo-Olivo S, Gadotti I, Warren S, Reid DC, Magee DJ. Reliability of scapular positioning measurement procedure using the Palpation Meter (PALM). *Physiotherapy.* 2010;96(1):59–67.
45. Gibson MH, Goebel GV, Jordan TM, Kegerreis S, Worrell TW. A reliability study of measurement techniques to determine static scapular position. *J Orthop Sports Phys Ther.* 1995;21(2):100–106.
46. Odom CJ, Taylor AB, Hurd CE, Denegar CR. Measurement of scapular asymmetry and assessment of shoulder dysfunction using the Lateral Scapular Slide Test: a reliability and validity study. *Phys Ther.* 2001;81(2):799–809.
47. McKenna L, Cunningham J, Straker L. Inter-tester reliability of scapular position in elite swimmers. *Phys Ther Sport.* 2004;5:146–155.

48. Shadmehr A, Bagheri H, Ansari NN, Sarafraz H. The reliability measurements of Lateral Scapular Slide Test at three different degrees of shoulder joint abduction. *Br J Sports Med.* 2010;44(4):289–293.
49. Borstad JD, Ludewig PM. The effect of long versus short pectoralis minor resting length on scapular kinematics in healthy individuals. *J Orthop Sports Phys Ther.* 2005;35(4):227–238.
50. Hart DL, Carmichael SW. Biomechanics of the shoulder. *J Orthop Sports Phys Ther.* 1985;6(4):1.
51. Culham E, Peat M. Functional anatomy of the shoulder complex. *J Orthop Sports Phys Ther.* 1993;18(1):342–350.
52. Johnson MP, McClure PW, Karduna AR. New method to assess scapular upward rotation in subjects with shoulder pathology. *J Orthop Sports Phys Ther.* 2001;31(2):81–89.
53. Borsa PA, Timmons MK, Sauers EL. Scapular-positioning patterns during humeral elevation in unimpaired shoulders. *J Athl Train.* 2003;38(1):12–17.
54. Nijs J, Roussel N, Vermeulen K, Souvereyns G. Scapular positioning in patients with shoulder pain: a study examining the reliability and clinical importance of 3 clinical tests. *Arch Phys Med Rehabil.* 2005;86(7):1349–1355.
55. Borstad JD. Measurement of pectoralis minor muscle length: validation and clinical application. *J Orthop Sports Phys Ther.* 2008;38(4):169–174.
56. Warner JJ, Micheli LJ, Arslanian LE, Kennedy J, Kennedy R. Scapulothoracic motion in normal shoulders and shoulders with glenohumeral instability and impingement syndrome: a study using Moiré topographic analysis. *Clin Orthop Relat Res.* 1992;285:191–199.
57. Koslow PA, Prosser LA, Strony GA, Suchecki SL, Mattingly GE. Specificity of the lateral scapular slide test in asymptomatic competitive athletes. *J Orthop Sports Phys Ther.* 2003;33(6):331–336.
58. Kibler WB, Sciascia A, Dome D. Evaluation of apparent and absolute supraspinatus strength in patients with shoulder injury using the Scapular Retraction Test. *Am J Sports Med.* 2006;34(10):1643–1647.
59. Tate AR, McClure PW, Kareha S, Irwin D. Effect of the Scapula Reposition Test on shoulder impingement symptoms and elevation strength in overhead athletes. *J Orthop Sports Phys Ther.* 2008;38(1):4–11.
60. Merolla G, De Santis E, Campi F, Paladini P, Porcellini G. Infraspinatus scapular retraction test: a reliable and practical method to assess infraspinatus strength in overhead athletes with scapular dyskinesis. *J Orthop Traumatol.* 2010;11(2):105–110.
61. Michener LA, Boardman ND, Pidcoe PE, Frith AM. Scapular muscle tests in subjects with shoulder pain and functional loss: reliability and construct validity. *Phys Ther.* 2005;85(11):1128–1138.
62. Ludewig PM, Hoff MS, Osowski EE, Meschke SA, Rundquist PJ. Relative balance of serratus anterior and upper trapezius muscle activity during push-up exercises. *Am J Sports Med.* 2004;32(2):484–493.
63. Cools AM, Witvrouw EE, Mahieu NN, Danneels LA. Isokinetic scapular muscle performance in overhead athletes with and without impingement symptoms. *J Athl Train.* 2005;40(2):104–110.
64. Lukasiewicz AC, McClure P, Michener L, Pratt N, Sennett B. Comparison of 3-dimensional scapular position and orientation between subjects with and without shoulder impingement. *J Orthop Sports Phys Ther.* 1999;29(10):574–586.
65. Peat M, Grahame RE. Electromyographic analysis of soft tissue lesions affecting shoulder function. *Am J Phys Med.* 1977;56(5):223–240.
66. Wadsworth DJ, Bullock-Saxton JE. Recruitment patterns of the scapular rotator muscles in freestyle swimmers with subacromial impingement. *Int J Sports Med.* 1997;18(8):618–624.
67. Cools AM, Dewitte V, Lanszweert F, et al. Rehabilitation of scapular muscle balance: which exercises to prescribe? *Am J Sports Med.* 2007;35(10):1744–1751.
68. Dvir Z, Berme N. The shoulder complex in elevation of the arm: a mechanism approach. *J Biomech.* 1978;11(5):219–225.
69. Ludewig PM, Cook TM, Nawoczenski DA. Three-dimensional scapular orientation and muscle activity at selected positions humeral elevation. *J Orthop Sports Phys Ther.* 1996;24(2):57–65.
70. Rabin A, Irrgang JJ, Fitzgerald GK, Eubanks A. The intertester reliability of the Scapular Assistance Test. *J Orthop Sports Phys Ther.* 2006;36(9):653–660.
71. Ekstrom RA, Bifulco KM, Lopau CJ, Andersen CF, Gough JR. Comparing the function of the upper and lower parts of the serratus anterior muscle using surface electromyography. *J Orthop Sports Phys Ther.* 2004;34(5):235–243.
72. Hislop H, Montgomery J, Connelly B. *Daniels and Worthingham's: Muscle Testing: Techniques of Manual Examination.* 6th ed. Philadelphia, PA: WB Saunders; 1995.
73. Riemann BL, Davies GJ, Ludwig L, Gardenhour H. Hand-held dynamometer testing of the internal and external rotator musculature based on selected positions to establish normative data and unilateral ratios. *J Shoulder Elbow Surg.* 2010;19(8):1175–1183.
74. Goldbeck TG, Davies GJ. Test-retest reliability of the Closed Kinetic Chain Upper Extremity Stability Test: a clinical field test. *J Sport Rehabil.* 2000;9:35–45.

IV-2

Rehabilitation of Scapular Dyskinesia

Bryce W. Gaunt, PT, SCS

CHAPTER CONTENTS

Clinical pearls are highlighted in yellow throughout the text.

Pain in the region of the scapula is a challenging condition to diagnose accurately and treat effectively. It can originate from many structures and can be affected by many factors. Table 1 lists some factors that can contribute to scapular pain. Scapular dyskinesia is one common condition that is associated with shoulder girdle pain and often treated by rehabilitation professionals. In this chapter, I discuss a step-by-step rehabilitation progression to correct scapular dyskinesia, emphasizing motor learning. I underscore the rationale to support an easy-to-follow clinical exercise progression that emphasizes motor learning to correct scapular dyskinesia during active forward elevation.

EVALUATION OF SCAPULAR DYSKINESIA

Scapular dyskinesia has been defined as alternations in the position and movement of the scapula.[1] Precise evaluation of both the resting scapular position and dynamic scapular movement to determine if scapular dyskinesia is present is the first step in formulating appropriate treatment. Determining if the resting position of the scapula on the thorax is normal or abnormal is important because an altered resting position tends to lead to abnormal dynamic movement. If one starts movement in an incorrect position, it is hard for the scapula to be in the correct position while moving dynamically. In addition, an abnormal resting position of the scapula can result in pain and functional limitations because incorrect positioning of the scapula with the upper extremity by the side places abnormal forces on muscles and neurovascular structures. Evaluation of the resting scapular position and normal scapular mechanics is detailed in chapter IV-1; however, normal scapular motion with active elevation of the upper extremity has been shown to be about 40° to 50° of upward rotation, 20° to 30° of posterior scapular tilt, and 2° to 24° of external rotation.[2,3]

If scapular dyskinesia is identified at rest or with movement, the next step in patient management is to determine if the dyskinesia is related to that patient's clinical signs and symptoms. This is difficult to determine because not all scapular dyskinesias are caused by or are causing the patient's pain or functional limitations. Comparing scapular positioning and movement of the affected extremity with that of the contralateral side, considering the clinical diagnosis, performing symptom-altering tests, and relying on clinical experience help the rehabilitation provider determine the relationship among scapular dyskinesia, pain, and functional limitations.

Table 1. Factors That Can Contribute to Pain in the Region of the Scapula

Systemic disease
Disorders of the spine
Acromioclavicular and/or sternoclavicular joint dysfunction
Muscle imbalances
Soft tissue disorders
Pectoralis minor tightness
Posterior shoulder tightness
Nervous system dysfunction or injury
Abnormal posture
Activities of daily living

Rehabilitation of Scapular Dyskinesia

Conflicting evidence exists regarding the symmetry of dynamic movement of the scapula in healthy people during active elevation of the shoulder. For example, Yoshizaki et al[4] demonstrated nearly symmetric movement and no difference in scapular movement when comparing dominant and nondominant upper extremities in 18 healthy individuals with a mean age of 24 years. However, other researchers have demonstrated asymmetric scapular motion or asymmetric scapular resting positions in healthy participants.[5–7] Uhl et al[6] reported that 71% (n = 21) of asymptomatic participants showed asymmetric scapular motion during 3-dimensional motion analysis.

The diagnosis of impingement,[8–10] instability,[11,12] and a limited glenohumeral internal rotation range of motion (GIRD)[13–15] have the most clinical evidence suggesting that they sometimes are associated with scapular dyskinesia. Symptom-altering tests, such as the scapular assistance test[16] (Figure 1), scapular retraction test,[17] and scapula reposition test (Figure 2),[18] can be used to help determine if the scapular dyskinesia that is appreciated is associated with a patient's pain. Each of these tests uses manual assistance to reposition the scapula in a more correct biomechanical position to see if symptoms are improved or alleviated. More details about these tests can be found in chapter IV-1.

Taken together with clinical experience, these factors are very helpful for determining if a scapular dyskinesia is associated with a patient's pain and functional limitation. For example, I screen for scapular dyskinesia in all patients with shoulder conditions, realizing that some asymmetry can be expected and might not be related to their clinical problems. However, in a patient with impingement, instability, or GIRD, less dyskinesia will make me postulate that his or her dyskinesia is clinically relevant. If I suspect that the dyskinesia is part of the cause of the patient's clinical signs and symptoms, I then use at least one of the symptom-altering tests to confirm my belief. If symptoms are minimized or resolved by these tests, then I assume a positive relationship exists between the clinical problem and the scapular dyskinesia. If symptoms are not affected by these tests, then I am less likely to believe the dyskinesia is associated with the patient's problem unless the dyskinesia is especially large.

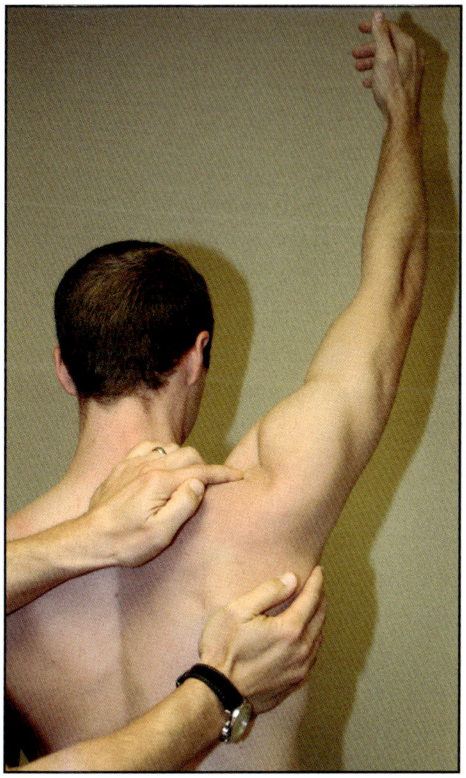

Figure 1. The scapular assistance test. The clinician applies posterior tilting force through grasping the superior border of the scapula and applies upward rotation force through the inferior angle of the scapula as the patient elevates his upper extremity.

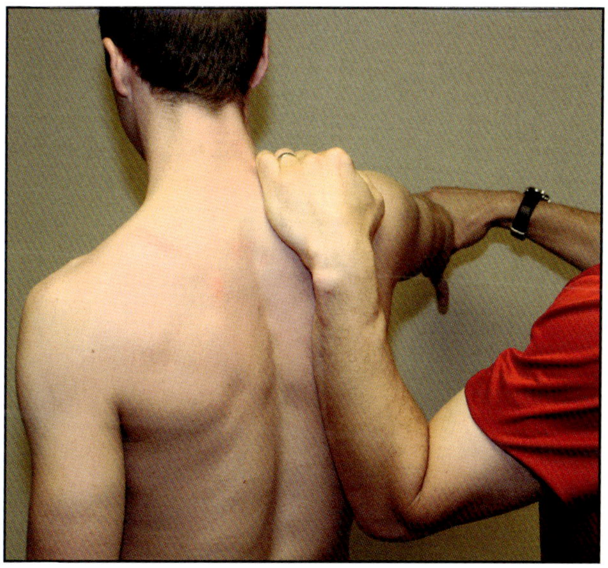

Figure 2. The scapula reposition test. The clinician grasps the acromioclavicular joint superiorly and scapula posteriorly then applies a posterior tilting and external rotation force to further approximate the scapula to the thorax. This is done during performance of the Jobe empty-can test. Diminished pain or a substantial increase in strength is considered a positive test result.

WHAT SHOULD BE THE EMPHASIS OF SCAPULAR REHABILITATION AND WHY?

To determine appropriate treatment for scapular dyskinesia, examining the job of the scapula is wise. A common definition is that the *scapula* provides a stable base for force transfer and efficient movement of the upper extremity. Over the past decade, the "stable base" part of this definition seems to have been the emphasis of scapular rehabilitation to a success in many patients. As related to scapular dyskinesia, recognizing that the purpose of the stable scapular base is for "efficient movement of the upper extremity" is important. As detailed in chapter IV-1, efficient movement of the upper extremity requires that the scapula moves a great deal, upwardly rotating approximately 40° to 50°, posteriorly tilting 20° to 30°, and externally rotating 2° to 24°[2,3] during active overhead elevation of the extremity (Figure 3). This much movement of the scapula is required to ensure proper alignment between the glenoid and humerus and to ensure that an optimal length-tension relationship of the rotator cuff, deltoid, and scapular musculature is present. Because of this, in my opinion, the emphasis of rehabilitation to correct scapular dyskinesia should be to restore correct movement of the scapula so that it efficiently and effectively can do its job. Isolated strength and endurance training and an emphasis on scapular stability in the resting position should be a secondary emphasis of rehabilitation.

To correct scapular dyskinesia so the scapula can move correctly, I prefer to emphasize motor learning during the rehabilitation process in a method similar to that suggested by Caldwell et al.[19] Faulty motor programs have been discussed as one possible cause of scapular dyskinesia; however, seldom do scapular rehabilitation programs seem to emphasize motor learning to correct scapular dyskinesia during forward elevation movements. Why should we emphasize motor learning to correct scapular dyskinesia? Early in my career, my primary method of treating patients with scapular dyskinesias, such as winging, was isolated strengthening of the weakened muscle. Although this was helpful, I remember several occasions in which the strength of a weakened scapular muscle greatly improved (from a manual muscle testing grade of 2+/5 to 5/5), but the dyskinesia (in this case scapular winging) remained unchanged. I then recognized that improved strength of the scapular muscles did not necessarily equal a resolution of the dyskinesia. Instead, I began to understand that actively elevating the upper extremity overhead is a complex task similar to riding a bicycle. Although riding a bicycle does take a certain amount of strength, the primary component needed for success is not strength but is coordination and the correct movement pattern. When I approached correcting scapular dyskinesia this same way and began to emphasize motor learning to correct movement patterns, I noticed that in some patients, dramatic improvements in scapular mechanics were evident after 5 to 10 minutes of training. Obviously, an increase in strength does not occur in this short time, but an improvement in coordination and movement patterns can occur. These things taken together solidified my belief that a motor-learning emphasis to correct scapular dyskinesia should be a primary focus of rehabilitation for this problem.

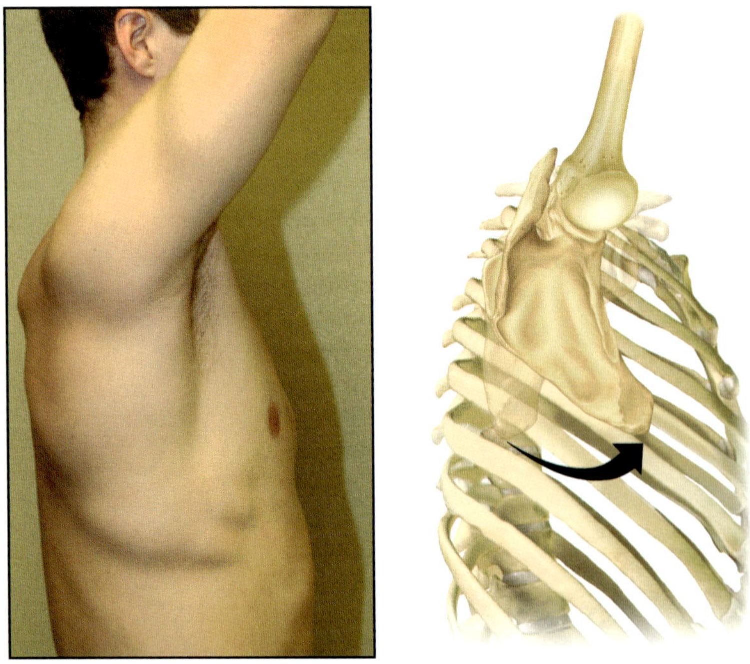

Figure 3. Typical ending position of the scapula during overhead active forward elevation.

THE 5-STEP CLINICAL REHABILITATION PROGRAM TO CORRECT SCAPULAR DYSKINESIA

1. Normalize the Static Resting Position of the Scapula

This emphasis in motor learning is part of my 5-step clinical rehabilitation program to correct scapular dyskinesia (Table 2). The first step of the progression is to normalize the static resting position of the scapula if any dyskinesia is present. The assessment of the resting position of the scapula is detailed in chapter IV-1. The specific interventions used depend on the dyskinesia found, but excess scapular internal rotation (sometimes called *scapular winging*) and excess anterior tilt are common static abnormalities. Both of these dyskinesias are associated with pectoralis minor tightness,[20] so an assessment of the pectoralis resting length is needed. Pectoralis minor length commonly is assessed by 1 of 2 methods. Borstad[21] validated a direct measurement technique using a tape measure or Vernier caliper. Sahrmann[22] recommended measuring the distance from the posterolateral angle of the scapula to the examination table of a patient lying supine, with distances greater than 2.54 cm (1 in) suggesting pectoralis minor tightness. If the pectoralis minor is tight and requires stretching, it can be stretched manually by the rehabilitation provider (Figure 4) or very effectively with home-based stretching. My preferred self-stretch is shown in Figure 5[23] and often restores the length of the pectoralis minor to normal within 2 weeks if 5 to 8 repetitions of the stretch are performed 4 to 6 times each day. Upper extremity weight-bearing

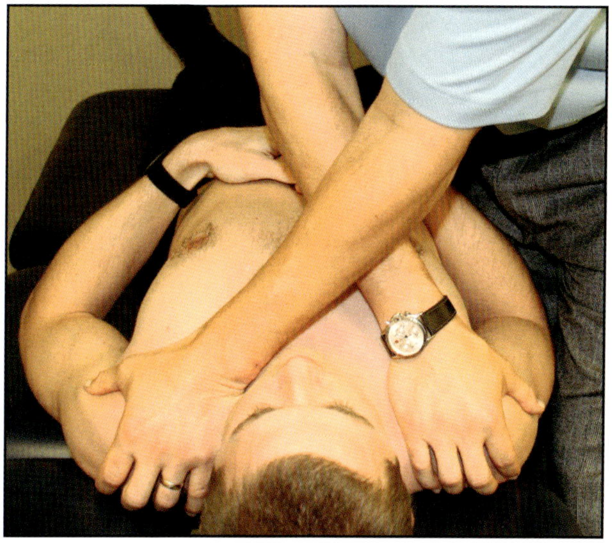

Figure 4. Manual pectoralis minor stretching in which the scapulae are retracted and elevated through the coracoid process.

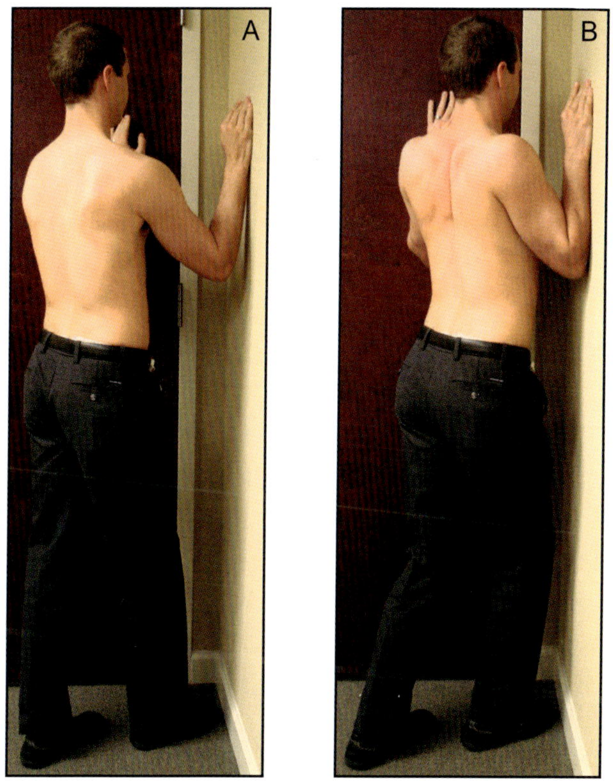

Figure 5. The author's preferred method of home pectoralis minor stretching. A, The correct starting position includes an upright torso and 1 foot forward. B, The scapulae are retracted and elevated by a force moving through the upper extremity while the shoulder is in 30° of flexion, as recommended and validated by Muraki et al.[23] Ensure that the torso stays upright and moves forward as a unit in unison with the pelvis and both knees.

Table 2. The St. Francis Rehabilitation Center's 5-Step Rehabilitation Program to Correct Scapular Dyskinesia

1. Normalize the static resting position of the scapula.
2. Look for and fix associated problems.
3. Normalize scapular mechanics during active elevation of the upper extremity.
4. Include isolated muscle strengthening.
5. Normalize scapular mechanics with advanced functional positions.

exercises in the quadruped, triped, and biped positions can be very helpful in correcting resting scapular position because these positions facilitate scapular posterior tilting and scapular external rotation (Figure 6). These are also advantageous positions to work on serratus anterior recruitment and to provide either manual resistance (Figure 7) or facilitation by the rehabilitation provider to correct the abnormal scapular position (Figure 8).

The final component used to correct the static position of the scapula is the posterior scapular tilt exercise, which is a motor-control drill (Figure 9). When learning this exercise, the patient almost always needs oral, visual, and/or manual cueing to tilt the scapula posteriorly with a slight amount of scapular elevation (Figure 10). This is a complex task involving activation of many muscles but usually is learned successfully in a short period with the oral cue, "tilt the top part of your shoulder blade back while you bring the bottom part of your shoulder blade toward your ribs." This position slightly overcorrects excessive scapular

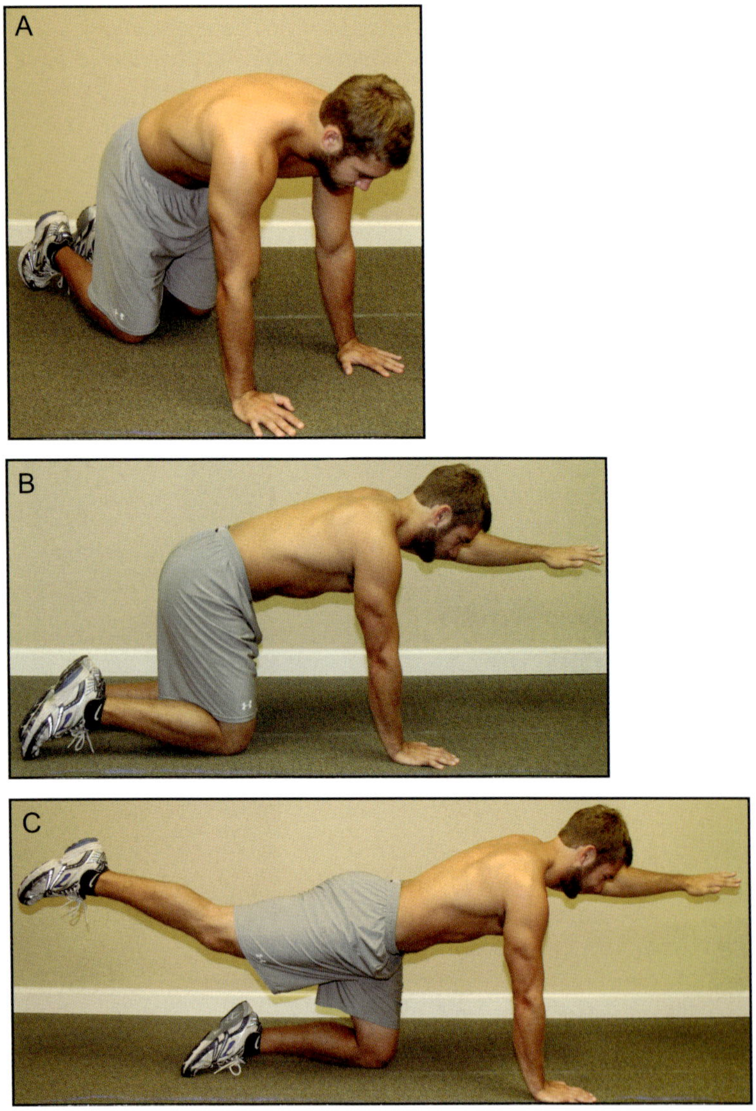

Figure 6. The quadruped, A, triped, B, and biped, C, positions facilitate scapular posterior tilting and scapular external rotation.

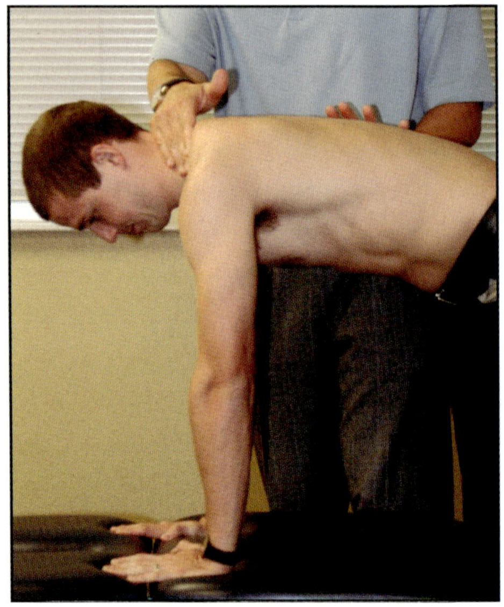
Figure 7. Manual pertubations to challenge maintaining the correct static scapular position.

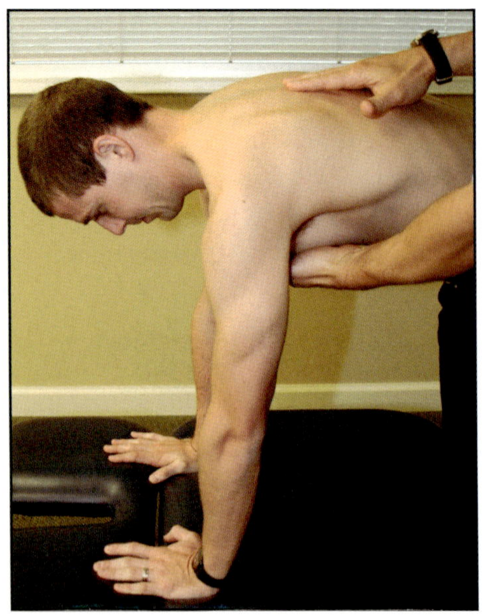
Figure 8. The patient is facilitated into the correct resting position of the scapula through oral, visual, or manual cues then maintains the correct position for a progressive length of time during the exercise.

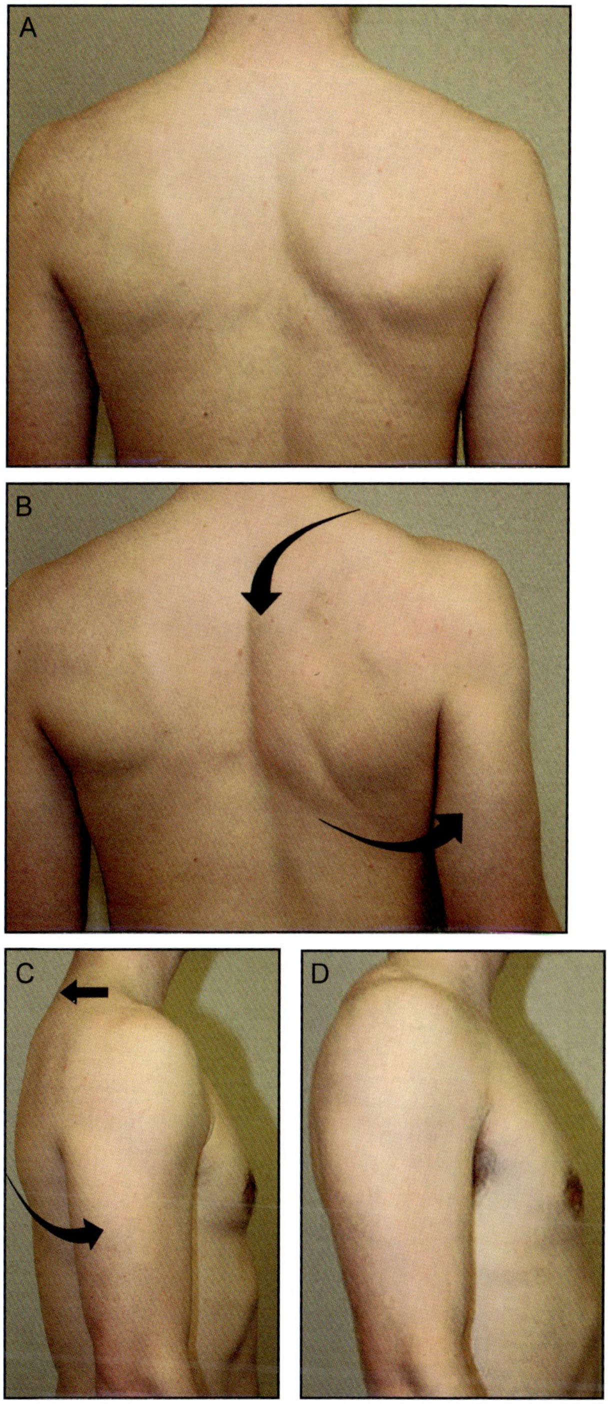

Figure 9. The starting, A and C, and ending, B and D, positions of the posterior scapular tilt exercise. The patient starts in his normal resting position and is instructed to tilt the scapula posteriorly with a small amount of scapular elevation.

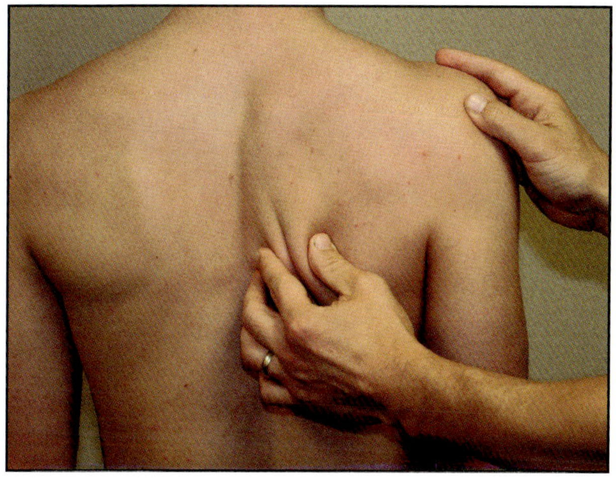

Figure 10. Manual cueing is provided to assist the patient in retracting and elevating the top part of the scapula and in moving the inferior angle of the scapula forward against the ribs.

anterior tilt and internal rotation. Next, the patient is instructed to hold this position as long as comfortable, which is usually until fatigue begins. Often, this initially is less than 5 seconds. The patient is instructed to perform 3 to 5 repetitions of this exercise 7 to 10 times each day, each time attempting to increase the comfortable length of hold up to 2 minutes. This frequently can be achieved within 2 to 3 weeks with regular practice. I have found that after this criterion is achieved, the normal resting position of the scapula often is restored as long as the flexibility of the shoulder girdle muscles, especially the pectoralis minor and latissimus dorsi, are within normal limits. If the patient has a hard time performing the posterior scapular tilt exercise correctly in an upright position, he or she typically has an easier time learning it in the side-lying position (Figure 11).

2. Look for and Fix Associated Problems

The second step of my 5-step clinical rehabilitation program to correct scapular dyskinesia is to look for and fix associated problems that might be contributing to the scapular dyskinesia or to the patient's clinical signs and symptoms. A partial list of things to consider is shown in Table 1. The bigger picture of what can be causing a patient's symptoms in addition to scapular dyskinesia is very important to consider. Whereas assessing and treating these other problems in the early stages of rehabilitation is most effective, generally these factors can be evaluated and treated in conjunction with any of the other steps of the scapular rehabilitation program. The assessment of specific problems listed in Table 1 is initiated as needed based on clinical reasoning. Depending on your findings, referral to another professional might be needed, or the focus of

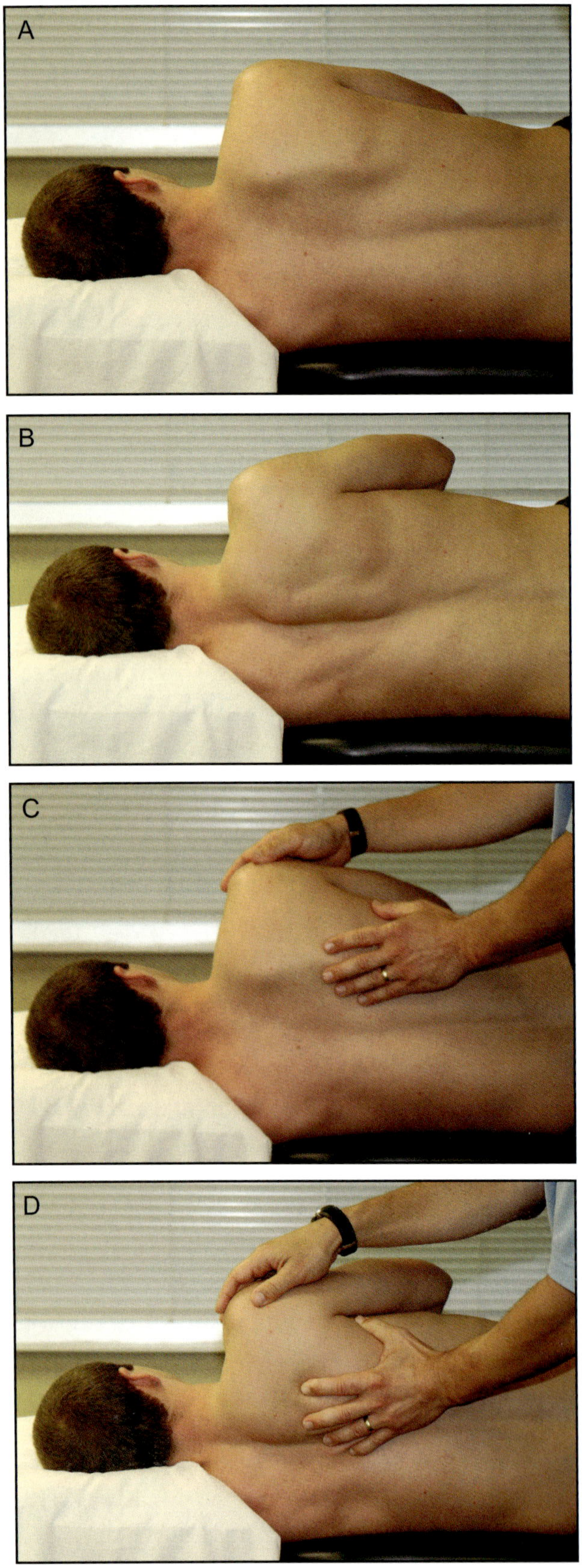

Figure 11 A-D. The posterior scapular tilt exercise performed in the side-lying position without, A and B, and with, C and D, manual facilitation.

treatment might change from scapular dyskinesia to another area, such as myofascial release or treatment of a spinal dysfunction.

3. Normalize Scapular Mechanics During Active Elevation of the Upper Extremity

The third step of my 5-step clinical rehabilitation program to correct scapular dyskinesia is to normalize the scapular mechanics during active elevation of the upper extremity. This is the stage of scapular rehabilitation that is best treated by emphasizing motor learning. To emphasize motor learning to correct scapular dyskinesia, I train the elevation movement but provide assistance to make learning the correct coordinated movement pattern easier on the patient. This assistance is akin to using training wheels when learning how to ride a bicycle. During scapular rehabilitation, this assistance is best provided both in the clinic and during the home exercise program. The rehabilitation provider can provide this assistance directly with tactile, oral, or visual cues.

Perhaps more important than this direct assistance by the rehabilitation provider is to decrease the load that the scapular muscles must overcome when elevating or moving the upper extremity. I consistently have noticed that decreasing the load to the upper extremity during active movement tends to improve scapular mechanics. Evidence has suggested the reason a decreased load to the shoulder girdle can improve scapular mechanics. Several investigators have shown that weighted active elevation of the upper extremity results in more scapular dyskinesia than unweighted elevation of the extremity.[1,9,24] Fatigue also has been shown consistently to result in abnormal scapular motion.[24,25] Unpublished work conducted by us in conjunction with the University of Kentucky has demonstrated that the load to the scapular muscles can be reduced during elevation activities (as evidenced by decreased electromyographic [EMG] activity) by supporting the upper extremity during either gravity-minimized exercises (Figure 12) or upright active-assistive exercises (Figure 13) compared with unsupported active elevation of the extremity (Figure 14). If we know that extra load to or fatigue of the scapular muscles tends to cause more dyskinesia, then we reasonably can assume that a decrease in load by using

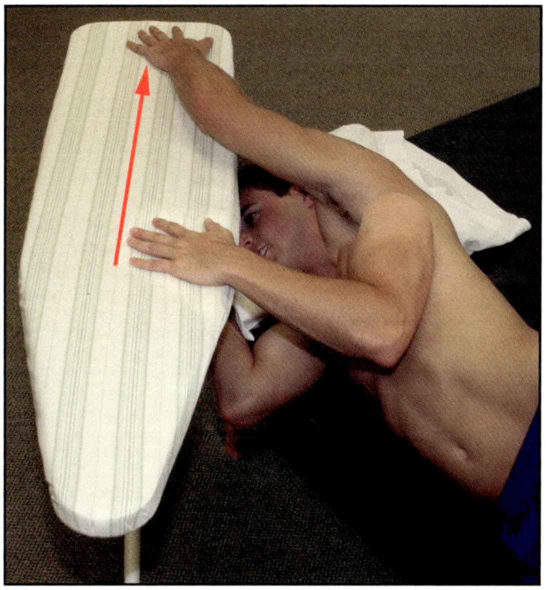

Figure 12. Side-lying active elevation is a gravity-minimized exercise.

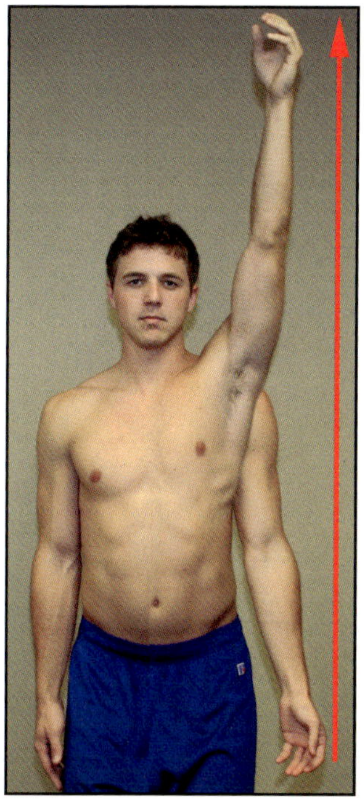

Figure 14. Active forward elevation.

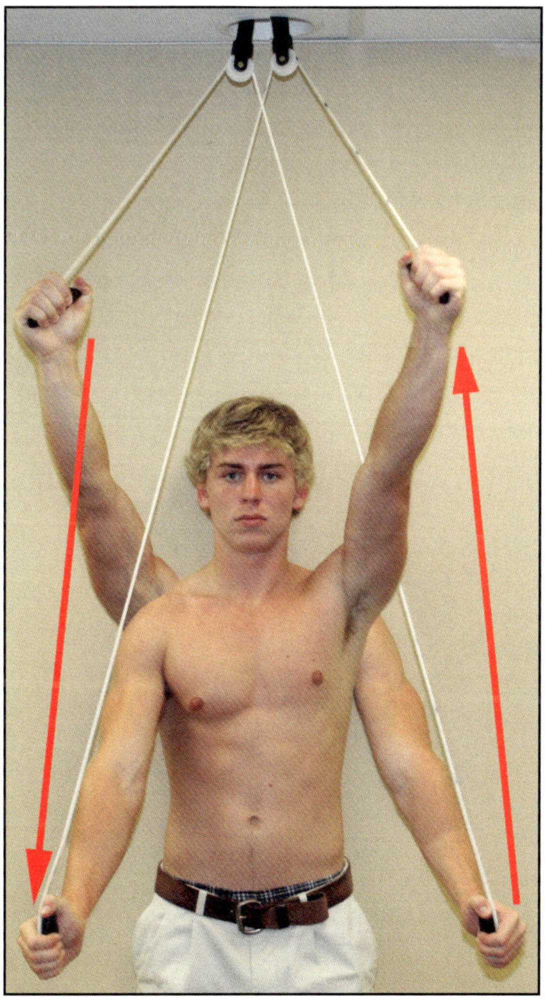

Figure 13. Rope-and-pulley assistive forward elevation is an upright assistive exercise.

either gravity-minimized exercises or upright assistive exercises might reduce or eliminate scapular dyskinesia. This matches our clinical experience; using these forms of assistive exercise to train the forward elevation movement seems to be less work for the scapular force couples, which makes the correct movements easier to practice and learn. In turn, this tends to result in a rapid improvement of scapular dyskinesia first in a position of decreased load and second in normal unweighted and weighted conditions. Our motor-learning-based retraining progression for the forward elevation movement is to progress from gravity-minimized exercises to upright assistive exercises, to upright active exercise, and to upright resistive exercise (Table 3). We clinically use many exercise progressions; a sample progression is shown in Figures 12–14, and a different progression is shown starting with Figure 15, progressing to Figure 16, to Figure 17, then to Figure 14. More details about gravity-minimized and upright assistive exercises can be found in chapter I-4.

When using this exercise progression, the patient moves from one exercise level to the next when 30 to 50 repetitions of the exercises in the easier level can be completed with normal scapular and glenohumeral mechanics and without pain or fatigue. The patient then performs exercises in the more difficult level, usually with a smaller number of repetitions, until fatigue begins but without abnormal mechanics. If scapular

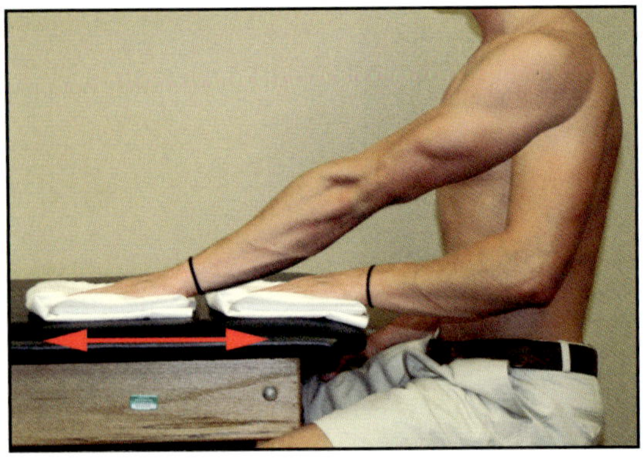

Figure 15. Horizontal dusting.

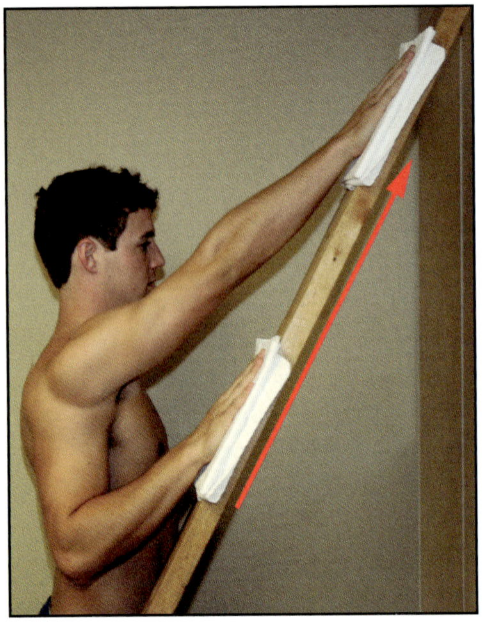

Figure 16. Incline dusting.

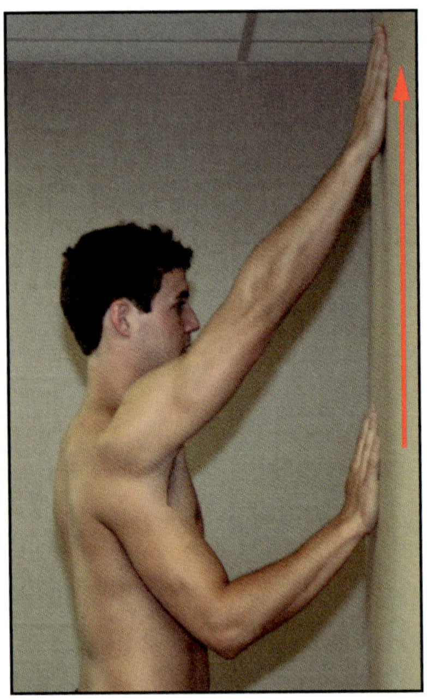

Figure 17. Wall slides.

Table 3. St. Francis Rehabilitation Center's Motor-Learning-Based Functional Elevation Strengthening Progression for the Scapular Rotators

Step 1	Gravity-minimized elevation exercises
Step 2	Upright assistive elevation exercises
Step 3	Upright active elevation
Step 4	Upright resistive elevation

dyskinesia is present during all repetitions even with facilitation and cueing, then a different exercise is chosen. Taken together, this provides a functional elevation strengthening progression to the shoulder girdle with a motor-learning emphasis that facilitates correct scapular mechanics. A bonus to using this progression is that after the correct motor program is re-established, the patient might have immediate carryover to normal scapular mechanics in a much more advanced level, such as resisted elevation, if his or her primary cause of dyskinesia was not strength but an incorrect motor program.

Some authors have suggested that the preferred exercises for scapular rehabilitation should be exercises that promote scapular muscle balance, meaning that the muscle activity of the lower trapezius (LT), middle trapezius, and/or serratus anterior (SA) is increased compared with the muscle activity of the upper trapezius (UT).[26,27] Cools et al[26] suggested this could be quantified by examining the ratio of EMG activity between the upper trapezius and each of the other muscles listed. They advocated a ratio of 60% or less provided "excellent" scapular muscle balance, with a lower ratio indicating better balance. In unpublished work, my colleagues and I evaluated selected gravity-minimized and selected upright assistive exercises that were detailed in another study of ours[28] and found that side-lying active

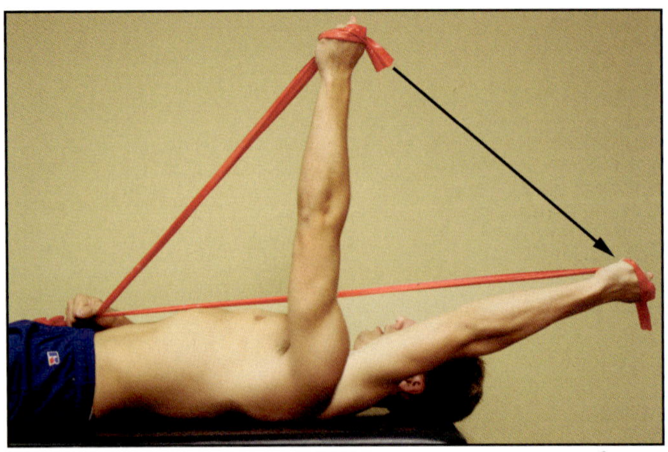

Figure 18. Supine elevation with elastic resistance.

elevation (Figure 12) has a UT to SA ratio of 19% and supine elevation with elastic resistance (Figure 18) has a UT to SA ratio of 29% and a UT to LT ratio of 50%. Therefore, these exercises might be good choices to use in the early stages of rehabilitation if the rehabilitation provider chooses to emphasize improving scapular muscle balance.

4. Include Isolated Muscle Strengthening

The fourth step of my 5-step clinical rehabilitation program to correct scapular dyskinesia is to include isolated muscle strengthening but to use these interventions only as needed to correct specific muscle deficits. As mentioned, contrary to other scapular rehabilitation programs, we generally use these exercises as a secondary rather than a primary rehabilitation focus. Although this is the fourth step of our rehabilitation program, isolated strengthening exercises can begin at any point in the rehabilitation progression and often are begun in the early stages of rehabilitation as long as the exercises can be performed correctly and are not painful.

The 3 exercises I use most frequently for this purpose are scapular retractions with elastic resistance (Figure 19), active forward elevation (AFE) (Figure 14), and forward reaching with elastic resistance (Figure 20). Although not often thought of as a scapular rehabilitation exercise, the AFE exercise is vital to include in scapular rehabilitation. Active forward elevation above 120° demonstrates very high serratus anterior recruitment, including greater EMG activity than resisted scapular protraction.[29] In another study, AFE above 120° resulted in the highest EMG activity of the lower serratus anterior compared with any exercise

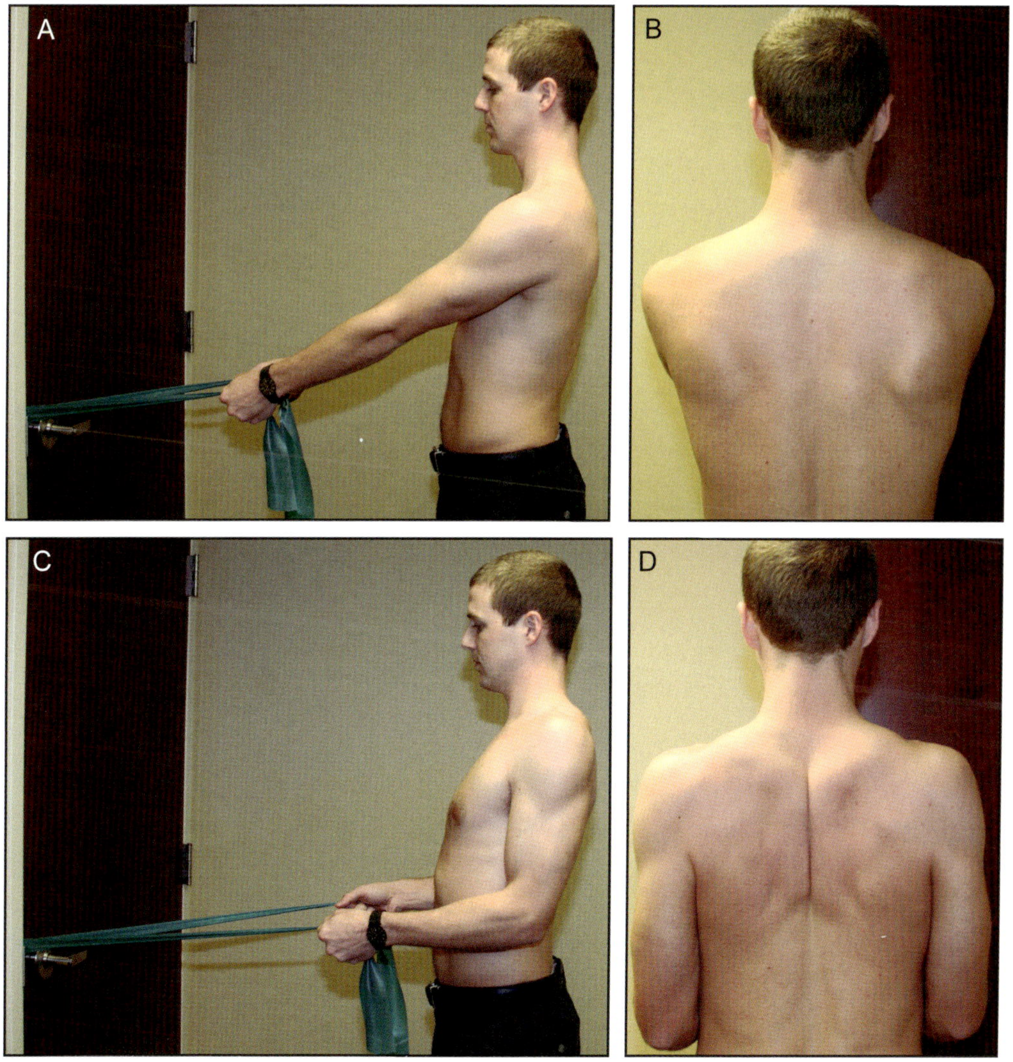

Figure 19. The starting, A and B, and ending, C and D, positions for scapular retraction with elastic resistance. Note that the elbow stops even with the midline of the torso in the ending position.

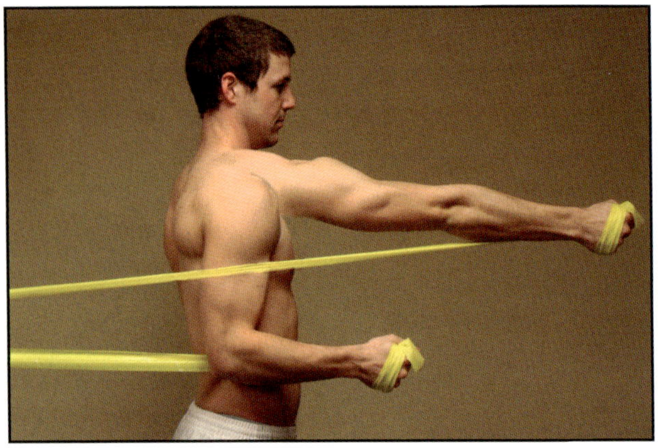

Figure 20. Forward reaching with elastic resistance.

tested, including push-up plus.[30] It also improves the strength and endurance of the very functional movement pattern of overhead reaching, as detailed in step 3 of our rehabilitation program. I recommend building up the patient's endurance to a point that 30 repetitions can be achieved easily then adding light weight to this exercise. From 1 pound (0.45 kg) to 3 pounds (1.35 kg) is the maximum weight I use with most patients depending on their body sizes and the functional goals they want to achieve. I have found that unless heavy lifting, repetitive overhead activities, or sports activities are desired, repetitive AFE with 2 pounds (0.90 kg) usually allows patients to return to their normal daily activities without symptoms. Remember that if a patient has scapular dyskinesia with AFE, then gravity-minimized or upright assistive exercises, as detailed in phase 3 of our rehabilitation progression, are used until AFE can be performed with normal scapular mechanics.

5. Normalize Scapular Mechanics With Advanced Functional Positions

The final step of my clinical rehabilitation program to correct scapular dyskinesia is to normalize scapular mechanics with advanced functional positions besides AFE. This is usually necessary for patients who use their upper extremities repetitively at shoulder level or overhead, regularly perform heavy lifting, or are overhead athletes with dyskinesia in their dominant extremities. Patients whose jobs require regular heavy lifting or who use their upper extremities repetitively at shoulder level or overhead require a large amount of endurance and strength beyond what is provided in a standard rehabilitation program. A work-reconditioning program or work-hardening program that emphasizes job-specific movements provides the progressive strength and endurance training necessary to meet these demanding needs. Beginning these programs is appropriate after dyskinesia is resolved during repetitive AFE using 2 pounds (0.90 kg) to 3 pounds (1.35 kg) and after the patient is asymptomatic with basic activities of daily living.

Overhead athletes also require specialized scapular training. The scapula must retract properly while the extremity is in the abducted and externally rotated position in overhead athletes during activities, such as the tennis serve or the late cocking phase of throwing (Figure 21). Inability to properly retract the scapula during the late cocking phase of throwing requires extra horizontal abduction at the glenohumeral joint. This combination has been shown to decrease throwing performance[16] and decrease glenohumeral rotation strength.[31] It has been associated with subacromial and internal impingement syndrome,[32,33] labral injury,[34] and increased stress to the anterior glenohumeral ligaments.[16,35]

In these athletes, resolving any posterior shoulder tightness or GIRD that is related to forward shoulder posture and shoulder pain is especially important. Normal pectoralis minor flexibility is emphasized along with basic (Figure 19) and advanced exercises (Figure 22) to strengthen the middle and lower trapezius. In addition, the rehabilitation provider must observe the scapular mechanics of the athlete during the throwing motion or tennis serve and must examine the amount of scapular retraction. If it appears decreased, then oral, visual, or tactile cues can be given to the athlete to purposely emphasize the amount of scapular retraction while in the abducted and externally rotated position (Figure 23) to help correct any faulty motor programs that exist. A thorough assessment of the lower extremity and core stabilizers, correcting any deficiencies that are found, is also prudent in these athletes with scapular dyskinesia.

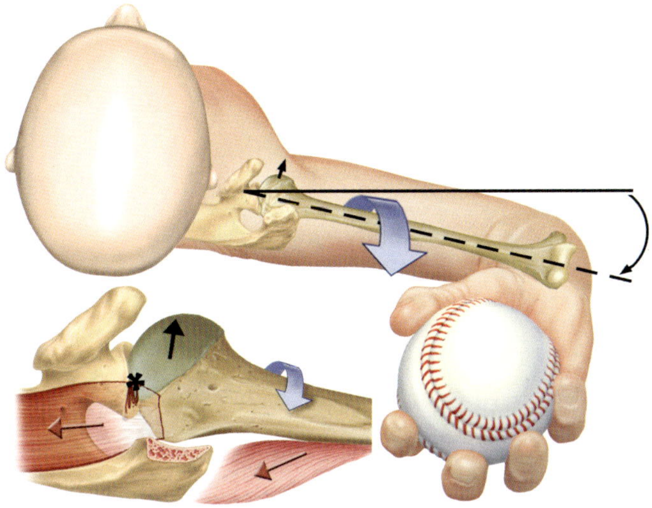

Figure 21. Limited scapular retraction during the late cocking phase of throwing, which is thought to lead to internal impingement and anterior shoulder laxity among other things.

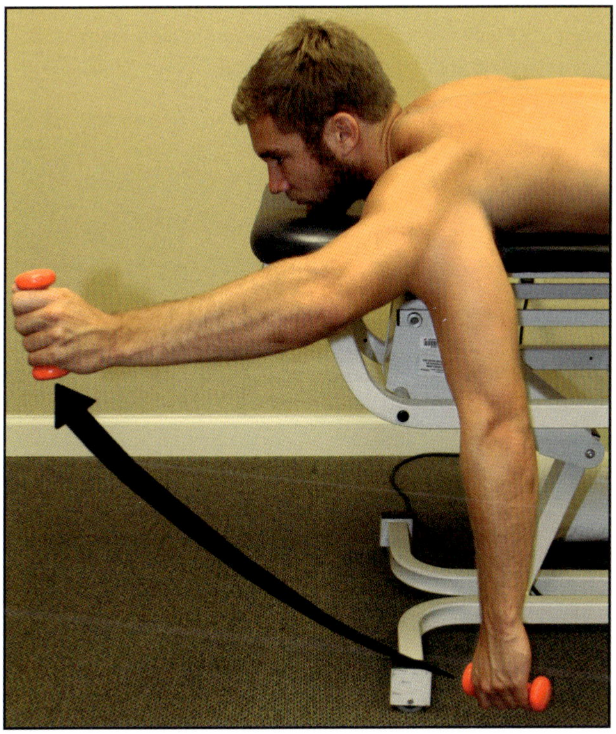

Figure 22. Prone horizonatal abduction at 100° of elevation.

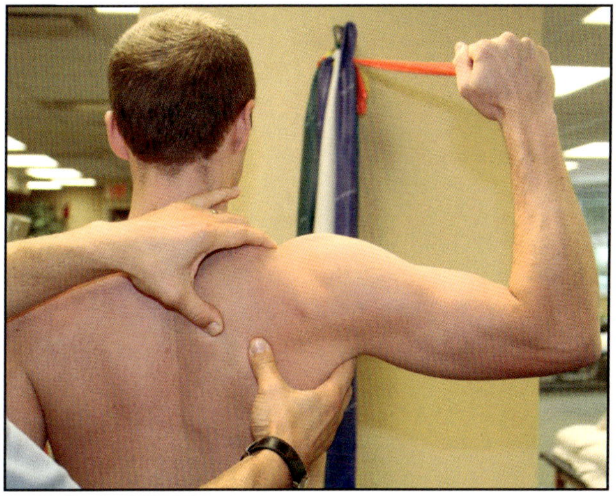

Figure 23. Facilitation to promote increased scapular retraction while the patient performs external rotation strengthening at 90° of abduction with an elastic band.

REFERENCES

1. Warner JJ, Micheli LJ, Arslanian LE, Kennedy J, Kennedy R. Scapulothoracic motion in normal shoulders and shoulders with glenohumeral instability and impingement syndrome: a study using Moiré topographic analysis. *Clin Orthop Relat Res*. 1992;285:191–199.
2. Ludewig PM, Phadke V, Braman JP, Hassett DR, Cieminski CJ, LaPrade RF. Motion of the shoulder complex during multiplanar humeral elevation. *J Bone Joint Surg Am*. 2009;91(2):378–389.
3. McClure PW, Michener LA, Sennett BJ, Karduna AR. Direct 3-dimensional measurement of scapular kinematics during dynamic movements in vivo. *J Shoulder Elbow Surg*. 2001;10(3):269–277.
4. Yoshizaki K, Hamada J, Tamai K, Sahara R, Fujiwara T, Fujimoto T. Analysis of the scapulohumeral rhythm and electromyography of the shoulder muscles during elevation and lowering: comparison of dominant and nondominant shoulders. *J Shoulder Elbow Surg*. 2009;18(5):756–763.
5. Matsuki K, Matsuki KO, Mu S, et al. In vivo 3-dimensional analysis of scapular kinematics: comparison of dominant and nondominant shoulders. *J Shoulder Elbow Surg*. 2011;20(4):659–665.
6. Uhl TL, Kibler WB, Gecewich B, Tripp BL. Evaluation of clinical assessment methods for scapular dyskinesis. *Arthroscopy*. 2009;25(11):1240–1248.
7. Oyama S, Myers JB, Wassinger CA, Daniel Ricci R, Lephart SM. Asymmetric resting scapular posture in healthy overhead athletes. *J Athl Train*. 2008;43(6):565–570.
8. Lukasiewicz AC, McClure P, Michener L, Pratt N, Sennett B. Comparison of 3-dimensional scapular position and orientation between subjects with and without shoulder impingement. *J Orthop Sports Phys Ther*. 1999;29(10):574–586.
9. Ludewig PM, Cook TM. Alterations in shoulder kinematics and associated muscle activity in people with symptoms of shoulder impingement. *Phys Ther*. 2000;80(3):276–291.

10. Endo K, Ikata T, Katoh S, Takeda Y. Radiographic assessment of scapular rotational tilt in chronic shoulder impingement syndrome. *J Orthop Sci*. 2001;6(1):3–10.
11. Ogston JB, Ludewig PM. Differences in 3-dimensional shoulder kinematics between persons with multidirectional instability and asymptomatic controls. *Am J Sports Med*. 2007;35(8):1361–1370.
12. Paletta GA Jr, Warner JJ, Warren RF, Deutsch A, Altchek DW. Shoulder kinematics with two-plane x-ray evaluation in patients with anterior instability or rotator cuff tearing. *J Shoulder Elbow Surg*. 1997;6(6):516–527.
13. Borich MR, Bright JM, Lorello DJ, Cieminski CJ, Buisman T, Ludewig PM. Scapular angular positioning at end range internal rotation in cases of glenohumeral internal rotation deficit. *J Orthop Sports Phys Ther*. 2006;36(12):926–934.
14. Thomas SJ, Swanik KA, Swanik CB, Kelly JD IV. Internal rotation deficits affect scapular positioning in baseball players. *Clin Orthop Relat Res*. 2010;468:1551–1557.
15. Thomas SJ, Swanik KA, Swanik C, Huxel KC, Kelly JD IV. Change in glenohumeral rotation and scapular position after competitive high school baseball. *J Sport Rehabil*. 2010;19(2):125–135.
16. Kibler WB. The role of the scapula in athletic shoulder function. *Am J Sports Med*. 1998;26(2):325–337.
17. Kibler WB, Sciascia A, Dome D. Evaluation of apparent and absolute supraspinatus strength in patients with shoulder injury using the scapular retraction test. *Am J Sports Med*. 2006;34(10):1643–1647.
18. Tate AR, McClure PW, Kareha S, Irwin D. Effect of the Scapula Reposition Test on shoulder impingement symptoms and elevation strength in overhead athletes. *J Orthop Sports Phys Ther*. 2008;38(1):4–11.
19. Caldwell C, Sahrmann S, Van Dillen L. Use of a movement system impairment diagnosis for physical therapy in the management of a patient with shoulder pain. *J Orthop Sports Phys Ther*. 2007;37(9):551–563.
20. Borstad JD, Ludewig PM. The effect of long versus short pectoralis minor resting length on scapular kinematics in healthy individuals. *J Orthop Sports Phys Ther*. 2005;35(4):227–238.
21. Borstad JD. Measurement of pectoralis minor muscle length: validation and clinical application. *J Orthop Sports Phys Ther*. 2008;38(4):169–174.
22. Sahrmann SA. *Diagnosis and Treatment of Movement Impairment Syndromes*. St Louis, MO: Mosby; 2002.
23. Muraki T, Aoki M, Izumi T, Fujii M, Hidaka E, Miyamoto S. Lengthening of the pectoralis minor muscle during passive shoulder motions and stretching techniques: a cadaveric biomechanical study. *Phys Ther*. 2009;89(4):333–341.
24. McQuade KJ, Dawson JD, Smidt GL. Scapulothoracic muscle fatigue associated with alterations in scapulohumeral rhythm kinematics during maximum resistive shoulder elevation. *J Orthop Sports Phys Ther*. 1998;28(2):74–80.
25. Ebaugh DD, McClure PW, Karduna AR. Scapulothoracic and glenohumeral kinematics following an external rotation fatigue protocol. *J Orthop Sports Phys Ther*. 2006;36(8):557–571.
26. Cools AM, Dewitte V, Lanszweert F, et al. Rehabilitation of scapular muscle balance: which exercises to prescribe? *Am J Sports Med*. 2007;35(10):1744–1751.
27. Ludewig PM, Hoff MS, Osowski EE, Meschke SA, Rundquist PJ. Relative balance of serratus anterior and upper trapezius muscle activity during push-up exercises. *Am J Sports Med*. 2004;32(2):484–493.
28. Gaunt BW, McCluskey GM, Uhl TL. An electromyographic evaluation of subdividing active-assistive shoulder elevation exercises. *Sports Health*. 2010;2(5):424–432.
29. Ekstrom RA, Donatelli RA, Soderberg GL. Surface electromyographic analysis of exercises for the trapezius and serratus anterior muscles. *J Orthop Sports Phys Ther*. 2003;33(5):247–258.
30. Moseley JB Jr, Jobe FW, Pink M, Perry J, Tibone J. EMG analysis of the scapular muscles during a shoulder rehabilitation program. *Am J Sports Med*. 1992;20(2):128–134.
31. Smith J, Dietrich CT, Kotajarvi BR, Kaufman KR. The effect of scapular protraction on isometric shoulder rotation strength in normal subjects. *J Shoulder Elbow Surg*. 2006;15(3):339–343.
32. Solem-Bertoft E, Thuomas KA, Westerberg CE. The influence of scapular retraction and protraction on the width of the subacromial space: an MRI study. *Clin Orthop Relat Res*. 1993;296:99–103.
33. Cools AM, Witvrouw EE, Declercq GA, Vanderstraeten GG, Cambier DC. Evaluation of isokinetic force production and associated muscle activity in the scapular rotators during a protraction-retraction movement in overhead athletes with impingement symptoms. *Br J Sports Med*. 2004;38(1):64–68.
34. Burkhart SS, Morgan CD, Kibler WB. The disabled throwing shoulder: spectrum of pathology part III. The SICK scapula, scapular dyskinesis, the kinetic chain, and rehabilitation. *Arthroscopy*. 2003;19(6):641–661.
35. Weiser WM, Lee TQ, McMaster WC, McMahon PJ. Effects of simulated scapular protraction on anterior glenohumeral stability. *Am J Sports Med*. 1999;27(6):801–805.

Rehabilitation of the Cervical Spine in Relationship With the Shoulder

Thomas Boers, PT, MT

Today's medical profession is increasingly specialized, and this movement to specialize has affected the rehabilitation provider. Specialization by orthopaedic surgeons and rehabilitation providers in the treatment of shoulder disorders has had a positive effect on the technological advancement of surgical procedures and rehabilitation approaches.

Shoulder pain is complex; the anatomic structures involve not only the shoulder, but also the cervical spine. The scapular stabilizers (Figure 1), such as the trapezius, levator scapulae, and rhomboids, have origins at the cervical and thoracic spine. Although any of these areas could be involved in shoulder pain, the cervical spine is the most overlooked area when shoulder surgeons and rehabilitation providers evaluate shoulder pain. Spine specialists, neurosurgeons, and orthopaedic surgeons typically are trained to recognize the problems of the spine, including herniated nucleus pulposus, spinal stenosis, and other degenerative problems that can cause impingement on the neural structures and might require operative treatment. Authors of almost all spine-related articles have stated that 80% of the spinal problems are undiagnosed. Many of those undiagnosed problems are mechanical facet dysfunctions. Spine specialists typically do not evaluate segmentally the range of motion of the facet joints. The task of evaluating the range of motion of the cervical spine lies much more on the path of a specifically trained physical therapist (manual therapist).

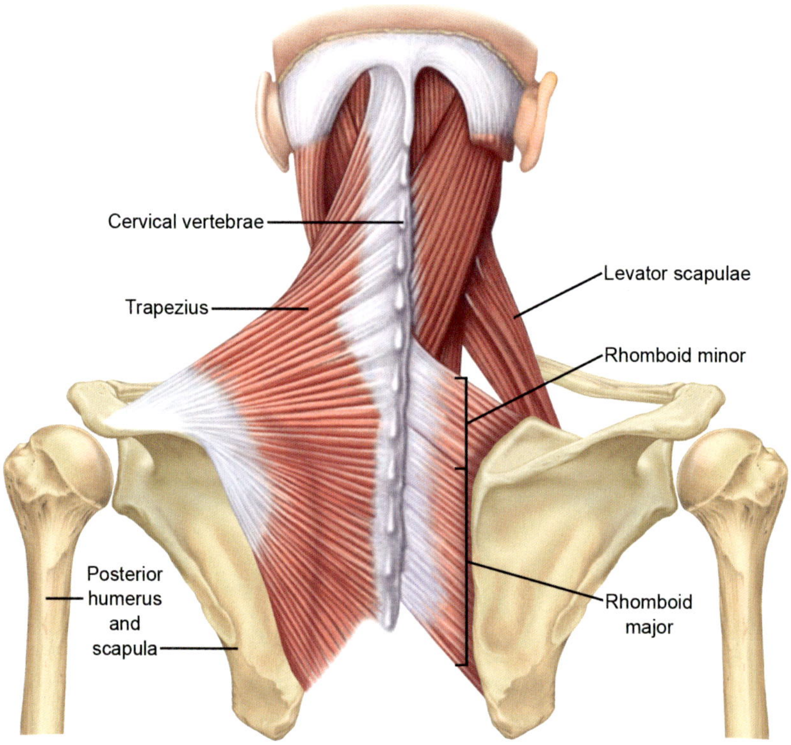

Figure 1. Scapular stabilizers.

The cause of shoulder disorders can be multifactoral. Segmental examination of the facet joints in the cervical and thoracic spine is often absent from the evaluation. The attitude of "what we do not know or what we cannot see (eg, with magnetic resonance imaging or computed tomography scans) does not exist" can limit the diagnosis and prolong the rehabilitation process. In this article, I only highlight the orthopaedic evaluation of the cervical facet joints.

The cervical spine includes 2 separate areas: (1) upper cervical spine, including the atlanto-occipital and atlantoaxial junction, and (2) lower cervical spine, including the C2 inferior facet to T4. The upper cervical junction has no disc-bearing junction. The ranges of motion are flexion, extension, lateral side-bending, and rotation. Flexion and extension roughly are divided evenly between C0-C1 and C1-C2. Lateral side-bending occurs mainly in the C0-C1 junction, and rotation is much

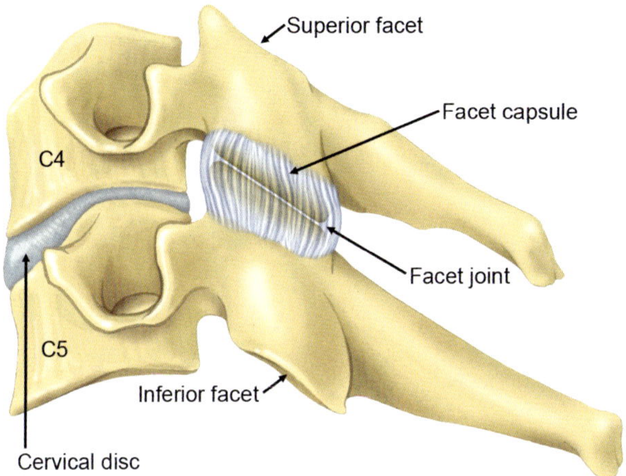

Figure 2. Cervical facet joint.

more dominant in the C1-C2 junction. In combination, the C0-C1-C2 has 3-dimensional (3-D) function and has some similarities to the combined function of the ankle joint and the subtalar joint. This construction provides excellent 3-D range of motion with adequate stabilization and without major muscle mass. The excellent motion of the upper cervical spine makes it vulnerable to dysfunction.

The lower cervical spine has all disc-bearing junctions and has a 3-D function in all segments (Figure 2). The function in these zygoapophyseal joints is limited to approximately 4° to 6° per segment. This is probably the main obstacle to segmental evaluation. The lower cervical spine, especially the C5-C6-C7 segments, develop the most substantial degenerative changes. These changes typically occur because of static pressure that is poorly tolerated by cartilage and disc-type structures. The degenerative processes (spurs, disc-space narrowing, uncovertebral arthrosis) are seen as restabilization activities and, therefore, are not necessarily abnormal unless they interfere with nerve tissue.

The symptoms accompanying cervical dysfunction and shoulder pain can overlap. Typically, the patient has a combination of muscle and joint pain with or without referred or radicular pain. The superomedial border of the scapula is often a painful site in both cervical and shoulder dysfunction. Cervical dysfunction often is accompanied by a hypertone levator scapulae, trapezius, splenius, etc, that elevates the scapula and negatively affects shoulder function. Recognizing and resolving the cervical dysfunction and, therefore, normalizing the muscle tone, could be a valuable part of rehabilitating the patient with shoulder dysfunction.

A patient with mechanical dysfunction in the spine demonstrates a protective reflex. Wyke[1] described this reflex mechanism that is based on Hilton's Law. Overloaded zygoapophyseal joints (ie, capsule) are protected by the stabilizing activity of the muscles in that area, causing stiffness. Compensation for the loss of function occurs in other areas. This can explain the variety of areas of pain depending on where the compensation occurs. For example, a forward head position is typically a compensation to avoid upper cervical rotation. Patients who have substantial degenerative changes in the lower cervical segments might have difficulty using that area to compensate for the loss of rotation in the upper cervical spine. Pain and inflammation might result. In this instance, pain in the distribution of the lower cervical spine (C5-C6-C7) actually results from stiffness in C1-C2.

Evaluating the cervical spine can be challenging because the zygoapophyseal joints are asymmetrical and the spine has multidirectional curves (Figures 3A and 3B). The rotation of the neck, therefore, is not necessarily symmetrical to the right and left. The mechanical evaluation assesses segmentally the function of the zygoapophyseal joints in a 3-D fashion. Normal facet range is recognized by end-point feel, which should be without muscle interference. The protective reflex (arthrokinematic reflex) causing a limitation

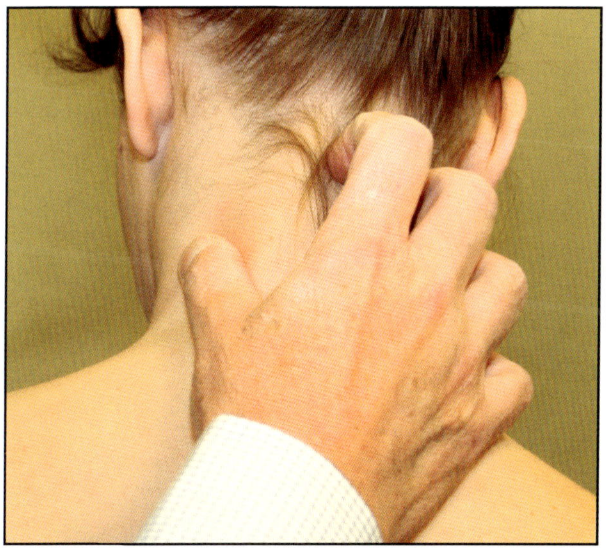

Figure 3A. Manual muscle testing of the cervical spine in flexion.

in the facet joint indicates dysfunction. The cervical dysfunction can be treated effectively by a specifically directed manual technique of the involved segment or segments to restore the lost function. Resolving the reflex mechanism results in instantaneous recovery of full range of motion of the involved facet joint. The patient should maintain the cervical range of motion with specific exercises.

In conclusion, cervical evaluation by a specifically trained physical therapist could help the orthopaedic surgeon and the shoulder rehabilitation provider more efficiently treat patients with shoulder dysfunction. The specific manual techniques instantly resolve arthrokinematic reflex without the use of force (high-velocity thrust manipulation). They have been shown to be safe and have been used for more than 25 years. The manual techniques to examine and treat the facet are a logical consequence based on anatomy and current biomechanical data.

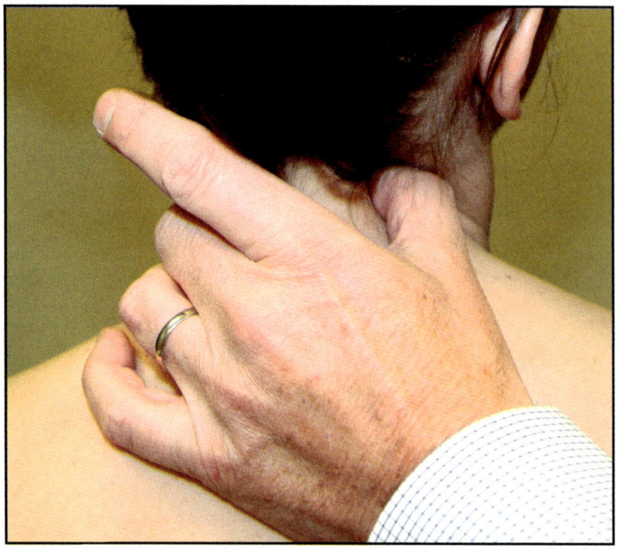

Figure 3B. Manual muscle testing of the cervical spine in extension.

REFERENCES

1. Wyke B. The neurology of joints. *Ann R Coll Surg Engl*. 1967;41(1):25–50.

IV-4

Modified Weight-Training Program

Joseph H. Kostuch, PT, SCS

CHAPTER CONTENTS

Clinical pearls are highlighted in yellow throughout the text.

For many patients, a full return to their preinjury levels of function includes working back to a weight-training routine. This step might be their final goal or the last step in reaching a full return to their previous sport or occupational demands. The weight-training program is an important piece of the strengthening puzzle. Rehabilitation providers must have a working knowledge of weight-training exercises so they safely can educate their patients as they initiate the program. In this chapter, I provide the groundwork and basic science behind an upper extremity weight-training program after shoulder injury or surgery and provide suggested exercises.

APPROPRIATE PATIENT SELECTION

Some patients have weight-training experience, and some do not. Experienced patients might have superior body awareness and might express their limitations and variables clearly. With their experience, however, they can have poor pre-existing exercise technique and a tendency to revert back too quickly to a preinjury training level with certain types and intensities of exercise. Patients who have no weight-training experience can be receptive to the correct technique from the start and might be more willing than experienced patients to adhere to a rehabilitation provider's guidelines. However, these inexperienced patients can have decreased or poor body awareness, difficulty differentiating between pain and muscle soreness, and a tendency to train too much or too little because of poor body awareness. The rehabilitation provider must account for all of these variables in the planning stages of a weight-training program to ensure a successful outcome.

WHEN IS IT SAFE TO INITIATE?

Before initiating a weight-training program after shoulder injury or surgery, allow the patient's tissues ample time to heal and mature. In addition, the referring physician should be consulted about the appropriate timing for a weight-training program. With this in mind, gradually integrate different areas of the body into the weight-training program. Begin with the legs and trunk. To decrease recruitment of the shoulder muscles, add the back and arms next, then add the chest and shoulders. These patients must have adequate flexibility and strength to initiate a weight-training program for the upper extremity. Range of motion in the affected extremity must equal range of motion in the unaffected extremity in all ranges, including any limited joint mobility that is more likely to predispose the patient to injury. The rehabilitation provider specifically should assess external rotation at 90° of abduction, internal rotation with extension, and horizontal abduction and adduction. Patients must demonstrate 5/5 strength on manual muscle testing of the rotator cuff muscles along with appropriate endurance. They also must be able to tolerate closed kinetic chain (CKC) activities and must have adequate overhead strength. This CKC tolerance can be assessed by following a push-up progression. Patients progress from performing push-ups against the wall to push-ups against a table or counter, to push-ups on their knees, and to full push-ups on their toes (Figure 1). The rehabilitation provider can assess overhead strength by having the patient perform a dumbbell press for overhead shoulder strength with a weight proportional to his or her body size.

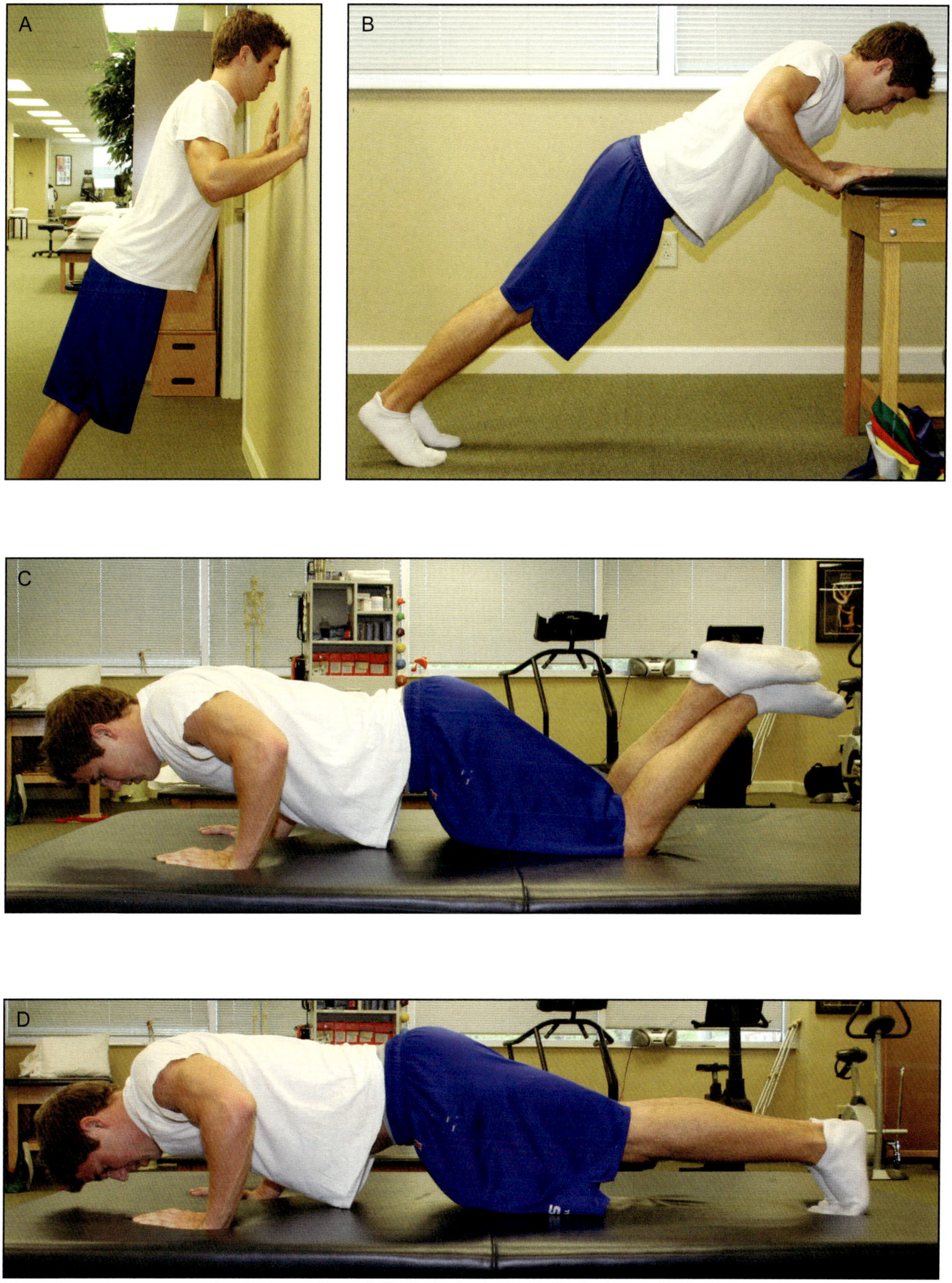

Figure 1. Push-up progression. A, Against a wall. B, Against a table. C, On the knees. D, On the toes.

EQUIPMENT SELECTION

With all weight training, either weight machines or free weights are used. The advantages of using weight machines include increased safety because of built-in range-of-motion stops; preset arc of motion that eliminates patients creating their own exercises; built-in spotter, which is safer initially; better isolation of a specific muscle group; and ease of use because they have a pin weight selector and multiple adjustments for seat, upper extremity, and lower extremity positions. The disadvantages of weight machines include fair replication of the natural strength curve and universal fit that does not fit every body type. With their advantages, weight machines can be a good initial option for inexperienced patients.

Using free weights also carries advantages and disadvantages. They provide more muscle recruitment with less external stabilization than weight machines provide. The smaller stabilizing muscles can help control the proximal joints. They also are more functional because the patient strengthens movements rather than just specific muscle groups. Muscles are recruited at multiple joints, and proximal muscles and the trunk are stabilized. However, more freedom of movement enables initiation of multiple substitution patterns from the trunk or proximal muscle groups. In addition, momentum or inertia can decrease the work of the targeted muscle group. Free weights might be a better option for the later stages of weight training or for patients who have previous weight-training experience.

PROGRAM DESIGN

When discussing the specific points of a weight-training program, introduce periodization to the patient. *Periodization* is the principle of gradual cycling of specificity, intensity, and volume of training to achieve peak levels of fitness for competition. During these phases, the weight-training methods change to reflect specific periods of training, which include the off season, preseason, and in season. When initiating the upper extremity weight-training program after a shoulder injury or surgery, patients will enter the preparatory phase of off-season training. In addition, early in the planning phases, the rehabilitation needs to develop the end goal and set realistic timeframes in which those training goals can be achieved.

When designing a specific program, teach patients that exercise order plays an important role. Active warm-up and stretching must be performed before beginning a training session. This can consist of using an upper body bicycle for a few minutes along with performing 1 set of light resistance rotator cuff exercises. Next, patients perform the more difficult exercises first in the routine because their muscles are the most rested. They also perform multiple-joint exercises before single-joint exercises, enabling the more complex patterns of movements to occur with rested muscles. For example, patients perform a cable row, which includes the scapula, shoulder, and elbow joints, before a biceps curl, which includes the elbow joint only. Initially, patients need to avoid advanced training techniques, such as supersetting, compound setting, or pre-exhaustion training. These advanced training techniques could prematurely fatigue the muscles and increase the risk of injury regardless of the patient's weight-training history. Circuit training initially is acceptable because this technique trains alternating muscle groups and provides a built-in rest time for the muscle previously worked.

Selecting Mode of Training

A patient's specific goals will also help dictate the mode of exercise used. Three basic modes of weight training include increasing strength, increasing size, and increasing endurance. To increase strength, patients use heavy weights to perform a small number of repetitions and include high rest (from 2 to 4 minutes between sets). To increase size, they use medium weights to perform a large number of repetitions and include medium rest (2 minutes between sets). To increase endurance, they use light weights to perform a large number of repetitions and include low rest (less than 1 minute between sets). Most general-fitness patients use a combination of the 3 modes. A sport-specific training program focuses on increasing strength and endurance. When initiating a weight-training program, explain the Specific Adaptation to Imposed Demands (or SAID) principle. It states that the type of demand placed on the body controls the type of adaptation that occurs.[1] That is, if you want to jump higher, practice jumping. Patients need to train the body for what they want it to do. This again emphasizes the importance of having specific and predetermined training goals in place.

Frequency, Duration, and Intensity

When discussing the frequency of weight training, teach patients that optimal results from early strength training are obtained from incorporating a minimum of 1 day of rest between sessions in which the same muscle group is worked. This concept is different for patients who typically during rehabilitation exercised at least 1 to 2 times each day. Teach them that as the intensity of the exercises increases, the rest time becomes just as important as the training itself. Training the same muscle group at higher intensity 2 to 3 days each week has been shown to yield the best results. In addition, early strength training increases damage to the muscle-tendon unit because of the eccentric load, so patients will need more rest to perform optimally.

The goal of the preparatory phase of training is to develop a strength and endurance foundation. Patients use lighter weights and a larger number of repetitions, working to achieve 3 to 4 sets of 12 to 15 repetitions. The ideal speed is to maintain a 6-second cycle for each repetition and an overall timeframe of 50 to 70 seconds for each exercise set because the muscles train anaerobically at this speed. Patients should continue this phase for as long as possible to develop a strong foundation for advanced strengthening.

EXERCISE SELECTION

I describe a 3-tiered system of exercise selection (Table). The first tier includes green-light exercises, which are safe to perform early in a weight-training program with minimal precautions (Figure 2). The second tier of exercises includes yellow-light exercises, which can be performed cautiously in later, more advanced stages of the program after a baseline level of strength has been achieved without experiencing any problems with the program. These exercises are mechanically safe but must be performed with strict limitations. In addition, they might not be safe to perform until 3 to 6 months after the weight-training program begins. These yellow-light exercises might put the patient at risk for injury, and this risk often outweighs the benefits of a specific exercise. The third tier includes red-light exercises, which should be avoided indefinitely for any patient who has had a shoulder injury or surgery (Figure 3).

Exercise Movements to Avoid

Although the reasons vary slightly depending on the exercise, several exercises or movements are too demanding for the shoulder and should be avoided indefinitely. Any exercise movement performed in an impingement position places undue stress on the shoulder, restricts blood flow within the rotator cuff, and mechanically pinches the rotator cuff. These positions generally include any movement in the frontal plane (abduction) of the body or any movement in the sagittal plane accompanied by internal rotation.

Any weighted or resisted movement into excessive humeral extension beyond the plane of the body should be avoided. This includes both concentric and eccentric movements. This position places abnormally high loads through the static anterior restraints, including the capsular complex, labrum, and biceps attachment. It also places the rotator cuff muscles on a severe stretch. The stretch creates a poor length-tension relationship for the cuff and, therefore, makes stabilizing the humeral head very difficult. Because of this mechanical disadvantage, the rotator cuff has to work excessively hard, which can leave it prone to a strain or tearing injury. With the cuff unable to adequately stabilize the humeral head, the anterior translation of the humeral head shifts an abnormally high load though the anterior static restraints, thus also making them susceptible to injury. These specific exercises are labeled as red-light exercises in the Table and should be avoided indefinitely.

Cardiovascular, Lower Extremity, and Core Exercises

Cardiovascular exercise initially also is limited after shoulder injury or surgery. Because of both the jarring and repetitive (although unweighted) upper extremity movements that occur with this cardiovascular exercise, patients do not tolerate these movements well, and they are generally unsafe for the healing shoulder. A patient's ability to safely advance into the base strengthening program also should allow safe initiation into cardiovascular exercise. The intensity of these workouts needs to be monitored to ensure the patient's comfort.

Table. The 3-Tiered System of Exercises for an Upper Extremity Weight-Training Program After Shoulder Injury[a]

Body Area	Exercises		
	Green Light	Yellow Light	Red Light
Back	Rows with a narrow or a neutral grip on a weight machine (**A**), with a pulley (**A**), or bent over with dumbbells (**B**)	Pull-ups with the bar grip anterior to the head	Lateral pull-downs or lateral pull-ups performed behind the neck (**A**)
	Lateral pull-downs from anterior to the head with a machine or pulley (**C**)		
Upper extremities	Standing curls with barbells, dumbbells, or pulley (**A**)	Preacher curls with weight machine, barbells, or dumbbells	Dips with body mass or on a weight machine (**A**)
	Triceps extensions (**B**)	Overhead triceps press	
	Triceps kickbacks with a pulley or a free weight (**C**)		
Shoulders	Overhead press in front of the head with a neutral grip and the humeral angle remaining in scaption, progressing from dumbbells to weight machines and to barbells (**A**)	Deltoid raises to the front or side with very light weight and the extremity below the shoulder level	Upright rows (**A**)
	Shrugs with a dumbbell or barbell (**B**)	Reverse flies with the elbow in front of the body	Overhead press behind the neck (**B**)
	Deltoid raises in a position of scaption with the weight below the shoulder level (**C**)		
Chest	Push-up progression from wall to table, to knees, and to toes (**Figure 1**)	Flys initiated on weight machines and progressed to dumbbells or pulleys with the position of the extremity not extending beyond the plane of the body	Decline chest press (**A**)
	Chest press on an incline or flat bench with weight machines, barbells, or dumbbells (**A, B**)		Dips

[a] Letters in parentheses refer to the lettered parts of the corresponding color-coded areas of Figures 2 and 3.

Modified Weight-Training Program

Figure 2. Green-light exercises. Letters refer to the descriptions of green-light exercises provided in the Table.

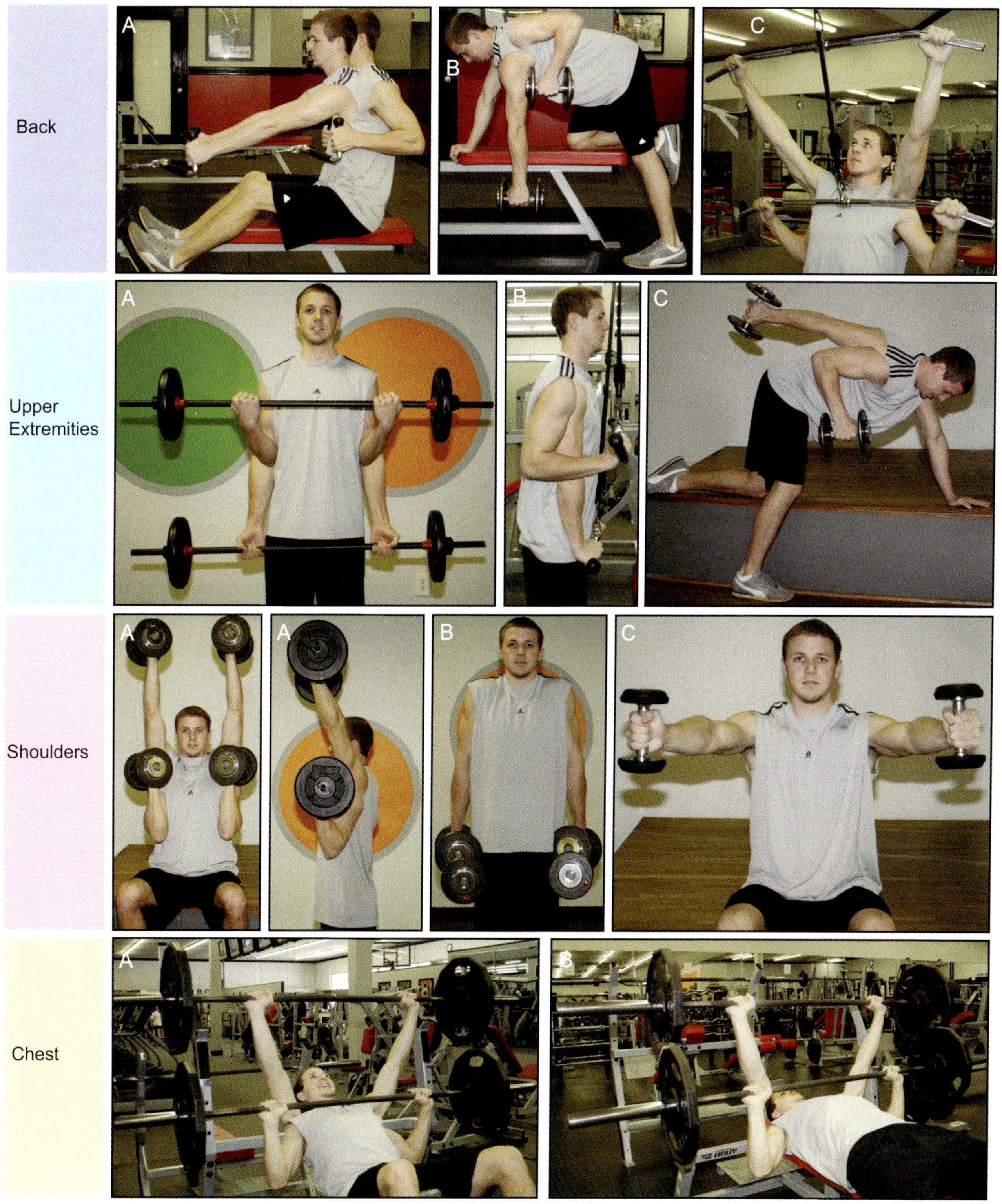

Figure 3. Red-light exercises. Letters refer to the descriptions of red-light exercises provided in the Table.

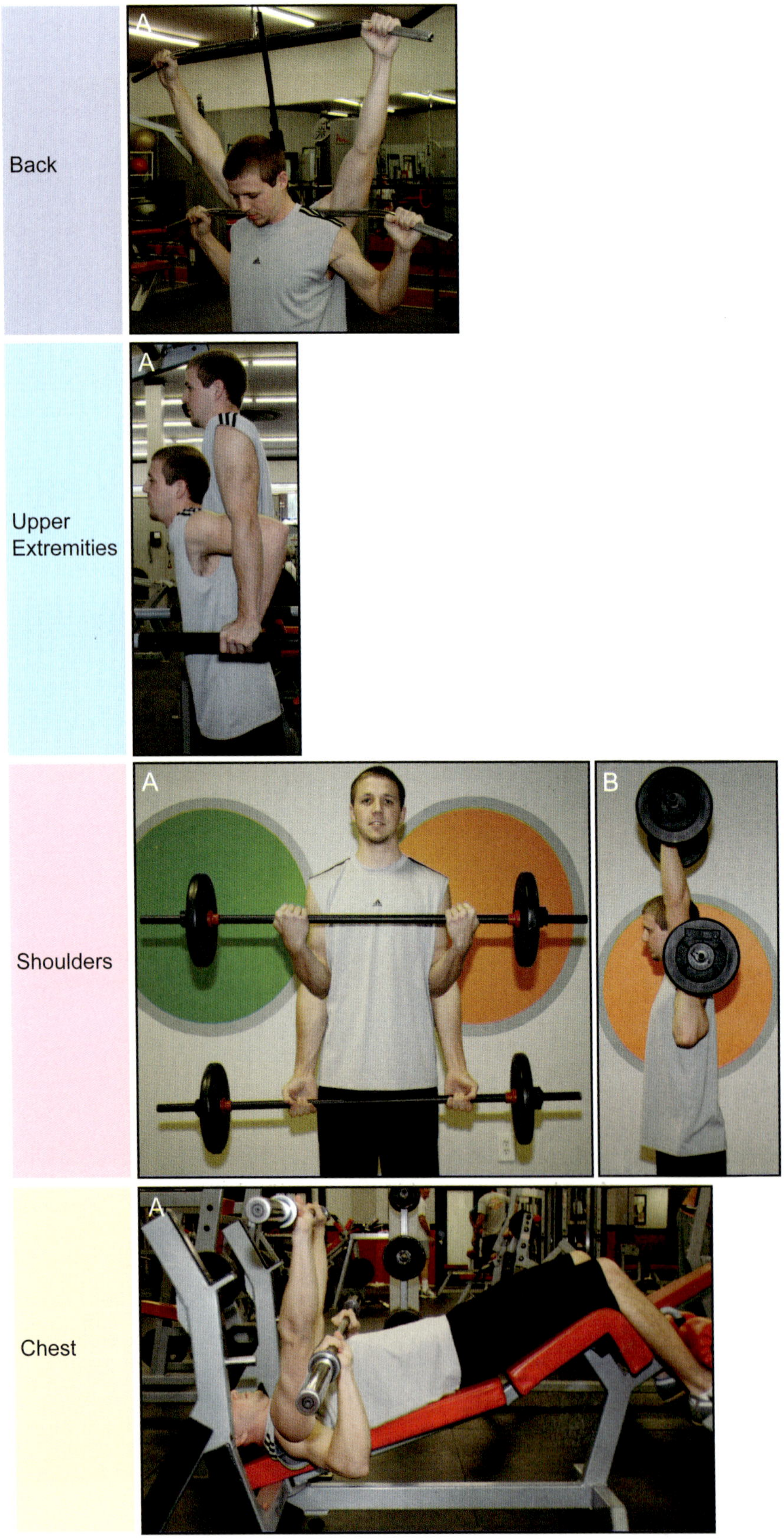

Lower extremity and core exercises also must be limited initially. When comfortable active range of motion has been achieved, most lower extremity exercises can be introduced, with the exception of squats or leg presses. These 2 exercises place increased pressure on the shoulder because of the set-up and placement of the weight directly on the shoulder. In addition, holding any weights for resistance during a lower extremity or core exercise is not permitted initially. When performing both core and lower body exercises, a strong isometric shoulder contraction often occurs to help stabilize the body. The intensity of this contraction can be damaging; therefore, lower extremity and core exercises also must be started at very low intensity. Focus needs to be placed on technique and muscle recruitment rather than on heavy weights or exhaustion training.

Warm-Up Exercises

Before starting shoulder exercises, the patients must warm up the shoulders by doing light rotator cuff exercises along with some specific stretching. These rotator cuff exercises warm up, but do not fatigue, the muscle group. Patients use a very light weight (10–20% of maximum) and perform 1 set of a large number of repetitions. The stretching includes primarily the posterior capsule of the shoulder, which can be addressed by either the sleeper stretch or the cross-body stretch.

Modified Weight-Training Program

In conclusion, the rehabilitation provider has many factors to consider when prescribing an upper extremity weight-training program after shoulder injury or surgery. Some important items to address include previous weight-training experience, access to equipment, and training goals and timeframes. By appropriately addressing these issues, the rehabilitation provider can better ensure a safe return to the weight room and a step closer to the patient's functional goals.

REFERENCE

1. Fleck SJ, Kraemer WJ. *Designing Resistance Training Programs*. Champaign, IL: Human Kinetics; 1987.

RECOMMENDED READING

Baechle TR, Earle RW, eds. *Essentials of Strength and Conditioning*. Champaign, IL: Human Kinetics; 1994:345–401.

Braith RW, Graves JE, Pollock ML, Leggett SL, Carpenter DM, Colven AB. Comparison of 2 vs 3 days/week of variable resistance training during 10- and 18-week programs. *Int J Sports Med*. 1989;10(6):450–454.

Chargina A, Stone M, Piedmonte J, et al. Periodization roundtable. *NSCA Journal*. 1986;8(5):12–23.

Garhammer J. Weight lifting and training. In: Vaughn CL, ed. *Biomechanics of Sport*. Boca Raton, FL: CRC Press; 1989:169–212.

Harman E. Resistive torque analysis of 5 Nautilus exercise machines. *Med Sci Sports Exerc*. 1983;15(2):113.

Johnson JH, Colodny S, Jackson D. Human torque capability versus machine resistive torque for four Eagle resistance machines. *J Appl Sport Sci Res*. 1990;4(3):83–87.

Lander JE, Bates BT, Sawhill JA, Hamill J. A comparison between free-weight and isokinetic bench pressing. *Med Sci Sports Exerc*. 1985;17(3):344–353.

IV-5

Arm Care Exercises for Youth Baseball

Kevin G. Laudner, PhD, ATC, FACSM

CHAPTER CONTENTS

- Warm-up
- Stretching guidelines
- Shoulder and elbow stretches
- Strengthening guidelines
- Shoulder and elbow strengthening guidelines
- Sensorimotor training
- Plyometric training
- Other considerations
- Cool-down

Clinical pearls are highlighted in yellow throughout the text.

Millions of youths annually participate in organized baseball. With the increased occurrence of year-round participation, it is not surprising that injury rates among these athletes have increased steadily.[1] Approximately 15% of game appearances by youth baseball pitchers result in shoulder or elbow pain, and 50% of youth pitchers report shoulder or elbow pain at some point during the competitive baseball season.[2]

Throwing a baseball is one of the most physically demanding athletic motions. This motion places a tremendous amount of force on the throwing shoulder and elbow,[3] often resulting in altered range of motion.[4] The accumulation of such forces among youth athletes can be devastating because of their skeletal and structural immaturity. Therefore, baseball players must have good flexibility and muscular endurance to help elicit proper biomechanics, elevate performance, and decrease the risk of injury. As such, stretching and strengthening exercises aimed at soft tissue lengthening and increasing dynamic stability, respectively, should be incorporated into any baseball player's physical training routine. When an appropriate level of these characteristics has been obtained, the program should be continued with maintenance as the goal.

Although baseball is primarily a unilateral upper extremity sport, performing the following stretching and strengthening exercises bilaterally can be beneficial. This bilateral focus will maintain equilibrium in muscle size and tone between sides, thereby minimizing any asymmetries that can lead to dysfunction. To limit any increases in duration of the arm care exercises by adding the nonthrowing side, athletes should be encouraged to perform the stretching and strengthening exercises for the nonthrowing arm during the rest periods of the throwing arm.

WARM-UP

A warm-up activity should be performed before any stretching and strengthening exercises. The warm-up is designed to bring oxygenated blood to specific areas of the body that will be stressed during the primary workout.

When focusing on arm care exercises, an appropriate warm-up should include exercises involving the upper extremity, such as jumping rope, use of an upper body ergometer, or upper extremity exercises with light resistance tubing.[5] However, if preferred, an athlete can complete a warm-up that does not specifically involve the upper extremity, such as jogging or stationary bicycling, and can still receive some of the same benefits as those of an upper extremity activity, but this might not be as effective.

Regardless of the activity chosen, the warm-up should be performed at a level of intensity high enough to elicit perspiration and an elevated heart rate (70–85% of maximum heart rate) or a feeling of being "out of breath." The duration of the warm-up is generally 10 to 15 minutes.

STRETCHING GUIDELINES

Immediately after completing the warm-up, the athlete should stretch to maximize the benefits for the muscles being stretched. Benefits include increased tissue temperature, elasticity, and extensibility of various soft tissue structures, such as muscle, tendon, ligament, and capsule.

Stretching can be performed daily and should be conducted without pain. Painful stretching indicates soft tissue trauma and should always be avoided. Rather, a gentle, comfortable stretch should be sustained for approximately 15 to 30 seconds for 3 or 4 sets.

The type of stretch used can be determined by the resources of the athlete and the ability to perform techniques with correct form. Strict form should be used during all stretching exercises to avoid injury and maximize gains. Performing any stretch incorrectly can cause serious soft tissue damage and lead to time missed from competition. The following sections include several stretching techniques that should be considered. The athlete should work with a rehabilitation provider to determine which technique is most appropriate for his or her specific characteristics.

Active Stretching

Active stretching involves the synergistic relationship between agonist (contracting) muscle and antagonist (lengthening) muscle. As the agonist muscle contracts or shortens, the antagonist muscle must stretch or lengthen an equal amount. For example, if the goal is to conduct an active stretch for the glenohumeral external rotators, the rehabilitation provider instructs the athlete to contract his or her internal rotators. Moving the glenohumeral joint into internal rotation by shortening the subscapularis subsequently lengthens the external rotators (infraspinatus, teres minor). Because of the contraction of the opposing muscle during active stretching, the muscle to be stretched is relaxed completely, which is known as *reciprocal inhibition*. However, the muscle only can lengthen as far as the shortening capability of the opposing muscle and is a limitation of this type of stretching.

Static Stretching

Static stretching is one of the most popular types of stretching. This stretching technique requires an external force that is applied to a body segment to lengthen a muscle more than an active stretch can. This type of stretching has the benefit of using an external force to produce a good stretch, but complete relaxation of the muscle is not always achieved.

Upon initial stretch of a muscle, the muscle spindles send sensory information to the central nervous system indicating that a stretch is occurring. The initial motor response from the central nervous system to the muscle is to reflexively contract. Therefore, the initial resistance felt during a static stretch is the body's protective mechanism attempting to prevent overstretching and is known as the *stretch reflex*. When a gentle stretch is maintained in a comfortable position for approximately 6 seconds, the initial protective resistance caused by the muscle spindles is overridden by the Golgi tendon organs of the muscle, resulting in relaxation of the muscle[6,7] and allowing for increased lengthening of the desired muscle or muscle group. This sequence of events adds to the benefits of using a gentle and comfortable stretch compared with using a painful stretch.

One of the most effective methods for lengthening soft tissue involves a combination of active and static stretching that is known as *active-assistive stretching*. This technique involves the contraction of the agonist muscle, which causes reciprocal inhibition and relaxation of the antagonist muscle, combined with a static stretch from an external source, allowing for lengthening beyond the shortening capabilities of the agonist. Therefore, this technique of combining active and static stretching provides all the benefits of both stretches without the negative effects.

Ballistic Stretching

Ballistic stretching uses momentum as an external force to increase lengthening of the chosen muscle. This technique is often used by athletes and mimics some of the motions and forces that are produced during a specific sports movement. However, the momentum is difficult, if not impossible, to control and can result in excessive stretching or tearing of the soft tissue. Therefore, ballistic stretching should be used with care or not at all.

Proprioceptive Neuromuscular Facilitation Stretching

Proprioceptive neuromuscular facilitation (PNF) stretching uses a series of contraction and relaxation cycles to elicit a stretch. It includes several variations using different methods of stretching (static, active-assistive) and contracting (isometric, isotonic), but I describe the hold-relax method for simplicity and an easily adaptable technique that an athlete can use without a partner. Begin with a static stretch of the antagonist muscle (15 to 30 seconds) followed by an isometric contraction (hence the term *hold*) then another static stretch (15 to 30 seconds).

The isometric contraction of the hold-relax PNF stretch should be held for approximately 3 to 10 seconds[8] in the middle range of motion rather than at the end range. Conducting the isometric contraction portion of the stretch at the end range of motion may elicit a protective reflex contraction of the muscle being stretched that is similar to the one described during static stretching.

Muscle Energy Technique

The concept and procedures of muscle energy techniques (METs) are similar to PNF and, therefore, often are used interchangeably. Both require a muscular contraction producing a movement in the opposite direction of the stretch followed by a stretch, and both use the reflex muscle relaxation cycle,[9] which immediately follows a muscle contraction, to promote maximum lengthening of the soft tissue. However, METs use strict guidelines regarding the production of force by the athlete.

The isometric contraction produced during an MET is individually based. Determinants of muscle contraction force include the size of the muscle being stretched and the injury status of the athlete.[10] For the purposes of healthy youth baseball players interested in preventative MET, I recommend isometric contractions of approximately 25% of the maximum force that can be produced. I suggest this amount because it is often more comfortable for the athlete, so the likelihood of muscle guarding and pain are reduced. For large muscles, such as the latissimus dorsi, 25% to 50% of maximum force can be used.

When an athlete has been shown how to conduct various PNF and MET stretches and is comfortable with the procedures, he or she should be taught how to perform such stretches without the assistance of a rehabilitation provider. Using external tools, such as a wall or doorway, the resistance provided by the opposite extremity, or resistance straps or tubing, can be very effective. This also allows the athlete to perform the stretches on a regular basis rather than just when a partner is present.

SHOULDER AND ELBOW STRETCHES

Although stretching should be conducted for the upper and lower extremities and for the core, stretching of several specific muscles, which cross the throwing shoulder and elbow, are critical for injury prevention.

Posterior Shoulder Stretches

The deceleration phase of the throwing motion is a major contributor in the development of soft tissue tightness in the posterior aspect of the shoulder. As the humerus internally rotates during the follow-through phase of the throwing motion, the posteroinferior glenohumeral capsule can be placed in a primary location to resist the deceleration forces.[11] Dynamic restraints, such as the posterior deltoid, infraspinatus, teres minor, and latissimus dorsi, work eccentrically to decelerate the humerus during this phase of throwing.[12] The loads placed on these static and dynamic tissues have been linked empirically to soft tissue shortening[11] and subsequent alterations in shoulder range of motion, such as decreased internal rotation, increased tightness in the posterior aspect of the shoulder (limited glenohumeral horizontal adduction),[4] and increased external rotation.[11] Furthermore, tightness in the posterior aspect of the shoulder can alter a player's throwing mechanics, and it has been associated with subacromial impingement,[13] superior labrum anterior-posterior lesions,[14] and internal impingement.[15]

Sleeper Stretch. The sleeper stretch is one of the most common stretches for the posterior aspect of the shoulder that overhead athletes use. It is performed with the athlete in a side-lying position on the side of the upper extremity to be stretched. In this position, the lateral border of the scapula is stabilized, and isolated glenohumeral movement can occur. The shoulder and elbow are placed in 90° of flexion. The opposite hand grasps the distal aspect of the forearm and produces passive internal rotation, moving the extremity toward the treatment table (Figure 1A).

Modified Sleeper Stretch. The sleeper stretch also can be modified to enable increased lengthening of the posterior shoulder. This is accomplished by increasing the amount of glenohumeral horizontal adduction while still applying internal rotation. The increase in glenohumeral horizontal adduction can be achieved by elevating the humerus off the table with folded towels placed under the posterior distal humerus (Figure 1B) or by rotating the athlete's body forward (Figure 1C). This increased stress on structures of the posterior aspect of the shoulder should be incorporated when the traditional sleeper stretch does not elicit the stretch that the athlete initially feels. The sleeper stretch also can be easily modified as an MET or PNF stretch by using resistive force that the opposite extremity provides.

Cross-Body Stretch. Athletes and rehabilitation providers might be inclined to stretch the posterior aspect of the shoulder by simply performing a cross-body stretch or shoulder horizontal adduction. However, the side-lying position of the sleeper stretch stabilizes the scapula against the upper body and the treatment surface, thereby enabling more isolation of the posterior glenohumeral joint. I recommend performing both the cross-body stretch and the sleeper stretch to lengthen the soft tissue structures at the scapulothoracic and glenohumeral articulations.

Pectoralis Major and Minor Stretch

Rounded shoulders is a common postural dysfunction in many overhead athletes, especially baseball players. Although the pectoralis minor is a relatively small muscle and often overlooked, excessive shortening can produce serious scapular dyskinesis, such as increased scapular anterior tilt and internal rotation,[16] as produced with rounded shoulders. Furthermore, this postural deformity and subsequent scapular deviations are often present in patients with various shoulder injuries.[17,18]

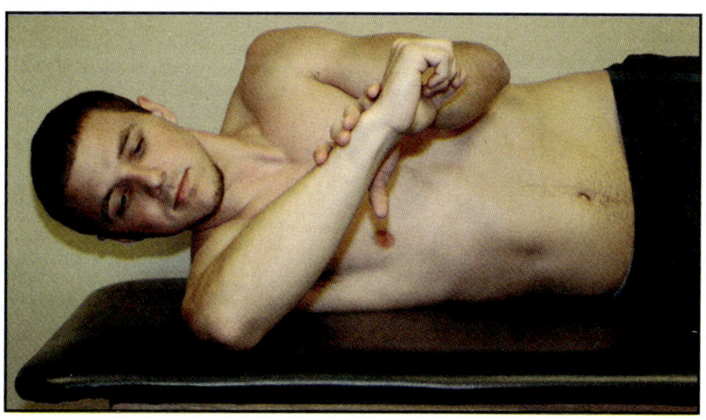

Figure 1A. Sleeper stretch.

Excessive scapular protraction partially might explain the visibly depressed appearance of the dominant shoulder in baseball players. As the scapula protracts, it is essentially abducting, internally rotating, and translating anteriorly along the contours of the thoracic cage, which angles inferiorly. Therefore, the scapula follows this same path inferiorly, leading to a depressed appearance. Because the pectoral muscles frequently are tight among baseball players and because several shoulder injuries are associated with this contracture, I strongly recommend pectoralis minor and major stretching.

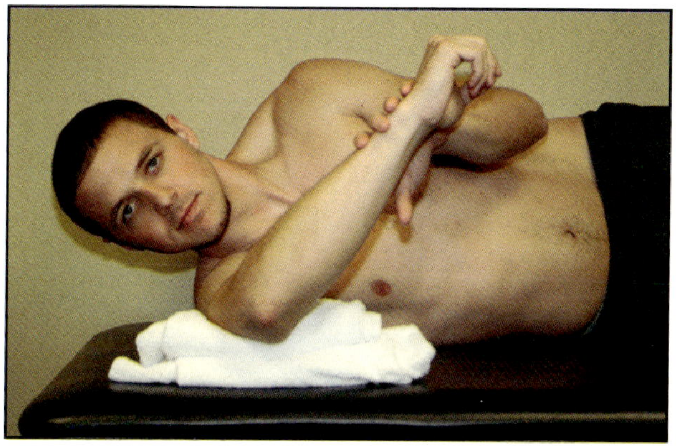

Figure 1B. Modified sleeper stretch. Add towels or a bolster under the distal humerus to increase horizontal adduction.

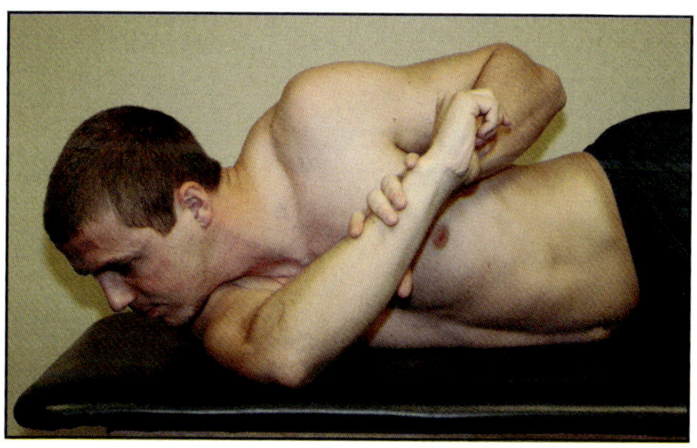

Figure 1C. Modified sleeper stretch. Rotate the body forward to increase horizontal adduction.

Numerous techniques can be used to stretch the pectoral muscles, and each technique generally produces the same motion using different variations and aides, such as a doorway or assistance from a partner. A chair is used to perform 1 stretch in this category and is very effective. For this stretch, the athlete sits in a chair and places his or her extremities over the back of the chair so the shoulders are in an extended position. Sometimes, it is advantageous for the athlete to grasp the opposite hand behind the chair. Placing the extremities behind the chair stabilizes the scapula for the pectoralis minor and the humerus for the pectoralis major. Next, the athlete gently leans forward with the trunk, pulling the thorax away from the scapula and humerus to stretch both muscles (Figure 2). This technique also lengthens the anterior deltoid, which plays a large role in the development of subacromial impingement when it is tight. The stretch also can be performed with the extremities over the top of a bench or a fence while standing, so it can be adapted easily for use at a baseball field.

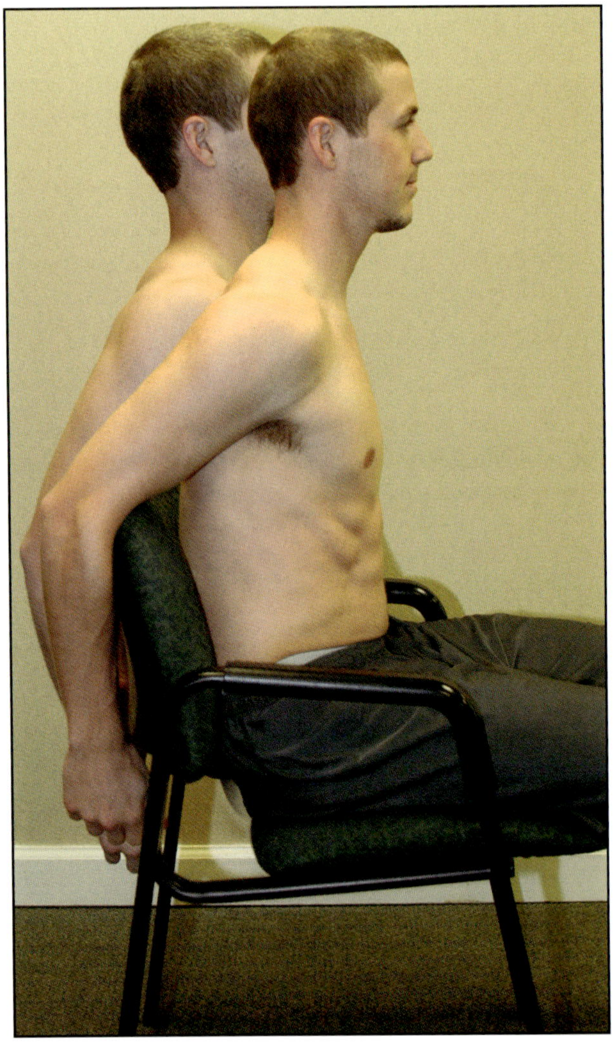

Figure 2. Pectoralis major and minor stretch.

Wrist Flexors Stretch

To stretch the wrist flexor muscles, a simple movement of passive wrist extension is sufficient. The athlete should be in a position of elbow extension, wrist supination and extension, and extension of the digits. Next, he or she uses the opposite hand to grasp the digits of the extremity to be stretched and passively extend the wrist until feeling a comfortable stretch (Figure 3).

STRENGTHENING GUIDELINES

Muscular endurance is necessary among baseball players to promote increased performance through better ball control, improved velocity, and sustained performance over a 2- to 3-hour game and to minimize stress placed on the static restraints. General strength programs should be designed with 2 primary goals. First, choose a program that can be completed in a relatively short time. Longer-duration strengthening programs usually result in athletes using improper form because they are attempting to finish the program or result in decreased interest in the program because of unrealistic time demands. Remember, these exercises are used as a supplement to the athlete's normal time demands of baseball practices and games. Second, choose exercises that promote injury prevention and enhanced athletic performance. If the rehabilitation provider can show athletes how a specific exercise

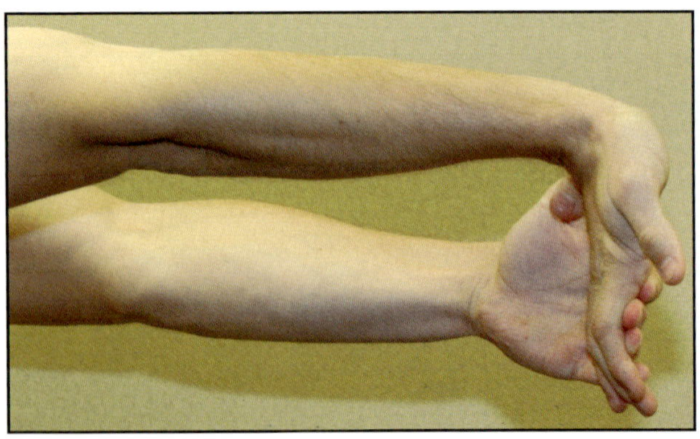

Figure 3. Wrist flexors stretch.

will benefit their baseball skills, they are generally much more likely to participate in the program.

Types of Resistance

Resistance used during exercises can come from several sources. Common resistance methods that baseball players use include movement against gravity, dumbbells, the athlete's body mass, isotonic exercise equipment, and resistive pulley systems. Another commonly used piece of strength equipment is resistance tubing. The athlete can use not only a commercially developed product, but also ordinary surgical tubing that can be purchased at a medical equipment store. Resistance tubing is inexpensive, can be used virtually anywhere, and is relatively safe. However, this equipment varies in the resistive force provided. Much as a rubber band, resistance tubing provides increased resistance as the band lengthens. Therefore, maximum resistance is provided at the end range of motion, and very little resistance is provided in the early ranges of motion. This can result in strengthening in only a portion of the full range of motion. As such, if feasible, choosing resistance equipment that provides equal force through a full range of motion is advantageous.

Muscular Endurance

Because of the repetitive nature of throwing during a baseball game or practice, muscular endurance is extremely important. Muscular fatigue causes altered biomechanics[19] and subsequent increased stress placed on the various restraints of the shoulder and elbow, leading to injury. Therefore, the focus of strengthening exercises in youth baseball players primarily should be on improving or maintaining muscular endurance.

With the primary goal of increasing muscular endurance, the athlete and rehabilitation provider should consider using exercises with a smaller amount of resistance and a larger number of repetitions. For all the exercises described in this section, the athlete should use a resistance that enables him or her to complete approximately 15 to 20 repetitions. Furthermore, these repetitions should be conducted using strict form. Athletes are very resourceful and, when not monitored and educated correctly, often use improper form, recruiting accessory muscles to conduct exercises where the intended muscle or muscle group is weak. Athletes should aim for performing 2 to 3 sets of each exercise with little rest between sets (approximately 30–45 seconds) to further emphasize muscular endurance.

Because of the smaller amount of resistance used during muscular endurance strength training, recovery of the body generally is quicker than recovery with heavier resistance training. Most baseball players can perform these exercises every other day or every 48 hours, if necessary. Strength training should not be conducted before an intense throwing session.

Strength Program Progression

A timed progression of the strengthening program should be strongly discouraged. I routinely hear athletes discuss adding resistance to an exercise on a weekly or biweekly basis regardless of their physical progression. This type of progression can lead to faulty mechanics and overuse injuries. The only progression guideline for strengthening is the physical condition of the athlete. When an athlete can perform all repetitions and sets of a given exercise using correct form and without having pain or delayed-onset muscle soreness, he or she should be allowed to increase the resistance.

SHOULDER AND ELBOW STRENGTHENING GUIDELINES

Exercises for increasing muscular endurance in the youth baseball player should focus on 3 key areas: the glenohumeral joint stabilizers, scapulothoracic joint stabilizers, and medial elbow joint stabilizers. All exercises should be performed at a smooth and controlled pace for both the concentric and eccentric portions of the motion.

Posterior Shoulder Strengthening

Blackburn exercises were developed to strengthen the scapular retractors and posterior rotator cuff muscles.[20] These exercises provide an easy sequence of 6 movements that can be completed in a short period yet hit several key areas of concern, including strengthening of the scapular retractors, shoulder external rotators, horizontal abductors, and extensors. All 6 of these exercises are performed in the prone position. The prone position places the upper extremities in an against-gravity position. Athletes should perform these exercises either against gravity only or with additional resistance, such as light hand weights or resistance tubing. Athletes also can be instructed to include a short pause at the transition between the concentric and eccentric phases to provide further strength gains.

Prone Horizontal Abduction With Neutral Rotation. From the prone position and with the upper extremities hanging toward the ground and in neutral rotation, the athlete horizontally abducts the extremities, squeezing the scapulae together at the end range of motion (Figure 4A).

Prone Horizontal Abduction With External Rotation. From the prone position and with the upper extremities hanging toward the ground and in full shoulder external rotation, the athlete horizontally abducts the extremities, squeezing the scapulae together at the end range of motion (Figure 4B).

Prone Horizontal Scaption With Neutral Rotation. This exercise is performed in the prone position and with the upper extremities hanging toward the ground but in the scapular plane, which is approximately 30° anterior to the frontal plane and in neutral rotation. From this starting position, the athlete horizontally abducts the extremities while maintaining the scapular plane, squeezing the scapulae together at the end range of motion (Figure 4C).

Prone Horizontal Scaption With External Rotation. From the prone position and with the upper extremities hanging toward the ground but in the scapular plane and in shoulder external rotation, the athlete horizontally abducts the extremities while maintaining the scapular plane, squeezing the scapulae together at the end range of motion (Figure 4D).

Prone Horizontal External Rotation. This exercise is performed in the prone position with the shoulders horizontally abducted until in alignment with the athlete's trunk and with the elbows in 90° of flexion. From this starting position, the athlete externally rotates the shoulders until reaching the end range of motion (Figure 4E).

Prone Horizontal Extension. This exercise is performed in the prone position with the athlete's upper extremities hanging toward the ground. From this starting position, the athlete extends the shoulders until reaching the end range of motion (Figure 4F).

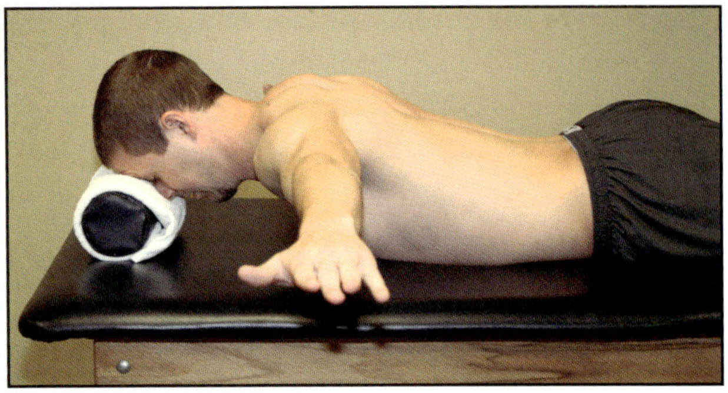

Figure 4A. Prone horizontal abduction with neutral rotation.

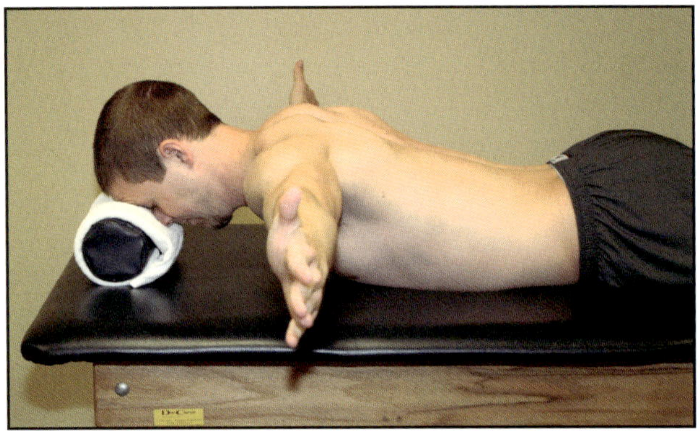

Figure 4B. Prone horizontal abduction with external rotation.

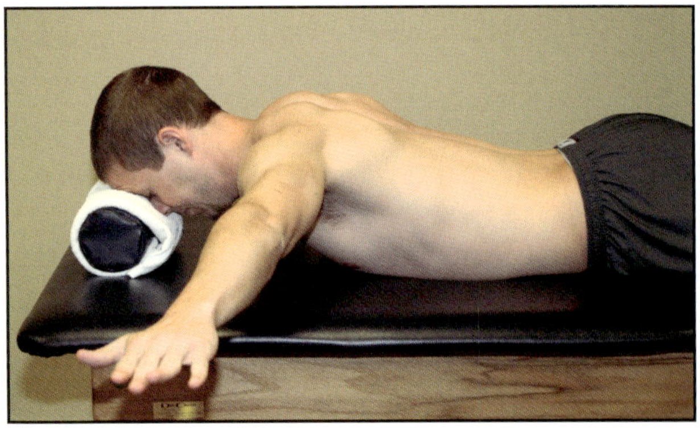

Figure 4C. Prone horizontal scaption with neutral rotation.

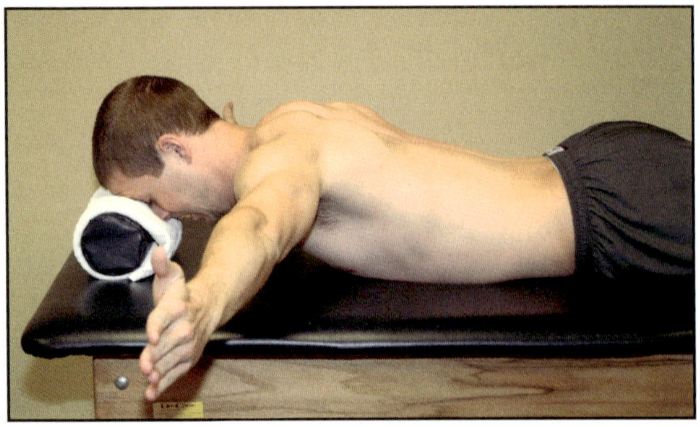

Figure 4D. Prone horizontal scaption with external rotation.

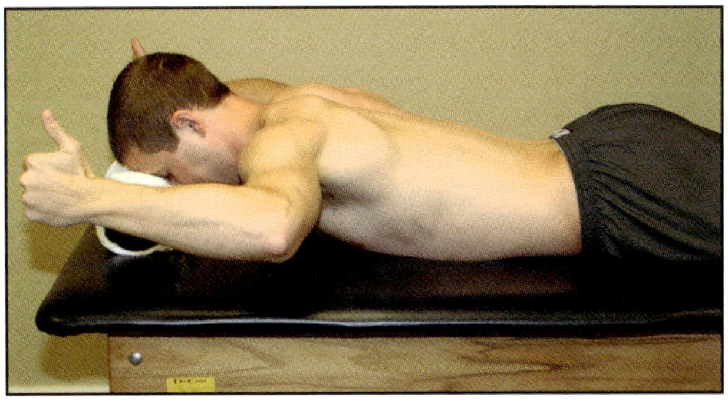

Figure 4E. Prone horizontal external rotation.

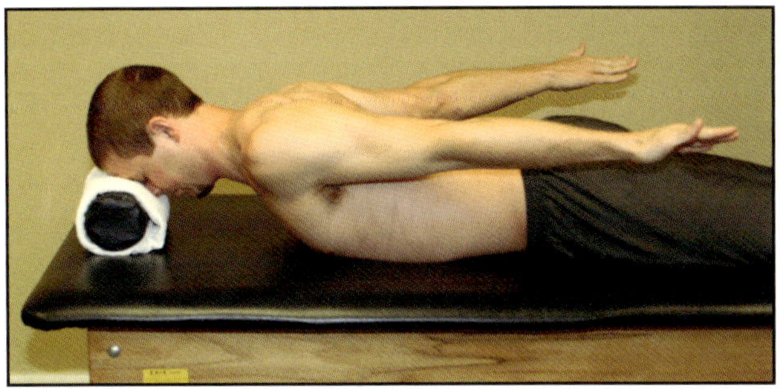

Figure 4F. Prone horizontal extension.

Eccentric Posterior Shoulder Strengthening

To minimize the force placed on the posterior glenohumeral capsule during the deceleration phase of the throwing motion, eccentric strengthening of the shoulder external rotators and horizontal abductors is beneficial.

Over-the-Shoulder Ball Toss. Several methods can be used to strengthen the musculature of the posterior aspect of the shoulder. The first method requires a light medicine ball or a baseball and a partner. Skeletally immature athletes should practice caution when using a medicine ball for this exercise because it places a large force on the shoulder and elbow. To avoid such concerns, use of a baseball or similarly weighted ball might be warranted. The athlete should kneel on 1 knee (throwing side) with the opposite limb in 90° of hip and knee flexion and with the foot flat on the ground. The throwing shoulder initially should be positioned in 90° of shoulder abduction and elbow flexion. The partner stands behind and slightly toward the throwing side of the athlete and softly tosses the ball over the dominant shoulder of the athlete. The athlete must catch the ball while eccentrically controlling the motion as the weight and momentum of the ball bring his or her shoulder into internal rotation and horizontal adduction (Figure 5). This exercise attempts to repli-

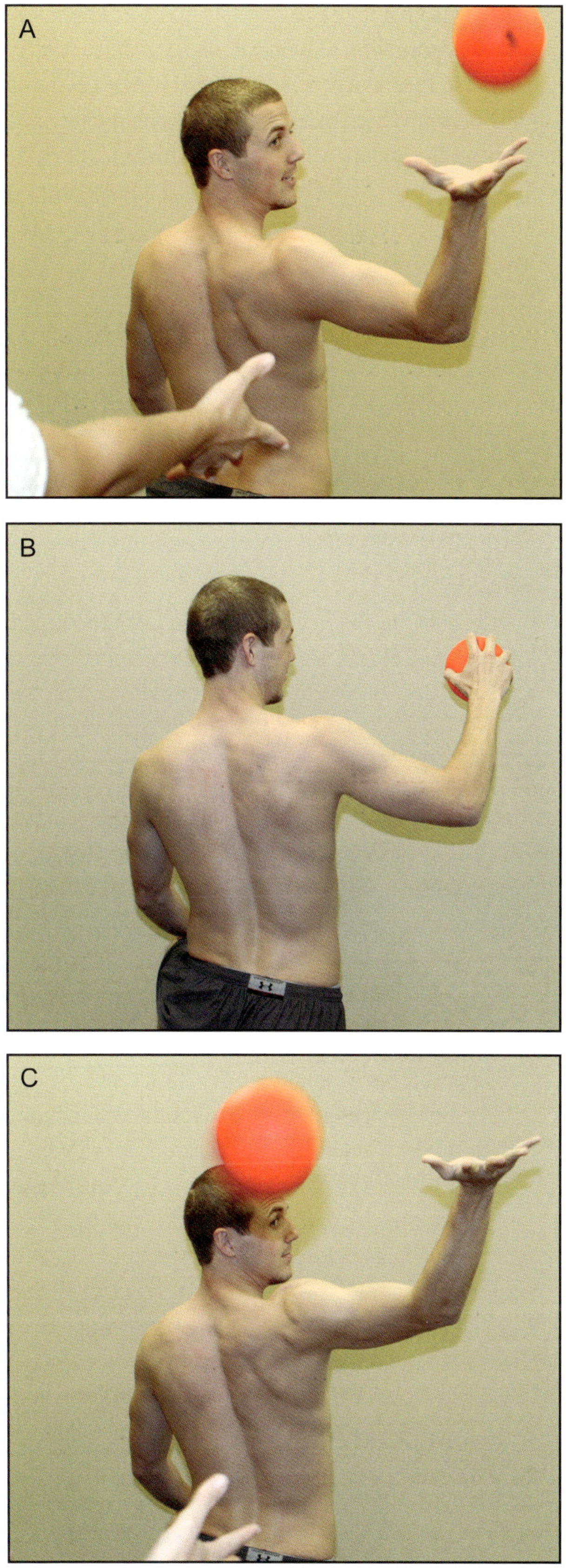

Figure 5 A–C. Over-the-shoulder ball toss to strengthen the posterior aspect of the shoulder.

cate the motion of the shoulder during the deceleration phase of the throwing sequence (chapter IV-6) and, therefore, mimics the eccentric control necessary during this phase. When the upper extremity has ceased movement, the athlete can reverse the motion (external rotation and horizontal abduction), working the same muscles concentrically as the ball is tossed behind him or her to the partner.

Throwing Deceleration Exercise. The second technique for eccentric strengthening the muscles of the posterior aspect of the shoulder mimics the over-the-shoulder ball toss, but it can be performed without a partner and requires either resistance tubing or a pulley system. For simplicity, I describe this exercise using resistance tubing, which can be secured to an object, such as a treatment table or chain-link fence. The resistance band should be secured at a low position, just off the ground and on the nonthrowing side of the athlete. The athlete faces the secured resistance tubing, kneeling on the knee of the throwing side with the opposite limb in 90° of hip and knee flexion and the foot flat on the ground. Next, the athlete grabs the band with the upper extremity in approximately 90° of forward flexion. In this position, the athlete should be far enough away from the band's attachment site so the band has no slack yet little tension. He or she then externally rotates and horizontally abducts the shoulder in a concentric manner (Figure 6), mimicking the cocking phase of the throwing motion (chapter IV-6). After reaching maximum shoulder external rotation, the athlete moves into shoulder internal rotation and horizontal adduction, working eccentrically to control the speed of the motion as the upper extremity is returned to the starting position.

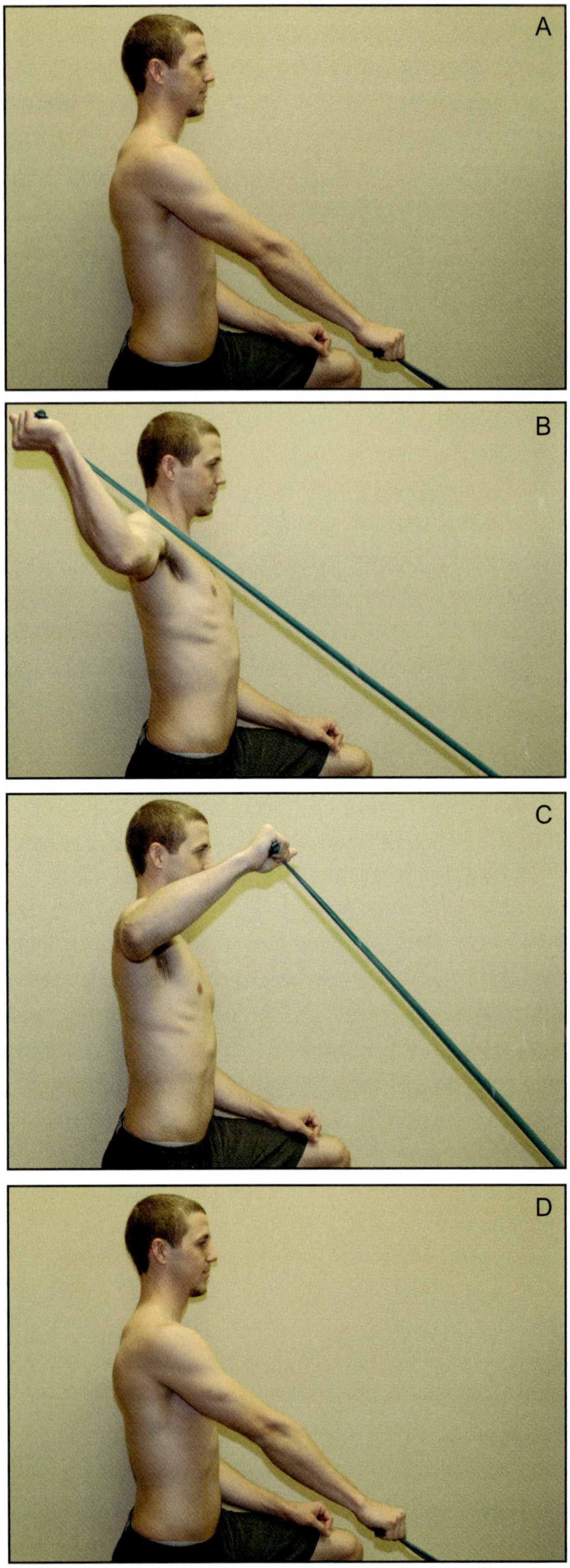

Figure 6 A–D. Throwing deceleration exercise to strengthen the posterior aspect of the shoulder.

Pectoral and Shoulder Internal Rotation Strengthening

I often see baseball players spending most of their strength-training time emphasizing the pectoral muscles while performing exercises, such as the bench press and dumbbell flies; however, this is an area that is best left alone. There is little if any reason to strengthen this area because of the problems associated with tight chest muscles, including increased scapular anterior tilt and protraction and their associated shoulder injuries, and because pectoral muscle strength has little to no relationship with improved throwing performance in baseball.

Shoulder internal rotation strengthening is another area that does not necessarily need to be addressed during arm care exercises. Most baseball players have good internal rotation strength simply from the repetitive throwing motion, so subsequent strengthening of these muscles provides little benefit. The real focus should be on increasing the strength of the shoulder external rotators to equalize the strength ratio of these 2 opposing muscle groups. Excessive shoulder internal rotation strengthening causes an imbalance of forces between the shoulder internal and external rotators, resulting in decreased stability.

Wrist Flexors Strengthening

The accumulation of valgus torque at the elbow during the throwing motion can lead to medial ulnar collateral ligament damage. In fact, the throwing motion commonly produces valgus forces exceeding the amount of force that the medial ulnar collateral ligament can resist.[3] The flexor-pronator muscle mass of the elbow assists in the dissipation of this force.[21] Therefore, strengthening of the flexor-pronator muscle mass of the elbow in baseball players is critical to preventing injury.

Wrist Flexors Strengthening With Forearm Supported. Numerous variations of medial elbow strengthening emphasize wrist flexion. One wrist flexors exercise is performed with the athlete in a seated position, the posterior aspect of the forearm resting on a table or his or her thighs, and the hand hanging over the edge and unsupported. While gripping a hand weight, the athlete slowly moves into wrist flexion until reaching the end range of motion before returning to the starting position in a controlled manner (Figure 7A).

The athlete also can be instructed to work the wrist extensors during the rest period for the wrist flexors, thereby maximizing his or her time. To strengthen the wrist extensors, the athlete simply places the anterior portion of the forearm on the table and moves the wrist into extension while holding the hand weight.

Wrist Flexors Strengthening in 90° of Forward Shoulder Flexion. Wrist flexors strengthening also can be performed using a piece of rope with one end tied to a small bar and the other end secured to an appropriately sized weight. The athlete stands with the shoulders in 90° of forward flexion and the wrists in supination and holds the bar with the rope elongated so the weight is slightly off the ground. The athlete then repeatedly flexes the wrist, which subsequently draws the weight away from the ground as the rope wraps around the bar (Figure 7B). This exercise not only works the wrist flexors, but also causes an isometric contraction of the anterior deltoids and long head of the biceps brachii because the shoulder is held in 90° of flexion.

Some athletes tend to extend or "rock" the lower back during this exercise to bring the weight up while reducing the concentration on the wrist flexors. Therefore, instruct the athlete to avoid this motion. If further measures are necessary to minimize this accessory motion, the athlete can be instructed to perform the exercise with his or her back against a wall to ensure proper spinal alignment. In addition to increased movement at the spine, the athlete can use accessory shoulder forward flexion to raise the weight. If accessory motion is noted at any time, the weight should be reduced until correct form can be maintained.

Grip Strengthening. A third option is to improve grip strength with the use of a soft, pliable ball or putty or with the use of a grip-strength device. For this exercise, the athlete can simply squeeze the ball or putty in a slow controlled manner, with each squeeze constituting 1 repetition. Muscular endurance also can be stressed by using a sustained isometric contraction

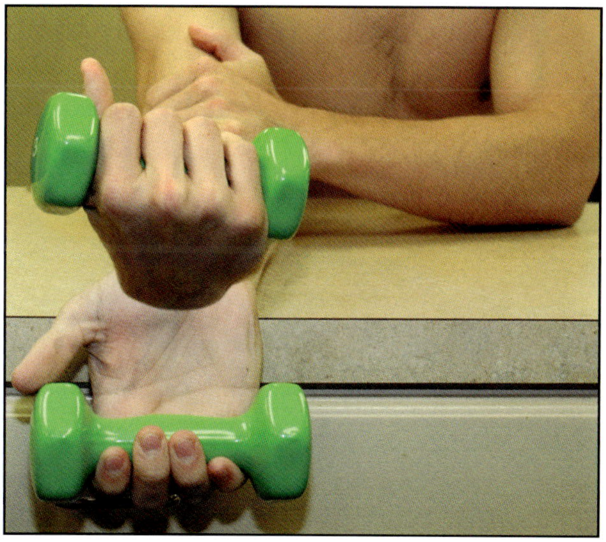

Figure 7A. Wrist flexors strengthening with the forearm supported.

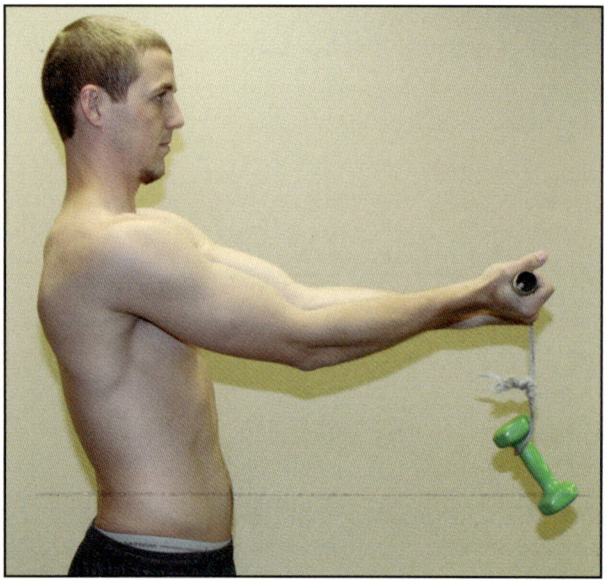

Figure 7B. Wrist flexors strengthening in 90° of shoulder forward flexion.

for 1 minute and repeating this contraction for 2 to 3 sets with 30 to 45 seconds of rest between each set.

Wrist Pronators Strengthening

To strengthen the wrist pronators, the athlete assumes the same position as for wrist flexors strengthening but should grip the end of a hand weight or small bar with weights attached to the opposite end (Figures 8A and 8B). With the wrist starting in a position of full supination, the athlete moves through a full range of pronation motion in a controlled manner before returning to the starting position. During this exercise, the athlete moves from supination to pronation and returns to a supinated position. Therefore, both the pronator and supinator muscles are strengthened.

SENSORIMOTOR TRAINING

A diagonal 2 (or D2) upper extremity flexion and extension PNF pattern can be very useful for baseball players because of this exercise's similarity to the throwing motion and the increased interaction between the sensory and motor facilitators responsible for joint motion and stability. This exercise can be performed either standing or supine and requires resistance tubing, a pulley system, or a partner. The athlete starts in a position of shoulder horizontal adduction, internal rotation, extension, and adduction with forearm pronation similar to the follow-through phase of the throwing motion (Figure 9). Next, the athlete moves the shoulder into horizontal abduction, external rotation, flexion, and abduction while supinating the forearm (Figure 10). Because of the complex combination of motions, this can be figuratively described to the athlete as an action similar to pulling a sword out of a sheath on the opposite hip, raising it overhead, then putting it back in the sheath.

PLYOMETRIC TRAINING

Plyometric training is an effective strengthening exercise for many sports, including baseball, because it mimics the quickness and power of many sport-specific motions. It involves 3 phases. The first phase

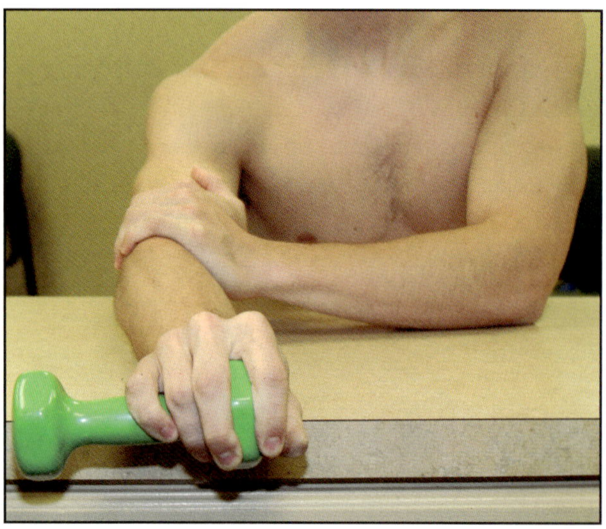

Figure 8A. Wrist pronators strengthening with the forearm supported in internal rotation.

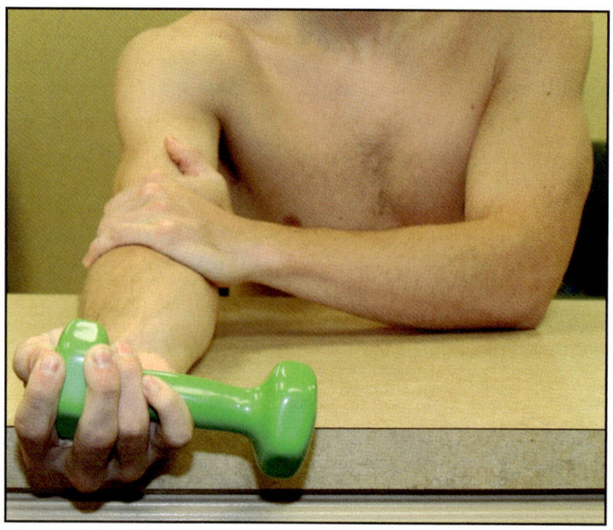

Figure 8B. Wrist pronators strengthening with the forearm supported in external rotation.

is termed *eccentric* because it involves a rapid eccentric contraction as the muscles lengthens, thereby activating the stretch reflex. The second phase, which is termed *amortization*, describes the elapsed time between the end of the eccentric contraction and the beginning of a *concentric* contraction, which is the third phase.

The most important factor of plyometrics is the time spent during the amortization phase. The stretch reflex that is initiated at the end of the eccentric phase helps create a powerful concentric contraction. However, as more time is spent in the amortization phase, this reflex becomes less effective in creating the powerful concentric contraction, resulting in dissipation of

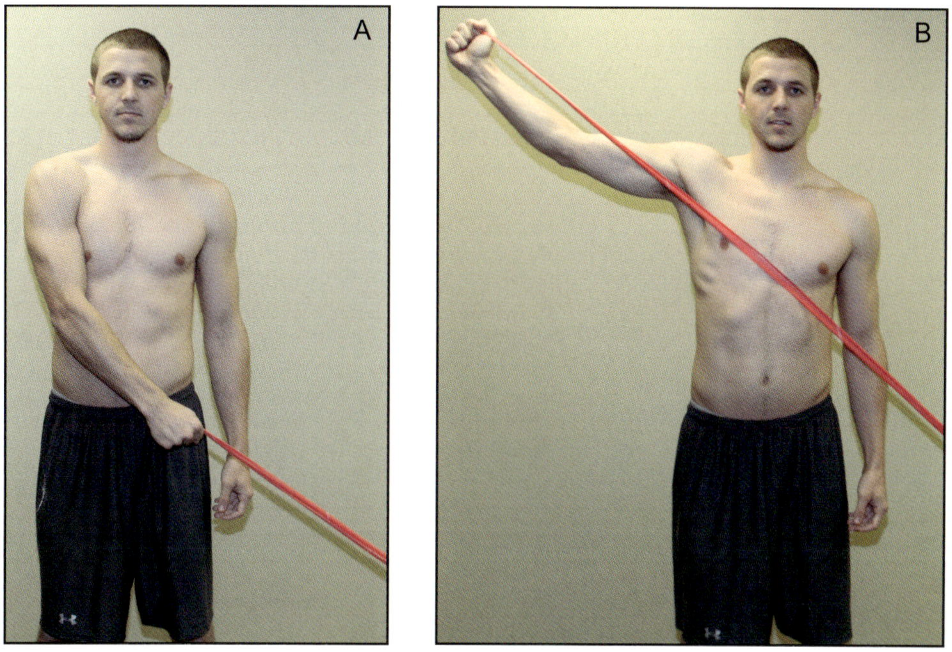

Figure 9 A and B. Diagonal 2 extension proprioceptive neuromuscular facilitation patterns.

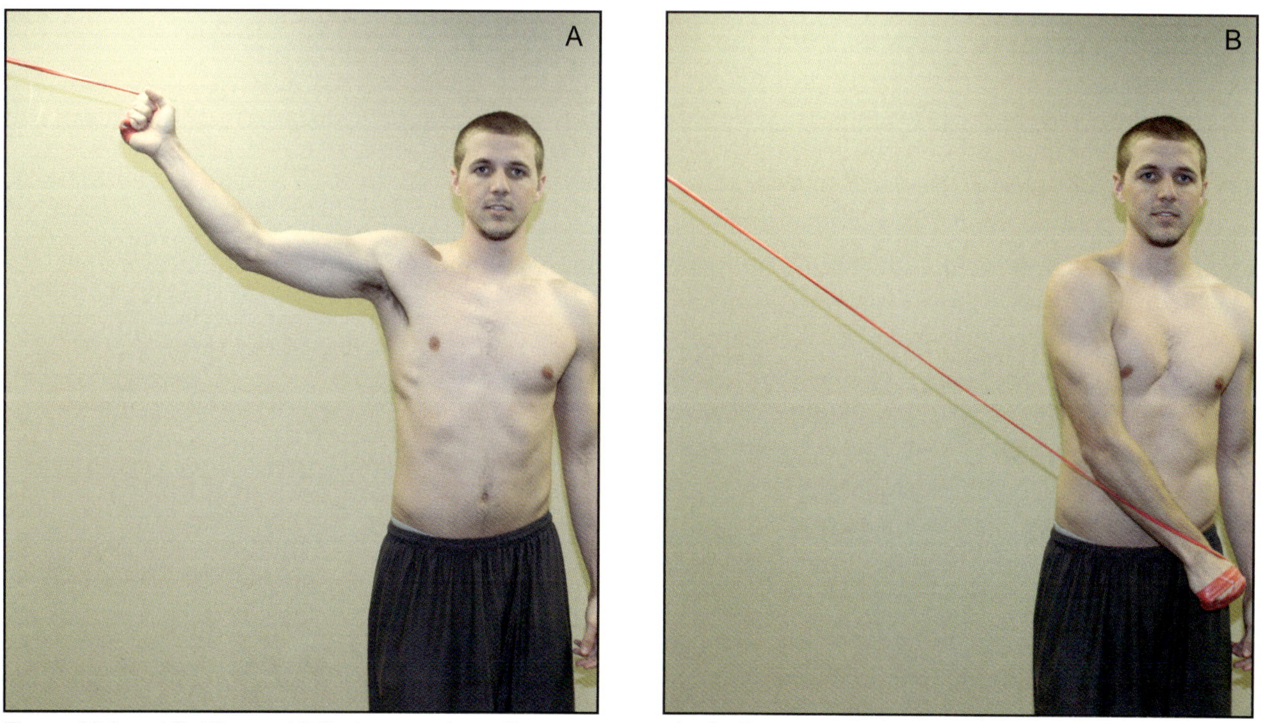

Figure 10 A and B. Diagonal 2 flexion proprioceptive neuromuscular facilitation patterns.

the elastic energy as heat rather than as a contraction. Therefore, athletes should be instructed to minimize the time of the amortization period as much as possible.

Any exercise can essentially be transformed into a plyometric exercise by controlling the speed of the eccentric, amortization, and concentric phases of the motion. However, plyometrics should be performed only if the rehabilitation provider confirms that the athlete has good flexibility, strength, and reflexes. Because of the large forces placed on the bony and soft tissue restraints of the shoulder and elbow during upper extremity plyometric training, physically immature youth athletes should use caution when performing these exercises. Furthermore, plyometrics often are performed with medicine balls. These weighted balls provide increased lengthening during the eccentric phase, but they also increase the amount of force on the athlete's body. Therefore, the weight of the medicine ball used is extremely important. I recommend that when using a medicine ball for plyometric exercises, the youth athlete always should start with the lightest ball, which is typically 1 kg (approximately 2 pounds). The athlete can progress in ball weight when he or she has completed each exercise for the desired repetitions and sets with proper form and no signs of pain or delayed-onset muscle soreness.

OTHER CONSIDERATIONS

Although this chapter pertains to arm care exercises, note that the core and lower extremity play a major role in the throwing motion. During the throwing sequence, an effective transfer of momentum from the forces developed by the lower extremity during the initial throwing phases to the core can assist in protecting the shoulder and elbow from additional stress and ultimately can lead to greater ball velocity.[22] More specifically, flexibility and strength of the hip abductors and rotators, as well as trunk motion in the sagittal and transverse planes, are critical to leg drive, resulting in optimal throwing mechanics, increased performance, and reduced likelihood of injury.[23,24] Therefore, exercises aimed at increasing flexibility and strength of the hip and trunk also should be incorporated into a youth baseball player's conditioning and maintenance programs.

COOL-DOWN

A cool-down should be performed after each strength-training session to minimize pooling of lactic acid in the muscles involved during the session. The removal of lactic acid is believed to decrease the risk of delayed-onset muscle soreness that can hinder the progression of a training program. The cool-down mimics the warm-up in intensity and duration but reverses the physiologic process assisting in returning blood from specific muscles to the heart.

REFERENCES

1. Olsen SJ II, Fleisig GS, Dun S, Loftice J, Andrews JR. Risk factors for shoulder and elbow injuries in adolescent baseball pitchers. *Am J Sports Med.* 2006;34(6):905–912.
2. Lyman S, Fleisig GS, Andrews JR, Osinski ED. Effect of pitch type, pitch count, and pitching mechanics on risk of elbow and shoulder pain in youth baseball pitchers. *Am J Sports Med.* 2002;30(4):463–468.
3. Fleisig GS, Andrews JR, Dillman CJ, Escamilla RF. Kinetics of baseball pitching with implications about injury mechanisms. *Am J Sports Med.* 1995;23(2):233–239.
4. Laudner KG, Stanek JM, Meister K. Assessing posterior shoulder contracture: the reliability and validity of measuring glenohumeral joint horizontal adduction. *J Athl Train.* 2006;41(4):375–380.
5. Myers JB, Pasquale MR, Laudner KG, Sell TC, Bradley JP, Lephart SM. On-the-field resistance-tubing exercises for throwers: an electromyographic analysis. *J Athl Train.* 2005;40(1):15–22.
6. McHugh MP, Magnusson SP, Gleim GW, Nicholas JA. Viscoelastic stress relaxation in human skeletal muscle. *Med Sci Sports Exerc.* 1992;24(12):1375–1382.
7. Taylor DC, Dalton JD Jr, Seaber AV, Garrett WE Jr. Viscoelastic properties of muscle-tendon units: the biomechanical effects of stretching. *Am J Sports Med.* 1990;18(3):300–309.
8. Bonnar BP, Deivert RG, Gould TE. The relationship between isometric contraction durations during hold-relax stretching and improvement of hamstring flexibility. *J Sports Med Phys Fitness.* 2004;44(3):258–261.
9. Moore MA, Kukulka CG. Depression of Hoffmann reflexes following voluntary contraction and implications for proprioceptive neuromuscular facilitation therapy. *Phys Ther.* 1991; 71(4):321–333.
10. Chaitow L. *Muscle Energy Techniques*. 3rd ed. New York, NY: Churchill Livingstone; 2006.
11. Burkhart SS, Morgan CD, Kibler WB. The disabled throwing shoulder: spectrum of pathology, part I. Pathoanatomy and biomechanics. *Arthroscopy.* 2003;19(4):404–420.
12. DiGiovine NM, Jobe FW, Pink M, Perry J. An electromyographic analysis of the upper extremity in pitching. *J Shoulder Elbow Surg.* 1992;1(1):15–25.
13. Tyler TF, Nicholas SJ, Roy T, Gleim GW. Quantification of posterior capsule tightness and motion loss in patients with shoulder impingement. *Am J Sports Med.* 2000;28(5):668–673.

14. Grossman MG, Tibone JE, McGarry MH, Schneider DJ, Veneziani S, Lee TQ. A cadaveric model of the throwing shoulder: a possible etiology of superior labrum anterior-to-posterior lesions. *J Bone Joint Surg Am.* 2005;87(4):824–831.

15. Myers JB, Laudner KG, Pasquale MR, Bradley JP, Lephart SM. Glenohumeral range of motion deficits and posterior shoulder tightness in throwers with pathologic internal impingement. *Am J Sports Med.* 2006;34(3):385–391.

16. Borstad JD, Ludewig PM. The effect of long versus short pectoralis minor resting length on scapular kinematics in healthy individuals. *J Orthop Sports Phys Ther.* 2005;35(4):227–238.

17. Solem-Bertoft E, Thuomas KA, Westerberg CE. The influence of scapular retraction and protraction on the width of the subacromial space: an MRI study. *Clin Orthop Relat Res.* 1993;296:99–103.

18. Weiser WM, Lee TQ, McMaster WC, McMahon PJ. Effects of simulated scapular protraction on anterior glenohumeral stability. *Am J Sports Med.* 1999;27(6):801–805.

19. Murray TA, Cook TD, Werner SL, Schlegel TF, Hawkins RJ. The effects of extended play on professional baseball pitchers. *Am J Sports Med.* 2001;29(2):137–142.

20. Burkhart SS, Morgan D, Kibler WB. The disabled throwing shoulder: spectrum of pathology, part III: The SICK scapula, scapular dyskinesis, the kinetic chain, and rehabilitation. *Arthroscopy.* 2003;19(6):641–661.

21. Lin F, Kohli N, Perlmutter S, Lim D, Nuber GW, Makhsous M. Muscle contribution to elbow joint valgus stability. *J Shoulder Elbow Surg.* 2007;16(6):795–802.

22. Wight J, Richards J, Hall S. Influence of pelvis rotation styles on baseball pitching mechanics. *Sports Biomech.* 2004;3(1):67–83.

23. Dillman CJ, Fleisig GS, Andrews JR. Biomechanics of pitching with emphasis upon shoulder kinematics. *J Orthop Sports Phys Ther.* 1993;18(2):402–408.

24. Fleisig GS, Escamilla RF, Barrentine SW. Biomechanics of pitching: mechanism and motion analysis. In: Andrews JR, Zarins B, Wilk KE, eds. *Injuries in Baseball.* Philadelphia, PA: Lippincott Williams & Wilkins; 1998:3–22.

RECOMMENDED READING

Carroll W. *Saving the Pitcher: Preventing Pitching Injuries in Modern Baseball.* Chicago, IL: Ivan R. Dee; 2004.

Pretz R. "Ballistic Six" plyometric training for the overhead throwing athlete. *Strength Cond J.* 2004;26(6):62–66.

IV-6

Interval Throwing Program

Kevin G. Laudner, PhD, ATC, FACSM

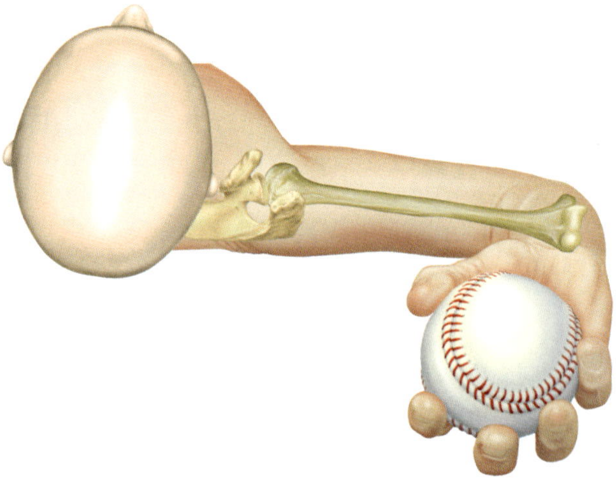

Clinical pearls are highlighted in yellow throughout the text.

The shoulder rehabilitation of a throwing athlete is never complete until a specific interval throwing program has been accomplished. This is the final step before releasing the athlete to full participation in sport and is critical to determining total physical and psychological recovery after injury.

The repetitive nature of throwing for athletes, such as baseball players, softball players, and football quarterbacks, places tremendous stress on the shoulder restraints,[1,2] resulting in functional alterations that can lead to decreased performance[3] and shoulder dysfunction.[4] Therefore, proper biomechanics must be used when throwing, and specific criteria must be used before, during, and after any throwing session. The following program details several areas of concern that should be addressed during an interval throwing program.

REQUIREMENTS FOR INITIATING AN INTERVAL THROWING PROGRAM

Before initiating an interval throwing program, the throwing athlete must have completed a successive rehabilitation program targeting several areas. These athletes should be screened to ensure that they have full range of motion, cardiovascular fitness, muscular strength, power, muscular endurance, and sensorimotor control. During the throwing program, players also must use appropriate biomechanics and regulate the quantity and quality of throws performed daily. As such, players should be cleared by a physician before the initiation of a throwing program and subsequently should work with a baseball coach or other expert to ensure proper throwing biomechanics.

Special caution should be used when working with youth throwing athletes whose shoulders are still skeletally immature and more prone to soft tissue and bony adaptations that can cause harm.[5] Many youth athletes do not have direct access to highly skilled coaches capable of correcting faulty biomechanics. Therefore, particularly when working with these athletes, the rehabilitation provider should have good knowledge of appropriate throwing biomechanics.

The last, but often overlooked, requirement for initiating an interval throwing program is the psychological status of the athlete. At times, players might be reluctant to begin or progress during a throwing program because they fear injury and have decreased confidence in their performance. The psychological aspect is just as important as the physical aspect in the athlete's progression. This hesitation and fear lead to increased muscle tension and altered biomechanics, which lead to an increased risk of injury. Such adverse psychological manifestations must be addressed before the initiation of an interval throwing program. In this case, I strongly recommend that an athlete address such issues with a sports psychologist or other health care professional.

WARM-UP

The athlete should always warm-up before throwing. Because throwing requires contribution from the entire body, a full-body activity should be used for this warm-up. The warm-up should be performed at an intensity and duration that produces an elevated heart rate and perspiration. The specificity of the warm-up can be individualized to the interest of the athlete and can include techniques, such as jogging, stationary bicycling, using an upper body ergometer, or jumping rope. The key is that the effort should be completed at a submaximal level, usually around 70% to 85% of the athlete's maximum heart rate, and sustained for approximately 10 to 15 minutes. Activities that require total-body effort are optimal for preparing the athlete for the total-body effort necessary for throwing. Some athletes prefer performing upper extremity strengthening exercises with light resistance tubing. Several exercises that have been shown to elicit strong muscle activity of the glenohumeral muscles and the scapulothoracic muscles include glenohumeral external rotation at 90° of abduction, a motion that mimics the deceleration phase of the throwing motion, glenohumeral flexion and extension, low angle rows, throwing acceleration motion, and scapular punches.[6]

STRETCHING AND STRENGTHENING

The athlete should stretch immediately after the warm-up routine. Stretching after a proper warm-up allows for maximum benefits from the increased blood flow to the muscles, resulting in increased extensibility and elasticity. A warm-up also allows for increased relaxation of muscles, resulting in less resistance during a stretch and ultimately greater muscle-lengthening capability.[7]

The throwing motion requires good range of motion from the entire body, so the upper body, core, and lower body all should be addressed. Specific areas that should be targeted include the neck, shoulder, elbow, trunk, hips, and knees. For specific stretches and guidelines, please refer to chapter IV-5.

A strength maintenance program should focus on high-repetition and low-intensity exercises that target both the upper and lower extremities and the core (chapter IV-5).[8] Strengthening exercises should be performed 3 times per week and preferably after a throwing session. Weight training before throwing can fatigue muscles and lead to altered kinematics and kinetics of the shoulder, thereby increasing the risk of injury. Days in between throwing and weight-training sessions should be used for recovery of microtrauma that has occurred in the muscles and other soft tissue restraints. Stretching should be performed more often, including before and after throwing sessions and on rest days.

THROWING MECHANICS

Fleisig et al[9] showed that few biomechanical differences exist between the various ages and levels of competitive baseball. However, although no kinematic differences exist, a distinct difference exists in the amount of force created at the various segments during the throwing motion between these different skill levels.[9] Therefore, youth baseball players should be required to produce biomechanics that are similar to those of baseball players at higher skill levels. Holding youth baseball players to these same biomechanical standards is critical for decreasing the risk of reinjury and can result in proper muscle education and biomechanics that can be used throughout the athletes' careers, thereby increasing performance. However, because force production varies between levels of athletes, the interval throwing program should vary slightly based on throwing experience. The following description provides information regarding proper mechanics for the throwing athlete (Figure 1).

Wind-Up

The wind-up is responsible for initiating the rhythm, which is followed throughout the remaining phases of the throwing motion.[10] The wind-up begins as the trail leg, which is the lower extremity on same side as the throwing arm, steps backward and the lead leg, which is the lower extremity on the opposite side of the throwing arm, begins to flex at the hip and knee. Next, the athlete must balance on the trail leg as the throwing shoulder abducts and the trunk begins to rotate away from the intended target. The forces on the shoulder in the wind-up phase are predominantly low[11] and, therefore, are not usually a source of pain for most athletes. However, faulty mechanics in the wind-up phase can

Figure 1. Pitch sequence by phase.

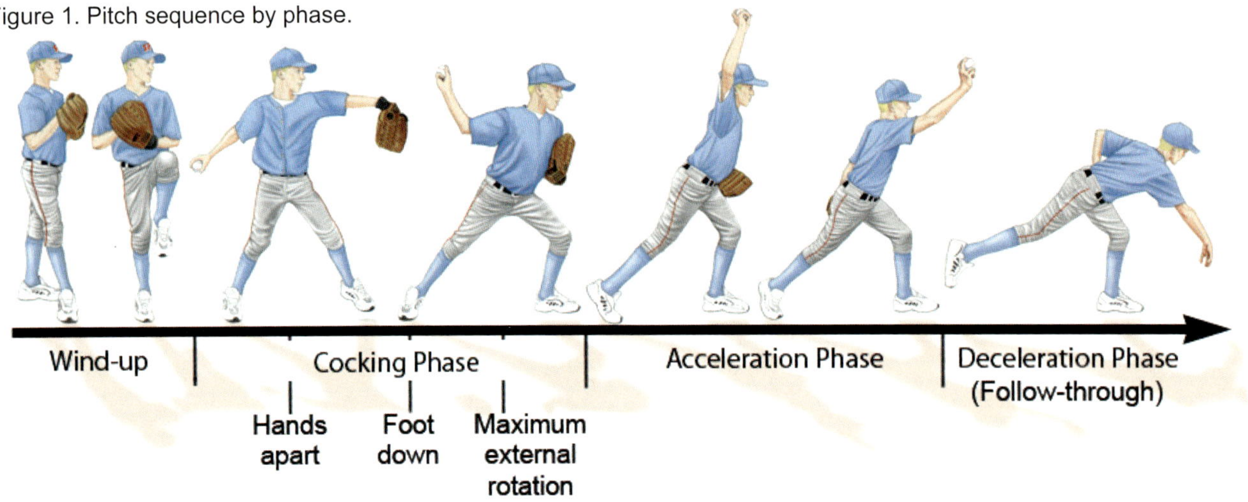

place increased stress on the shoulder during the later phases. Therefore, this phase should not be neglected during biomechanical evaluation.

Cocking

During the cocking phase, the athlete attempts to bring the upper extremity and ball back as far as possible through a contribution of continued trunk rotation, shoulder external rotation and retraction, and elbow flexion. This allows for an optimal position to begin the acceleration of the extremity and subsequent increase in ball velocity. During this phase, the shoulder continues to abduct until approximately 90° and also starts to externally rotate. Before the lead leg contacts the ground, the body is propelled forward during a stride that is approximately the length of the athlete's height.[1] During the stride, the trunk rotates toward the intended target.

When the foot of the lead leg contacts the ground, it should be pointed approximately toward the intended target. Too much rotation of the lower limb can lead to the body "opening up," which places excessive stress on the anterior shoulder restraints. Insufficient hip rotation results in the athlete throwing across his or her body, which subsequently reduces the power initially developed in the lower extremities and trunk and places increased stress on the upper extremity to generate power.

The cocking phase continues until maximum shoulder external rotation is achieved. This shoulder external rotation is typically very large in throwing athletes. However, excessive amounts of shoulder external rotation can be considered hazardous, placing unwarranted stress on the restraints of the anterior aspect of the shoulder.[12] During observation, the rehabilitation provider may note that the forearm often rotates to a point past horizontal, giving the appearance of excessive shoulder external rotation. This shoulder external rotation can appear to be more than 180°; however, this is a combination of motions from various articulations, including scapulothoracic retraction and trunk rotation away from the intended target. If excessive glenohumeral external rotation or diminished scapulothoracic or trunk rotation is noted, the alteration should be addressed before the initiation of an interval-based throwing program.

Acceleration

The acceleration phase is a violent motion that produces shoulder internal rotation speeds in excess of 10,000°/s.[2] The shoulder begins to horizontally adduct and internally rotate while the trunk forward flexes and the elbow extends at 2500°/s.[2] Essentially, all the force developed in the lower extremities and trunk during the previous phases are transferred in progressive order to the shoulder, to the elbow, to the wrist, and finally to the hand as the ball is released toward the intended target.

Deceleration and Follow-Through

After all the forces have been produced in the lower extremities, trunk, and upper extremity during the wind-up, cocking, and acceleration phases and the ball has been released toward the intended target, the body must decelerate the upper extremity and resist an extremely large amount of glenohumeral distraction force.[2] This deceleration and follow-through phase begins after ball release as the shoulder continues to horizontally adduct the upper extremity across the body while the shoulder internally rotates and the elbow extends.[1]

THROWING GUIDELINES

Many throwing programs discourage decelerating the speed of the upper extremity despite varying distances; rather, the rehabilitation provider instructs the athlete to throw "through" the intended target. This instruction primarily is given to limit the negative performance effects of decelerating the extremity during an interval throwing program. Throwing through the target might be an appropriate technique for interval throwing programs involving most athletes; however, when using a throwing program during the rehabilitation of a shoulder injury, the distances provided are designed specifically to gradually increase the stress placed on the shoulder restraints, allowing for an appropriate progression. Therefore, the interval throwing program that I describe should be conducted initially so that each throw just reaches the target at the set distance (Figure 2). This method will minimize the stress placed on the shoulder during the initial phases of the program and gradually increase the distance of throws, thereby increasing the stress placed on the shoulder in a logical progressive manner.

In conjunction with the biomechanics described in this chapter, athletes should be encouraged to use the "crow-hop" method at the beginning of the throwing motion when they are not throwing from a pitching

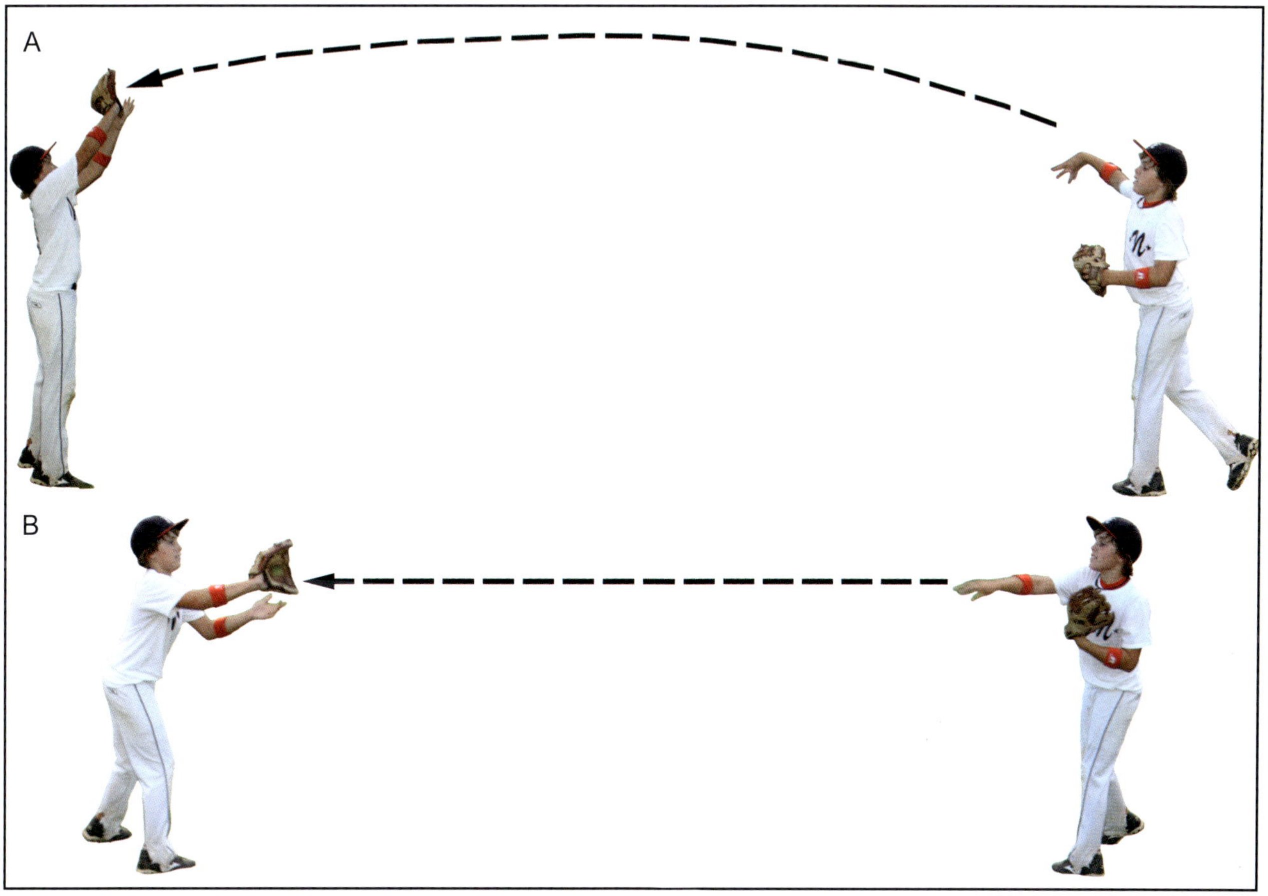

Figure 2. A, Recommended flight path of the ball during initial phases of an interval throwing program. B, Throwing "through" the intended target should be discouraged.

mound. When using this method, the athlete skips then hops directly into the throwing motion (Figure 3). The combination of movements during the crow hop allows for muscle re-education of proper throwing mechanics, leading to increased efficiency and decreased risk of injury.

Drills in which athletes throw flatfooted place an increased emphasis on the motion of the upper extremity. However, they also place unwarranted stress on the upper extremity and encourage improper throwing mechanics. As such, athletes recovering from a shoulder injury should be discouraged from partaking in these types of throwing drills.

INTERVAL THROWING PROGRAM

The following interval throwing program provides a general return-to-participation progression and is designed for the throwing athlete (Table 1). The program should not be used as the sole basis for conditioning. Rather, it should be used in conjunction with an appropriate flexibility and strengthening maintenance program for the upper and lower body (chapter IV-5). Alterations of this interval throwing program might be necessary based on the ages, positions played, and the competitive levels of different players.

To minimize the risk of injury and reinjury, USA Baseball[13] has proposed specific restrictions regarding the throwing volume of youth baseball

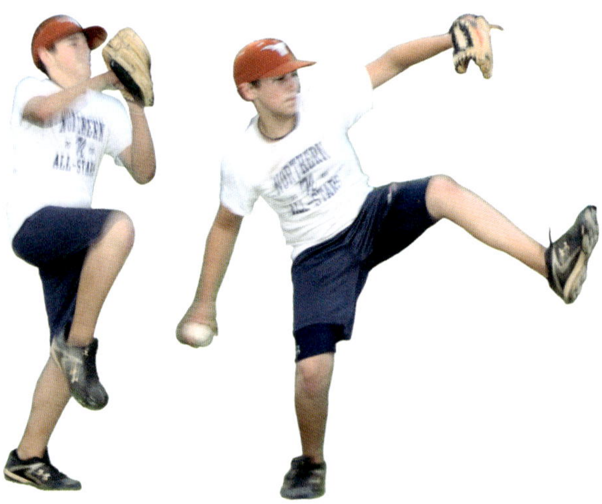

Figure 3. "Crow-hop" method of throwing.

Table 1. Interval Throwing Program

	Step	
Phase	Step 1	Step 2
1	Throwing warm-up 20 throws at 45 ft Rest 20 throws at 45 ft Throwing cool-down	Throwing warm-up 20 throws at 45 ft Rest 20 throws at 45 ft Rest 20 throws at 45 ft Throwing cool-down
2	Throwing warm-up 20 throws at 60 ft Rest 20 throws at 60 ft Throwing cool-down	Throwing warm-up 20 throws at 60 ft Rest 20 throws at 60 ft Rest 20 throws at 60 ft Rest Throwing cool-down
3	Throwing warm-up 20 throws at 90 ft Rest 20 throws at 90 ft Throwing cool-down	Throwing warm-up 20 throws at 90 ft Rest 20 throws at 90 ft Rest 20 throws at 90 ft Throwing cool-down
4	Throwing warm-up 20 throws at 120 ft Rest 20 throws at 120 ft Throwing cool-down	Throwing warm-up 20 throws at 120 ft Rest 20 throws at 120 ft Rest 20 throws at 120 ft Throwing cool-down
5	Throwing warm-up 20 throws at 150 ft Rest 20 throws at 150 ft Throwing cool-down	Throwing warm-up 20 throws at 150 ft Rest 20 throws at 150 ft Rest 20 throws at 150 ft Throwing cool-down

Interval Throwing Program

Table 2. USA Baseball Recommendations for Youth Baseball Pitchers[a]

	No. of Pitches			
Pitcher Age, y	Per Game	Per Week	Per Season	Per Year
9–10	50	75	1000	2000
11–12	75	100	1000	3000
13–14	75	125	1000	3000

[a]These pitch count restrictions pertain to throws during a game only.
Adapted with permission from USA Baseball.[13]

players. These guidelines should be followed when the youth baseball pitcher returns to participation (Table 2).

Youth throwing athletes who are classified as position players, such as catchers, infielders, and outfielders, also should be monitored for an excessive volume of throws. These athletes should be encouraged to participate in 1 league at a time and different sports over the year rather than to participate in year-round baseball or other throwing or overhead motion sports. This alteration of sport participation enables the youth athlete to rest and psychologically and physiologically recover from the stresses placed on the soft tissue and bony restraints during the competitive baseball season.

Athletes, coaches, and rehabilitation providers should recognize the individual progression requirements of each athlete to determine when to advance the program and when to back off of it. Progression is determined through mutual agreement of the athlete, coach, and rehabilitation provider. If the athlete can complete an entire phase of the program 2 to 3 times without pain during or after a throwing session, without delayed onset muscle soreness, and with good biomechanics, he or she should be encouraged to progress with the program. Some athletes might require extra days of rest between throwing sessions. Most athletes require approximately 4 to 6 weeks to develop a solid throwing base.

The interval throwing program should be discontinued or delayed when any of the following symptoms or conditions occurs: any pain, continued loss of control or velocity, feelings of faulty mechanics, or psychological regression of physical status.

In addition to the warm-up and stretching exercises that should be completed before throwing, each athlete should also perform a throwing warm-up. This portion of the interval throwing program is designed to gradually activate the various muscles and to stress the soft tissue restraints involved during the throwing motion. Therefore, this throwing warm-up should be conducted before throwing at the specified distances and after each throwing session to minimize delayed-onset muscle soreness.

The throwing warm-up consists of throwing at a distance of approximately 10 feet for 3 to 5 throws and then increasing the distance by 10 feet every 3 to 5 more throws until the desired distance is reached. During the throwing cool-down, this process should simply be reversed by decreasing the distance by 10 feet every 3 to 5 throws. The throwing cool-down is the last exercise for each step of the interval throwing program. After throwing, the athlete always should perform stretching and cool-down exercises.

Baseball pitchers should complete a pitching simulation phase after finishing the interval throwing program (Table 3). During this phase, the athlete uses pitching mechanics rather than the crow hop and progresses from throwing on flat ground to throwing off a pitching mound. After the athlete has completed the initial mound pitching phases, he or she can begin throwing other types of pitches, such as curveballs, sliders, and change-ups, based on the preinjury preference and the coach's preference. Pitches should be limited or restricted based on age and skill level because of the various kinematic and kinetic differences that can increase the risk of injury.[11,14,15] When the athlete is comfortable with all the necessary types of pitches, a simulated game can be initiated. These simulation games should include throwing 5 to 7 innings for starting pitchers and 2 to 3 innings for relievers. Each inning should consist of the recommended number of pitches and approximately 7 minutes of rest between innings.

Table 3. Pitching Recommendations for the Interval Throwing Program

	Fastball		Curveball[a]	
	No. of Throws	Maximum Velocity, %	No. of Throws	Maximum Velocity, %
Phase 1: Flat ground				
Simulated pitching motion				
Step 1	20	50		
Step 2	35	50		
Step 3	50	50		
Step 4	20	75		
Step 5	35	75		
Step 6	50	75		
Step 7	20	100		
Step 8	35	100		
Step 9	50	100		
Phase 2: Pitching mound				
Simulated pitching motion				
Step 1	20	50		
Step 2	35	50		
Step 3	50	50		
Step 4	20	75		
Step 5	35	75		
Step 6	50	75		
Step 7	20	100		
Step 8	35	100		
Step 9	50	100		
Phase 3: Simulated game				
Step 1	35	50	20	50
Step 2	35	75	20	50
Step 3	35	75	20	75
Step 4	35	100	20	75
Step 5	35	100	20	100

[a] Indicates that the curveball is not introduced until Phase 3.

REFERENCES

1. Dillman CJ, Fleisig GS, Andrews JR. Biomechanics of pitching with emphasis upon shoulder kinematics. *J Orthop Sports Phys Ther.* 1993;18(2):402–408.
2. Werner SL, Gill TJ, Murray TA, Cook TD, Hawkins RJ. Relationships between throwing mechanics and shoulder distraction in professional baseball pitchers. *Am J Sports Med.* 2001;29(3):354–358.
3. Kibler WB. The role of the scapula in athletic shoulder function. *Am J Sports Med.* 1998;26(2):325–337.
4. Fleisig GS, Andrews JR, Dillman CJ, Escamilla RF. Kinetics of baseball pitching with implications about injury mechanisms. *Am J Sports Med.* 1995;23(2):233–239.
5. Meister K, Day T, Horodyski M, Kaminski TW, Wasik MP, Tillman S. Rotational motion changes in the glenohumeral joint of the adolescent/Little League baseball player. *Am J Sports Med.* 2005;33(5):693–698.
6. Myers JB, Pasquale MR, Laudner KG, Sell TC, Bradley JP, Lephart SM. On-the-field resistance-tubing exercises for throwers: an electromyographic analysis. *J Athl Train.* 2005; 40(1):15–22.
7. Shellock FG, Prentice WE. Warming-up and stretching for improved physical performance and prevention of sports-related injuries. *Sports Med.* 1985;2(4):267–278.
8. Hirashima M, Kadota H, Sakurai S, Kudo K, Ohtsuki T. Sequential muscle activity and its functional role in the upper extremity and trunk during overarm throwing. *J Sports Sci.* 2002;20(4):301–310.
9. Fleisig GS, Barrentine SW, Zheng N, Escamilla RF, Andrews JR. Kinematic and kinetic comparison of baseball pitching among various levels of development. *J Biomech.* 1999;32(12): 1371–1375.
10. Pappas AM, Zawacki RM, Sullivan TJ. Biomechanics of baseball pitching: a preliminary report. *Am J Sports Med.* 1985; 13(4):216–222.
11. Fleisig GS, Kingsley DS, Loftice JW, et al. Kinetic comparison among the fastball, curveball, change-up, and slider in collegiate baseball pitchers. *Am J Sports Med.* 2006;34(3):423–430.
12. Miyashita K, Urabe Y, Kobayashi H, et al. Relationship between maximum shoulder external rotation angle during throwing and physical variables. *J Sports Sci Med.* 2008;7(1):47–53.
13. *USA Baseball Medical & Safety Advisory Committee Position Statement on Youth Baseball Injuries November 2008.* http://mlb.mlb.com/usa_baseball/article.jsp?story=medsafety11. Accessed December 12, 2008.
14. Dun S, Loftice J, Fleisig GS, Kingsley D, Andrews JR. A biomechanical comparison of youth baseball pitches: is the curveball potentially harmful? *Am J Sports Med.* 2008;36(4): 686–692.
15. Lyman S, Fleisig GS, Andrews JR, Osinski ED. Effect of pitch type, pitch count, and pitching mechanics on risk of elbow and shoulder pain in youth baseball pitchers. *Am J Sports Med.* 2002;30(4):463–468.

RECOMMENDED READING

Axe MJ, Wickham R, Snyder-Mackler L. Data-based interval throwing programs for Little League, high school, college, and professional baseball pitchers. *Sports Med Arthrosc Rev.* 2001;9(1):24–34.

Borsa PA, Laudner KG, Sauers EL. Mobility and stability adaptations in the shoulder of the overhead athlete: a theoretical and evidence-based perspective. *Sports Med.* 2008;38(1):17–36.

Carroll W. *Saving the Pitcher: Preventing Pitching Injuries in Modern Baseball*. Chicago, IL: Ivan R. Dee; 2004.

Hutchinson MR, Ireland ML. Overuse and throwing injuries in the skeletally immature athlete. *Instr Course Lect.* 2003;52:25–36.

Meister K. Injuries to the shoulder in the throwing athlete, part one: biomechanics/pathophysiology/classification of injury. *Am J Sports Med.* 2000;28(2):265–275.

IV-7

Interval Golf Program

Brian J. Phillips, PT, DPT

CHAPTER CONTENTS

- Risk of injury
- Injury and reinjury prevention
- Special considerations
- General tips
- Interval golf program

Clinical pearls are highlighted in yellow throughout the text.

For many patients seeking physical therapy to rehabilitate an injured or surgically repaired shoulder, their ultimate goal is to return to sport participation. Surgery might be necessary to treat an orthopaedic condition that limits sport participation because of pain, weakness, or limited range of motion (ROM). In a study of 75 patients who underwent total shoulder arthroplasty, McCarty et al[1] reported that one reason 64% (n = 48) of these patients underwent surgery was so they could return to playing sports. In this chapter, I provide information about golfing injuries, provide information about injury and reinjury prevention, highlight key concepts to returning to golf participation after rehabilitation, and discuss an interval golf program.

RISK OF INJURY

Although it is a low-intensity activity, golf is not an injury-free sport. Common injuries in golf include back, elbow, shoulder, and wrist injuries.[2] For the amateur golfer, the shoulder is the fourth most commonly injured part of the body.[3] For the professional golfer, the shoulder is the third most commonly injured part of the body.[3] Professional golfers have a higher rate of injury than amateur golfers.[2] Male and female golfers are equally affected by golf injuries. When comparing male and female European golfers, investigators found no difference in the number, anatomic distribution, or severity of golf-related injuries.[2]

For the healthy athlete, a deficit in strength, endurance, ROM, and proper mechanics places the individual at risk for an initial injury. Failure to address these impairments places the athlete at greater risk for further injury. Rehabilitation of injured athletes should focus on addressing any deficit in strength, endurance, ROM, and proper mechanics before returning to active sport participation.

INJURY AND REINJURY PREVENTION

The rehabilitation provider must consider many different issues when assisting a patient or athlete with returning to golf participation. A key consideration is injury and reinjury prevention. The rehabilitation provider not only must focus on preventing reinjury of the specific body part being treated during rehabilitation, but also must consider all aspects of golf participation to prevent new injuries from occurring.

Two aspects of injury and reinjury prevention that many golfers do not consider are the effects of warming up and the effects of carrying a golf bag. In a study of 703 golfers, Gosheger et al[2] noted that 570 (81.0%) golfers did not warm-up for more than 10 minutes before playing a round of golf. Golfers whose warm-ups lasted more than 10 minutes had significantly fewer injuries per player (0.41) than golfers whose warm-ups lasted 10 minutes or less (1.02 injuries per player) ($P < .05$).[2]

Gosheger et al[2] also studied the effects of golfers carrying their own golf bags. They reported that 221 (31.4%) of the 703 golfers regularly carried their bags on their backs, whereas 482 (68.6%) of the golfers used either a caddy or a golf trolley. Those who regularly carried their own bags had significantly more injuries to their shoulders, low backs, and ankles than those who did not carry their bags ($P < .05$).[2] Based on the information presented in this study, rehabilitation providers should educate patients about the relationship between injury prevention and properly warming up for at least 10 minutes before golfing. They also should teach patients that using a caddy, golf trolley, or golf cart to carry the golf bag might prevent injury.

SPECIAL CONSIDERATIONS

The mechanism of injury, timeframe since the injury, previous treatments received, and recent history of surgery are just a few things that the rehabilitation provider needs to consider when returning a patient to golf participation. In this section, I discuss key points to consider during rehabilitation of various shoulder disorders that have been treated operatively or nonoperatively.

Unlike other overhead sports, golf does not demand extreme ranges of motion of the shoulder.[4,5] Mitchell et al[6] found that for both college-aged and middle-aged (aged 25 to 49 years) golfers, the *lead arm*, which was defined as the left upper extremity for the right-handed golfer, was elevated above 90° for more than 30% of the entire motion of the swing. This is important because the period when it is typically above shoulder level (during the backswing) is also the period when the lead arm is most horizontally adducted. This combination of elevation and horizontal adduction is a common mechanism for the development of shoulder impingement, particularly with the large number of repetitions required during practice and play.[6] In fact, subacromial impingement and rotator cuff disorders are among the most common problems of the lead shoulder for golfers.[3] Special considerations for patients with impingement or rotator cuff disorders include giving attention to posterior shoulder flexibility,[7] establishing adequate rotator cuff and scapular muscle strength,[3,8] and limiting repetitive movements of the extremities above shoulder level. Adjustments in swing mechanics might be necessary to address these issues and might help to prevent repetitive microtrauma of the rotator cuff and other soft tissues. Left untreated, such injuries can lead to more debilitating shoulder injuries.

For the patient who has undergone shoulder surgery, the type of surgery and details of the operation are important factors to consider when implementing a program to return to golf participation. In the following paragraphs, I discuss special considerations for the patient returning to golf after surgery. These are generalizations based on the type of surgery performed, and exceptions to these generalizations might exist. Contact with the referring physician is required if the surgery included concomitant procedures or other specialized techniques that are unfamiliar to the rehabilitation provider.

Rotator Cuff Repair

Shoulder pain in golfers who are middle-aged or older frequently is associated with rotator cuff impairment.[5] These types of dysfunctions often can be treated with physical therapy. If nonoperative therapy is unsuccessful or if the rotator cuff condition is too severe, surgery might be warranted. Chapter III-1 provides a specific treatment protocol for routine rotator cuff repairs. As noted in the protocol, patients generally can begin light chipping and putting by 3 months after surgery. Irons and drivers can be used at 4 to 5 months after surgery. Note that these timeframes are intended for routine rotator cuff repairs only and not for large or massive repairs. Reinold et al[8] encouraged patients returning to playing golf to "begin using each club with a tee to avoid the deleterious forces that may be produced during a divot." In a study of 29 golfers who underwent rotator cuff repair, Vives et al[5] found no difference in presymptomatic handicaps or driving distances compared with those reported at follow-up (average = 37 months). Ninety percent (n = 26) of the 29 golfers studied returned to playing golf, with 88% (n = 23 of 26) of these golfers reporting that they were able to return to their former competitive levels.[5]

Total Shoulder Arthroplasty

The desire to return to pain-free golf participation can be one of the main reasons that a patient undergoes shoulder joint replacement surgery. McCarty et al[1] reported that the ability to participate in sports can be curtailed by the condition that eventually necessitates the joint replacement. In a retrospective review of 24 patients who underwent total shoulder replacement, Jensen and Rockwood[9] found that 23 patients (96%) were able to resume playing golf. Eighteen of these patients were able to report their preoperative handicaps and noted an average improvement of almost 5 strokes.[9]

A special consideration for the patient who has undergone shoulder replacement is the protection of the subscapularis muscle, which is often taken down or bisected so the surgeon can access the shoulder joint. Electromyography (EMG) studies performed on golfers have shown that the subscapularis is the most active rotator cuff muscle in both the lead and trail arms during a golf swing.[3] The rehabilitation provider should consider adequate healing time and proper strengthening progression of the subscapularis before allowing these patients to return to golf participation. In chapter III-7, Gaunt describes a postoperative protocol for patients who have had shoulder replacement surgery. Postoperatively, chipping and putting with progression to light wedge shots typically can begin 9 to 12 weeks after surgery. Progression to an interval golf program can be initiated during months 3 to 5. McCarty et al[1] found that the average time for patients to return to full participation in sport after total shoulder arthroplasty was 5.8 months.

GENERAL TIPS

In this section, I highlight general tips and make recommendations for patients wanting to return to golf after shoulder injury or surgery. Strengthening and toning of the entire shoulder complex can be just as important as training the specific muscles of the rotator cuff. In their EMG study, Kim et al[3] noted that the latissimus dorsi and pectoralis major demonstrated the most activity of all shoulder muscles during a golf swing. Moynes et al[4] also noted high electromyographic levels of the latissimus dorsi, pectoralis major, and subscapularis in both the lead and trail arms during the acceleration phase of the golf swing before ball strike.

Strengthening of the scapular stabilizers should be included as part of a global strengthening program of the shoulder. Kim et al[3] noted the activation of the trapezius, rhomboids, serratus anterior, and levator scapulae muscles in both the lead and trail arms during multiple phases of a golf swing. Increased electromyographic activation especially was noted during the downswing and acceleration phases.[3] Reinold et al[8] suggested that any strengthening program for an overhead athlete should emphasize strengthening the posterior rotator cuff and scapular musculature.

Finally, the rehabilitation provider also should focus on improvement of overall flexibility, core strengthening, proprioception, and balance in individuals wanting to return to golf. Lephart et al[10] recommended an 8-week golf-specific training program to increase strength, flexibility, and balance to improve golf performance. Improving a golfer's base of support and flexibility can allow for greater upper body rotational velocities, resulting in greater club head velocity and potentially leading to longer drive distances.[10]

INTERVAL GOLF PROGRAM

Interval sports programs are used to methodically return patients to sport participation by slowly progressing them through graduated sport-specific activities.[8] Before starting an interval golf program, the patient should receive clearance from the referring physician and should have adequate ROM, strength, and muscle endurance. The rehabilitation provider should give special attention to each patient's specific disorder or type of surgery so potential damaging stress is not placed on the shoulder. Because each individual is different, there is no specific timeframe in which the patient must complete each section or the entire program.[8]

Reinold et al[8] developed and published a 5-week interval golf program. Although the program follows a 5-week progression, this can be modified to meet each patient's specific needs and ability level. The program is designed for golfing 3 days each week on Monday, Wednesday, and Friday. Week 1 consists of chipping and putting, with short irons introduced at the end of the week. During week 2, the patient continues chipping and using short irons and begins using medium irons by Friday of that week. In week 3, long irons and 3-wood and 5-wood clubs are introduced. Week 4 begins with the introduction of drivers, and the patient attempts playing 9 holes of golf by the middle of the week. By week 5 of the program, the patient is playing between 9 and 18 holes of golf as tolerated. As mentioned, Reinold et al[8] recommended the initial use of a tee with each club to prevent potential damaging forces produced by a divot. Patients also are encouraged to begin swings at partial effort, progressing to full effort as tolerated as long as it is pain-free. If the patient experiences pain while progressing through the program, he or she is encouraged to return to the most recent portion of the program that could be completed without pain. Next, the golfer should continue with the interval golf program from that point of pain-free activity. If pain continues, a follow-up examination by the referring physician might be warranted.

In conclusion, close communication among the patient, rehabilitation provider, and physician is essential to ensuring a safe and effective return to sport. The combination of a supervised rehabilitation program and an interval golf program can allow patients to return to golfing after shoulder injury or surgery.

REFERENCES

1. McCarty EC, Marx RG, Maerz D, Altchek D, Warren RF. Sports participation after shoulder replacement surgery. *Am J Sports Med*. 2008;36(8):1577–1581.
2. Gosheger G, Liem D, Ludwig K, Greshake O, Winkelmann W. Injuries and overuse syndromes in golf. *Am J Sports Med*. 2003;31(3):438–443.
3. Kim DH, Millett PJ, Warner JJ, Jobe FW. Shoulder injuries in golf. *Am J Sports Med*. 2004;32(5):1324–1330.
4. Moynes DR, Perry J, Antonelli DJ, Jobe FW. Electromyography and motion analysis of the upper extremity in sports. *Phys Ther*. 1986;66(12):1905–1911.
5. Vives MJ, Miller LS, Rubenstein DL, Taliwal RV, Becker CE. Repair of rotator cuff tears in golfers. *Arthroscopy*. 2001;17(2): 165–172.
6. Mitchell K, Banks S, Morgan D, Sugaya H. Shoulder motions during thc golf swing in male amateur golfers. *J Orthop Sports Phys Ther*. 2003;33(4):196–203.
7. Tyler TF, Nicholas SJ, Roy T, Gleim GW. Quantification of posterior capsule tightness and motion loss in patients with shoulder impingement. *Am J Sports Med*. 2000;28(5):668–673.
8. Reinold MM, Wilk KE, Reed J, Crenshaw K, Andrews JR. Interval sport programs: guidelines for baseball, tennis, and golf. *J Orthop Sports Phys Ther*. 2002;32(6):293–298.
9. Jensen KL, Rockwood CA. Shoulder arthroplasty in recreational golfers. *J Shoulder Elbow Surg*. 1998;7(4):362–367.
10. Lephart SM, Smoliga JM, Myers JB, Sell TC, Tsai YS. An eight-week golf-specific exercise program improves physical characteristics, swing mechanics, and golf performance in recreational golfers. *J Strength Cond Res*. 2007;21(3):860–869.

IV-8

Interval Tennis Program

Joel B. Stenslie, PT

CHAPTER CONTENTS

Clinical pearls are highlighted in yellow throughout the text.

Millions of people in the United States enjoy tennis. They often start playing as early as 4 years of age and possibility can play for 90 years or more. Many communities around the country have tennis clubs and leagues that allow for all levels of play and year-round competition. Given the repetitive overhead activity of tennis, many players seek medical attention, such as physical therapy, because of pain and restricted play. Priest and Nagel[1] found that more than 50% of the world's top tennis players had experienced shoulder pain, especially with the serve and smash strokes, during their careers. In this chapter, I describe the risk of injury, briefly explain the rehabilitation guideline for a tennis player, and detail an interval tennis program.

INJURY IN TENNIS PLAYERS

The most common injuries in overhead athletes include rotator cuff disorders with secondary bursitis and microtraumatic instability.[2,3] Tennis is a repetitive activity involving the entire kinetic chain. The foot and ground forces that act on the knee, hip, trunk, scapula, shoulder, elbow, and wrist joints influence the racket angle and speed of a tennis shot. Pain within the kinetic chain can alter proper mechanics, leading to compensatory movements. These compensatory movements can result in shoulder conditions that cause restricted motion, increased pain, and decreased strength of the dynamic stabilizers of the shoulder and can trigger a cascade of events leading to other conditions. Detecting and properly diagnosing disorders of the shoulder early is important to prevent further destruction of its static and dynamic stabilizers.

Precursors to injury along the kinetic chain include internal rotation deficits, imbalances between strength of internal and external rotation, poor scapular stability with serratus anterior and trapezius weakness, faulty body mechanics during overhead activity, and lack of flexibility and strength of the trunk and lower extremities.[2] An overload to the compromised shoulder can lead to tendinitis of the supraspinatus and external rotators. Mismanagement can result in further overload of the static stabilizers, causing tears along the capsule and labrum of the shoulder. Properly differentiating among inflammation, chronic tendinitis, and chronic tendonosis and addressing any deficits or functional impairments are imperative for early return of the athlete to sport participation.

WHAT SHOULD BE THE EMPHASIS OF REHABILITATION AND WHY?

The primary goal of rehabilitation is reducing the symptoms associated with pathologic conditions, such as inflammation, decreased range of motion (ROM), and muscle atrophy. The focus of the acute phase, or phase 1, of rehabilitation is the restoration of pain-free ROM and scapular stability. Nonsteroidal anti-inflammatory medication; modalities, such as cryotherapy and high-voltage electrical stimulation; and bursal injections can be used to help decrease pain and inflammation.

During the intermediate phase, or phase 2, of rehabilitation, strengthening exercises are initiated after restoration of pain-free ROM. Restoring full activation and recruitment of muscle groups requires the elimination of nociceptive signals from inflamed tissues. The emphasis of phase 2 is regaining sport-related end range of mobility along with functional strengthening in multiplanar motions. These motions include eccentric and concentric activity with the shoulder in the cocked or loaded position. Elastic-resistance bands are used to strengthen the posterior aspect of the shoulder to mimic the deceleration phase of the serve and forehand.

The goal of phase 3 rehabilitation is to return the patient to full participation in sporting activities. At this point in the rehabilitation process, full functional ROM should be established, and upper extremity strength and endurance and scapular stability are maintained through weight-bearing and resistance exercises. If the patient has undergone surgery, physician approval is required before he or she can return to sport participation or can start an interval tennis program. For all patients, close supervision from the referring physician and from the rehabilitation provider will enable a safe and efficient return to sport participation.

GENERAL REHABILITATION TIPS FOR TENNIS PLAYERS

In this section, I provide tips for patients returning to tennis after injury or surgery. Dynamic strengthening of the entire kinetic chain is important for performance and injury prevention. Dynamic lower limb joint motion, speed, and power combined with trunk rotation are paramount and are associated with developing high hitting speeds.[4] High angular velocities with upper extremity internal rotation developed through large ROMs play a similarly positive and substantial role in developing racket velocity in selected strokes.[5] Stabilization of the scapula via increased activation of the serratus anterior and lower trapezius is essential to control the kinetic forces created from the lower extremity traveling through the trunk to the upper extremity. As Kibler[6] described, the scapula balances the humerus as a seal balances a ball on its nose (Figure 1). Without the control of the dynamic scapular thoracic stabilizers, the humeral head will have improper joint position and altered mechanics during elevated activity.[6] Given the nature of the anterior strokes of tennis, the proximal aspect of the shoulder develops excessive internal rotation strength; therefore, emphasis should be placed on improving the strength of the external rotators.[7] For issues of flexibility, areas that need focus include the pectoralis major, posterior capsule, and levator scapulae.

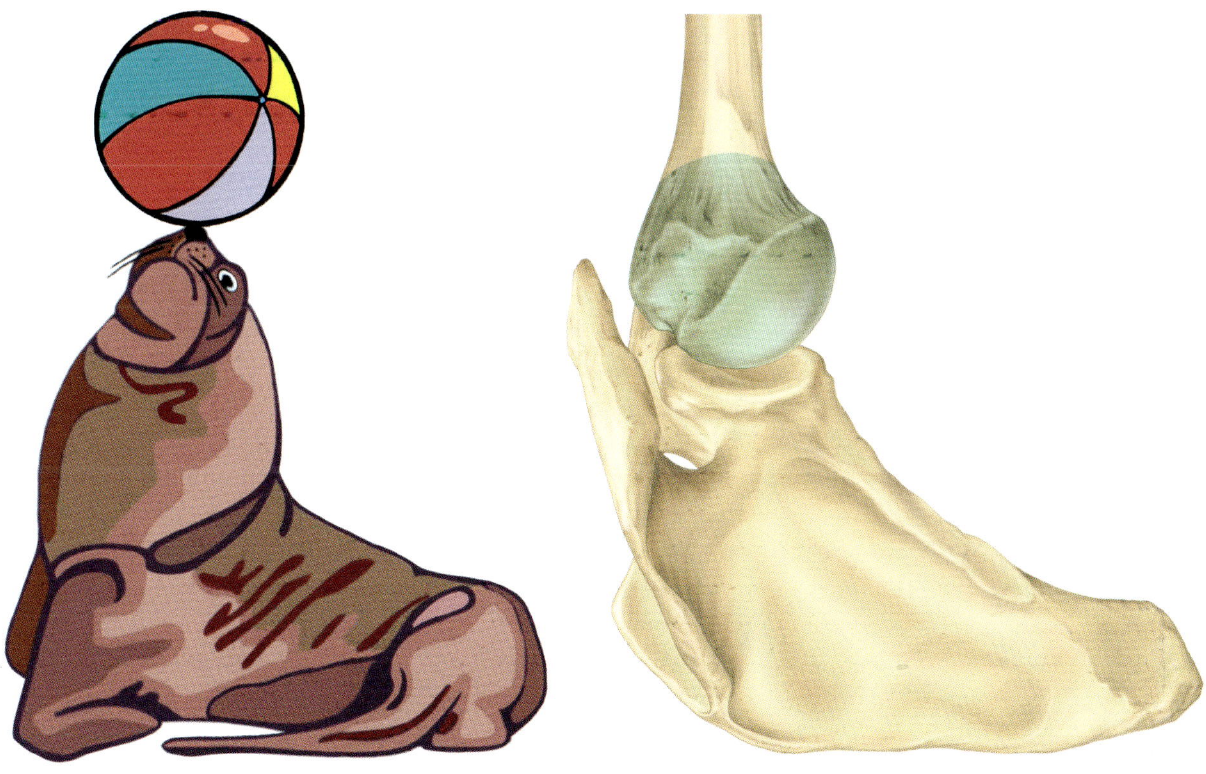

Figure 1. Kibler's[7] "ball and seal" concept illustrating similar glenohumeral dynamic balance.

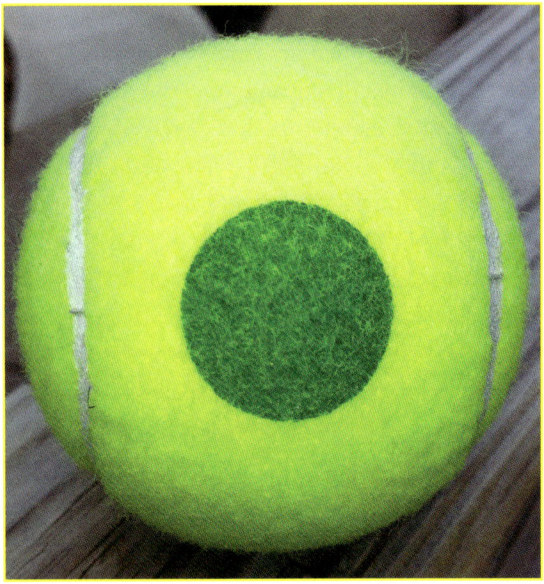

Figure 2. Low-compression green-dot ball.

THE 6-WEEK INTERVAL TENNIS PROGRAM

Interval sport programs are used to methodically return patients to sport participation by slowly progressing them through graduated sport-specific activities.[8] Before starting an interval sport program, the patient should have clearance from the referring physician and should have adequate ROM, strength, and muscle endurance. Given the nature of injuries and timeframes of healing, the rehabilitation provider should progress each patient according to his or her functional level and not by a set timeframe. Progressing too fast might cause undue soreness and further injury, delaying full return to sport.

The Appendix provides a 6-week return-to-tennis program that involves the athlete being on the court 1 to 3 times per week. During weeks 1 through 3, he or she needs to maintain full swing and follow-through, starting with 50% effort and progressing by 25% each week. During the early weeks, athletes start with a short game within the service box as a warm-up along with short volleys. To decrease overall vibration and speed of the ball, the patient can hit low-compression green-dot balls (Figure 2). Using low-compression balls will allow proper setup and less apprehension when swinging through the ball, which does not bounce high into the area of impingement. Weeks 3 and 4 involve progression of racket speed along with initiating overhead swings. The patient starts overhead smashes, serving at 50% of effort and proper technique and progressing by 25% at each practice. During weeks 5 and 6, the athlete can progress to playing 3 to 5 games to 2 sets if he or she has no pain. Each week, the athlete needs to progress with strength and confidence. If the player experiences lasting soreness or pain with mobility of the swing, he or she decreases the volume, strength, and overhead activity. If pain persists, the athlete should return for physical therapy.

REFERENCES

1. Priest JD, Nagel DA. Tennis shoulder. *Am J Sports Med.* 1976;4(1):28–42.
2. Gokeler A, Lehmann M, Mathijs O, Kentsch A. Tennis: rehabilitation, training, and tips. *Sports Med Arthrosc Rev.* 2001;9(1):105–113.
3. Elliott B, Fleisig G, Nicholls R, Escamilia R. Technique effects on upper limb loading in the tennis serve. *J Sci Med Sport.* 2003;6(1):76–87.
4. Reid M, Schneiker K. Strength and conditioning in tennis: current research and practice. *J Sci Med Sport.* 2008;11(3):248–256.
5. Elliott BC, Marshall RN, Noffal G. Contribution of upper limb segment rotations during the power serve in tennis. *J Appl Biomech.* 1995;11(4):433–442.
6. Kibler WB. The role of the scapula in athletic shoulder function. *Am J Sports Med.* 1998;26(2):325–337.
7. Chandler TJ, Kibler WB, Stracener EC, Ziegler AK, Pace B. Shoulder strength, power, and endurance in college tennis players. *Am J Sports Med.* 1992:20(4):455–458.
8. Reinold MM, Wilk KE, Reed J, Crenshaw K, Andrews JR. Interval sport programs: guidelines for baseball, tennis, and golf. *J Orthop Sports Phys Ther.* 2002;32(6):293–298.

Appendix.

THE 6-WEEK INTERVAL TENNIS PROGRAM

Week	Warm-Up	Forehands	Backhands	Overhead Slams	Serves	Games or Sets
1	5 min on short court	2 sets of 10–20 strokes with rest between sets	2 sets of 10–20 strokes with rest between sets	None	None	None
2	5–8 min on short court	3 sets of 10–20 strokes with rest between sets	3 sets of 10–20 strokes with rest between sets	None	None	None
3	10 min on short court	3–4 sets of 20–30 strokes and progress only without pain	3–4 sets of 20–30 strokes and progress only without pain	1 set of 10 strokes at 50% effort	None	None
4	10 min on short court	3–5 sets of 20–30 strokes	3–5 sets of 20–30 strokes	2 sets of 10 strokes at 50–75% effort	1 set of 10 strokes at 50–75% effort	None
5	10 min on short court	3–5 sets of 20–30 strokes	3–5 sets of 20–30 strokes	2 sets of 10 strokes at 75–100% effort	2 sets of 20 strokes at 75–100% effort	3–6 games
6	10 min on short court	3–6 sets of 20–30 strokes	3–6 sets of 20–30 strokes	3 sets of 10 strokes at 75–100% effort	2–3 sets of 20 strokes at 75–100% effort	1–3 sets

IV-9

Aquatic Rehabilitation

Shannon B. Lucas, PTA

CHAPTER CONTENTS

Clinical pearls are highlighted in yellow throughout the text.

Water has been used for centuries for rehabilitation. The muscles use less energy to counteract the force of gravity when exercises are performed in water than when they are performed on land. Therefore, in the early stages of rehabilitation after shoulder injury or surgery, recovery can occur more easily, more safely, and with less pain when water is used as an exercise medium.

The primary goal of any rehabilitation program is to return patients to their preinjury or preoperative activity levels as quickly as possible. Water therapy can be initiated immediately after an injury or surgery when all incisions have closed completely. Investigators have reported that 3 weeks of inactivity can lead to a great loss of cardiovascular fitness, and 6 weeks of rest can lead to a decrease of as much as 14% to 16% of maximum oxygen consumption.[1–3] Regardless of the activity level of the patient before the injury or surgery, minimizing the loss of endurance and strength is critical in shortening the time of rehabilitation.

In this chapter, I focus on shoulder rehabilitation in an aquatic setting and discuss the physical properties of water, the physiologic effects of water, therapeutic effects of exercising in the water, the contraindications and precautions for aquatic rehabilitation, aquatic equipment, and a staged aquatic program for shoulder rehabilitation.

PHYSICAL PROPERTIES OF WATER

The physical properties of water include buoyancy, specific gravity or relative density, hydrostatic pressure, viscosity, and fluid dynamics. I discuss each of these separately.

Buoyancy

Buoyancy is the upward thrust that a fluid exerts on an object less dense than itself. The Greek mathematician, Archimedes, described this force, which is referred to as the *Archimedes Principle*. This principle states that when a body is partially or completely submerged in a fluid at rest, it experiences an upward thrust equal to the weight of the fluid displaced. What does this mean for aquatic exercise? Buoyancy decreases the effect of weight-bearing and gravitational forces on the muscles, joints, and connective tissues. As the patient is submerged deeper into the water, he or she experiences a greater unloading effect. When submerged to the C7 vertebra, weight-bearing forces decrease by 0% to 25%; from the axilla to the C7 vertebra, 25% to 50%; from the diaphragm to the axilla, 50% to 75%; and below the diaphragm, 75% to 100%.[4]

Buoyancy can be used to assist, resist, or support our movements. Buoyancy-assisted movements, such as shoulder flexion performed in the standing position, occur in the same direction as the force of buoyancy (Figure 1). The movement raises the extremities or trunk toward the surface of the water.

Buoyancy-resisted movements, such as shoulder extension and adduction in standing, occur in the opposite direction of the force of buoyancy (Figure 2).

The movement pushes the body part down away from the surface of the water.

Buoyancy-supported movements, such as shoulder horizontal abduction and adduction in standing, occur perpendicular to the force of buoyancy (Figure 3). The movement is parallel to the water's surface.

Specific Gravity or Relative Density

Specific gravity or *relative density* of an object is the property that determines whether an object sinks or floats when immersed in a fluid. It is the ratio of the weight of an object to the weight of an equal volume of water. If the object has a relative density of 1.0 or more, it sinks. If it has a relative density of less than 1.0, it floats. The relative density of the human body is between 0.97 and 0.95. It is slightly less than that of water, which is 1.0,[3] so most patients float.

Factors that affect relative density of the human body include lean body mass, bone density, and respiratory capacity. Fatty tissue has a relative density of 0.90. Increased body fat decreases the relative

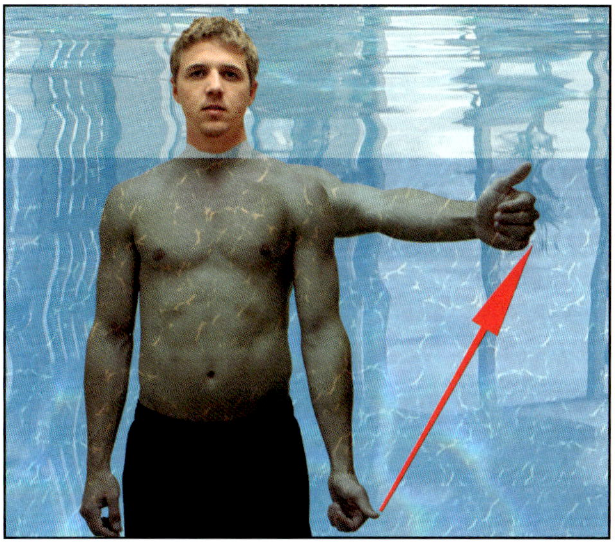

Figure 1. The patient performs active forward elevation in the plane of the scapula. He stands in water up to neck level and prevents all portions of the affected upper extremity from breaking the surface of the water.

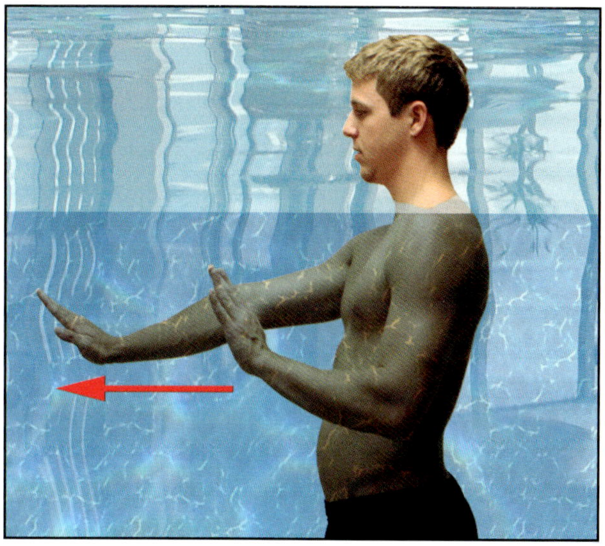

Figure 3. Standing in water up to neck level, the patient performs the push-pull motion at chest level while standing in water up to neck level.

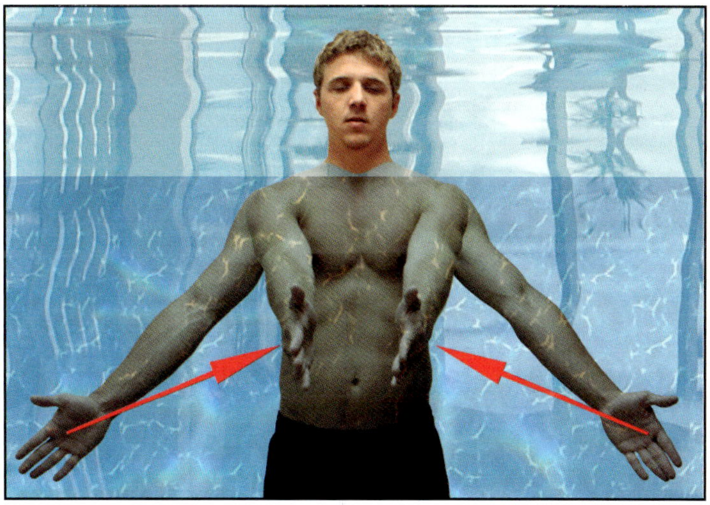

Figure 2. Standing in water up to neck level, the patient performs active horizontal abduction and adduction at waist level from a neutral position to about 45° horizontal of abduction.

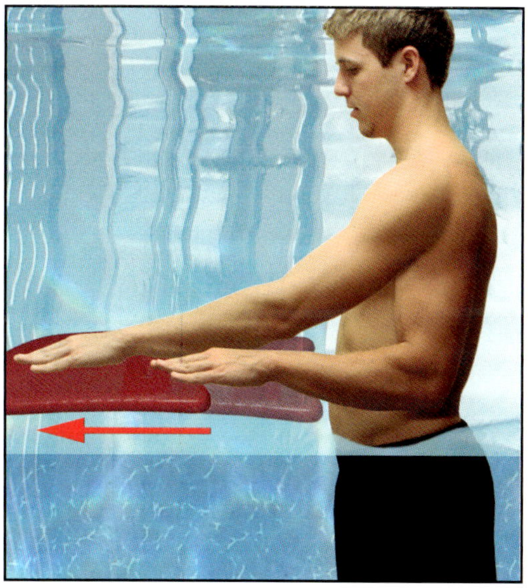

Figure 4. The patient performs W dusting while supporting the hand on a kickboard and standing in water just below chest level.

density and increases a patient's ability to float. Bones, muscles, and connective tissues have a relative density of 1.10; therefore, a lean, fit patient might require a floatation device to increase his or her ability to float. A patient with decreased respiratory capacity has increased relative density, so he or she has a decreased ability to float and also might need a floatation device (Figure 4).

Hydrostatic Pressure

Hydrostatic pressure is the pressure exerted by the thrust of fluid molecules on the submerged parts of the body. Pascal's Law states that fluid pressure is felt equally on all submerged surface areas at rest at a given depth. Hydrostatic pressure increases as the depth of the water increases. It is related directly to the density of the fluid and is responsible for the cardiovascular changes that occur with aquatic-based rehabilitation. It causes a centralization of blood flow away from the extremities. Because of this redirection of blood flow, hydrostatic pressure might be used in rehabilitation to help reduce effusion or to enable patients to exercise an injured extremity without increasing effusion.

Viscosity

Viscosity is the internal friction between molecules that causes a resistance to flow. This resistance to flow is known as *drag*. Viscosity is directly proportional to drag. When viscosity increases, drag increases, and when viscosity decreases, drag decreases. Changing the temperature of the water affects the viscosity. Increasing the temperature decreases viscosity and drag. Other factors influencing viscosity are speed of movement, surface area of movement, and lever-arm length. Slow movements, increased surface area, and increased lever-arm length increase drag and viscosity.

Fluid Dynamics

The 2 types of water flow are laminar flow and turbulent flow. *Laminar flow* is the smooth flow of water molecules. It carries the least amount of resistance because the molecules are flowing in the same direction and at the same speed. An example of this is exercising in a pool with the jets turned off. When the jets are turned on, they create more turbulent or interrupted flow of water and more resistance for the patient to overcome. When the water molecules are bouncing off one another in multiple directions, exercising becomes more challenging.

Equipment choices and body positioning affect turbulent flow. A tapered object causes laminar flow, whereas an untapered object creates turbulent flow. Performing shoulder internal and external rotation with the elbows at the sides and palms down (forearms pronated) produces little resistance (laminar flow) compared with performing the same exercise with the palms facing each other (neutral forearm position), which creates much resistance (turbulent flow).

PHYSIOLOGIC EFFECTS OF AQUATIC EXERCISE

Certain physiologic changes occur both at rest and during exercise when a patient is submerged in water. Resting changes result from hydrostatic pressure and include a cephalad redistribution of blood flow. Immersion to the neck causes a central shift of peripheral blood flow and can result in a 700-mL increase in central blood volume.[2] It also causes a 180- to 250-mL increase in blood volume of the heart. As the heart rate increases, right atrial pressure increases by 8 to 12 mmHg. The increased pressure increases the shunting of blood flow into the central circulation and causes increased venous return (up to 700 cm^3) into the great vein of the thorax and into the heart. It also causes increased right atrial pressure, increased stroke volume, increased cardiac output, and potentially decreased heart rate (Table).[2] This shunting of blood is known as the *Frank-Starling mechanism*. Submersion in water to shoulder level reduces vital capacity by 10%, which can cause difficulty breathing secondary to the increased pressure on the chest cavity; therefore, patients with vital capacities less than 1.5 L should not exercise in water this deep.

Several studies have been conducted to determine what changes occur when exercising in water. Christie et al[5] studied 10 men performing bicycle ergometry on land and in water to the suprasternal notch. Participants in both groups exercised at 40%, 60%, 80%, and 100% of maximum oxygen consumption. The researchers observed the participants' cardiac responses

Table. Cardiovascular Responses to Immersion to the Neck at Rest

Measure	Response
Right atrial pressure	Increase (8–12 mmHg)
Heart blood volume	Increase (180–250 mL)
Cardiac output	Increase (25+ %)
Stroke volume	Increase (25+ %)
Central venous pressure	Increase
Heart rate	Remain the same or decrease slightly
Systemic blood pressure	Remain the same or increase slightly

Reprinted with permission from the *Journal of Athletic Training*.[2]

to the exercise, and although they found no differences in the maximum oxygen consumption between the 2 groups, they noted differences in the cardiac responses. Cardiac response was greater among the water-based group. Cardiac preload was elevated both at rest and with exercise in water, suggesting the centralization of peripheral blood flow exists despite the redistribution of blood flow known to occur during exercise.

Sheldahl et al[6] conducted a similar study using 2 groups of 9 men. The 2 groups performed supervised bicycle ergometry 3 times each week for 12 weeks: one group on land and the other group in water up to the suprasternal notch. They found an increase in stroke volume, a decrease in heart rate and blood pressure, and a similar increase in maximum oxygen consumption in both groups. The authors concluded that exercise training is not affected by the cephalad shift in blood volume during water exercise.

Because of the cardiovascular changes that occur when submerged in water, the training heart rate should be established in water and not on land. In general, heart rates are approximately 17 beats per minute lower during deep-water exercise than during comparable land-based exercise.

Warm water can place additional strain on the cardiovascular system as it tries to prevent overheating. Intense water exercise should take place from 81°F to 83°F to prevent any heat-related problems. However, for basic shoulder rehabilitation, patients can safely exercise in water temperatures ranging from 91°F to 93°F. These warmer water temperatures have numerous therapeutic effects, including

- muscle relaxation, which leads to decreased guarding and spasms;
- improved tissue flexibility;
- reduced gravitational pressure;
- increased circulation through injured tissue, which aids in delivery of vital nutrients and the removal of harmful metabolites to facilitate the healing process; and
- sensory input that can help to block pain receptors in the brain.

Regardless of the temperature of the water, aquatic exercise has many benefits. Beyond those mentioned, aquatic-based exercise promotes

- early, improved mobility of injured joints or muscles;
- early cardiovascular training;
- core body strengthening;
- stretching;
- resistive training; and
- improved proprioception and balance.

CONTRAINDICATIONS AND PRECAUTIONS FOR AQUATIC EXERCISE

Contraindications

- Cardiac conditions, such as unstable angina
- Peripheral vascular disease with increased blood pressure
- Open wounds
- Infections, such as urinary, respiratory, blood, eye, ear, nose, and throat
- Fever
- Tracheostomies, including plugged tracheostomies
- Bowel and bladder incontinence
- Menstruation unless using internal protection
- Dermatosis, such as active psoriasis, rashes, and athlete's foot
- Uncontrolled seizure disorders
- Infectious diseases
- Active joint diseases, such as rheumatoid arthritis
- Great mental confusion

Precautions

- Diabetes
- Ostomy, colostomy, ilieostomy, and frostily corked tracheotomy

- Vital capacity of 1 to 1.5 L
- Autonomic dysreflexia
- Orthostatic hypotension and hypertension
- Seizure disorder that is controlled medically
- Cardiac conditions
- Absence of cough reflex or mouth closure deficits
- Chemical sensitivity
- Ear sensitivity
- Hearing aids
- Contact lens
- Behavior problems
- Fear of water

For patients with diabetes, monitor their responses to immersion and exercise and keep sugar and medications poolside. Monitor the responses to immersion and exercise for patients with cardiac conditions and keep medications poolside. Patients with cough reflex or mouth closure deficits should keep their faces away from the water. Chemical-sensitive patients should shower in lukewarm water and regularly moisturize the skin. Patients with ear sensitivity should wear ear plugs. Contact lenses and hearing aids should be removed and left in the locker room to prevent coming into contact with the water. When working with children or adults with traumatic brain injury, the rehabilitation provider might need the assistance of additional staff for safety. With patients who fear water, progress slowly and provide physical contact throughout the session or until fear subsides.

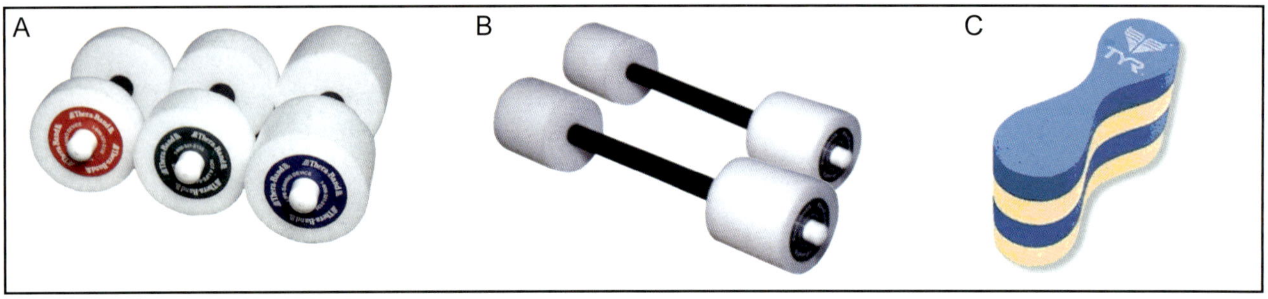

Figure 5. Buoyant equipment. A, Barbells. B, Pool buoys. C, Kickboard.

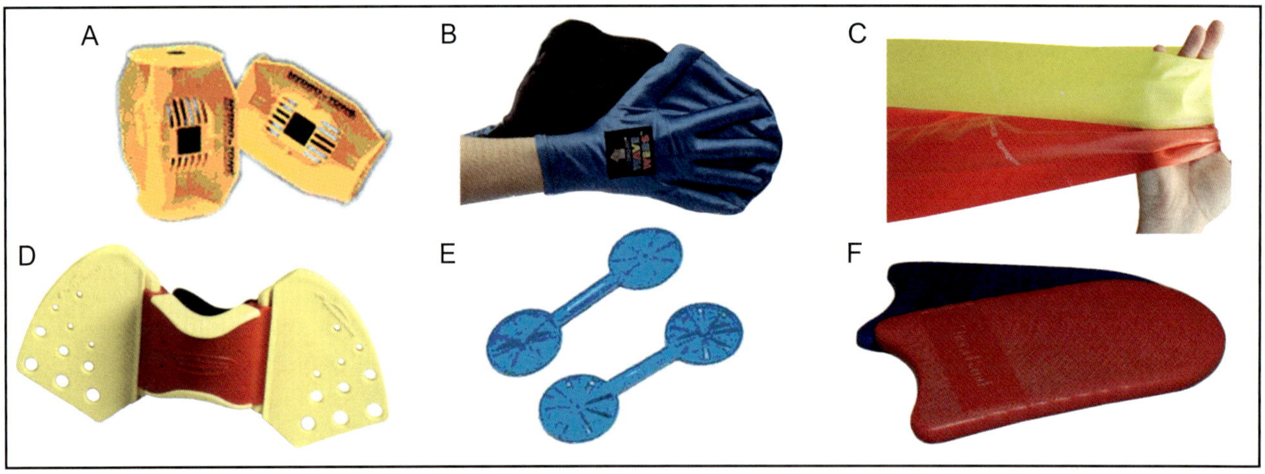

Figure 6. Resistive equipment. A, Barbells. B, Webbed gloves. C, Elastic-resistance bands. D, Fins. E, Paddles. F, Kickboard.

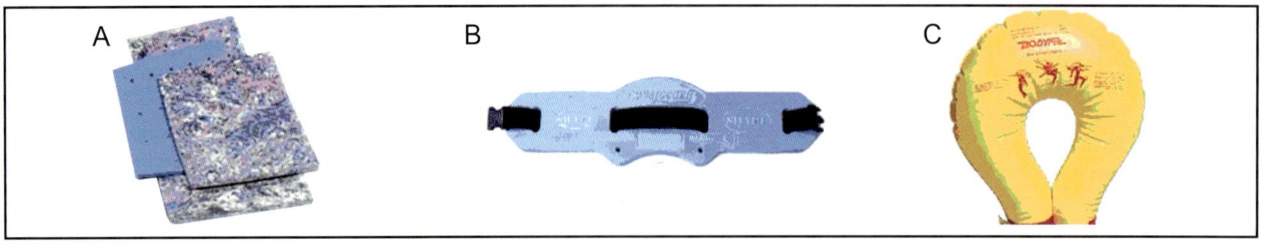

Figure 7. Supportive equipment. A, Flowmats. B, Jog belt. C, Inflatable collar.

AQUATIC THERAPY EQUIPMENT

Aquatic therapy equipment provides a quantifiable means to achieve a patient's goals as established in the plan of care. The rehabilitation provider uses equipment to design an individualized rehabilitation program for the patient and to show progressions in his or her strength, range of motion, endurance, and flexibility. The 3 main types of aquatic equipment are buoyant, resistive, and supportive. Buoyant equipment includes barbells, pool buoys, and kickboards (Figure 5). Resistive equipment includes barbells, webbed gloves, elastic-resistance bands, fins, paddles, and kickboards (Figure 6). Supportive equipment includes flowmats, jog belts, and inflatable collars (Figure 7).

AQUATIC REHABILITATION OF THE SHOULDER

Kelly et al[4] studied 6 nonimpaired participants to determine muscle activation of the nondominant shoulder during exercises on dry land and in water. They applied waterproof, intramuscular indwelling wire electrodes to the supraspinatus, infraspinatus, and subscapularis muscles and placed waterproof surface-adhesive electrodes on the anterior, middle, and posterior deltoid muscles. The participants performed shoulder elevation in the plane of the scapula (0°–90°) with neutral humeral head rotation while on land and while submerged in water up to their necks. The exercise was performed at 30°/s, 45°/s, and 90°/s. They performed 3 trials on dry land and in water. At 30°/s of elevation, all 6 muscles had less activation when tested in water than when tested on dry land. With the exception of the middle deltoid, all muscles had less activation at 45°/s of elevation when tested in water than when tested on dry land. The subscapularis muscle was the only muscle that showed more relative activation at 90°/s of elevation when tested in water than when tested on dry land.

Before patients begin aquatic rehabilitation after surgery, they must have their sutures removed and must have complete closure of their incisions, which typically occurs by postoperative week 2. Next, a 2-phase aquatic program for the shoulder can begin. Phase 1 aquatic exercises are used to rehabilitate patients after injury or surgery, such as rotator cuff repair, that requires passive range of motion only for a period. In this phase, all exercises requiring glenohumeral range

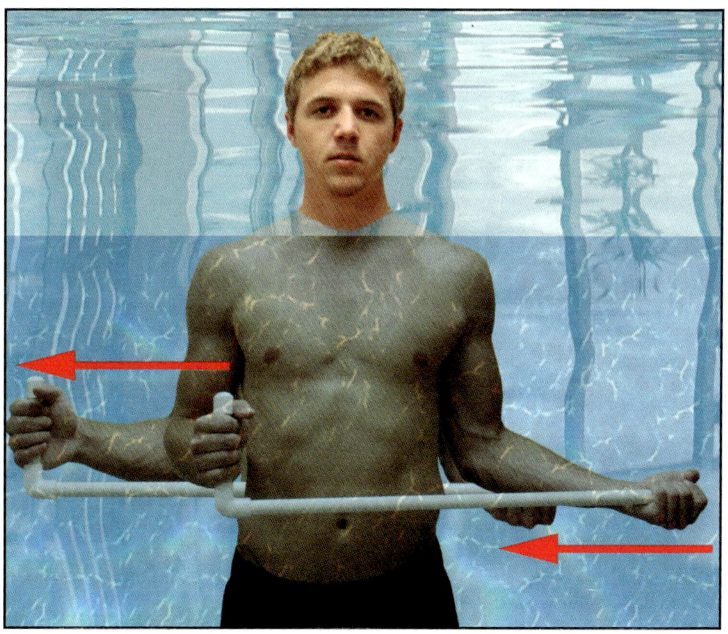

Figure 8A. With the entire shoulder submerged in water, the patient performs passive external rotation using a T-bar.

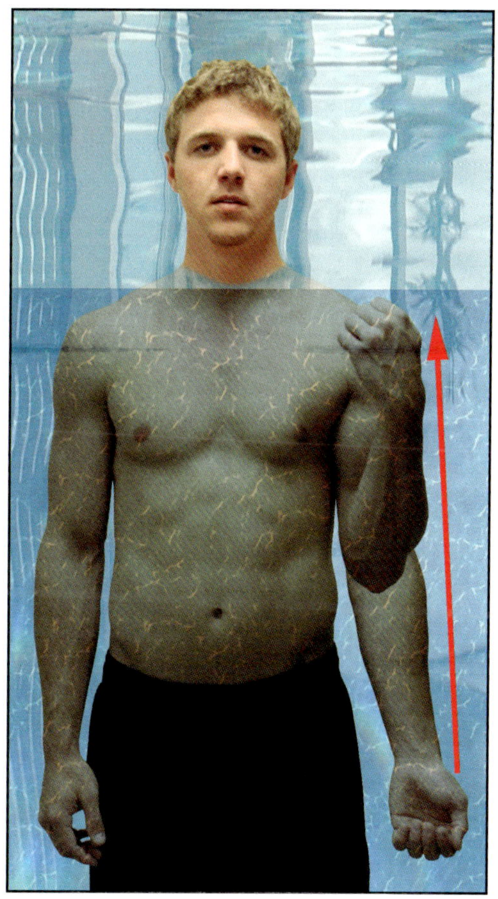

Figure 8B. Standing in water up to neck level, the patient performs active biceps curls.

of motion are either buoyancy-supported or buoyancy-assisted. Typically, phase 1 exercises include W dusting with the patient standing in waist-level water and the hand resting on a kickboard with the elbow at the side; passive external rotation with a T-bar with the patient submerged to the neck; active biceps curls with the patient standing in neck-level water; and float-supported passive forward elevation with the patient standing in waist-level water with both hands resisting on a kickboard and squatting to the point of a gentle, pain-free stretch (Figures 4 and 8).

Phase 2 aquatic exercises begin when the physician allows glenohumeral active range of motion and strengthening, typically at postoperative weeks 4 to 6. In this phase, the patient progresses from buoyancy-assisted to buoyancy-resisted exercises that include active horizontal abduction and adduction at waist level from a neutral position to about 45° of horizontal abduction, push-pull motion at chest level, and active external and internal rotation at 0° of abduction (Figures 1–3 and 9). All exercises in phase 2 can be made easier by spreading the fingers apart or by moving the upper extremities slowly, which decreases viscosity and drag. They can be made harder by keeping the fingers closed, increasing the speed of the motion, or adding resistive equipment.

In conclusion, regaining early range of motion, regaining normal kinematics, and returning normal function are important after shoulder injury or surgery. Aquatic therapy can be used to achieve these goals early in an environment that does not adversely affect the healing tissues. Buoyancy helps to support the extremity and results in passive-assistive to active-assistive range of motion that yields movement with little muscle activity.

Figure 8C. To perform passive forward elevation, the patient stands in waist-level water and supports both upper extremities on a float. Passive forward elevation is achieved when the patient squats in the water while keeping the upper extremities and hands resting on the float.

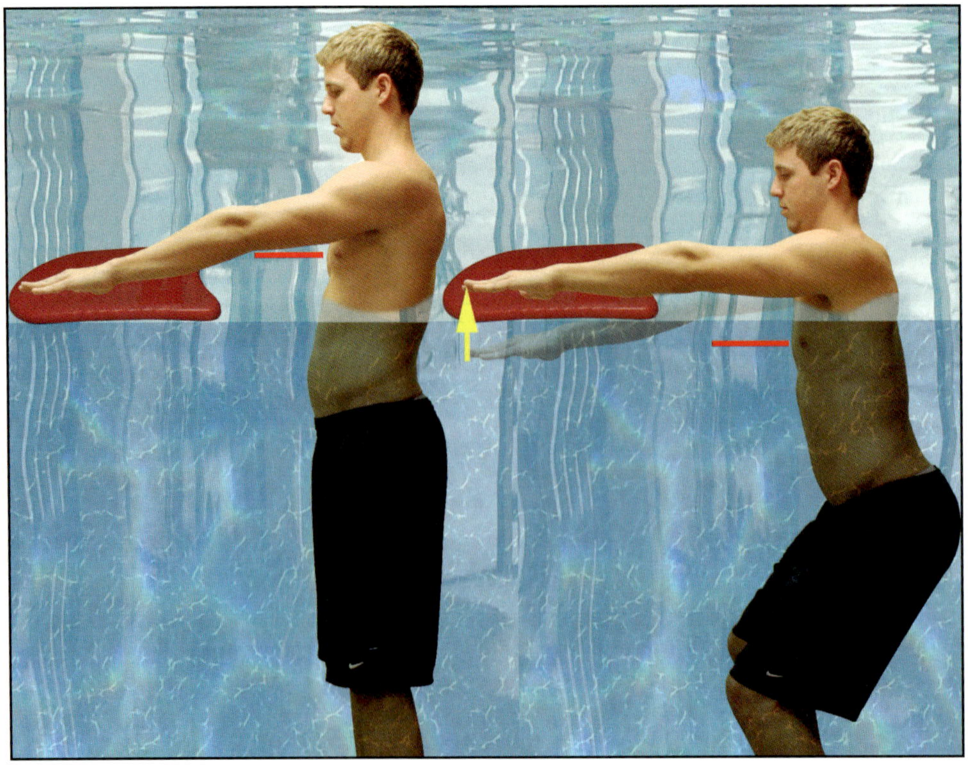

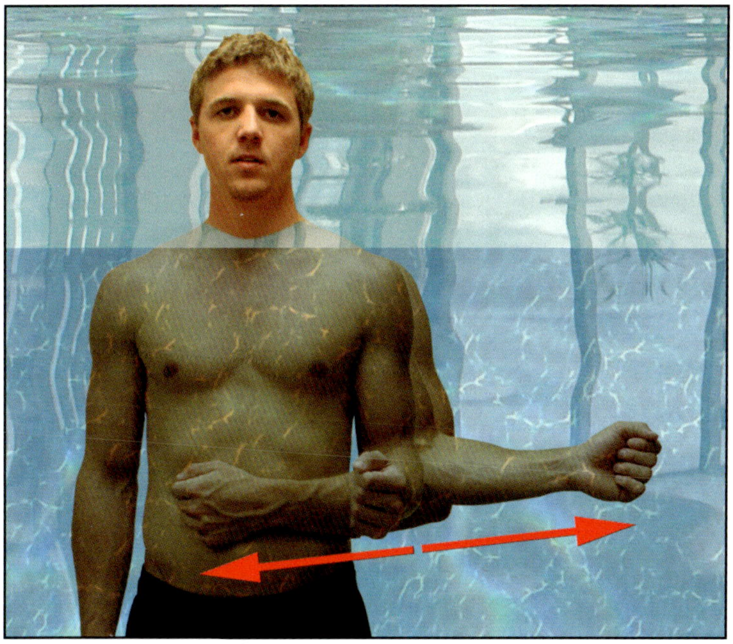

Figure 9. While standing in water up to neck level, the patient performs active external and internal rotation at 0° of abduction.

REFERENCES

1. Brody LT. Current trends in therapeutic exercise for the rehabilitation of the athlete: aquatic physical therapy for the athlete. *Sports Phys Ther Sect Home Study Course.* 1997;1:1–20.
2. Thein JM, Brody LT. Aquatic-based rehabilitation and training for the shoulder. *J Athl Train.* 2000;35(3):382–389.
3. Thein J, Brody LT. Aquatic-based rehabilitation and training for the elite athlete. *J Orthop Sports Phys Ther.* 1998;27(1):32–41.
4. Kelly BT, Kirkendall DT, Roskin LA, Speer KP. Shoulder muscle activation during aquatic and dry land exercises in nonimpaired subjects. *J Orthop Sports Phys Ther.* 2000;30(4):204–210.
5. Christie JL, Sheldahl LM, Tristani FE, et al. Cardiovascular regulation during head-out water immersion exercise. *J Appl Physiol.* 1990;69(2):657–664.
6. Sheldahl LM, Tristani FE, Clifford PS, Kalbfleisch JH, Smits G, Hughes CV. Effect of head-out water immersion on response to exercise training. *J Appl Physiol.* 1986;60(6):1878–1881.

IV-10

Functional Capacity Evaluations and Impairment Ratings: Tools for Closing Worker's Compensation Claims

Jo A. Barker, PT

CHAPTER CONTENTS

- Funtional Capacity Evaluations
- Impairment Ratings
  - Case History
  - Options

Clinical pearls are highlighted in yellow throughout the text.

The US Department of Labor[1] defines *musculoskeletal disorder* as an injury or disorder of the muscles, nerves, tendons, joints, cartilage, and spinal discs. They continue to dominate the type of occupational injury or illness occurring in all workers. Recent declines have been noted in the manufacturing, transportation, and construction industries likely due to the economic downturn and higher unemployment in these occupational categories.[2] However, the number of cases reported for light or delivery service truck drivers, restaurant cooks, landscapers/groundskeepers, and registered nurses have increased, resulting in a continued demand for health care services.[2]

Accepting the injured worker for treatment presents several variables not present with the patient who has private insurance. Whereas the ultimate goal for all patients is to maximize improvement and function, returning a worker to his or her previous status is easier said than done because of the entities to be satisfied, including the employer; the worker's compensation case manager or adjustor; legal representation for either or both parties; and of course, the worker. Clearly, health care providers who participate in industrial medicine serve many masters, but ultimately we serve the injured employee first. The health care provider or the administrator responsible for managing these patients should expect to facilitate communication among all parties to ensure everyone has the same information.

Several "truths" exist in industrial medicine, and all affect those involved in caring for an injured worker:

- **Focus on case resolution.** Return to work is not the only resolution for the injured employee. The referral source needs more options, particularly when the worker's injury is catastrophic or when questions of effort or reliability present themselves.
- **Ask the questions.** Make certain of expectations from the worker and the referral source.
- **Answer the referral source's questions.** Specifically, what is the worker's concern? Is the worker progressing as expected? What is the likelihood of returning to his or her previous job? How long is the worker expected to be out of the workplace?
- **Address issues of effort and reliability.** Documentation should demonstrate clearly if the worker's subjective and objective information are congruent. Documentation from the treating physician and rehabilitation providers should reflect evidence of compliance or noncompliance and of progression with treatment programs.
- **Be prepared to respond to anger or depression, or both.** Both might appear for various reasons and can include physical limitations, financial concerns, altered work ethic, or friction between the worker and the employer or the worker and the worker's compensation case manager. Identifying and addressing these issues earlier rather than later will assist the process.

At the end of the treatment process for the injured employee, the physician of record will be faced with the question of disposition. As a rule, a physician's goal is not to predict a person's ability or inability to perform the essential elements of work but to determine if the medical condition has become permanent because it has reached a stable plateau. *Stable* is defined as a state in which no medical reason exists to expect that the individual will gain or lose future functional ability.[3] At this point, the physician should request a functional capacity evaluation (FCE).

FUNCTIONAL CAPACITY EVALUATIONS

A registered nurse and an assembly line worker share many essential functions: standing tolerance, walking, dexterity (or fingering), and lifting and carrying. The difference exists in the frequency of these tasks and forces associated with them.

Matheson et al[3] published the *Physical Demands Characteristic Chart*, which describes frequency and weight tolerances and describes anticipated energy requirements expressed as metabolic equivalents (Table 1). This chart is based on the *Dictionary of Occupational Titles*,[4] which provides force and postural requirements for job descriptions in all industries.

The FCE is a full-body assessment designed to evaluate the essential functions of work, including force testing (lift, carry), sustained positioning (standing, sitting), repetitive movement, and fingering. Certain test activities are required for all clients; job-specific tasks (identified by a formal job description or client's report) can be added to improve validity and ensure safety. The FCE also captures objective measurements, such as range of motion, girth (edema or atrophy, or both), strength, balance, and sensation. For the worker with a musculoskeletal disorder, testing ideally should be performed by a physical or occupational therapist, but certified athletic trainers and kinesiologists also are trained to perform the testing.

Test activities are performed in a structured manner, with the examiner monitoring movement patterns, heart rate, and objective signs of increased effort and increased pain. Time required to perform each lift and carry activity is recorded. Oral communication with the client to monitor pain and fatigue is initiated.

The FCE also identifies level of effort and reliability of client reports (RCR) through consistency of performance in similar activities (eg, repetitive squats and floor-to-waist lift) and distraction-based testing. Additional testing, including coefficients of variance and questionnaires pertaining to pain and function (eg, the Ransford Pain Drawing,[5] the Neck Disability Index,[6] and the Modified Somatic Perception Questionnaire[7]), might be included to specifically clarify issues of reliability and effort. These components of testing are not intended to imply motive or intent; they are intended only to identify the existence of these behaviors. In addition, a cluster of testing rather than 1 test should be used to confirm issues of validity and reliability.

Table 1. Physical Demand Characteristics of Work

Physical Demand Level	Occasional 0–33% of Workday	Frequent 34–66% of Workday	Constant 67–100% of Workday	Typical Energy Required
Sedentary	10 lb	Negligible	Negligible	1.5–2.1 METS
Light	20 lb	10 lb and/or Walk/stand/ push/pull of arm/leg controls	Negligible push/pull of arm/leg controls while seated	2.2–3.5 METS
Medium	20–50 lb	10–25 lb	10 lb	3.6–6.3 METS
Heavy	50–100 lb	25–50 lb	10–20 lb	6.4–7.5 METS
Very heavy	>100 lb	>50 lb	>20 lb	>7.5 METS

Abbreviation: METS, metabolic equivalents.
Adapted with permission from Leonard N. Matheson, PhD, CRC, CVE.[3]

Generally, the FCE will have 1 of 4 possible outcomes: full effort and good RCR, full effort and poor RCR, poor effort and good RCR, and poor effort and poor RCR. When effort and reliability of reporting are submaximal or variable, the return-to-work determination is expressed as what the employee was willing to perform and not as the full capability of the employee.

The first rule for any examiner performing FCEs is safety. As noted, the examiner monitors movement patterns and heart rate throughout testing and does not leave the client unsupervised. Because this examination is function-based and not diagnosis-based, the client must be stable medically not just from the perspective of the isolated injury but for the entire body. Uncontrolled hypertension, overlying orthopaedic problems not related to the injury, or chronic systemic disease in periods of exacerbation (eg, rheumatoid arthritis, sickle cell disease, systemic lupus erythematosus) will limit or prevent testing.

For the employee who has an injury requiring extensive intervention (>3 months of limited activity, multiple procedures), the decline in physical activity reasonably can be assumed to lead to weight gain; a loss of physical conditioning; and at times, a new onset of hypertension or diabetes. A medical clearance from a general practitioner is **strongly** recommended for clients who are in high-risk categories for such physiologic diseases. If any physical restrictions are currently in place, the referring physician should differentiate an absolute restriction (one that is related directly to the surgical intervention and will not be lifted in any scenario) from a relative restriction (one that is in place for transitioning to the workplace).

The second rule, which is a close second, for an examiner is to provide an objective assessment of the injured worker's function. The assessment is based purely on the performance of the worker; conclusions regarding maximum effort and consistency of concerns or abilities can be made and should be reported. The examiner should not speculate the "why" of performance as it pertains to motivation, which is best evaluated from a psychosocial aspect. Ideally, the worker's individual job description and notation of any specific areas of concern as verbalized by the referral source or sources will be available. The report will contrast the worker's FCE performance against the job description to specifically identify areas of deficiency.

Some debate exists in the reliability and validity of FCEs; in other words, does an FCE accurately predict the ability to return to work? Researchers have examined this topic from many angles, including validity of test items, interrater and intrarater reliability, and systems used.[8–12] In addition to the factors inherent to the test system and the examiner, one must consider the test subject when contemplating validity.

In light of this discussion, we should consider other examiner-patient testing performed, such as manual muscle testing, goniometry, and gait analysis.[13,14] Investigators have demonstrated that interrater reliability with goniometric testing can vary from 5° to 7° among practitioners.[15] Repetition improves performance, and the same skills used for evaluation and treatment of the acutely injured patient also are performed in FCEs. I would argue that the reliability and validity of the FCE are rooted in the examiner rather than in the test system and its components particularly because all test systems contain the same basic activities to assess work (material handling or force testing, sustained postures, fingering).

The FCE can be useful in directing further care and serve as an entry point to a work-hardening or work-reintegration program. As mentioned, workers with injuries requiring extensive interventions (generally >3 months) most certainly will become deconditioned. For the worker who performs at or higher than a medium level of physical demand[4] or is required to meet productivity goals, it would be reasonable to assume that he or she would lack the endurance needed to maintain a production pace in addition to losses of strength and power. In this instance, the FCE would serve as a starting point for entry to a work-hardening or work-reintegration program.

A work-conditioning program is also appropriate for the worker who demonstrates submaximal effort or poor reliability in reporting pain or function. Work hardening allows the client to perform essential elements of his job in a supervised environment over the course of several weeks. The practitioner supervising the client is able to discern factors, such as fear, lack of confidence, or lack of conditioning, and address them in treatment. If the client has demonstrated poor effort and poor reliability in FCE, these behaviors are addressed during work hardening. If successful, the client will overcome deficiencies and successfully return to work. If unsuccessful, the program will help identify further treatment options or, in the case of poor effort and reliability, identify a lack of engagement in the recovery process and lead to case closure.

Ideally, the examiner will return the report within 2 business days. The FCE report includes, at the very least, a summary of physical examination; a grid expressing the client's performance in terms of weight and frequency; and a summary with statements regarding current level of physical demand, cooperation and effort, and return-to-work options. Areas of critical concern can be communicated in a more immediate fashion, such as by telephone or e-mail.

IMPAIRMENT RATINGS

An impairment rating (IR) differs from the FCE in that the IR is not function-based at all; rather, specific measures, such as range of motion, electromyographic and nerve conduction velocity findings, girth, and radiographic examination are used to arrive at a percentage of impairment. All IRs are performed in accordance with guidelines in *Guides to the Evaluation of Permanent Impairment, 5th ed.*[16] The worker's condition must be considered stable, which also is known as *maximum medical improvement*, before the rating is performed. The average healing time for a rotator cuff repair is 1 year; with adherence to a home exercise program, active range of motion in the shoulder often improves from the time of discharge from physical therapy to the 1-year postoperative mark. Preferably, the impairment rating should not be performed until this time to ensure that maximum medical improvement has been achieved. Unfortunately, the surgeons and the worker's compensation carriers will not wait that long to achieve case closure.

Impairment ratings require physician orders to perform and are the final approval for the rating. Again, physical and occupational therapists, as well as certified athletic trainers, can perform the data collection for musculoskeletal disorders, but the results cannot be discussed with anyone except the referring physician until approved because this is the practitioner who must justify the percentage of impairment. Nonphysicians cannot assign permanent or partial impairment ratings; they only can gather accurate data to help the physician determine this.

Typically, the ratings are used for settlement or job reassignment at the time of case closure. It is not considered a statement of ability or function because the rating might be artificially high or low in comparison. This is particularly true in orthopaedic medicine where reconstructive and salvage procedures have increased in complexity to restore basic function but have not allowed heavy demands on the joint. A good example of this situation is the person requiring a reverse total shoulder arthroplasty.

Case History

A 52-year-old man underwent 2 rotator cuff repairs, both of which failed, followed by a total shoulder replacement and major rotator cuff reconstruction in 1990. He required a reverse total shoulder arthroplasty in 2011. His ultimate active range of motion was limited severely. An impairment rating could be performed using 1 of 2 methods noted in *Guides to the Evaluation of Permanent Impairment, 5th ed.*[16] Following are both methods and a rating using a proposed method that considers the advances in this area of practice.

Options

Option 1 (Range-of-Motion Method). The examination revealed elevation to 70°, extension to 30°, abduction to 50°, adduction to 22°, internal rotation to 50°, and external rotation to 45°. The impairment rating was 18% for the upper extremity and 11% for the whole person.

Option 2 (After Arthroplasty). After total shoulder arthroplasty, the impairment rating was 24% for the upper extremity and 14% for the whole person. This patient underwent 3 separate operative repairs to address his limitations and pain, eventually requiring a salvage operation to allow basic personal tasks and alleviate pain. He could not return to his former occupation (unloading trucks for a big box store). Arguably, 24% of upper extremity impairment does not adequately represent the extent of loss for this extremity.

In collaboration with a shoulder therapist, Table 2 was devised as a possible means of addressing more complicated operative procedures and the permanent limitations that result. It incorporates range of motion and also addresses loss of anatomic structure and permanent restriction based on the repair itself. Table 2 has not been approved for use in assigning impairment ratings in lieu of those guidelines set forth in *Guides to the Evaluation of Permanent Impairment, 5th ed*,[16] and should not be considered a valid instrument. Guidelines for use of Table 2 include (1) no use of the Guide's range-of-motion or diagnosis-related, estimate-based impairments; (2) impairment per category is based on the number of points met (2% per point); (3) pain cannot be separated out for additional impairment; and (4) activity limitations must be documented by the treating surgeon and not per patient report; likewise, difficulty performing activities of daily living must be documented by the treating rehabilitation provider.

Option 3. The examination revealed category III (salvage procedure), greater than 30% loss of motion in multiple planes, moderate levels of pain (average of 5/10 with use), moderate limitation or difficulty with personal activities of daily living (no overhead reaching or cross-body reaching based on motion limitations), and sedentary work only (absolute or permanent restriction due to the procedure). The impairment rating was 50% for the upper extremity and 30% for the whole person. As mentioned, this is one possible modification to the impairment rating criteria that could better express the loss after a complex or catastrophic work injury. Certainly, an injury of a magnitude to warrant extensive measures of treatment would prohibit return to the previous occupation and also would warrant a greater rating of impairment than the current system allows.

Table 2. Potential Way to Address Complicated Operative Procedures and the Resulting Permanent Limitations[a]

Category	Examination	Upper Extremity Impairment Rating, %
I	20% Loss of motion in elevation (compared with the contralateral limb) Completes personal and basic activities of daily living without difficulty Limited outdoor activities of daily living Lifting <30 lb (13.5 kg) from the floor and occasional elevated work allowed Anatomic repair performed	20–30
II	30% Loss of motion in multiple planes (compared with the contralateral limb) Minimal difficulty and modification in completing personal and basic activities of daily living Revision procedure Lifting <15 lb (6.75 kg) from the floor Repair via nonanatomic means	30–40
III	>30% Loss of motion in multiple planes (compared with the contralateral limb) Moderate difficulty and modification for personal and basic activities of daily living Sedentary work only Moderate pain levels (average pain rating of 4/10–6/10) Irreparable, salvage, or pain management procedure	40–50

[a] Guidelines for use include (1) client is independent of range-of-motion or diagnosis-related estimate-based impairments; (2) impairment per category is based on the number of points met (2% per point); (3) no additional ratings for pain; and (4) activity limitations must be documented by the treating surgeon and not per patient report; likewise, difficulty in performing activities of daily living must be documented by the treating rehabilitation provider.

REFERENCES

1. Bureau of Labor Statistics, US Department of Labor. *Injuries, Illnesses, and Fatalities: Frequently Asked Questions (FAQs).* http://www.bls.gov/iif/oshfaq1.htm. Accessed November 22, 2011.
2. Bureau of Labor Statistics, US Department of Labor. *Nonfatal Occupational Injuries and Illnesses Requiring Days Away From Work, 2009.* November 2010:1–37. http:/www.bls.gov/news.release/archives/osh2_11092010.pdf. Accessed November 22, 2011.
3. Matheson L, Langford K, Enright W, Kyi MT, Reynolds J, Lynch L. *The Functional Capacity Evaluation Certification Program.* Keene, NH: Roy Matheson and Associates, Inc; 2001.
4. National Academy of Sciences, Committee on Occupational Classification and Analysis. Dictionary of Occupational Titles (DOT): part I. Current Population Survey, April 1971, Augmented With DOT Characterisitcs. Part II. 4th ed Dictionary of DOT Scores for 1970 Census Categories [computer file]. Washington, DC: US Department of Commerce, Bureau of the Census [producer], 197?. Ann Arbor, MI: Inter-university Consortium for Political and Social Research [distributor], 1981. http://www.occupationalinfo.org. Accessed November 22, 2011.
5. Ransford AO, Cairns D, Mooney V. The pain drawing as an aid to the psychologic evaluation patients with low-back pain. *Spine (Phila Pa 1976).* 1976;1(2):127–134.
6. Vernon H, Mior S. The Neck Disability Index: a study of reliability and validity. *J Manipulative Physiol Ther.* 1991;14(7):409–415.
7. Main CJ. The Modified Somatic Perception Questionnaire (MSPQ). *J Psychosom Res.* 1983;27(6):503–514.
8. Gibson L, Strong J, Wallace A. Functional capacity evaluation as a performance measure: evidence for a new approach for clients with chronic back pain. *Clin J Pain.* 2005;21(3):207–215.
9. Reneman MF, Soer F. Was predictive validity for a job-specific FCE established? *J Occup Environ Med.* 2010;52(12):1145–1146.
10. Lemstra M, Olszynski WP, Enright W. The sensitivity and specificity of functional capacity evaluations in determining maximal effort: a randomized trial. *Spine (Phila Pa 1976).* 2004;29(9):953–959.
11. Reneman MF, Jaegers SM, Westmaas M, Göeken LN. The reliability of determining effort level of lifting and carrying in a functional capacity evaluation. *Work.* 2002;18(1):23–27.
12. Gouttebarge V, Wind H, Kuijer PP, Frings-Dresen MH. Reliability and validity of Functional Capacity Evaluation methods: a systematic review with reference to Blankenship system, Ergos work simulator, Ergo-Kit and Isernhagen work system. *Int Arch Occup Environ Health.* 2004;77(8):527–537.
13. Nussbaumer S, Leunig M, Glatthorn JF, Stauffacher S, Gerber H, Maffiuletti NA. Validity and test-retest reliability of manual goniometers for measuring passive hip range of motion in femoroacetabular impingement patients. *BMC Musculoskelet Disord.* 2010;31(11):194.
14. Nadeau S, Kovacs S, Gravel D, et al. Active movement measurements of the shoulder girdle in healthy subjects with goniometer and tape measure techniques: a study on reliability and validity. *Physiother Theory Pract.* 2007;23(3):179–187.
15. Gajdosik RL, Bohannon RW. Clinical measurement of range of motion: review of goniometry emphasizing reliability and validity. *Phy Ther.* 1987;67(12):1867–1872.
16. Cocchiarella L, Andersson GBJ. *Guides to the Evaluation of Permanent Impairment.* 5th ed. New York, NY: American Medical Association; 2001.

IV-11

The Basics of Ordering and Interpreting Electromyography and Nerve Conduction Studies of the Shoulder Girdle

Jeff R. Fraser, PT, MS, ECS, CNIM, and Andrew Beach, PT, ECS

CHAPTER CONTENTS

- Why test
- Key nerve conduction findings
- Key electromyography findings
- Reaction of the peripheral nervous system to injury
- Case studies

Clinical pearls are highlighted in yellow throughout the text.

Electromyography (EMG) and nerve conduction studies (NCS) are used to detect pathologic conditions and function of the nerve root, brachial plexus, peripheral nerves, neuromuscular junction, and muscle tissue. Generally, no test is complete without the performance of both parts. Nerve conduction studies involve collecting information related to the transmission of an action potential along a specific nerve. The EMG component of the test provides additional information about the function of the peripheral nerve by placing a needle recording electrode in a muscle and analyzing various electrical characteristics of that particular muscle.

Our discussion focuses on the use of EMG/NCS as it applies to the evaluation, diagnosis, and treatment of shoulder and upper extremity conditions. The EMG/NCS should be used to evaluate potential pathologic conditions that can mimic symptoms related to glenohumeral disorders or any other disorder, such as cervical radiculopathy, focal neuropathy (eg, carpal tunnel or cubital tunnel), injury to the brachial plexus, and generalized peripheral neuropathy, that might coexist with various shoulder conditions. A properly performed EMG/NCS can be an invaluable part of a complete upper extremity assessment.

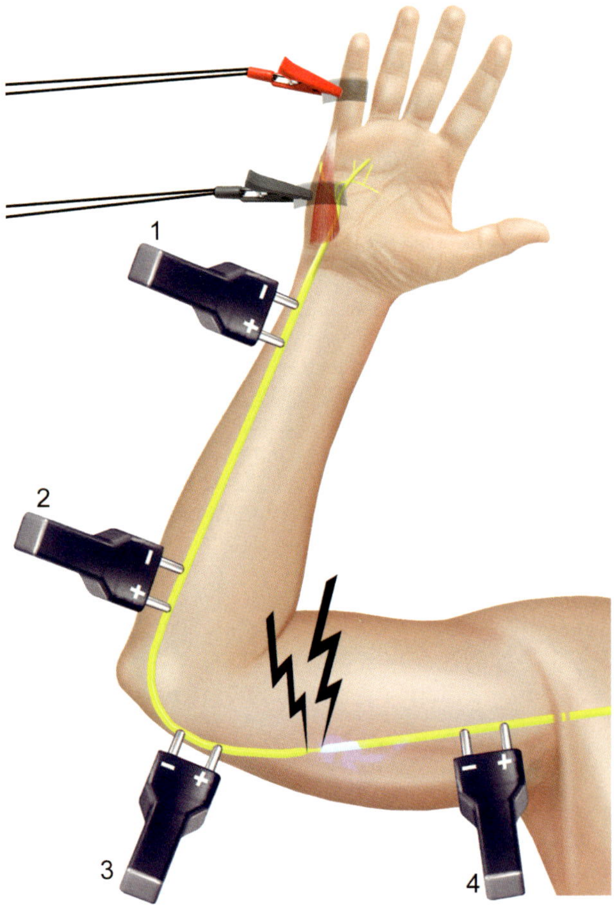

Figure 1. Nerve conduction study of the ulnar nerve. Electrodes are placed on the abductor digiti minimi, and the nerve is stimulated at various locations (1–4 starting distal to proximal) along the nerve. This figure depicts a lesion of the nerve in the arm that is discussed later in the chapter.

WHY TEST

The EMG/NCS enables the clinician to determine if nerve involvement is present; to identify which nerve is involved; and to provide information about the chronicity, severity, and type of nerve injury. This information is invaluable when assessing and treating the shoulder. A properly performed examination can help clarify the symptoms that do not necessarily fit the glenohumeral diagnosis. For instance, a winged scapula could be due to generalized muscle weakness of the rhomboids or serratus anterior, a C7 radiculopathy, or injury to the long thoracic nerve or spinal accessory nerves. Another common presentation is weakness of the external rotator muscles and anterior shoulder pain. This weakness could be due to a tear or tendinitis in the infraspinatus, a suprascapular neuropathy, or C5-C6 radiculopathy. Even a positive magnetic resonance imaging (MRI) scan for a tear in the infraspinatus or supraspinatus might not explain the weakness found on clinical examination. In this instance, a properly performed EMG/NCS examination gives the clinician certainty about whether the weakness in external rotation (ER) is purely muscular or whether a nerve injury is causing some or most of the muscle weakness.

The time at which EMG/NCS is performed in relation to the onset of the patient's symptoms is critical to have meaningful results. To increase understanding of when to refer a patient for EMG testing, we will briefly review some of the key findings from an EMG examination and the reaction of the peripheral nervous system to injury.

KEY NERVE CONDUCTION FINDINGS

When performing an NCS, a peripheral nerve is stimulated at some point along its length, and the response is recorded from electrodes, which generally are placed distal to the stimulation site on either a sensory nerve or a muscle when testing motor nerves (Figure 1). A sensory nerve action potential (SNAP) is generated when recording from a sensory nerve, and a compound muscle action potential (CMAP) is generated when recording over a muscle. These responses are not isolated action potentials from 1 nerve fiber but are the summation of multiple nerve fibers that compose the entire peripheral nerve. Testing generally occurs at multiple sites along the nerve, and multiple CMAPs or SNAPs are generated (Figure 2).

The variables of the SNAP or CMAP that generally are measured include the latency, amplitude, and nerve conduction velocity (NCV). The *latency* is the time in milliseconds needed for a nerve impulse to travel from the point of stimulation to the recording site. A prolonged latency (ie, a nerve that is conducting slower

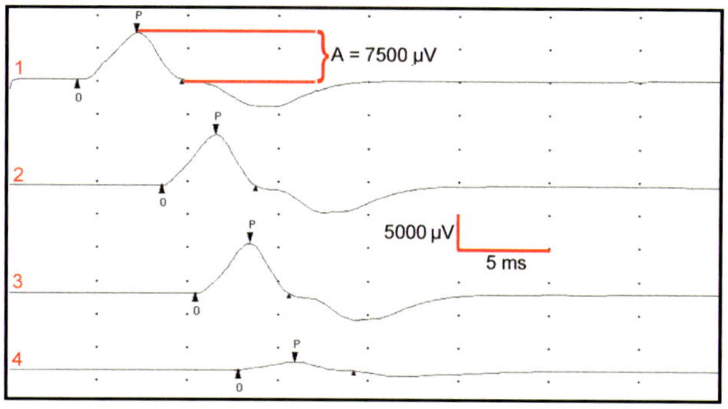

Figure 2. Ulnar nerve conduction block. The ulnar nerve compound muscle action potentials recorded from the abductor digiti minimi to ulnar nerve stimulation at the wrist, 1, below the elbow, 2, above the elbow, 3, and in the axilla, 4. Note the reduced amplitude of the fourth response compared with the other responses. This is an indication of motor conduction block in the arm. See Figure 1. Abbreviations: O, onset of the response; P, peak of the response; and A, amplitude.

than predicted) is generally an indication of demyelination. The *amplitude*, measured in microvolts, is the height of the response from the baseline to the peak; it represents an approximation of the total number of individual nerve fibers that are contributing to the response. For instance, a reduced amplitude would indicate the loss of axons due to injury or disease or a failure of an action potential to conduct past a certain point along the nerve (ie, conduction block) (Figure 2). The *NCV*, measured in meters per second, is the speed at which the action potential travels over a given nerve segment. This can be calculated by dividing the distance of a nerve segment by the latency between 2 stimulation points. Slow NCV indicates demyelination either at a specific location (focal demyelination) or along the course of the nerve (general or segmental demyelination).

KEY ELECTROMYOGRAPHY FINDINGS

The EMG portion of the examination includes inserting a needle recording electrode in various muscles and analyzing the resulting electrical activity. The needle electrode is typically in the vicinity of several individual motor units. A *motor unit* is the individual motor axon and all of the muscle fibers it innervates. Some of the key variables in this portion of the examination include electrical activity of the muscle at rest, motor unit recruitment, the structure and appearance of the motor unit, and motor unit amplitude (Table 1).

Table 1. Summary of Key Electromyography and Nerve Conduction Variables

Examination	Key Variable	Importance
Nerve conduction	Latency	Slow = demyelination
	Amplitude	Reduced = axonal loss
	Nerve conduction velocity	Slow = demyelination or conduction block
Electromyography	Resting activity	Fibrillation potentials and positive sharp waves = axonal loss[a]
	Motor unit recruitment	Reduced = axonal loss or conduction block
	Motor unit amplitude	Large = chronic axonal loss
	Motor unit morphology (polyphasic)	Large amplitude = collateral sprouting Small amplitude = axonal regeneration

[a] Indicates that it can be seen in other conditions that are beyond the scope of this chapter.

When the EMG needle is inserted and is no longer moving through muscle tissue and the muscle is relaxed, it should be electrically silent. Abnormal resting activity, such as fibrillation potentials and positive sharp waves, are seen with motor axonal loss. When an injury to a motor axon is severe enough, the distal portion of the axon undergoes wallerian degeneration, and the muscle fibers that it supplied become denervated. After approximately 4 weeks, the denervated muscle fibers begin to fibrillate spontaneously, and this appears electrically as fibrillation potentials or positive sharp waves. The precise time that these potentials can be seen depends on the distance of the muscle from the site of the nerve lesion. For example, with lumbar radiculopathy, they would be seen first in the paraspinal muscles (closer to the lesion site) and last in the most distal muscle (innervated by that particular myotome). These potentials are one of the hallmark findings of denervation. They also can be seen in other conditions, but that is beyond the scope of this chapter.

After analysis of resting activity, the patient is instructed to minimally contract the targeted muscle. With a minimal contraction, it is possible to see only 1 motor unit potential firing on the display screen. With increasing muscle force, the firing frequency of the motor unit increases until another motor unit is activated or "recruited." It continues with additional motor unit potentials being activated until the display screen is filled with motor unit potentials. This is called *motor unit recruitment analysis*. In cases of axonal loss or conduction block, the neuromuscular system compensates for fewer motor units by having the initial motor unit potential fire at an abnormally fast rate with recruitment of fewer than expected additional motor unit potentials. This is referred to as *reduced motor unit recruitment*.

The structure, appearance, and amplitude of the individual motor unit potential can provide useful information about the nerve that supplies a particular muscle. Normal motor unit potentials are biphasic and triphasic (Figure 3). Small-amplitude polyphasic motor unit potentials are seen as a nerve fiber regenerates. As the regenerating nerve fiber comes into contact with the muscle it once supplied, the sprouts at the end of the axon reaching the individual muscle fibers initially are immature and do not conduct a nerve impulse normally. The nerve impulse in a normal motor unit reaches each muscle fiber relatively synchronously, resulting in a biphasic or triphasic motor unit potential. However, in a regenerating axon, conduction across this segment is much more variable, meaning that the nerve transmission to the individual nerve fibers occurs over a longer period and results in a polyphasic response.

Large-amplitude motor unit potentials can be seen in cases of chronic axonal loss. When some of the axons to a given muscle die, the remaining intact axons in the area send out collateral sprouts and incorporate the previously denervated muscle fibers into its motor unit. This results in a motor unit potential with an increased number of muscle fibers, which manifests electrically as a large-amplitude motor unit potential. During the process of collateral sprouting, the axonal sprouts

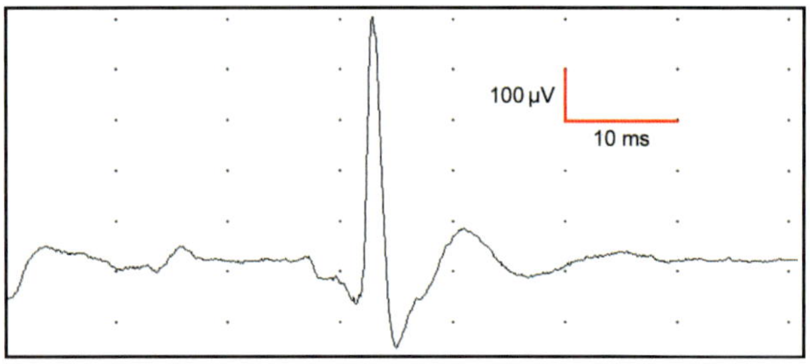

Figure 3. Triphasic motor unit potential.

from the intact nerves reaching the denervated muscle are immature, which is similar to those of regenerating axons. This results in a motor unit potential with a large amplitude that is also polyphasic. As these axonal sprouts mature, the number of phases is reduced and leaves a biphasic or triphasic large-amplitude motor unit potential.

REACTION OF THE PERIPHERAL NERVOUS SYSTEM TO INJURY

A peripheral nerve comprises individual axons (nerve fibers) surrounded by a myelin sheath. This nerve fiber travels through a connective tissue framework called the *endoneural tube*. All of the axons are supported by additional connective tissue framework. Wallerian degeneration takes place with an axon that has been damaged and dies distal to the site of the injury (Figure 4).

Three types of peripheral nerve injuries are important to understand when analyzing results of EMG/NCS (Figure 5). Neurapraxia, or conduction block, is the mildest type of nerve injury in which nerve conduction is blocked temporarily due to local ischemia and damage to the myelin sheath. Axonal integrity is maintained, and wallerian degeneration does not take place. Neurapraxia usually resolves within 6 to 8 weeks. A patient presenting with a neurapraxia has numbness and weakness along the distribution of that nerve distal to the lesion. Nerve conduction testing shows an amplitude reduction when stimulating above the lesion because of the blocked fibers but a normal amplitude when stimulating distal to the lesion because

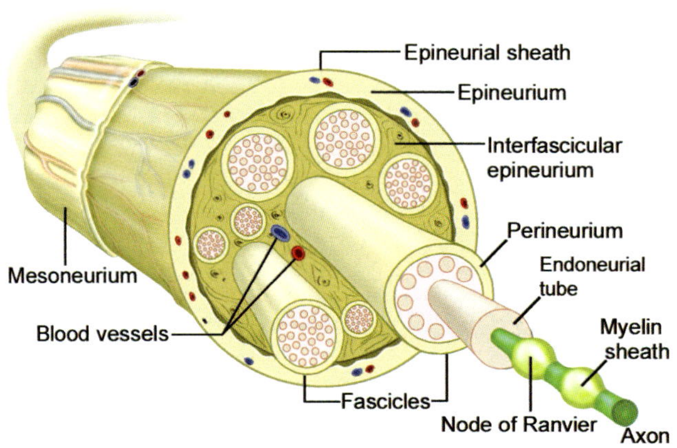

Figure 4. Peripheral nerve anatomy.

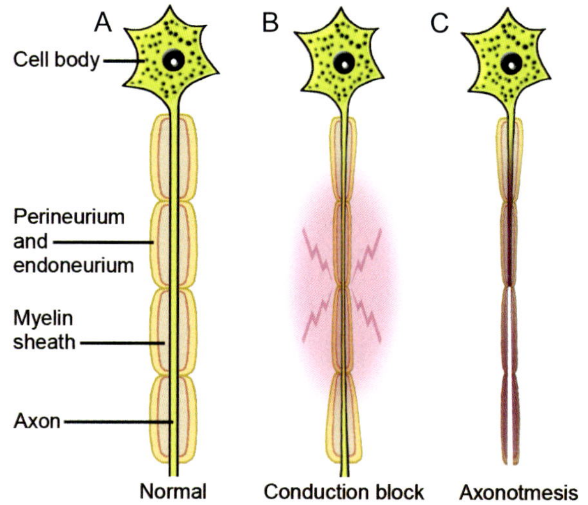

Figure 5. Types of peripheral nerve injuries. A, Normal axonal and connective tissue integrity. B, Conduction block due to local ischemia causes the nerve transmission to fail although the axonal integrity is maintained. C, The axon is damaged and undergoes wallerian degeneration distal to the lesion, but the endoneural tube remains as a guide to direct the axon as it regenerates.

the axon is intact (Figure 2). Depending on the severity of the injury, EMG might show reduced motor unit recruitment. Fibrillation potentials and positive sharp waves are not expected because the muscle is not denervated. As the conduction block resolves, the NCS and EMG findings return to normal.

Axonotmesis is a progressively more severe type of nerve injury in which the axonal integrity is disrupted and the axon distal to the lesion undergoes wallerian degeneration, resulting in denervation. However, the endoneural tube remains intact. This is important because a channel exists through which the regenerating nerve fiber can travel to eventually resupply the target end organ. If enough individual nerve fibers within the peripheral nerve are involved, an axonotmesis injury manifests clinically as weakness or numbness, or both. Nerve conduction studies show a reduced amplitude distal **and** proximal to the axonal injury (Figure 6). Electromyography reveals reduced motor unit recruitment, and after 4 to 6 weeks, fibrillation potentials and positive sharp waves would be expected.

Neurotmesis describes disruption of the axon, endoneural tube, and other portions of the connective tissue framework of the peripheral nerve. This also leads to wallerian degeneration of the affected axons and

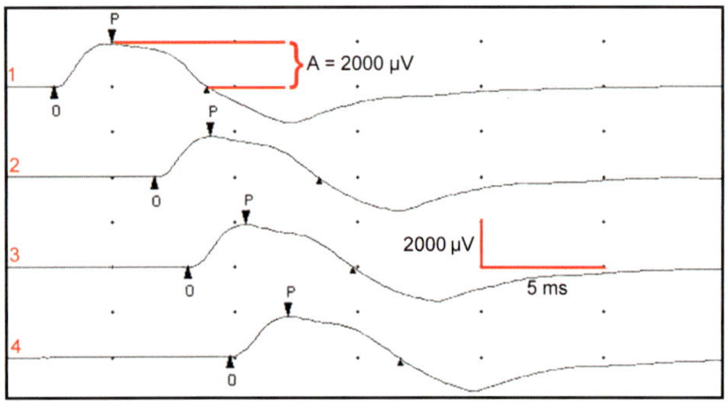

Figure 6. Ulnar nerve axonal loss. The amplitude of these responses are approximately 2000 µV but should be more than 5000 µV. Because all responses are reduced, this is an indication of an axonal loss lesion at some point along the nerve, plexus, or nerve root. A detailed electromyographic examination will be invaluable in determining the location of the lesion. Abbreviations: O, onset of the response; P, peak of the response; and A, amplitude.

denervation. In this case, however, no clear path exists for a regenerating nerve fiber to travel, which leads to only partial or incomplete recovery. Unfortunately, an axonotmesis lesion is electrophysiologically indistinguishable from a neurotmesis. Although distinguishing between the 2 might be important from a clinical standpoint, the only conclusion that can be made electrophysiologically is whether axonal loss is present.

Table 2 shows that immediately after a nerve injury, neurapraxia and axonal loss lesions are indistinguishable. After 3 to 5 days, an axonal loss lesion would be expected to demonstrate decreased amplitude with NCSs. After 4 to 6 weeks, fibrillation potentials would be expected in involved muscles. If a test is performed too soon without a clear understanding of how these changes occur over time, erroneous conclusions can be made.

Consider a scenario in which the ulnar nerve is lacerated in the proximal arm. Clinically, one would expect weakness and numbness in an ulnar nerve distribution. On NCS testing, if the ulnar nerve is stimulated proximal to the lesion, no response would be recorded from the ulnar-innervated abductor digiti minimi in the hand. This is obviously because the action potential traveling on the individual nerve fibers composing the ulnar nerve simply would stop at the site of the laceration. However, if the nerve is stimulated distal to the lesion, a response would be present for the first few days because the distal portion of the nerve continues to conduct normally. However, over the next 3 to 5 days as the nerve undergoes wallerian degeneration, the amplitude of the response to distal stimulation would decrease, and eventually, no response would be recorded either proximally or distally.

As discussed, conduction block looks clinically and electrophysiologically identical to an axonal loss lesion immediately after a nerve injury. Consider again the ulnar nerve lesion mentioned previously. However, instead of knowing the nerve has been lacerated, assume that a patient has sustained a blow to the arm and it is unclear if the nerve fibers are intact. Stimulation proximal to the lesion would result in no response because the conduction is "blocked" at the lesion site. Stimulation distally would result in a normal response.

However, after waiting 3 to 5 days for wallerian degeneration to occur, a reduced amplitude to both proximal and distal stimulation would indicate axonal loss (Figure 6), whereas conduction block would continue to show a normal response to distal stimulation. After 4 to 6 weeks, fibrillation potentials and positive sharp waves would be expected in an ulnar nerve distribu-

Table 2. Neurapraxia Versus Axonal Loss

	Conduction Block			Axonal Loss		
Examination	Day 1[a]	>5 d	4–6 wk	Day 1	>5 d	4–6 wk
Nerve conduction study						
Distal stimulation	Normal	Normal	Normal	Normal	Abnormal	Abnormal
Proximal stimulation	Abnormal	Abnormal	Improving	Abnormal	Abnormal	Abnormal
Electromyography						
Recruitment	Reduced	Reduced	Improving	Reduced	Reduced	Reduced
Fibrillation potentials and positive sharp waves	No	No	No	No	No	Yes

[a] Note that on day 1, a conduction block lesion looks identical to an axonal loss lesion. As time progresses, different findings are manifest with electromyography and nerve conduction studies. A test that is performed too soon without knowledge of these changes can lead to erroneous conclusions about the type of nerve injury and prognosis for recovery.

tion if axonal loss were present. Unless some type of intervention is going to be contemplated in the interim, waiting 4 to 6 weeks after a suspected axonal loss injury to perform EMG/NCS might be prudent. This would allow time for all electrophysiologic abnormalities to be fully manifest and avoid the possibility of making clinical decisions based on incomplete results.

To further illustrate the importance of when an EMG is done in relation to the onset of symptoms, consider a patient with a suspected brachial plexopathy or a radiculopathy. Because of the proximal location of the lesion, reliably stimulating both proximal and distal to the lesion to determine if any change in amplitude is present might not be possible. If a test is done too early after the onset of the symptoms, substantial findings, such as fibrillation potentials and positive sharp waves that take time to develop, might be missed. In this case, one would conclude that the study was normal when in fact sufficient time had not elapsed to detect abnormalities with EMG.

CASE STUDIES

Consider the following case studies that further illustrate the usefulness of EMG/NCS testing for the upper extremity.

Case 1

A 63-year-old man with a 20-year history of left upper extremity pain and numbness noticed increased neck, left shoulder, and upper extremity pain and numbness and tingling into the hand over the past 6 months. He had surgical excision of an extracranial tumor on the left side more than 20 years before this examination and surgical excision of a left parietal tumor 6 months before this examination. He reported that his symptoms became worse after the latter procedure.

Pretest physical examination showed reduced cervical rotation to the left. Active range of motion in the left shoulder was limited into forward elevation (FE) with pain on end range. He had strength limitations in the left upper extremity, including 4/5 ER, 4/5 FE with pain, and less grip strength with his left than his right upper extremity. Sensation along the median nerve distribution in the hand in the C8-T1 dermatome was decreased. He had a positive Tinel sign at the carpal tunnel region.

Nerve conduction findings included the following: (1) prolonged median motor latency proximal to the wrist with slowed conduction velocity through the carpal tunnel region and (2) amplitude in the median antebrachial cutaneous sensory nerve that was decreased greater than 50% compared with the right side (Tables 3 and 4). Electromyography findings included the fol-

Table 3. Upper Extremity Sensory Nerve Conduction Data Summary[a]

Site	Latency Peak, ms	Normal Peak, ms	O–P Amplitude μV[b]	Norm O–P Amplitude[b]
Left all sensory				
Median digit 3 above wrist	**4.0**[d]	<3.2	30	>15
Median digit 3 below wrist	1.7		32	>15
Ulnar digit 5	3.0	<3.2	21	>10
Median digit 1	**3.4**[d]	<3.0	18	>15
Radial digit 1	2.7	<3.0	12	>5
Left medial antebrachial cutaneous nerve	2.4	3.2	**5**[e]	8
Right medial antebrachial cutaneous nerve[c]	2.6	3.2	16	8

[a] Abnormal values are shown in bold.
[b] Amplitude is measured from the onset (O) to the peak (P) of the response.
[c] The medial antebrachial cutaneous nerve is a branch from the medial cord of the brachial plexus.
[d] The median sensor latency to digits 1 and 3 is prolonged and indicates a focal lesion at the carpal tunnel area.
[e] The left medial antebrachial cutaneous amplitude is reduced compared with the right and is an indication of axonal loss. A sensory amplitude that is reduced 50% or greater compared with the contralateral side is considered significant and is an indication of axonal loss. These findings are in agreement with the abnormal electromyographic data, showing chronic axonal loss (large-amplitude motor unit potentials) in muscles innervated by the medial cord.

lowing: (1) large-amplitude motor unit potentials in the flexor carpi ulnaris, first dorsal interosseous, abductor pollicis brevis, and flexor pollicis longus and (2) reduced motor unit recruitment noted in the abductor pollicis brevis and first dorsal interosseous (Table 5).

The findings showed evidence of (1) a moderate focal neuropathy of the left median nerve at the carpal tunnel and (2) a chronic, moderate injury to the medial cord of the left brachial plexus with no evidence of acute axonal injury observed.

This patient's pretest examination gave rise to suspicions of carpal tunnel syndrome, a C8-T1 radiculopathy, and/or a medial cord plexopathy. The EMG/NCS examination was constructed to explore these possibilities. A prolonged latency proximal to the wrist and conduction velocity slowing across the segment of the median nerve that traverses the carpal tunnel region was positive evidence of carpal tunnel syndrome and was consistent with pretest findings. The large-amplitude motor unit potentials observed in the C8-T1 myotome or myotomes was evidence of a chronic or previous axonal injury in this distribution. The decreased amplitude in the medial antebrachial cutaneous nerve on the left indicated axonal loss to this nerve. This finding coupled with the large-amplitude motor unit potentials in the C8-T1 indicated previous injury to the medial cord of the brachial plexus.

Table 4. Motor Summary

Site	Latency Onset, ms	Norm Onset, ms	O–P Amplitude, μV[a]	Norm O–P Amplitude[a]	Distance, cm	Velocity, m/s
Left median motor (recording from abductor pollicis brevis)						
Below wrist	1.8	<2.0	8.1	>5	6.0	17
Above wrist	**5.6**[b]	<4.3	8.3	>5	25.0	53
Elbow	10.3	NA	8.0	>5	NA	NA
Left ulnar motor (recording from abductor digiti minimi)						
Wrist	3.1	<3.2	7.3	>5	23.0	52
Below wrist	7.5	NA	7.6	>5	11.0	55
Above wrist	9.5	NA	7.5	>5	NA	NA

[a] Amplitude is measured from the onset (O) to the peak (P) of the response.

[b] The median motor distal latency (above the wrist) stimulation site is prolonged at the carpal tunnel. Median and ulnar nerve conduction otherwise are normal.

Abbreviation: NA, not applicable.

Table 5. Left Upper Extremity Electromyographic Data[a]

Muscle	Nerve	Origin From Plexus: Cord	Root	Amplitude[b]	Recruitment
Biceps	Musculocutaneous nerve	Lateral	C5-6	Normal	Normal
Deltoid	Axillary	Posterior	C5-6	Normal	Normal
Triceps	Radial	Posterior	C7-8	Normal	Normal
Extensor carpi radialis	Radial	Posterior	C6-7	Normal	Normal
Flexor carpi radialis	Median	Medial/lateral	C6-7	Normal	Normal
Flexor carpi ulnaris	Ulnar	Medial	C7-T1	Large	Normal
First dorsal interosseous	Ulnar	Medial	C8-T1	Large	Reduced
Abductor pollicis brevis	Median	Medial	C8-T1	Large	Reduced
Extensor indicis	Radial	Posterior	C7-8	Normal	Normal
Extensor carpi ulnaris	Radial	Posterior	C7-8	Normal	Normal
Anconeus	Radial	Posterior	C7-8	Normal	Normal
Flexor pollicis longus	Anterior indicis	Medial	C8-T1	Large	Normal
Cervical paraspinal	Dorsi rami	Not applicable	C4-T1	Normal	Normal

[a] Variables, such as insertional activity, resting activity, and duration, were omitted from the Table but were normal.

[b] The large-amplitude motor unit potentials noted in the muscles are consistent with a chronic medial cord brachial plexopathy. A C8-T1 radiculopathy or lower trunk plexopathy is not indicated because other C8-T1 muscles that are innervated by the nonmedial cord are normal.

Case 2

A 13-year-old boy who was a Little League Baseball pitcher developed insidious pain and weakness in his throwing shoulder that persisted for 5 months despite nonoperative treatment and rest. His pain was located at the deltoid insertion in the anterior and posterior aspect of the glenohumoral joint and trapezius. The MRI was positive for a superior labrum anterior-posterior lesion.

His pretest physical examination revealed pain with palpation on the proximal aspect of the biceps tendon, pain with active ER and FE, and strength limitations of 3/5 ER with pain and 4-/5 FE with pain. Nerve conduction findings included the following: (1) evaluation of the right suprascapular motor nerve showed a prolonged latency (slow nerve conduction) through the spinoglenoid notch, and (2) all remaining nerves as indicated in Tables 6 and 7 were within normal limits. All examined muscles showed no evidence of electrical instability (Table 8).

This examination revealed electrophysiologic evidence of a moderate focal neuropathy (focal demyelination) of the right suprascapular nerve likely at the spinoglenoid notch region. No evidence of a cervical radiculopathy or brachial plexopathy was observed.

Table 6. Right Upper Extremity Sensory Summary[a]

Site	Latency Peak, ms	Norm Peak, ms	O–P Amplitude, μV[b]	Norm O–P Amplitude[b]
Median to digit 3	2.6	<3.2	46	>15
Ulnar to digit 5	2.5	<3.2	41	>10
Median to digit 1	2.7	<3.0	29	>15
Radial to digit 1	2.3	<3.0	16	>5

[a] All values are normal.

[b] Amplitude is measured from the onset (O) to the peak (P) of the response.

Table 7. Right Motor Summary Table

Site	Latency Onset, ms	Norm Onset, ms	O–P Amplitude, μV[a]	Norm O–P Amplitude[a]	Distance, cm	Velocity, m/s
Right median motor (recording from abductus pollicis brevis)						
Above wrist	3.8	<4.3	6.6	>5	23.0	59
Elbow	7.7	NA	6.6	>5	NA	NA
Right suprascapular motor						
Supraspinatus	2.7[b]	<3.7	NA[c]	NA	NA	NA
Infraspinatus	**7.7**[d]	<4.7	NA[c]	NA	NA	NA

[a] Amplitude is measured from the onset (O) to the peak (P) of the response.

[b] Because the latency to the supraspinatus is normal, this indicates that the lesion is at the spinoglenoid notch.

[c] Indicates amplitude was recorded with a needle electrode (NA, not applicable).

[d] The latency was prolonged when recording from the infraspinatus.

Table 8. Right Upper Extremity Electromyographic Data[a]

Muscle	Nerve	Nerve Root
Deltoid	Axillary	C5-6
Triceps	Radial	C7
Extensor carpi radialis	Radial	C6-7
Flexor carpi radialis	Median	C6-7
Flexor carpi ulnaris	Ulnar	C7-T1
Supraspinatus	Suprascapular	C5-6
Infraspinatus	Suprascapular	C5-6
Biceps	Musculocutaneous	C5-6
Cervical paraspinal	Dorsal rami	C5-T1
First dorsal interosseous	Ulnar	C8-T1

[a] Indicates variables, such as insertional activity, resting activity, amplitude, recruitment, and duration, were omitted from the Table but were normal.

The pretest examination of this patient gave rise to suspicions of a brachial plexopathy, suprascapular nerve palsy, axillary nerve injury, and cervical radiculopathy. The EMG/NCS examination was constructed to examine these possibilities. The slow nerve conduction in the suprascapular nerve recording from the infraspinatus indicated injury to the myelin sheath at the spinoglenoid notch. Normal findings with EMG ruled out any acute or chronic axonal injury to the cervical nerve roots, brachial plexus, or other peripheral nerves.

RECOMMENDED READING

Dumitru D. *Electrodiagnostic Medicine*. Philadelphia, PA: Hanley & Belfus; 1995.

Cummins CA, Messer TM, Nuber GW. Suprascapular nerve entrapment. *J Bone Joint Surg Am*. 2000;82(3):415–424.

Kimura J. *Electrodiagnosis in Diseases of Nerve and Muscle: Principles and Practice*. 3rd ed. New York, NY: Oxford University Press; 2001.

Katirji B. *Electromyography in Clinical Practice: A Case Study Approach*. 2nd ed. Philadelphia, PA: Mosby Elsevier; 2007.

IV-12

Evidence-Based Use of Modalities in the Shoulder Girdle

Kristine Jankowski, PT, DPT, CPI, and Michael T. Lebec, PT, PhD

CHAPTER CONTENTS

Clinical pearls are highlighted in yellow throughout the text.

In this chapter, we focus on the most common therapeutic modalities that rehabilitation providers use to manage pathologic conditions affecting the shoulder joint. It is a summary and is not considered to be a complete reference. The reader is assumed to have general knowledge of the modalities described.

With respect to commentary on the evidence that guides the use of these modalities, the following concepts should be kept in mind. In the profession of physical therapy, evidence-based practice is important for streamlining decisions regarding the most effective and appropriate interventions. Whereas the use of evidence is extremely important in the profession, this approach in isolation is often controversial because of several limitations, including a clinician's interpretive skills, the inability of research findings to translate into clinical settings, time constraints, inconsistent research methods, and the hierarchy of studies.[1] Therefore, whereas the use of evidence is essential, it is equally important to remember that evidence-based practice demands that the practitioner also rely on his or her clinical experience and the unique values and perspectives of the individual patient when determining how to apply the best research evidence in a given situation.[2]

Bélanger[1] devised a classification system for the current body of evidence using a grading system of I, II, or III (Table 1). These resources were published in English and contained in peer-reviewed journals. All 3 grades are used to classify studies regardless of the level of randomization and blinding. Grade I classification is for controlled studies of humans, grade II is for noncontrolled studies of humans, and grade III is based on human case studies.

THERMOTHERAPY

Definition

Thermotherapy as related to physical therapy applications is the application of superficial heat sources to the skin surface to elevate tissue temperatures. The most common superficial heat source used to treat conditions affecting the shoulder joint is the moist hot pack.

Proposed Mechanism and Therapeutic Effects

Superficial heat is heat that penetrates to within 1 cm of the skin's surface, whereas *deep thermotherapy* is heat that penetrates more than 1 cm.[1] Superficial

Table 1. Bélanger's[1] Classification System on Evidence-Based Practice

Grade[a]	Evidence
I	Based on controlled studies of humans regardless of the level of randomization and blindness
II	Based on noncontrolled studies of humans regardless of the level of randomization and blindness
III	Based on case studies of humans regardless of the level of randomization and blindness[1]

[a] Indicates grade I is stronger than grade II and grades I and II are stronger than grade III.

heating via application of a moist hot pack is proposed to produce numerous therapeutic effects by increasing blood flow, elevating cell metabolism, elevating tissue temperature, decreasing pain, increasing tissue elasticity, and decreasing muscle spasm.[3] Increased blood flow occurs via vasodilatation of superficial blood vessels, which might result in enhanced delivery of nutrients and healing agents to the injured area. Raising tissue temperatures can increase metabolic effects and result in increased activity within cells, producing therapeutic substances.

Application of superficial heat potentially can decrease the perception of pain through gate theory mechanisms. This system often is described in a simplified manner as the gate from the peripheral nervous system being "open" or "closed" to the higher centers of the brain. When the gate is closed, neural impulses initiated by painful stimuli do not reach the brain, and thus the perception of pain is reduced.[1,4] Because heat might reduce sensitivity of muscle spindles, it also might result in increased muscle relaxation or decreased muscle spasm. Lastly, when elevated by 3°C to 5°C, collagen tissue becomes more extensible and susceptible to stretch, which might lead to an increase in range of motion (ROM) of the shoulder.[5]

Relevant Treatment Variables

Unlike other modalities used in the management of shoulder conditions, there are few relevant variables to consider. Of greatest importance are sufficient preheating of moist hot packs, treatment duration, and efficient layering to avoid injury. Hot packs should be immersed for 30 minutes or longer before application for proper heating and therapeutic effects.[1] Application for at least 20 minutes is recommended for maximum heating of soft tissues,[6] and a coupling thickness of approximately 5 to 8 layers of towels should be used to avoid superficial burning of the skin.[1] Many clinicians use thick reusable terry cloth covers in the cervical size to accommodate the varying angles of the shoulder. Injury during heat therapy or application of hot packs ranked fourth and accounted for 10% of physical therapy liability claims from December 1993 to March 2006.[7] Therefore, because of variations in sensitivity, skin, and comfort levels, each patient should be monitored frequently.

Practical Treatment Considerations

Whereas research regarding the use of superficial heat supports the therapeutic claims presented, the context within which these occur is somewhat limited. Because direct energy emitted by superficial heat does not penetrate to depths of greater than 1 cm, therapeutic effects typically are limited to tissues located within these layers. Although tissue temperature in deeper layers might be elevated when the blood within superficial vessels becomes heated and penetrates to lower layers, the degree to which this occurs is minimal with respect to temperature changes necessary for therapeutic effects. Abramson et al[8] demonstrated this when examining changes in tissue temperature. They showed that after 30 minutes of moist heat application, intramuscular forearm temperatures increased to a maximum of 1°C.[8] Such changes are the bare minimum necessary to increase cellular metabolism but are not sufficient to produce any other therapeutic effects associated with elevated tissue temperatures that require increases of 2°C to 5°C.[9] The exception of course might be in patients who have ectomorphic body types and might have much more superficially located anatomic structures.

Specific Indications

Based on this information, thermotherapy via moist hot packs is indicated most for the following purposes. Enhanced healing through increased blood flow and cellular metabolism is likely only possible in conditions affecting very superficial tissues, such as sprains of the acromioclavicluar joint or conditions of the biceps. These effects also might be possible in slightly deeper tissues in individuals with very slight builds and smaller frames. Whereas many clinicians might describe using superficial heat to increase the extensibility of connective tissues found within joint capsules, ligaments, and rotator cuff tendons, these tissues are located much too deeply in most individuals to allow sufficient heating for these purposes. Therefore, most patients who have developed contractures or capsular restrictions might not benefit substantially from the use of moist heat to increase the elastic properties of the affected tissues.

Perhaps the best use for superficial heat in patients with conditions of the shoulder is for increasing relaxation and decreasing pain and spasm. Patients with osteoarthritis, bursitis, and tendinitis of the shoulder structures might benefit from application of moist heat before engaging in exercise or undergoing manual therapy because it helps reduce sensitivity to pain or existing muscle spasm. Although an individual with shortening of the shoulder's connective tissues probably will not benefit from superficial heat to increase tissue elasticity, he or she might benefit from its use to maximize relaxation of the surrounding musculature to minimize guarding during joint mobilization.

Summary of the Evidence

Table 2 illustrates research of grade II evidence on the shoulder, showing therapeutic benefits of hot packs is limited. Grade II studies show therapeutic benefits for treating neck and shoulder pain, adhesive capsulitis, and rheumatoid arthritis in the shoulder and for increasing shoulder ROM.

Lentell et al[13] reported that shoulder flexibility increased more in a group that received superficial heat with low-load prolonged stretch than in the control group that did not receive superficial heat. Miller et al[11] used a combination of moist heat, home exercise program, and anti-inflammatory medication that resulted in all 50 patients with adhesive capsulitis gaining a significant amount of ROM.

Overall Conclusions

Hot packs have been used for more than 80 years, yet a small amount of research about them has been performed.[1] Moist heat is beneficial for shoulder conditions and is best used in conjunction with other appropriate interventions, such as therapeutic exercise, ROM, and patient education. Hot packs are best used to supply superficial heat to increase relaxation and to decrease pain and spasm in superficial tissues equal to or less than 1 cm. These therapeutic effects might allow for an increase in shoulder ROM and a decrease in pain for many pathologic conditions, including adhesive capsulitis and rheumatic diseases of the shoulder.

CRYOTHERAPY

Definition

Cryotherapy is the removal of heat or lowering of soft tissue temperature.[1] The most commonly used forms of cryotherapy for the shoulder are surface agents, such as ice packs and gel packs. These cooling agents lower tissue temperatures by absorbing heat energy from warmer tissues when placed in contact with the body part.[5]

Proposed Mechanism and Therapeutic Effects

Cryotherapy interventions produce several therapeutic effects that might supplement treatment for conditions affecting the shoulder joint. Perhaps the greatest value of cold modalities is in their ability to control acute inflammation.[5] Decreasing tissue temperature results in vasoconstriction of blood vessels. A decrease in overall blood flow to inflamed tissues results and limits the delivery of some chemical mediators that perpetuate the inflammatory response.[9] Because cellular metabolism also slows when tissues are cooled sufficiently, fewer inflammatory chemical mediators also are produced.

Reducing cell metabolism has the added benefit of limiting secondary trauma associated with hypoxic cell death. In other words, by slowing metabolic processes, cells within damaged tissues receiving less oxygen secondary to the presence of edema are less likely to die due to hypoxia. This prevents the release of additional interstitial proteins from these cells, and with less accumulation of such proteins, further formation

Table 2. Evidence-Based Research on Thermotherapy[1]

Thermotherapy Research	Benefit	Evidence Grade	Reference
Neck and shoulder pain	Yes	II	Cordray and Krusen, 1959[10]
Adhesive capsulitis	Yes	II	Miller et al, 1966[11]
Shoulder with rheumatoid arthritis	Yes	II	Williams et al, 1986[12]
Increase in shoulder range of motion	Yes	--	Lentell et al, 1992[13]

of edema is prevented.[14] The combined effect of less vascular supply through vasoconstriction and reduced hypoxic cell death potentially can limit the accumulation of additional edema in damaged tissues during the acute inflammatory response phase of healing. Although cryotherapy often is used to reduce existing edema, researchers have suggested that it is not always effective for this purpose.[15,16]

Other common rationales for using cryotherapy include reducing pain and muscle spasm.[9] By slowing the conduction of impulses that nociceptive neurons carry, application of cold potentially can produce an analgesic effect. Similarly, cryotherapy treatments can raise the threshold of muscle spindles, making them less reactive. This results in a reduction of existing muscle spasm. The combination of these effects results in an interruption of the pain-spasm-pain cycle that further reduces both symptoms.[5]

Relevant Treatment Variables

Relevant variables associated with cryotherapy for shoulder conditions include application method, treatment duration, and often coupling method. Again, the most common cryostatic agents used on the shoulder are ice packs and gel packs because these are inexpensive, effective, and reusable.[1] Ice massage is another viable option for reducing temperatures of shoulder tissues because the size of the treatment area in patients is often small. Cryocompression-controlled and cryotemperature-controlled devices are effective but more expensive. A cryocompression-controlled device combines cold and compression, whereas a cryotemperature-controlled device administers cold at constant temperatures.[1] The Cryocuff (Aircast; DJO, LLC, Vista, CA) is an example of a cryocompression-controlled device. This product has an accessory that is custom fitted for shoulder joints and allows for the simultaneous application of cold and compression.[9]

Treatment duration varies depending on the cryoagent used. Cryostatic agents, such as ice and gel packs, typically are applied for 12 to 30 minutes.[1] Whereas applications of cryotherapy for more than 30 minutes has been commonly believed to potentially increase edema formation through cold-induced vasodilation, this phenomenon is no longer thought to hold true.[3] Otte et al[17] showed that the decrease in intramuscular temperature using cryostatic cryotherapy depended on subcutaneous adipose thickness. Adipose tissue equal to or less than 20 mm required 25 minutes of cryostatic cryotherapy, 21 to 30 mm required 40 minutes, and between 30 and 40 mm required 60 minutes to decrease intramuscular temperature by 7°.[17] Nonetheless, longer applications should be monitored in superficial joints to prevent frostbite and to permit necessary movement. In addition, any cryostatic agents applied to the axilla region should be monitored closely and kept within these limits to avoid damage to superficial nerves of the brachial plexus, which might occur with prolonged exposure.[14] Many cryocompression devices might be applied for as long as 2 hours. Durations associated with cryotemperature devices might be several hours to 10 hours with water temperatures between 7.2°C (45°F) and 12.8°C (55°F).[1] Note that duration times are not specific to the shoulder.

With the exception of the gel pack,[1] the agents described do not need a coupling agent to maximize cooling of soft tissue.[18–20] A damp cloth can be used as a coupling medium with gel packs, and application should be limited to 30 minutes.[1,18]

Practical Treatment Considerations

Compared with superficial heat sources, cryotherapy treatments potentially can produce greater changes in tissue temperature and also can generate such changes in deeper tissues. For example, Martin et al[21] demonstrated that ice packs can decrease intra-articular temperatures as much as 7°C. Because heat and cold therapies have some common physiologic effects, rehabilitation providers often need to choose between these modalities. However, the depth of the target tissues and degree of temperature change needed might determine the rehabilitation approach. Cryotherapy might be a more efficient approach to effect temperature changes in deeper shoulder structures, such as the rotator cuff, the shoulder capsule, or the subacromial bursa. Heat might be a viable option for cutaneous or superficial shoulder anatomy, such as the acromioclavicular joint or superficial muscle layers.

Furthermore, the stage of the healing process within which the patient with a shoulder condition presents also should guide the rehabilitation provider's choice of treatment.[9] During acute inflammation, heat should be avoided because of its potential to accelerate the inflammatory response, and cryotherapy is likely of greater benefit. During the repair phase, use of both modalities might be possible. Finally, for superficial tissues in the remodeling phase, heat might be indicated more than cold to maximize elastic properties. Heat also might be beneficial in this phase to promote relaxation, enabling patients to better tolerate mobilization and stretching of shoulder tissues.

Specific Indications

Given its ability to control processes associated with inflammation, cryotherapy is valuable for such conditions during the early stages of healing. Acute inflammatory conditions of the shoulder (subacromial bursitis, bicipital tendinitis, tendinitis affecting the rotator cuff tendons, or capsulitis) might benefit from cold interventions during acute presentation.

Cryotherapy also might be of important benefit after treatment is provided for any condition that is prone to exacerbation. A strong analgesic effect can be obtained via cryotherapy; however, again this approach likely is best for relieving pain after shoulder interventions. Applying cryotherapy treatments before activity or manual therapy might decrease sensation and prevent patients from perceiving whether activity during treatment is excessive, causing additional tissue damage.

Summary of the Evidence

The evidence shows strong support for the use of cryotherapy after shoulder surgery but only grade II and III for the shoulder with rheumatoid arthritis and bicipital tendinitis, respectively (Table 3). Singh et al[22] showed continuous cryotherapy after shoulder surgery decreased the severity and frequency of pain during sleep and with rehabilitation. Speer et al[23] demonstrated decreased intensity and frequency of pain, improved sleep, decreased use of pain medicine, decreased swelling, and decreased pain with shoulder movement during rehabilitation after shoulder surgery.

Overall Conclusions

Strong evidence exists for the beneficial use of cryotherapy after shoulder surgery. Unfortunately, researchers predominantly have focused on ankle sprains, spasticity, and total knee arthroplasty,[1] and more research on shoulder cryotherapy needs to be performed. Investigators have shown that cryotherapy for the shoulder reduces pain and muscle spasm and controls acute inflammation by slowing cellular metabolism and decreasing inflammatory chemical mediators. A practitioner should feel confident treating acute inflammatory conditions, such as subacromial bursitis, bicipital tendinitis, and rotator cuff tendinitis or capsulitis, with cryotherapy. Pay attention to any indication of cold urticaria; this allergic reaction from the exposure of a cold stimulus results in hives or welts.[25]

CONVENTIONAL ULTRASOUND

Definition

Ultrasound as typically is used in the practice of physical therapy is the delivery of acoustic energy to human tissue to create a therapeutic effect.[9,26] In this section, we focus on conventional ultrasound, which involves using the moveable direct contact applicator. This acoustic energy, which also is known as *sound waves*, is generated through the reversed piezoelectric effect in which an electrical current is passed across a piezoelectric crystal located within the moveable soundhead of the ultrasound unit.[1,9]

Proposed Mechanism and Therapeutic Effects

Ultrasound waves are proposed to produce 2 general types of therapeutic effects: thermal benefit, in which sound energy is used to elevate tissue temperature, and nonthermal benefits, which result from mechanical effects produced by ultrasound waves with properties

Table 3. Evidence-Based Research on Cryotherapy[1]

Cryotherapy Research	Benefit	Evidence Grade	Reference
Postoperative shoulder	Yes	I	Singh et al, 2001[22]
	Yes	I	Speer et al, 1996[23]
Shoulder with rheumatoid arthritis	Yes	II	Williams et al, 1986[12]
Bicipital tendinitis	Yes	III	Lane, 1971[24]

that do not produce heating effects.[3] Heating of tissue occurs when sound waves are absorbed within tissues and cause microcellular vibration that results in generation of frictional heat. Increases in temperature then might lead to therapeutic effects associated with elevated tissue temperature, such as an increase in blood flow, cellular metabolism, and tissue extensibility; analgesia; and reduced muscle spasm.[26] The physiologic mechanisms by which elevated tissue temperature produces these effects were described in greater detail in the Thermotherapy section.

Nonthermal benefits of conventional ultrasound waves include mechanical effects known as *cavitation* and *acoustic microstreaming*.[3] Cavitation occurs when the vibration of the tissue causes microscopic air bubbles to form within tissue and to vibrate, which in turn directly stimulates cell membranes. Similarly, acoustic microstreaming occurs when sound waves cause pressure changes that result in the movement of fluids around cellular membranes. This physical stimulation enhances membrane permeability, which promotes soft tissue healing through increased cell motility, synthesis, and secretion. Ultimately, these processes potentially can enhance cellular and tissue repair.[27]

Relevant Treatment Variables

Rehabilitation providers must understand and consider several variables when using conventional ultrasound as a component of the plan of care for patients with conditions affecting the shoulder joint. Correct choice of variables can be the difference between an effective treatment that accomplishes the desired physiologic effects and an inefficient effort. These variables and associated rationale are described.

Frequency. *Frequency* refers to the number of cycles per second through which the ultrasound waves move. For conventional ultrasound, the choice of frequency is typically 1 MHz or 3.3 MHz.[1] A frequency of 1 MHz is indicated to produce therapeutic effects in deeper soft tissues (between approximately 2 and 5 cm).[1,28,29] For superficial soft tissues, the 3-MHz setting is recommended.[1] Although sources describing the depth at which 3-MHz ultrasound energy is absorbed vary, researchers recently have suggested that this frequency might be used to affect tissues at depths of up to 2.5 cm.[26]

Intensity. The *intensity* of ultrasound waves refers to the amount of overall energy delivered per unit of area, typically is expressed in watts per square centimeter, and is related directly to the amount of energy emitted by the transducer.[3] Intensity usually ranges from 0.1 to 3 W/cm^2.[1] In general, a higher intensity of the ultrasound waves results in a greater potential for heating tissues.

Duty Cycle. Most contemporary, conventional ultrasound units offer a choice of delivering continuous or pulsed sound waves. The continuous setting provides a nonstop flow of acoustic energy, whereas the pulsed mode emits an interrupted flow of ultrasound waves.[1] In other words, *duty cycle* is an expression of the period in percentage over the course of a treatment during which acoustic energy is delivered[1]: Duty Cycle = (ON time/[ON time + OFF time])100. Therefore, a lower duty cycle often is used when the rehabilitation provider wants to limit the overall energy delivered to tissues. Commonly available duty-cycle settings include choices of pulsing sound waves during 10%, 20%, 50%, and 100% of the treatment.[1]

Duration. Treatment *duration* considers the overall length in minutes of the ultrasound treatment. Although this might vary based on time constraints and other practical considerations, the principle consideration for choosing a duration should be the degree to which the rehabilitation provider wants to increase tissue temperature.

Practical Treatment Considerations

Many practical considerations for implementing an ultrasound treatment in the shoulder region are related directly to the rehabilitation provider's choice of variables. The estimated depth of the target tissues should determine whether a frequency of 1 MHz or 3 MHz is used. This might vary based on the relevant anatomy or build of the individual patient. Tissue depth in shoulders is extremely variable depending on upper extremity size, adipose tissue, and bulk of the deltoid and trapezius.

The rehabilitation provider also needs to understand that ultrasound energy is absorbed selectively by collagen fibers found within the connective tissue. Thus, ligaments, joint capsules, tendons, fascia, and scar tissue are more likely to be the target of physiologic ef-

Table 4. Temperature Increases Required to Achieve Specific Therapeutic Goals

Desired Effect	Required Temperature Increase, °C
Acceleration of metabolic rate	1
Reduction of muscle spasm	2–3
Pain control and increase in blood flow	2–3
Increase in collagen extensibility	3–5

fects, whereas muscle fibers, adipose, and intracellular and extracellular fluids will be less affected.[1]

Perhaps the most important clinical decisions regarding the use of ultrasound concerns the selection of the appropriate combination of variables to achieve either thermal or nonthermal effects. The correct combination of intensity and duty cycle will greatly influence the degree of tissue heating. For the most pronounced heating effect, a combination of a continuous duty cycle and higher intensities (approximately 1.0–2.0 W/cm^2) should be chosen. For mechanical effect of cavitation and acoustic microstreaming without heating of tissue, investigators have recommended a pulsed duty cycle with a normal intensity (0.75–1.25 W/cm^2) or a continuous duty cycle with a very low intensity (≤0.3 W/cm^2). The latter approach is advocated by Johns[30] for producing more stable and prolonged mechanical therapeutic effects associated with healing.

Although typical durations of treatment have been described as between 5 and 15 minutes[1,31] when thermal effects are desired, duration should be considered carefully based on (1) the desired amount of temperature change and (2) the combination of frequency and intensity selected. Tables 4 and 5 illustrate these concepts. For example, as shown in Table 4, an increase in tissue temperature of 3°C to 5°C might be seen as necessary to produce an increase in collagen fiber extensibility.[32,33] When using a frequency of 1 MHz at an intensity of 1.5 W/cm^2, selecting an absolute minimum duration of 10 minutes is necessary to achieve the desired effect (duration of 10 minutes equals the needed change of 3°C multiplied by a rate of heating of 0.3°C/min).[34]

Furthermore, considering that tissue temperatures begin to decrease as soon as the treatment is terminated, the rehabilitation provider likely needs to achieve an even longer duration to ensure that temperatures remain elevated long enough for the tissues to benefit from enhanced elastic properties after treatment.[35,36] This phenomenon, which is known as the *stretching window*, suggests that the temperature of tissues heated using an ultrasound treatment with a 3-MHz frequency will remain elevated sufficiently to enhance stretching for approximately 3 minutes. The temperature of tissues heated using a treatment with a 1-MHz frequency will remain sufficiently elevated to increase extensibility slightly longer (approximately 5 minutes). Thus, using the variables in the given example, the rehabilitation provider should perform an ultrasound treatment lasting 13 to 14 minutes to ensure that tissue temperatures stay elevated long enough to maintain increased extensibility to enhance stretching or mobilization after the ultrasound is completed. Therefore, depending on the treatment goal, the chosen frequency, and the tolerated sound-wave intensity, achieving substantial thermal effects often requires relatively longer durations than those to which many rehabilitation providers are accustomed.

Specific Indications

A primary indication for using ultrasound might be in its potential to create therapeutic effects in tissues at depths of up to 5 cm. Although superficial heat generates similar effects, this modality cannot elevate tissue temperatures as substantially or as deeply as ultrasound. Therefore, in patients who have developed contractures affecting the flexibility of deeper shoulder structures, such as joint capsules, ligaments, and rotator cuff tendons, thermal ultrasound is a viable option to increase tissue extensibility before mobilization or stretching, or both, if the rehabilitation provider follows the given recommendations for selecting the correct variables.

Table 5. Ultrasound Rate of Heating per Minute

Intensity, W/cm^2	1 MHz, °C	3 MHz, °C
0.5	0.04	0.3
1.0	0.20	0.6
1.5	0.30	0.9
2.0	0.40	1.4

Evidence-Based Use of Modalities in the Shoulder Girdle

The stage of healing within which the patient presents also should guide the rehabilitation provider's clinical decision regarding the use of ultrasound. In the acute phase, nonthermal protocols should be used. Variables producing thermal effects might elevate tissue temperatures and might produce and further accelerate the inflammatory response. Mechanical effects, on the other hand, can enhance therapeutic cellular events associated with inflammation and allow a faster progression to the proliferative stage.[37] Within the proliferative stage, thermal or nonthermal effects might be beneficial depending on the rehabilitation provider's treatment goal. Thermal effects might increase blood flow and mitigate pain.[9] Certain shoulder structures, such as the supraspinatus tendon, have a limited blood supply and, during healing, might benefit from improved vascular supply.[38] Nonthermal effects might provide a needed boost in fibroblast activity for healing connective tissues. Finally, within the remodeling stage, thermal protocols sufficient to increase elastic properties might allow greater stress on newly developed connective tissue without additional tissue damage.

Summary of the Evidence

As summarized in Table 6, Bélanger's[1] rationale indicates ultrasound displays "fair-good" strength of evidence-based practice for shoulder conditions. Researchers have indicated that ultrasound might contribute to the healing of calcific tendinitis, shoulder pain, and bursitis. However, the data presented in Table 6 span more than 60 years of research on ultrasound, with authors of 4 grade I studies indicating that it was not a statistical benefit for the proposed pathologic condition. As discussed, variables and duration of ultrasound application are crucial to affect the targeted pain source. If proper variables are not used (ie, too short duration to raise tissue temperature), then the full benefits might not be accomplished.

Overall Conclusions

Ultrasound potentially can provide a number of therapeutic effects for both superficial and deep tissues up to 5 cm. Research findings vary with respect to effectiveness, and high-quality studies are limited. However, authors of animal studies have confirmed that ultrasound waves do produce desired physiologic responses in healing tissue.[37] Important considerations for the rehabilitation provider are to choose thermal or nonthermal effects; desired temperature increases; depth of penetration; proper treatment variables of frequency, intensity, duty cycle, and adequate duration; and proper use of the stretching window.

Table 6. Evidence-Based Research on Ultrasound[1]

Ultrasound Research	Benefit	Evidence Grade	Reference
Calcific tendinitis	Yes	I	Ebenbichler et al, 1999[31]
Painful shoulders	Yes	I	Munting, 1978[39]
Calcific tendinitis	Yes	II	Ebenbichler et al, 1997[40]
Subdeltoid bursitis	Yes	II	Aldes et al, 1954[41]
Subdeltoid bursitis	Yes	II	Aldes and Klaras, 1954[42]
Calcific bursitis	Yes	II	Cline, 1963[43]
Adhesive subacromial bursitis	Yes	II	Roden, 1952[44]
Shoulder disorders	Yes	II	Grynbaum, 1954[45]
Peritendinitis calcerea	Yes	II	Flax, 1964[46]
Painful shoulder	Yes	II	Herrera-Lasso et al, 1993[47]
Periarticular shoulder pain	Yes	II	Shehab and Adham, 2000[48]
Supraspinatus bursitis	Yes	III	Bundt, 1958[49]
Subacromial bursitis	Yes	III	Bearzy, 1953[50]
Subacromial bursitis	Yes	III	Gorkiewicz, 1984[51]
Subacromial bursitis	No	I	Downing and Weinstein, 1986[52]
Shoulder pain	No	I	Ainsworth et al, 2007[53]
Calcific tendinitis	No	I	Perron and Malouin, 1997[54]
Painful shoulder with hemiplegia	No	I	Inaba and Piorkowski, 1972[55]
Painful shoulder	No	II	Nykänen, 1995[56]
Bicipital tendinitis	Yes	II	Echternach, 1965[57]

Although reimbursement for ultrasound is limited,[58] cost is also minimal. When used appropriately and effectively, it carries few side effects and various potential benefits that might supplement and complement other interventions, such as manual therapy and therapeutic exercise.

TRANSCUTANEOUS ELECTRICAL NERVE STIMULATION FOR PAIN MODULATION

Definition

Transcutaneous electrical nerve stimulation (TENS) uses electrical current to stimulate or depolarize nerve fibers through the skin.[1,59] This intervention approach uses 2 or more surface electrodes to deliver current. Although *TENS* technically refers to the use of an electrical current to stimulate nerve fibers for any purpose, we focus on the colloquially accepted use of the term, which describes the use of electrical current to stimulate sensory nerves for pain relief.[9]

Proposed Mechanism and Therapeutic Effects

The primary pain modulation system activated by TENS treatments is the gate control system,[1,4,60,61] which was described in the Thermotherapy section. More specifically, the gate system works as follows. A-β neurons, which are large-diameter afferent nerve fibers that carry signals from mechanical stimuli toward the brain, activate an area within the spinal cord that is known as the *substantia gelatinosa*. In turn, the substantia gelatinosa inhibits the transmission of A-Δ and C nerve fibers; these small-diameter nerve fibers carry pain signals toward the central nervous system. Therefore, when a TENS current is applied, it causes the depolarization of A-β fibers, sets the gate mechanism in motion, and results in closing of the gate by preventing A-Δ and C fibers from synapsing in the spinal cord.[5]

Some TENS protocols activate another pain modulation system known as the *descending endogenous opiate system*. The mechanism by which this system acts to produce analgesia is quite complex but is summarized as follows. Certain TENS variables generate a current that directly depolarizes nociceptive A-Δ and C fibers. As might be hypothesized, the patient often perceives such currents as uncomfortable. These neural signals travel to the higher brain centers and activitate opioid mechanisms that provide pain relief by releasing beneficial endogenous opiate substances (endorphins).[1,62]

Table 7. Description of Specialized Currents for Pain Modulation

Current	Unique Characterisitcs	Unique Advantages	Summary
Interferential current	Amplitude-modulated biphasic current created by 2 interfering currents; 4-electrode setup	Stimulate larger treatment area	Other than larger treatment area, no additional advantages supported by evidence
Premodulated current	Amplitude-modulated biphasic current; 2-electrode setup	None additional	2-electrode option similar to interferential current
High-volt pulsed current	Monophasic, twin-peak current with large interpulse interval; 2-electrode setup	Penetrates deeply; because of large interval, can achieve high intensities with patient comfort	Deeply penetrating, high-intensity current
Microcurrent	Low-frequency, long-pulse-duration current with very low intensity (<1mA); biphasic or monophasic; 2-electrode setup	None additional	Although proposed for pain control, minimal supportive theory or evidence for this purpose

Table 8. Common Variables for Custom Transcutaneous Electrical Nerve Stimulation Currents

Variable	Description
Pulse duration and width	The time interval that elapses between the beginning and end of each electrical pulse. Pulse durations associated with pain-control protocols commonly range from 50 to 400 μs.[1]
Frequency and pulse rates	The number of pulses per second measured in hertz. It typically ranges from 1 to 200 Hz for pain-control models.[1]
Current intensity and amplitude	The magnitude or strength of the current necessary to depolarize sensory peripheral nerve fibers. It varies from 0 to 120 mA.[1]
Polarity	The direction of current flow between surface electrodes. *Monophasic polarity* refers to unidirectional flow, and *biphasic polarity* implies bidirectional flow.

Relevant Treatment Variables

Variable selection differs based on whether the rehabilitation provider chooses to use a custom or specialized current. For custom-designed currents, the provider usually needs to set all variables that determine the properties of the waveform. Specialized currents are currents with many preset variables.[9] These include currents with common names, such as interferential, premodulated, microcurrent, and high-volt pulsed current (HVPC) (Table 7). Because many of the waveform properties associated with specialized currents are predetermined, the variables that the rehabilitation provider needs to set often only include basic considerations, such as current intensity, on and off times, and treatment duration. Nonetheless, both custom and specialized currents can produce analgesia in patients with painful shoulders. A detailed explanation concerning the physics associated with all TENS variables is beyond the scope of this text; however, Table 8 contains a brief description of the most relevant custom-selected settings.

Practical Treatment Considerations

Various combinations of the given custom variables have been identified for producing analgesia via the previously described pain modulation systems. These combinations of variables often are known as *protocols* or *modes*. The protocols or modes described in this chapter include conventional, low-frequency, and brief-intense TENS (Table 9).[3,9,63]

Conventional TENS uses the gate mechanism to depolarize A-β nerves for the rapid onset of pain relief. It is used most often to treat acute pain. Of all protocols listed here, it tends to be the most comfortable current for the patient because it only stimulates A-β sensory fibers.[1,63]

Low-frequency or acupuncture-like TENS uses the opiate system for analgesic effects. It also is versatile and is cited as appropriate for either acute or chronic pain. Other advantages include long-lasting analgesic effects and minimal adaptation to the stimulus. A disadvantage is that the use of a current often is perceived as uncomfortable to the patient. In addition, Brotzman and Wilk[63] stated that treatments should be limited to 60-minute daily sessions.

Brief-intense TENS uses the depolarization of A-Δ and C fibers to activate the opiate system.[1,63] This protocol is beneficial for both acute and chronic pain. Onset of analgesia is rapid and long lasting.[1] As its title stipulates, the disadvantage of this protocol is that the current can be uncomfortable for many patients.

Table 9. Custom Transcutaneous Electrical Nerve Stimulation Protocols for Pain Modulation

Transcutaneous Electrical Nerve Stimulation Protocols and Modes[1,3,9,63]	Conventional	Low-Frequency or Acupuncture-Like	Brief-Intense
Pulse duration	Short (50–125 ms)	Long (150–500 ms)	Long (>150 ms)
Frequency	High (80–150 Hz)	Low (<10 Hz)	High (>80 Hz)
Current amplitude	Comfortable Sensory level	Comfortable and tolerable Sensory and motor level	Tolerable Noxious level
Nerve fibers depolarized	A-β	A-Δ and C	A-Δ and C
Pain modulation system	Gate	Opiate	Opiate

Specialized Currents for Pain Control

Specialized currents with the potential to provide pain modulation for the shoulder include interferential and premodulated currents, HVPC, and microcurrent.[3,9] An in-depth description of the theory describing each specialized waveform is also beyond the scope of this chapter. Table 7 provides a brief description of each current's unique characteristics and advantages. As mentioned, many variables are preset in these currents. For this reason, many rehabilitation providers prefer these currents for their ease of use. Although some advantages associated with these currents have been proposed in the literature, authors of controlled studies have suggested that they provide few substantial benefits over custom protocols.[1]

Practical Treatment Considerations and Specific Indications

Because pain is an impairment associated with most shoulder conditions, we describe treatment considerations and specific indications together in this section of the chapter. Recommendations for the type of TENS to be used might be associated with whether the patient presents with acute or chronic pain. These recommendations were summarized in the discussion of custom variables.

One consideration for choice of TENS currents or protocols concerns the size of the treatment area. An interferential current setup requires 4 electrodes, so current can be delivered over the largest area. However, because the average patient with shoulder pain reports symptoms concentrated within a specific area (commonly anterior, posterior, or superior), delivering current over a wide expanse often is not necessary. For this reason, use of interferential current that requires placing 4 electrodes around the shoulder complex often is not the best choice. The exception is in a much larger patient or unusually expansive treatment area. A more common choice is any of the available biphasic currents, such as premodulated current, or any custom biphasic protocol. With biphasic currents, electrodes alternate polarity and thus equally are capable of depolarizing sensory nerves, so efficient pain relief might occur throughout the area between them. For very small treatment areas approximately the size of 1 electrode, monophasic currents are most appropriate because they result in unidirectional current flow, meaning that only 1 of the 2 electrodes per channel is most capable of nerve depolarization. In these cases, the cathode is placed directly over the painful area. These ideas not only create the most efficient method of current delivery, but save costs by avoiding the use of unnecessary electrode supplies.

As with other modalities, the depths of the targeted structures in the shoulder are important to consider when administering TENS. For pain generated by deeper structures (eg, labrum, capsule, rotator cuff) or in individuals with considerable muscle mass, deeper penetrating currents are recommended. Although interferential current has been described as having the capability to reach deeper tissues, most researchers do not support this claim.[1] However, HVPC seems to have greater potential for depolarizing deeper nerves because it is a waveform with a high, but well-tolerated, intensity.

A related treatment consideration concerns electrode placement. Electrodes placed closely together will result in a more superficial flow of current. Alternately, placing electrodes farther apart will cause the current to be concentrated deeper in tissue.[9] Another placement consideration when the treatment goal is pain modulation is elicitation of muscle contractions. For patients experiencing higher levels of pain, involuntary muscle contraction might increase muscle spasm or decrease relaxation. This then might result in less overall analgesic effects.

Table 10. Evidence-Based for Grade I, II, and III Studies on Transcutaneous Electrical Nerve Stimulation[1]

Transcutaneous Electrical Nerve Stimulation	Benefit	Evidence Grade	Reference
Pain due to stroke	Yes	I	Sonde et al, 1998[64]
Pain due to stroke	Yes	II	Tekeoğlu et al, 1998[65]
Pain due to hemiplegia	Yes	I	Leandri et al, 1990[66]
Brachial plexus pain	Yes	III	Frampton, 1996[67]

Summary of the Evidence

Table 10 illustrates evidence for grade I, II, and III studies of TENS. All sources indicated a statistical benefit for using TENS for pain in the upper extremity due to stroke, pain in the shoulder due to hemiplegia, and brachial plexus pain. These results show promising benefit for the use of TENS with shoulder conditions.

Overall Conclusions

A general understanding of the various TENS currents and protocols might guide their efficient use in patients with shoulder conditions. Mode selection primarily should be based on patient comfort because researchers have not shown that one mode is superior to others for reducing pain.[1] In reviews of TENS evidence, investigators have indicated an insubstantial amount of evidence, suggesting it enhances long-term outcomes in patients with shoulder pain of musculoskeletal origin.[1,68,69] However, they have shown TENS therapy is beneficial in providing short-term analgesic effects and thus is a viable treatment adjunct for modulating shoulder pain.[1,68,69]

IONTOPHORESIS

Definition and Proposed Mechanism

Iontophoresis is a method of transferring ionized medicated and nonmedicated substances transdermally via an electrical current known as *direct current*. Direct current is a type of monophasic electrical current that has constant amplitude. Iontophoresis delivers substances transdermally through the following mechanism. With direct current, a positively charged electrode (anode) and a negatively charged electrode (cathode) are applied to complete the circuit. The active electrode containing the medication is placed over the area of treatment, whereas the other electrode is placed at a distance longer than the diameter of the smallest electrode.[1,70–72] Negatively charged ions are placed under the cathode (negative), and positively charged ions are placed under the anode (positive). The repelling forces of anode and cathode then facilitate the penetration of this therapeutic substance into the skin. The electrical current makes skin pathways (hair follicles, pores, and sebaceous [oil] glands) permeable for the ions to penetrate the various layers of the integument.[1] After this is achieved, passive diffusion allows for the further penetration of the applied substance to achieve greater depths.[1]

Iontophoresis can be delivered through traditional wired devices and transportable patches. Benefits of delivering substances via iontophoresis include bypassing the gastrointestinal and liver systems in a noninvasive manner with minimal risk of infection.[1]

Proposed Therapeutic Effects

Therapeutic effects vary based on the medication or substance being administered. The most commonly administered substances are dexamethasone, lidocaine, and acetic acid, which are proposed to produce anti-inflammatory, analgesic, and decalcifying effects, respectively.[3] Of these, dexamethasone is the most frequently used in contemporary physical therapy practice. Table 11 outlines the proposed effects of

Table 11. Iontophoresis Claims and Ions

Therapeutic Claims[1]	Ions
Anti-inflammatory	Dexamethasone,[a] hydrocortisone, prednisone, and salicylate
Analgesic	Lidocaine[a] and salicylate
Decalcifying	Acetic acid[a]
Antiseptic	Iodine and zinc oxide
Sclerolytic	Chlorine and iodine
Antiedema	Hyaluronidase
Anesthetic	Lidocaine
Muscle relaxant	Magnesium sulfate
Membrane stabilizing	Calcium chloride
Antisweating	Tap water
Anticholinergic	Glycoperronium bromide, poldine methosulfate

[a] Indicates most commonly used in physical therapy.

several substances that have been reported for use with iontophoresis.

Relevant Treatment Variables

Current intensity and dosage are the most important variables for rehabilitation providers to understand when administering iontophoresis to the shoulder region. Intensity is typically available in a range from 0 to 4 mA or 5 mA.[9] At higher intensities, the medication will be delivered faster. However, as with other forms of electrical stimulation, higher intensities often are less well tolerated.

Dosage (D) is an expression of the total medication to be delivered. It is equal to the current magnitude (A) of intensity in milliamperes multiplied by the total application duration (T) in minutes. Therefore, dosage is expressed in milliampere minutes and is calculated as $D = AT$.[1,3] Typical dosages range from 1 to 80 mA min, when the maximum amplitude is 4 mA. A commonly reported dosage of dexamethasone is 40 mA min. This is based on recommendations for providing the treatment with minimal skin irritation. However, when using buffered electrodes, dosages of up to 80 mA min might be administered safely.

Current density (CD) is the magnitude of the applied current (A) in milliamperes divided by the conductive surface area (S) of the electrode in square centimeters: $CD = A/S$.[1] To minimize skin irritation and burns, do not exceed 0.5 mA/cm^2 for the cathode and do not exceed 1.0 mA/cm^2 for the anode.[1]

Practical Treatment Considerations

The primary consideration when administering an iontophoresis treatment in the shoulder region is the depth of the target structures. Researchers have suggested that substances delivered via iontophoresis rarely penetrate deeper than 1.5 cm into tissue.[3,9,73] Because few anatomic structures of the shoulder are located this superficially, situations in which iontophoresis might be valuable for patients with shoulder conditions are limited. Again, the rehabilitation provider must consider the individual patient's build and the depth of the tissue that he or she hopes to reach through phoretic action.

Another relevant treatment consideration concerns the potential for each patient to absorb the medication being administered. Evidence has suggested that the degree to which medications, such as dexamethasone, are absorbed in human tissue is highly variable, with some individuals absorbing large amounts of medication via iontophoresis and others absorbing minimal amounts.[74] Based on this finding, Gurney et al[74] recommended that when minimal progress has been noted over 2 to 3 iontophoresis treatments, the rehabilitation provider might consider other alternatives.

Specific Indications

Indications for iontophoresis largely are based on the depths of the target structures and the medication used. Considering the limited potential for iontophoresis to deliver medications to tissues deeper than 1.5 cm, this modality is indicated only for conditions affecting very superficial anatomic structures. For many patients, using iontophoresis to deliver medications to rotator cuff tendons, bursae, the glenoid labrum, and other deep structures is not recommended. Superficially located anatomy is a more feasible target.

Considering these ideas, the most commonly used iontophoresis medication, dexamethasone, is indicated for managing inflammatory conditions associated with superficial structures, such as acute bicipital tendinitis or sprains of the acromioclavicular joint. Acetate might be used to break down calcium deposits that form in patients with calcific tendinitis or myositis ossificans affecting the shoulder complex. Lidocaine might help reduce pain but again only in relatively superficial structures.

Table 12. Evidence-Based Research on Shoulder Conditions and Iontophoresis[1]

Shoulder Conditions and Iontophoresis	Ion	Benefit	Grade	Reference
Calcifying tendinitis	Acetic acid	Yes	II	Psaki and Carroll, 1955[75]
	Acetic acid	No	I	Perron and Malouin, 1997[54]
	Acetic acid	No	I	Leduc et al, 2003[76]
Subdeltoid bursitis	Magnesium sulfate	Yes	II	Weinstein and Gordon, 1958[77]

Index

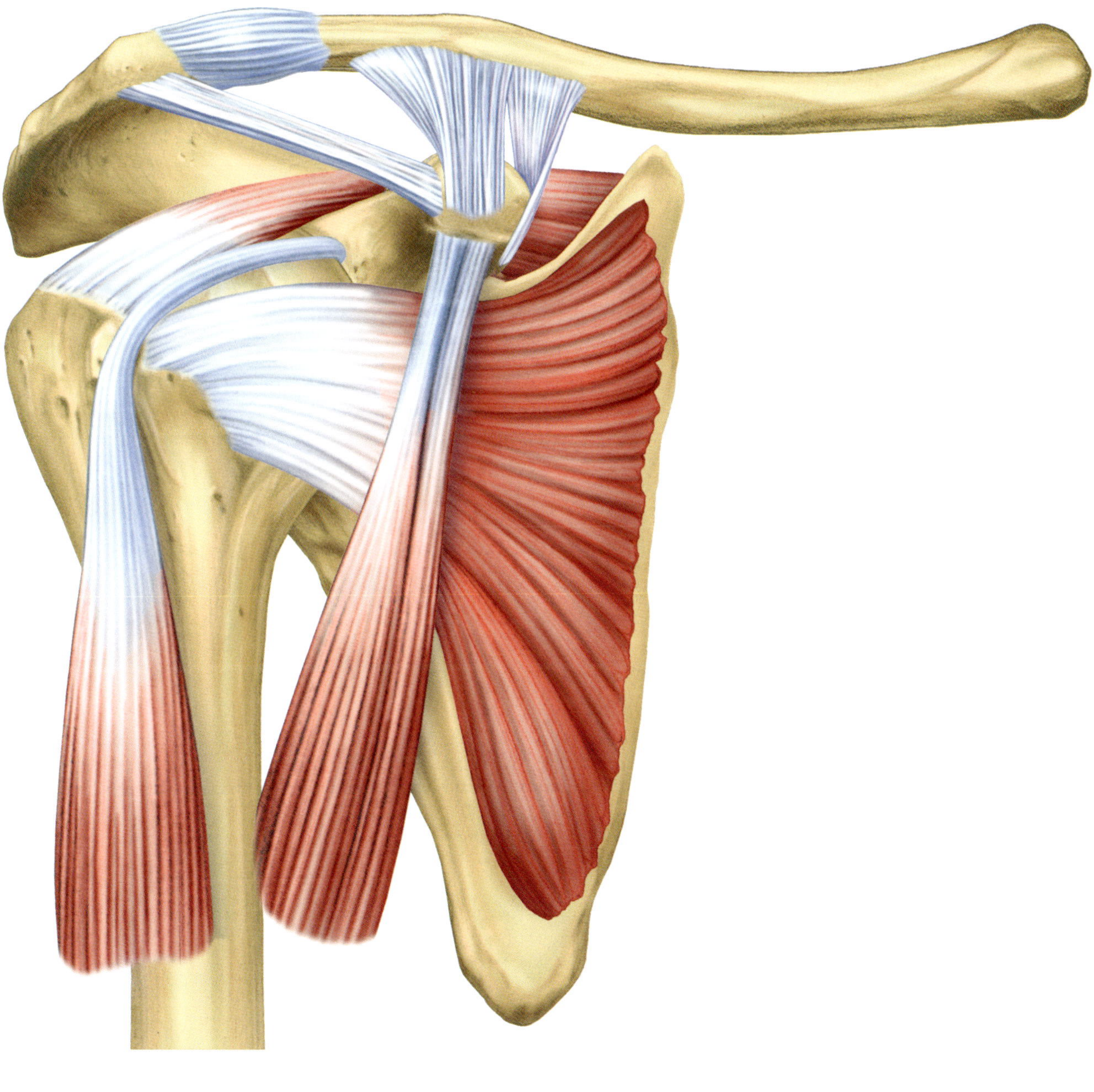

Index

Page references followed by t and f indicate tables and figures, respectively.

A

B

C

D

E

F

G

H

I

J

K

L

M

N

O

P

Q

R

S

T

U

V

W

Y

Z